# Atlas of Emergency Imaging from Head-to-Toe

Michael N. Patlas • Douglas S. Katz •
Mariano Scaglione

Editors

# Atlas of Emergency Imaging from Head-to-Toe

With 864 Figures and 55 Tables

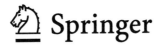 Springer

*Editors*
Michael N. Patlas
Department of Radiology
McMaster University
Hamilton, ON, Canada

Douglas S. Katz
NYU Langone Hospital - Long Island and the NYU Long
Island School of Medicine
Mineola, NY, USA

Mariano Scaglione
Department of Medical, Surgical and Experimental Sciences
University of Medicine and Surgery
Sassari, Italy

Department of Radiology
James Cook University Hospital
Middlesbrough, UK

Teesside University School of Health and Life Sciences
Middlesbrough, Tees Valley, UK

Department of Radiology
Pineta Grande Hospital
Castel Volturno, Italy

ISBN 978-3-030-92110-1      ISBN 978-3-030-92111-8 (eBook)
https://doi.org/10.1007/978-3-030-92111-8

*To Nataly Patlas, my wife, my best friend, my smartest adviser, and love of my life.*

*Michael N. Patlas*

*This book is dedicated to my father, my grandmother Sadie aka Bobby, and my aunt Elinor. I hope that current and future advances in medicine, including medical imaging and emergency radiology, will prolong the lives of the loved ones of all who are reading this book, which was a team effort with numerous contributions from around the world.*

*Douglas S. Katz*

*To my parents, Pietro and Ida, and to my sons, Pietro and Ruben, my past, my present, my future...*

*Mariano Scaglione*

# Foreword

At a time when there is a plethora of information available to radiologists instantaneously at their fingertips, it remains particularly important, especially in a field as rapidly changing as radiology, that trusted sources of evidence-based material be available for those looking to optimize their practice of radiology. In their Atlas of Emergency Radiology, Drs. Michael Patlas, Douglas Katz, and Mariano Scaglione, renowned radiologists, educators, and colleagues who have devoted their careers to the education of radiologists in training and in practice, with a long-standing major interest in emergency radiology in particular, provide an expansive and beautifully illustrated text that offers a verified resource for radiologists, emergency physicians, and professionals responsible for the diagnosis and care of the acutely ill or injured patient.

In assembling the material for this textbook, Drs. Patlas, Katz, and Scaglione have turned to other acknowledged leaders in the radiology subspecialties, who contribute their experience and expertise in emergency imaging. The first section of the book, edited by Drs. Patlas, Katz, and Scaglione, provides an overview of emergency and trauma imaging, including the evolving role of artificial intelligence in patient triage and diagnosis. An important aspect in the evaluation of the acutely ill or traumatized patient is deciding when to engage an interventional radiologist in the patient management, an issue addressed by Dr. S. Mafeld. Imaging, particularly CT, is central to the neurologic evaluation of those presenting with traumatic head injuries or stroke, and the section on neuroradiologic emergencies edited by Professor Carlos Torres amply addresses these and related emergency head, neck, and spine topics. Thoracic trauma, acute aortic syndromes, and pulmonary infections are common emergency chest issues and comprise the thoracic section of the textbook edited by Dr. Constantine Raptis. In particular, this section provides an update on the evolving concept of thoracic aortic dissection and its variants, which are important entities where the radiologist plays a crucial role in diagnosis and patient triage. A unique feature of this section is the chapter on the imaging of breast emergencies, an uncommon but important topic that receives scant coverage in most emergency radiology textbooks. The extensive abdomen and pelvis section of the book, edited by Dr. Vincent Mellnick from the Mallinckrodt Institute of Radiology at Washington University in St. Louis, reviews the spectrum of non-traumatic and traumatic solid organ, peritoneal, abdominal wall, and bowel conditions commonly encountered in the emergency setting. Important chapters addressing emergency imaging of the bariatric or pregnant patient, and abdominal emergencies in cancer patients, provide insight into the challenges of imaging these select groups of emergency patients with their particular challenges. Traumatic musculoskeletal conditions are addressed using an anatomic approach in the section edited by Drs. Kumaravel and Beckmann. The chapter on non-traumatic musculoskeletal emergencies is particularly appreciated. The final section, edited by Dr. Elka Miller, offers a system-based review of pediatric emergency imaging, including a chapter on the role of interventional radiology in pediatric emergencies. The material and insights provided in this section are particularly useful for those of us who may encounter the occasional pediatric emergency patient but do not have the extensive experience with the unique aspects of imaging pediatric emergency patients provided by the authors in these chapters.

While larger North American medical centers designated by the U.S. American Trauma Society or the Trauma Association of Canada's Accreditation Canada Trauma Distinction Program as Level 1 Trauma Centers may be able to provide 24/7 emergency imaging care utilizing a dedicated core of radiologists with broad emergency radiology training and multi-system imaging expertise, the majority of facilities in North America do not have the staffing to dedicate to this task, primarily because they do not see a large enough volume or experience a broad spectrum of conditions afflicting traumatized or acutely ill patients. As a result, the rapid interpretation of emergency imaging examinations often falls to residents, emergency department physicians, other advanced practice providers, on-call attendings with subspecialty radiology training but perhaps not necessarily emergency radiology expertise, or perhaps teleradiology services in situations where local after-hours radiology is unavailable. For this reason, a resource such as this textbook becomes an important source of information and should prove invaluable to those working in the acute care and trauma setting. By assembling this wealth of up-to-date material, Drs. Patlas, Katz, and Scaglione have provided a practical and easily accessible resource which should help those responsible for imaging this vulnerable population, thereby positively contributing to improved patient outcomes.

Burlington, USA                                                                                       Jeffrey S. Klein

# Preface

People choose careers in medicine in general and in radiology in particular to make a difference. Imaging has a tremendous role in all facets of modern medicine. However, there is no imaging subspecialty with so much immediate impact on the lives of acutely ill patients and also the potential for devastating consequences if errors are made, as does emergency and trauma imaging. Emergency imagers detect strokes in a timely fashion, effectively triage patients with acute chest pain, and advise surgeons regarding the need for laparotomy in victims of major trauma. Enormous technological advances and trust in the skills of emergency radiologists have caused continuous growth in emergency department (ED) imaging volumes in multiple countries around the world. Therefore, these critical decisions should be made quickly and quite often happen in the middle of the night or at the last hour of a 12-h shift.

The coeditors-in-chief of this book have over 80 years of combined frontline imaging experience and enjoy teaching emergency and trauma imaging across the globe. During discussions with attendees at multiple conferences as well as at weekly rounds with our own trainees and colleagues, we had been repeatedly asked whether there is a practical, updated, and comprehensive emergency radiology textbook for beginners as well as for seasoned professionals. The *Atlas of Emergency Imaging from Head-to-Toe* was conceived as a "one-stop source" for residents, fellows, and junior attendings dealing with challenging cases on call, and also as a reference for experts looking for refreshers on challenging topics. We have tried to avoid esoteric entities more suitable for a film panel at a national or international meeting, and have focused on familiar conditions which can be encountered when you cover the ED as an emergency or general radiologist. According to the common expression, "a picture is worth a thousand words," so this book is richly illustrated and the chapters have been kept concise by the editors, to provide essential information which can be quickly digested in the stressful environments of the ED and the trauma suite.

We have used a classical head-to-toe approach, with a few exceptions. The book starts with an overview of modalities used by emergency imagers, followed by a chapter describing the role of artificial intelligence in emergency imaging, and then two chapters defining the place of the interventional radiologist (IR) in the diagnosis and management of patients with vascular and non-vascular emergencies. Timely communication has particularly paramount importance in emergency imaging. For this reason, both interventional chapters describe when to call IR to avoid compromising the outcome of the emergency and/or trauma patient's management. Imaging of acutely ill children is routinely performed by pediatric radiologists at major children's hospitals. However, emergency radiologists are required to perform imaging interpretation in patients with pediatric emergencies in the community setting with some degree of regularity. Therefore, the book contains a full section describing acute pediatric conditions pertinent for the practice of emergency imager. In the editors' opinion, there are two additional groups of patients with unique imaging presentations justifying dedicated chapters: pregnant patients and bariatric patients.

We are indebted to our outstanding Section Editors. Dr. Carlos Torres from the University of Ottawa served as the Section Editor for Neurological Emergencies. Dr. Constantine Raptis from the Mallinckrodt Institute of Radiology/Washington University in Saint Louis has edited the Thoracic Emergencies Section. Dr. Vincent Mellnick, also from Mallinckrodt, served as the Section Editor for Abdominal and Pelvic Emergencies. Drs. Manickam Kumaravel and Nicholas Beckmann from the University of Texas at Houston edited the section on Musculoskeletal Emergencies. Dr. Elka Miller from the University of Ottawa served as a Section Editor for Pediatric Emergencies. The book draws on the vast clinical experience of contributors from the largest medical centers across North America and Europe. It has been a privilege to work with our stellar team and with all of our contributing authors.

Hamilton, Canada                                                                Michael N. Patlas
Long Island, USA                                                               Douglas S. Katz
Sassari, Italy                                                                Mariano Scaglione
June 2022

# Contents

## About the Editors

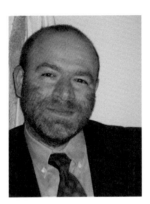

**Michael N. Patlas,** is a Professor of Radiology and Emergency/Trauma Imaging Section Chief in the Department of Radiology, McMaster University. He is an Editor-in-Chief for *Canadian Association of Radiologists Journal* and five radiology books, author of over 150 peer-reviewed papers, editorials, and book chapters; Vice President of Canadian Emergency, Trauma and Acute Care Radiology Society, Program Committee Chair for Canadian Association of Radiologists; and an honored fellow of the American Society of Emergency Radiology, the Canadian Association of Radiologists, and the Society of Abdominal Radiology.

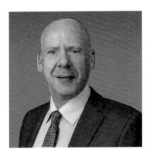

**Dr. Douglas S. Katz** is Vice-Chair for Research at NYU (New York University) Langone Hospital – Long Island and Professor of Radiology at the NYU Long Island School of Medicine (on the Scholar Track - Clinical Arm). He has held essentially the same position since 1999 and has been attending what was formerly Winthrop-University Hospital since 1996. He has co-authored over 900 peer-reviewed publications and abstracts, and multiple books, syllabi, book chapters, and other publications. He has held a variety of positions in organized academic radiology regionally, nationally, and internationally over his three-decade career; has been awarded top honors from his hospital and medical school; and has been Attending of the Year six times, two of which for internal medicine (although he is board certified only in diagnostic radiology). With diverse interests and extensive writing and reviewing and editorial experience, his focus since residency has been on various aspects of emergency radiology, as well as on cross-sectional imaging in general.

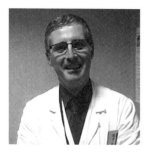

**Mariano Scaglione,** is an Associate Professor of Radiology at the University of Sassari, Honorary Professor at Tesside University, and Consultant Radiologist at the James Cook University Hospital at Middlesbrough, UK.

He was the Chairman for the Emergency Radiology Subcommittee for ECR in 2012, President of the Italian College of Emergency Radiology SIRM (2010–2014), and ESER President (2015–2017). He has been a member of the Emergency Radiology subcommittee of the Scientific Program for RSNA (2012–2018).

He is a seasoned speaker having delivered more than 150 presentations at international meetings and published author, publishing more than 160 papers, editing 12 books, and primary author for 32 book chapters. He was also appointed Lead Editor for the Emergency Radiology Trilogy books, and his article "Role of contrast-enhanced helical CT in the evaluation of acute thoracic aortic injuries" is one of the most cited articles in the *Eur Radiol Journal* in the last 25 years. He is an Editorial Board Member in many Radiology journals including "Emergency Radiology" the official journal of the ASER since 2005.

He was awarded the "Gold Medal" 2014 and Honorary Member 2019 for ESER.

# Contributors

**Laura Acosta-Izquierdo** Medical Imaging Department, CHEO, Department of Radiology, University of Ottawa, Ottawa, ON, Canada

**Jake M. Adkins** UTHealth – McGovern School of Medicine, Houston, TX, USA

**Abdullah Alabousi** Department of Radiology, McMaster University, St. Joseph's Healthcare Hamilton, Hamilton, ON, Canada

**Mostafa Alabousi** Department of Radiology, McMaster University, Hamilton, ON, Canada

**Abdullah O. Alenezi** Division of Interventional Radiology, University Health Network, Toronto General Hospital, Toronto, ON, Canada

**Joao Amaral** Division of Image-Guided Therapy (IGT), Department of Diagnostic Imaging, The Hospital for Sick Children, Medical Imaging department, University of Toronto, Toronto, ON, Canada

**G. Annamalai** Division of Interventional Radiology, Department of Medical Imaging, University Health Network, Toronto, ON, Canada

**Armonde Baghdanian** Department of Radiology, Keck School of Medicine, University of Southern California, Los Angeles, CA, USA

**Arthur Baghdanian** Department of Radiology, Keck School of Medicine, University of Southern California, Los Angeles, CA, USA

**David H. Ballard** Mallinckrodt Institute of Radiology, Washington University School of Medicine, St. Louis, MO, USA

**Raffaella Basilico** Department of Neuroscience, Imaging and Clinical Sciences, G. d'Annunzio University of Chieti, Chieti, Italy

**David D. B. Bates** Department of Radiology, Memorial Sloan Kettering Cancer Center, New York, NY, USA

**Pritish Bawa** Department of Diagnostic and Interventional Imaging, McGovern Medical School at UT Health, Houston, TX, USA

**Gregg W. Bean** University of Texas Health San Antoni, San Antonio, TX, USA

**Nicholas M. Beckmann** UTHealth – McGovern School of Medicine, Houston, TX, USA

**Sanjeev Bhalla** Mallinckrodt Institute of Radiology, St. Louis, MO, USA

**Colin Brown** University of California Davis Health Department of Radiology and Shriners Hospital for Children Northern California, Sacramento, CA, USA

**Kimberley N. Brown** UTHealth – McGovern School of Medicine, Houston, TX, USA

**Martin Bunge** Section of Pediatric Radiology, Children's Hospital, Department of Radiology, University of Manitoba, Winnipeg, MB, Canada

**John F. Burke** Brain and Spine Injury Center, Zuckerberg San Francisco General Hospital and Trauma Center, San Francisco, CA, USA

Department of Neurological Surgery, University of California, San Francisco, CA, USA

**Suzanne C. Byrne** Division of Thoracic Imaging, Department of Radiology, Brigham and Women's Hospital, Harvard Medical School, Boston, MA, USA

**Andrew Callen** Department of Radiology, University of Colorado Anschutz Medical Campus, Denver, CO, USA

**Mauricio Castillo** Division of Neuroradiology, Department of Radiology, University of North Carolina School of Medicine, Chapel Hill, NC, USA

**Pamela I. Causa Andrieu** Department of Radiology, Memorial Sloan Kettering Cancer Center, New York, NY, USA

**Victoria Chernyak** Beth Israel Deaconess Medical Center, Boston, MA, USA

**Vaeman Chintamaneni** Department of Diagnostic and Interventional Imaging, McGovern Medical School at UT Health, Houston, TX, USA

**Charlotte Y. Chung** Department of Radiology and Imaging Sciences, Emory University School of Medicine, Atlanta, GA, USA

**Roberta Cianci** Department of Neuroscience, Imaging and Clinical Sciences, G. d'Annunzio University of Chieti, Chieti, Italy

**Petra Cimflova** Department of Medical Imaging, St. Anne's University Hospital Brno and Faculty of Medicine, Masaryk University, Brno, Czech Republic

Departments of Radiology and Clinical Neurosciences, University of Calgary, Foothills Medical Centre, Calgary, AB, Canada

**Kayla Cort** University of California Davis health and Shriners Hospitals for Children Northern California, Sacramento, CA, USA

**Ginevra Danti** Department of Radiology, Azienda Ospedaliero Universitaria Careggi, Florence, Italy

**Michael A. Davis** University of Texas Health San Antoni, San Antonio, TX, USA

**Sanjay S. Dhall** Brain and Spine Injury Center, Zuckerberg San Francisco General Hospital and Trauma Center, San Francisco, CA, USA

Department of Neurological Surgery, University of California, San Francisco, CA, USA

**Marco Di Maurizio** Department of Radiology, Azienda Ospedaliero Universitaria Meyer, Florence, Italy

**Austin X. Dixon** Department of Radiology, Duke University Medical Center, Durham, NC, USA

**Adam A. Dmytriw** Neuroradiology and Image Guided Therapy, Diagnostic Imaging, The Hospital for Sick Children, and University of Toronto, Toronto, ON, Canada

**Prachi Dubey** Houston Methodist Hospital, Houston Radiology Associated, Houston, TX, USA

**Birgit B. Ertl-Wagner** Division of Neuroradiology, The Hospital for Sick Children, Toronto, ON, Canada

Department of Medical Imaging, University of Toronto, Toronto, ON, Canada

**Jonathan Flug** Mayo Clinic Arizona, Department of Radiology, Phoenix, AZ, USA

**T. J. Fraum** Department of Abdominal Imaging and Nuclear Medicine, Mallinckrodt Institute of Radiology, Washington University School of Medicine, Barnes-Jewish Hospital, St. Louis, MO, USA

**Daniel Furlanetto** Department of Radiology, Vancouver General Hospital/University of British Columbia, Vancouver, BC, Canada

**Mayank Goyal** Departments of Radiology and Clinical Neurosciences, University of Calgary, Foothills Medical Centre, Calgary, AB, Canada

**Joshua Gu** UTHealth – McGovern School of Medicine, Houston, TX, USA

**Angela Guarnizo** Department of Radiology, Division of Neuroradiology, University of Ottawa, Ottawa, ON, Canada

**Baher R. A. Guirguis** Department of Radiology, University of Kentucky, Lexington, KY, USA

**Brian M. Haas** Zuckerburg San Francisco General Hospital and University of California San Francisco, San Francisco, CA, USA

**Scott A. Hamlin** Emory University School of Medicine, Atlanta, GA, USA

**Mark M. Hammer** Division of Thoracic Imaging, Department of Radiology, Brigham and Women's Hospital, Harvard Medical School, Boston, MA, USA

**Travis S. Henry** Duke University School of Medicine, Durham, NC, USA

**Shivaprakash Hiremath** Department of Radiology, Division of Neuroradiology, University of Ottawa, Ottawa, ON, Canada

**Mark J. Hoegger** Mallinckrodt Institute of Radiology, Washington University School of Medicine, St. Louis, MO, USA

**F. Iacobellis** Department of General and Emergency Radiology, "A. Cardarelli" Hospital, Naples, Italy

**Arash Jaberi** Division of Interventional Radiology, University Health Network, Toronto General Hospital, Toronto, ON, Canada

**Gayatri Joshi** Department of Radiology and Imaging Sciences, Emory University School of Medicine, Atlanta, GA, USA

**Amy Juliano** Massachusetts Eye and Ear, Harvard Medical School, Boston, USA

**Marc Jutras** Department of Radiology, Vancouver General Hospital/University of British Columbia, Vancouver, BC, Canada

**Douglas S. Katz** NYU Langone Hospital - Long Island and the NYU Long Island School of Medicine, Mineola, NY, USA

**Shekhar D. Khanpara** Department of Diagnostic and Interventional Imaging, University of Texas Health Science Center at Houston, Houston, TX, USA

**Claudia F. E. Kirsch** Department of Radiology Northwell Health, Zucker Hofstra School of Medicine at Northwell, North Shore University Hospital, Manhasset, NY, USA

**Peter G. Kranz** Department of Radiology, Duke University Medical Center, Durham, NC, USA

**Supriya Kulkarni** Department of Medical Imaging, University of Toronto, Princess Margaret Hospital, Toronto, ON, Canada

**Manickam Kumaravel** UTHealth – McGovern School of Medicine, Houston, TX, USA

**Christina A. LeBedis** Boston University Medical Center, Boston, MA, USA

**James T. Lee** Department of Radiology, University of Kentucky, Lexington, KY, USA

**John Lee** Boston University Medical Center, Boston, MA, USA

**Jeffrey Levine** Department of Radiology, Memorial Sloan Kettering Cancer Center, New York, NY, USA

**Brittany T. Lewis** Emergency and Trauma Imaging, Emory University School of Medicine, Atlanta, GA, USA

**Jonathan Liu** Mallinckrodt Institute of Radiology, St. Louis, MO, USA

**Jeremiah Long** Mayo Clinic Arizona, Department of Radiology, Phoenix, AZ, USA

**Meghan Lubner** University of Wisconsin School of Medicine and Public Health, Madison, WI, USA

**Daniel R. Ludwig** Mallinckrodt Institute of Radiology, Washington University School of Medicine, St. Louis, MO, USA

**Sebastian Mafeld** Division of Interventional Radiology, Department of Medical Imaging, University Health Network, Toronto, ON, Canada

**Kaitlin M. Marquis** Mallinckrodt Institute of Radiology, St. Louis, MO, USA

**Claudia Martinez-Rios** Medical Imaging Department, CHEO, Department of Radiology, University of Ottawa, Ottawa, ON, Canada

**Vincent M. Mellnick** Mallinckrodt Institute of Radiology, Washington University School of Medicine, St. Louis, MO, USA

**Christine O. Menias** Mayo Clinic Department of Radiology, Scottsdale, AZ, USA

**Vittorio Miele** Department of Radiology, Azienda Ospedaliero Universitaria Careggi, Florence, Italy

**Elka Miller** Medical Imaging Department, CHEO, Department of Radiology, University of Ottawa, Ottawa, ON, Canada

**Aaron Mintz** Mallinckrodt Institute of Radiology, St. Louis, MO, USA

**Arash Mir-Rahimi** Division of Interventional Radiology, University Health Network, Toronto General Hospital, Toronto, ON, Canada

**Hayley Moffatt** Section of Pediatric Radiology, Children's Hospital, Department of Radiology, University of Manitoba, Winnipeg, MB, Canada

**Gul Moonis** New York University Langone Health, NYU Grossman School of Medicine, New York, NY, USA

**Yunib H. Munir** UTHealth – McGovern School of Medicine, Houston, TX, USA

**Nicolas Murray** Department of Radiology, Vancouver General Hospital/University of British Columbia, Vancouver, BC, Canada

**Prakash Muthusami** Neuroradiology and Image Guided Therapy, Diagnostic Imaging, The Hospital for Sick Children, and University of Toronto, Toronto, ON, Canada

**Muhammad Naeem** Mallinckrodt Institute of Radiology, Washington University School of Medicine, St. Louis, MO, USA

**Jared Narvid** Department of Radiology and Biomedical Imaging, UCSF and Zuckerberg San Francisco General Hospital and Trauma Center, San Francisco, CA, USA

**Arash Nazeri** Mallinckrodt Institute of Radiology, St. Louis, MO, USA

**Kevin Neal** Mallinckrodt Institute of Radiology, St. Louis, MO, USA

**Savvas Nicolaou** Department of Radiology, Vancouver General Hospital/University of British Columbia, Vancouver, BC, Canada

**R. Niola** Department of Diagnostic and Interventional Radiology, "A. Cardarelli" Hospital, Naples, Italy

**Diego B. Nunez** Department of Radiology, Brigham and Women's Hospital, Harvard Medical School, Boston, MA, USA

**Devang Odedra** Department of Radiology, McMaster University, Hamilton, ON, Canada

**Daniel Oppenheimer** Abdominal Imaging Division, Department of Imaging Sciences, University of Rochester Medical Center, Rochester, NY, USA

**G. Oreopoulos** Division of Interventional Radiology, Department of Medical Imaging, University Health Network, Toronto, ON, Canada

Department of Surgery, Division of Vascular Surgery, University Health Network, Toronto, ON, Canada

**Johanna Maria Ospel** Department of Radiology, University Hospital Basel, University of Basel, Basel, Switzerland

Departments of Radiology and Clinical Neurosciences, University of Calgary, Foothills Medical Centre, Calgary, AB, Canada

**Neeral R. Patel** Division of Interventional Radiology, University Health Network, Toronto General Hospital, Toronto, ON, Canada

**Saagar Patel** UTHealth – McGovern School of Medicine, Houston, TX, USA

**Michael N. Patlas** Department of Radiology, McMaster University, Hamilton, ON, Canada

**Thuy-Huong Pham** Department of Surgery, Indiana University School of Medicine, Indianapolis, IN, USA

**Andrea Delli Pizzi** Department of Neuroscience, Imaging and Clinical Sciences, G. d'Annunzio University of Chieti, Chieti, Italy

**Jordan R. Pollock** Mayo Clinic Alix School of Medicine, Scottsdale, AZ, USA

**Christopher A. Potter** Department of Radiology, Brigham and Women's Hospital, Harvard Medical School, Boston, MA, USA

**Paulo Puac** Department of Radiology, Division of Neuroradiology, University of Ottawa, Ottawa, ON, Canada

**E. Qazi** Division of Interventional Radiology, Department of Medical Imaging, University Health Network, Toronto, ON, Canada

**Mohamed Z. Rajput** Mallinckrodt Institute of Radiology, Washington University School of Medicine, St. Louis, MO, USA

**Constantine A. Raptis** Mallinckrodt Institute of Radiology, St. Louis, MO, USA

**Varun Razdan** University of Wisconsin School of Medicine and Public Health, Madison, WI, USA

**Martin H. Reed** Section of Pediatric Radiology, Children's Hospital, Departments of Radiology and of Pediatrics and Child Health, University of Manitoba, Winnipeg, MB, Canada

**Roy F. Riascos** Department of Diagnostic and Interventional Imaging, University of Texas Health Science Center at Houston, Houston, TX, USA

**Francisco Rivas-Rodriguez** Department of Radiology, University of Michigan, Ann Arbor, MI, USA

**L. Romano** Department of General and Emergency Radiology, "A. Cardarelli" Hospital, Naples, Italy

**Enrica Rossi** Department of Radiology, Azienda Ospedaliero Universitaria Meyer, Florence, Italy

**Katya Rozovsky** Section of Pediatric Radiology, Children's Hospital, Department of Radiology, University of Manitoba, Winnipeg, MB, Canada

**Mariano Scaglione** Department of Medical, Surgical and Experimental Sciences, University of Medicine and Surgery, Sassari, Italy

Department of Radiology, James Cook University Hospital, Middlesbrough, UK

Teesside University School of Health and Life Sciences, Middlesbrough, Tees Valley, UK

Department of Radiology, Pineta Grande Hospital, Castel Volturno, Italy

**Barbara Seccia** Department of Neuroscience, Imaging and Clinical Sciences, G. d'Annunzio University of Chieti, Chieti, Italy

**Vinil Shah** Department of Radiology and Biomedical Imaging, UCSF and Zuckerberg San Francisco General Hospital and Trauma Center, San Francisco, CA, USA

**Gali Shapira-Zaltsberg** Department of Medical Imaging, CHEO, Ottawa, University of Toronto, Toronto, ON, Canada

**Donghoon Shin** Boston University Medical Center, Boston, MA, USA

**Manohar M. Shroff** Neuroradiology and Image Guided Therapy, Diagnostic Imaging, The Hospital for Sick Children, and University of Toronto, Toronto, ON, Canada

**Scott D. Steenburg** Department of Radiology and Imaging Sciences, Indiana University School of Medicine, Indianapolis, IN, USA

**Kacie L. Steinbrecher** Mallinckrodt Institute of Radiology, St. Louis, MO, USA

**Rebecca Stein-Wexler** University of California Davis Health Department of Radiology and Shriners Hospital for Children Northern California, Sacramento, CA, USA

**Jason F. Talbott** Department of Radiology and Biomedical Imaging, UCSF and Zuckerberg San Francisco General Hospital and Trauma Center, San Francisco, CA, USA

Brain and Spine Injury Center, Zuckerberg San Francisco General Hospital and Trauma Center, San Francisco, CA, USA

**M. J. Tao** Division of Interventional Radiology, Department of Medical Imaging, University Health Network, Toronto, ON, Canada

**Alessio Taraschi** Department of Neuroscience, Imaging and Clinical Sciences, G. d'Annunzio University of Chieti, Chieti, Italy

**Sara R. Teixeira** Radiology Department, Children's Hospital of Philadelphia, University of Pennsylvania, Philadelphia, PA, USA

**Michael Temple** Division of Image-Guided Therapy (IGT), Department of Diagnostic Imaging, The Hospital for Sick Children, Medical Imaging department, University of Toronto, Toronto, ON, Canada

**Richard Thomas** Department of Radiology, Lahey Hospital & Medical Center, Burlington, MA, USA

**Carlos Torres** Department of Radiology, Division of Neuroradiology, University of Ottawa, Ottawa, ON, Canada

**Ngoc-Anh Tran** Department of Radiology, Brigham and Women's Hospital, Harvard Medical School, Boston, MA, USA

**Margherita Trinci** Department of Emergency Radiology, Azienda Ospedaliera S. Camillo-Forlanini, Rome, Italy

**Jennifer F. True** Department of Radiology, University of Kentucky, Lexington, KY, USA

**F. Eymen Ucisik** Department of Diagnostic and Interventional Imaging, University of Texas Health Science Center at Houston, Houston, TX, USA

**Jennifer W. Uyeda** Department of Radiology, Division of Emergency Radiology, Brigham and Women's Hospital/Harvard Medical School, Boston, MA, USA

**Matthias W. Wagner** Division of Neuroradiology, The Hospital for Sick Children, Toronto, ON, Canada

**Walter F. Wiggins** Department of Radiology, Duke University Medical Center, Durham, NC, USA

**Thomas Wong** Vanderbilt University Medical Center, Department of Radiology, Nashville, TN, USA

**Jens Wrogemann** Section of Pediatric Radiology, Children's Hospital, Department of Radiology, University of Manitoba, Winnipeg, MB, Canada

**Motoyo Yano** Mayo Clinic Department of Radiology, Scottsdale, AZ, USA

**HeiShun Yu** Department of Radiology, Division of Emergency Radiology, Brigham and Women's Hospital/Harvard Medical School, Boston, MA, USA

**Nader Zakhari** Department of Radiology, Division of Neuroradiology, University of Ottawa, Ottawa, ON, Canada

**Carlos Zamora** Division of Neuroradiology, Department of Radiology, University of North Carolina School of Medicine, Chapel Hill, NC, USA

**Maria Zulfiqar** Mallinckrodt Institute of Radiology, Washington University School of Medicine, St. Louis, MO, USA

# Emergency and Trauma Imaging

## General Principles, Modalities, Challenges, and Opportunities

Michael N. Patlas, Douglas S. Katz, and Devang Odedra

## Contents

### Abstract

There has been a steady increase in emergency department (ED) visits worldwide over the past decade. Correspondingly, the utilization of the imaging in the ED is on the rise. The ED clinician today has a multitude of imaging modalities at his or her disposal, depending on the appropriateness of the modality for the presentation and on availability. Radiography and ultrasound are the most widely available modalities and often are part of the initial assessment of the patient. Point-of-care ultrasound (POCUS) has gained increasing attention and become more prevalent in the ED (and is used by both ED personnel and radiology) as a screening tool. Computed tomography (CT) has become the workhorse of advanced imaging in the ED given its growing availability, excellent anatomical resolution, and speed. Substantial advances have been made in CT technology, allowing for even faster image acquisition, reduction in dose, and analysis of tissue characteristics. Magnetic resonance imaging (MRI) and nuclear medicine have a more limited role in the initial assessment in the ED, are less readily available after hours, and often serve as second- or third-line modalities for problem-solving purposes, although for selective indications MRI is increasingly being used emergently in some regions and practices, if available. Choosing the correct modality with the highest yield and avoiding potential harm to the patient as well as limiting costs to the system is a joint effort between the ED clinician and the radiologist.

### Keywords

Emergency medicine · Emergency radiology · Radiography · Ultrasound · Computed tomography · Magnetic resonance imaging · Nuclear medicine · Dual-energy computed tomography · Point-of-care ultrasound

## Epidemiology

Emergency departments (EDs) around the world are getting busier. There were 10 million ED visits in Canada in 2014–2015 reported to the National Ambulatory Care Reporting System, which only represented approximately

M. N. Patlas · D. Odedra (✉)
Department of Radiology, McMaster University, Hamilton, ON, Canada
e-mail: patlas@hhsc.ca; devang.odedra@medportal.ca

D. S. Katz
NYU Langone Hospital - Long Island and the NYU Long Island School of Medicine, Mineola, NY, USA

63% of all ED visits [1]. In the USA, there were 137.8 million ED visits in 2014, which increased 14.8 percent from 2006 [2]. In England, approximately 70,000 patients visited an ED daily in 2019, a number that has been rising steadily as compared to 59,000 in 2012–2013 [3].

The top 3 reasons for visiting the ED are fever, cough, and abdominal pain in the pediatric population; abdominal pain, chest pain, and back pain in the adult population; and chest pain, abdominal pain, and shortness of breath in those over 65 years of age [1, 2]. While not one of the most common presentations, trauma carries a significant morbidity and mortality risk as well as a burden on the ED, given its requirement for acute and team-based management. In the year 2015, there were a total of 861,888 cases of trauma registered to the combined USA/Canada Trauma Registry, with a mortality rate of 4.4% [4]. Fall was the most common mechanism (44%), followed by motor vehicle collisions (26%). Firearm and penetrating trauma accounted for 8% collectively. Similarly, there were a total 33 million injury-related ED visits, resulting in 5 million hospital admissions and 230,000 deaths in the European Union (EU), between the years 2013 and 2015 [5].

Imaging plays an increasingly important role in the initial assessment, disposition, and follow-up of ED patients. There has been a steady increase in the utilization of imaging in the ED. The ED clinician now has a multitude of imaging modalities at his or her disposal, depending on the appropriateness and accessibility (Table 1). A recent patient-based survey showed that there was a significant increase in the utilization of advanced imaging with CT or MRI, while the utilization of radiography and ultrasound remained relatively stable. In particular, 14 of the 16 common clinical presentations to the ED were associated with CT or MRI in >10% of the visits in 2014 [6]. In another study, the number of cross-sectional imaging examinations (US, CT, or MRI) ordered increased from 400/1000 patients in 2006 to 550/1000 patients in 2011 [7]. An analysis of 595,895 ED visits in the USA from 2003 to 2012 demonstrated a steady increase in CT utilization with 142 CT scans per 1000 ED visits in 2003 to 169.2 scans in 2012 [8]. Efforts are underway worldwide for curbing the use of excessive imaging in the ED and in healthcare in general as exemplified by campaigns such as "Choosing Wisely" and the American College of Radiology Appropriateness Criteria [9, 10].

## Radiography

Initial assessment for many of the commonly presenting clinical complaints often begins with radiographs. It is the most commonly available imaging modality in the ED, and its relative ease of use for both the operator and the patient make it the most widely used one [11].

Chest radiography is the most frequently performed radiographic examination in the ED. It is the initial test of choice for the assessment of pneumonia, pneumothorax, or pleural effusions and is also the primary examination in the imaging workup of generalized complaints such as fatigue or weakness in the elderly. While the modality has good performance in certain situations, such as a sensitivity of up to 82% for the depiction of pneumonia, it has poor performance in other clinical scenarios, with a sensitivity range of only 10–22% for various radiographical signs of pulmonary embolism [12, 13]. Hence, chest radiography often serves as a screening modality, with more advanced imaging reserved for more definitive evaluation.

Abdominal radiographs are often the first line of investigation in patients with abdominal signs and symptoms including pain, vomiting, or change in bowel habits. There has been a mounting body of evidence against the diagnostic utility of abdominal radiographs in the ED setting, with limited sensitivity profile as the major drawback. Abdominal radiographs have been replaced with low-dose non-contrast CT protocols with much improved diagnostic utility at some centers around the world [14].

Radiographs are indispensable in the diagnosis and assessment of acute musculoskeletal injuries. They are the first line and often the most definitive modality in the management of extremity fractures, with further cross-sectional imaging reserved for more complex injury patterns. In contrast, radiography has a limited role in the assessment of certain anatomical regions, particularly the spine and the paranasal sinuses [15, 16]. The former presents a great challenge to ED clinicians, as back pain is one of the most common reasons for visiting the ED.

Radiography is based on ionizing radiation, which is a major drawback of the modality. However, the range of typical radiography is well below the generally accepted threshold of 10 mSv, above which the cancer risk from radiation exposure is believed to become more substantial [17]. For example, a standard two-view posteroanterior/lateral radiograph of the chest contributes 0.1 mSv of effective dose, and a single-view abdominal radiograph contributes 0.7 mSv of effective dose. In comparison, the average background radiation to an individual per year would amount to an equivalent of approximately 30 standard chest radiographs (3 mSv) [18]. However, as with other ionizing radiation modalities, the risk accumulates over the patient's lifetime with each additional imaging examination, and hence caution should be practiced, particularly in children, adolescents, and pregnant patients.

## Ultrasound

Ultrasound (US) is the second most widely utilized imaging modality in the ED. It benefits from absence of ionizing radiation, low cost, and widespread availability.

**Table 1** Relative costs, benefits, and common usages of imaging modalities in the ED [59, 60]

|  | Radiography | Ultrasound | CT | MRI | Nuclear medicine |
|---|---|---|---|---|---|
| Availability | ++++ | +++ | +++ | + | + |
| Relative cost | + | ++ | +++ | ++++ | ++++ |
| Radiation exposure | + | − | +++ | − | +++ |
| Operator variability | + | +++ | + | + | + |
| Common uses | MSK<br>Chest<br>Abdomen | Abdomen<br>Pelvis<br>Obstetrical<br>Vascular | Head<br>Chest<br>Abdomen<br>Pelvis<br>MSK | MSK<br>Neuro<br>Abdomen | Abdomen<br>Neuro<br>MSK |

MSK: musculoskeletal

US is particularly helpful in the assessment of solid abdominal and pelvic organs and also allows excellent assessment of the biliary system, urinary tract, and pelvic organs. US is the most definitive test for the acute assessment of cholecystitis, ovarian torsion, or testicular torsion [19]. It is also the first-line modality in the assessment of soft tissue lumps and bumps presenting in the ED. Vascular ultrasound also plays an important role in the ED, for example, in assessing for internal carotid artery stenosis or suspected deep vein thrombus.

In the recent years, point-of-care ultrasound (POCUS) has evolved into almost a separate imaging examination, which is often incorporated into the clinician's initial workup of the patient [20]. Many ED physicians now have completed certifications or diploma programs to enhance their competency in POCUS. POCUS has become a core competency in many of the current ED training programs [21]. There are now workshops and conferences dedicated to POCUS. The sensitivity of POCUS has been shown to be high for specific bedside indications, such as up to 100% for at least moderate-grade hydronephrosis [22] and up to 90% for cholelithiasis [23]. It can also be utilized for real-time guidance of bedside procedures including paracentesis, thoracentesis, or vascular access. However, the technique is highly dependent on the experience and ability of the operator, as well as the equipment [24]. It often serves to diagnose or exclude certain conditions and to organize patient disposition while the patient awaits a formal ultrasound in the radiology department.

One particular use of POCUS is the focused abdominal sonographic examination in trauma (FAST) examination. The FAST scan is a rapid and relatively easy tool at the bedside for the detection of free fluid within the pericardium and in three potential spaces: the right upper quadrant, the left upper quadrant, and in the rectovesical/rectouterine pouches. The sensitivity of FAST has been shown to be 85–96%, with a specificity of 98%. It has become a standard of practice in up to 96% of level I trauma centers [25]. It can also be readily extended for detection of hemothorax.

Ultrasound offers a real-time anatomical evaluation without the downside of associated radiation. However, there are also certain limitations of ultrasound. While the visualization of superficial structures is excellent, the image quality quickly degrades with depth in a large body habitus or with intervening bowel gas. This limitation affects an increasingly large number of patients with the rising trend in obesity worldwide. In addition, ultrasound is a highly operator-dependent modality, producing a great deal of variability in different hands depending on the level of experience and skill [26].

## Computed Tomography

CT has become the workhorse of emergency radiology over the last two decades. The greater spatial resolution, widespread availability, and rapid throughput afforded by CT have taken this modality to a new height.

From diagnosis of acute stroke to the evaluation of an ischemic limb, CT has truly emerged as a head-to-toe imaging modality in modern emergency medicine. A recent patient-based survey based on common conditions for presenting to the ED demonstrated a significant increase in CT utilization over the last decade. In 2014, 12 out of the 16 common conditions were associated with >10% of visits in the utilization of CT or MRI. For urinary calculus and headache, the utilization was up to 48.5% and 33.3% of the visits, respectively [6]. In 2008, a survey of a random sample of 5% of US EDs showed that 96% of the institutions had 24/7 access to a CT unit [27]. A study of trends of CT usage in the ED demonstrated a mounting growth in the number of ED visits involving a CT scan, with an annual growth of 16%. The percentage of ED visits resulting in a CT also grew exponentially, with up to 16.8% of ED visits resulting in a CT by 2007 [28, 29]. In another study, the authors analyzed the CT relative value units (RVUs) between 1993 and 2012 in the ED, demonstrating that the CT RVUs increased to 493% until 2007 and then decreased by 33% until 2012 [30].

CT is often the first screening examination for neurological presentations, particularly acute stroke. It has become the imaging modality of choice for acute respiratory conditions including pulmonary embolism, as well as for better assessment of parenchymal and pleural findings. It is the main modality for assessment of an acute abdomen. It has nearly replaced conventional angiography for the assessment of acute vascular pathologies such as aortic dissection [31] or critical limb ischemia. It permits better visualization and characterization of complex fracture patterns or hardware elements. Lastly, CT is at the epicenter of acute assessment in a multisystem trauma [32].

The major drawback of a CT is the ionizing radiation risk to the patient. A non-contrast CT of the brain contributes 2 mSv, which is equivalent to the exposure from 100 chest radiographs. A CT of the chest typically has a radiation exposure of 10–15 mSv and an abdominal single-phase CT of up to 10 mSv [33]. While the benefits of performing the examination almost always outweigh the theoretical risk of developing a cancer from a single CT examination, the risk becomes significant in patients who undergo multiple CT examinations during their lifespan. The collective burden of this risk may not be inconsequential with the aging demographics and a longer life expectancy [34].

There has been an abundance of technological innovation in CT. Advances on both software and hardware fronts have led to improvements in image quality and reduction in radiation dose. On the hardware side, the vast majority of current CT scanners are equipped with a two-dimensional array of detector elements, called multi-detector CT (MDCT). In contrast to the early scanners with a single linear array of detector elements, these newer MDCT scanners allow acquisition of a larger volume in a shorter amount of time [35]. The latest scanners are now capable of up to 320 detector rows, allowing them to capture better images of the beating heart. On the software front, advances in image reconstruction algorithms have led to radiation dose reduction and improvement in image quality. Iterative reconstruction techniques utilize several cycles of image construction and incorporate the use of photon statistics such as Poisson distribution and system hardware details to minimize image noise at lower dose levels [36].

Recently, momentum has been building for dual-energy CT (DECT). DECT is a newer technique where images are acquired simultaneously at two different energy levels. The attenuation differences in materials are utilized for deriving valuable information, including virtual monochromatic images, artifact suppression, and material characterization of various tissues. It has multiple applications in emergency radiology, ranging from improving the detection of pulmonary emboli, reducing metallic streak artifacts in penetrating trauma, subtracting plaques to better characterize vessels, and permitting analysis of composition of renal calculi [37, 38].

## Magnetic Resonance Imaging

The role of MRI has traditionally been limited in the ED due to its lack of access, high cost, and long study duration. Additionally, the acute management in most patients is guided by other modalities including radiography, ultrasound, and CT. In a very select number of patients, MRI is the first-line modality. In most patients, it is often the third- or fourth-line imaging test used to narrow the differential or to help make a specific diagnosis.

Brain and spine imaging are the most commonly performed MRI examinations in the ED [39]. MRI plays a key role in the diagnosis and monitoring of ischemic stroke, following initial assessment with non-contrast CT and CT angiography [40, 41]. Additionally, it also has utility in the diagnosis and recognition of complications of intracranial infections. MRI is a first-line test in a patient suspected of spinal cord compression, as it allows better visualization of the nerve roots and any compressive etiologies than any other modality. Similarly, MRI plays an important role in the assessment of any spinal pathology (such as a neoplasm or infection) which could lead to spinal cord compression [39, 42–44].

The other major use of MRI in the ED is in the assessment of acute musculoskeletal injuries such as hip or scaphoid fractures which can be occult on the initial radiographic or CT assessment, and missed diagnosis can lead to serious complications [45–47]. MRI also has a role in body imaging in the assessment of pediatric and pregnant patients, such as for assessment of possible appendicitis [48–51].

Aside from the overall lack of availability, there are certain limitations that hinder the use of MRI in the ED. Any history of MRI-unsafe metallic objects, including foreign bodies or implants, is a contraindication to MRI. Eliciting this history is especially challenging in the ED, where patients are seen very briefly and often without any previous documented records. Additionally, although affecting fewer than 1% patients, claustrophobia can prevent patients from undergoing MRI or can degrade image quality, reducing the utility of the modality [52]. Finally, the relatively longer duration of an MRI examination requires the patient to be away from optimal medical supervision for an extended period, which is a patient safety concern especially in the critically ill.

## Nuclear Medicine

Nuclear medicine is currently infrequently utilized in the evaluation of an ED patient. This is due to a multitude of variables including the sparse availability of nuclear medicine services after hours, its somewhat high cost, and more widespread availability of alternative imaging modalities. However, in certain scenarios where other modalities have failed to answer the clinical question, nuclear medicine techniques provide a superior role in diagnosis and management. The ability of the modality to image the physiological and functional aspects of disease processes lends itself a unique advantage over other modalities.

Some of the examples of nuclear medicine applications in acute presentations include a tagged red blood cell scan for acute gastrointestinal bleeding, which can reveal hemorrhage at a rate of as low as 0.1 mL/s, cholescintigraphy for otherwise equivocal cases of cholecystitis, ventilation/perfusion scans for pulmonary embolism, a brain perfusion examination for assessment of brain death (often for consideration of organ donation), a bone scan for acute musculoskeletal emergencies such as osteomyelitis or fractures, and a myocardial perfusion examination for ischemic heart disease [53–55].

Similar to radiography and CT, there is a potential risk of radiation from nuclear medicine examinations. For example, the effective radiation dose can be up to 2.5 mSv for a lung $^{133}$Xe/$^{99m}$Tc-MAA ventilation/perfusion scan, 7.8 mSv for a $^{99m}$Tc-labeled RBC scan, 3.1 mSv for a $^{99m}$Tc-disofenin biliary scan, 6.3 mSv for a $^{99m}$Tc-MDP bone scan, and 6.9 mSv for a $^{99m}$Tc-HMPAO-exametazime brain scan [56]. Additionally, a nuclear medicine division/operation requires adherence to a myriad of regulations, access to advanced expertise, and high operating costs [57]. Many of the radiopharmaceuticals utilized in nuclear medicine have complex and costly production processes and limited half-lives. A survey conducted by the Society of Nuclear Medicine in 2004 reported that only 29% out of the 983 responding institutions offered nuclear medicine over weekends [58]. Particularly in the hospitals with "0–125 beds" category, 65% were only open for 45 hours or less per week [58].

## Conclusion

The role of emergency radiology has evolved greatly over the last decade. An emergency clinician now has a gamut of multi-modality imaging at his or her disposal for rapid and accurate assessment of an acutely ill patient. While radiographs and ultrasound form the basis of initial imaging assessment in many patients, CT has become a cornerstone of the modern ED due to its universal accessibility, rapid operability, and excellent anatomical detail. MRI and nuclear medicine are often reserved for more delayed imaging for problem-solving purposes. Consequently, the emergency radiologist plays a key role at all stages of an ED patient's visit, providing valuable input on the appropriate selection of modality and interpretation of images.

**Key Points**
- Utilization of imaging in the ED is on the rise, particularly in the use of cross-sectional advanced imaging modalities (CT or MRI) for the evaluation of multiple parts of the human body.
- Plain radiography and ultrasound are the imaging cornerstone of the initial assessment of the ED patient.
- CT is the "workhorse" of definite imaging in the acutely ill patient, with numerous protocols and indications.
- MRI and nuclear medicine have a more selective and often problem-solving role in the ED.

## References

1. Emergency Department Visits in 2014–2015. Toronto: Canadian Institute for Health Information, 2015.
2. Moore BJ, Stocks C, Owens P. Trends in emergency department visits, 2006–2014. Agency for healthcare research and quality. 2017; Statistical Brief #227.:1–20.
3. Baker C. NHS key statistics: England February 2020. London: House of Commons Library; 2020.
4. Chang MC. National trauma data bank 2016 annual report. American College of Surgeons, 2016.
5. Kisser R, Walters A, Rogmans W, Turner S, Lyons R. Injuries in the European Union: 2013–2015. Amsterdam: EuroSafe; 2017.
6. Rosenkrantz AB, Hanna TN, Babb JS, Duszak R Jr. Changes in emergency department imaging: perspectives from national patient surveys over two decades. J Am Coll Radiol. 2017;14(10):1282–90.
7. Chaudhry S, Dhalla I, Lebovic G, Rogalla P, Dowdell T. Increase in utilization of afterhours medical imaging: a study of three Canadian academic centers. Can Assoc Radiol J. 2015;66(4):302–9.
8. Bellolio MF, Bellew SD, Sangaralingham LR, Campbell RL, Cabrera D, Jeffery MM, et al. Access to primary care and computed tomography use in the emergency department. BMC Health Serv Res. 2018;18(1):154.
9. Levinson W, Kallewaard M, Bhatia RS, Wolfson D, Shortt S, Kerr EA, et al. 'Choosing Wisely': a growing international campaign. BMJ Qual Saf. 2015;24(2):167–74.
10. Sistrom CL. The ACR appropriateness criteria: translation to practice and research. J Am Coll Radiol. 2005;2(1):61–7.
11. Levin DC, Rao VM, Parker L, Frangos AJ. Continued growth in emergency department imaging is bucking the overall trends. J Am Coll Radiol. 2014;11(11):1044–7.
12. Moore AJE, Wachsmann J, Chamarthy MR, Panjikaran L, Tanabe Y, Rajiah P. Imaging of acute pulmonary embolism: an update. Cardiovasc Diagn Ther. 2018;8(3):225–43.
13. Karimi E. Comparing sensitivity of ultrasonography and plain chest radiography in detection of pneumonia; a diagnostic value study. Arch Acad Emerg Med. 2019;7(1):e8.
14. Alshamari M, Norrman E, Geijer M, Jansson K, Geijer H. Diagnostic accuracy of low-dose CT compared with abdominal radiography in non-traumatic acute abdominal pain: prospective study and systematic review. Eur Radiol. 2016;26(6):1766–74.
15. Patel ND, Broderick DF, Burns J, Deshmukh TK, Fries IB, Harvey HB, et al. ACR appropriateness criteria low back pain. J Am Coll Radiol. 2016;13(9):1069–78.
16. Burke TF, Guertler AT, Timmons JH. Comparison of sinus x-rays with computed tomography scans in acute sinusitis. Acad Emerg Med. 1994;1(3):235–9.

17. Lin EC. Radiation risk from medical imaging. Mayo Clin Proc. 2010;85(12):1142–6. quiz 6
18. Jones JG, Mills CN, Mogensen MA, Lee CI. Radiation dose from medical imaging: a primer for emergency physicians. West J Emerg Med. 2012;13(2):202–10.
19. Michalke JA. An overview of emergency ultrasound in the United States. World J Emerg Med. 2012;3(2):85–90.
20. Leger P, Fleet R, Maltais-Giguere J, Plant J, Piette E, Legare F, et al. A majority of rural emergency departments in the province of Quebec use point-of-care ultrasound: a cross-sectional survey. BMC Emerg Med. 2015;15:36.
21. Galdamez LA. The evolving role of ultrasound in emergency medicine. Subhy A, editor: InTech Open; 2018.
22. Riddell J, Case A, Wopat R, Beckham S, Lucas M, McClung CD, et al. Sensitivity of emergency bedside ultrasound to detect hydronephrosis in patients with computed tomography-proven stones. West J Emerg Med. 2014;15(1):96–100.
23. Ross M, Brown M, McLaughlin K, Atkinson P, Thompson J, Powelson S, et al. Emergency physician-performed ultrasound to diagnose cholelithiasis: a systematic review. Acad Emerg Med. 2011;18(3):227–35.
24. Chawla TP, Cresswell M, Dhillon S, Greer MC, Hartery A, Keough V, et al. Canadian association of radiologists position statement on point-of-care ultrasound. Can Assoc Radiol J. 2019;70(3): 219–25.
25. Bloom BA, Gibbons RC. Focused Assessment with Sonography for Trauma (FAST). Treasure Island (FL): StatPearls; 2019.
26. Roberts S. Ultrasound-pros and cons [cited 2020 February 15]. Available from: https://www.euroespa.com/science-education/spe cialized-sections/espa-pain-committee/us-regional-anaesthesia/ultra sound-pros-and-cons/.
27. Ginde AA, Foianini A, Renner DM, Valley M, Camargo CA Jr. Availability and quality of computed tomography and magnetic resonance imaging equipment in U.S. emergency departments. Acad Emerg Med. 2008;15(8):780–3.
28. Larson DB, Johnson LW, Schnell BM, Salisbury SR, Forman HP. National trends in CT use in the emergency department: 1995–2007. Radiology. 2011;258(1):164–73.
29. Zhang X, Kim J, Patzer RE, Pitts SR, Chokshi FH, Schrager JD. Advanced diagnostic imaging utilization during emergency department visits in the United States: a predictive modeling study for emergency department triage. PLoS One. 2019;14(4): e0214905.
30. Raja AS, Ip IK, Sodickson AD, Walls RM, Seltzer SE, Kosowsky JM, et al. Radiology utilization in the emergency department: trends of the past 2 decades. AJR Am J Roentgenol. 2014;203(2): 355–60.
31. Meng J, Mellnick VM, Monteiro S, Patlas MN. Acute aortic syndrome: Yield of computed tomography angiography in patients with acute chest pain. Can Assoc Radiol J. 2019;70(1):23–8.
32. Pandharipande PV, Reisner AT, Binder WD, Zaheer A, Gunn ML, Linnau KF, et al. CT in the emergency department: a real-time study of changes in physician decision making. Radiology. 2016;278(3): 812–21.
33. Trattner S, Pearson GDN, Chin C, Cody DD, Gupta R, Hess CP, et al. Standardization and optimization of CT protocols to achieve low dose. J Am Coll Radiol. 2014;11(3):271–8.
34. Puts MTE, Hsu T, Szumacher E, Sattar S, Toubasi S, Rosario C, et al. Meeting the needs of the aging population: the Canadian Network on Aging and Cancer—report on the first Network meeting, 27 April 2016. Curr Oncol. 2017;24(2):e163–e70.
35. Horton KM, Sheth S, Corl F, Fishman EK. Multidetector row CT: principles and clinical applications. Crit Rev Comput Tomogr. 2002;43(2):143–81.
36. Padole A, Ali Khawaja RD, Kalra MK, Singh S. CT radiation dose and iterative reconstruction techniques. AJR Am J Roentgenol. 2015;204(4):W384–92.
37. Aran S, Shaqdan KW, Abujudeh HH. Dual-energy computed tomography (DECT) in emergency radiology: basic principles, techniques, and limitations. Emerg Radiol. 2014;21(4):391–405.
38. Aran S, Daftari Besheli L, Karcaaltincaba M, Gupta R, Flores EJ, Abujudeh HH. Applications of dual-energy CT in emergency radiology. AJR Am J Roentgenol. 2014;202(4):W314–24.
39. Sanchez Y, Yun BJ, Prabhakar AM, Glover M, White BA, Benzer TI, et al. Magnetic resonance imaging utilization in an emergency department observation unit. West J Emerg Med. 2017;18(5): 780–4.
40. Wintermark M, Sanelli PC, Albers GW, Bello JA, Derdeyn CP, Hetts SW, et al. Imaging recommendations for acute stroke and transient ischemic attack patients: a joint statement by the American Society of Neuroradiology, the American College of Radiology and the Society of NeuroInterventional Surgery. J Am Coll Radiol. 2013;10(11):828–32.
41. Lev MH. CT versus MR for acute stroke imaging: is the "obvious" choice necessarily the correct one? AJNR Am J Neuroradiol. 2003;24(10):1930–1.
42. Long A. The utility of MRI in the emergency department. 2017 [cited 2020 February 23]. Available from: http://www.emdocs.net/ utility-mri-emergency-department/.
43. Davis DP, Wold RM, Patel RJ, Tran AJ, Tokhi RN, Chan TC, et al. The clinical presentation and impact of diagnostic delays on emergency department patients with spinal epidural abscess. J Emerg Med. 2004;26(3):285–91.
44. Seidenwurm DJ, Wippold FJ 2nd, Cornelius RS, Angevine PD, Angtuaco EJ, Broderick DF, et al. ACR Appropriateness Criteria ((R)) myelopathy. J Am Coll Radiol. 2012;9(5):315–24.
45. Hakkarinen DK, Banh KV, Hendey GW. Magnetic resonance imaging identifies occult hip fractures missed by 64-slice computed tomography. J Emerg Med. 2012;43(2):303–7.
46. Ramasubbu B, Mac Suibhne E, El-Gammal A, Sheehy N, Shields D. Utilising magnetic resonance imaging as the gold-standard in management of suspected scaphoid fractures in the emergency department setting. Ir Med J. 2017;110(2):515.
47. Alabousi M, Gauthier ID, Li N, Dos Santos GM, Golev D, Patlas MN, et al. Multi-detector CT for suspected hip fragility fractures: a diagnostic test accuracy systematic review and meta-analysis. Emerg Radiol. 2019;26(5):549–56.
48. Furey EA, Bailey AA, Pedrosa I. Magnetic resonance imaging of acute abdominal and pelvic pain in pregnancy. Top Magn Reson Imaging. 2014;23(4):225–42.
49. Long SS, Long C, Lai H, Macura KJ. Imaging strategies for right lower quadrant pain in pregnancy. AJR Am J Roentgenol. 2011;196 (1):4–12.
50. Rosines LA, Chow DS, Lampl BS, Chen S, Gordon S, Mui LW, et al. Value of gadolinium-enhanced MRI in detection of acute appendicitis in children and adolescents. AJR Am J Roentgenol. 2014;203(5):W543–8.
51. Aspelund G, Fingeret A, Gross E, Kessler D, Keung C, Thirumoorthi A, et al. Ultrasonography/MRI versus CT for diagnosing appendicitis. Pediatrics. 2014;133(4):586–93.
52. Dewey M, Schink T, Dewey CF. Claustrophobia during magnetic resonance imaging: cohort study in over 55,000 patients. J Magn Reson Imaging. 2007;26(5):1322–7.
53. Amini B, Patel CB, Lewin MR, Kim T, Fisher RE. Diagnostic nuclear medicine in the ED. Am J Emerg Med. 2011;29(1): 91–101.
54. McGlone BS, Balan KK. The use of nuclear medicine techniques in the emergency department. Emerg Med J. 2001;18(6):424–9.

55. Behnia F, Gross JA, Ragucci M, Monti S, Mancini M, Elman S, et al. Nuclear medicine and the emergency department patient: an illustrative case-based approach. Radiol Med. 2015;120(1):158–70.
56. Mettler FA Jr, Huda W, Yoshizumi TT, Mahesh M. Effective doses in radiology and diagnostic nuclear medicine: a catalog. Radiology. 2008;248(1):254–63.
57. Adedapo KS, Onimode YA, Ejeh JE, Adepoju AO. Avoidable challenges of a nuclear medicine facility in a developing nation. Indian J Nucl Med. 2013;28(4):195–9.
58. Merlino DA. Nuclear medicine facility survey: SNM 2003 survey reporting on 2002 cost and utilization. J Nucl Med Technol. 2004;32 (4):215–9.
59. Brant WE. In: Brant WE, Helms CA, editors. Diagnostic imaging methods. Philadelphia: Lippincott, Williams and Wilkins; 2007.
60. Bushberg JT. In: Bushberg JT, Seibert JA, Leidholdt EM, Boone JM, editors. Introduction to medical imaging. Philadephia: Lippincott, Williams and Wilkins; 2011.

# Role of Artificial Intelligence in Emergency Radiology

**2**

Jonathan Liu, Arash Nazeri, and Aaron Mintz

## Contents

### Abstract

Advances in the field of artificial intelligence (AI), and in computing in the past decade, have made possible artificial neural networks that can "learn" to perform tasks previously reserved exclusively for humans. AI-enabled applications are already being deployed in radiology to assist in the detection and classification of diseases. The emergency department (ED), where timely and accurate diagnosis is critical, is an area of great interest for application of AI-driven solutions. AI algorithms offer great promise for addressing the challenges posed by increasing imaging volumes, increasing case complexity, and the need for rapid turnaround of results. Many products have already received US FDA clearance for clinical use. This chapter provides an introduction to key AI concepts, explores applications of AI in emergency radiology, and considers implications that AI will have for the field.

### Keywords

Artificial intelligence · AI · Deep learning · Machine learning · AI in radiology · AI in the emergency department

## Introduction

Advances in the field of artificial intelligence (AI), and in computing in the past decade, have made possible artificial neural networks that can "learn" to perform tasks previously reserved exclusively for humans. AI-enabled applications are already being deployed in radiology to assist in the detection and classification of diseases. The emergency department (ED), where timely and accurate diagnosis is critical, is an area of great interest for application of AI-driven solutions. AI algorithms offer great promise for addressing the challenges posed by increasing imaging volumes, increasing case complexity, and the need for rapid turnaround of results. Many products have already received US FDA clearance for clinical use. This chapter provides an introduction to key AI concepts and explores applications of AI in emergency radiology.

J. Liu · A. Nazeri · A. Mintz (✉)
Mallinckrodt Institute of Radiology, St. Louis, MO, USA
e-mail: jonathanliu@wustl.edu; a.nazeri@wustl.edu; mintza@wustl.edu

© Springer Nature Switzerland AG 2022
M. N. Patlas et al. (eds.), *Atlas of Emergency Imaging from Head-to-Toe*,
https://doi.org/10.1007/978-3-030-92111-8_2

## A Brief Overview of Artificial Intelligence

The idea of machines performing intelligent tasks dates to the origins of the field of computer science itself. It was not until 1956, however, at the Dartmouth conference on artificial intelligence (AI) that the field as we have come to know it was named [1]. AI has grown to be a broad, multidisciplinary field, encompassing the development of intelligent systems with the potential to impact nearly every aspect of modern life. From self-driving cars to doorbell cameras that recognize homeowners, AI-enabled applications are no longer the realm of science fiction. These developments have been made possible by a branch of computer science known as machine learning. Machine learning is a subset of artificial intelligence which deals with computer programs that can "learn" from data [2]. In a conventional algorithm, the variables that determine the algorithm's output given a set of inputs is fixed. These must be determined at the time of software writing. Machine learning algorithms, however, can learn from data to modify their variables so that their performance improves with training.

This difference is best illustrated with a high-level example. Consider the problem of detecting spiculated breast malignancies. A hard-coded computer program might take into account variables such as spicule length, central mass density, and the presence of calcification, and if these variables fall within or above a certain range, the program will flag the finding as concerning for malignancy. A machine learning approach would involve taking those same features (spicule length, mass density, and the presence of calcification), and training an algorithm on images of findings labeled as malignant or benign. The machine learning algorithm will modify its parameters to achieve a best fit to the training data, in the same way that a linear regression will achieve a best fit for a given two-dimensional dataset (in fact, linear regression is itself a machine learning algorithm). The result is improved performance for breast cancer detection. This machine learning approach is often referred to as "classical" machine learning [3]. Algorithms such as support vector machines, K-means clustering, and random forest classifiers fall into this category, a discussion of which is beyond the scope of this chapter.

In general, these algorithms require training features to be hand selected: spicule length, density, and the presence of calcification in our case. The massive breakthrough in artificial intelligence in the past decade has been made possible by a more general approach known as deep learning. Deep learning is built on neural networks, the same framework that underlies human cognition. In the case of breast malignancy detection, rather than relying on human selected features for training, deep learning methods allow for neural networks to identify the best features, and nonlinear relationships among those features, to "learn" how to classify abnormalities as benign or malignant (see Fig. 1). "Deep learning" refers to layers of neurons in between the input and output neurons, termed "hidden layers." These hidden layers are composed of interconnected nodes, and are where the "magic" happens (see Fig. 2). As a network is trained the weights between nodes are adjusted until, given an input, the network outputs the correct solution. Although artificial neural networks are not new, rapid development in graphical processing units (GPUs) which can perform certain types of mathematical operations much faster than central processing units (CPUs) has been the catalyst for accelerated advancement in this field starting around 2010 [2]. In that year a convolutional network, AlexNet, demonstrated the power of GPUs for implementing large complex neural networks with multiple layers [4]. Convolutional neural network (CNN) is a type of deep learning technique that lends itself very well to image-based problems. At a high level, CNNs build layers of filters which can be applied across a given image (Figs. 3 and 4). Low-level filters in the first layers of the network detect

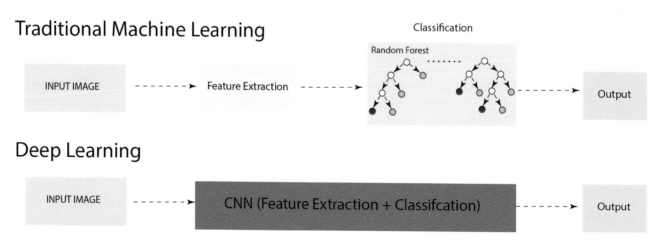

**Fig. 1** Depiction of "classical/traditional" machine learning vs deep learning: Historically, machine learning algorithms have required human-selected features. Deep learning techniques, in most cases, let the neural network identify the best features to learn for improved task performance

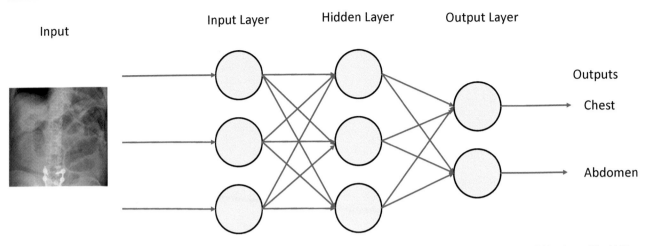

**Fig. 2** Deep learning neural network example: An artificial neural network (ANN) with input layer, output layer, and a hidden layer. The hidden layer(s) manage the complex computations that the network performs and differentiate the approach from ANNs with only input and output layers

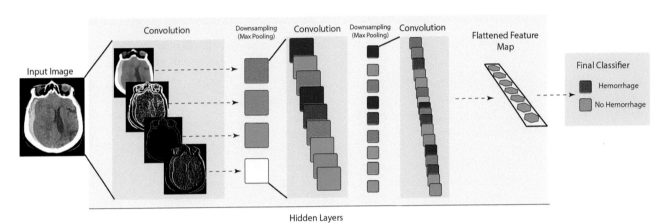

**Fig. 3** Depiction of a convolutional neural network (CNN): Deep learning network uses filters which are convolved across an image. Each subsequent layer in the network defines higher-level features (i.e., sharp edge vs spiculated shape). The filters are "learned" through training to optimize network performance

image features such as sharp edges or curves, while high-level filters make up the last layers of the network, and are activated when presented with more complex patterns. The process of applying a filter over an image is termed "convolving," which is where the technique gets its name [5, 6].

Applications of artificial intelligence in radiology are often categorized by task: detection, classification, and segmentation [2]. Detection refers to algorithms which identify the presence or absence of a finding on a given image, and in most cases the location of the finding; classification refers to algorithms that given an image will assign a class or category (i.e., benign or malignant), while segmentation algorithms delineate portions of an image on a pixel-by-pixel level (i.e., segmenting the left ventricular myocardium). These tasks may be implemented independently or as part of integrated workflows to detect and classify pathology, and form the basis for much of what we have come to know as artificial intelligence in radiology. There is also a great deal of interest

in image generation, which in the context of radiology refers to algorithms designed to improve image quality (for example, denoising low-dose CT images) [7].

As with any technology, the potential reach of deep learning is not limitless. Training neural networks is both computationally intensive and data intensive. Large datasets and, in most cases, labeled datasets are needed to train models to achieve acceptable performance. As a result, detecting and classifying rare pathologies present a challenge for current approaches [8]. Additionally, the quality and breadth of the training data utilized will determine the performance of the network. If the training dataset is not representative of the patient population where the algorithm is to be deployed, the network may not generalize well to real-world application, a problem known as overfitting. For example, an algorithm trained to reduce image artifact trained only on images generated by GE CT scanners may not perform well on Philips products. Likewise, an algorithm for fracture detection

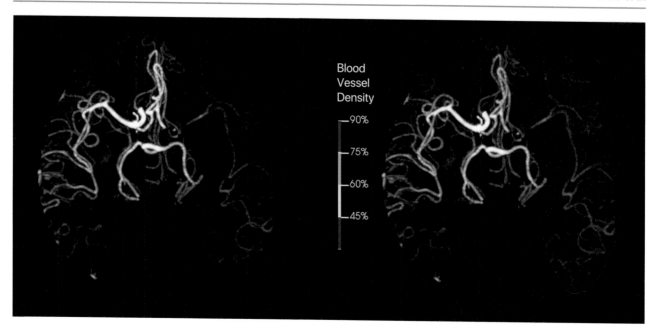

**Fig. 4** Depiction of RapidAI-automated ischemic stroke detection and perfusion analysis. (rapidai.com with permission)

trained on younger patients may perform poorly on patients with osteopenia. As a result, approval of AI algorithms necessitates that both training datasets, and datasets used for validation, have sufficient breadth, and are representative of the broader patient population.

Many radiologists have already interacted with tools that use machine learning for detection tasks. Breast imaging has been using computer-aided detection since the early 2000s [9]. Historically, CAD applications were built using classical machine learning algorithms with hand-crafted features [5]. While early studies showed a benefit to CAD in mammography, subsequent large trials in the mid-2010s did not realize an improvement in radiologist performance or patient outcomes [10]. With the advent of deep learning, these same tools have improved substantially, offering the promise of improving radiologist efficiency and patient outcomes [11]. In the past 2 years there has been accelerated progress in the field with deep learning enabled solutions now available for use in clinical practice. AI has made its way into every subspecialty of radiology, ranging from solutions for pediatric bone age assessment to classifying interstitial lung disease, and to detecting pulmonary emboli.

## AI Application in the ED

The emergency department (ED), where timely and accurate diagnosis is critical, is an area of great interest for application of AI-driven solutions. AI algorithms offer great promise for addressing the challenges posed by increasing imaging volumes, increasing case complexity, and the need for rapid turnaround of results. Beyond imaging applications uses, artificial intelligence has shown promise in several other domains including facilitating communication with ordering providers, creating prioritized worklists, and improving speech detection/prediction, among others. Although a thorough survey of all new algorithms is not possible within the scope of this chapter, a summary of currently US FDA-approved algorithms is provided to highlight the variety of applications currently or soon to be available in radiology (see Table 1) [12].

## Neuroimaging

Perhaps the earliest application of AI in the ED setting has been in the field of stroke imaging. With the advent of CT perfusion imaging and with multiple clinical trials demonstrating the benefit of even delayed intervention for large vessel occlusions in ischemic stroke, automated detection of perfusion abnormalities is now commonplace and a routine part of the clinical workflow in many radiology practices and academic institutions [13]. Several companies have created US FDA-approved AI systems to estimate or detect various features including infarct core/ischemic penumbra size, ASPECTS scores, presence of large vessel occlusions, and intracranial hemorrhage. The most well known is the Rapid Platform (https://www.rapidai.com/) which has been in clinical use with FDA approval since early 2019. At the time of writing, more than ten companies have submitted machine learning algorithms to the FDA for approval, all capable of sensitivity and specificities of detecting various intracranial

**Table 1** FDA-approved AI algorithms: Selected FDA-approved algorithms by application, modality, indication, and performance [12]

| Company | Area of interest | Modality | Pathology | Sensitivity (%) | Specificity (%) |
|---|---|---|---|---|---|
| **AIDoc** | Brain | CT | Large vessel occlusion | 89 | 87 |
| **AVICENNA. AI** | Brain | CT | Large vessel occlusion | 88 | 90 |
| **Viz.ai** | Brain | CT | Large vessel occlusion | 88 | 90 |
| **AIDoc** | Brain | CT | Intracranial hemorrhage | 94 | 92 |
| **AVICENNA. AI** | Brain | CT | Intracranial hemorrhage | 94 | 92 |
| **Curacloud** | Brain | CT | Intracranial hemorrhage | 91 | 93 |
| **Deep01** | Brain | CT | Intracranial hemorrhage | 94 | 92 |
| **RapidAI** | Brain | CT | Intracranial hemorrhage, ASPECTS score | 90 | 94 |
| **Qure.ai** | Brain | CT | Intracranial hemorrhage, fracture, mass effect, midline shift | 98 | 91 |
| **Zebra Medical** | Brain | CT | Intracranial hemorrhage | 95 | 93 |
| **Icometrix** | Brain | CT | Perfusion mapping | n/a | n/a |
| **AIDoc** | Spine | CT | Fracture | 92 | 89 |
| **Zebra Medical** | Spine | CT | Fracture | 90 | 87 |
| **Zebra Medical** | Chest | XR | Pleural effusion | 93 | 94 |
| **Behold.AI** | Chest | XR | Pneumothorax | 95 | 88 |
| **GE** | Chest | XR | Pneumothorax | 84 | 94 |
| **RadLogics** | Chest | XR | Pneumothorax | 92 | 90 |
| **Zebra Medical** | Chest | XR | Pneumothorax | 93 | 93 |
| **Qure.ai** | Chest | XR | Tuberculosis | 93–95 | 67–78 |
| **AIDoc** | Chest | CT | Pulmonary embolism | 91 | 90 |
| **AIDoc** | Abdomen | CT | Free intraabdominal air | 91 | 89 |

pathology at approximately 90%. It remains to be seen if this excellent performance in clinical trial settings is realized in clinical use. Nevertheless, accurate and reproducible detection of any of these findings represents an important time-saving measure, one that can markedly alter patient management. On average, these automated systems aim to cut down the time to notification from an hour after the examination has been performed to less than 5 min. Such prompt notification is paramount when treatment for ischemic stroke or an intracranial hemorrhage must occur within hours of symptom onset to avoid patient morbidity or mortality.

## Radiography

One of the most commonly ordered imaging examination in the emergency department is the chest radiograph. Often a screening tool ordered at the time of patient presentation, there may be a substantial delay between radiography acquisition and interpretation, particularly during off hours. Important findings including pneumothoraces, mediastinal hematoma, pleural effusions, and pneumonia may not be identified in some cases up to several hours later (depending on overnight radiologist availability). With the large amounts of data available to train machine learning algorithms, several

algorithms have been developed to detect these critical findings. In fact, many of the currently US FDA-approved algorithms as applied to chest radiographs aim to provide a similar level of sensitivity and accuracy to what is provided by board-certified radiologists. Currently, US FDA-approved algorithms exist to detect pneumothoraces or pleural effusions with over 90% sensitivity and specificity and receiver operating characteristics of over 0.95, a figure comparable, if not superior, to board certified radiologists. A second use for feature detection in ED is for the detection of bacterial and atypical pneumonia, most notably pulmonary tuberculosis. Machine learning algorithms have been developed to detect the developing cavitary foci or consolidations that may signal primary or reactivated tuberculosis with receiver operating characteristics approaching 0.90. Such a machine learning algorithm is particularly attractive in low-resource settings, where patients may not have access to further cross-sectional imaging, yet accurate diagnosis is required.

While some AI applications render a diagnosis or the presence of a finding, other algorithms can modify the appearance of the examination itself, either accentuating or masking certain attributes of the examination. This application is particularly useful in the setting of identifying misplaced lines or tubes. Currently, several companies have developed methods to highlight the tip of central venous catheters and cardiac leads, facilitating the detection of aberrantly placed or malpositioned devices. This application is an example of a broader category of applications utilizing image generation, where the output of the software is a new image or series of images to assist in study interpretation (denoising and quality enhancement).

## Cross-Sectional Body Imaging

One particularly common indication for CT is the detection of pulmonary emboli (PE). Currently, US FDA-approved algorithms boast nearly 90% sensitivity and specificity for PE detection. Again, in addition to accurate detection of critical findings, the automated nature of pulmonary embolism detection allows for timely notification to the ordering providers. Depending on the speed of the machine learning algorithm and presence of infrastructure for communication through the hospital's existing EMR, an emergency room physician may be notified within 5–10 min after performing the scan. Alternatively, the algorithm may be integrated into the radiology worklist to prioritize the examination for interpretation. Similar performance metrics have been reported for detection of free intrabdominal gas on abdominal CT and spinal fractures on spine CT scan.

US FDA-approved segmentation algorithms have much promise in the ED radiology setting, including, for example, in the diagnosis and surveillance of aortic aneurysms. A change in the diameter or shape of an aortic aneurysm may signal an impending rupture or other acute aortic injury. Algorithms are now available which are able to recognize aortic landmarks and to render measurements that are accurate to the order of 1.5 mm. Reliable, reproducible measurement is often a time-consuming process, especially when multiplanar reformatting is unavailable or cumbersome. Automating this process can potentially lead to improvements in report turnaround time and reproducibility of measurements. Future directions will likely involve developing automated monitoring strategies of these critical findings or structures (e.g., aortic aneurysm size, metastatic findings, or location of implanted devices).

Image generation applications show great promise for emergency radiology. Currently, algorithms exist to reduce the quantum mottle present in a low-dose CT for lung cancer screening. Denoising an image improves the accuracy with which radiologists can detect small abnormalities, such as pulmonary nodules, or findings which require high resolution, such as coronary angiography. Poor-quality images occur frequently in the emergency department setting either because of patient motion or large body habitus, resulting in photon starvation. When used in conjunction with high-pitch imaging, there is great potential for reducing both radiation dose and motion artifact while maintaining adequate contrast and spatial resolution.

## Non-image-Based Applications

AI-enabled language processing algorithms are also becoming ubiquitous. Many companies are working on software to improve speech recognition, prioritize the imaging worklist, and implement automatic decision support such as recommending the appropriate screening or management guidelines for incidental findings and notify ordering providers [14].

## Implementation Challenges

There are many paths currently to integrating AI algorithms into existing workflows. Many vendor solutions receive images from the modality (either via on-site or cloud applications running their algorithms), process the data, and send the output directly to a picture archival and communication system (PACS) or radiology information system (RIS) for annotations to be reviewed, and/or worklist prioritization to be updated [15]. To the extent that an organization wishes to integrate multiple algorithms, this offers a challenge to IT departments, as each vendor will require DICOM and HL7 integration independently. To solve for this challenge, vendors such as Nuance communications (nuance.com), the maker of Powerscribe dictation software, are building app marketplaces similar to the Apple app store. By defining standards for integration, these marketplaces will make it easier for hospitals and radiology practices to identify AI applications of interest, and to integrate them into existing IT workflows.

## Implications for ED Radiology

AI is advancing rapidly in the field of radiology. Many US FDA-approved algorithms are either targeted specifically toward indications common to the ED, or have potential application in ED radiology. This is primarily a reflection of the need to detect discrete pathology in a timely fashion to rule in or rule out potentially life-threatening conditions (PE, pneumothorax, cerebral hemorrhage, etc.). As it currently stands, these products are designed to support the ED radiologist, prioritizing cases with critical findings, highlighting detected pathology on images within the PACS, or improving image quality. Taken as a whole, these systems seek to make radiologists more efficient and more accurate. The scope of the applications is limited, however. Although the technology continues to evolve rapidly, availability of high-quality labeled data will continue to be a significant challenge as researchers and companies try to build AI systems that go beyond the above-described detection and classification tasks. Although unsupervised learning, a technique not requiring labeled data, may offer hope for addressing this challenge, it is unlikely to completely alleviate it. Were one to compare the current list of approved algorithms with an exhaustive list of diagnoses that may be made in ED imaging, it becomes clear that AI is in no danger of replacing radiologists in the emergency department anytime in the foreseeable future.

# References

1. Buchanan BG. A (very) brief history of artificial intelligence. AI Mag. 2005;26:53.
2. Chartrand G, Cheng PM, Vorontsov E, Drozdzal M, Turcotte S, Pal CJ, et al. Deep learning: a primer for radiologists. Radiographics. 2017;37(7):2113–31.
3. van Ginneken B. Fifty years of computer analysis in chest imaging: rule-based, machine learning, deep learning. Radiol Phys Technol. 2017;10:23–32.
4. Krizhevsky A, Sutskever I, Hinton GE. Imagenet classification with deep convolutional neural networks. Adv Neural Inf Process Syst. 2012;25:1097–105.
5. Do S, Song KD, Chung JW. Basics of deep learning: a radiologist's guide to understanding published radiology articles on deep learning. Korean J Radiol. 2020;21:33–41.
6. Giger ML. Machine learning in medical imaging. J Am Coll Radiol. 2018;15(3):512–20.
7. Higaki T, Nakamura Y, Tatsugami F, Nakaura T, Awai K. Improvement of image quality at CT and MRI using deep learning. Jpn J Radiol. 2019;37(1):73–80.
8. Yasaka K, Abe O. Deep learning and artificial intelligence in radiology: current applications and future directions. PLoS Med. 2018;15(11):e1002707.
9. Baker JA, Rosen EL, Lo JY, Gimenez EI, Walsh R, Soo MS. Computer-aided detection (CAD) in screening mammography: sensitivity of commercial CAD systems for detecting architectural distortion. Am J Roentgenol. 2003;181(4):1083–8.
10. Fenton JJ, Abraham L, Taplin SH, Geller BM, Carney PA, D'Orsi C, et al. Effectiveness of computer-aided detection in community mammography practice. J Natl Cancer Inst. 2011;103(15):1152–61.
11. Gao Y, Geras KJ, Lewin AA, Moy L. New frontiers: an update on computer-aided diagnosis for breast imaging in the age of artificial intelligence. Am J Roentgenol. 2019;212(2):300–7.
12. FDA Cleared AI Algorithms | American College of Radiology [Internet]. [Cited 2020, Aug 10]. Available from: https://www.acrdsi.org/DSI-Services/FDA-Cleared-AI-Algorithms
13. Campbell BCV, Mitchell PJ, Kleinig TJ, Dewey HM, Churilov L, Yassi N, et al. Endovascular therapy for ischemic stroke with perfusion-imaging selection. N Engl J Med. 2015;372(11):1009–18.
14. Sorin V, Barash Y, Konen E, Klang E. Deep learning for natural language processing in radiology – fundamentals and a systematic review. J Am Coll Radiol. 2020;17(5):639–48.
15. Dikici E, Bigelow M, Prevedello LM, White RD, Erdal BS. Integrating AI into radiology workflow: levels of research, production, and feedback maturity. J Med Imaging. 2020;7(01):1.

# Vascular Emergencies

## When to Call an Interventional Radiologist

E. Qazi, M. J. Tao, G. Oreopoulos, G. Annamalai, and Sebastian Mafeld

**3**

## Contents

E. Qazi · M. J. Tao · G. Annamalai · S. Mafeld (✉)
Division of Interventional Radiology, Department of Medical Imaging,
University Health Network, Toronto, ON, Canada
e-mail: SebastianCharles.Mafeld@uhn.ca

G. Oreopoulos
Division of Interventional Radiology, Department of Medical Imaging,
University Health Network, Toronto, ON, Canada

Department of Surgery, Division of Vascular Surgery, University Health
Network, Toronto, ON, Canada

© Springer Nature Switzerland AG 2022
M. N. Patlas et al. (eds.), *Atlas of Emergency Imaging from Head-to-Toe*,
https://doi.org/10.1007/978-3-030-92111-8_3

### Abstract

Interventional radiology is in a unique position to provide both expert image interpretation and treatment for vascular emergencies. With a general shift toward becoming a more clinical specialty, many interventional radiologists appreciate being contacted early in a patient's care pathway. The authors have witnessed many instances where interventional radiology was contacted late in a patient's management which can compromise the outcome. With varied provision of interventional radiology on-call services globally, "when to call the interventional radiologist" is heavily dependent upon an individual institution's logistical setup. Another Factor to consider is that many on-call interventional radiology services are based around a team that is "off-site," and requires advanced notice before a case can be initiated. Again, this further emphasizes the importance of contacting interventional radiology early in a patient's care pathway. In the cases below we have sought to highlight specific conditions where interventional radiology can assist in providing both expert vascular imaging interpretation as well as management. The vascular emergencies that have been highlighted include ruptured abdominal aortic aneurysm, aortic dissection, liver/kidney/spleen/pelvic trauma, acute limb ischemia, hemoptysis, gastrointestinal bleeding, and postpartum hemorrhage.

### Keywords

Vascular emergencies · Endovascular management · Abdominal aortic aneurysm · Aortic dissection · Visceral trauma · Limb ischemia · Hemoptysis · GI bleeding and post partum hemorrhage

## Ruptured Abdominal Aortic Aneurysm (RAAA)

### Epidemiology

RAAA is a life-threatening complication with a mortality of 80–90%, with three-fourth of these occurring outside of a hospital [1]. Risk factors for rupturing an aneurysm include aneurysm size, expansion rate, the presence of symptoms, and patient factors (Fig. 1).

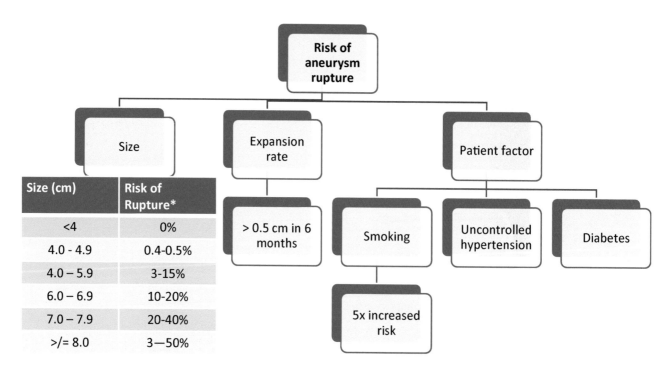

| Size (cm) | Risk of Rupture* |
|-----------|------------------|
| <4 | 0% |
| 4.0 - 4.9 | 0.4-0.5% |
| 4.0 – 5.9 | 3-15% |
| 6.0 – 6.9 | 10-20% |
| 7.0 – 7.9 | 20-40% |
| >/= 8.0 | 3—50% |

* Brewster DC, Cronenwett JL, Hallett JW, Johnston KW, Krupski WC, Matsumura JS, et al. Guidelines for the treatment of abdominal aortic aneurysms. Report of a subcommittee of the Joint Council of the American Association for Vascular Surgery and Society for Vascular Surgery. J Vasc Surg. 2003 May;37(5):1106–17.

**Fig. 1** Ruptured abdominal aortic aneurysm risk factors [1]

## Clinical Features

RAAA can present with acute onset of severe abdominal or back pain, hypotension, and shock. A clinical diagnosis of ruptured abdominal aortic aneurysm should be considered in patients >50 years old who present with back pain and hypotension, particularly if they have a known AAA [2]. Large aneurysms or thin patients may have a pulsatile mass [2].

## Diagnostic Investigation

Ultrasound has a limited role in the evaluation of RAAA. The aorta may not be visualized due to overlying bowel gas or body habitus, and while US may confirm the presence of an AAA, it cannot be used to reliably exclude or confirm rupture [3]. CT angiography (CTA) is the imaging modality of choice, and should include a noncontrast scan in addition to post IV contrast imaging. Many of the symptoms of RAAA are nonspecific, and can be seen with other causes of abdominal pain. As such, RAAA may be diagnosed on CT performed for other indications.

The most common finding of RAAA is a retroperitoneal hematoma adjacent to an AAA (Fig. 2). On CTA, active extravasation of contrast may be visualized. Signs suggesting acute or impending rupture also include the "crescent sign," "draped aorta" sign, and interruption of circumferential calcifications (Fig. 3) [3].

## Management

RAAA is a surgical emergency. High perioperative morbidity and mortality risks remain in patients who survive to undergo repair. Emergency vascular surgery and interventional radiology/ consultation should be obtained, and immediate transfer to a center with expertise in aortic repair may be required [3]. "Permissive hypotension" (systolic 60–70 mmHg and not above 100 mmHg) should be maintained as aggressive fluid resuscitation can worsen hemorrhage by overcoming the tamponade. Resuscitation goals are to maintain consciousness, prevent ischemic cardiac changes on ECG, as well to maintain an adequate urine output (>0.5 cc/kg/h).

Both open surgical repair (OSR) and EVAR are acceptable options for RAAA depending on aneurysm characteristics. Decision-making is often complex. Temporary aortic balloon occlusion can be used to control hemodynamic instability. Relative exclusion criteria for EVAR are listed in Table 1. Evolving evidence suggests a survival advantage and reduced hospital length of stay for patients undergoing EVAR for RAAA ("REVAR") compared with OSR [4].

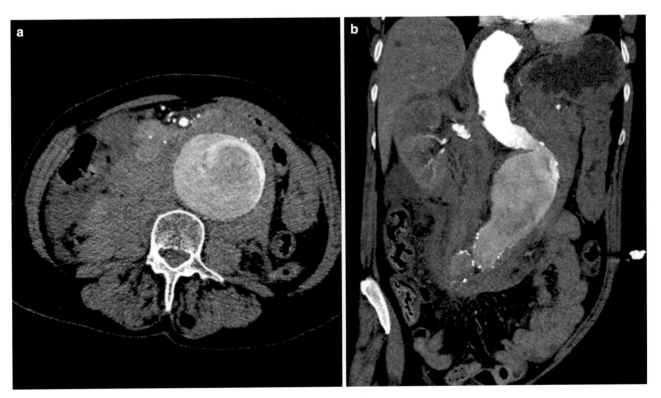

**Fig. 2** Axial (**a**) and coronal (**b**) CT angiogram of a ruptured abdominal aortic aneurysm. Extensive perianeurysmal retroperitoneal hematoma is present. No active extravasation of contrast

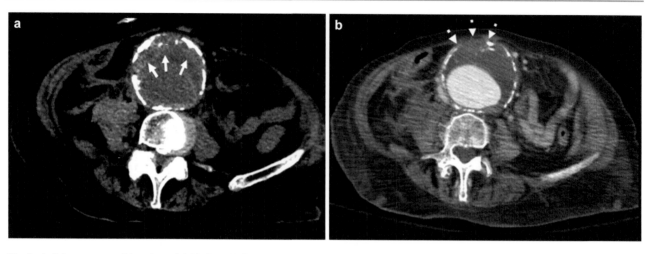

**Fig. 3** Axial noncontrast (**a**) and arterial (**b**) CT with features of a ruptured abdominal aortic aneurysm as demonstrated by a hyperdense crescent sign (arrows), disruption of calcification (arrowheads), and retroperitoneal hemorrhage

**Table 1** Relative exclusion criteria for infrarenal endovascular aneurysm repair (EVAR)

| Relative Exclusion criteria for EVAR |
| --- |
| Aneurysm neck length <1 cm |
| Neck diameter >3.2 cm |
| Aortic aneurysm neck angulation greater than 60 ° |
| Common iliac diameter >2.0 cm or <0.6 cm |

Exclusions depend on type of endograft and are manufacturer dependent

**Key Points**

- CTA is the imaging modality of choice to investigate RAAA in the stable patient.
- RAAA is a life-threatening emergency. <u>Immediate</u> consultation with an aortic (vascular) service should be obtained.
- Interventional radiologists are often key members of an aortic service, and should be consulted early as part of a multidisciplinary approach to managing a RAAA.
- **R**EVAR and OSR are both viable treatment options for ruptured AAA, with REVAR offering a survival advantage.

## Aortic Dissection (AD)

### Epidemiology

AD is a life-threatening condition with an incidence of 2–3.5/ 100,000 people [5]. Mortality is reported in one-third of hospitalized patients [6]. Risk factors for AD include hypertension, connective tissue diseases (e.g., Marfans, Loey Dietz, and Ehlers-Danlos), trauma, penetrating aortic ulcer, and illicit drugs. Early diagnosis and treatment are critical to improve outcomes [7]. Prognosis depends on the type of dissection, extent of branch vessel involvement, and associated complications [7].

Multiple classification systems exist for AD, including DeBakey, Stanford, and the recent SVS classification (Fig. 4) [7]. A Stanford type A dissection involves the ascending aorta, while the ascending aorta is spared in a type B dissection, and the intimal tear originates distal to the left subclavian artery. The distinction between type A and B dissections is important, as type A dissections have a worse prognosis and are treated emergently with surgical repair by cardiovascular surgery [7]. DeBakey and Stanford classifications have been subject to critique due to confusion surrounding how to classify dissections that extend into the aortic arch but spare the ascending aorta (Fig. 5) [8]. While the Stanford classification defined type A and type B by their location relative to the left subclavian artery, the new SVS guidelines classify a dissection by location of the entry tear along with the extent of the dissection defined by aortic zone (Fig. 4). Any dissection with an entry tear involving zone 0 is considered type A, while if the entry tear is in zone 1 or beyond it is classified as type B [7]. For example, a type A dissection with its entry tear in zone 0 extending to zone 9 of the aorta (see Fig. 4 SVS classification) is now classified as A9. A type B with an entry tear in zone 3 but with proximal extent of the dissection from zone 1 and distal extent to zone 9 would be categorized B1,9. If the entry tear cannot be identified but the dissection involves zone 1 or beyond, the dissection is still classified as type B. If the dissection involves zone 0 but the entry tear cannot be seen, in theory it could be a type A or type B, therefore by the new SVS guidelines this dissection would be classified as Indeterminate "I."

## Clinical Features

The most common presentation of AD is pain [5, 7]. It typically presents as abrupt onset tearing abdominal or chest

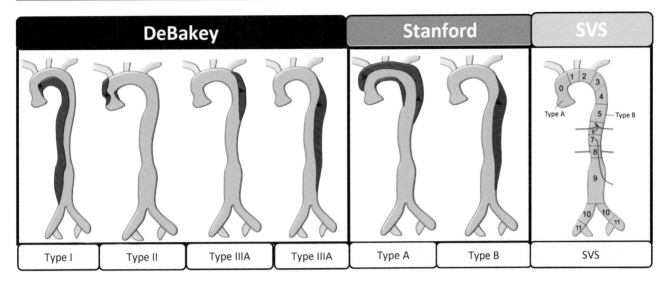

**Fig. 4** Debakey, Stanford, and Society of Vascular Surgery (SVS) classifications of aortic dissections. Stanford type A aortic dissections involve the proximal ascending aorta, while type B dissections involve the aorta distal to the left subclavian. The SVS classification classifies aortic dissections by location of the entry tear along with its proximal and distal extent. (Adapted from Lombardi et al. [7])

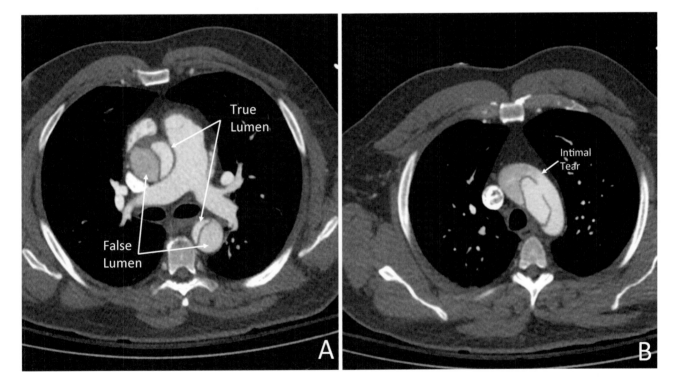

**Fig. 5** Axial CT angiogram demonstrating aortic dissection with intimal tear originating in the aortic arch (**a–b**). There is retrograde extension of the dissection flap into the proximal ascending aorta. The distal extent of the dissection flap is to the common iliac arteries (not shown). This is in keeping with a Stanford type A dissection, and B 0, 10, according to the SVS guidelines

pain that radiates to the back [5]. Type A dissections can present with cardiac complications including tamponade, or aortic regurgitation, if the dissection flap extends to the aortic root. Cerebrovascular, mesenteric, renal, and limb ischemia can result from branch involvement of the dissection flap, or if there is obliteration of the true lumen by the false lumen. A dissection flap can extend into a branch vessel with resultant narrowing or occlusion (static obstruction). Alternatively, with changes in pressurization of the true and false lumen, the intimal flap can transiently occlude the orifices of visceral branches (dynamic obstruction). Identifying dynamic obstruction on CT can be challenging, therefore relying on imaging findings alone to diagnose malperfusion is insufficient.

## Diagnostic Investigations

ECG evaluation may be normal unless there is involvement of the coronary arteries by the dissection [6]. Transthoracic echocardiography (TTE) can be used to assess the ascending aorta, with a sensitivity of 59-83% and specificity of 63–93% [6]. Transesophageal echocardiography has a sensitivity of 94–100% and a specificity of 77–100% to identify an intimal flap [6]. However, the distal aorta and its branching vessels are not well assessed on echocardiography [6].

Evaluation of the entire aorta, branch vessels, iliacs, and proximal femoral arteries is required when there is clinical suspicion of an AD. CTA of the thorax, abdomen, and pelvis is used to identify the intimal entry tear and the extent of the dissection flap. Magnetic resonance angiography (MRA) is not typically used for acute AD, although in stable patients dynamic MRA can be considered to determine entry tear location and treatment planning [6].

## Management

Management of AD is complex, and should involve a multidisciplinary team. Type A dissections are typically treated by cardiothoracic surgical repair. Type B dissections can be uncomplicated or complicated. An uncomplicated dissection demonstrates no evidence of rupture, malperfusion, or high-risk features (Table 2) [7]. Treatment of type B dissections is dictated by patient presentation (i.e., uncomplicated versus complicated) [7]. Acute uUncomplicated type B dissections are managed medically with antihypertensives in an ICU [7]. Complicated type B dissections can be treated with thoracic endovascular aortic repair (TEVAR) or open surgical repair [9–12]. With favorable anatomy, TEVAR is the first choice, and advantages include lower perioperative morbidity/mortality, shorter hospitalization, and avoidance of aortic cross-clamping and cardiopulmonary bypass [11, 13]. Closure of the primary intimal tear can result in aortic remodeling, defined as regression of the false lumen and expansion of the

**Table 2** High-risk features in aortic dissections [7]

| High-risk features |
| --- |
| Refractory pain |
| Refractory hypertension |
| Bloody pleural effusion |
| Aortic diameter >40 mm |
| Radiographic malperfusion |
| Readmission, entry tear in lesser curve location |
| False lumen diameter >22 mm |

true lumen [14]. This is associated with improved long-term survival, and fewer aortic-related adverse events [14].

### Key Points
- Acute AD is a complex, life-threatening condition, with outcomes improved by early diagnosis and management.
- AD has traditionally been classified by the DeBakey and Stanford classification systems. The new 2020 SVS classification classifies a dissection by the location of the entry tear, along with the proximal and distal extent, by aortic zone.
- Type B dissections can be complicated or uncomplicated. Uncomplicated dissections are generally treated with medical management, while complicated dissections are treated with TEVAR (or surgical repair).
- Interventional radiologists are key members of a multidisciplinary aortic service who can assist in determining the extent of AD as well as the endovascular management for complicated type B AD.

## Trauma: Spleen, Liver, Kidney, and Pelvis

Traumatic injuries are a major cause of morbidity and mortality. Initial assessment and management follow advanced trauma life support (ATLS) principles. For stable patients, diagnostic investigations include radiographs (chest and pelvis), bedside-focused ultrasound (FAST), and multiphasic CT panscan using the institutional trauma protocol. Embolization may be considered for stabilization of patients with solid organ or pelvic injury in the absence of indications for immediate surgery. IR thus plays a pivotal role in the multidisciplinary management algorithm.

Commonly injured visceral organs include the spleen, liver, kidneys, small bowel, and/or mesentery, bladder, colon and/or rectum, diaphragm, pancreas, and major vessels [15]. The American Association for the Surgery of Trauma (AAST) scale is an accepted classification system for visceral organ injuries (Table 3) [16, 17].

## Spleen

The spleen is highly vascular making untreated injuries potentially fatal. Its main arterial supply is the splenic artery, and also has abundant collaterals (short gastric and gastroepiploic arteries). IV contrast-enhanced CT is the reference standard for diagnosis and grading of splenic injuries, with a sensitivity and specificity of 96–100% (Fig. 6) [18].

Splenectomy is often required for hemodynamically unstable patients and in patients with associated injuries or peritonitis. For hemodynamically stable patients without peritonitis, nonoperative management with splenic preservation is the standard of care.

**Table 3** American Association for the Surgery of Trauma (AAST) scale of the spleen, liver, and kidneys [17]

| | Spleen | Liver | Kidney |
|---|---|---|---|
| Grade I | Subcapsular hematoma <10% surface area | Subcapsular hematoma <10% surface area | Subcapsular hematoma or contusion, without laceration |
| | Parenchymal laceration <1 cm | Parenchymal laceration <1 cm depth | |
| | Capsular tear | | |
| Grade II | Subcapsular hematoma 10–50% surface area | Subcapsular hematoma 10–50% surface area | Hematoma: nonexpanding perirenal confined to renal retroperitoneum |
| | Intraparenchymal hematoma <5 cm | Intraparenchymal hematoma <10 cm in diameter | Laceration: ≤1 cm depth not involving the collecting system |
| | Parenchymal laceration 1–3 cm | Laceration 1–3 cm in depth and ≤10 cm length | |
| Grade III | Subcapsular hematoma >50% surface area | Subcapsular hematoma >50% surface area; ruptured subcapsular or parenchymal hematoma | Laceration >1 cm not involving the collecting system |
| | Ruptured subcapsular or intraparenchymal hematoma ≥5 cm | Intraparenchymal laceration >10 cm | Vascular injury or active bleeding contained within Gerota fascia |
| | Parenchymal laceration >3 cm | Laceration >3 cm depth | |
| | | Any injury in the presence of a liver vascular injury or active bleeding contained within liver parenchyma | |
| Grade IV | Vascular injury or active bleeding confined within the capsule | Parenchymal disruption involving 25–75% of a hepatic lobe | Parenchymal laceration extending into urinary collecting system with urinary extravasation |
| | Parenchymal laceration involving segmental or hilar vessels producing >25% devascularization | Active bleeding extending beyond the liver parenchyma into the peritoneum | Renal pelvis laceration and/or complete ureteropelvic disruption |
| | | | Segmental renal vein or artery injury |
| | | | Active bleeding beyond Gerota fascia into the retroperitoneum or peritoneum |
| | | | Segmental or complete kidney infarction(s) due to vessel thrombosis without active bleeding |
| Grade V | Completely shattered spleen | Parenchymal disruption >75% of hepatic lobe | Main renal artery or vein laceration or avulsion of hilum |
| | Vascular injury with active bleeding extended beyond the spleen into the peritoneum | Juxtahepatic venous injury to include retrohepatic vena cava and central major hepatic veins | Devascularized kidney with active bleeding |
| | | | Shattered kidney with loss of identifiable parenchymal renal anatomy |

Vascular injury: defined as pseudoaneurysm or arteriovenous fistula and appears as a focal collection of vascular contrast that decreases in attenuation with delayed imaging

Active bleeding presents as vascular contrast, focal or diffuse, that increases in size or attenuation in delayed phase

**When to Call IR?** The Society of Interventional Radiology recommends embolization be considered for hemodynamically stable patients with grade IV/V injuries or any grade of injury with imaging or clinical suspicion for ongoing hemorrhage [19]. Overall success rate for endovascular management is up to 90% [20]. Complications have been reported in up to 19% of cases with splenic infarction, persistent hemorrhage requiring splenectomy, and splenic abscesses being the most frequently encountered [21].

source of bleeding demonstrated on CT, or in the setting of suspicion for ongoing bleeding, or persistent source of arterial bleeding despite operative intervention (Fig. 7) [19]. The technical success rate for embolization has been reported to be as high as 97%, with major complications being hepatic ischemia (8.6%), abscess (6.8%), gallbladder necrosis (3.6%), and biloma (2.8%) [22].

## Kidneys

Surgical management of renal injuries with nephrectomy is increasingly rare and is typically reserved for grade V injuries or patients who require surgical exploration, such as in the setting of penetrating injuries. Grade I/II renal injuries are generally self-limiting and managed conservatively. **When to**

## Liver

Surgical interventions remain the standard of care for hemodynamically unstable patients regardless of injury grade. **When to call IR?** Embolization is indicated for an arterial

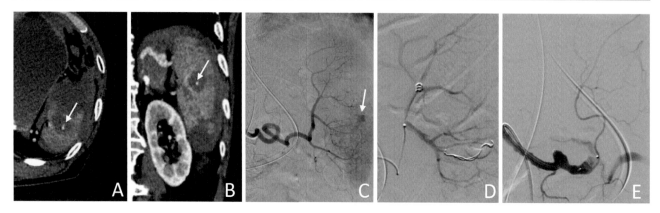

**Fig. 6** History of trauma with significant hemoglobin drop (40 Hgb). Axial and coronal CT angiogram demonstrates a splenic laceration (7.5 cm), pseudoaneurysm (arrow), intraparenchymal hematoma, and perisplenic hematoma (**a–b**). Conventional angiogram demonstrated a pseudoaneurysm (arrow) (**c**). Multiple splenic artery branches were super subselected and embolized, and an Amplatzer plug was placed proximally with the splenic artery (**d–e**). Adequate hemostasis was achieved

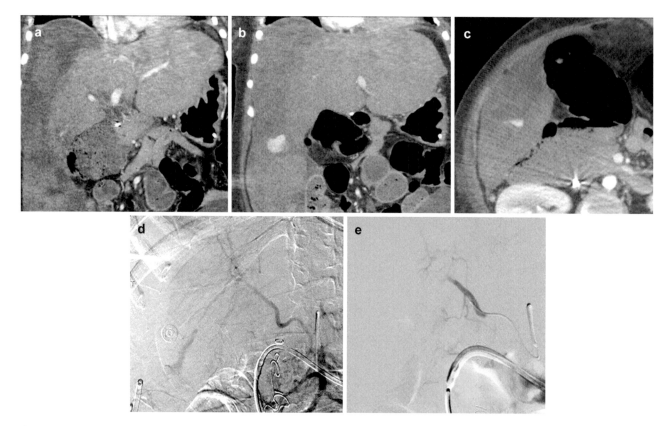

**Fig. 7** Coronal (**a–b**) and axial (**c**) CECT of a patient post-CPR demonstrating a liver laceration of segment 6 extending into the liver capsule. Extensive adjacent perihepatic hematoma with contrast bush (arrow) is in keeping with active extravasation. This is compatible with a grade IV injury. Conventional angiography demonstrates active extravasation of contrast of the distal replaced right hepatic artery, which originates from the SMA (**d**). This was embolized using 355–550 micron PVA

**call IR?** Embolization should be considered in grade III/IV renal injuries when surgical exploration is not warranted and when an arterial source of bleeding has been demonstrated on CT (Fig. 8) [19]. It is important to differentiate arterial extravasation from contrast extravasation secondary to a collecting system injury as this may influence treatment approach (arterial embolization vs ureteric stenting).

## Pelvis

Life-threatening hemorrhage relating to pelvic fractures may originate from venous, osseous, and/or arterial sources. Venous and osseous hemorrhage are often treated with external fixation and stabilization. On the other hand, arterial hemorrhage is the leading cause of death attributable to

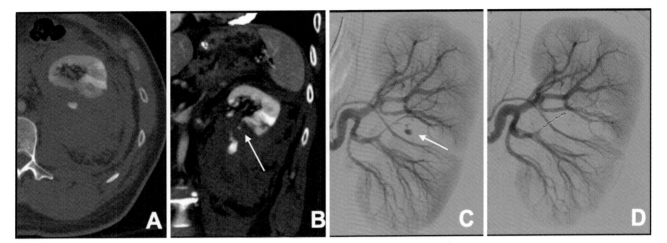

**Fig. 8** Axial and coronal CTA images of a trauma patient demonstrating a large left perinephric hematoma. A small pseudoaneurysm (arrow) is seen in the interpolar region of the kidney, with active extravasation of contrast inferiorly (**b**; arrow). Conventional angiogram re-demonstrates the pseudoaneurysm (arrow), which was embolized using coils (**c–d**)

pelvic fractures, and can often be predicted based on the mechanism and site of injury. Anterior-posterior compression fractures often result in injuries to the posterior division of the iliac arteries [23]. In particular, the iliolumbar arteries are prone to injury given its location in relation to the anterior sacroiliac joint, and the superior gluteal arteries are subjected to sheering between the sharp piriformis fascial layer and the greater sciatic foramen as it exits the pelvis [23]. Lateral compression fracture often results in injuries to the anterior division of the internal iliac artery [24].

**When to Call IR?** Embolization for pelvic trauma is the first-line therapy and the standard of care over surgery, even in hemodynamically unstable patients with pelvic ring fractures in whom intrathoracic and/or intra-abdominal sources have been excluded [19]. Additional indications for IR referrals include evidence of vascular injuries such as active contrast extravasation, large-volume pelvic hematoma, pseudoaneurysm, arterial stretch injury, or a vascular "cutoff" sign implying thrombosis, or transection of the involved artery on the IV contrast-enhanced CT.

**Key Points**

- Embolization as an adjunct to nonoperative management should be considered for high-grade, isolated splenic injuries in hemodynamically stable patients, or if there is high suspicion for ongoing hemorrhage.
- Embolization for hepatic trauma is indicated in stable patients with active arterial contrast extravasation.
- Usually conservative management for grade I/II blunt renal injuries. Whereas, embolization may be considered for high-grade injuries with arterial extravasation.
- Embolization is often the first-line therapy for unstable patients with pelvic ring fracture when intrathoracic and/or intra-abdominal sources have been excluded.

## Thrombolysis

### Acute Limb Ischemia

Acute limb ischemia (ALI) is defined as sudden decrease in limb perfusion resulting in potential threat to limb viability (Fig. 9) [25]. Common etiologies include thromboembolism, atherosclerosis, and trauma. The Rutherford classification (Table 4) serves to stratify severity and prognosis based on physical examination and Doppler evaluation [26].

Imaging provides essential information on the location/size of areas of stenosis or occlusion, revascularization targets, and degree of collateralization. However, time to imaging should be weighed against urgency of revascularization. CTA is often the first-line modality given its relative ease of access and characterization of the arterial system, which can be used to identify not only location of occlusion, but may also demonstrate potential underlying embolic sources. Ultrasound and MRA have limited utility in the setting of acute ischemia.

In general, therapeutic strategy depends on type of occlusion (thrombus or embolus), location, Rutherford class, duration of symptoms, medical comorbidities, and therapy-related risks [28]. Surgical revascularization is often reserved for patients with Rutherford III disease, native artery occlusions, and symptoms lasting longer than 14 days [29].

**When to Call IR?** Thrombolytic therapy can be used in the setting of acute occlusions (less than 14 days), bypass graft occlusions, and long occlusions without adequate runoff vessel suitable for surgical bypass (Fig. 9) [29]. Patients with Rutherford grade IIa disease should be considered for catheter-directed thrombolysis (CDT), an alternative to

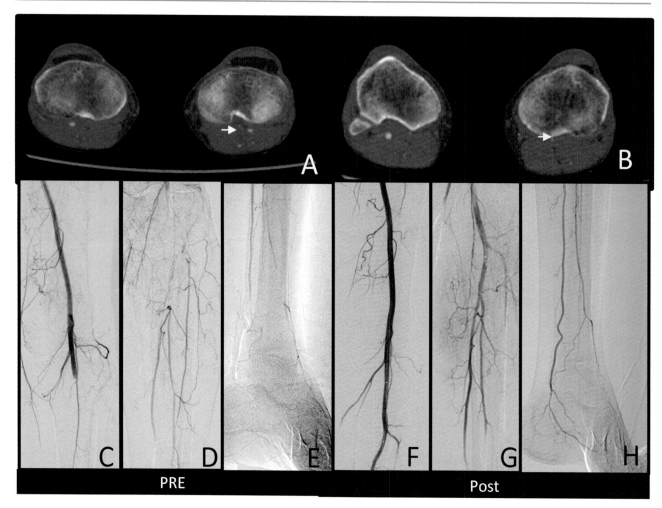

**Fig. 9** Patient with acute limb ischemia of the left leg secondary to atrial fibrillation. Axial CT and conventional angiogram demonstrate occlusion of the left popliteal artery extending into the trifurcation (**a–e**). Post-mechanical embolectomy and thrombolysis, the left popliteal artery is patent with a two-vessel runoff (**f–h**)

**Table 4** Rutherford classification for acute limb ischemia [26]

| Category | Description/prognosis | Findings | | Doppler signals | |
|---|---|---|---|---|---|
| | | Sensory loss | Muscle weakness | Arterial | Venous |
| I. Viable | Not immediately threatened | None | None | Audible | Audible |
| II. Threatened | | | | | |
| (a) Marginally | Salvageable if promptly treated | Minimal (toes) or none | None | Inaudible | Audible |
| (b) Immediately | Salvageable with immediate revascularization | More than toes, associated with rest pain | Mild, moderate | Inaudible | Audible |
| III. Irreversible | Major tissue loss or permanent nerve damage inevitables | Profound, anesthetic | Profound, paralysis (rigor) | Inaudible | Inaudible |

surgery, whereas Rutherford grade IIb disease may be considered for thrombolysis only in the setting of high perioperative risks, although this needs to be balanced against increased time to reperfusion [6].

## Pulmonary Embolism

Acute pulmonary embolism (PE) is classified into three risk categories based on the presence or absence of right heart

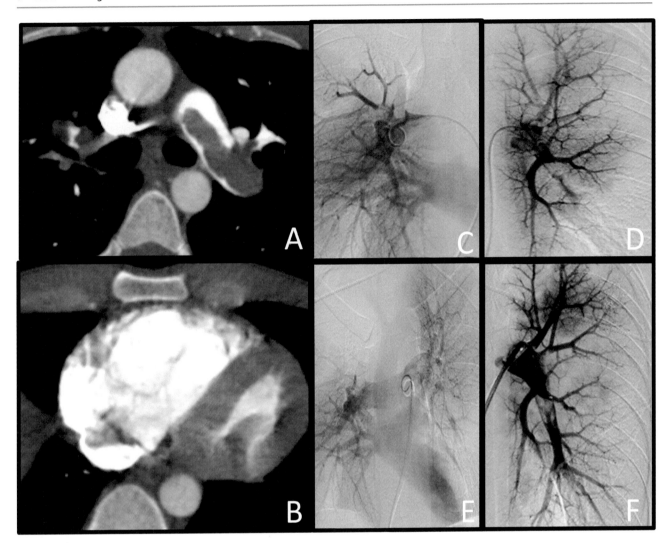

**Fig. 10** Axial CT pulmonary angiogram demonstrates extensive pulmonary embolism with enlargement of the right atrium and ventricle and leftward deviation of the intraventricular septum (**a** and **b**). Conventional angiography demonstrated nonopacification of the left main pulmonary artery and multiple segmental branches (**c–f**). The patient underwent catheter-directed embolectomy and thrombolysis. Post-treatment there is a persistent nonocclusive thrombus in the left posterior basal segmental branch

strain and systemic hemodynamic instability (Fig. 10 and Table 5) [30, 31]. Massive PE has a high mortality (25–65%) [30]. Aggressive measures including systemic

**Table 5** Risk categories for pulmonary embolisms [31]

| | Right heart strain | Systemic arterial hypotension |
|---|---|---|
| Low risk | No | No |
| Intermediate risk (Submassive) | Yes | No |
| High risk (Massive) | Yes | Yes (systolic blood pressure <90 mmHg for at least 15 min or requiring inotropic support) |

thrombolysis, CDT, and/or surgical embolectomy should be considered.

CDT can have a role in the management of massive PE with stabilization of hemodynamic parameters, resolution of hypoxia, and survival to hospital discharge [32]. However, current data are insufficient to support the routine use of CDT for patients with submassive PE to our knowledge. The decision-making for intervention in PE is becoming increasingly multidisciplinary, with the creation of pulmonary embolism response (PERT) teams. The role and evidence for mechanical devices used to extract pulmonary emboli/thrombus is evolving. **When to call IR?** This is perhaps best represented by the recent recommendations from the Society of Interventional Radiology as is outlined in Table 6.

**Table 6** Society of Interventional Radiology Position Statements on Pulmonary Embolisms [31]

| |
|---|
| 1. Supports catheter-directed thrombolysis in carefully selected patients with proximal acute massive PE, especially in highly compromised or rapidly deteriorating PE patients who have failed systemic thrombolysis |
| 2. Insufficient evidence to date supporting the routine use of CDT for patients with submassive PE; however close monitoring encouraged for rapid progression to massive PE |
| 3. Close monitoring and precautions of patients who undergo CDT |
| 4. Supports ongoing and new research on the use of CDT for acute PE, particularly for submassive PE |

## Deep Vein Thrombosis

CDT as an adjunct to anticoagulation therapy for patients with acute iliofemoral deep vein thrombosis (DVT) is controversial to our knowledge. The **ATTRACT trial** (Acute Venous Thrombosis: Thrombus Removal with Adjunctive Catheter-Directed Thrombolysis) reported no reduction in the incidences of post-thrombotic syndrome (PTS) in patients with acute, proximal DVTs in those treated with CDT compared to anticoagulation alone, but it did increase the bleeding complications [33]. However, further subanalysis of 391 participants with iliofemoral DVT showed that CDT led to a 35% reduction in the incidence of moderate-or-severe PTS compared to 28% in the control group [34]. Hence, there may still be a potential role for CDT in well-selected patients with severe symptoms, although careful review of bleeding risks is required (Fig. 11).

Venous thrombolysis may also be indicated for a **venous thoracic outlet/Paget Schroetter syndrome**, which results from extrinsic compression of the subclavian vein as it passes through the superior thoracic aperture (Fig. 12). Technical success for thrombolysis ranges from 62–84%, with lower success seen in cases of high disease burden and delayed time to treatment [35].

### Thrombolysis Key Points
- CDT to be considered for patients with:
  - Acute arterial occlusion Rutherford grade IIa disease
  - Acute massive proximal/saddle PE, particularly in highly compromised or rapidly deteriorating patients who have failed systemic thrombolysis
  - Venous thoracic outlet/Paget Schroetter syndrome
- Controversy continues with respect to CDT for acute iliofemoral deep vein thrombosis, but may be beneficial in carefully selected patients.

## Hemoptysis

## Epidemiology

Massive hemoptysis is a potentially life-threatening condition. While there is no clear consensus on quantifying the definition of "massive hemoptysis," thresholds ranging from 100–1000 mL over 24 h have been proposed [36–38]. In practice, relevant factors including bleeding rate, airway patency, hemodynamic stability, and underlying physiological reserve determine morbidity and mortality. Common etiologies are summarized in Table 7.

## Diagnostic Investigations

CTA is recognized as the best noninvasive imaging modality given its capability to identify the underlying cause and delineation of vascular anatomy. Normal bronchial arteries are less than 2 mm at their origin, and 0.5 mm as they enter into the bronchopulmonary segment [39]. Optimal evaluation of these vessels requires a high-volume (80–100 mL) intravenous contrast media, high flow rate (3–4 mL/s), and thin reformations (<1 mm) [39]. Furthermore, CTA is important in the evaluation of nonbronchial collateral supplies, which will appear as arteries running along the pleural surface [40]. Imaging features suggestive of nonbronchial systemic artery supply include pleural thickening of more than 3 mm, and tortuous enhancing vascular structures within hypertrophic extrapleural fat [41].

Bronchial artery anatomy has varying origins and branching patterns. Most commonly, bronchial arteries originate from the proximal descending aorta between the upper T5 vertebrae and lower T6 vertebrae [39]. Bronchial arteries which originate from elsewhere on the aorta or other vessels are referred as *ectopic origins,* and potential donor sites include the inferior aortic arch, descending thoracic aorta, subclavian artery, brachiocephalic trunk, thyrocervical trunk, internal mammary artery, and even coronary arteries [39]. There are four classical branching patterns depicted on Fig. 13 [39, 40]. **Type I** has a single right bronchial artery arising from an intercostal bronchial trunk (ICBT) and two left bronchial arteries. **Type II** has a right artery arising from an ICBT and a single left bronchial artery. **Type III** has a right artery arising from an ICBT, a second right artery at the aortic origin, and two left bronchial arteries. **Type IV** has a right artery arising from an ICBT, a second right artery of aortic origin, and a single left artery.

**When to Call IR?** Bronchial artery embolization (BAE) is often recognized as a first-line treatment option for massive hemoptysis (Fig. 14) [36]. Angiographic manifestations of abnormal bronchial arteries include increased tortuosity,

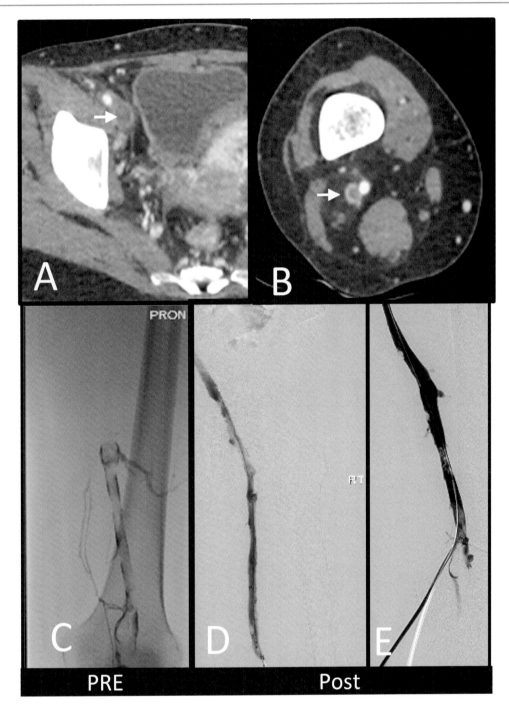

**Fig. 11** Axial CT angiogram and selected angiogram demonstrates extensive deep vein thrombosis involving the right internal iliac to the popliteal vein (arrow) (**a–c**). Patient was treated with catheter-directed thrombolysis and angioplasty with recanalization of the femoral and popliteal veins (**d** and **e**)

dilatation, hyper- and/or neovascularity, aneurysms, and shunting, with active contrast extravasation only seen in rare cases [39]. Visualization of the anterior medullary artery (artery of Adamkiewicz) is a relative contraindication given the potential risk of transient or permanent paraparesis or paraplegia due to spinal cord ischemia, a rare but serious complication that occurs in 0.6–4.4% of cases [42]. The rate of major complications is minimal, with a median incidence of 0.1% (0–6.6%) [42]. Immediate clinical success defined as complete cessation or clinical significant reduction in hemoptysis within 24 h varies from 70–99% [42]. Rate of recurrence ranges from 12–57%, often relating to the presence of non-bronchial systemic collaterals, bronchopulmonary shunting, aspergillomas, and multidrug-resistant tuberculosis [42].

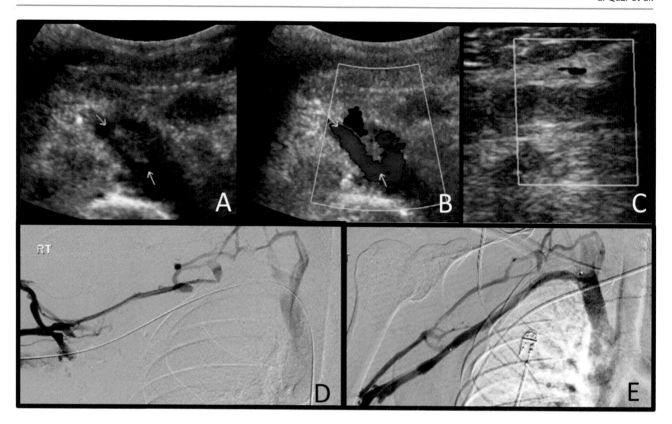

**Fig. 12** Ultrasound and conventional angiogram demonstrating occlusion of the right subclavian vein in a patient with thoracic outlet syndrome (**a–d**). Recanalization with catheter-directed thrombolysis using tPA (**e**)

**Table 7** Common etiologies for hemoptysis [38]

| Airway disease | Parenchymal disease | Cardiovascular disease | Others |
|---|---|---|---|
| Bronchitis | Infection (tuberculosis, pneumonia, aspergilloma, and lung abscess) | Pulmonary vascular malformations | Coagulopathy |
| Bronchiectasis (i.e., cystic fibrosis) | Inflammatory (sarcoidosis, Goodpasture's syndrome, and granulomatosis with polyangiitis) | Pulmonary embolism | Foreign body |
| Neoplasm: primary bronchogenic carcinoma, endobronchial metastatic carcinoma, and bronchial carcinoid | Iatrogenic (biopsy, radiation, chest tube, or thoracentesis) | Elevated pulmonary capillary pressure | Trauma |
| Tracheo-aortic fistula | | Traumatic pulmonary artery pseudoaneurysms | Cocaine |
| | | Vasculitis – granulomatosis with polyangiitis, Takayasu's, and Bechet's | |
| | | Mitral stenosis | |

**Key Points**

- Bronchial artery embolization (BAE) can be a first-line therapy for massive hemoptysis after initial resuscitation.
- Evaluation of bronchial artery anatomy and nonbronchial supplies is important for procedural planning.
- High immediate clinical success rate (70–99%) with a low major complication incidence (median 0.1%); however, there is a variable recurrence rate (12–57%).

# Gastrointestinal Bleeding

## Epidemiology

Acute gastrointestinal bleeding (GIB) can be life threatening, and lead to significant morbidity if not treated [43, 44]. A bleeding source proximal to the ligament of Treitz is considered an upper GIB, while a source distal to the ligament and

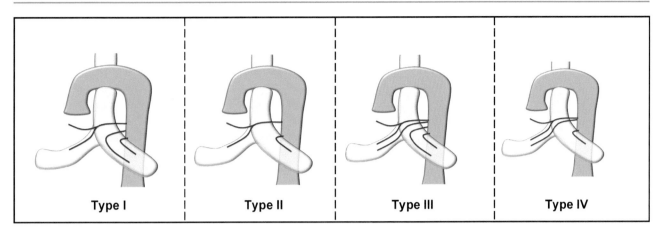

**Fig. 13** Classical branching patterns of the bronchial arteries. (Adapted from Chung et al. [40])

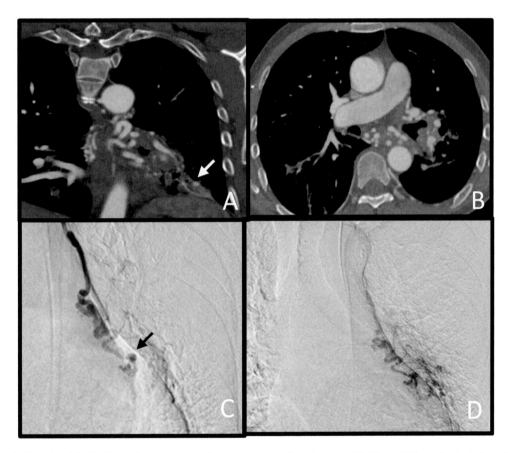

**Fig. 14** Coronal (**a**) and axial (**b**) CT angiogram in a patient with history of tuberculosis presenting with hemoptysis demonstrating multiple hypertrophied bronchial and internal thoracic arteries extending into the left lower lobe. Conventional angiogram demonstrates prominent hypertrophied bronchial arteries (not shown). Angiographic run of the internal thoracic artery demonstrated a pseudoaneurysm (**c**) with active extravasation (**d**). This was embolized using PVA 250–350 microns until stasis was achieved

beyond the duodenojejunal flexure is a lower GIB. There are multiple causes of GIB (Table 8). The most common cause of UGIB is peptic ulcer disease. The annual incidence is approximately 40–150 cases/10,000 for UGIB, and 20–27 cases/100,000 for LGIB, with mortality ranging from 4–10% [43].

### Clinical Features

UGIB can present with frank hematemesis, coffee-ground emesis, melena, or hematochezia in the cases of brisk bleeds. LGIB often presents with hematochezia but can present with

**Table 8** Causes of gastrointestinal bleeding [45, 46]

| Type of bleed | Etiology | |
|---|---|---|
| Upper gastrointestinal bleeding | Peptic ulcer disease (duodenal and gastric) | 35% |
| | Varices (esophageal, gastric, duodenal, etc.) | 25% |
| | Gastritis/esophagitis | 15% |
| | Mallory-Weiss tears | 5% |
| | Benign and malignant tumors | 5% |
| | Dieulafoy lesions | |
| | Vascular malformations (AVMS) | |
| | Aortoenteric fistulas | |
| Lower gastrointestinal bleeding | Diverticulosis/diverticulitis | 28% |
| | Angiodysplasia | 15% |
| | Erosive disease | 17% |
| | Infection/ischemia | 14% |
| | Malignancy | 13% |
| | Other | 8% |
| | No cause | 5% |

melena if the bleeding source is the small bowel. On physical examination, patients may exhibit signs of hemodynamic instability depending on the severity of hemorrhage, including tachycardia and hypotension.

## Diagnostic Investigation

First-line endoscopy is performed to localize the source of bleeding. If the bleeding site is not identified, CTA may be used to localize the source of bleeding and identify the underlying etiology. CT can depict bleeding rates as low as 0.3 mL/min, with a sensitivity of 50–86% and specificity 92–95% [45, 46]. On noncontrast CT, hyperattenuation within the bowel lumen may signify recent hemorrhage or "sentinel clot." The hallmark of bleeding is active extravasation of contrast. It appears as a blush of contrast on arterial phase, which progressively increases in size on the later portal venous phase images. The CTA can also provide important information regarding the vascular anatomy for endovascular or surgical planning.

Nuclear scintigraphy with Tc-99m-labeled RBCs can help detect the source of gastrointestinal bleeding. It is utilized when the patient is stable and the source of bleeding cannot be identified through endoscopy or CTA. It can depict rates as low as 0.1–0.35 mL/min, with a sensitivity of 95% and a specificity of 93% [45]. Patients who demonstrate an immediate blush on RBC scintigraphy are more likely to require urgent intervention when compared to patients who have a delayed blush. These are likely to have low yield on angiography.

## Management

For emergent cases, endoscopy is generally the first-line treatment for both UGIB and LGIB [45, 47]. It offers both diagnostic and therapeutic options. Patients with upper GI bleeding are investigated with esophagogastroduodenoscopy (EGD), which has a sensitivity of 92% in identifying the source of bleeding, as well as a high specificity for identifying the underlying etiology. For lower GI bleeding, patients are investigated with colonoscopy [47]. The sensitivity of colonoscopy in identifying the source of bleeding is 90% in LGIB, with a PPV of 87% in identifying LGI foci. Approximately, 10–15% of patients with symptoms of a LGIB may have a bleeding source in the upper GI tract, and EGD can be considered if colonoscopy is negative. General factors that predict treatment failure with endoscopy include patients who present in shock, Hb <10, >6 units of blood transfused, and significant comorbidities [47]. In particular for UGIB, a large size of ulcer and location along the posterior wall of the duodenal bulb are associated with technical failure. Endoscopic therapeutic options largely depend on etiology. These include epinephrine injection, sclerotherapy, metal clip placement, and band ligation of varices. In emergencies, endoscopic balloon tamponade or covered stent can be placed for temporary control of variceal bleeding [48].

**When to Call IR?** In cases of failed endoscopic management for upper GI bleeding, if a clear source of nonvariceal hemorrhage is identified, then consideration of transfer directly to angiography can be considered. The goal of angiography is to identify the bleeding vessel and perform transarterial embolization [49]. An advantage of angiography is that it is not hampered by impaired visualization due to intraluminal blood. It can depict bleeding rates as low as 0.5 mL/min [49]. However, only arterial or capillary bleeding is identified. Digital subtraction angiography features of active bleeding include active extravasation of contrast and mucosal blushes with abnormal neovessels [49]. In cases of a UGIB, if the source is not identified but a clear location has been established from endoscopy, empiric embolization can be considered. In these cases if the bleed is suspected to be from the fundus of the stomach, then the left gastric artery is embolized [49]. If the bleeding is suspected to be from the gastric antrum or proximal duodenum, then the GDA is empirically embolized [49]. If endovascular options are unavailable or have failed, then surgical resection can be considered [49].

The value of endoscopy and pre-procedural imaging is helpful for the interventional radiologist to localize and help classify GI bleeding as variceal or nonvariceal. While arterial bleeding can be managed with embolization, variceal bleeding may require other forms of management such as transjugular portosystemic shunt (TIPS) insertion, transvisceral, or retrograde transvenous variceal embolization.

## Key Points

- Endoscopy should be considered as first-line treatment of both UGIB and LGIB.
- CTA with noncontrast, arterial, and venous phases can depict bleeding rates as low as 0.3 mL/min.
- For nonvariceal UGIB and LGIB in the context of failed endoscopic management, interventional radiology can provide further management with transarterial embolization.

## Postpartum Hemorrhage

### Epidemiology

Postpartum hemorrhage (PPH) is a major cause of maternal death, with an estimated 1 % mortality rate [50]. It is defined as blood loss greater than 500 mL following vaginal delivery. Primary PPH is hemorrhage within 24 h of delivery. Secondary PPH is hemorrhage occurring >24 h postdelivery. Primary PPH has a higher mortality rate. It can be minor (500–1000 mL) or major (>1000 mL). Clinically any volume of blood loss resulting in hemodynamic instability is considered PPH [51, 52]. Risk factors for developing PPH include a preexisting bleeding disorder, anticoagulation, chorioamnionitis, augmented labor, abnormal placenta variation (placenta acreta and placenta previa), fetal macrosomia, material anemia, prolonged labor, and preeclampsia. Excessive bleeding postpartum affects approximately 5–15% of women giving birth [53]. The most common etiology of PPH includes the 4Ts (tone, tissue, trauma, and thrombin). Tone refers to when the uterus is unable to contract to arrest bleeding at the placental site [53]. Coagulation abnormalities (thrombin), retained products of conception (tissue), or lacerations (trauma) during delivery, can all result in hemorrhage postpartum.

### Clinical Features

Clinical features depend on the degree of blood loss. Excessive bleeding results in hemodynamic instability [53]. Generally, blood loss between 500 and 1000 mL is tolerated with patients developing palpitations, dizziness, and tachycardia. Greater than 1000 mL blood loss results in hypotension, and

>1500 mL results in oliguria and marked hypotension [53]. However, patients with risk factors including gestational hypertension with proteinuria, underlying anemia, or small stature will become symptomatic with smaller volumes of blood loss [53].

### Management

Endovascular or surgical approaches to management can be considered. Surgical options include uterine artery ligation, internal artery ligation, abdominal packing, or emergency hysterectomy.

**When to Call IR?** For a patient who is actively bleeding, no imaging is typically required and interventional radiology can provide the endovascular option of pelvic arterial embolization of the uterine or internal iliac arteries (Fig. 15). It has a high technical success rate of 89.6% [54]. The advantage of embolization is that it is minimally invasive, can be performed under local anesthetic, allows for prompt hemostasis, and has the possibility of preserving fertility.

### Key Points

- The most common causes of PPH include the 4Ts (tone, tissue, trauma, and thrombin).
- Direct surgical or endovascular treatment should be considered in patients with persistent PPH despite medical treatment or hemodynamic instability.
- Embolization is a minimally invasive effective treatment option for PPH with a high success rate and possibility of fertility preservation.

## Summary

This chapter has summarized the role of interventional radiology in the diagnosis and management of vascular emergencies including ruptured abdominal aortic aneurysm, aortic dissection, liver/kidney/spleen/pelvic trauma, acute limb ischemia, hemoptysis, gastrointestinal bleeding, and postpartum hemorrhage. While the evidence for treatments such as endovascular aneurysm repair are well established, the evidence in other areas such as the endovascular management of DVT and PE is evolving. Interventional radiologists are key members of the multidisciplinary team needed to manage patients with the aforementioned conditions and should therefore be consulted early in the patient's care pathway.

| Right | Left |
|---|---|

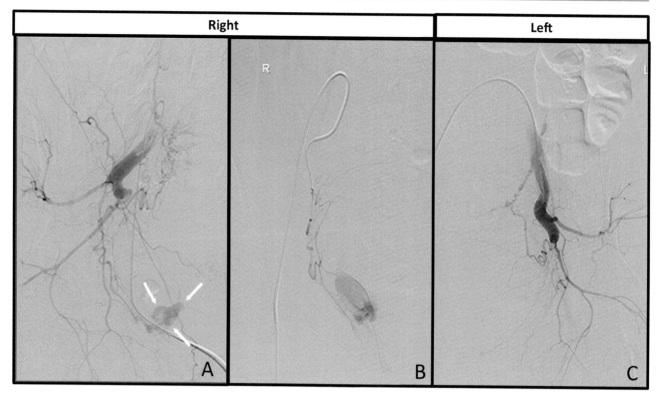

**Fig. 15** Conventional angiogram demonstrates selected images of the right internal iliac artery (**a**) and uterine artery (**b**) with a pseudo-aneurysm of the uterine artery (arrow) in a woman with severe postpartum hemorrhage. The contralateral uterine arteries demonstrate vasospasm of the internal iliac branches but no extravasation, pseudoaneurysm, or AV fistula (**c**). Both sides were embolized using Gelfoam and coils (not shown)

## References

1. Hoornweg L, Storm-Versloot M, Ubbink D, Koelemay M, Legemate D, Balm R. Meta analysis on mortality of ruptured abdominal aortic aneurysms. Eur J Vasc Endovasc Surg. 2008;35 (5):558–70.
2. Mell MW, Starnes BW, Kraiss LW, Schneider PA, Pevec WC. Western Vascular Society guidelines for transfer of patients with ruptured abdominal aortic aneurysm. J Vasc Surg. 2017;65(3): 603–8.
3. Rakita D, Newatia A, Hines JJ, Siegel DN, Friedman B. Spectrum of CT findings in rupture and impending rupture of abdominal aortic aneurysms. Radiographics. 2007;27(2):497–507.
4. Investigators. Endovascular or open repair strategy for ruptured abdominal aortic aneurysm: 30 day outcomes from IMPROVE randomised trial. BMJ. 2014;348:f7661.
5. Hiratzka LF, Bakris GL, Beckman JA, Bersin RM, Carr VF, Casey DE, et al. 2010 ACCF/AHA/AATS/ACR/ASA/SCA/SCAI/SIR/STS/SVM guidelines for the diagnosis and management of patients with thoracic aortic disease. J Am Coll Cardiol. 2010;55(14):e27–e129.
6. McMahon MA, Squirrell CA. Multidetector CT of aortic dissection: a pictorial review. Radiographics. 2010;30(2):445–60.
7. Lombardi JV, Hughes GC, Appoo JJ, Bavaria JE, Beck AW, Cambria RP, et al. Society for Vascular Surgery (SVS) and Society of Thoracic Surgeons (STS) reporting standards for type B aortic dissections. Ann Thorac Surg. 2020;
8. Lempel JK, Frazier AA, Jeudy J, Kligerman SJ, Schultz R, Ninalowo HA, et al. Aortic arch dissection: a controversy of classification. Radiology. 2014;271(3):848–55.
9. Trimarchi S, Jonker FHW, Muhs BE, Grassi V, Righini P, Upchurch GR, et al. Long-term outcomes of surgical aortic fenestration for complicated acute type B aortic dissections. J Vasc Surg. 2010;52 (2):261–6.
10. Rong D, Ge Y, Liu J, Liu X, Guo W. Combined proximal descending aortic endografting plus distal bare metal stenting (PETTICOAT technique) versus conventional proximal descending aortic stent graft repair for complicated type B aortic dissections. Cochrane Database Syst Rev. 2019;10
11. Kouvelos GN, Vourliotakis G, Arnaoutoglou E, Papa N, Avgos S, Peroulis M, et al. Endovascular treatment for isolated acute abdominal aortic dissection. J Vasc Surg. 2013;58(6):1505–11.
12. Sachs T, Pomposelli F, Hagberg R, Hamdan A, Wyers M, Giles K, et al. Open and endovascular repair of type B aortic dissection in the Nationwide Inpatient Sample. J Vasc Surg. 2010;52(4):860–6.
13. Hogendoorn W, Hunink MM, Schlösser FJ, Moll FL, Sumpio BE, Muhs BE. Endovascular vs. open repair of complicated acute type B aortic dissections. J Endovasc Ther. 2014;21(4): 503–14.
14. Watanabe Y, Shimamura K, Yoshida T, Daimon T, Shirakawa Y, Torikai K, et al. Aortic remodeling as a prognostic factor for late aortic events after thoracic endovascular aortic repair in type B aortic dissection with patent false lumen. J Endovasc Ther. 2014;21(4):517–25.
15. Soto JA, Anderson SW. Multidetector CT of blunt abdominal trauma. Radiology. 2012;265(3):678–93.
16. Madoff DC, Denys A, Wallace MJ, Murthy R, Gupta S, Pillsbury EP, et al. Splenic arterial interventions: anatomy, indications, technical considerations, and potential complications. Radiographics. 2005;25(suppl_1):S191–211.

17. Kozar RA, Crandall M, Shanmuganathan K, Zarzaur BL, Coburn M, Cribari C, et al. Organ injury scaling 2018 update: spleen, liver, and kidney. J Trauma Acute Care Surg. 2018;85(6):1119–22.

18. Coccolini F, Montori G, Catena F, Kluger Y, Biffl W, Moore EE, et al. Splenic trauma: WSES classification and guidelines for adult and pediatric patients. World J Emerg Surg. 2017;12(1):40.

19. Padia SA, Ingraham CR, Moriarty JM, Wilkins LR, Bream PR Jr, Tam AL, et al. Society of interventional radiology position statement on endovascular intervention for trauma. JVIR. 2020;31(3):363.

20. Rong J-J, Liu D, Liang M, Wang Q-H, Sun J-Y, Zhang Q-Y, et al. The impacts of different embolization techniques on splenic artery embolization for blunt splenic injury: a systematic review and meta-analysis. Mil Med Res. 2017;4(1):17.

21. Haan JM, Biffl W, Knudson MM, Davis KA, Oka T, Majercik S, et al. Splenic embolization revisited: a multicenter review. J Trauma Acute Care Surg. 2004;56(3):542–7.

22. Virdis F, Reccia I, Di Saverio S, Tugnoli G, Kwan S, Kumar J, et al. Clinical outcomes of primary arterial embolization in severe hepatic trauma: a systematic review. Diagn Interv Imaging. 2019;100(2):65–75.

23. Yoon W, Kim JK, Jeong YY, Seo JJ, Park JG, Kang HK. Pelvic arterial hemorrhage in patients with pelvic fractures: detection with contrast-enhanced CT. Radiographics. 2004;24(6):1591–605.

24. Kachlik D, Vobornik T, Dzupa V, Marvanova Z, Toupal O, Navara E, et al. Where and what arteries are most likely injured with pelvic fractures? The influence of localization, shape, and fracture dislocation on the arterial injury during pelvic fractures. Clin Anat. 2019;32(5):682–8.

25. Norgren L, Hiatt WR, Dormandy JA, Nehler MR, Harris KA, Fowkes FGR. Inter-society consensus for the management of peripheral arterial disease (TASC II). J Vasc Surg. 2007;45(1):S5–S67.

26. Rutherford RB, Baker JD, Ernst C, Johnston KW, Porter JM, Ahn S, et al. Recommended standards for reports dealing with lower extremity ischemia: revised version. J Vasc Surg. 1997;26(3):517–38.

27. Working party on thrombolysis in the management of limb ischemia. Thrombolysis in the management of lower limb peripheral arterial occlusion-a consensus document. Am J Cardiol. 1998;81(2):207–18.

28. Olinic D-M, Stanek A, Tătaru D-A, Homorodean C, Olinic M. Acute limb ischemia: an update on diagnosis and management. J Clin Med. 2019;8(8):1215.

29. Björck M, Earnshaw JJ, Acosta S, Gonçalves FB, Cochennec F, Debus ES, et al. Editor's choice–European society for vascular surgery (ESVS) 2020 clinical practice guidelines on the management of acute limb ischaemia. Eur J Vasc Endovasc Surg. 2020;59(2):173–218.

30. Jaff MR, McMurtry MS, Archer SL, Cushman M, Goldenberg N, Goldhaber SZ, et al. Management of massive and submassive pulmonary embolism, iliofemoral deep vein thrombosis, and chronic thromboembolic pulmonary hypertension: a scientific statement from the American Heart Association. Circulation. 2011;123(16):1788–830.

31. Kuo WT, Sista AK, Faintuch S, Dariushnia SR, Baerlocher MO, Lookstein RA, et al. Society of interventional radiology position statement on catheter-directed therapy for acute pulmonary embolism. JVIR. 2018;29(3):293.

32. Kuo WT, Gould MK, Louie JD, Rosenberg JK, Sze DY, Hofmann LV. Catheter-directed therapy for the treatment of massive pulmonary embolism: systematic review and meta-analysis of modern techniques. J Vasc Interv Radiol. 2009;20(11):1431–40.

33. Vedantham S, Goldhaber SZ, Julian JA, Kahn SR, Jaff MR, Cohen DJ, et al. Pharmacomechanical catheter-directed thrombolysis for deep-vein thrombosis. N Engl J Med. 2017;377(23):2240–52.

34. Comerota AJ, Kearon C, Gu C-S, Julian JA, Goldhaber SZ, Kahn SR, et al. Endovascular thrombus removal for acute iliofemoral deep vein thrombosis: analysis from a stratified multicenter randomized trial. Circulation. 2019;139(9):1162–73.

35. Tsekouras N, Comerota AJ. Current trends in the treatment of venous thoracic outlet syndrome: a comprehensive review. Interv Cardiol. 2014;6(1):103–18.

36. Radchenko C, Alraiyes AH, Shojaee S. A systematic approach to the management of massive hemoptysis. J Thorac Dis. 2017;9(Suppl 10):S1069–S86.

37. Davidson K, Shojaee S. Managing massive hemoptysis. Chest. 2020;157(1):77–88.

38. Andersen PE. Imaging and interventional radiological treatment of hemoptysis. Acta Radiol. 2006;47(8):780–92.

39. Walker CM, Rosado-de-Christenson ML, Martínez-Jiménez S, Kunin JR, Wible BC. Bronchial arteries: anatomy, function, hypertrophy, and anomalies. Radiographics. 2015;35(1):32–49.

40. Chun J-Y, Morgan R, Belli A-M. Radiological management of hemoptysis: a comprehensive review of diagnostic imaging and bronchial arterial embolization. Cardiovasc Intervent Radiol. 2010;33(2):240–50.

41. Yoon W, Kim JK, Kim YH, Chung TW, Kang HK. Bronchial and nonbronchial systemic artery embolization for life-threatening hemoptysis: a comprehensive review. Radiographics. 2002;22(6):1395–409.

42. Panda A, Bhalla AS, Goyal A. Bronchial artery embolization in hemoptysis: a systematic review. Diagn Interv Radiol. 2017;23(4):307.

43. Ramaswamy RS, Choi HW, Mouser HC, Narsinh KH, McCammack KC, Treesit T, et al. Role of interventional radiology in the management of acute gastrointestinal bleeding. World J Radiol. 2014;6(4):82.

44. Singh-Bhinder N, Kim DH, Holly BP, Johnson PT, Hanley M, Carucci LR, et al. ACR Appropriateness Criteria nonvariceal upper gastrointestinal bleeding. J Am Coll Radiol. 2017;14(5):S177–S88.

45. Zuccaro G. Epidemiology of lower gastrointestinal bleeding. Best Pract Res Clin Gastroenterol. 2008;22(2):225–32.

46. Ghassemi KA, Jensen DM. Lower GI bleeding: epidemiology and management. Curr Gastroenterol Rep. 2013;15(7):333.

47. Hwang JH, Fisher DA, Ben-Menachem T, Chandrasekhara V, Chathadi K, Decker GA, et al. The role of endoscopy in the management of acute non-variceal upper GI bleeding. Gastrointest Endosc. 2012;75(6):1132–8.

48. Escorsell À, Pavel O, Cárdenas A, Morillas R, Llop E, Villanueva C, et al. Esophageal balloon tamponade versus esophageal stent in controlling acute refractory variceal bleeding: a multicenter randomized, controlled trial. Hepatology. 2016;63(6):1957–67.

49. Andersen PE, Duvnjak S. Endovascular treatment of nonvariceal acute arterial upper gastrointestinal bleeding. World J Radiol. 2010;2(7):257.

50. AbouZahr C. Global burden of maternal death and disability. Br Med Bull. 2003;67(1):1–11.

51. Kirby JM, Kachura JR, Rajan DK, Sniderman KW, Simons ME, Windrim RC, et al. Arterial embolization for primary postpartum hemorrhage. J Vasc Interv Radiol. 2009;20(8):1036–45.

52. Leduc D, Senikas V, Lalonde AB. No. 235-Active management of the third stage of labour: prevention and treatment of postpartum hemorrhage. J Obstet Gynaecol Can. 2018;40(12):e841–e55.

53. Anderson JM, Etches D. Prevention and management of postpartum hemorrhage. Am Fam Physician. 2007;75(6):875–82.

54. Lee HY, Shin JH, Kim J, Yoon H-K, Ko G-Y, Won H-S, et al. Primary postpartum hemorrhage: outcome of pelvic arterial embolization in 251 patients at a single institution. Radiology. 2012;264(3):903–9.

# Nonvascular Emergencies

## When to Call an Interventional Radiologist

**4**

Abdullah O. Alenezi, Neeral R. Patel, Arash Mir-Rahimi, Arash Jaberi, and Sebastian Mafeld

## Contents

**Abstract**

Nonvascular emergencies involving the abdomen are common and represent areas where interventional radiology (IR) can add value in patient care. Familiarity with the common emergency conditions which may require IR input related to intra-abdominal and visceral abscess drainage, biliary obstruction, urological obstruction, as well as large bowel obstruction stenting is essential given the radiologist may be the first physician to contact IR. Appreciation of the features of nonvascular procedure complications is also imperative. Clinicians will often contact radiologists with queries regarding tubes and catheters IRs have inserted; this chapter also serves to provide an overview to deal with such inquiries.

A. O. Alenezi · N. R. Patel · A. Mir-Rahimi · A. Jaberi
Division of Interventional Radiology, University Health Network, Toronto General Hospital, Toronto, ON, Canada

S. Mafeld (✉)
Division of Interventional Radiology, Department of Medical Imaging, University Health Network, Toronto, ON, Canada
e-mail: sebastiancharles.mafeld@uhn.ca

© Springer Nature Switzerland AG 2022
M. N. Patlas et al. (eds.), *Atlas of Emergency Imaging from Head-to-Toe*,
https://doi.org/10.1007/978-3-030-92111-8_4

**Keywords**

Nonvascular · Interventional radiology · Renal · Biliary · Gastrointestinal

## Introduction

Nonvascular emergencies involving the abdomen are common and represent areas where interventional radiology (IR) can add value in patient care. Familiarity with the common emergency conditions which may require IR input and an understanding of the procedures that can be offered, the imaging findings pre- and post-procedure, as well as potential complications are essential for radiologists to be aware of in day-to-day practice. Indeed, a radiologist may be the first physician to consult IR for an emergent procedure having reviewed a scan.

The majority of the nonvascular interventions performed involve percutaneous drain insertion under image guidance. Central to many of the complications of percutaneous tube insertion, including leakage, dislodgement, and subsequent ease of reinsertion, is the concept of tract formation, the thin fibrous capsule that forms around the catheter; this is a normal response by the body to implanted foreign bodies [1]. Tract formation is a complex process and is dependent upon a normal immune response; patients taking immunosuppressants, those who are malnourished, or those with underlying malignancy have an impaired ability to form a tract and are at higher risk of developing tube-related complications [2]. Tract maturation generally takes in the order of 2 to 4 weeks prior to which the risk of tube-related complications is highest. This chapter aims to serve as a guide for radiologists to understand the most common pathologies where image-guided procedures can have an impact in the acute setting and also when an IR opinion should be sought.

## Abdominal Abscess Drainage

### Epidemiology

Abdominal collections may involve nearly every organ and/or potential space Pyogenic hepatic abscesses constitute approximately 50% of abdominal visceral abscesses [3]. Abscesses can occur in a wide range of conditions such as appendicitis, diverticulitis , biliary obstruction, and postoperative status [3, 4]. Intraperitoneal abscesses form due to localized inflammation and infection and are most commonly seen in postoperative patients due to anastomotic leak, infected hematoma, or biliarye collection, as well as in patients with a perforated viscus [5, 6].

## Clinical Features

Patients will generally present with fever, chills, and pain localized to the organ and abdominal space involved.

## Radiological Findings

Ultrasound (US) may be performed to assess collection size, complexity, and post treatment follow-up. Portable US examination is valuable in critically unwell patients with clinical evidence of intra-abdominal collections who cannot be transferred for cross-sectional imaging. Contrast-enhanced computed tomography (CT) in the portal venous phase can be performed for suspected intra-abdominal peritoneal and retroperitoneal collections. Infected fluid collections may exert mass effect on adjacent structures and demonstrate rim enhancement as well as internal gas locules [6, 7]. US and CT can also be used to assess the feasibility of percutaneous drainage of abdominal collections and plan routes for procedural access.

## Role of Interventional Radiology

### Indications

Urgent drainage is performed in patients with sepsis refractory to antibiotic therapy [8]. Furthermore, patients who are septic with hemodynamic compromise should be considered for emergent drainage. It is important to keep in mind that a collection may not require emergent intervention; in a hemodynamically stable patient who is responding to antibiotics, it may be prudent to treat conservatively. The clinical condition of the patient is paramount in determining the need for an intervention and its urgency.

### Techniques

Interventional radiologists can perform drainage via a percutaneous or transorifical (transvaginal and transrectal) approach, depending on the location of the collection. For collections that are challenging to access safely via the aforementioned routes, for example, in the lesser sac, endoscopic transgastric drainage may be a therapeutic option.

Whether a liver abscess, peritoneal, or retroperitoneal collection is targeted, there are two basic techniques used for drain placement, namely, Seldinger and trocar techniques. The Seldinger technique involves more steps than the trocar technique, although it is considered safer. The size of drain chosen is dependent on the consistency of the abscess contents. If serous, an 8-French drain is usually sufficient, whereas if the contents are thick, a larger 10-French or 12-French drain is more appropriate. Once the tract has been dilated, the selected drain is advanced over a wire and the pigtail (Cope loop) formed within the collection cavity. The contents of the collection can be aspirated and the catheter connected to a drainage bag.

## Liver Abscess Drainage

In the last two decades, percutaneous liver abscess drainage has superseded surgery as the mainstay treatment for liver abscess. Specific to liver abscess, the transhepatic route is required to reach intrahepatic collections, via the subcostal or intercostal approach (Fig. 1). Aspiration alone may be beneficial for smaller liver abscesses, but percutaneous drainage is more effective in achieving maximal cavity collapse [9, 10]. A systematic review and meta-analysis performed showed percutaneous drainage as having a higher success rate and greater reduction in abscess cavity size in comparison with needle aspiration alone [11].

## Peritoneal and Retroperitoneal Collection Drainage

Most peritoneal and retroperitoneal collections will be amenable to percutaneous drainage if clinically appropriate. Peritoneal collections, for example, appendiceal or diverticular abscesses can often be drained with the patient in a supine position, (Fig. 2). When abdominal structures, such as bowel, obscure a direct percutaneous path to the collection, simple maneuvers such as placing the patient in the lateral decubitus position may cause the bowel to move and allow drainage to be performed; discussion with an IR is therefore imperative to determine whether collections are technically amenable to drainage. For retroperitoneal collections such a psoas abscess, the patient will usually be positioned prone (Fig. 3).

## Pelvic Collection Drainage

Deep pelvic collections, usually related to gynecological pathology, such as a tubo-ovarian abscess or collections

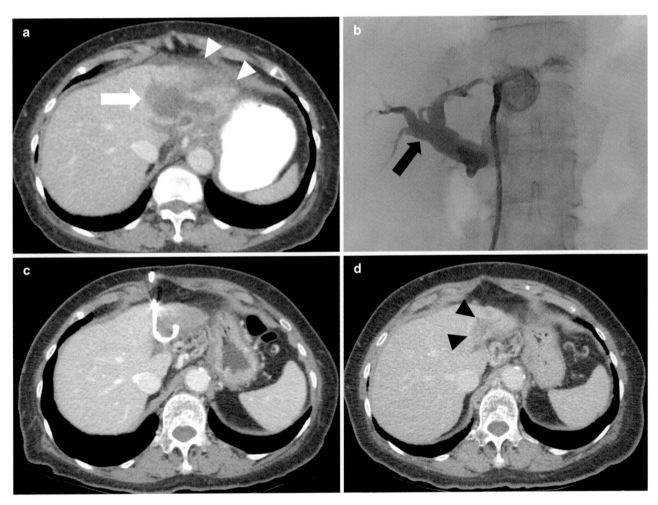

**Fig. 1** (a–d) Patient with Hepatitis C liver cirrhosis presented 3 weeks post microwave ablation of segment 2 HCC with abdominal pain and fever. (a) Contrast-enhanced CT of the abdomen and pelvis demonstrated an oval hypoattenuating segment 2 lesion with an adjacent hypodense tract and perihepatic fat stranding, consistent with abscess formation within the ablation zone. (b) Fluoroscopic image with contrast injected through abscess drain showed opacification of the biliary tree suggesting fistulous tract formation. (c and d) Follow-up-contrast enhanced CT of the abdomen and pelvis showed decrease in abscess size before (c) and after drain removal (d)

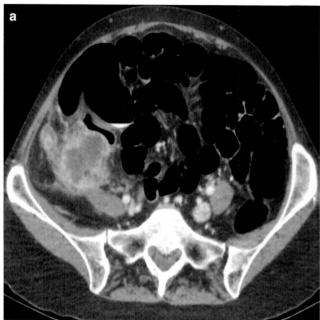 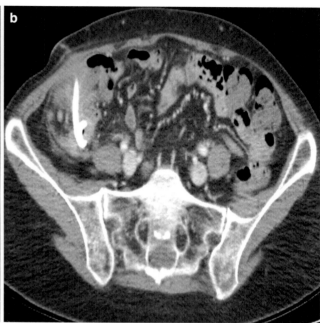

**Fig. 2** (**a** and **b**): Patient presented with 4-day history of abdominal pain localized to the right lower quadrant. (**a**) Contrast-enhanced CT of the abdomen and pelvis demonstrated acute appendicitis complicated by perforation and abscess formation. (**b**) Follow-up contrast enhanced CT of the abdomen and pelvis with percutaneous drain in situ demonstrated collapse of abscess cavity

associated with pelvic inflammatory disease may not be amenable to percutaneous drainage. The transvaginal route is often an option in centers in which there is an IR who offers this approach to drainage (Fig. 4).

### Post-procedure Care

To ensure adequate drainage, a catheter can be flushed regularly, for example, 10 cc of normal saline twice daily, to avoid tube occlusion. A frequent indication for follow-up cross-sectional imaging is to assess changes in intra-abdominal collections. For drain blockages and leakages, CT imaging alone may be of limited value, and consulting IR for a drain check, change, or manipulation should be considered. In the case of viscous contents, upsizing of the catheter may improve drainage. For blocked drains it is may be advisable to attempt gentle flushing on the ward. When there is drain leakage, a practical step prior to contacting IR is to assess the full length of the drain without dressings, particularly at the site of drainage bag connection. The aforementioned simple steps may prevent the patient from undergoing an unnecessary procedure or imaging investigation.

Drains should be removed as soon as possible to avoid being a source of infection. However, the cessation of drain output in itself is not sufficient to warrant drain removal; catheters may become blocked leading to false reassurance that a collection has resolved. Therefore, a combination of the clinical response, as well as imaging, if there is clinical uncertainty, should be utilized before drain removal is considered. A drain should also have minimal output (<10 mL/day) prior to removal being considered.

### Complications

The incidence of complications related to percutaneous drainage procedures is low (~10%) [12]. Adverse events may include septic storm, infecting otherwise sterile fluid, hemorrhage, and injury to the bowel or adjacent organs [8]. Given the liver is a vascular organ, there is an inherent risk of bleeding once the capsule has been breached in the case of liver abscess drainage. Iatrogenic vessel injury, pseudoaneurysm, and arteriovenous fistula formation may occur [13]. Bleeding from small hepatic vessels is usually self-limiting and can often be managed conservatively; however persistent bleeding may require embolization.

## Biliary Drainage and Cholecystostomy

### Epidemiology

Gallstones are a common pathology, affecting 15% of North Americans, and may obstruct the cystic duct, causing cholecystitis, or dislodge into the common bile duct (CBD) and cause biliary obstruction with or without cholangitis [14]. Biliary obstruction secondary to

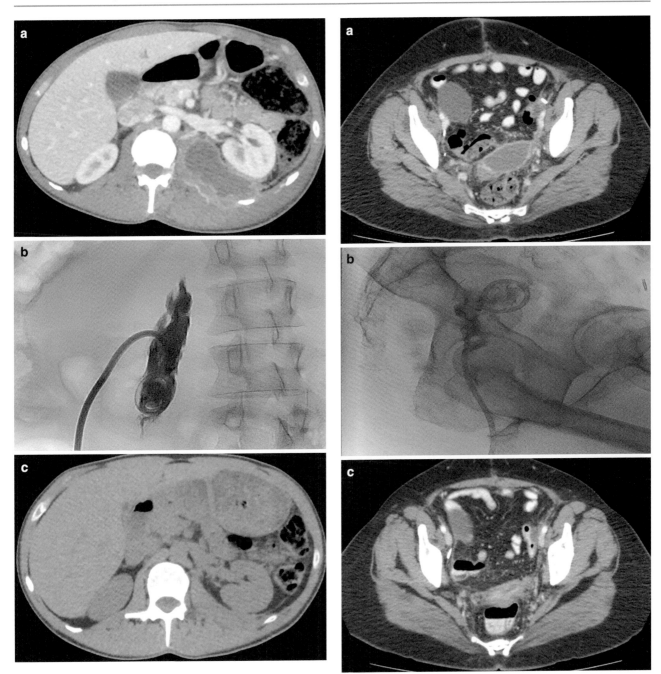

**Fig. 3** (**a**–**c**) Patient presented with left flank and hip pain. (**a**) Contrast-enhanced CT of the abdomen and pelvis showed a hypodense collection with peripheral enhancement within the left psoas muscle. (**b**) Fluoroscopic image in prone position confirmed drain placement within the collection. (**c**) Follow-up unenhanced CT of the abdomen and pelvis after drain removal demonstrated decrease in left psoas muscle size (nearly symmetrical) and resolution of the hypodense collection

**Fig. 4** (**a**–**c**) Patient post total abdominal hysterectomy and bilateral salpingo-oophorectomy for ovarian cancer presented with fever and pelvic pain. (**a**) Contrast-enhanced CT of the abdomen and pelvis demonstrated a hypodense collection with peripheral enhancement within the surgical cavity, incidental uncomplicated pelvic seroma adjacent to the right iliac vessels. (**b**) Oblique view fluoroscopic image demonstrating a transvaginal drain placement within the abscess. (**c**) Follow-up contrast-enhanced CT of the abdomen and pelvis after removal of the drain showed significant improvement in the abscess cavity.,

strictures may be due to either benign or malignant etiology. Benign biliary strictures typically occurs in response to biliary injury, whether traumatic (e.g., postsurgical; liver transplantation/cholecystectomy) or secondary to passage of biliary ductal stones, or conditions such as primary sclerosing cholangitis and pancreatitis [15]. On the other hand, malignant strictures can also occur and are estimated at 1.5/10,000 people per year in North America [16].

## Clinical Features

The clinical presentation of biliary obstruction is variable and depends on the presence or absence and acuity of and level of the obstruction. Patients may present with right upper quadrant pain, jaundice, pale stool, and dark urine in presence of obstruction. This can be abrupt in cases of choledocholithiasis or more indolent in benign and malignant obstructions [17]. Superimposed cholangitis may cause fever, chills, or overt sepsis and in severe cases, hemodynamic compromise [17].

## Radiological Findings

Ultrasound is usually the first modality for investigation in suspected cases of biliary colic or acute cholecystitis [18]. Evaluation of distal CBD obstruction may be limited by overlying bowel gas, though secondary signs of obstruction may be seen such as intrahepatic biliary duct or CBD dilatation [19]. While ultrasound alone is often sufficient in the diagnosis of cholecystitis, CT can be useful in the evaluation of complicated cholecystitis or identifying alternative causes of biliary tract obstruction [19]. Magnetic resonance cholangiopancreatography (MRCP) is the modality of choice for noninvasive evaluation of biliary tree dilatation and level and extent of obstruction. It is valuable in confirming the presence or absence of stones and determining the nature of biliary strictures [19].

## Biliary Obstruction: When to Call IR?

A common query which arises with regard to biliary obstruction management is whether the patient should undergo drainage via endoscopic retrograde cholangiopancreatography (ERCP) or if percutaneous biliary drainage should be performed. The decision will be dependent on local service provision; however, guidelines state ERCP is the recommended first-line therapeutic method whether obstruction is caused by choledocholithiasis or malignant common bile duct obstruction [20]. Percutaneous biliary drainage should however be first-line treatment in the case of hilar malignancy (Klatskin tumor) [20]. Percutaneous biliary interventions may also be required in situations where ERCP is unsuccessful, such as unfavorable anatomy for an endoscopic approach (Roux-en-Y anatomy) or if duodenal stents are in situ [20, 21].

IRs perform percutaneous biliary drainage through a combination of ultrasound and fluoroscopy guidance. In contrast to liver abscess drainage, a smaller caliber 21-gauge access needle is usually used to puncture the target biliary duct under US guidance. Once the level of concern is reached and traversed, an internal-external drain can be sited, the Cope loop formed and locked within the duodenum, with side holes proximal and distal to the level of obstruction; drainage can therefore occur in both an antegrade and retrograde manner (Fig. 5a). For at least 48 h (or until signs of sepsis resolve), the drain should be attached to bag drainage. After this time period, the tube can be capped to promote internal drainage of bile. In situations where the biliary duct system is grossly dilated, it can be difficult to manipulate a wire beyond the level of obstruction; an external drain may be left in situ to decompress the biliary system, and the patient can subsequently return to the IR suite for reattempt at inserting an internal-external biliary drain (Fig. 5b). There should be a low threshold for a staged procedure as excessive biliary manipulation during a single session may lead to bacteremia and sepsis.

## Percutaneous Cholecystostomy

For gallbladder disease, IRs are frequently consulted for percutaneous cholecystostomy tube insertion in high-risk surgical patients with acute calculous cholecystitis. A randomized controlled trial demonstrated a significantly increased risk of major complications and re-intervention rate in high-risk patients undergoing percutaneous cholecystostomy in comparison with laparoscopic cholecystectomy for acute cholecystitis [22]. Therefore, careful multidisciplinary decision-making is essential when selecting suitable patients for percutaneous cholecystostomy.

Laparoscopic cholecystectomy is the gold standard treatment for calculous gallbladder disease. In patients with acute cholecystitis caused by an obstructing calculus who are poor surgical candidates, percutaneous cholecystectomy can provide temporary drainage of the gallbladder (Fig. 6). Once a cholecystostomy tube has been placed, subsequent attempts can be made to extract gallbladder stones using either endoscopy, fluoroscopy, or a combination of both modalities.

Although percutaneous cholecystostomy is usually performed under US and fluoroscopic guidance, the latter is not essential, and the procedure may be achieved successfully solely under US guidance, particularly when performed in the intensive care unit on the critically ill patient. The operator may site a cholecystostomy tube via a transhepatic or transperitoneal route. Although there is a shorter time to tract maturation when performed using the transhepatic route (2 weeks versus 3 weeks), studies have shown no difference in short-term complications when either approach is used [23, 24].

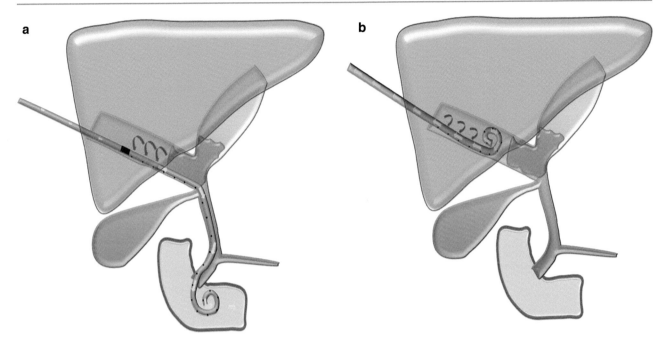

**Fig. 5** (**a** and **b**) Schematic drawing illustrating hilar obstruction. In cases where the obstruction can be traversed in a single session (**a**), an internal-external drain can be sited with drainage occurring into both an attached bag and also antegrade into the duodenum. If the biliary tree is grossly dilated, it may be difficult to cross the obstruction (**b**), and an external drain attached to a bag can be left in situ to allow the biliary system to decompress

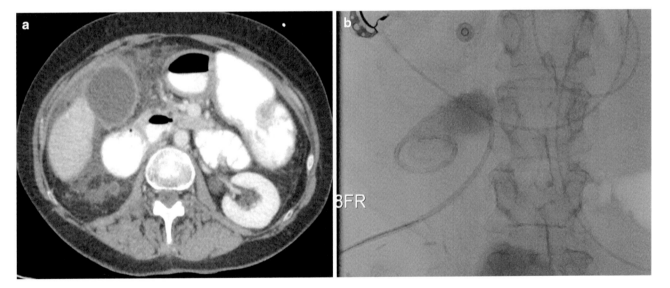

**Fig. 6** Patient with right upper quadrant pain, fever, and tenderness. (**a**) Contrast-enhanced CT of the abdomen and pelvis demonstrated features of acute cholecystitis. (**b**) Fluoroscopic image confirms position of an 8-French cholecystostomy tube in the gallbladder, inserted under ultrasound guidance through a transhepatic approach

## Complications of Biliary Drainage

Complications that occur as a result of percutaneous biliary drainage or cholecystostomy tube insertion may either be procedure or tube related. The quoted major complication rate for percutaneous biliary drainage and cholecystostomy is 10% and 5%, respectively [25]. Hemorrhage and sepsis are the most commonly occurring complications.

Bile leak along the tract can occur if there are drain side holes exposed outside of the biliary tree (Fig. 7). Peri-drain leak can also occur if the catheter becomes blocked; bile leaks via the side holes and in a retrograde manner through the tract

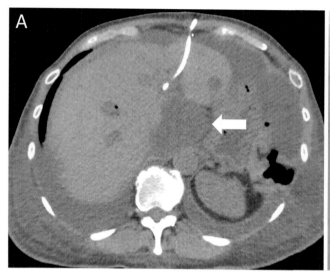 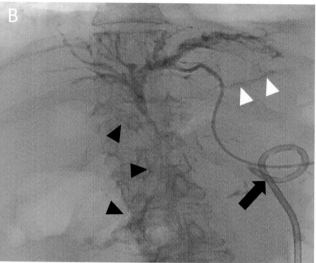

**Fig. 7** (**a** and **b**) Patient with metastatic pancreatic carcinoma, CBD stent, and external biliary drain presented with abdominal pain. (**a**) Unenhanced CT of the abdomen and pelvis demonstrated peritoneal ascites with an apparent fluid loculation (white arrow) and; external biliary drain check was suggested. (**b**) External biliary drain check demonstrated contrast leakage through a retracted side hole (white arrowhead) into the peritoneum, biliary stent (black arrowhead), and left upper quadrant drain (black arrow) are seen

along the path of least resistance. Conversely if the catheter slips too far into the duodenum, with no side hole proximal to the obstruction, there will be no drainage of the obstructed system. Although internal-external drains can be flushed, aspiration should generally be avoided given the possibility of forcing intestinal bacteria from the duodenum into the biliary tree with increased risk of ascending cholangitis. In all scenarios presented, an IR consult is necessary with a view to check and/or reposition or exchange the drain.

Both biliary drains and cholecystostomy tubes may dislodge completely. In scenarios where a mature tract has not formed (<2-4 weeks), a de novo procedure may be required. If a mature tract has formed, it may be possible to reinsert the catheter via the tract. In either case, IR should be contacted as soon as possible as there is a higher success rate of reinsertion in the setting of a mature tract if this occurs within 48 hours of tube dislodgement [26].

## Urological Obstruction

### Epidemiology

Urinary tract obstruction (UTO) prevalence ranges from 5/10,000 to 50/10,000 [27]. UTO can occur at various levels of the urinary tract (kidneys, ureters, bladder, and urethra) secondary to a multitude of causes including, but not limited to, calculi, transitional cell carcinoma, infection, and blood clot.

## Clinical Features

Patients may present with variable changes in urine characteristics (hematuria or pyuria) and reduced urine output [28]. Flank and abdominal pain are most commonly present in cases of ureteric calculi and infection. External ureteral compression leading to UTO is usually painless because of the slowly progressive course of obstruction.

## Radiological Findings

US is the first-line modality of choice with a negative predictive value of 98% [29]. A non-contrast-enhanced CT is the initial study of consideration when an obstructing calculus is suspected. Contrast-enhanced CT may be useful for characterization of the renal parenchyma., [30].

## Role of Interventional Radiology

### Indications
Percutaneous nephrostomy (PCN) for decompression of an obstructed kidney is a common urological intervention performed by IR [31]. PCN may be performed for urine drainage in obstruction and urinary diversion in cases of ureteric injury/urine leak and also serves as an access route to the collecting system for further interventions such as percutaneous nephrolithotomy (PCNL). Indications for urgent PCN include sepsis and acute renal dysfunction.

## Techniques

IR can offer two therapies for UTO caused by benign or malignant obstruction: PCN and antegrade ureteric stenting. PCN has a technical success rate of 96–99% by experienced operators [32]. The procedure is usually performed with the patient in the prone position. Using US guidance, the dilated collecting system is targeted with either a 21-gauge or 18-gauge access needle depending on the operator preference

and degree of hydronephrosis. A dilated posterior mid- or lower pole calyx is targeted as this presents the lowest risk of bleeding complications. Using Seldinger technique, an 8-French Cope-loop catheter is introduced under fluoroscopic guidance, the loop formed within the renal pelvis and the nephrostomy tube kept on free drainage (Fig. 8).

If internal drainage urinary drainage is desired, ureteric stenting can be considered to allow drainage past the site of

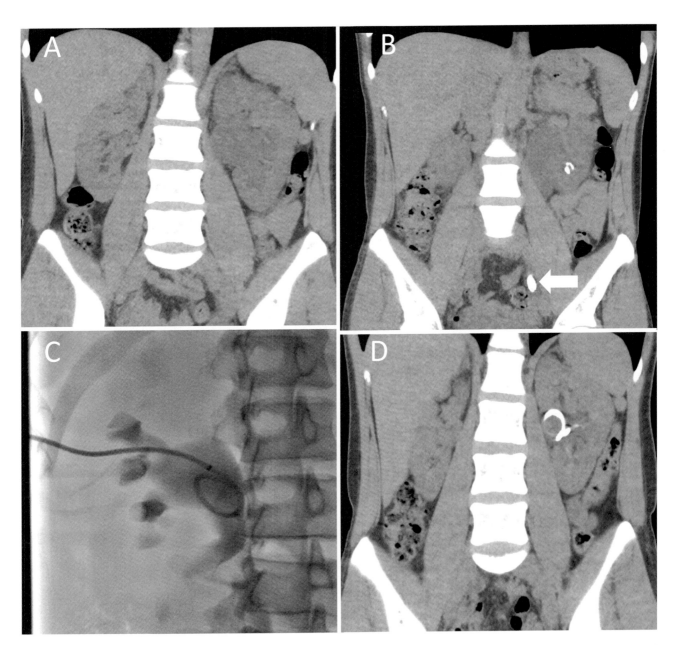

**Fig. 8** (**a**–**d**) Patient presented with left flank pain.(**a**) Unenhanced CT of the abdomen and pelvis demonstrated left moderate to severe hydronephrosis with left mid-ureteric stone (white arrow in (**b**)). (**c**) Contrast injection through the left nephrostomy tube confirmed placement of Cope loop in the left renal pelvis. (**d**) Follow-up CT of the abdomen and pelvis demonstrated the left nephrostomy tube in appropriate position along with a decompressed renal pelvis

obstruction and to the bladder. PCN In the acute setting, particularly if the patient is septic, it is usually favored to decompress the collecting system and have the patient return for antegrade stent insertion given the risk of septic storm. If the patient does not have signs of sepsis, attempts may be made to perform primary antegrade stenting with placement of a double J stent or nephroureterostomy.

### Precautious Antegrade vs Retrograde Intervention

The alternative to antegrade PCN or stenting in UTO is retrograde ureteroscopic management.. A randomized controlled trial comparing both management strategies for obstructing ureteric stone disease concluded equivalence between the two approaches, and ultimately patient management will depend upon local hospital service provision [33].

### Complications

PCN is a safe and well-tolerated procedure with a reported mortality rate of 0.04–0.3% [34, 35]. Overall complication rate related to PCN is less than 10% with most common minor complication related to tube dislodgement or dysfunction [36]. Major PCN-related complications include sepsis (1.8–2.2%), hemorrhage requiring transfusion or embolization, and visceral organ injury; complication rates are noted to be higher in patients with pyonephrosis and in cases performed emergently out of routine hours [34, 37].

Similar to percutaneous biliary drains, a PCN may become obstructed, retract, or become dislodged. In cases of PCN obstruction, which can occur when debris within the tip prevents urine flow, the patient may notice urine leak around the

catheter exit site at the level of the skin and minimal output into the drainage bag; this occurs as urine passes along the mature tract via the path of least resistance. Retraction may occur if the PCN is inadvertently pulled and may also result in reduced urine output and leakage. In both circumstances prompt IR consult is required for tube exchange to prevent urosepsis. If the tube becomes completely dislodged and is at least 2-4 weeks old (time for mature tract formation), a new tube may be inserted via the existing tract. If less than 2 weeks old, a de novo PCN may be required. Prompt IR consultation is required in these cases given the tract will begin to close once a tube has been dislodged [2].

## Gastrointestinal Interventions

### Percutaneous Radiologic Gastrostomy Complications

Enteral nutrition is the primary method of providing supplemental nutrition in patients who cannot tolerate oral intake. Patients with head and neck cancer, upper gastrointestinal malignancies, and neurological disease which impairs the swallowing mechanism are at particular risk of dysphagia resulting in weight loss and malnutrition. Furthermore, surgical treatments, chemotherapy, and/or radiotherapy in these patient groups can compound dysphagia, resulting in impairment of oral nutritional intake. Gastrostomy feeding tubes can be inserted either fluoroscopically, endoscopically, or surgically. Procedure-related complications such as hemorrhage, infection, and collection (Fig. 9) may occur; however, tube-related

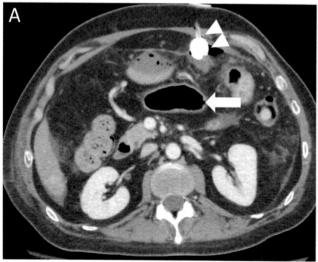
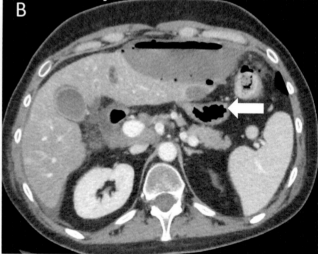

**Fig. 9** (**a** and **b**) Patient with head and neck cancer requiring gastrostomy tube insertion. (**a**) Contrast-enhanced CT of the abdomen demonstrated a malpositioned balloon-retention gastrostomy tube (white arrow head) outside of the stomach (white arrow). **b**) Contrast-enhanced CT of the abdomen more cephalad demonstrated a collection around the tube tip and displacing the liver and stomach (white arrow)

**Table 1** Summary of common gastrostomy tube insertion-related complications, conservative measures, and solutions

| Complication | Presentation | Solution |
|---|---|---|
| Pneumoperitoneum | Abdominal pain | Usually self limiting. If significant discomfort due to large pneumoperitoneum, may benefit from aspiration of the air. |
| | Free intraperitoneal gas on erect chest radiograph or on CT | Pneumoperitoneum post gastrostomy insertion may persist for several days with varying rates of resolution reported in the literature. Interpretation of imaging in conjunction with history and procedural details may be helpful. In the event of clinical concern, CT and/or a tube check can be helpful. |
| Collection | Abdominal pain | Consult IR |
| | Sepsis | Collection on imaging could be drained if symptomatic and technically amenable |
| Blocked tube | Inability to feed | Attempt gently flushing tube |
| | Leakage of tube at exit site | If not successful consult IR for tube check/exchange |
| | Usually occurs after attempting to instill crushed tablets through tube | Tube should be flushed with water or normal saline prior to and after routine use |
| Dislodged tube | Tube pulled back significantly or completely dislodged | Consult IR as soon as possible |
| | | If tube >4 weeks old and completely dislodged, attempt can be made to insert Foley catheter to prevent tract from closing |
| | | Tube reinsertion can be attempted by IR if a mature tract exists. |
| | | Evaluate external bolster to ensure not too tight |
| | | If not successful may need gastrostomy tube upsizing |
| Tube migration | Abdominal pain on feeding | IR consult for tube check/manipulation/exchange |
| | Diarrhea | |

complications occur far more frequently. A summary of common gastrostomy tube-related complications and solutions is shown in Table 1. Prior to contacting IR, it is useful for radiologists to be aware of the type of tube that has been inserted, the position of the tip of the tube on imaging, and integrity of the balloon (if imaging is available).

## Colonic Stenting

The most common cause of large bowel obstruction is colonic malignancy. Other causes include extrinsic malignant compression and benign causes such as post-radiation and inflammatory bowel-related strictures. Guidance states insertion of a self-expanding metal stent may be indicated in patients presenting with large bowel obstruction secondary to left-sided colonic malignancy, as an alternative to acute surgery in those who are high-risk operative candidates (Fig. 10) [38]. Colonic stenting may also be performed as a palliative measure. In either case, multidisciplinary decision-making is required between surgeons, oncologists, gastroenterologists, and interventional radiologists. Endoscopic guidance can be a useful adjunct to fluoroscopic colonic stent insertion, in particular if lesions are proximal to the rectosigmoid as these can be challenging to navigate with catheters/wires alone. Colonic stenting is typically reserved for left-sided colonic lesions. Access to strictures that are proximal to the splenic flexure can be technically challenging although there are reports of right-sided colonic stenting [39].

## Summary

Radiologists, particularly those dealing with acute imaging, will encounter pathologies for which IR can provide valuable patient care over a range of minimally invasive nonvascular interventions with a good safety profile. It is imperative that IRs are contacted in a timely manner to prevent further complications from ensuing. It is also essential that radiologists are aware of the imaging findings of potential complications related to nonvascular IR procedures.

## References

1. Coleman DL, King RN, Andrade JD. The foreign body reaction: a chronic inflammatory response. J Biomed Mater Res. 1974;8(5): 199–211.
2. Huang SY, Engstrom BI, Lungren MP, Kim CY. Management of dysfunctional catheters and tubes inserted by interventional radiology. Semin Intervent Radiol. 2015;32:67–77. Thieme Medical Publishers
3. Sharma A, Mukewar S, Mara KC, Dierkhising RA, Kamath PS, Cummins N. Epidemiologic factors, clinical presentation, causes, and outcomes of liver abscess: A 35-year Olmsted County Study. Mayo Clin Proc Innov Qual Outcomes. 2018 Mar;2(1):16–25.
4. Rahimian J, Wilson T, Oram V, Holzman RS. Pyogenic liver abscess: recent trends in etiology and mortality. Clin Infect Dis. 2004;39(11):1654–9. Available from: https://academic.oup.com/cid/article-lookup/doi/10.1086/425616
5. Hadley GP. Intra-abdominal sepsis-epidemiology, aetiology and management. Semin Pediatr Surg. 2014;23(6):357–62.
6. Pharaon KS, Trunkey DD. Abdominal abscess. In: Clinical infectious disease. 2nd ed. Cambridge University Press; 2015. p. 366–9.

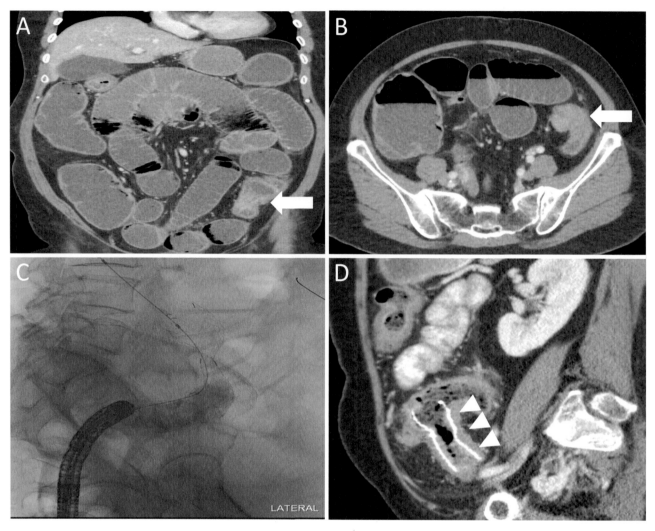

**Fig. 10** (**a–d**) Patient presented with nausea, vomiting and constipation (**a** and **b**) Contrast-enhanced CT of the abdomen and pelvis demonstrated dilated small and large bowel loops (incompetent ileocecal valve) with transition point seen at the sigmoid colon secondary to focal circumferential sigmoid wall thickening (white arrow) in (**a** and **b**). (**c**) Colonoscopic- and fluoroscopic-guided insertion of colonic stent with follow-up CT (**d**), demonstrating a patent stent (white arrowheads) with fecal matter within it and decompression of proximal small and large bowel

7. Heffner JE, Klein JS, Hampson C. Diagnostic utility and clinical application of imaging for pleural space infections [Internet]. 2010. Available from: www.chestjournal.org
8. Dariushnia SR, Mitchell JW, Chaudry G, Hogan MJ. Society of interventional radiology quality improvement standards for image-guided percutaneous drainage and aspiration of abscesses and fluid collections. J Vasc Interv Radiol. 2020;31(4):662–666.e4.
9. Dulku G, Mohan G, Samuelson S, Ferguson J, Tibballs J. Percutaneous aspiration versus catheter drainage of liver abscess: a retrospective review. Australas Med J. 2015;8(1):7–18.
10. Zerem E, Hadzic A. Sonographically guided percutaneous catheter drainage versus needle aspiration in the management of pyogenic liver abscess. AJR Am J Roentgenol. 2007;189(3)
11. Cai YL, Xiong XZ, Lu J, Cheng Y, Yang C, Lin YX, et al. Percutaneous needle aspiration versus catheter drainage in the management of liver abscess: a systematic review and meta-analysis, vol. 17, HPB. Blackwell Publishing Ltd; 2015. p. 195–201.
12. Wallace MJ, Chin KW, Fletcher TB, Bakal CW, Cardella JF, Grassi CJ, et al. Quality improvement guidelines for percutaneous drainage/Aspiration of abscess and fluid collections. J Vasc Interv Radiol. 2010;21(4):431–5.
13. Lorenz J, Thomas JL. Complications of percutaneous fluid drainage. Semin Intervent Radiol. 2006;23:194–204.
14. Stinton LM, Shaffer EA. Epidemiology of gallbladder disease: cholelithiasis and cancer. Edit Off Gut and Liver. 2012;6:172–87.
15. Dadhwal US, Kumar V. Benign bile duct strictures. Med J Armed Forces India. 2012;68(3):299–303.
16. Siegel R, Ma J, Zou Z, Jemal A. Cancer statistics, 2014. CA Cancer J Clin. 2014 Jan;64(1):9–29.
17. Diagnostic approach to the adult with jaundice or asymptomatic hyperbilirubinemia – UpToDate [Internet]. 2020. Available from: https://www.uptodate.com/contents/diagnostic-approach-to-the-adult-with-jaundice-or-asymptomatic-hyperbilirubinemia#H2
18. Shea JA, Berlin JA, Escarce JJ, Clarke JR, Kinosian BP, Cabana MD, et al. Revised estimates of diagnostic test sensitivity and specificity in suspected biliary tract disease. Arch Intern Med. 1994;154(22):2573–81.
19. Thomas S, Jahangir K. Noninvasive imaging of the biliary system relevant to percutaneous interventions. Semin Intervent Radiol. 2016;33(4):277–82.
20. Fairchild AH, Hohenwalter EJ, Gipson MG, Al-Refaie WB, Braun AR, Cash BD, et al. ACR appropriateness criteria ® radiologic

management of biliary obstruction. J Am Coll Radiol. 2019;16(5): S196–213.

21. Ma MX, Jayasekeran V, Chong AK. Benign biliary strictures: prevalence, impact, and management strategies. Clin Exp Gastroenterol. 2019;12:83–92. Available from: https://www.dovepress.com/benign-biliary-strictures-prevalence-impact-and-management-strategies-peer-reviewed-article-CEG

22. Loozen CS, Van Santvoort HC, Van Duijvendijk P, Besselink MG, Gouma DJ, Nieuwenhuijzen GA, et al. Laparoscopic cholecystectomy versus percutaneous catheter drainage for acute cholecystitis in high risk patients (CHOCOLATE): multicentre randomised clinical trial. BMJ. 2018;8:363.

23. Hatjidakis AA, Karampekios S, Prassopoulos P, Xynos E, Raissaki M, Vasilakis SI, et al. Maturation of the tract after percutaneous cholecystostomy with regard to the access route. Cardiovasc Intervent Radiol. 1998;21(1):36–40. Available from: http://link.springer.com/10.1007/s002709900208

24. Loberant N, Notes Y, Eitan A, Yakir O, Bickel A. Comparison of early outcome from transperitoneal versus transhepatic percutaneous cholecystostomy. Hepatogastroenterology. 2010;57(97):12–7.

25. Saad WEA, Wallace MJ, Wojak JC, Kundu S, Cardella JF. Quality improvement guidelines for percutaneous transhepatic cholangiography, biliary drainage, and percutaneous cholecystostomy. J Vasc Interv Radiol. 2010;21(6):789–95.

26. Collares FB, Faintuch S, Kim SK, Rabkin DJ. Reinsertion of accidentally dislodged catheters through the original track: what is the likelihood of success? J Vasc Interv Radiol. 2010;21(6): 861–4.

27. Preminger GM. Obstructive uropathy – genitourinary disorders – merck manuals professional edition [Internet]. 2020. Available from: https://www.merckmanuals.com/en-ca/professional/genitourinary-disorders/obstructive-uropathy/obstructive-uropathy?query=urinarytractobstruction

28. Urinary Tract Obstruction – Brenner and Rector's The Kidney, 8th ed [Internet]. 2020. Available from: https://doctorlib.info/nephrology/kidney/36.html

29. Ellenbogen PH, Scheible FW, Talner LB, Leopold GR. Sensitivity of gray scale ultrasound in detecting urinary tract obstruction. Am J Roentgenol. 1978;130(4):731–3.

30. Craig WD, Wagner BJ, Travis MD. From the archives of the AFIP. Pyelonephritis: radiologic-pathologic review. Radiographics. 2008;28:255–76. Radiological Society of North America

31. Goodwin WE, Casey WC, Woolf W. Percutaneous trocar (needle) nephrostomy in hydronephrosis. J Am Med Assoc. 1955;157(11): 891–4.

32. Pabon-Ramos WM, Dariushnia SR, Walker TG, Janne D'Othée B, Ganguli S, Midia M, et al. Quality improvement guidelines for percutaneous nephrostomy. J Vasc Interv Radiol. 2016;27(3):410–4.

33. Wang CJ, Hsu C, Sen CHW, Chang CH, Tsai PC. Percutaneous nephrostomy versus ureteroscopic management of sepsis associated with ureteral stone impaction: a randomized controlled trial. Urolithiasis. 2016;44(5):415–9.

34. Patel U. Emergency percutaneous nephrostomy: results and complications. J Vasc Interv Radiol. 1994;5(1):135–9.

35. Dyer RB, Regan JD, Kavanagh PV, Khatod EG, Chen MY, Zagoria RJ. Percutaneous nephrostomy with extensions of the technique: Step by step 1. Radiographics. 2002;22(3):503–25.

36. Kaskarelis IS, Papadaki MG, Malliaraki NE, Robotis ED, Malagari KS, Piperopoulos PN. Complications of percutaneous nephrostomy, percutaneous insertion of ureteral endoprosthesis, and replacement procedures. Cardiovasc Intervent Radiol. 2001;24(4):224–8.

37. Lewis S, Patel U. Major complications after percutaneous nephrostomy – lessons from a department audit. Clin Radiol. 2004;59(2):171–9.

38. Van Hooft JE, Van Halsema EE, Vanbiervliet G, Beets-Tan RGH, Dewitt JM, Donnellan F, et al. Self-expandable metal stents for obstructing colonic and extracolonic cancer: European Society of Gastrointestinal Endoscopy (ESGE) Clinical Guideline. Endoscopy. 2014;46(11):990–1002.

39. Saida Y. Current status of colonic stent for obstructive colorectal cancer in Japan; a review of the literature. J Anus Rectum Colon. 2019;3(3):99–105.

# Imaging of Traumatic Brain Injury

Walter F. Wiggins, Austin X. Dixon, and Peter G. Kranz

## Contents

## Abstract

Traumatic injury to the brain and head has several manifestations, including primary brain parenchymal injuries, secondary brain injury, extra-axial hemorrhage, and vascular injury. In this chapter, we review the mechanisms and imaging appearance of traumatic brain injury on CT, MRI, and cerebrovascular imaging. We also discuss the role of advanced imaging techniques in the investigation of brain trauma.

## Keywords

Trauma · Traumatic Brain Injury · Diffuse Axonal Injury · Epidural Hematoma · Subdural Hematoma · Cerebrovascular Injury

## Introduction

In this chapter, we will cover essential topics in the imaging of traumatic brain injury. Non-contrast-enhanced CT of the head (NECT) is the primary screening tool for patients with head trauma, but MRI and CT angiography (CTA) can also play an important role. The different patterns of injury are discussed, including injuries to the brain parenchyma, extra-axial hemorrhage, herniation syndromes, and intracranial vascular injury. We conclude with a brief discussion about the role of advanced imaging in brain trauma.

## Brain Parenchymal Injuries

Traumatic injuries to the brain parenchyma include non-hemorrhagic and hemorrhagic contusions, diffuse axonal injury (DAI), diffuse cerebral edema, and hypoxic-ischemic injury. These injury types occur via different mechanisms and result in differing patterns of neurologic deficit. Contusions and DAI are primary injuries to the brain parenchyma, the

W. F. Wiggins · A. X. Dixon · P. G. Kranz (✉)
Department of Radiology, Duke University Medical Center, Durham, NC, USA
e-mail: peter.kranz@duke.edu

© Springer Nature Switzerland AG 2022
M. N. Patlas et al. (eds.), *Atlas of Emergency Imaging from Head-to-Toe*,
https://doi.org/10.1007/978-3-030-92111-8_5

result of the deposition of kinetic energy related to the trauma. Contusions are local injuries caused by a direct impact to the brain, whereas DAI is a more widespread process resulting from shear forces generated due to rapid acceleration, deceleration, or rotation. Diffuse cerebral edema and hypoxic-ischemic injury are forms of secondary injury to the brain that can occur concurrently with the initial trauma or evolve in the subsequent hours to days. Each of these patterns of injury has typical locations and associated findings on non-enhanced CT imaging of the head (NECT). MRI may serve as an important adjunct in some cases, to assess the full extent of the injury, particularly when evaluating DAI.

## Parenchymal Contusions

Contusions of the brain parenchyma can occur anywhere along the outer surface of the brain, as a result of direct impact of the brain against the cranial vault, although certain locations are more common than others (Fig. 1). Frequent locations for contusions include the anterior frontal (frontal "pole"), orbital frontal (or subfrontal), and anterior temporal (temporal "pole") lobes (Fig. 2). A direct strike to the head or rapid deceleration causes the brain to impact against the anterior surfaces of the skull, especially along the floor of the anterior cranial fossa and middle cranial fossa, producing impact injuries to these characteristic locations. If the force of

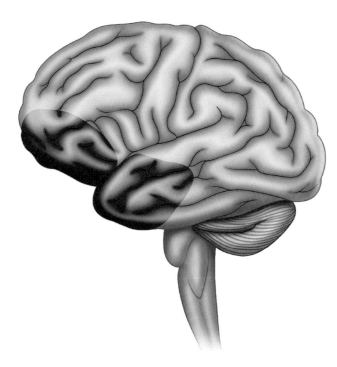

**Fig. 1** Typical location of brain contusions in trauma. The inferior frontal lobes and anterior temporal lobes (shaded in red) are the most location for contusions, particularly in high-speed injuries involving rapid deceleration

impact is sufficiently strong, the brain may rebound after impact and strike the opposite side of the skull, resulting in an additional contusion; such a pattern is referred to as a "coup-contrecoup" pattern of injury [1].

Contusions may be nonhemorrhagic (sometimes termed "bland" contusions) or hemorrhagic. On NECT, non-hemorrhagic contusions appear as focal regions of decreased attenuation at or close to the surface of the brain. These low-density areas represent edema of the brain parenchyma. Hemorrhagic contusions will appear as areas of increased attenuation (i.e., hemorrhage), often surrounded by a halo of low-attenuation edema. On MRI, nonhemorrhagic contusions are seen as focal regions of increased T2 signal located in the periphery of the brain. This peripheral location is a key feature in distinguishing contusions from shear-related injury, which occurs deep in the brain. Hemorrhagic contusions will show internal areas of blood, characterized by variable but often increased T1 signal, low T2 signal, and blooming (i.e., increased size of low T2 signal focus) on T2*-weighted sequences, including gradient recalled echo (GRE) or susceptibility-weighted imaging (SWI) (Fig. 3).

It is common for hemorrhagic contusions to expand over time or for contusions that are initially nonhemorrhagic to become hemorrhagic. This phenomenon, known as hemorrhagic progression of contusions (HPC), occurs in approximately half of cases where contusions are present [2]. At times, the increase in size of the hemorrhagic contusions may result in rapid clinical deterioration due to increasing mass effect (Fig. 4) and in some cases may require surgical decompression. New areas of hemorrhage may also appear in previously normal-appearing brain parenchyma (Fig. 5).

HPC may occur up to several days after the initial injury but most commonly occurs within the first 12 hours [2]. For this reason, a follow-up NECT is commonly obtained within 6–12 hours of the initial scan in order to evaluate for expansion of previous hemorrhage, the presence of new hemorrhage, or new mass effect or herniation [2–5]. Subsequent follow-up imaging after 12 hours may be performed if there are new or worsening neurologic deficits or for whom a reliable neurologic examination cannot be readily obtained (e.g., comatose or intubated/sedated patients) [4].

## DAI

Shear forces resulting from rapid acceleration or deceleration are the mechanism by which DAI occurs [6]. DAI may occur with or without a direct blow to the head and is frequently seen in the setting of severe head trauma, particularly cases involving high-speed motor vehicle collisions [7]. DAI is more commonly hemorrhagic but can also be non-hemorrhagic. The identification of DAI on imaging is important in explaining cases of head trauma where the degree of

**Fig. 2** Typical location of hemorrhagic contusions. Axial NECT images at the level of the inferior frontal lobes (**a**) and anterior temporal lobes (**b**) show hemorrhagic contusions in these typical locations following severe head trauma

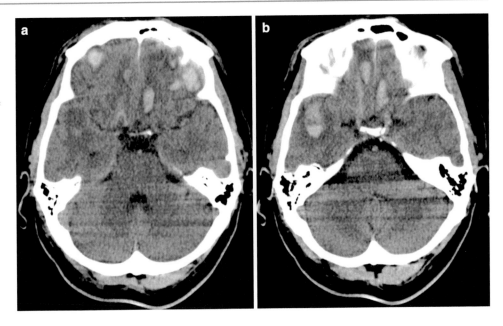

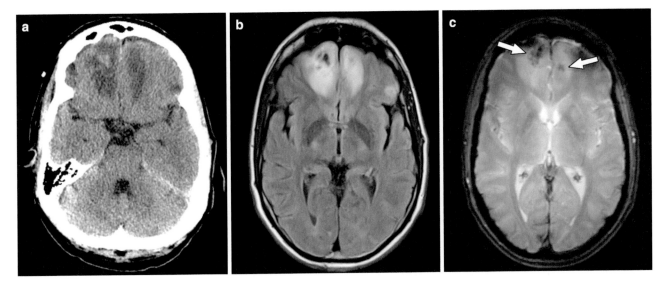

**Fig. 3** Appearance of contusions on MRI. Axial NECT image (**a**) shows bifrontal hypodense contusions, with a focus of hyperdense hemorrhagic component on the right. Axial FLAIR MR image (**b**) shows increased signal in the contusions due to edema, with internal areas of low-signal corresponding to the hemorrhage. Axial T2* (GRE) MR image (**c**) shows increased conspicuity of the low-signal areas of hemorrhage (arrows)

clinical deficit exceeds the apparent injury on initial imaging. DAI also serves as a prognostic indicator for both severity of head injury and persistent cognitive deficits after relatively mild head trauma [8].

MRI is the mainstay of diagnostic imaging in DAI. Hemorrhagic DAI foci will show small areas of susceptibility – or loss of signal – on GRE or SWI images (Fig. 6). Due to the additional information imparted by phase differences in addition to T2*-weighted effects, SWI imaging is more sensitive for the detection of small foci of hemorrhage compared to GRE imaging [9].

Some hemorrhagic foci may be seen on CT, although prospective diagnosis is often challenging because of the small size of these abnormalities (Fig. 7). Nonhemorrhagic DAI foci are best seen on diffusion-weighted imaging as areas of high signal, indicating decreased local diffusivity of water due to disruption of normal axonal pathways (Fig. 8).

Areas of injury related to DAI are frequently located at the interface of tissues of different density, differential motion of adjacent structures, and focal points of high torque in the setting of rapid acceleration or deceleration. DAI is most

**Fig. 4** HPC. Axial NECT image obtained after head trauma (**a**) shows a small hemorrhagic contusion (arrow). Diffuse edema is also seen, with effacement of the basal cisterns. Follow-up scan obtained 9 hours later (**b**) shows expansion of the initial hemorrhagic contusion, with new areas of hemorrhage visualized in wider area throughout the right temporal lobe

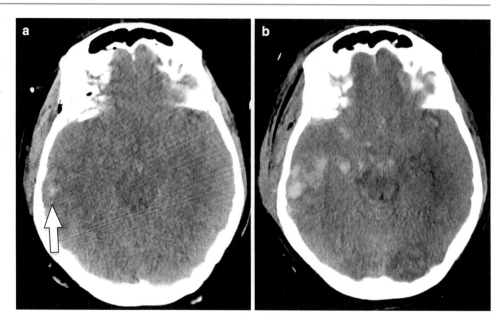

**Fig. 5** Delayed development of hemorrhagic contusions. Axial NECT image obtained after head trauma (**a**) shows no visible parenchymal injury to the right temporal lobe. A repeat scan obtained 7 hours later (**b**), prompted by neurologic deterioration, shows new large hemorrhagic contusions

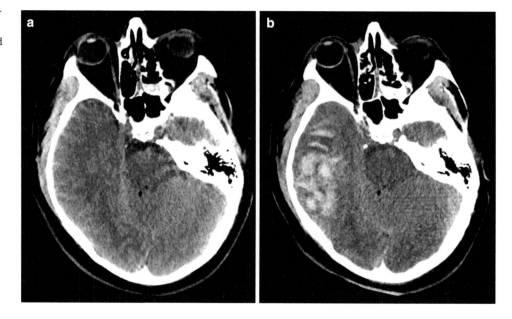

commonly seen at the gray-white junction in the frontal and temporal lobes and in the corpus callosum, particularly the splenium. It can also be seen in the deep white matter and occasionally involves the brainstem, often in the upper brainstem at its junction with the larger cerebral hemispheres.

## Secondary Injuries: Diffuse Edema and Hypoxic-Ischemic Injury

Brain injury in trauma is not limited to the primary injury caused by kinetic forces on the brain parenchyma. Biochemical processes triggered by contusions, hemorrhage, and shear injury, together with concomitant physiologic states including hypoperfusion, hypoxia, and seizures, may result in more widespread cellular damage [10].

Diffuse cerebral edema may develop within hours of the primary injury or even days later, causing increased intracranial pressure, which may in turn worsen brain perfusion [11]. Decreased blood oxygenation and decreased perfusion pressure to the brain can also occur as a result of trauma-related cardiac or respiratory arrest, resulting in hypoxic injury (in the setting of decreased blood oxygenation accompanying respiratory failure) or ischemic brain injury (in the

**Fig. 6** DAI. Axial NECT images (**a** & **b**) obtained after head trauma show trace blood in the atrium of the right lateral ventricle but no parenchymal injury. Axial T2* (GRE) MR images obtained at corresponding levels (**c** & **d**) show extensive small microhemorrhages (arrows) due to DAI. These microhemorrhages were occult on CT

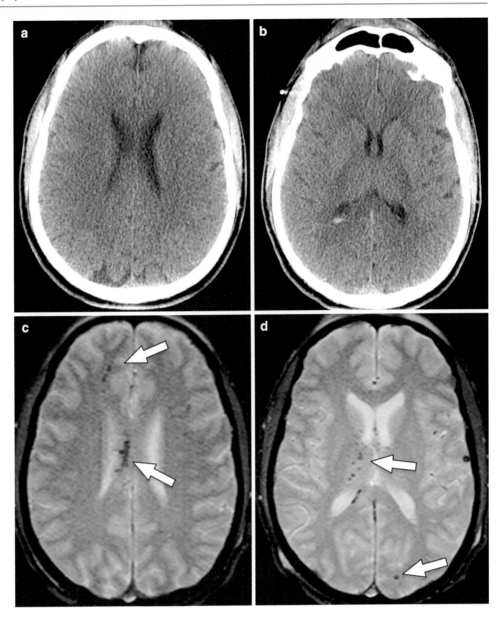

setting of decreased perfusion pressure accompanying cardiac dysfunction or hypovolemia) [12]. Diffuse cerebral edema and hypoxic-ischemic injury may occur together, producing a combination of both vasogenic and cytotoxic edema.

Imaging evidence of cerebral edema includes loss of sulci, effacement of the ventricles, and effacement of the cisterns surrounding the brain [13]. In the early stages, these changes may be difficult to recognize, particularly in young patients who have greater parenchymal volumes and less prominent cerebrospinal fluid (CSF) spaces at baseline. Regardless of patient age, however, patients typically have some visible CSF space in the quadrigeminal plate cistern, the suprasellar cistern, and the sulci over the convexities (Fig. 9). Loss of CSF in these spaces on imaging should raise concern for

cerebral edema. Severe edema can produce congestion or stasis in the veins on the brain surface, producing the appearance of hyperdensity in the sulci, known as the "pseudo-subarachnoid sign" for its similarity to the appearance of subarachnoid hemorrhage (SAH) [14].

Hypoxic-ischemic injury typically causes loss of gray-white differentiation on NECT. On MR, edema in the gray matter (characterized by increased T2 signal and swelling) is accompanied by diffusion restriction on DWI sequences. The pattern of gray matter involved depends on the severity and duration of hypoxia. Acute, profound hypoxia affects the deep gray nuclei of the brain because of their high rate of metabolic activity (Fig. 10). Partial-prolonged hypoxia may preferentially involve the cortical gray matter, with sparing of the deep gray nuclei (Fig. 11). In young children, the

**Fig. 7** Subtle DAI on CT. Axial NECT image (**a**) obtained after a high-speed motor vehicle collision shows subtle, small, punctate foci of increased density in the right frontal lobe (arrow). Axial SWI MR image at the corresponding level (**b**) confirms the presence of microhemorrhage along the gray-white junction, and in the deep white matter, due to shear injury. Although visible on CT, the extent of injury is better depicted on MR

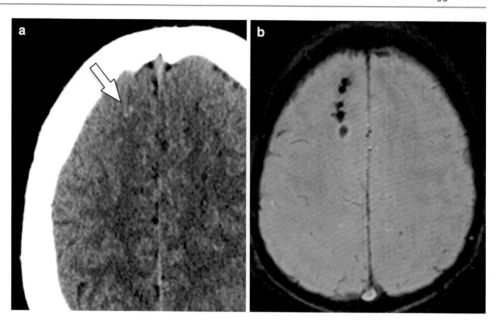

involvement of the supratentorial cortex may be even more pronounced, leading to a more conspicuous contrast in the density of the cerebellum compared to the injured cerebral hemispheres. This pattern is known as the "white cerebellum" sign (Fig. 12). If ischemia (rather than hypoxia) predominates, watershed zone infarctions may be seen. Infarction in the territory of specific arteries may be seen due to embolic phenomena, direct vascular injury, or herniation syndromes.

## Extra-axial Hemorrhage

Extra-axial hemorrhage is classified into three major types depending on the location of the hemorrhage relative to the three layers of the meninges. These types include epidural, subdural, and SAH [15]. The location of the hemorrhage influences the imaging appearance, clinical prognosis, and expected complications.

## Epidural Hematoma (EDH)

EDHs form in the potential space between the inner table of the skull and the dura. Because the dura is tightly connected to the inner surface of the skull at cranial sutures, EDHs typically do not cross suture lines [16, 17]. This limitation to spread results in localized accumulation of blood in a classically biconvex, or lentiform, collection (Fig. 13). Variations to this pattern can occur in the setting of skull fractures which cross cranial sutures, traumatic diastasis of sutures, or vertex location of an EDH [16, 18]. In the pediatric

population, EDHs often cross sutures given the frequency of skull fractures involving sutures and sutural diastasis.

EDHs are most commonly arterial in origin (approximately 90%) and usually are accompanied by an overlying skull fracture [19]. Injury to the middle meningeal artery, which can be lacerated when fractures resulting from blows to the side of the head involve the pterion or adjacent squamous temporal bone, is a common source of EDH [20]. Arterial EDHs can expand rapidly, producing rapid clinical deterioration, and are therefore closely monitored and often evacuated on an emergent basis [21].

Although less common than arterial injury, venous injury may also result in EDH. The bleeding vessels in venous EDH are under lower pressure than in arterial EDH, resulting in a lower likelihood that venous EDH will expand rapidly. Thus, they are more likely to be managed conservatively, with serial monitoring. Venous EDHs are typically associated with fractures which cross dural venous sinuses [18, 22]. The middle cranial fossa (adjacent to the anterior temporal lobe) is a common location for venous EDH and is caused when temporal or skull base fractures disrupt the sphenoparietal sinus (Fig. 14) [21]. EDH in this location should raise the possibility of a venous origin, which may prompt more conservative management. Other common locations for venous EDH include the posterior fossa (due to injury to the transverse dural venous sinus) or at the vertex (due to superior sagittal sinus injury) [23].

On NECT, acute EDH appears as a hyperdense lentiform collection, usually in association with an adjacent skull fracture, with local mass effect on the adjacent brain. In cases of ongoing active arterial bleeding, ovoid or irregular regions of low attenuation may be interspersed among the high-density blood, a finding known as the "swirl sign" [24]. Air may be

**Fig. 8** Nonhemorrhagic DAI. Axial NECT image (**a**) obtained in an obtunded patient after trauma shows only a small focus of hemorrhage in the right frontal white matter (arrow). Axial DW MR image (**b**) and ADC map (**c**) show extensive diffusion restriction in the corpus callosum in a nonvascular distribution due to shear injury. Axial T2* (GRE) MR image (**d**) shows a few foci of hemorrhage (arrows) but no hemorrhage in the corpus callosum where the diffusion restriction is seen

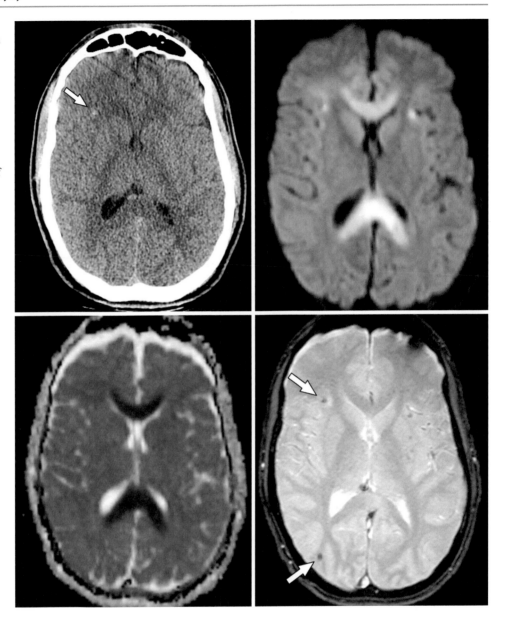

seen within the hematoma, particularly if the causative fracture traverses an aerated part of the skull, such as the mastoid air cells or paranasal sinuses. Diffuse low attenuation and peripheral dural thickening and enhancement suggest chronicity [25]. On MRI, the appearance of EDH varies depending on the age of the blood products. MR is not commonly used to evaluate acute EDH, but if MR is performed, signal characteristics of the hematoma would be expected to match those of acute blood (Table 1).

## Subdural Hematoma (SDH)

SDHs form in the potential space between the dura and arachnoid layers of the meninges. Most SDHs are the result of cortical veins that tear as these vessels course through the subdural space [20]. Consequently, SDHs are under lower pressure than arterial EDH and therefore do not expand as quickly. Unlike the epidural space, the subdural space is not limited by dural attachments at suture lines, allowing SDH to freely cross sutures, which can help distinguish them from EDH. Spread of SDH is limited at areas of dural reflection, however, such as the falx cerebri and tentorium. These factors contribute to the appearance of SDH as crescentic-shaped collections that can cross sutures but not the midline or tentorium. SDHs are most commonly supratentorial; infratentorial SDHs are encountered much less frequently and are often associated with occipital bone fractures [26, 27].

On NECT, acute SDHs are hyperdense. Small SDHs can be easily missed because their convex curvature matches the

**Fig. 9** Diffuse cerebral edema. Axial NECT image (**a**) and magnified image of the quadrigeminal plate cistern (**b**) obtained at the time of presentation in a patient with severe head trauma shows initial patency of the cistern (red oval). Follow-up NECT image obtained 10 hours later (**c**) and magnified image (**d**) show effacement of the quadrigeminal plate cistern (red oval) due to diffuse cerebral edema. A posterior parafalcine SDH and left anterior temporal hemorrhagic contusion are also seen

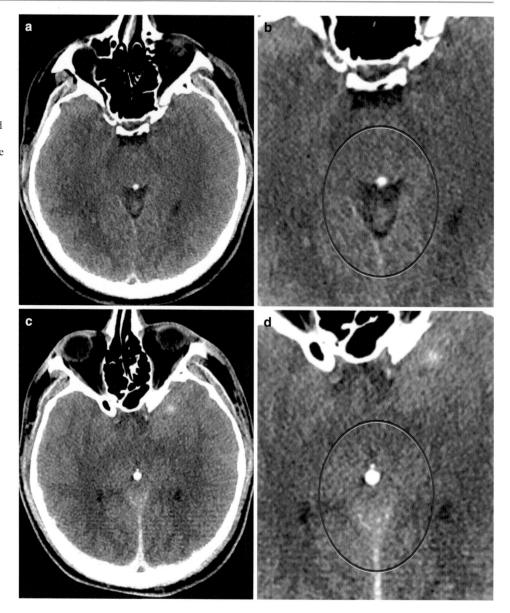

contours of the skull and their density may not be distinguished from the density of the bone if reviewed using standard window width settings. For this reason, the use of a "blood" or "subdural" window (typically using a width of 200 HU and a level of 80 HU) is an important part of the assessment of NECT done for trauma (Fig. 15) [28]. With time, the density of a SDH will decrease, eventually developing into a homogeneously low-density collection in the chronic stage. As the density decreases between the acute and chronic stages, the SDH will pass through a phase when it is isodense to brain cortex, making it difficult to visualize [15, 28]. These isodense subacute SDHs can be recognized as areas where the cortex appears abnormally wide (due to the

similar density of cortex and subacute blood) and the brain is displaced medially due to the mass effect of the SDH (Fig. 16) [28].

Occasionally, a traumatic tear in the arachnoid may allow CSF to enter the subdural space without associated hemorrhage. In this case, a low-density collection known as a subdural hygroma may appear in the acute setting (Fig. 17) [28]. These hygromas may be difficult to distinguish from chronic SDH unless recent prior brain imaging is available.

Areas of mixed density and fluid-fluid levels (i.e., hematocrit levels) can be seen in SDH under several conditions: (1) bleeding of varying ages (such as acute

**Fig. 10** Acute profound hypoxic injury. Axial NECT image (**a**) of a patient found down at the scene of trauma shows multifocal hemorrhagic contusions at the periphery of the brain. Axial DWI image (**b**) obtained at the same level shows restricted diffusion in the basal ganglia bilaterally. This pattern of abnormal signal on DWI indicates an acute, profound hypoxic episode

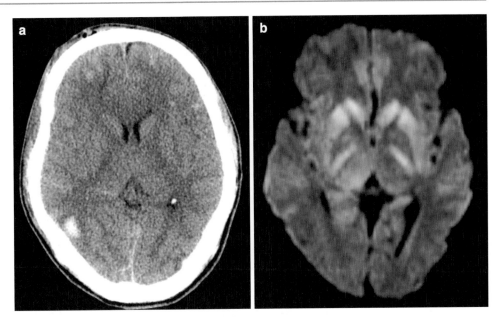

**Fig. 11** Partial-prolonged hypoxic injury. Axial NECT image (**a**) of a child who suffered non-accidental trauma shows diffuse loss of the gray-white differentiation of the cortex. Axial DWI image (**b**) shows diffusion restriction involving the cortex but sparing the basal ganglia, due to partial-prolonged hypoxia

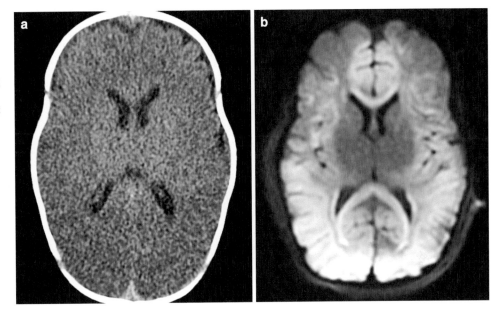

hemorrhage into preexisting chronic subdural hemorrhage); (2) separation of various components of unclotted blood, especially in the setting of underlying coagulopathy; or (3) mixing of blood with CSF in the subdural space due to a coexistent traumatic tear in the arachnoid layer [28, 29].

On MR, the signal characteristics of subdural collections vary depending on the age of the hematoma (Table 1). In general, acute blood is isointense on T1-weighted imaging and will be variable in signal on T2-weighed imaging. T1 signal will be hyperintense in the subacute to early chronic time frame, eventually becoming T1 hypointense in long-standing chronic collections [15, 30].

## SAH

The pathogenesis of traumatic SAH is likely multifactorial but primarily thought to be the result of injury to arteries on the surface of the brain and from blood entering the subarachnoid space from superficial brain contusions [31]. Although the volume and location of traumatic SAH depends on the

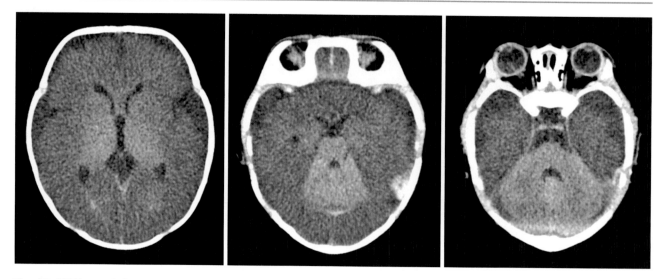

**Fig. 12** "White cerebellum" sign. Axial NECT images of a child obtained after trauma with partial-prolonged hypoxia show diffuse cortical hypodensity in the supratentorial brain, with preserved density of the deep gray nuclei and cerebellum. This "white cerebellum" sign is due to relative sparing of these structures from hypoxic injury due to preferential shunting of blood

**Fig. 13** EDH. Axial NECT image (**a**) shows the typical biconvex appearance of an EDH (arrow). The same axial image displayed using a bone window (**b**) shows a fracture (arrowhead) overlying the hematoma

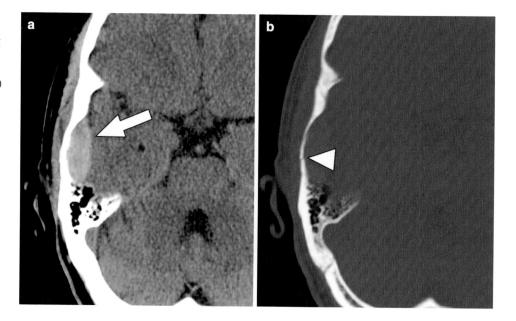

severity and nature of the inciting trauma, at initial presentation, it is commonly found over the convexities of the supratentorial brain.

This distribution distinguishes traumatic SAH, which arises from the cortical surfaces and small peripheral vessels, from aneurysmal SAH, which is more commonly found in the basal cisterns, close to the major arterial branch points and the circle of Willis, where aneurysms are most commonly found. Although convexal SAH is commonly encountered in the setting of trauma, layering SAH may also be found in the dependent portions of the subarachnoid spaces, including the interpeduncular cistern, the ambient cisterns, the posterior Sylvian fissures, and the dependent portions of the ventricular system, due to the fact that injured patients typically lie in the supine position and blood settles dependently.

On NECT, hyperdensity of the CSF filling sulci, fissures, and cisterns is seen (Fig. 18). In many instances, this SAH may be scattered widely over noncontiguous regions of the brain, again distinguishing it for aneurysmal SAH. On MRI, SWI and T2-weighted FLAIR imaging have the highest

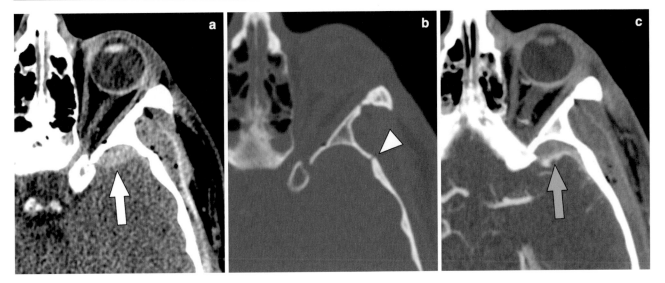

**Fig. 14** Venous EDH. Axial NECT (**a**) shows a biconvex hematoma (white arrow) at the anterior aspect of the middle cranial fossa. The same axial image displayed using a bone window (**b**) shows an overlying fracture (arrowhead). Axial CT angiogram (**c**) shows that the hematoma is displacing the injured sphenoparietal sinus (gray arrow). This location in the middle cranial fossa is typical of venous EDHs

**Table 1** Imaging manifestation of intracranial hemorrhage based on age of blood

| Time frame | T1-weighted MRI signal intensity | T2-weighted MRI signal intensity |
| --- | --- | --- |
| Acute | Dark to isointense | Dark |
| Early subacute | Bright | Dark |
| Late subacute | Bright | Bright |
| Chronic | Dark | Dark |

Modified from Brant and Helms [30]

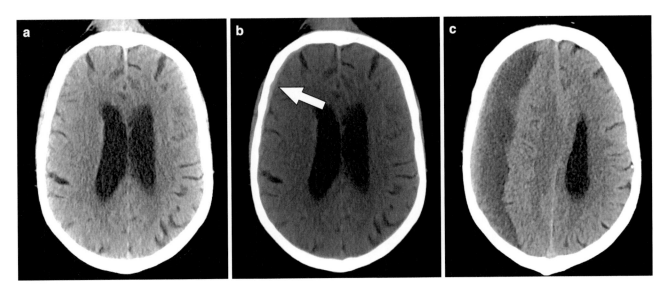

**Fig. 15** SDH. Axial NECT image displayed on standard window/level settings (**a**) shows a large forehead hematoma but no clear intracranial hemorrhage. The same axial image displayed using a subdural window (**b**) reveals the presence of a small SDH (arrow) that was not visible when displayed with narrower window settings. Follow-up NECT obtained 1 month later (**c**) shows expansion of the now chronic SDH and increased mass effect

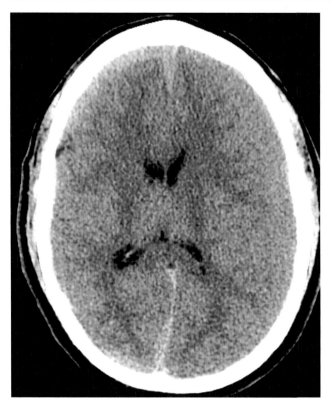

**Fig. 16** Isodense SDHs. Axial NECT image shows bilateral subacute SDHs. The left SDH and portions of the right SDH are isodense to the adjacent cortex, making the SDH harder to identify. Recognition that the cortex appears thicker than normal, because of the adjacent isodense blood, can help with detection of these subacute SDHs

sensitivity, demonstrating susceptibility artifact and hyperintensity, respectively [15]. Vasospasm due to traumatic SAH occurs less frequently than with aneurysmal SAH and tends to be less severe but has an earlier onset, sometimes occurring within 24 hours of the trauma [32].

## Herniation Syndromes

Herniation refers to the abnormal expulsion of brain parenchyma beyond its normal compartmental boundaries. There are five types of herniation encountered in head trauma: subfalcine, uncal, descending transtentorial, ascending transtentorial, and cerebellar tonsillar (Fig. 19) [33]. Each pattern of herniation results from a specific anatomic distribution of pathology and has its own potential for compromise of vessels, cranial nerves, or both.

Subfalcine herniation occurs when the frontal lobes and corpus callosum are pushed under the free margin of the falx. In the setting of head trauma, this most often occurs as a result of asymmetric, hemorrhagic frontal lobe contusion or extra-axial hemorrhage overlying the frontal lobe. On imaging, the interhemispheric fissure is displaced away from the midline. In severe cases, the anterior cerebral artery (ACA) may become kinked or compressed between the cingulate gyrus and the falx, resulting in vascular occlusion and medial frontal lobe infarction (Fig. 20).

Uncal herniation occurs when the uncus (the anteromedial portion of the parahippocampal gyrus, a part of the medial temporal lobe) is displaced medially. On imaging, crowding of the suprasellar cistern is observed. Resulting compression

**Fig. 17** Acute subdural hygromas. Axial NECT image obtained after head trauma (**a**) shows bilateral low-density subdural collections. Axial NECT obtained 1 week before (**b**) shows neither hygromas nor SDH, confirming that the new collections are acute hygromas

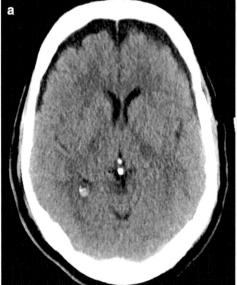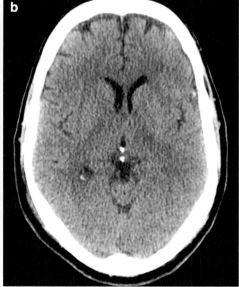

**Fig. 18** Traumatic SAH. Axial NECT images at the level of the basal ganglia (**a**) and at the vertex (**b**) show hyperdense subarachnoid blood filling the left Sylvian fissure, as well as sulci over the bilateral cerebral convexities (arrowheads). Multifocal and convexal distribution of SAH are patterns commonly seen with trauma

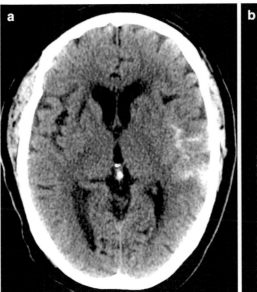
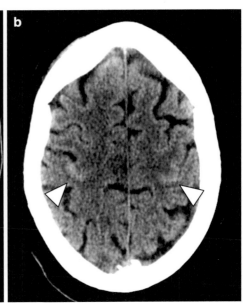

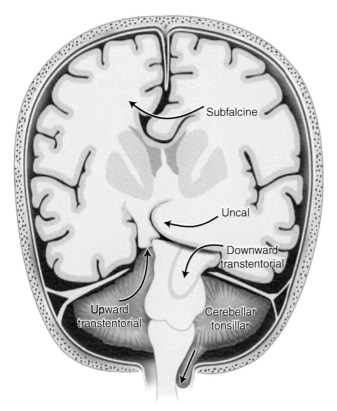

**Fig. 19** Major herniation patterns seen in trauma

of the third cranial nerve may result in a fixed and dilated (or "blown") pupil. The posterior cerebral artery (PCA) may be compressed against the tentorial margin, producing

ipsilateral infarction (Fig. 21). As uncal herniation progresses, midbrain torsion develops. As the brainstem is pushed away from the herniating uncus, the ipsilateral ambient cistern is widened, and the contralateral cerebral peduncle is forced against the tentorium on the opposite side of the brain, producing a characteristic indentation of the brain parenchyma known as Kernohan's notch, compression of motor fibers, and paralysis [34].

Descending transtentorial herniation occurs when downward central forces push the cerebrum downward over the tentorial incisura. This may occur bilaterally, due to diffuse cerebral edema or extra-axial hemorrhage. This type of herniation increases pressure within the posterior fossa and may compress the brainstem against the clivus. Stretching of the perforating arteries arising from the basilar artery may result in hemorrhages within the brainstem, known as Duret hemorrhages (Fig. 22), usually with fatal consequences [35].

In ascending transtentorial herniation, the cerebellum herniates upward past the tentorial incisura, typically due to cerebellar ischemia or massive hemorrhage in the posterior fossa. On NECT, there will be effacement of the quadrigeminal plate cistern and the CSF along the tentorial margin as the cerebellar vermis is forced upward [36].

Cerebellar tonsillar herniation is also seen due to increased mass effect in the posterior fossa and may be seen in combination with either descending or ascending transtentorial herniation. On NECT, the foramen magnum becomes effaced as cerebellar tissue is forced caudally. This type of herniation heralds a poor prognosis and may be accompanied by obstructive hydrocephalus of the fourth ventricle,

**Fig. 20** Subfalcine herniation. Axial NECT image (**a**) shows a large right SDH, producing herniation of the brain below the falx and across the midline (dashed line). Axial NECT image from the same scan, closer to the vertex and displayed on stroke windows (**b**), shows infarction of the ipsilateral ACA territory (arrow), a complication of subfalcine herniation

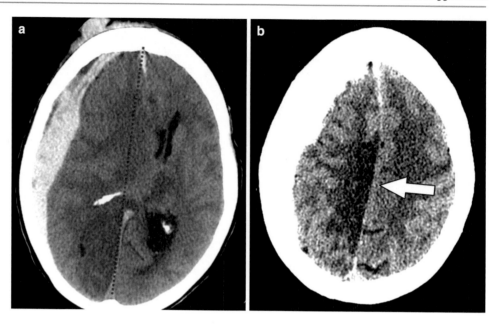

**Fig. 21** Uncal herniation. Axial NECT image (**a**) of the same patient shown in the previous figure shows herniation of the anteromedial temporal lobe (dashed line) – the uncus – past midline into the suprasellar cistern. Axial NECT image from the same scan, through the level of the occipital lobe and displayed on stroke windows (**b**), shows infarction of the PCA territory (arrow), a complication of uncal herniation

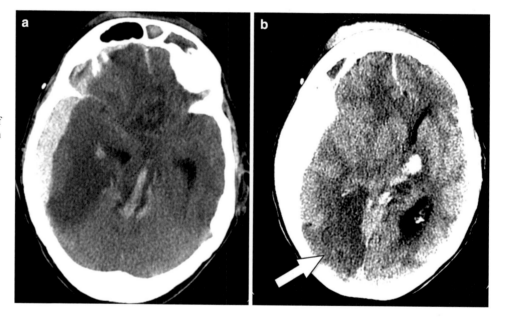

compression of the cervicomedullary junction, and the potential for spinal cord infarction due to compression of the anterior spinal arteries [33].

## Intracranial Vascular Injury

Although intracranial vascular injury is less commonly encountered than traumatic vascular injuries in the neck, they do occur due to both blunt and penetrating injury and are often associated with high levels of morbidity and mortality.

Internal carotid artery (ICA) injury may occur when fractures involve the skull base, either in the petrous segment in association with temporal bone fractures or in the lacerum or cavernous segments in association with fractures of the central sphenoid bone. When fractures are found that traverse the path of the ICA in these areas, CTA should be performed to evaluate for vascular injury [28, 37].

Vascular injuries can range from mild injury to the intima with irregularity of the vessel wall to the most severe injuries where there is vascular transection. The Biffl grading scale, described in detail in ▶ Chap. 11, "Imaging of Traumatic Vascular Neck Injuries," was developed to describe the

**Fig. 22** Descending transtentorial herniation and Duret hemorrhage. Axial NECT image (**a**) in a patient with a large right subdural hemorrhage shows herniation of the medial temporal lobe (dashed line) over the tentorial margin. Coronal reformatted NECT image (**b**) again shows downward and medial herniation of the temporal lobe (dashed line). A focus of hemorrhage is seen in the brainstem (arrow), which is termed a Duret hemorrhage

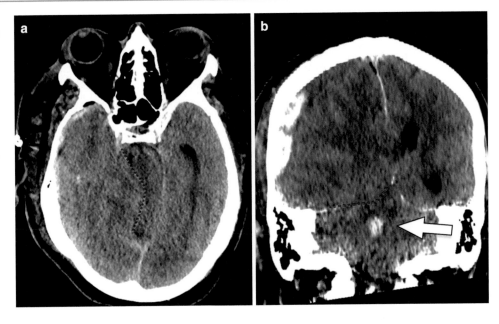

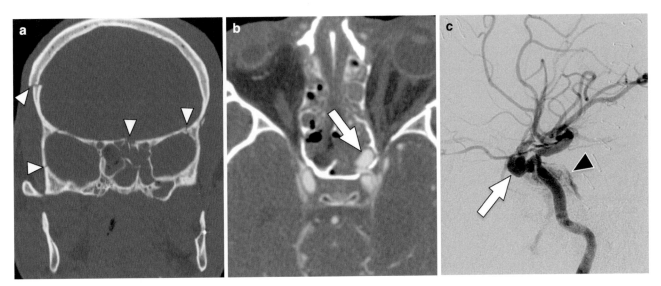

**Fig. 23** Traumatic pseudoaneurysm and CCF. Coronal reformatted NECT image (**a**) shows extensive facial, skull base, and calvarial fractures (arrowheads) in a patient involved in a high-speed motor vehicle collision. Axial CT angiogram image (**b**) shows a contrast-enhancing pseudoaneurysm (arrow) arising from the left ICA, with the neck of the pseudoaneurysm interposed between the fracture fragments of the sphenoid bone. Lateral projection from a digital subtraction angiogram during a left ICA injection (**c**) shows early venous filling of the cavernous sinus (arrowhead) due to the presence of a traumatic CCF. The pseudoaneurysm is also seen (arrow)

range of blunt carotid cerebrovascular injuries [38]. Increasing severity on this scale is correlated with increasing stroke risk and mortality.

When there is disruption of the cavernous segment of the ICA, a direct carotid-cavernous fistula (CCF) may be formed. In this entity, the cavernous sinus is subjected to arterial pressure transmitted across the fistula, which in turn can impair venous drainage from the orbit. Clinically, CCFs present with the triad of proptosis, bruit, and chemosis (i.e., a red, injected eye) [39]. On imaging, one or both superior ophthalmic veins may be enlarged due to the increased pressure [20, 40]. Although cross-sectional imaging can sometimes suggest the presence of a fistula, by demonstrating asymmetric enlargement and contrast opacification of the cavernous sinus ipsilateral to a vascular injury, catheter angiography is considered the reference standard for diagnosis, because the temporal resolution of angiography allows it to directly show shunting into the cavernous sinus during the arterial phase of contrast (Fig. 23).

Pseudoaneurysms can also be the result of penetrating trauma. The location of traumatic pseudoaneurysms is much more varied than in blunt injuries and is highly dependent on the path of the penetrating injury

[38, 41]. Pseudoaneurysms resulting from penetrating trauma carry a very high rate of mortality, with death rates of approximately 50% if left untreated [42].

## Advanced Imaging Techniques

Beyond standard imaging, research has revealed the potential of advanced approaches. These techniques include functional MRI (fMRI), perfusion imaging, diffusion-tensor imaging (DTI), and MRI spectroscopy (MRS) [43] [44]. Currently, there is not sufficient evidence to support the use of these techniques in routine clinical care [45].

fMRI measures oxygen utilization in the brain using a technique called blood-oxygen-level dependent (BOLD) contrast [46]. This oxygen utilization is correlated with neuronal activity and can be assessed during completion of specific functional tasks or during rest. Numerous studies have alterations in measures of task-based and resting state activation following TBI, raising the possibility that this technique may be useful in diagnosis and assessment of recovery following trauma [44, 47].

Perfusion imaging demonstrates how well a given area of brain is perfused based on measures including cerebral blood volume, cerebral blood flow, and mean transit time. Perfusion imaging modalities include CT perfusion, dynamic susceptibility-weighted contrast-enhanced perfusion MRI, and arterial spin-labeling MRI [48]. TBI may show changes on perfusion imaging because of associated alterations of blood-brain barrier integrity and cerebrovascular function [49, 50]. Several studies show positive correlation between perfusion and long-term functional outcome [48]. However, larger, more rigorous investigations are needed to determine if such differences between groups can be translated to prediction of individual prognosis [48, 51].

DTI has been used to examine structural connections within the brain, which can be injured in blunt TBI, using metrics including fractional anisotropy (FA) and mean diffusivity (MD). DTI may be useful in detecting injury not visible on anatomic imaging. Numerous studies have shown decreases in FA values in multiple brain regions in patients who had TBI and that these changes are more widespread with increasing severity of injury [52]. Currently, DTI is useful in comparing groups or assessing longitudinal changes in individuals as a research tool but is limited in application to individuals because of the lack of normative values and issues of repeatability [49].

MRS quantifies in vivo metabolite concentrations, which vary depending on changes in the surrounding cellular environment [44, 48]. TBI has been shown to alter this metabolic environment [53]. After moderate-to-severe acute TBI, various studies have shown decreased $N$-acetylaspartate (NAA) and increased choline that relate to worse injury/prognosis.

However, MRS currently suffers from low specificity and inconsistency with mild TBI [50].

In summary, advanced imaging techniques hold the prospect of improving detection, characterization, and prognosis prediction in TBI, although more work needs to be done to translate the differences that have been shown to exist in larger groups into individual patient-level information.

**Key Points**
- Brain parenchymal injury includes primary injuries such as contusions and diffuse axonal injury (DAI) and secondary injuries such as diffuse cerebral edema and hypoxic-ischemic injury.
- Recognition of these injury types helps inform subsequent imaging timing and selection of additional imaging modalities and helps define patient prognosis.
- Extra-axial hemorrhage including epidural hematomas (EDHs), subdural hematomas (SDHs), and subarachnoid hemorrhage (SAH) is common in trauma and can be distinguished based on imaging appearance.
- Patterns of cerebral herniation and associated complications are critical to recognize in the setting of trauma, as these injuries are associated with high morbidity and mortality.
- Intracranial vascular injuries can be the result of blunt or penetrating trauma. Familiarity with the types of injury and their grading can help facilitate management of these emergent conditions.

## References

1. Drew LB, Drew WE. The contrecoup–coup phenomenon: a new understanding of the mechanism of closed head injury. Neurocrit Care. 2004;1(3):385–90.
2. Kurland D, Hong C, Aarabi B, Gerzanich V, Simard JM. Hemorrhagic progression of a contusion after traumatic brain injury: a review. J Neurotrauma. 2012;29(1):19–31.
3. Brown CVR, Zada G, Salim A, Inaba K, Kasotakis G, Hadjizacharia P, et al. Indications for routine repeat head computed tomography (CT) stratified by severity of traumatic brain injury. J Trauma. 2007;62(6):1339–45.
4. Smith JS, Chang EF, Rosenthal G, Meeker M, Von Koch C, Manley GT, et al. The role of early follow-up computed tomography imaging in the management of traumatic brain injury patients with intracranial hemorrhage. J Trauma. 2007;63(1):75–82.
5. Sullivan TP, Jarvik JG, Cohen WA. Follow-up of conservatively managed epidural hematomas: implications for timing of repeat CT. AJNR Am J Neuroradiol. 1999;20(1):107–13.
6. Hammoud DA, Wasserman BA. Diffuse axonal injuries: pathophysiology and imaging. Neuroimaging Clin N Am. 2002;12(2):205–16.
7. Huisman TAGM, Sorensen AG, Hergan K, Gonzalez RG, Schaefer PW. Diffusion-weighted imaging for the evaluation of diffuse axonal injury in closed head injury. J Comput Assist Tomogr. 2003;27 (1):5–11.
8. Humble SS, Wilson LD, Wang L, Long DA, Smith MA, Siktberg JC, et al. Prognosis of diffuse axonal injury with traumatic brain injury. J Trauma Acute Care Surg. 2018;85(1):155–9.

9. Chavhan GB, Babyn PS, Thomas B, Shroff MM, Haacke EM. Principles, techniques, and applications of T2*-based MR imaging and its special applications. Radiographics. 2009;29(5): 1433–49.

10. Jha RM, Kochanek PM, Simard JM. Pathophysiology and treatment of cerebral edema in traumatic brain injury. Neuropharmacology. 2019;145(Pt B):230–46.

11. Winkler EA, Minter D, Yue JK, Manley GT. Cerebral edema in traumatic brain injury: pathophysiology and prospective therapeutic targets. Neurosurg Clin N Am. 2016;27(4):473–88.

12. Toth P, Szarka N, Farkas E, Ezer E, Czeiter E, Amrein K, et al. Traumatic brain injury-induced autoregulatory dysfunction and spreading depression-related neurovascular uncoupling: Pathomechanisms, perspectives, and therapeutic implications. Am J Physiol Heart Circ Physiol. 2016;311(5):H1118–H31.

13. Kubal WS. Updated imaging of traumatic brain injury. Radiol Clin N Am. 2012;50(1):15–41.

14. Given CA 2nd, Burdette JH, Elster AD, Williams DW 3rd. Pseudo-subarachnoid hemorrhage: a potential imaging pitfall associated with diffuse cerebral edema. AJNR Am J Neuroradiol. 2003;24(2): 254–6.

15. Altmeyer W, Steven A, Gutierrez J. Use of magnetic resonance in the evaluation of cranial trauma. Magn Reson Imaging Clin N Am. 2016;24(2):305–23.

16. Clement MO. Imaging of brain trauma. Radiol Clin N Am. 2019;57 (4):733–44.

17. Verma SK, Borkar SA, Singh PK, Tandon V, Gurjar HK, Sinha S, et al. Traumatic posterior fossa extradural hematoma: experience at level I trauma center. Asian J Neurosurg. 2018;13 (2):227–32.

18. Ramesh VG, Kodeeswaran M, Deiveegan K, Sundar V, Sriram K. Vertex epidural hematoma: an analysis of a large series. Asian J Neurosurg. 2017;12(2):167–71.

19. Khairat A, Waseem M. Epidural hematoma. Treasure Island: StatPearls; 2020.

20. Freeman WD, Aguilar MI. Intracranial hemorrhage: diagnosis and management. Neurol Clin. 2012;30(1):211–40, ix.

21. Gean AD, Fischbein NJ, Purcell DD, Aiken AH, Manley GT, Stiver SI. Benign anterior temporal epidural hematoma: indolent lesion with a characteristic CT imaging appearance after blunt head trauma. Radiology. 2010;257(1):212–8.

22. Araki T, Yokota H, Morita A. Pediatric traumatic brain injury: characteristic features, diagnosis, and management. Neurol Med Chir (Tokyo). 2017;57(2):82–93.

23. Prat R, Galeano I. Posterior fossa venous epidural hematoma. Based on 2 cases. Neurologia. 2003;18(1):38–41.

24. Selariu E, Zia E, Brizzi M, Abul-Kasim K. Swirl sign in intracerebral haemorrhage: definition, prevalence, reliability and prognostic value. BMC Neurol. 2012;12:109.

25. Hirsh LF. Chronic epidural hematomas. Neurosurgery. 1980;6(5): 508–12.

26. Takeuchi S, Takasato Y, Wada K, Nawashiro H, Otani N, Masaoka H, et al. Traumatic posterior fossa subdural hematomas. J Trauma Acute Care Surg. 2012;72(2):480–6.

27. Borzone M, Rivano C, Altomonte M, Baldini M. Acute traumatic posterior fossa subdural haematomas. Acta Neurochir. 1995;135 (1–2):32–7.

28. Lolli V, Pezzullo M, Delpierre I, Sadeghi N. MDCT imaging of traumatic brain injury. Br J Radiol. 2016;89(1061):20150849.

29. Stone JL, Lang RG, Sugar O, Moody RA. Traumatic subdural hygroma. Neurosurgery. 1981;8(5):542–50.

30. Brant WE, Helms CA. Fundamentals of diagnostic radiology. 3rd ed. Philadelphia: Lippincott, Williams & Wilkins; 2007. p. xix, 1559 p., ISBN: 0781761352.

31. Armin SS, Colohan AR, Zhang JH. Traumatic subarachnoid hemorrhage: our current understanding and its evolution over the past half century. Neurol Res. 2006;28(4):445–52.

32. Kramer DR, Winer JL, Pease BA, Amar AP, Mack WJ. Cerebral vasospasm in traumatic brain injury. Neurol Res Int. 2013;2013: 415813.

33. Johnson PL, Eckard DA, Chason DP, Brecheisen MA, Batnitzky S. Imaging of acquired cerebral herniations. Neuroimaging Clin N Am. 2002;12(2):217–28.

34. Dammers R, Volovici V, Kompanje EJ. The history of the Kernohan notch revisited. Neurosurgery. 2016;78(4):581–4.

35. Parizel PM, Makkat S, Jorens PG, Ozsarlak O, Cras P, Van Goethem JW, et al. Brainstem hemorrhage in descending transtentorial herniation (Duret hemorrhage). Intensive Care Med. 2002;28(1):85–8.

36. Osborn AG, Heaston DK, Wing SD. Diagnosis of ascending transtentorial herniation by cranial computed tomography. AJR Am J Roentgenol. 1978;130(4):755–60.

37. York G, Barboriak D, Petrella J, DeLong D, Provenzale JM. Association of internal carotid artery injury with carotid canal fractures in patients with head trauma. AJR Am J Roentgenol. 2005;184(5):1672–8.

38. Biffl WL, Moore EE, Offner PJ, Brega KE, Franciose RJ, Burch JM. Blunt carotid arterial injuries: implications of a new grading scale. J Trauma. 1999;47(5):845–53.

39. Fattahi TT, Brandt MT, Jenkins WS, Steinberg B. Traumatic carotid-cavernous fistula: pathophysiology and treatment. J Craniofac Surg. 2003;14(2):240–6.

40. Chen CC, Chang PC, Shy CG, Chen WS, Hung HC. CT angiography and MR angiography in the evaluation of carotid cavernous sinus fistula prior to embolization: a comparison of techniques. AJNR Am J Neuroradiol. 2005;26(9):2349–56.

41. Zanini MA, de Lima Resende LA, de Souza Faleiros AT, Gabarra RC. Traumatic subdural hygromas: proposed pathogenesis based classification. J Trauma. 2008;64(3):705–13.

42. Uzan M, Cantasdemir M, Seckin MS, Hanci M, Kocer N, Sarioglu AC, et al. Traumatic intracranial carotid tree aneurysms. Neurosurgery. 1998;43(6):1314–20; discussion 20–2.

43. Mutch CA, Talbott JF, Gean A. Imaging evaluation of acute traumatic brain injury. Neurosurg Clin N Am. 2016;27(4):409–39.

44. Koerte IK, Hufschmidt J, Muehlmann M, Lin AP, Shenton ME. Advanced neuroimaging of mild traumatic brain injury. In: Laskowitz D, Grant G, editors. Translational research in traumatic brain injury, Frontiers in neuroscience. Boca Raton: CRC Press; 2016.

45. Wintermark M, Sanelli PC, Anzai Y, Tsiouris AJ, Whitlow CT, American College of Radiology Head Injury Institute. Imaging evidence and recommendations for traumatic brain injury: advanced neuro- and neurovascular imaging techniques. AJNR Am J Neuroradiol. 2015;36(2):E1–E11.

46. Glover GH. Overview of functional magnetic resonance imaging. Neurosurg Clin N Am. 2011;22(2):133–9, vii.

47. Scheibel RS. Functional magnetic resonance imaging of cognitive control following traumatic brain injury. Front Neurol. 2017;8:352.

48. Smith LGF, Milliron E, Ho ML, Hu HH, Rusin J, Leonard J, et al. Advanced neuroimaging in traumatic brain injury: an overview. Neurosurg Focus. 2019;47(6):E17.

49. Douglas DB, Ro T, Toffoli T, Krawchuk B, Muldermans J, Gullo J, et al. Neuroimaging of traumatic brain injury. Med Sci (Basel). 2018;7(1)

50. Lee AL. Advanced imaging of traumatic brain injury. Korean J Neurotrauma. 2020;16(1):3–17.

51. Rostami E, Engquist H, Enblad P. Imaging of cerebral blood flow in patients with severe traumatic brain injury in the neurointensive care. Front Neurol. 2014;5:114.

52. Wallace EJ, Mathias JL, Ward L. Diffusion tensor imaging changes following mild, moderate and severe adult traumatic brain injury: a meta-analysis. Brain Imaging Behav. 2018;12(6):1607–21.

53. Ng TS, Lin AP, Koerte IK, Pasternak O, Liao H, Merugumala S, et al. Neuroimaging in repetitive brain trauma. Alzheimers Res Ther. 2014;6(1):10.

# Imaging of Skull Base Fractures and Complications

**6**

Ngoc-Anh Tran, Diego B. Nunez, and Christopher A. Potter

## Contents

## Abstract

Skull base fractures comprise a small but substantial portion of traumatic injuries with associated potential high morbidity and mortality. However, these injuries can often be difficult to detect both clinically and radiologically. This chapter aims to review the basic anatomy of the skull base, along with important anatomic considerations, mechanisms of injury, key clinical features, distinct fracture patterns, and associated complications.

## Keywords

Trauma · Skull base fractures · Temporal bone fractures · Occipital condyle fractures · Carotid-cavernous fistula · Cerebrospinal fluid leak

## Introduction

Traumatic head injury affects millions of Americans annually, and accounts for approximately 300,000 or 35–38% of trauma-related hospital admissions each year [26]. Fractures of the skull base comprise about 4–12% of overall head injuries, and 20–24% of all skull fractures [16]. Most occur in the setting of high-impact trauma, including motor vehicle collisions, blunt head trauma, sports injuries, falls, or assaults. Due to the proximity to critical neurovascular structures, these fractures are associated with high morbidity and mortality, and can include cranial neuropathy, cerebrovascular injury, intracranial hemorrhage, cerebrospinal fluid leak, meningitis, and even death [16].

Given the potential for severe complications, timely and accurate diagnosis is imperative in the management and outcome of skull base fractures. Although clinical signs including raccoon eyes, the Battle sign, hemotympanum, rhinorrhea, and otorrhea are classically associated with skull base fractures, these findings are not always present at initial evaluation [9, 12, 22]. Definitive diagnosis is therefore primarily achieved with imaging, which helps identify and

N.-A. Tran (✉) · D. B. Nunez · C. A. Potter
Department of Radiology, Brigham and Women's Hospital, Harvard Medical School, Boston, MA, USA
e-mail: ntran@bwh.harvard.edu; dnunez@bwh.harvard.edu; cpotter3@bwh.harvard.edu

© Springer Nature Switzerland AG 2022
M. N. Patlas et al. (eds.), *Atlas of Emergency Imaging from Head-to-Toe*,
https://doi.org/10.1007/978-3-030-92111-8_6

characterize fracture location, fracture morphology, extent of injury, and associated complications. Imaging findings ultimately help guide treatment decisions and surgical intervention.

## Imaging Modalities

Radiographs have a limited role, as most skull base fractures are obscured by overlapping bone and soft tissue. Multidetector computed tomography (CT) is the first-line and modality of choice in the trauma setting due to its speed and accessibility. When optimized with high spatial resolution thin slices, bone window reconstructions, and multiplanar reformations, CT can further improve the radiologic diagnosis of skull base fractures [5]. CT angiography (CTA) is an important adjunct in the setting of potential vascular injury to identify dissection, occlusion, frank extravasation, or pseudoaneurysms. Three-dimensional surface reconstructions may be helpful in better visualization of fracture morphology, and in surgical planning.

Magnetic resonance imaging (MRI) and angiography (MRA) are useful in the evaluation of inconclusive cases or specific complications. MRI has superior soft tissue resolution, and aids in the assessment of post-traumatic neuropathy, stroke, and other intracranial injuries, as well as cranio-cervical ligamentous injuries. CT or radionuclide cisternography following administration of intrathecal agents may be helpful in the evaluation for CSF leak or fistula.

## Skull Base Fractures

The skull base is a complex osseous structure that forms the floor of the cranial cavity. It is composed of five bones: frontal, ethmoid, sphenoid, temporal, and occipital. Three naturally contoured regions further divide the skull base into the anterior, middle, and posterior cranial fossae.

Fractures of the skull base most commonly involve the temporal bone (40%), followed by the orbital roof (24%), sphenoid bone (23%), occiput (15%), ethmoid sinus (11%), and clivus (1%) [16]. Numerous foramina and canals within the skull base transmit vital neurovascular structures which can be damaged in the setting of trauma (Table 1). This chapter aims to review the basic anatomy in each cranial fossa along with important anatomic considerations, mechanisms of injury, key clinical features, distinct fracture patterns, and associated complications.

**Table 1** Anterior, middle, and posterior cranial fossae with relevant structures and clinical presentation following traumatic injury [13, 23]

| Skull base subdivisions | Relevant structures | Clinical signs/Symptoms |
|---|---|---|
| Anterior fossa | Cribriform plate (ethmoid): CN I, anterior and posterior ethmoid vessels<br>Optic canal (lesser wing of sphenoid): CN II, ophthalmic artery, and retinal artery<br>Superior orbital fissure (between greater and lesser wings of sphenoid): CN III, IV, $V_1$, VI; superior ophthalmic vein | Anosmia, epistaxis, and CSF rhinorrhea<br>Vision loss, impaired pupillary reflex, raccoon eyes, and subconjunctival hemorrhage<br>Oculomotor palsies, mydriasis, diplopia, ptosis, impaired pupillary reflex, and anesthesia to forehead, brow, nose |
| Middle fossa: Central skull base Lateral skull base | Cavernous sinus: ICA; CN III, IV, $V_1$, $V_2$, VI<br>Foramen rotundum/pterygopalatine fossa: $V_2$<br>Foramen ovale: $V_3$<br>Foramen spinosum: middle meningeal artery<br>Carotid canal: ICA<br>External auditory canal and middle ear<br>Internal auditory canal: CN VII, VIII; labyrinthine (internal auditory) artery | ICA injury, CN palsies, CCF<br>Anesthesia to cheek, upper lip, and hard palate<br>Anesthesia to chin and impaired mastication<br>Epidural hematoma and temporal lobe injuries (impaired hearing and memory, seizures)<br>Cortical strokes resulting in weakness to face and upper/lower extremities<br>CSF otorrhea, hemotympanum, Battle sign, and conductive hearing loss<br>SNHL, facial paralysis, vestibular dysfunction, vertigo, tinnitus, dry eye, dry mouth |
| Posterior fossa | Jugular foramen: CN IX, X, XI, jugular vein, sigmoid sinus, and posterior meningeal artery<br>Hypoglossal canal: CN XII<br>Foramen magnum: brainstem/medulla, vertebrobasilar arteries, meninges, and spinal roots of CN XI | Dysphagia, loss of gag reflex, vocal cord paralysis, impaired parasympathetics, and limited neck flexion<br>Ipsilateral tongue deviation and atrophy<br>Cardiac and respiratory depression, death, and associated C-spine fractures |

Cranial nerve (CN): olfactory (I), optic (II), oculomotor (III), trochlear (IV), trigeminal (V), ophthalmic branch ($V_1$), maxillary branch ($V_2$), mandibular branch ($V_3$), abducens (VI), facial (VII), vestibulocochlear (VIII), glossopharyngeal (IX), vagus (X), spinal accessory (XI), hypoglossal (XII); cerebrospinal fluid (CSF); internal carotid artery (ICA); carotid-cavernous fistula (CCF); sensorineural hearing loss (SNHL)

## Anterior Cranial Fossa

*Anatomic considerations.* The anterior cranial fossa is formed anterolaterally by the posterior table of the frontal sinus and orbital plate of the frontal bone, inferiorly by the roof of the sinonasal cavity and the cribriform plate of the ethmoid bone, and posteriorly by the lesser wing of the sphenoid bone and the anterior clinoid process (Fig. 1). The ethmoid bone, lamina papyracea, orbital roof, and posterior wall of the frontal sinus are particularly thin bones which are prone to comminuted fractures [15]. Dense dural adhesions to the cribriform plate, fovea ethmoidalis (roof of the ethmoid sinus), and posterior table of the frontal sinus predispose to dural laceration and resultant CSF leak [15]. Several important neurovascular structures traversing their respective foramina are also prone to injury, including CN I, II, III, IV, $V_1$, and VI, as well as the retinal artery, ophthalmic artery, and superior ophthalmic vein. Injury to the anterior and posterior ethmoid vessels are a substantial source of epistaxis. In addition, close association with orbital structures risk injury to the orbital rim, globe, extraocular muscles, and lacrimal apparatus.

*Epidemiology and clinical features.* Anterior skull base fractures typically occur following severe direct trauma to the frontal region or midface, often in the presence of other facial or orbital fractures [25]. Various clinical signs and symptoms suggest injury to specific parts of the anterior cranial fossa, including epistaxis, anosmia, CSF rhinorrhea, periorbital ecchymosis (raccoon eyes), and retro-orbital hematoma [13].

*Diagnostic investigation.* Frontobasal fractures involve the upper third of the face (frontal bone and superior orbital rim) and the anterior cranial base (cribriform

plate, ethmoid roof, and planum sphenoidale) [2]. Several distinct fracture patterns have been described based on site of impact, force, and associated complications [4, 19, 20, 24]. Overall, they can be simplified into central, lateral, or combined fractures. Central fractures typically result from lower-impact trauma to the central frontal bone (Fig. 2), and feature fractures of the frontal sinus, paranasal sinuses, naso-orbital ethmoid, and cribriform plate, which may extend along the sella or petrous ridge toward the middle fossa. These fractures are associated with lowest rates of overall complication, though those that are closer to the midline and span more than 1 cm have higher risk of infection [24]. Lateral fracture patterns involve the lateral frontal bone, potentially extending to the supraorbital ridge, squamous temporal bone, orbital roof, or orbital apex. Combined medial and lateral frontobasal fractures are the most common type, often featuring comminution of the entire frontal bone, orbital roof, and lateral cranial vault. Fractures that are comminuted or farther from midline are associated with more substantial forceful trauma, mid-face fractures, CSF leak, and intracranial injuries including hemorrhage, contusion, and diffuse axonal injury [19, 20].

*Management and complications.* Less severe cranial neuropathies such as those affecting smell and extraocular motor function are often managed conservatively, with full or partial return of function within weeks to months [13]. High-risk injuries warranting potential intervention include those that are extensively comminuted or displaced greater than 7 mm, as well as those resulting in persistent or recurrent CSF leak, intracranial infection (meningitis, abscess, or empyema), optic nerve injury, carotid artery injury, and significant intracranial

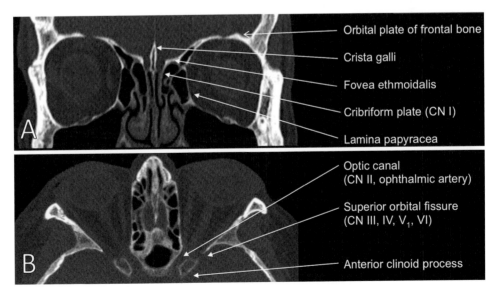

**Fig. 1** *Normal osseous anatomy of the anterior cranial fossa on CT in bone window in coronal (**a**) and axial (**b**) planes (Cranial nerve, CN)*

Orbital plate of frontal bone

Crista galli

Fovea ethmoidalis

Cribriform plate (CN I)

Lamina papyracea

Optic canal
(CN II, ophthalmic artery)

Superior orbital fissure
(CN III, IV, $V_1$, VI)

Anterior clinoid process

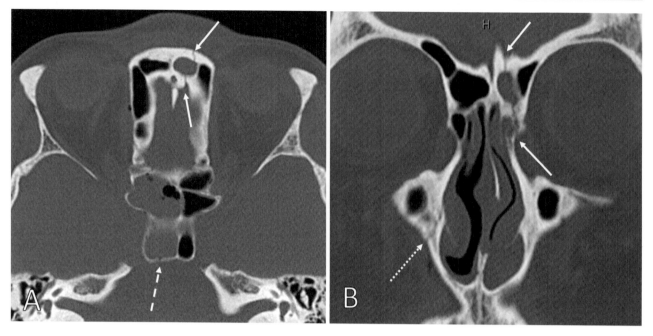

**Fig. 2** *Anterior skull base fracture with associated maxillofacial frac-tures* in a 34-year-old female following motor vehicle collision. Axial CT of the skull base in bone window (**a**) demonstrates fractures of frontal bone with extension into the ethmoid bone (solid arrows), and the posterior walls of the sphenoid sinus (dashed arrow). Coronal CT image of the face (**b**) demonstrates the frontal bone fracture extension into the ethmoid air cells (solid arrows). There is also fracture of the medial wall of the maxillary sinus (dotted arrows). CTA of the head and neck (not shown) demonstrated no vascular injury

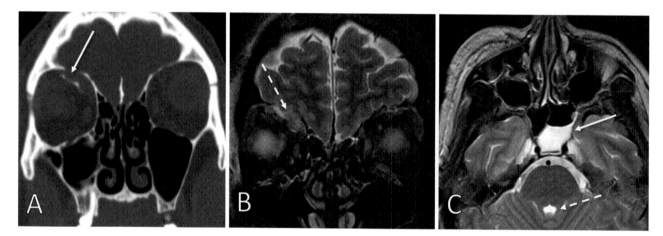

**Fig. 3** *Orbital roof fracture complicated by meningoencephalocele and CSF leak* in a 42-year-old female pedestrian struck by a motor vehicle. Coronal noncontrast CT image (**a**) shows a comminuted fracture of the right orbital roof with 7 mm inferior depression of the fracture fragment (solid arrow). There is a soft tissue component overlying the depressed fragment. Coronal T2-weighted MRI image (T2WI) (**b**) demonstrates inferior herniation of the brain (dashed arrow) with associated T2 hyperintensity of the right inferior frontal gyrus representing contusion. Axial T2WI (**c**) shows layering fluid in the sphenoid sinus (solid arrow) with signal isointensity to CSF in the fourth ventricle (dashed arrow), raising concern for CSF leak. A dural tear was confirmed at orbital roof repair

hematoma with mass effect or herniation [15]. Of partic-ular note, CSF leaks, which complicate 12–30% of skull base fractures, have been observed to spontaneously resolve in 85% of cases after one week of conservative management [10, 29]. Prolonged leaks persisting over one week, however, are at increased risk for meningitis, and

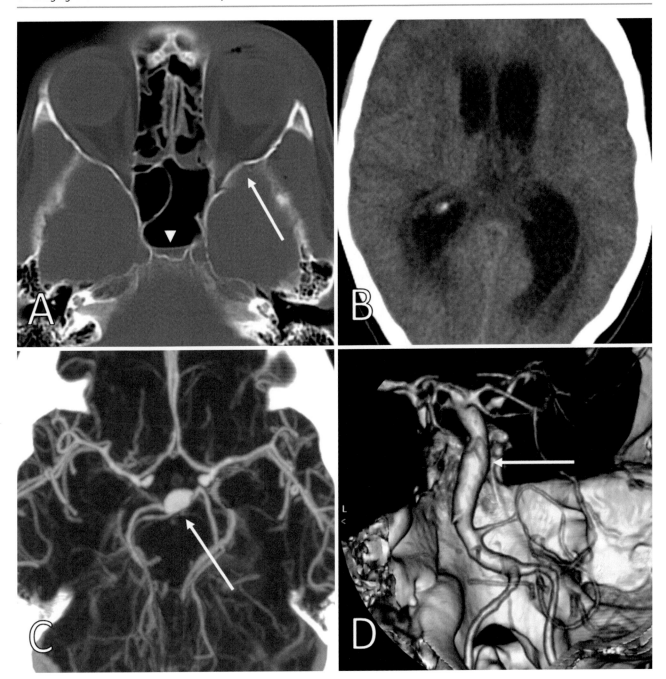

**Fig. 4** *Orbital wall fracture with sinus extension complicated by meningitis and mycotic basilar pseudoaneurysm* in a 45-year-old female with history of prior traumatic injury, presenting with intractable headaches, fever, and nuchal rigidity. Axial CT image in bone window (**a**) demonstrates slightly displaced fracture of the posterior lateral orbital wall (arrow). Note layering fluid in the sphenoid sinus (arrowhead).
Follow-up axial CT (**b**) and CTA (**c**) obtained 10 days after the initial trauma for subsequent intractable headaches, fever, and neck rigidity show new hydrocephalus related to meningitis, and a mycotic pseudoaneurysm of the basilar artery (arrow), fully seen on sagittal 3D reconstruction (**d**)

therefore warrant consideration for antibiotic initiation with CSF diversion via lumbar drainage or endoscopic repair [3, 7, 29]. Markedly displaced fractures with

resultant defects in the skull base risk the formation of meningoencephaloceles with herniation of the meninges, brain tissue, and CSF (Figs. 3 and 4).

**Fig. 5** *Normal osseous anatomy of the central portion of the middle cranial fossa on CT in bone window in coronal (**a**) and axial (**b**) planes*

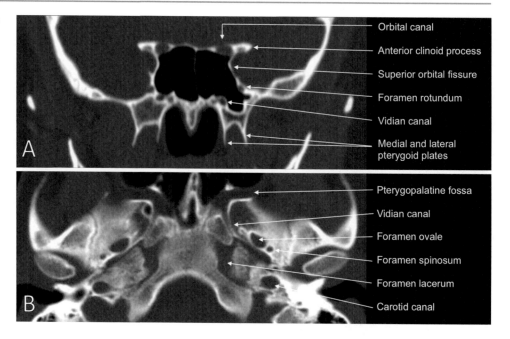

Orbital canal
Anterior clinoid process
Superior orbital fissure
Foramen rotundum
Vidian canal
Medial and lateral pterygoid plates

Pterygopalatine fossa
Vidian canal
Foramen ovale
Foramen spinosum
Foramen lacerum
Carotid canal

## Middle Cranial Fossa: Central Skull Base

*Anatomic considerations.* The middle cranial fossa, formed by the greater wing of the sphenoid and the anterior temporal bones, can be further subdivided into the central and lateral skull base (Fig. 5). The central skull base is mainly formed by the body of the sphenoid, and features the sella and pituitary gland, the sphenoid sinus, the cavernous sinus, and the basi-sphenoid portion of the clivus. The cavernous sinus, which extends from the orbital apex and superior orbital fissure to Meckel's cave, houses many important neurovascular structures, including cranial nerves III, IV, $V_1$, $V_2$, VI, and the internal carotid artery – all of which can be injured in the setting of trauma.

*Epidemiology and clinical features.* Many fractures of the central skull base result from direct extension of frontobasal fractures, and involve concomitant intracranial injuries including diffuse axonal injury, multicompartmental hemorrhage, and brain contusions [2, 23]. Fractures through the neural foramina or canals can transect or lacerate cranial nerves leading to neuropathies including ophthalmoplegia, anesthesia in the V1 and V2 distribution, and Horner's syndrome. Those involving the internal carotid artery may lead to symptoms of vascular compromise from dissection, transection, or entrapment.

*Diagnostic investigations.* Fractures may extend through the sella and sphenoid sinus, and are often described as being transverse or oblique in orientation [2]. Transverse fractures of the anterior central skull base often involve the posterior aspect of the anterior cranial fossa, the orbital apex, and the superior orbital fissure. Transverse fractures in the posterior central skull base may involve the temporal bones and clivus. Oblique fractures are more often associated with facial and frontobasal fractures, with an increased incidence of CSF leak [2].

*Management and complications.* Management is primarily dependent on associated complications. Injuries involving the cavernous internal carotid artery (ICA) can result in a rare, but clinically important carotid-cavernous fistula (CCF), a high-flow arteriovenous fistula between the ICA and cavernous sinus (Fig. 6). Patients present with exophthalmos, bruit, chemosis, ophthalmoplegia, and vision loss. Imaging reveals proptosis, intra-orbital fat stranding, enlarged superior ophthalmic veins, and asymmetric prominence or early filling of the cavernous sinus. Visualization of fistulous flow between the ICA and cavernous sinus on CTA or angiography confirms the diagnosis. Treatment is with endovascular repair or stent placement. Other notable vascular injuries include carotid occlusion (Fig. 7) and pseudoaneurysm formation (Fig. 8).

## Middle Cranial Fossa: Lateral Skull Base (Temporal Bones)

*Anatomic considerations.* The temporal bone features five osseous parts: tympanic (containing the external auditory canal), petrous (containing the middle and inner ear),

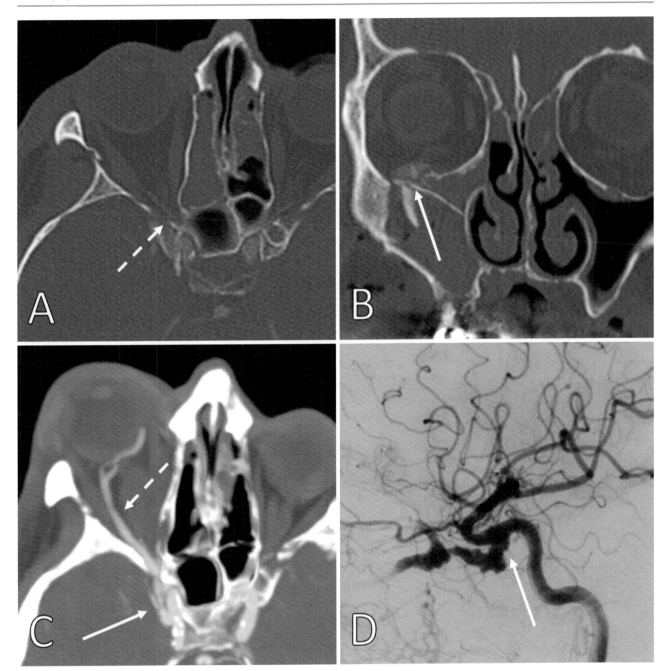

**Fig. 6** *Orbital apex and superior orbital fissure fractures with carotid-cavernous fistula* in a 64-year-old male following a fall from a 20-foot ladder. Axial (**a**) and coronal (**b**) CT images in bone window show comminuted fractures of the orbital floor (solid arrow in **b**), extending to the orbital apex and superior orbital fissure (dashed arrow in **a**). There is also a fracture of the lateral wall of the right maxillary sinus with associated maxillary sinus opacification and subcutaneous emphysema in the zygomaticomaxillary region. Follow-up axial CTA (**c**) demonstrates asymmetric prominence of the right cavernous sinus (solid arrow), as well as enlargement and early opacification of the dilated superior ophthalmic vein (dashed arrow) suggestive of arterial-venous mixing related to fistula formation. There is associated right-sided proptosis, pre-septal edema, and extraocular muscle enlargement. Lateral digital subtraction cerebral catheter angiogram (D) confirms the cavernous carotid fistula (arrow)

mastoid, squamous, and styloid. The most commonly involved in trauma are the petrous and mastoid portions. Important structures to scrutinize in the evaluation of temporal bone trauma include the external auditory canal, the ossicular chain (malleus, incus, and stapes), tegmen tympani (roof of the middle ear), otic capsule (cochlea,

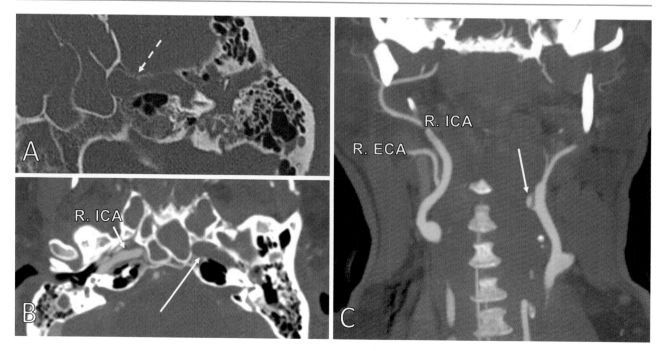

**Fig. 7** *Central skull base fracture involving the left carotid canal and petrous carotid* in a 53-year-old male following a 15-foot fall from a roof. Axial noncontrast CT image (**a**) demonstrates a linear mildly displaced fracture (dashed arrow) through the carotid canal. Axial CTA (**b**) and coronal CTA MIP (**c**) show normal opacification of the right internal and external carotid arteries (R. ICA, R. ECA), but non-opacification of the left internal carotid artery (solid arrow) from the bifurcation to the cavernous ICA. There is distal reconstitution of flow at the left supraclinoid segment (not shown)

vestibule, semicircular canals, and vestibular aqueduct), and the facial nerve canal (Fig. 9). In addition, it is equally important to evaluate the critical vascular structures, which include the internal carotid artery (petrous and cavernous segments), middle meningeal artery, and venous sinuses (transverse, sigmoid, and jugular bulb).

*Epidemiology and clinical features.* Temporal bone fractures are among the most common fractures of the skull base, usually resulting from high-energy blunt trauma with direct lateral blow to the temporoparietal skull, or indirectly from trauma to the frontal or occipital regions. Observable clinical signs include postauricular ecchymosis (Battle sign), hemotympanum (blood in the middle ear), and otorrhagia (blood in the external auditory canal) (Fig. 10). CSF leak can occur secondary to disruption of the tegmen tympani, with resultant CSF otorrhea when there is concomitant injury to the tympanic membrane. Symptoms include facial paralysis (CN VII), hearing loss, and vertigo (CN VIII).

*Diagnostic investigations.* Temporal bone fractures can be subtle on initial noncontrast CT head. Helpful indirect signs include opacification of mastoid and middle ear, contusions or hematomas of the temporal and occipital lobes, as well as air in the adjacent extra-axial space, internal auditory canal (pneumolabyrinth), or temporomandibular joint (Fig. 11). Dedicated temporal bone CT reconstruction allows detailed evaluation of the ossicular chain, otic capsule, and facial nerve.

Temporal bone fractures have been historically categorized by orientation, either longitudinal (parallel) or transverse (perpendicular) relative to the long axis of the petrous pyramid (Fig. 12). A more functional and clinically predictive classification system delineates fractures that spare or violate the otic capsule [6]. Longitudinal fractures comprise 70–90% of temporal bone fractures, and typically extend anteromedially to involve the external auditory canal and middle ear cavity, thereby sparing the otic capsule [8]. They are instead associated with tympanic membrane rupture, hemotympanum, and ossicular disruption – all of which can result in conductive hearing loss. The most common type of ossicular chain injury is incudomalleolar joint discontinuity (Fig. 13), with the incus being the most frequently affected, and likely related to its minimal ligamentous support. Facial nerve injury is found in 10–20% of longitudinal fractures and, when present, usually occurs at the geniculate ganglion [8, 13].

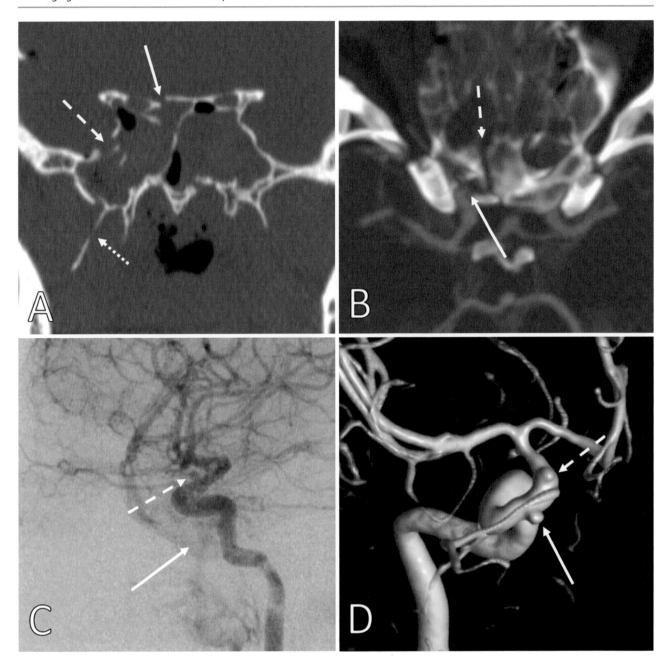

**Fig. 8** *Central skull base fractures complicated by CCF and pseudo-aneurysms* in a 33-year-old male following a fall from a 15-foot powerline. Coronal CT image in bone window (**a**) shows fractures of the planum sphenoidale (solid arrow), floor of the middle cranial fossa (dashed arrow), and lateral pterygoid plate (dotted arrow). Axial CTA MIP (**b**) shows a small focal outpouching in the ophthalmic segment of the right ICA (solid arrow), directly adjacent to a mildly displaced fracture of the sphenoid (dashed arrow). Cerebral angiogram (**c**) shows early venous opacification of the cavernous sinus (solid arrow) and focal superiorly directed outpouching within the cavernous ICA (dashed arrow). Three-dimensional rotational angiography (**d**) demonstrated 2 mm cavernous and ophthalmic segment pseudoaneurysms (solid and dashed arrows, respectively) in the region of cavernous sinus fistula seen on cerebral angiogram

In contrast, the less common transverse fractures comprise 10–30% of temporal bone fractures, and often involve the inner ear, bony labyrinth, and otic capsule (Fig. 14) [8]. Otic capsule-violating fractures course through the labyrinth, cochlea, vestibule, or semicircular canal are more clinically important due to increased risk of associated complications

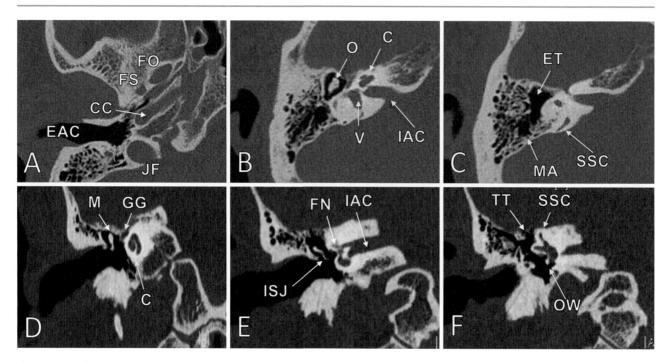

**Fig. 9** *Normal osseous anatomy of the temporal bone* on CT in bone window in axial plane from inferior to superior (**a**, **b**, and **c**) and coronal plane from anterior to posterior (**d**, **e**, and **f**). EAC, external auditory canal; CC, carotid canal; JF, jugular foramen; FS, foramen spinosum; FO, foramen ovale; O, ossicles; C, cochlea; V, vestibule; IAC, internal auditory canal; ET, epitympanum; MA, mastoid antrum/air cells; SCC, superior semicircular canal; M, malleus; GG, geniculate ganglion; FN, facial nerve; ISJ, incus-stapes junction; TT, tegmen tympani; OW, oval window

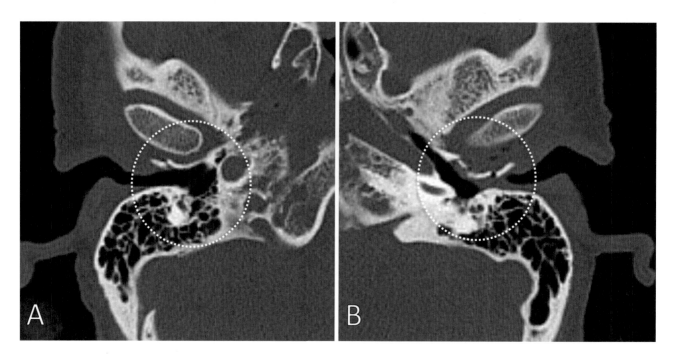

**Fig. 10** *Bilateral EAC fractures* in a 48-year-old female following fall off bicycle, presenting with bilateral otorrhagia. Axial CT of the bilateral temporal bones demonstrate fractures of the anterior wall of the right (**a**) and left (**b**) external auditory canals (EAC). There is resultant impaction of the mandibular condyles (not shown) and stenosis of the EAC

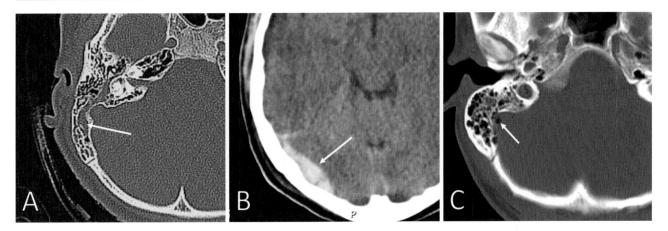

**Fig. 11** *Indirect signs of temporal bone fractures* in a 15-year-old male following a fall. Axial noncontrast head CT image in bone window (**a**) shows opacification of the right mastoid air cells (arrow) and middle ear.

Axial CT image in soft tissue window (**b**) demonstrates a small venous epidural hematoma in the right occipital region (arrow). Axial CT image in bone window (**c**) demonstrates adjacent extra-axial air (arrow)

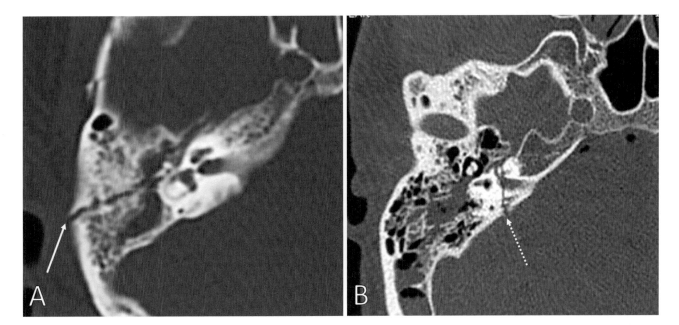

**Fig. 12** *Otic capsule-sparing and violating fractures of the temporal bone.* Axial CT images of the right temporal bone showing an otic capsule-sparing fracture (solid arrow in **a**), and an otic capsule-violating fracture (dotted arrow in **b**). These fracture patterns often correlate with

the classification of longitudinal and transverse fractures, respectively. Otic capsule-violating fractures have higher rates of severe complications, including SNHL and facial nerve injury

including sensorineural hearing loss (SNHL), CSF leak (4-8x), and facial nerve injury (2–5x) [6, 9, 18]. Facial nerve injury in transverse fractures tend to occur in the internal auditory canal or distal tympanic or mastoid segments of the facial canal, often resulting in immediate and complete facial paralysis (Fig. 15) [11, 28]. Intracranial complications including epidural hematoma and subarachnoid hemorrhage are also more common in otic capsule-violating fractures [6].

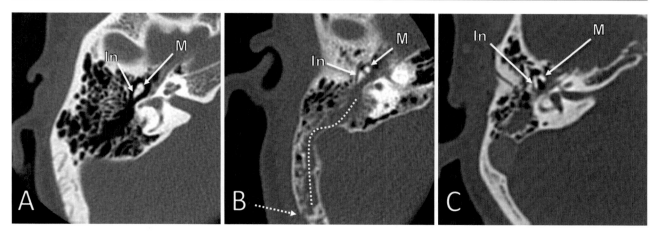

**Fig. 13** *Temporal bone fracture with ossicular chain disruption resulting in conductive hearing loss.* Axial CT image of the right temporal bone (**a**) shows a normal incudomalleolar junction with close apposition of the incus (In) and malleus (M). Axial CT image (**b**) shows an acute mildly displaced fracture at the squamosal region (middle image, dotted arrow) extending into the mastoid and middle ear (dotted line), with a small gap between the malleus and incus representing incudomalleolar dissociation. A different patient with frank ossicular chain disruption (**c**) shows an anteriorly displaced incus, and a displaced and abnormally angulated malleus

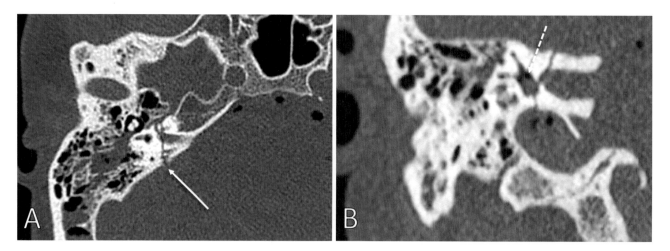

**Fig. 14** *Temporal bone fracture with otic capsule violation resulting in sensorineural hearing loss.* Axial CT image of the right temporal bone (**a**) shows an acute nondisplaced fracture through the otic capsule (solid arrow). Coronal CT (**b**) demonstrates pneumolabyrinth (dashed arrow), which is strongly suggestive of a perilymphatic fistula

*Management and complications.* Complications include conductive or sensorineural hearing loss, vestibular dysfunction, facial nerve paralysis, vascular injury, and CSF leak. Perilymphatic fistulas may occur as communication of perilymph between the inner and middle ears, most commonly at the oval or round window. Operative intervention is generally reserved for fractures with otic capsule violation, complete or immediate facial paralysis, and post-traumatic CSF fistulae with meningitis. Conductive hearing loss is often managed conservatively or with nonemergent elective repair, whereas SNHL has a poor prognosis, and typically warrants more aggressive management [9]. Patients with delayed facial paralysis have a better prognosis, with up to 90–94% achieving complete recovery [9, 14]. Vascular injury (Fig. 16) and intracranial hemorrhage are common in high-impact trauma, and may require surgical decompression if the associated mass effect is substantial. Venous epidural hematomas (typically related to sphenoparietal sinus injury), however, are benign, self-limited, and often do not require surgical intervention [2].

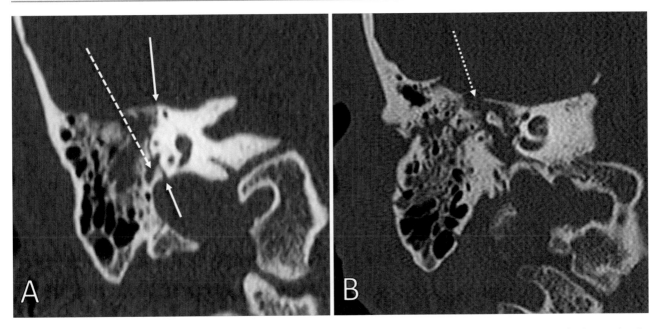

**Fig. 15** *Temporal bone fracture with facial nerve injury.* Coronal CT image shows a right temporal bone fracture (solid arrows in **a**) traversing the mastoid segment of the facial nerve (dashed arrow in A) and tegmen tympani (dotted arrow in **b**)

## Posterior Cranial Fossa

*Anatomic considerations.* The posterior skull base is formed by the posterior temporal and occipital bones, with osseous landmarks including the basi-occiput portion of the clivus, the occipital condyles, and the squamous portion of the occipital bone. The fossa itself holds the cerebellum and brainstem. Major foramina include the foramen magnum transmitting the medulla oblongata, vertebral arteries, and spinal portion of CN XI; the jugular foramen transmitting CN IX, X, and XI; and the hypoglossal canal transmitting CN XII (Fig. 17). Fractures involving the jugular foramen can cause CN IX-XI neuropathies, as well as vascular injury or thrombosis. Fractures of the occipital condyle can extend to involve the hypoglossal canal.

*Epidemiology and clinical features.* Posterior cranial fossa fractures are low in incidence (0.39–1.2%), usually occurring in the setting of severe, high-energy blunt trauma with multisystem injury [9]. Presentation is highly variable, but most frequently feature lower cranial nerve deficits (dysphagia, loss of gag reflex, hoarseness, tongue atrophy, or deviation), hemi- or quadriparesis, and signs and symptoms of brainstem injury or vertebrobasilar ischemia [17].

*Diagnostic investigations.* Two distinct types of fractures involve the clivus and the occipital condyles. Clival fractures

are especially rare, but carry a high mortality rate of 24–31% given proximity to the brainstem and pons (Fig. 18) [27]. They can be described as longitudinal, oblique, or transverse – with more propensity for posterior circulation (basilar artery) and brainstem compromise in longitudinal fractures, and damage to the anterior circulation (ICA) and surrounding cranial nerves in oblique or transverse fractures [27].

Occipital condyle fractures are most commonly classified by the Anderson and Montesano system, with three distinct fracture types based on radiologic appearance and presumed mechanism of injury (Fig. 19) [1]. Type I is the least common, and results from axial loading injury, featuring an impacted and comminuted occipital condyle without displacement. Type II typically results from direct blow to the skull, and features fracture of the occipital condyle extending from a basilar skull fracture. Type III fractures are the most common, comprising 75% of occipital condyle fractures, and usually resulting from severe contralateral flexion or rotation. It features an avulsion fracture of the inferomedial condyle with associated disruption of the tectorial membrane and contralateral alar ligament, resulting in potential joint instability [17]. Both the tectorial membrane and alar ligaments provide major mechanical stability to the joint, with the former limiting extension and the latter limiting lateral flexion or axial rotation. Types I and II are generally considered stable, whereas type III is generally considered unstable.

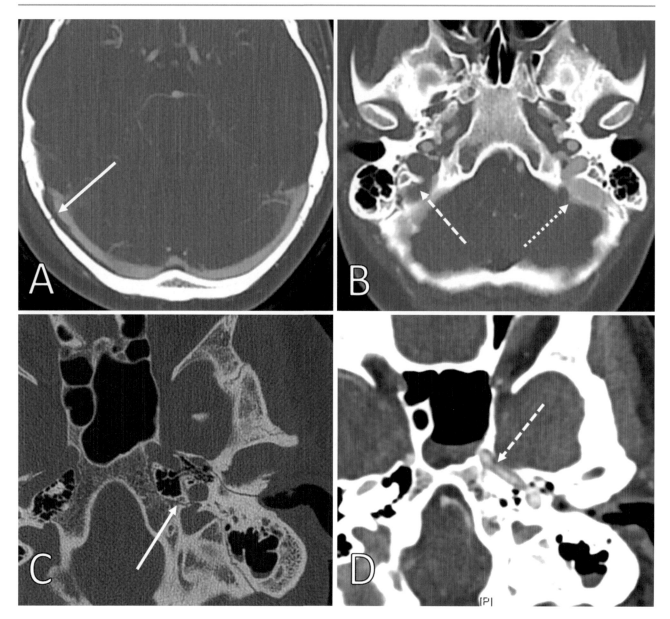

**Fig. 16** *Temporal bone fractures with associated vascular complications.* Axial images of a CTA of the head at the level of the circle of Willis (**a**) and skull base (**b**) show a nondisplaced fracture of the occipital bone with adjacent narrowing of the transverse sinus (solid arrow in **a**) and nonopacification of the right sigmoid sinus (dashed arrow in B). Note the normal opacification of the left sigmoid sinus (dotted arrow in **b**). Axial noncontrast CT (**c**) and CTA images (**d**) show an acute longitudinal fracture of the left temporal bone adjacent to the carotid canal (solid arrow in **c**), with irregularity of the internal carotid artery (dashed arrow in **d**) representing vascular injury

*Management and complications.* Posterior fossa fractures have high morbidity and mortality given close proximity to the brainstem. They are frequently associated with intracranial injuries, including parenchymal and extra-axial hemorrhage. Venous epidural hematomas from injury to the transverse sinus, sigmoid sinus, or jugular bulb can predispose to venous sinus thromboses, and warrant evaluation with CT venography when suspected. Clival fractures have an especially high rate of cranial neuropathy, most commonly and classically involving CN VI palsy due to the location of Dorello's canal in the clivus [2, 21]. Additional associated injuries of the craniocervical junction and cervical spine, with varying degrees of ligamentous compromise, can further complicate survival.

**Fig. 17** *Normal osseous anatomy of the posterior cranial fossa in axial plane on CT in bone window.* The jugular foramen consists of the larger more posterior pars vascularis and the more anteromedial pars nervosa (inferior petrosal sinus and glossopharyngeal nerve)

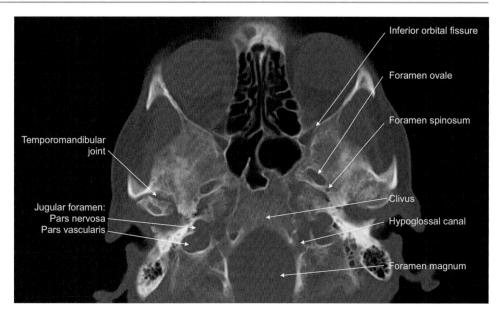

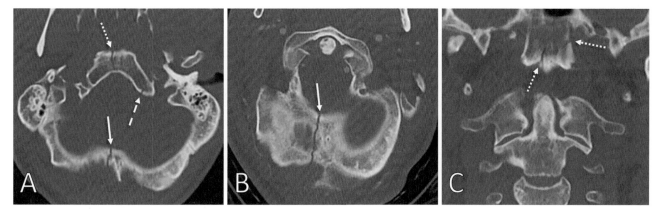

**Fig. 18** *Posterior cranial fossa fracture involving the clivus* in a 49-year-old male pedestrian struck by a car. Axial CT image of the skull base (**a**) shows nondisplaced fractures of the right paramedian occipital bone (solid arrow), left occipital condyle (dashed arrow), and basi-occiput of the clivus at the pharyngeal tubercle (dotted arrows).

Axial CT image (**b**) more inferiorly shows the fracture extending to the posterior foramen magnum (solid arrow). Coronal CT image (**c**) shows the longitudinal fractures through the clivus. No dural sinus thrombosis was detected on CTV (not shown)

## Conclusion

Skull base injuries are important entities in the setting of head trauma with potential for a wide range of sensory, neurologic, vascular, and infectious complications. The structural and neurovascular complexity of the skull base further complicates radiographic evaluation of fractures in this region. As such, thorough understanding of the clinical presentation, anatomy, fracture patterns, associated complications, and treatment indications are essential in the evaluation and management of these injuries.

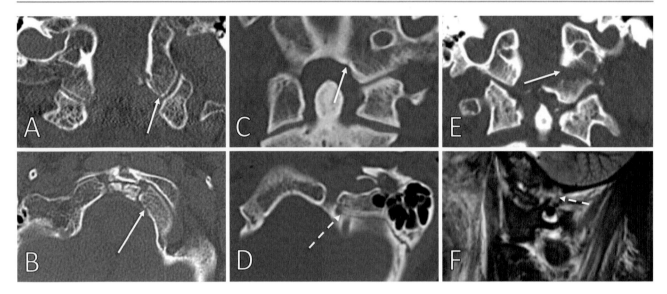

**Fig. 19** *Types of occipital condyle fractures. Type I occipital condyle fracture* in an 84-year-old female following a ground-level fall. Coronal (**a**) and axial CT (**b**) show nondisplaced comminuted fracture of the left occipital condyle, likely due to an axial loading injury following an unwitnessed fall. *Type II occipital condyle fracture* in a 52-year-old female with polytrauma following an assault. Coronal (**c**) and axial CT (**d**) show fracture of the left mastoid air cells and temporal bone (dashed arrow) extending along the lambdoid suture and into the ipsilateral occipital condyle (solid arrow). *Type III occipital condyle fracture* in a 44-year-old female following a motorcycle accident. Coronal CT (**e**) shows a comminuted and displaced fracture of the left occipital condyle with 7 mm diastases (**f**). Sagittal STIR MRI (bottom image) shows signal hyperintensity surrounding the atlantoaxial joint (dashed arrow) due to ligamentous injury

## Key Points

- Skull base fractures comprise a small but substantial portion of all head injuries, with the potential for high morbidity and mortality.
- Radiologic evaluation of skull base injuries is often challenging and subtle, necessitating thorough understanding of the intrinsic anatomic complexities and key neurovascular structures.
- Each cranial fossa features distinct fracture patterns and associated complications, differing in management strategies and outcomes.

## References

1. Anderson PA, Montesano PX. Morphology and treatment of occipital condyle fractures. Spine. 1988; https://doi.org/10.1097/00007632-198807000-00004.
2. Baugnon KL, Hudgins PA. Skull base fractures and their complications. In: Neuroimaging clinics of North America; 2014. https://doi.org/10.1016/j.nic.2014.03.001.
3. Bernal-Sprekelsen M, Alobid I, Mullol J, Trobat F, Tomás-Barberán M. Closure of cerebrospinal fluid leaks prevents ascending bacterial meningitis. Rhinology. 2005;43(4):277–81. PMID: 16405272.
4. Bobinski M, Shen PY, Dublin AB. Basic imaging of skull base trauma. J Neurol Surg, Part B: Skull Base. 2016;77(5):381–7. https://doi.org/10.1055/s-0036-1583540.
5. Connor SEJ, Flis C. The contribution of high-resolution multiplanar reformats of the skull base to the detection of skull-base fractures. Clin Radiol. 2005; https://doi.org/10.1016/j.crad.2005.04.003.
6. Dahiya R, Keller JD, Litofsky NS, Bankey PE, Bonassar LJ, Megerian CA. Temporal bone fractures: otic capsule sparing versus otic capsule violating clinical and radiographic considerations. J Trauma – Injury Infect Crit Care. 1999; https://doi.org/10.1097/00005373-199912000-00014.
7. Daudia A, Biswas D, Jones NS. Risk of meningitis with cerebrospinal fluid rhinorrhea. Ann Otol Rhinol Laryngol. 2007;116(12):902–5. https://doi.org/10.1177/000348940711601206.
8. De Foer B, Bali A, Bernaerts A, van Dinther J, Offeciers E, Casselman JW. Temporal bone trauma. In: Skull base imaging. Elsevier Inc.; 2018. https://doi.org/10.1016/b978-0-323-48563-0.00007-6.
9. Feldman JS, Farnoosh S, Kellman RM, Tatum SA. Skull base trauma: clinical considerations in evaluation and diagnosis and review of management techniques and surgical approaches. Semin Plast Surg. 2017;31(4):177–88. https://doi.org/10.1055/s-0037-1607275.
10. Friedman JA, Ebersold MJ, Quast LM. Post-traumatic cerebrospinal fluid leakage. World J Surg. 2001;25(8):1062–6. https://doi.org/10.1007/s00268-001-0059-7.
11. Go JL, Acharya J, Branchcomb JC, Rajamohan AG. Traumatic neck and skull base injuries. Radiographics. 2019; https://doi.org/10.1148/rg.2019190177.
12. Guyer RA, Turner JH. Delayed presentation of traumatic cerebrospinal fluid rhinorrhea: case report and literature review. Allergy Rhinol. 2015;6(3):188–90. https://doi.org/10.2500/ar.2015.6.0132.
13. Katzen JT, Jarrahy R, Eby JB, Mathiasen RA, Margulies DR, Shahinian HK. Craniofacial and skull base trauma. J Trauma. 2003;54(5):1026–34. https://doi.org/10.1097/01.TA.0000066180.14666.8B.
14. Kennedy TA, Avey GD, Gentry LR. Imaging of temporal bone trauma. Neuroimaging Clin N Am. 2014;24(3):467–86. https://doi.org/10.1016/j.nic.2014.03.003.
15. Kienstra MA, Van Loveren H. Anterior skull base fractures. Facial Plast Surg. 2005;21(3):180–6. https://doi.org/10.1055/s-2005-922857.

16. Lemole M, Behbahani M. Retrospective study of skull base fracture: a study of incidents, complications, management, and outcome overview from trauma-one-level institute over 5 years. J Neurol Surg Part B: Skull Base. 2013;74:S01. https://doi.org/10.1055/s-0033-1336362.

17. Leone A, Cerase A, Colosimo C, Lauro L, Puca A, Marano P. Occipital condylar fractures: a review. Radiology. 2000;216(3):635–44. https://doi.org/10.1148/radiology.216.3.r00se23635.

18. Little SC, Kesser BW. Radiographic classification of temporal bone fractures. Arch Otolaryngol–Head Neck Surg. 2006;132(12):1300. https://doi.org/10.1001/archotol.132.12.1300.

19. Madhusudan G, Sharma RK, Khandelwal N, Tewari MK. Nomenclature of frontobasal trauma: a new clinicoradiographic classification. Plast Reconstr Surg. 2006;117(7):2382–8. https://doi.org/10.1097/01.prs.0000218794.28670.07.

20. Manson PN, Stanwix MG, Yaremchuk MJ, Nam AJ, Hui-Chou H, Rodriguez ED. Frontobasal fractures: anatomical classification and clinical significance. Plast Reconstr Surg. 2009;124(6):2096–106. https://doi.org/10.1097/PRS.0b013e3181bf8394.

21. Menkü A, Koç RK, Tucer B, Durak AC, Akdemir H. Clivus fractures: clinical presentations and courses. Neurosurg Rev. 2004;27(3):194–8. https://doi.org/10.1007/s10143-004-0320-2.

22. Pretto Flores L, De Almeida CS, Casulari LA, Andrioli G, De Divitiis E, Foroglou G. Positive predictive values of selected clinical signs associated with skull base fractures. J Neurosurg Sci. 2000;44(2):77–83.

23. Raut AA, Naphade PS, Chawla A. Imaging of skull base: pictorial essay:[PAUTHORS ], Indian Jo ... Imaging of skull base: Pictorial essay full text imaging of skull base: Pictorial essay:[ PAUTHORS ],

24. Sakas DE, Beale DJ, Ameen AA, Whitwell HL, Whittaker KW, Krebs AJ, Abbasi KH, Dias PS. Compound anterior cranial base fractures: Classification using computerized tomography scanning as a basis for selection of patients for dural repair. J Neurosurg. 1998;88(3):471–7. https://doi.org/10.3171/jns.1998.88.3.0471.

25. Slupchynskyj OS, Berkower AS, Byrne DW, Cayten CG. Association of skull base and facial fractures. Laryngoscope. 1992;102(11):1247–50. https://doi.org/10.1288/00005537-199211000-00008. PMID: 1405985.

26. Stewart RM, Rotondo MF, Nathens AB, Neal M, Caden-Price C, Lynch J, Chang MC, Burd RS, Chung KC, Cuschieri J, Della Rocca GJ, Ellenbogen RG, Fantus RJ, Gibran NS, Hartsock LA, Hemmila MR, Bradford Henley FM, Hunt JP, Mccarthy M, ... Weinand M. National trauma data bank report 2016. American College of Surgeons (ACS). 2016. Retrieved 29 Apr 2020 from https://www.facs.org/quality-programs/trauma/tqp/center-programs/ntdb/docpub

27. Winkler-Schwartz A, Correa JA, Marcoux J. Clival fract bures in a level I trauma center. J Neurosurg. 2015;122(1):227–35. https://doi.org/10.3171/2014.9.JNS14245.

28. Zayas JO, Feliciano YZ, Hadley CR, Gomez AA, Vidal JA. Temporal bone trauma and the role of multidetector CT in the emergency department. Radiographics. 2011;31(6):1741–55. https://doi.org/10.1148/rg.316115506.

29. Ziu M, Savage JG, Jimenez DF. Diagnosis and treatment of cerebrospinal fluid rhinorrhea following accidental traumatic anterior skull base fractures. Neurosurg Focus. 2012;32(6) https://doi.org/10.3171/2012.4.FOCUS1244.

Indian Jo ... Important Anatomical Landmarks in Central Skull Base. 2012;1:4–13.

# Imaging of Midfacial and Orbital Trauma

Claudia F. E. Kirsch

## Contents

**Abstract**

The midface's central location, nasal projection anteriorly, and zygomas laterally make it commonly involved in trauma. The midface has singular bony elements including the vomer, ethmoid, sphenoid, mandible and paired bony maxilla, inferior nasal concha, palatine, nasal, lacrimal, and zygomatic bones. The bones form the facial skeleton with four transverse and four paired vertical buttresses. Fractures of the midfacial bones usually involve the nasal bones, followed by zygomatic complex fractures, and often occur from blunt trauma secondary to falls, altercations, or motor vehicle collisions and less commonly in penetrating trauma from gunshots or foreign bodies. Computed tomography (CT) is the imaging modality of choice to delineate fractures and can be used for orbital volumetric measurements and preoperative planning. MRI can be used to supplement CT in assessing intracranial and optic nerve involvement. Although utilized for over a century, the Le Fort classification of midfacial trauma is anachronistic and less relevant for high-speed trauma and does not include orbital and zygomaticofacial complex involvement; therefore, more recent classification schemes may be more relevant for surgical planning. This chapter reviews midface and orbit anatomy, key radiographic features from trauma including the importance of multi-

C. F. E. Kirsch (✉)
Department of Radiology Northwell Health, Zucker Hofstra School of Medicine at Northwell, North Shore University Hospital, Manhasset, NY, USA
e-mail: ckirsch@Northwell.edu

© Springer Nature Switzerland AG 2022
M. N. Patlas et al. (eds.), *Atlas of Emergency Imaging from Head-to-Toe*,
https://doi.org/10.1007/978-3-030-92111-8_7

planar imaging, and awareness of critical adjacent structures including the nasolacrimal ducts, orbital musculature, and sinonasal passageways that may be become displaced or obstructed. Importantly, this chapter highlights relevant fracture patterns in midfacial subunits including the nose, naso-orbito-ethmoidal region (NOE), orbital complex, and zygomaticomaxillary complex (ZMC). For each subunit, there is a brief review of relevant epidemiology, clinical features, and critical anatomy affected, highlighting radiographic findings that should be assessed, with a summary of key points, to facilitate optimal treatment.

### Keywords

Midface · Orbit · Trauma · Fracture · Computed tomography · Magnetic resonance imaging · Preoperative planning

## Introduction

The midface triangular region contains the middle third facial skeleton, which is delineated superiorly by a line connecting the bilateral zygomaticofrontal sutures tangential to the skull base and inferiorly at the maxillary dental occlusal margin or in edentulous patients the upper alveolar ridge (Fig. 1a–f). The midface nose protrudes anteriorly from the face, and the midface posterior margin extends to the sphenoethmoidal junction including the sphenoid pterygoid lamina inferiorly. Bones of the midface include the single ethmoid, vomer, mandible, and sphenoid bone and the paired, maxilla, inferior nasal concha, palatine, nasal, lacrimal, and zygomatic bones. The midface bones form four transverse and four paired vertical buttresses, acting like bumpers when impacted by trauma (Fig. 1e). According to the Global Burden of Disease Study (GBD), the first study to measure the prevalence of facial fractures, in 2017, there were 7,538,662 new cases of facial trauma, with falls being the most common etiology [1]. Causes of midfacial and orbital trauma also include assaults, motor vehicle collisions, occupational accidents, and gunshot wounds [2, 3]. The majority of facial trauma patients are men aged 25–51 years [1, 4, 5]. Facial fractures may be simple, involving one anatomic subunit, or complex with multiple units. Although the "Le Fort subcranial" system [6] has been used for over a century, it is anachronistic and ineffective for high-velocity trauma and is limited in delineating complex fractures of the zygoma and orbit [7–10]. However, it is a good starting point to understand how fractures are transmitted and is briefly outlined below, followed by a detailed description of the current AOCMF/AOCMG system (which stands for

Arbeitsgemeinschaft für Osteosynthesefragen, kraniomaxillofaziale Fachdisziplinen). In short, AO is German for "Association for the Study of Internal Fixation," and the CMF system is used for classification of maxillofacial trauma based on previous classifications combined with an intuitive imaging approach. AO is a Swiss study nonprofit organization founded in 1958 [11, 12], which is dedicated to improving outcomes for trauma patients. Importantly, the CMF classification of midfacial trauma is composed of three levels: levels 1 and 2 localize the fracture, and level 3 adds detailed morphology on fragmentation and dislocation [7, 13, 14].

Using the AOCMF as a reference guide, this chapter focuses on the radiographic features of trauma resulting in fractures of the nasal bones, naso-orbito-ethmoidal (NOE) region, zygomaticomaxillary complex (ZMC), maxillary occlusion- bearing region, and internal orbits, briefly discussing the epidemiology and relevant anatomic bony, arterial, and neural anatomy affected and focusing on the critical patterns of trauma in diagnostic imaging, with key clinical and radiographic points highlighted.

## Classification of Midfacial Trauma

In 1901, the French surgeon Rene Le Fort applied blunt force to cadaver skulls and described three fracture types (Fig. 2), occurring because air-filled sinus cavities provided points of least resistance, with all fractures in this system involving the pterygoid plates [6, 7]. A Le Fort l fracture is a floating palate with a horizontal fracture from the piriform aperture through lateral maxillary and the lateral nasal walls that separates the teeth from the upper face, with a fracture via the alveolar ridge, lateral nose, and inferior wall maxillary sinus. Le Fort type II is a floating maxilla with a pyramidal fracture, and the teeth are at the pyramid base, with the nasofrontal suture at the fracture apex through nasal bones, posterior alveolar ridge, maxillary sinus lateral walls, inferior orbital rim, and uppermost fracture line at the nasofrontal junction or maxillary frontal process. Le Fort III is a floating face with craniofacial disjunction. The transverse fracture extends along the nasofrontal suture, maxillo-frontal suture, orbital wall, zygomaticofrontal suture, and zygomatic arch. Because Le Fort created these fractures with relatively low-velocity injury, by smashing the skulls with clubs and iron rods or throwing them on a table, the schematic may not be relevant for the high-velocity trauma seen with many motor vehicle collisions, and the AOCMF classification (Fig. 2b) below may be more relevant for current evaluation of midface trauma [ 7, 13, 14].

In the AOCMF fracture classification, level 1 determines if the fracture location is part of the mandible (code 91), midface (code 92), skull base (code 93), or cranial vault

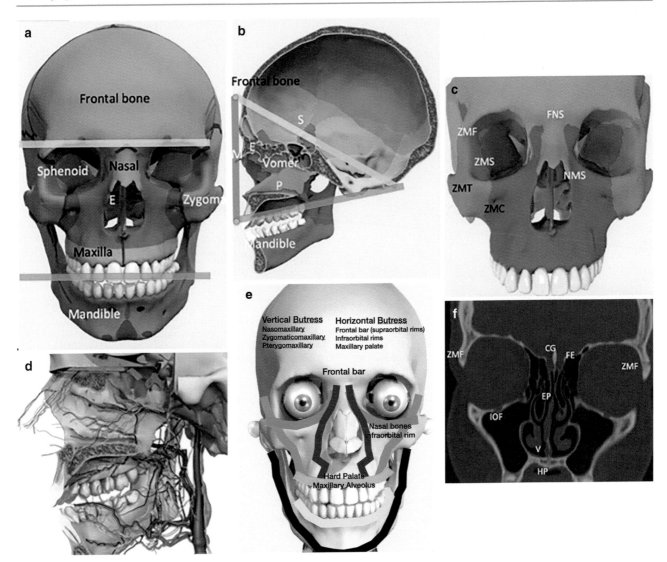

**Fig. 1** a,b,c,d. (**a**) Skull midface between yellow line along bilateral zygomaticofrontal sutures and the blue line, along the inferior maxillary occlusal margin: E, ethmoid; M, maxilla; P, hard palate; S, sphenoid; V, vomer. (**b**) Lines from 1A converge posteriorly creating a midface triangle, the largest portion shown with a green line along the anterior midface. (**c**) Coronal midface suture lines: ZMC, zygomaticomaxillary; ZMT, zygomaticotemporal; ZMF, zygomaticofrontal; ZMS, zygomaticosphenoid; FNS, frontonasal; and NMS, nasomaxillary suture. (**d**) Note the internal and external carotid artery supply to the midface with terminal vessels that run from lateral to medial supplying the nasal septum. (**e**) The midface is composed of four transverse and vertical buttresses that act like a bumper. (**f**) Corresponding coronal CT scan: CG, crista galli; FE, fovea ethmoidalis; IOF, infraorbital foramen for the infraorbital nerve division V2; HP, hard palate; V, vomer; EP, perpendicular plate of the ethmoid

(code 94) [ 7] (Table 1). Level 2 classification is useful for all craniomaxillofacial specialties and refers to the midface anatomic subregions, and level 3 assesses the fractures. This chapter focuses only on level 92, the midface. As in Fig. 2b, per the AOCMF, the midface is subdivided into upper, intermediate, and lower regions. The central midface is formed by stacking of the upper, intermediate, and lower central midface units. The UCM – or upper central midface – contains the upper frontomaxillary processes forming the anterior medial orbital margins and two nasal bones. The lateral midface is formed by the zygoma and the zygomatic arch; however, of note, anatomically, the zygomatic orbital surface or lateral orbital flange is considered part of the lateral internal orbit or anterior lateral orbital wall.

Centrally, as in Fig. 2b, the UCM is demarcated inferiorly by a line at the lower lacrimal fossa margin and contains the nasal skeleton, bones, and nasofrontal maxilla. The ICM – or intermediate central midface – is the infraorbital maxilla and maxillary antrum and middle nasal meatus. Boundaries for the ICM include the zygomaticofrontal suture and superior medially the infraorbital margin and orbital rim, above and piriform aperture inferiorly. The inferior aspect of the ICM is the maxillary buttress convergence in the nasal cavities, to the base of the zygomaticomaxillary crest and the upper

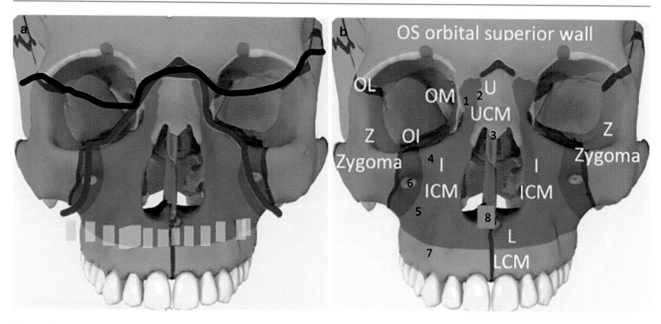

**Fig. 2** a,b. Le Fort classification, Le Fort I: Dotted yellow line, fracture extends from piriform aperture to lateral nasal and maxillary walls posteriorly including pterygoid plate segments creating a floating maxilla. Le Fort II: Red line, rarely occurs by itself, usually with other fractures, fracture through the naso-orbital ethmoid and nasofrontal bone to pterygoid plate. Le Fort III: Black line, fracture through the frontozygomatic suture, lateral orbit, sphenozygomatic suture, inferior orbital fissure, medial orbital floor, and nasal dorsum, causing craniofacial disjunction 2B. AOCMF classification, the central midface is divided into UCM (upper central midface), ICM (intermediate central midface), and LCM (lower central midface). UCM includes (1) frontonasal maxillary process/medial orbital rim, (2) nasal bone, and (3) upper nasal septum/ethmoid perpendicular plate. ICM includes (4) medial inferior orbital rim/infraorbital maxillary margin, (5) anterior maxillary antrum bony wall and parapiriform buttress, and (6) zygomaticomaxillary crest. LCM includes (7) maxillary alveolar process upper margin, if patient edentulous bony resorption and lower margin, and (8) lower nasal septum and vomer

maxillary tuberosity, and contains the inferior orbital fissure and the pterygomaxillary junction. The ICM contains the para-piriform maxilla and the infraorbital maxilla. The LCM or lower central midface contains the maxillary solid body, alveolar process, maxillary tuberosity to the inferior orbital fissure, and sphenopalatine foramen, and the posterior aspect is the pterygomaxillary fissure. Within the LCM is the infra-zygomatic maxilla, zygoma and zygomatic arch, pterygoid process, palate, and the medial, lateral, and inferior orbital walls [13–17]. In this classification, the midface is located below the frontozygomatic sutures laterally and the frontonasal suture medially, divided centrally into the upper jaw composed of two maxillary bodies surrounding the piriform aperture and the superior frontal processes extending to the anterior skull base. Laterally, the frontal bone orbital roofs and supraorbital rims form the orbital upper margin as the anterior skull base.

Essentially the UCM comprises the nasal skeleton and medial orbital rims, medially containing the paired nasal bones above the nasal aperture between the frontonasal maxillary processes that create the nasal bony lateral margins/medial orbital rims. Centrally is the nasal septum formed by the quadrangular cartilage, ethmoid perpendicular plate, vomer, and palatine bone. The lateral midface as seen in Fig. 2b contains the zygoma and zygomatic arch, which are easily demarcated by their suture lines. However, the posterior zygomatic arch is located along the temporal bone glenoid fossa, and the orbital surface of the zygoma or lateral orbital flange is part of the lateral internal orbit, and the posterior thin lateral orbital wall is from the greater wing of the sphenoid [7, 13–17]. The AOCMF subdivides the midface into clinically relevant anatomic subunits, traumas, and fractures, and these subunits are then delineated if there is fragmentation, displacement, or bone loss. Fragmentation is classified as 0 (non-fragmented with a single straight or twisted fracture line) or 1 (fragmented with more than one fracture line); the terms "multi-fragmentary" or "comminuted" are more out of date. Therefore, bones which have multiple fragments are considered a 1. Displacement refers to fragments which are not in their original, normal location, regardless of how far or little change in position. Traumatic bone loss or defects are denoted either 0 (no bone loss) or 1 (bone loss) [13–18].

## Nasal Trauma and Naso-ethmoidal Injury

Because the nose is front and center and protrudes anteriorly from the face, nasal bone fractures are the most common facial fracture, occurring in up to 50% of facial trauma, and are the third most common fracture of the bony skeleton [18–20, 24–26]. Fractures of the thin nasal bones are extremely common in athletes, as well as in pediatric and elderly patients, and constitute up to approximately one-third of pediatric facial fractures [26–30]. Of note, the use of airbag technology and seat belts substantially reduces the likelihood of facial fractures in motor vehicle collisions [29]. Identification of nasal fractures is critical, as untreated fracture deformities may result in nasal valve collapse, obstruction of airflow, cosmetic deformities, and sinusitis, and missed nasal septal hematomas can result in a "saddle nose" deformity. Imaging is recommended for high-energy trauma as well as in low-energy injury with isolated trauma to the nose. CT is the modality of choice with non-contrast thin sections that can be reformatted into multi-planar sagittal, coronal, and 3D reconstructions, as radiographs are often noncontributory [30–37].

The centrally located nasal cavities, frontal sinuses above, maxillary sinuses and orbits located laterally with the hard palate, and the oral cavity inferiorly, form a triangular pyramid split in half by the nasal septum, containing the upper lateral and lower lateral nasal cartilages (Fig. 3a). When trauma occurs to the midface, the force of external impact is transmitted from the nasal bones to the midline septum. Inferiorly the two nares (nostrils) are separated by the nasal septum, the outer round margin of the nares is the ala nasi which is mobile, and inferiorly in the midline is the nasomaxillary spine that may be fractured in severe trauma [ 31–17]. The nasion is where the superior frontonasal suture line anchors the two superior two nasal bones and is thicker superiorly above the intercanthal line where they join the suture. Laterally, there is a nasomaxillary suture line with the nasal bones abutting the maxillary ascending process, with an internasal suture line in the midline. The rhinion is the osseocartilaginous junction of the thinner inferior nasal bone beveled edge articulating with connective tissue to upper lateral nasal cartilages, whose inferior margin forms the anterior septal angle and articulates with the lower lateral

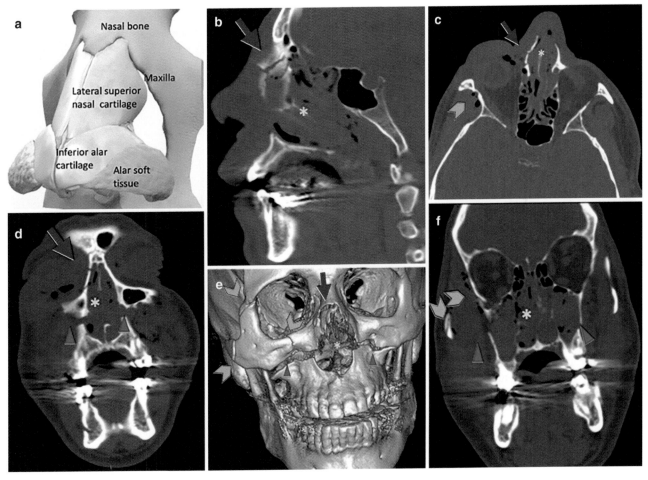

**Fig. 3** a–f. (**a**) Schematic of normal nasal bones and cartilage. (**b–f**) (**b**) Sagittal, (**c**) axial, (**d,f**) coronal, and (**e**) 3D-reconstructed CT, 55-year-old man following assault with orbital and subcutaneous emphysema, multiple facial fractures including comminuted right nasal bone fractures (red arrow), nasal septal fractures with nasal septal hematoma (yellow asterisk), bilateral Le Fort 1 fractures (blue arrowheads), and a right zygomaticomaxillary (ZMC) fracture (green chevron)

cartilage. The transition point between the thicker superior nasal bone and thinner inferior margin is a common site for fractures [35–39] (Fig. 3a).

The nasal septum is formed by the quadrangular cartilage anteriorly functioning as a central support wall that articulates with the perpendicular plate of the ethmoid posteriorly and vomer inferiorly, with the inferior vomer articulating with the nasal crest of the maxilla anteriorly and nasal crest of the palatine bone posteriorly. The nasal blood supply is the only location where blood flows from lateral to medial with supply from the internal and external carotid artery branches [39–43] (Fig. 1d). The majority of the nasoseptal blood supply arises from external carotid maxillary artery greater palatine, infraorbital, and sphenopalatine branches, with the facial artery supplying a superior labial branch and with anterior and posterior ethmoidal branches arising from the internal carotid artery. These are terminal vessels without substantial collateral blood supply. Trauma to the nasal cartilage, mucosa, or hematoma disrupting the highly vascular mucoperichondrium can lead to septal necrosis and collapse, resulting in a saddle nose deformity. Epistaxis from minor trauma can damage to the highly vascular plexus and is one of the most common ENT emergencies [39–42].

The nasal region is innervated by the trigeminal nerve (CN V) V1 ophthalmic and V2 maxillary divisions. Superiorly the olfactory nerve (CN 1) terminates in the olfactory bulb that lies above the nasal cavity in the olfactory groove of the anterior cranial fossa. The olfactory bulb contains mitral cells synapsing with synaptic glomeruli whose axons from the fila olfactoria form small nerves extending through ethmoid bone cribriform plate foramina to enter the nasal cavity.

Trauma to the nose may result in fractures of the nasal bones and septum (Fig. 3b–f). Currently, no standard worldwide classification is present, to my knowledge, although various classification schemes have been proposed. Broad categories include whether the fracture is lateral versus frontal, as frontal injuries are more likely to involve the nasal septum [43–45]. In 1989, Murray et al. [46]dropped weights on cadaver noses and described seven types of fracture lines and septal involvement, as either unilateral or bilateral, open book with splayed bones, impacted, greenstick, or comminuted. Harrison [47] defined fractures as follows:

Class 1: Chevallet fracture, presenting with depression over the nasal bones with tenderness and crepitus over fractured nasal bones with the fracture line parallel to dorsum and nasomaxillary sutures joining at thickest point of the nasal bone

Class 2: Jaraway fracture with cosmetic deformity with nasal bone and frontonasal process of the maxilla fractures

Class 3: Even if the ethmodial labyrinth and orbits are intact, high velocity trauma clinically often leads to a telecanthus and disruption of the medial canthal ligament from the lacrimal crest, with epiphora if associated with a lacrimal crest injury involving the naso-orbital and naso-ethmodial regions [47]

The high-velocity fractures may result in a Le Fort fracture of the maxilla with the force of impact transmitted to nasal bones and cartilages, resulting in buckling and interlocking of the fracture deformities [39–47]. CT is the imaging modality of choice in identifying the fractures (Fig. 3b–f), assessing spatial alignment or lack thereof, the presence or absence of a nasal septal hematoma or cribriform plate fracture, and resultant cerebrospinal fluid (CSF) leak, with a sensitivity of up to 88–95% for revealing the site of leakage [49–52]. In some cases, MRI may also be utilized for further evaluation using MRI cisternography [49–54].

CT should be optimized to define the fracture deformities. [58-60] Because axial CT images may not reveal up to a quarter of nasal pyramid fractures, and transverse minimally displaced fractures may be overlooked in the axial plane, it is imperative that multi-planar sagittal and coronal reformations are routinely obtained and carefully reviewed [59] (Fig. 3b–f). The CT report should comment on the presence or absence of a nasal septal hematoma, nasofrontal duct injury, ocular or brain injury, and presence (or absence) and site of cerebrospinal leak [14, 57–61]. Because septal fractures and dislocations may lead to the upper nasal cartilage deformation of nasal bones when healing, up to half of patients with a successful closed nasal reduction may have malunion and then require a septorhinoplasty [6].

## Takeaway Points

Nasal septal fractures may be overlooked in the axial plane on CT, so multi-planar sagittal and coronal images should be routinely obtained and carefully evaluated.

Septal fractures may exert deforming forces to the nasal cartilages, and up to half of patients with closed nasal reductions may require septorhinoplasty to treat malunion.

Carefully assess the nasolacrimal ducts and the nasal septal cartilage on CT images, as mucosal injury and hematoma can result in a nasal septal hematoma and saddle nose injury.

## Central Midface-Naso-orbito-ethmoid (NOE) Fractures

Nasal fractures involving the frontal bone, cribriform plate, and orbit are complex fractures that may have intracranial or orbital involvement and warrant imaging with CT of the brain and facial bones [55]. Using the Markowitz and Manson classification, [56] these can be divided into type 1 (single fragment, most common type of injury), type 2 (comminuted with intact medial canthal tendon insertion), or type 3 (comminuted with medial canthal lateral displacement or avulsion)

(Fig. 3b–e). On CT, the bones to which the medial canthal tendon is attached, including the orbital rim and wall and the nasolacrimal bones, should be assessed for fractures which may affect the medial canthal tendon. The actual mobility of the medial canthal tendon may be better assessed under anesthesia. Fractures to the nasolacrimal duct can result in epiphora, dacryocystoceles, or cysts forming along the inferomedial orbital canthus from duct obstruction or dacyrocystitis, which is an inflammation along the nasolacrimal duct and medial orbital canthus [14, 47, 55–57]. Anatomically, naso-orbito-ethmoidal fractures have a single or comminuted fracture along five critical fracture lines or "cardinal tracts," [60-66] namely:

1. The lateral nose and piriform aperture
2. Nasomaxillary buttress
3. Inferior orbital rim and floor
4. Medial orbital wall
5. Frontomaxillary suture

Anatomically, the anterior and posterior portions of the medial canthal tendon form from the fusion of the tarsal plates and orbicularis oculi muscles, inserting on the lacrimal crests bordering the lacrimal fossa (Fig. 4a, b). When a fracture displaces the bony central fragment laterally, the medial canthal tendon is displaced (Fig. 3c), causing a telecanthus with a shortened truncated medial palpebral fissure. Lateral bony displacement of the NOE fragment can cause globe displacement with hypertelorism and dorsal nasal collapse [59–64]. Although CT does not completely delineate the medial canthal tendon, it can demonstrate the degree of fracture comminution along the medial orbital wall at the lacrimal fossa and may aid surgical planning for the tendon repair. Because NOE fractures may affect the nasolacrimal duct located in the maxillary frontal process, extending anteriorly along the ethmoidal labyrinth into the inferior meatus, assessment for trauma that impairs drainage is important, as disruption can lead to blockage, resulting in epiphora or a dacryocystocele. Trauma to the anterior ethmoidal complex and frontonasal duct, best seen on sagittal CT, can involve the frontal sinus floor through the ethmoidal labyrinth to the ostiomeatal complex and hiatus semilunaris and lead to obstruction and impaired mucociliary clearance. In the AOCMF classification, NOE fractures involve the UCM (upper central midface) and ICM (intermediate central midface) similar to a Le Fort II fracture of the midface, involving the medial inferior orbital rim, facial antral wall, and para-piriform buttress

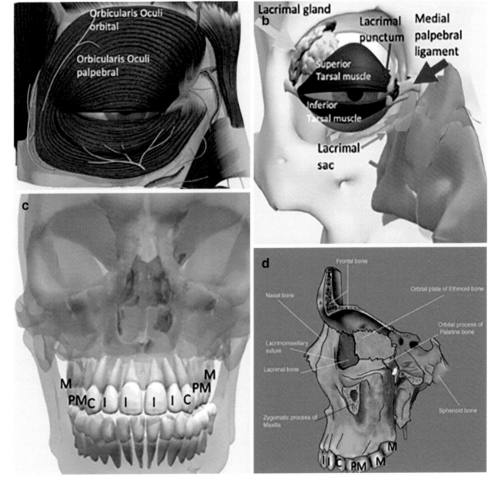

**Fig. 4** (a) Normal coronal schematic of orbicularis oculi; the thin muscle sheet covers upper and lower eyelids with palpebral, orbital, and lacrimal portions. (b) Superior and inferior tarsal plates attach to the medial palpebral ligament extending to the maxilla's anterior lacrimal crest. The ligament extends anterior to the lacrimal sac. (c) Schematic of maxillary alveolus and teeth. I, incisors; C, canines; PM, premolars; M, molars. (d) Schematic in the sagittal plane showing lacrimal bone and adjacent suture lines

[14, 17, 57]. The fracture line can also be assessed for extension to the zygomaticomaxillary suture and the zygoma, along the ICM. The more inferior LCM (lower central midface) fractures are akin to Le Fort I type fractures, with the fracture extending through the solid maxilla, maxillary tuberosity, and upper alveolar process containing maxillary teeth roots.

Regarding the maxillary dentition and the hard palate (Fig. 4c, d), tooth loss at the maxillary alveolar ridge causes bony resorption with decreased bone height (Fig. 6e), classified as 0 (no or mild loss of vertical alveolar height > 11 mm), 1 (moderate, loss of bone height 6–10 mm), and 2 (severe atrophy, loss of vertical height < 5 mm). Fractures through the maxillary alveolus can result in tooth avulsion or loosening. The bony palate is composed of the premaxilla, maxillary palatine processes, and palatine bone horizontal plate. Fractures in the palate per the AOCMF are classified as 1 (one transverse fracture line), 2 (one para- or midsagittal fracture line), and 3 (two or more fracture lines), and bone loss can be denoted by a d= bone defect. Extending posteriorly in this region are the pterygoid processes of the sphenoid bone; in the AOCMF classification, these are considered separate anatomic units and are classified as either fractured or not fractured and whether or not it is separated vertically from the maxilla.[18, 59, 60]

## Takeaway Points

NOE fractures involve posterior disruption of the medial orbital canthal regions, ethmoids, and medial orbital walls. Although the tendons in the medial orbital canthal regions are not well seen on CT, the nasal profile in NOE fractures is lost in the sagittal plane, and the distance between the the inner eyes will be altered in the coronal plane.

Radiologists interpreting CT should comment on degree of bony disruption of medial vertical maxillary buttresses, especially in the region of the lacrimal fossa, where the medial canthus attaches.

In NOE fractures, adjacent nasolacrimal and nasofrontal ducts may be affected, impairing drainage of tears and mucociliary clearance, with the potential development of a dacryocystocele or mucocele.

## Lateral Midface, Zygoma, and Zygomaticomaxillary Complex (ZMC) Fractures

The zygomatic bones or "cheek bones" (Fig. 5a) have a quadripod appearance defining the midface height and width. The word zygomatic is from the Greek word "zygon," meaning a yoke or crossbar that two animals could be hitched to; these bones project laterally and are seen in up to 17% of facial fracture deformities

[59–66]. The bony zygomas are attached via four suture lines including the zygomaticotemporal, zygomaticofrontal, zygomaticosphenoid, and zygomaticomaxillary and form the lateral orbital floors and margins that helps define the orbital volume [55, 61–64]. Together the ZMC has an upper transverse maxillary buttress along the zygomaticomaxillary and zygomaticotemporal sutures and a lateral vertical maxillary buttress along the zygomaticomaxillary and frontozygomatic sutures (Fig. 5a, b). Because fractures often involve three of these suture-related buttresses, the term "tripod" fracture is sometimes used to describe zygomaticomaxillary complex (ZMC) fractures; however, this is a misnomer as it misses the sphenoid suture attachment, and ZMC fractures are really quadripod fractures (Figs. 5c–f). Because the zygoma forms the lateral orbital wall and floor rotation of the ZMC fracture alters the orbital volume and can result in a cosmetic facial deformity and enophthalmos, that may be harder to correct if there is bony malunion or if the mandibular coronoid is impinged resulting in difficulty with jaw movements [60–66]. CT is the imaging modality of choice and can display the fracture lines and inferior orbital rim step-off. In low- to moderate-impact trauma, the zygoma may have retrusion from internal rotation at the zygomaticomaxillary buttress and posterior displacement of the zygomatic crest. Trauma can lead to offset of the zygomaticosphenoid suture cause medial or lateral angulation with orbital rim step-off. Higher-impact injuries may widen the midface with trauma at the zygomaticosphenoid suture causing posterolateral displacement and external rotation [65].

Zingg et al. [67] classified zygoma fractures into three types. Zingg type A fractures only involve the zygomatic arch (type A1), lateral orbital rim or wall (type A2), or inferior orbital rim (type A3). After closed reduction, these fractures are stable; types A2 and A3 may be able to be repaired with closed manipulation. Zingg type B fractures are the classic "quadripod" fractures with a zygomatic bony fragment which is no longer attached, and approximately 17% of these Zingg type B fractures may be able to be repaired with closed reduction. The majority of type B fractures are not stable and require internal fixation, such as with single-point fixation with plate and screws. Zingg type C fractures are comminuted fractures requiring open reduction with internal fixation (ORIF), with plate stabilization.

Importantly, fractures at the zygomaticomaxillary sutures often go through the infraorbital foramen and affect the infraorbital nerve, a continuation of the V2 maxillary nerve, even when the nerve appears intact with patients experiencing numbness or impaired sensation along the cheek, midface, or upper lip [60–67]. Areas the radiologist needs to "double-check" include the upper transverse maxillary buttress at the temporal bone, as fractures in this region can be easily missed.

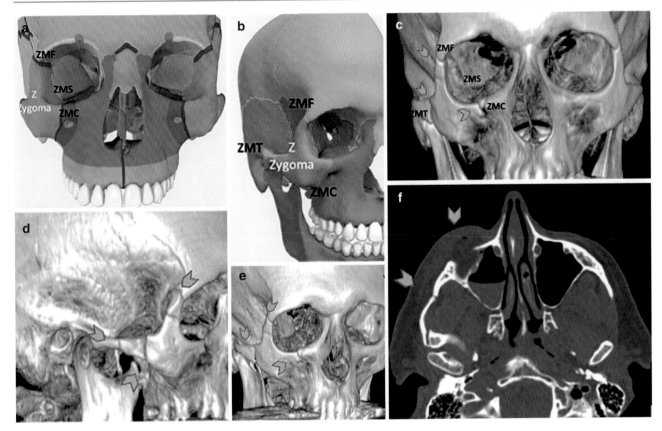

**Fig. 5** a–f. (**a,b**) Schematic of zygoma: There are four suture lines as in Fig. 1c, (**c**) coronal, (**d**) lateral, (**e**) oblique, 3D CT reconstruction, (**f**) axial CT of right ZMC "quadripod" fracture in a 69-year-old woman with a traumatic fall. The quadripod ZMC fracture (green chevron) extends through four suture lines including the ZMC, zygomatico-maxillary; ZMT, zygomaticotemporal; ZMF, zygomaticofrontal; ZMS, zygomaticosphenoid sutures, completely disarticulating the zygoma. (**f**) Axial CT of the same patient: The fractured right zygomatic arch impinges on right temporalis muscle. The fracture involves the right V2 infraorbital nerve, and there is a hemorrhagic air-fluid level in the right maxillary sinus

## Takeaway Points

The zygomas as their name implies are like the yokes surrounding the eyes and create facial width, with four attachment points to the temporal bone, maxilla, sphenoid, and frontal bone; thus, ZMC fractures are "quadripod" fractures, and all sites need to be assessed on CT.

Because the zygoma forms the lateral wall and floor of the orbit, ZMC fractures with displacement will alter orbital volumes, and increased volumes result in posterior globe displacement or enophthalmos.

Fractures along the zygomaticomaxillary suture may affect the V2 infraorbital nerve, even when the nerve appears intact on imaging.

## Orbits

In facial trauma, up to 55% of patients may have associated ocular or orbital injuries, requiring careful orbital assesment [68, 69]. The bony orbit has seven bones including the maxillary, palatine, zygomatic, lacrimal, ethmoidal, sphenoid, and frontal bones, creating a pyramidal pear-shaped cavity protecting the orbital globe (Fig. 6b). The orbits are a transitional zone between the midface and anterior and middle skull base. Anatomically orbital bones encase the globe with a four-sided pyramid measuring approximately 4 cm wide by 3.5 cm high, rotated laterally, exposing the lateral globe margin [71]. The globe extends approximately 1 cm behind the bony rim, and the bony orbital apex is narrowed to a three-sided pyramid approximately 44–50 cm posterior to the globe because of the foreshortened orbital floor [7, 68].

The orbital apex contains critical neurovascular structures including the optic nerve, CNS III, IV, and VI, and branches of V and VII. The orbital medial walls are parallel at approximately 2.5 cm apart, separated by ethmoid sinuses. Lateral bony orbital walls are at a 45-degree angle to the medial wall, creating an orbital volume of about 30 ml; the globe is approximately 7 ml [71]. The orbital globe is encased by three outer layers (Fig. 6a). The retina, the innermost sensory layer, has rods and cones. The middle uveal layer has vascular choroid posteriorly and the ciliary body anteriorly. The outer fibrous sclera continues as the cornea anteriorly. The lens is attached to the sclera by the zonular fibers with an

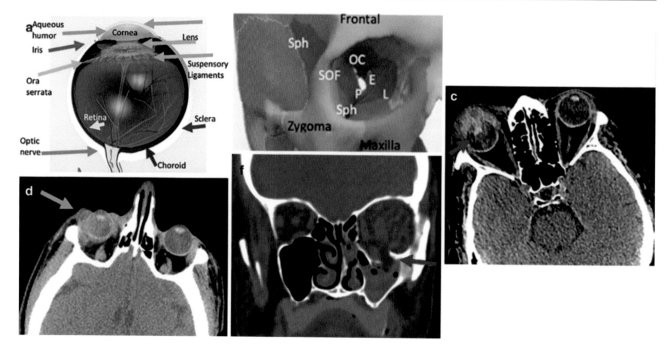

**Fig. 6** a-e. (**a**) Globe anatomy, (**b**) seven bones form bony orbital cone, E, ethmoid; L, lacrimal; P, palatine; Sph, sphenoid, along with frontal, maxilla, and zygoma. (**c**) A 60-year-old woman following a fall. Axial non-contrast CT image shows right globe rupture, with decreased globe volume and posterior lens displacement (red arrow). (**d**) Axial non-contrast CT, 49-year-old man with globe rupture, vitreous hemorrhage, and posterior lens displacement compared to the left side.

(**e**) Coronal CT of an elderly man with edentulous maxilla following a fall with a fractured left orbital floor, orbital conal fat downward herniation, and inferior displacement left inferior rectus muscle. There is loss of normal retrobulbar fat planes and opacification of the left maxillary sinus. The patient is edentulous with maxillary alveolar bony resorption and artificial dental hardware in situ

anterior segment with aqueous humor and posterior segment with viscous vitreous humor. Within the anterior chamber, the iris divides the anterior segment into the anterior and posterior chambers. The orbital cone is formed by the six extraocular muscles with the fascial membranes and contains orbital fat.

Traumatic disruption of ciliary body or iris blood vessels may lead to bleeding in the anterior chamber, with a blood-fluid level, which is referred to as a hyphema [72] (Fig. 6c). Trauma may disrupt the zonular lens attachments resulting in lens dislocation. Orbital lenses usually dislocate posteriorly, as the iris limits anterior dislocations. Spontaneous or minimally nontraumatic lens dislocations may occur in connective tissue disorders including Ehlers Danlos, Marfan's, or homocystinuria [72–76]. In orbital trauma, careful assessment for foreign bodies is necessary as they may lead to infection or disruption of the globe, especially with glass fragments, with the caveat that wood or plastic can resemble air [77]. Ruptured sclera can demonstrate vitreous humor extruding through the defect and loss of orbital volume or intraocular air. In difficult cases with overlying soft tissue swelling, globe disruption may demonstrate decreased posterior segment volume, and the lens on the affected side may move posteriorly by a few millimeters, enlarging the anterior chamber, a subtle but important imaging clue that rupture has

occurred [78, 79]. Trauma may separate globe layers including the inner retinal layer loosely attached to the choroid and tightly attached anteriorly at the anterior ora serrata and posterior optic disk. In a subretinal detachment, vitreous fluid and hemorrhage track into the subretinal space, creating a V-shaped "tulip"-like subretinal fluid collection [80–82]. This finding in pediatric patients requires particularly careful attention as it may result from non-accidental trauma [83]. Because the choroid vortex veins are firmly attached to the ora serrata along the margins, choroid detachments with suprachoroidal transudative fluid or hemorrhage have a biconvex "baseball"-like appearance (Fig. 6d). Severe traumatic injury may also result in carotid cavernous fistulas or optic nerve injuries and may require more advanced imaging with CT angiography, MRI/MRA, or dedicated cerebral angiography.

## Orbital Fractures

Orbital fractures may occur in association with the NOE and ZMC fractures and may also occur in isolation (Fig. 3b–f, 6d). An orbital blowout fracture is a displaced fracture of the orbital wall, which is considered a pure fracture if no rim involvement and impure when the rim is involved [84]. The inferior orbital bony floor is thin, measuring less than 0.5 mm in maximum thickness. Because the thin inferior orbital floor is also weakened by the inferior orbital fissure, it is the most frequent orbital fracture, followed by the thin medial orbital wall, with superior orbital roof fractures occurring least often [85]. Orbital blowout fractures may occur from increased posteriorly oriented hydraulic forces and increased intraorbital pressure, leading to fracture of the weakest orbital margin for pressure relief, with herniation of extraconal fat through the fracture defect [58, 84, 85]. If there is defect in the orbital floor, coronal CT may aid in assessing the fascial sling and inferior rectus displacement into the fracture defect [58, 60, 83–91] (Fig. 6d). Importantly, a "trapdoor" fracture occurs when the inferior rectus muscle herniates through the fracture defect entrapping the inferior rectus muscle. Because the bone fragment may spring back like a trapdoor to its appropriate position, the fracture can therefore be easily overlooked on CT, with the risk of subsequent damage to the inferior rectus muscle. Trapdoor fractures of the orbit with an entrapped inferior rectus muscle require urgent treatment to minimize permanent damage to ocular motility [58, 84–90]. Medial orbital wall fractures may also result in entrapment of the medial rectus musculature and diplopia. Less commonly superior orbital roof fractures may occur, which can result in a dural tear, cerebrospinal fluid leak, or brain herniation, and may best be visualized on coronal CT images. Although orbital apex fractures are less common, these are highly critical cases if there is optic nerve impingement. CT findings including traumatic damage to the globe, retrobulbar hematoma, impingement from bony fragments, or some combination of these findings require urgent communication to the treating physicians and surgeons [58, 82–91]. Traumatic proptosis and increased pressure causing posterior tenting of the globe margin, narrowing it from the normal approximately 160 degrees, is a surgical emergency. Because trauma is the second leading cause of blindness, fast and accurate reliable orbital imaging in the setting of facial trauma is critical. In these cases, computed tomography (CT) in midfacial and orbital trauma is the reference standard for rapid 3D assessment [90, 91].

## Takeaway Points

Facial trauma may have associated orbital trauma greater than 50% of the time, so assess the globes carefully, and be wary of wood or plastic foreign bodies that can mimic air on CT.

Carefully assess the appearance of inferior and medial rectus muscles on CT, especially in the coronal plane.

Pediatric "trapdoor" orbital fractures are surgical emergencies, so as not to lose ocular motility.

Retinal hemorrhages in pediatric patients may be a sign of non-accidental trauma.

## Maxillary Alveolar Process and Teeth

In the maxilla, fractures of the maxillary alveolar process are the most common and may result in disruption of the underlying teeth (Fig. 3f). Dental injury is extremely common, with up to one-third of the population experiencing dental injury in their lifetime in the US population. Anatomically, teeth in the maxillary alveolar ridge have a root covered by the alveolar bone and a crown with an outer hard layer of enamel and deeper layer of dentin surrounding the pulp, with the crown extending above the bony margin where it can be visualized on oral inspection [92] (Fig. 4c). The dentin and central pulp containing the neurovascular component form the root and have a surrounding layer of cementum. The junction of the tooth crown and root is termed the cementoenamel junction or neck. Dental trauma can be classified as either luxation, the most common dental injury in primary dentition, or fracture, which is the most common injury in adult teeth usually involving the crown, with traumatic injury usually affecting the maxillary incisors. Fractures are defined by the affected tooth segment, and if involving the underlying alveolar bone referred to as a dentoalveolar fracture. Fractures of the pulp put the tooth at greatest risk for being nonviable and carry the worst prognosis [92–95].

Classification of dental trauma includes the Ellis system, in which class I trauma only involves enamel and the patient can be followed by a dentist as an outpatient; class II, where yellow dentin is exposed requiring a dressing of calcium hydroxide and wrapping in dental foil, with avoidance of solid food until dental follow-up; and class lll, with dental pulp exposure requiring emergent dental evaluation within 48 hours. Any tooth avulsion ideally should be treated within 2 hours, and reimplantation is more likely to be successful if performed within 1 hour of injury [96]. Dental injury can involve tooth luxation, intrusion, extrusion, or fractures of the root or crown or avulsion of the tooth from the alveolar ridge [92–99].. Because alveolar ridge fractures are open fractures in addition to splinting because of the risk of infection, antibiotics are often needed. If a tooth avulsion occurs, care must be taken that it has not been aspirated with risk for airway obstruction or secondary infection. CT scans may be obtained using either multispiral scanners or cone-beam CT (CBCT) scanners. CBCT is based on a conical beam projected onto one sensor or panel rotating around the subject. Although there is less radiation dose with CBCT, it is limited for tissue assessment; therefore in cases of severe facial trauma that likely affect adjacent soft tissues, a multi-planar CT is a more appropriate imaging modality than a CBCT [98, 99].

## Takeaway Points

Alveolar ridge fractures are open fractures and require antibiotic coverage.

In patients with tooth avulsion, the faster the treatment, the better the outcome, ideally within the first hour after trauma.

Although cone-beam CT has a lower radiation dose and can identify osseous fractures, it has limited ability assessing soft tissue injury; therefore, with complex trauma, a conventional CT is more appropriate.

## Conclusion

The midface triangular region contains the ethmoid, vomer, mandible, and sphenoid bone and the paired, maxilla, inferior nasal concha, palatine, nasal, lacrimal, and zygomatic bones. The "Le Fort subcranial" system is ineffective for high-speed trauma, with limitations in delineating complex zygoma and orbital fractures. This chapter discussed midfacial region fractures and the Le Fort l, ll, and lll classifications, which all involve pterygoid plates, and the current AOCMF classifications of midfacial trauma, which is composed of three levels. The AOCMF levels 1 and 2 localize fractures, and level 3 adds detailed morphology on fragmentation and dislocation [7, 13, 14]. This chapter has also discussed the fractures involving the nasal bones, naso-orbito-ethmoidal (NOE) region, zygomaticomaxillary complex (ZMC), maxilla, and orbit highlighting key anatomical, clinical, and radiographic findings.

## References

1. Lalloo R, Lucchesi LR, Bisignano C, et al Epidemiology of facial fractures: incidence, prevalence and years lived with disability estimates from the Global Burden of Disease 2017 study *Injury Prevention* Published Online First: 08 January 2020. https://doi.org/10.1136/injuryprev-2019-043297
2. Erdmann D, Follmar KE, Debruijn M, et al. A retrospective analysis of facial fracture etiologies. Ann Plast Surg. 2008;60(4):398–403.
3. Allareddy V, Allareddy V, Nalliah RP. Epidemiology of facial fracture injuries. J Oral Maxillofac Surg. 2011;69(10):2613–8.
4. Al-Hassani A, Ahmad K, El-Menyar A, et al. Prevalence and patterns of maxillofacial trauma: a retrospective descriptive study. Eur J Trauma Emerg Surg. 2019; https://doi.org/10.1007/s00068-019-01174-6.
5. Arslan ED, et al. Assessment of maxillofacial trauma in emergency department. World J Emerg Surg: WJES. 2014;9(1):13. https://doi.org/10.1186/1749-7922-9-13.
6. Le Fort R. Etude experimental sur les fractures de la machoire superieure. Rev Chir. 1901;23:208–27.
7. Mast G, Ehrenfeld M, Cornelius CP, Litschel R, Tasman AJ. Maxillofacial fractures: midface and internal orbit-part I: classification and assessment. Facial Plast Surg. 2015;31(4):351–6. https://doi.org/10.1055/s-0035-1563692.
8. Buitrago-Téllez CH, Schilli W, Bohnert M, Alt K, Kimmig M. A comprehensive classificatión of craniofacial fractures: postmortem and clinical studies with two- and three-dimensional computed tomography. Injury. 2002;33(8):651–68.
9. Catapano J, Fialkov JA, Binhammer PA, McMillan C, Antonyshyn OM. A new system for severity scoring of facial fractures: development and validation. J Craniofac Surg. 2010;21(4):1098–103.
10. Zhang J, Zhang Y, El-Maaytah M, Ma L, Liu L, Zhou LD. Maxillofacial injury severity score: proposal of a new scoring system. Int J OralMaxillofac Surg. 2006;35(2):109–14.
11. https://www.aofoundation.org/who-we-are
12. Schlich T (2002). Starting the network. Surgery, science and industry. pp. 28–45. https://doi.org/10.1057/9780230513280_3. ISBN 978-1-349-43181-6
13. Mast G, Ehrenfeld M, Cornelius CP, Tasman AJ, Litschel R. Maxillofacial fractures: midface and internal orbit-part II: principles and surgical treatment. Facial Plast Surg. 2015;31(4):357–67. https://doi.org/10.1055/s-0035-1563693.
14. Gómez Roselló E, Quiles Granado AM, Artajona Garcia M, et al. Facial fractures: classification and highlights for a useful report. Insights Imaging. 2020;11(1):49. Published 2020 Mar 19. https://doi.org/10.1186/s13244-020-00847-w
15. Buitrago-Téllez CH, Cornelius CP, Prein J, Kunz C, di Ieva A, Audigé L. The comprehensive AOCMF classification system: radiological issues and systematic approach. Craniomaxillofac Trauma Reconstr. 2014;7(Suppl 1):S123–30. https://doi.org/10.1055/s-0034-1389565.
16. Kunz C, Audigé L, Cornelius CP, et al. The comprehensive AOCMF classification system: midface fractures – level 2 tutorial. Craniomaxillofac Trauma Reconstr. 2014;7(Suppl 1):S059–S67. https://doi.org/10.1055/s-0034-1389560.
17. Cornelius CP, Audigé L, Kunz C, Buitrago-Téllez CH, Rudderman R, Prein J. The comprehensive AOCMF classification system: midface fractures – level 3 tutorial. Craniomaxillofac Trauma Reconstr. 2014;7(Suppl 1):S068–S91. https://doi.org/10.1055/s-0034-1389561.
18. Kraft A, Abermann E, Stigler R, et al. Craniomaxillofacial trauma: synopsis of 14,654 cases with 35,129 injuries in 15 years. Craniomaxillofac Trauma Reconstr. 2012;05(01):41–50.
19. Mourouzis C, Koumoura F. Sports-related maxillofacial fractures: retrospective study of 125 patients. Int J Oral Maxillofac Surg. 2005;34(6):635–8.
20. Kühne CA, Krueger C, Homann M, Mohr C, Ruchholtz S. Epidemiologie und Behandlungsmanagement bei Schockraum patienten mit Gesichtsschädelverletzungen. Mund Kiefer Gesichts Chir. 2007;11(4):201–8.
21. Erol B, Tanrikulu R, Gorgün B. Maxillofacial fractures. Analysis of demographic distribution and treatment in 2901 patients (25-year experience). J Craniomaxillofac Surg Surg. 2004;32(5):308–13.
22. Motamedi MH. An assessment of maxillofacial fractures: a 5-year study of 237 patients. J Oral Maxillofac Surg. 2003;61(1):61–4.
23. Westfall E, Nelson B, Vernon D, et al. Nasal bone fractures and the use of radiographic imaging: an otolaryngologist perspective. Am J Otolaryngol. 2019;40(6):102295. https://doi.org/10.1016/j.amjoto.2019.102295.
24. Alvi A, Doherty T, Lewen G. Facial fractures and concomitant injuries in trauma patients. Laryngoscope. 2003;113(1):102–6. https://doi.org/10.1097/00005537-200301000-00019.
25. Henry M, Hern HG. Traumatic injuries of the ear, nose and throat. Emerg Med Clin North Am. 2019;37(1):131–6. https://doi.org/10.1016/j.emc.2018.09.011.

26. Holt GR. Biomechanics of nasal septal trauma. Otolaryngol Clin N Am. 1999;32(4):615–9. https://doi.org/10.1016/s0030-6665(05)70159-6.

27. Borner U, Anschuetz L, Kaiser N, Rieke A, Dubach P, Caversaccio M. Blunt nasal trauma in children: a frequent diagnostic challenge. Eur Arch Otorhinolaryngol. 2019;276(1):85–91. https://doi.org/10.1007/s00405-018-5183-1.

28. Marston AP, O'Brien EK, Hamilton GS 3rd. Nasal Injuries in Sports. Clin Sports Med. 2017;36(2):337–53. https://doi.org/10.1016/j.csm.2016.11.004.

29. Hyman DA, Saha S, Nayar HS, Doyle JF, Agarwal SK, Chaiet SR. Patterns of facial fractures and protective device use in motor vehicle collisions from 2007 to 201. JAMA Facial Plast Surg. 2016:455–61. https://doi.org/10.1001/jamafacial.2016.0733.

30. Chou C, Chen CW, Wu YC, Chen KK, Lee SS. Refinement treatment of nasal bone fracture: a 6-year study of 329 patients. Asian J Surg. 2015;38(4):191–8.

31. Nigam A, Goni A, Benjamin A, Dasgupta AR. The value of radiographs in the management of the fractured nose. Arch Emerg Med. 1993;10(4):293–7. https://doi.org/10.1136/emj.10.4.293.

32. Li S, Papsin B, Brown DH. Value of nasal radiographs in nasal trauma management. J Otolaryngol. 1996;25(3):162–4.

33. Ogle OE, Weinstock RJ, Friedman E. Surgical anatomy of the nasal cavity and paranasal sinuses. Oral Maxillofac Surg Clin North Am. 2012;24(2):155–vii. https://doi.org/10.1016/j.coms.2012.01.011.

34. Klinginsmith M, Katrib Z. Nasal septal fracture. In: Stat Pearls. Treasure Island: StatPearls Publishing; 2020.

35. Adnot J, Desbarats C, Joly LM, Trost O. Nasomaxillary fracture: retrospective review of 11 consecutive patients and literature review. J Stomatol Oral Maxillofac Surg. 2019;120(6):534–9. https://doi.org/10.1016/j.jormas.2019.03.003.

36. Hwang K, Wu X, Kim H, Kang YH. Localization of the maxillary ostium in relation to the reduction of depressed nasomaxillary fractures. J Craniofac Surg. 2018;29(5):1358–62. https://doi.org/10.1097/SCS.0000000000004449.

37. Lu GN, Humphrey CD, Kriet JD. Correction of nasal fractures. Facial Plast Surg Clin North Am. 2017;25(4):537–46. https://doi.org/10.1016/j.fsc.2017.06.005.

38. Murray JA, Maran AG, Busuttil A, et al. A pathological classification of nasal fractures. Injury. 1986;17(5):338–44.

39. Holt GR. Biomechanics of nasal septal trauma. Otolaryngol Clin N Am. 1999;32(4):615–9.

40. Kelley BP, Downey CR, Stal S. Evaluation and reduction of nasal trauma. Semin Plast Surg. 2010;24(4):339–47. https://doi.org/10.1055/s-0030-1269763.

41. Puricelli MD, Zitsch RP 3rd. Septal hematoma following nasal trauma. J Emerg Med. 2016;50(1):121–2. https://doi.org/10.1016/j.jemermed.2015.07.016.

42. Landis BN, Borner U. Septal hematoma: always think about it! J Pediatr. 2013;163(4):1223. https://doi.org/10.1016/j.jpeds.2013.06.006.

43. Lee M, Inman J, Callahan S, Ducic Y. Fracture patterns of the nasal septum. Otolaryngol Head Neck Surg. 2010;143(6):784–8. https://doi.org/10.1016/j.otohns.2010.08.027.

44. Imahara SD, Hopper RA, Wang J, Rivara FP, Klein MB. Patterns and outcomes of pediatric facial fractures in the United States: a survey of the National Trauma Data Bank. J Am Coll Surg. 2008;207(5):710–6.

45. Rowe NL. Maxillofacial injuries–current trends and techniques. Injury. 1985;16(8):513–25. https://doi.org/10.1016/0020-1383(85)90076-2.

46. Murray JA, Maran AG, Busuttil A, Vaughan G. A pathological classification of nasal fractures. Injury. 1986;17(5):338–44. https://doi.org/10.1016/0020-1383(86)90159-2.

47. Harrison DH. Nasal injuries: their pathogenesis and treatment. Br J Plast Surg. 1979;32(1):57–64. https://doi.org/10.1016/0007-1226(79)90063-8.

48. Carvalho TB, Cancian LR, Marques CG, Piatto VB, Maniglia JV, Molina FD. Six years of facial trauma care: an epidemiological analysis of 355 cases. Braz J Otorhinolaryngol. 2010;76(5):565–74.

49. Shetty VS, Reis MN, Aulino JM, et al. ACR appropriateness criteria head trauma. J Am Coll Radiol. 2016;13(6):668–79. https://doi.org/10.1016/j.jacr.2016.02.023.

50. Reddy M, Baugnon K. Imaging of cerebrospinal fluid rhinorrhea and otorrhea. Radiol Clin N Am. 2017;55(1):167–87. https://doi.org/10.1016/j.rcl.2016.08.005.

51. Hiremath SB, Gautam AA, Sasindran V, Therakathu J, Benjamin G. Cerebrospinal fluid rhinorrhea and otorrhea: a multimodality imaging approach. Diagn Interv Imaging. 2019;100(1):3–15. https://doi.org/10.1016/j.diii.2018.05.003.

52. Mostafa BE, Khafagi A. Combined HRCT and MRI in the detection of CSF rhinorrhea. Skull Base. 2004;14(3):157–61.

53. Algin O, Hakyemez B, Gokalp G, et al. The contribution of 3D-CISS and contrast-enhanced MR cisternography in detecting cerebrospinal fluid leak in patients with rhinorrhoea. Br J Radiol. 2014;83(987):225–32.

54. Zapalac JS, Marple BF, Schwade ND. Skull base cerebrospinal fluid fistulas: a comprehensive diagnostic algorithm. Otolaryngol Head Neck Surg. 2002;126(6):669–76.

55. Uzelac A, Gean AD. Orbital and facial fractures. Neuroimaging Clin N Am. 2014;24(3):407–vii. https://doi.org/10.1016/j.nic.2014.03.008.

56. Markowitz BL, Manson PN, Sargent L, et al. Management of the medial canthal tendon in nasoethmoid orbital fractures: the importance of the central fragment in classification and treatment. Plast Reconstr Surg. 1991;87(5):843–53.

57. Langner S. Optimized imaging of the midface and orbits. GMS Curr Top Otorhinolaryngol Head Neck Surg. 2015;14:Doc05. Published 2015 Dec 22. https://doi.org/10.3205/cto000120.

58. Wikner J, Riecke B, Gröbe A, Heiland M, Hanken H. Imaging of the midfacial and orbital trauma. Facial Plast Surg. 2014;30(5):528–36. https://doi.org/10.1055/s-0034-1394098.

59. Dreizin D, Nam AJ, Diaconu SC, Bernstein MP, Bodanapally UK, Munera F. Multidetector CT of midfacial fractures: classification systems, principles of reduction, and common complications. Radiographics. 2018;38(1):248–74. https://doi.org/10.1148/rg.2018170074.

60. Hopper RA, Salemy S, Sze RW. Diagnosis of midface fractures with CT: what the surgeon needs to know. Radiographics. 2006;26(3):783–93. https://doi.org/10.1148/rg.263045710.

61. Winegar BA, Murillo H, Tantiwongkosi B. Spectrum of critical imaging findings in complex facial skeletal trauma. Radiographics. 2013;33(1):3–19. https://doi.org/10.1148/rg.331125080.

62. Remmler D, Denny A, Gosain A, Subichin S. Role of three-dimensional computed tomography in the assessment of nasoorbitoethmoidal fractures. Ann Plast Surg. 2000;44(5):553–62. discussion 562–563

63. Leipziger LS, Manson PN. Nasoethmoid orbital fractures: current concepts and management principles. Clin Plast Surg. 1992;19(1):167–93.

64. Manson PN. Three-dimensional CT diagnosis of maxillofacial trauma [comment]. N Engl J Med. 1994;330(1):69.

65. Marinho RO, Freire-Maia B. Management of fractures of the zygomaticomaxillary complex. Oral Maxillofac Surg Clin North Am. 2013;25(4):617–36.

66. Lee EI, Mohan K, Koshy JC, Hollier LH Jr. Optimizing the surgical management of zygomaticomaxillary complex fractures. Semin Plast Surg. 2010;24(4):389–97.

67. Zingg M, Chowdhury K, Lädrach K, Vuillemin T, Sutter F, Raveh J. Treatment of 813 Zygoma-lateral orbital complex fractures: new aspects. Arch Otolaryngol Head Neck Surg. 1991;117(6):611–20. https://doi.org/10.1001/archotol.1991.01870180047010.

68. Poon A, McCluskey PJ, Hill DA. Eye injuries in patients with major trauma. J Trauma. 1999;46:494–9.

69. Bord SP, Linden J. Trauma to the globe and orbit. Emerg Med Clin North Am. 2008;26:97–123.

70. Long J, Tann T. Orbital trauma. Ophthalmol Clin N Am. 2002;15(2):249–viii. https://doi.org/10.1016/s0896-1549(02)00015-9.

71. René C. Update on orbital anatomy. Eye. 2006;20:1119–29. https://doi.org/10.1038/sj.eye.6702376.

72. Kubal WS. Imaging of orbital trauma. Radiographics. 2008;28(6):1729–39. https://doi.org/10.1148/rg.286085523.

73. NovellineRA LT, Jordan J, et al. Computed tomography of ocular trauma. Emerg Radiol. 1994;1:56–67.

74. Netland KE, Martinez J, LaCour OJ, Netland PA. Traumatic anterior lens dislocation. J Emerg Med. 1999;17:637–9.

75. Hardjasudarma M, Rivera E, Ganley JP, McClellan RL. Computed tomography of traumatic dislocation of the lens. Emerg Radiol. 1994;1:180–2.

76. Joseph DP, Pieramici DJ, Beauchamp NJ. Computed tomography in the diagnosis and prognosis of open globe injuries. Ophthalmology. 2000;107:1899–906.

77. Gor DM, Kirsch CF, Leen J, Turbin R, Von Hagen S. Radiologic differentiation of intraocular glass: evaluation of imaging techniques, glass types, size, and effect of intraocular hemorrhage. AJR Am J Roentgenol. 2001;177(5):1199–203. https://doi.org/10.2214/ajr.177.5.1771199.

78. Arey ML, Mootha VV, Whittemore AR, et al. Computed tomography in the diagnosis of occult open globe injuries. Ophthalmology. 2007;114:1448–52.

79. Weissman JL, Beatty RL, Hirsch WL, Curtin HD. Enlarged anterior chamber: CT finding of a ruptured globe. AJNR Am J Neuroradiol. 1995;16:936–8.

80. Mafee MF, Karimi A, Shah J, et al. Anatomy and pathology of the eye: role of MR imaging and CT. Neuroimaging Clin N Am. 2005;15:23–47.

81. Pieramici DJ. Vitreo retinal trauma. Ophthalmol Clin N Am. 2002;15:225–34.

82. Dalma-Weiszhausz J, Dalma A. The uvea in ocular trauma. Ophthalmol Clin N Am. 2002;15:205–13.

83. Garcia TA, McGetric BA, Janik JS. Spectrum of ocular injuries in children with major trauma. J Trauma. 2005;59:169–74.

84. Winegar BA, Gutierrez JE. Imaging of orbital trauma and emergent non-traumatic conditions. Neuroimaging Clin N Am. 2015;25(3):439–56. https://doi.org/10.1016/j.nic.2015.05.007.

85. Vujcich N, Gebauer D. Current and evolving trends in the management of facial fractures. Aust Dent J. 2018;63(Suppl 1):S35–47. https://doi.org/10.1111/adj.12589.

86. Betts AM, O'Brien WT, Davies BW, Youssef OH. A systematic approach to CT evaluation of orbital trauma. Emerg Radiol. 2014;21(5):511–31. https://doi.org/10.1007/s10140-014-1221-5.

87. Chazen JL, Lantos J, Gupta A, Lelli GJ Jr, Phillips CD. Orbital soft-tissue trauma. Neuroimaging Clin N Am. 2014;24(3):425–vii. https://doi.org/10.1016/j.nic.2014.03.005.

88. Go JL, Vu VN, Lee KJ, Becker TS. Orbital trauma. Neuroimaging Clin N Am. 2002;12(2):311–24. https://doi.org/10.1016/s1052-5149(02)00012-6.

89. Felding UNA. Blowout fractures – clinic, imaging and applied anatomy of the orbit. Dan Med J. 2018;65(3):B5459.

90. Caranci F, Cicala D, Cappabianca S, Briganti F, Brunese L, Fonio P. Orbital fractures: role of imaging. Semin Ultrasound CT MR. 2012;33(5):385–91. https://doi.org/10.1053/j.sult.2012.06.007.

91. Sung EK, Nadgir RN, Fujita A, et al. Injuries of the globe: what can the radiologist offer? [published correction appears in Radio-graphics. 2014 Jul-Aug;34(4):8A]. Radiographics. 2014;34(3):764–76. https://doi.org/10.1148/rg.343135120.

92. Loureiro RM, Naves EA, Zanello RF, Sumi DV, Gomes RLE, Daniel MM. Dental emergencies: a practical guide. Radiographics. 2019;39(6):1782–95. https://doi.org/10.1148/rg.2019190019.

93. Andreasen JO, Lauridsen E, Gerds TA, Ahrensburg SS. Dental Trauma Guide: a source of evidence-based treatment guidelines for dental trauma. Dent Traumatol. 2012;28(5):345–50. https://doi.org/10.1111/j.1600-9657.2011.01059_1.x.

94. Alimohammadi R. Imaging of dentoalveolar and jaw trauma. Radiol Clin N Am. 2018;56(1):105–24. https://doi.org/10.1016/j.rcl.2017.08.008.

95. Chauhan R, Rasaratnam L, Alani A, Djemal S. Adult dental trauma: what should the dental practitioner know? Prim Dent J. 2016;5(3):70–81.

96. Ka Louis M, Agrawal N, Truong TA. Midface fractures II. Semin Plast Surg. 2017;31(2):94–9. https://doi.org/10.1055/s-0037-1601373.

97. Kamburoğlu K, Ilker Cebeci AR, Gröndahl HG. Effectiveness of limited cone-beam computed tomography in the detection of horizontal root fracture. Dent Traumatol. 2009;25(3):256–61. https://doi.org/10.1111/j.1600-9657.2009.00770.x.

98. Khan L. Dental care and trauma management in children and adolescents. Pediatr Ann. 2019;48(1):e3–8. https://doi.org/10.3928/19382359-20181213-01.

99. Malmgren B, Andreasen JO, Flores MT, et al. Guidelines for the management of traumatic dental injuries: 3. injuries in the primary dentition. Pediatr Dent. 2017;39(6):420–8. https://doi.org/10.1111/j.1600-9657.2012.01146.x.

# Stroke Imaging

8

Johanna Maria Ospel, Petra Cimflova, and Mayank Goyal

## Contents

### Abstract

Imaging is essential for accurate diagnosis and timely treatment of acute ischemic stroke (AIS), which is caused by an occlusion of an intracranial artery. There are typical findings on imaging that lead toward correct and timely diagnosis. The two major treatment options for AIS patients are endovascular treatment and intravenous thrombolysis, both of which are highly time-dependent.

J. M. Ospel
Department of Radiology, University Hospital Basel, University of Basel, Basel, Switzerland

Departments of Radiology and Clinical Neurosciences, University of Calgary, Foothills Medical Centre, Calgary, AB, Canada

P. Cimflova
Department of Medical Imaging, St. Anne's University Hospital Brno and Faculty of Medicine, Masaryk University, Brno, Czech Republic

Departments of Radiology and Clinical Neurosciences, University of Calgary, Foothills Medical Centre, Calgary, AB, Canada

M. Goyal (✉)
Departments of Radiology and Clinical Neurosciences, University of Calgary, Foothills Medical Centre, Calgary, AB, Canada
e-mail: mgoyal@ucalgary.ca

Thus, the overarching goal of acute stroke imaging is to allow for accurate and fast diagnosis, which, in turn, results in faster treatment and ultimately in better patient outcomes. This chapter will outline the typical imaging findings of AIS and point out some of the pitfalls in acute stroke imaging, with special emphasis on the imaging findings that are of relevance for treatment decision-making and patient management.

### Keywords

Acute stroke · Ischemic stroke · Endovascular treatment · Intravenous alteplase

## Introduction: Acute Ischemic Stroke Epidemiology and Role of Imaging in Acute Ischemic Stroke Management

In the setting of acute ischemic stroke (AIS), imaging is essential for diagnosis and treatment. Based on imaging findings, physicians decide whether and how to treat the patient. AIS is caused by an occlusion of an intracranial artery (approximately 85% of all acute strokes) [1]. There are varying underlying causes of such vessel occlusions, the most common ones being large-artery atherosclerosis (arterial plaques from the aortic arch, an extracranial or a major intracranial vessel, embolize distally, thereby leading to downstream occlusion of an intracranial vessel, so-called arterio-embolic strokes) or cardioembolic (cardiac thrombus fragments, e.g., from a left atrial appendix thrombus, embolize distally). The Trial of Org 10,172 in Acute Stroke Treatment (TOAST) criteria are the most commonly used classification system to categorize AIS etiology and subdivide AIS causes into cardioembolism, small-vessel occlusion, large-artery atherosclerosis, and stroke of undetermined etiology [2]. However, TOAST criteria have recently been challenged, since in many cases that are classified as "stroke of undetermined etiology," a stroke cause can actually be identified with modern imaging tools [3]. Furthermore, the TOAST criteria require a stenosis >50% for large-artery atherosclerosis, but there is increasing evidence that carotid plaques with less than 50% stenosis are an important source of AIS as well [4]. Less frequent causes of AIS include vasculitis, systemic inflammatory diseases, and iatrogenic embolization during surgery or endovascular procedures. While in acute hemorrhagic stroke, the deficits are never fully reversible, and therapy is mainly supportive and targeted at prevention and management of complications, AIS patients can fully recover when recanalization of the occluded vessel is achieved quickly. The two treatment options for AIS are medical treatment with intravenous tissue plasminogen activator (alteplase) and endovascular thrombectomy (EVT) [5]. While the former is quite effective at opening smaller vessel occlusions, recanalizing medium-sized and large vessel occlusions almost always requires mechanical recanalization, that is, EVT [6]. A typical AIS patient with a large vessel occlusion loses 1.9 million neurons per minute if left untreated [7]. In other words, the condition is highly time-critical, and fast treatment leads to better outcomes. How can one decide based on imaging whether a patient suffers from a stroke and which type of stroke it is? How can imaging guide physicians in their treatment decisions? The following paragraphs will provide a practical summary as well as examples of imaging findings in acute stroke, highlighting the key imaging features that need to be recognized in an acute stroke patient. We will mostly focus on CT imaging, since it is widely available, fast, and inexpensive and has almost no contraindications. MRI imaging, which is more time-consuming and less often available in the acute stroke setting, will be briefly addressed as well.

## Imaging Findings of Acute Ischemic Stroke

### Non-contrast Imaging

On non-contrast head CT (NCCT), ischemic tissue appears swollen and slightly hypodense compared to the unaffected parenchyma, and there is loss of the differentiation between gray matter (i.e., the cortex and basal ganglia) and white matter. The Alberta Stroke Program Early CT Score (ASPECTS) can be used to quantify the extent of hypo-attenuation in middle cerebral artery (MCA) strokes (aspectsinstroke.com, Fig. 1). In brief, the MCA territory is divided into ten distinct regions: seven at the ganglionic and three at the supra-ganglionic level. For each area with hypodensity, swelling, and/or loss of gray-white matter differentiation, one point is subtracted; the lower the ASPECTS score, the more extensive the ischemic changes and the higher the risk of intracranial hemorrhage and poor functional outcome despite treatment with IV alteplase or EVT [8]. It is however important to know that not all signs of early ischemic changes on NCCT represent irreversible injury. Some of these changes are reversible if fast and complete reperfusion of the occluded vessel can be achieved [9]. Diffusion-weighted MR imaging (DWI-MRI) relies on cytotoxic edema, which occurs in severely ischemic brain parenchyma, leading to an increase in intracellular volume with a subsequent decrease in extracellular volume. This results in reduced diffusivity of water molecules in the extracellular space, which results in a high DWI signal [10]. Therefore, areas affected by cytotoxic edema appear bright (hyperintense) on DWI and dark on apparent diffusion coefficient (ADC) sequences (Fig. 2). Diffusion restriction is very specific for irreversible tissue damage (DWI-reversible lesions in the context of AIS may occur but are uncommon [11]), and the volume of diffusion-restricted tissue is an independent predictor for outcome following EVT and IV alteplase. DWI imaging turns positive within minutes and is particularly helpful for detection of acute lacunar infarcts and small posterior circulation strokes, which are oftentimes hard to detect on NCCT. However, DWI negative infarcts have been described, especially in the posterior circulation [12].

### Vascular Imaging

By visualizing the vessel occlusion, the diagnosis of AIS can be confirmed, and the clot location can be determined (Fig. 3a), which in turn will guide treatment decisions. Large- and medium-sized vessel occlusions of the intracranial arteries (i.e., terminal internal carotid artery (Fig. 3b), M1 segment (Fig. 3c), A1 and proximal A2 segments (Fig. 3d),

**Fig. 1 ASPECTS regions.** The ten regions of the ASPECTS include the M1, M2, M3 territory, internal capsule (IC), caudate nucleus (C), lentiform nucleus (L) and insula (I) at the ganglionic level (top row), and the M4, M5, and M6 territory at the supraganglionic level (bottom row). For a detailed explanation of ASPECTS and interactive examples, see aspectsinstroke.com

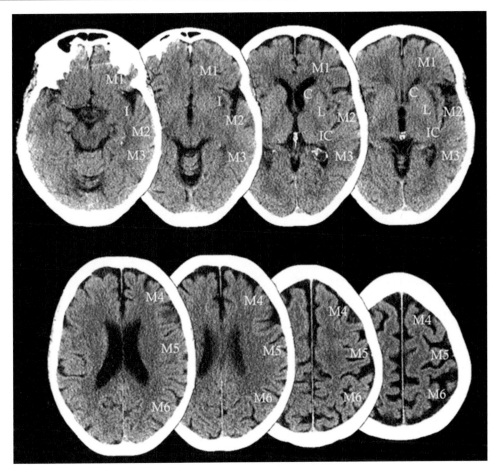

**Fig. 2 AIS on MRI.** An acute infarct in the left middle cerebral artery territory appears hyperintense (bright) on DWI (**a**) and dark on the corresponding ADC map (**b**)

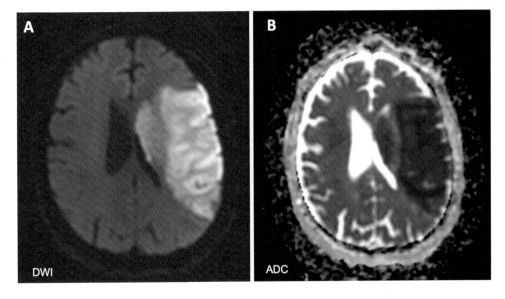

proximal M2 segment (Fig. 3e), basilar artery (Fig. 3f), P1 and proximal P2 segments) are less likely to recanalize with IV tPA alone. These patients will almost always require EVT [6, 13–18]. Distal vessel occlusions have a higher probability to recanalize with IV tPA than large- and medium-sized vessel occlusions. Accurate localization of the vessel

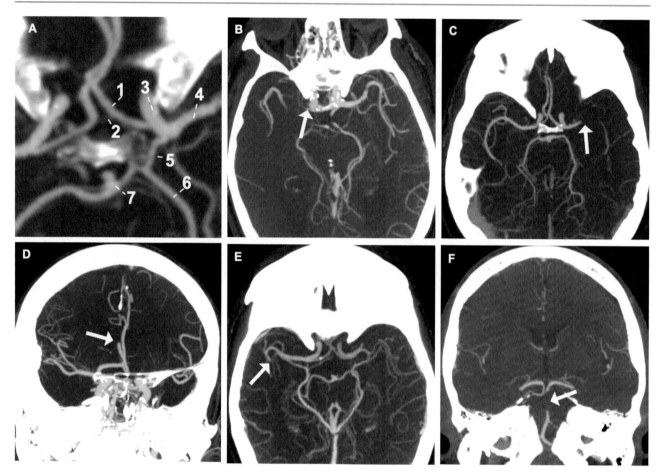

**Fig. 3** **CTA overview of intracranial arteries with examples of large vessel occlusions.** (**a**) Schematic overview of the circle of Willis; (1) anterior cerebral artery (ACA), (2) anterior communicating artery (ACom), (3) terminal internal carotid artery (ICA), (4) middle cerebral artery (MCA), (5) posterior communicating artery (PCom), (6) posterior cerebral artery (PCA), (7) tip of the basilar artery (BA). (**b**) Right-sided terminal ICA occlusion. (**c**) Left-sided M1 segment MCA occlusion. (**d**) Right A2 segment ACA occlusion. (**e**) Right-sided M2 segment MCA occlusion. (**f**) Mid-basilar artery occlusion

occlusion is vital to decide whether a patient is an EVT candidate or not. It is also important to assess the extracranial arterial vasculature in order to choose the appropriate endovascular treatment access and devices. Vascular imaging of intra- and extracranial vasculature (arch-to-vertex) is routinely obtained in AIS patients, which provides useful information about extracranial vessel tortuosity, atherosclerotic disease, and anatomic variants. In CT angiography (CTA), a bolus of iodinated contrast is injected, and a single aortic arch-to-vertex angiography is obtained. In multiphase CTA (mCTA), the same contrast bolus is used to obtain two additional series during the peak-venous and late-venous phase, which cover only the intracranial vasculature (skull base to vertex, Fig. 4). CTA has a sensitivity and specificity of around 97% for large vessel occlusion detection, with high

inter-rater reliability [19]. It can easily be combined with NCCT, is easy to interpret, and is inexpensive. Centers using MRI for acute stroke imaging perform time-of-flight MR angiography (TOF-MRA) to image the intracranial vessels. TOF-MRA relies on the signal of inflowing spins to visualize the intracranial vasculature (Fig. 5a and b). Large vessel occlusions can easily be detected on TOF-MRA, but diagnostic accuracy for medium-sized and distal occlusions is low [20, 21], and it cannot be used to image the extracranial vessels. This is done by contrast-enhanced MRA (CE-MRA), which requires gadolinium-based contrast media. Gadolinium shortens the T1 relaxation time, thereby leading to a high signal in the vessel lumen on T1-weighted sequences (Fig. 5c). Most centers perform CTA rather than MRA, since it is much faster and less susceptible to motion, and as

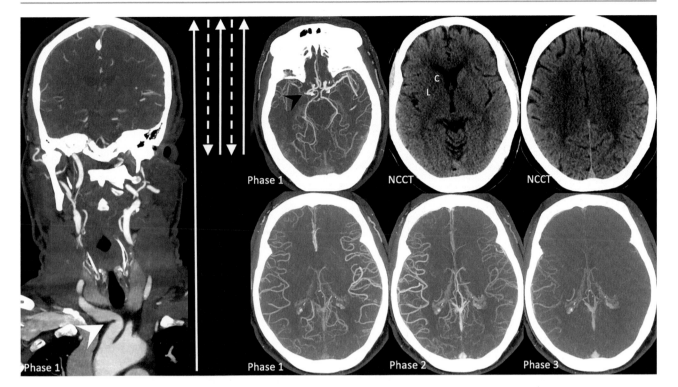

**Fig. 4 CT imaging protocol for AIS.** The non-contrast head CT (NCCT) which is obtained first to rule out hemorrhage and provide a rough estimate about ischemic core shows hypodensity of the right caudate nucleus (C) and lentiform nucleus (L), consistent with a small ischemic core (ASPECTS 8). mCTA (see next section for more details) is then obtained. The first phase that covers the intra- and extracranial vasculature from skull base to vertex (long white arrow in the coronal image of phase 1) shows a right-sided M1 middle cerebral artery segment occlusion (black arrowhead in the axial image of phase 1). It also provides useful information about endovascular treatment access, such as the sharp kink in the proximal brachiocephalic trunk (white arrowhead). The second and third phases cover the intracranial vasculature from skull base to vertex (short white arrows) and show good collateral opacification (for more details on collateral assessment, see Sect. 2.3)

opposed to MRA [22], it is possible to image the extra- and intracranial vasculature at the same time in one sequence.

## "Advanced" Imaging

"Advanced" or "functional" stroke imaging relies on the pathophysiological concept of an ischemic "core" (i.e., irreversibly damaged brain tissue) that is surrounded by the so-called penumbra or tissue at risk, i.e., ischemic tissue that is kept alive through collateral blood flow and not irreversibly damaged yet (tissue which can be salvaged if blood flow is restored/ the occluded vessel is recanalized). In theory, reperfusion of the ischemic "core" will not save the "core" tissue but carries an increased risk of reperfusion hemorrhage [23]. In the early years of advanced imaging, it was thought that reopening the occluded blood vessel is only helpful when the "core" is small and the penumbra is large (so-called target mismatch profile). However, it is increasingly recognized that we lack the ability to accurately identify infarct "core" and that even patients with large infarct "core" can benefit from vessel recanalization with EVT [24].

Multiphase CT angiography (mCTA) is an advanced imaging technique that improves the assessment of collateral flow and severity of ischemia. It is obtained after single phase CTA by adding two additional phases, a peak-venous and late-venous phase that covers the head and intracranial vessels from the skull base to the vertex (Fig. 4). It uses the same contrast bolus that is administered for the single-phase CTA and therefore does not require any additional contrast media. Collaterals on mCTA can be graded with a scoring system (Fig. 6). mCTA collateral score predicts patient outcomes following IV alteplase and EVT, and it can help to select patients for EVT. This was shown in the ESCAPE trial [15], a landmark randomized trial that showed benefit of EVT compared to medical management in AIS patients with proven large vessel occlusion. Collateral scoring on mCTA has good

**Fig. 5 MR angiography imaging in AIS.** (**a**) TOF-MRA, used to visualize the intracranial arteries, shows a right-sided M1 segment MCA occlusion (arrow). (**b**) Post-processed coronal 3D TOF-MRA images of the same patient show the occlusion more clearly (arrow). (**c**) CE-MRA of another patient shows a left-sided cervical internal carotid artery occlusion (arrow)

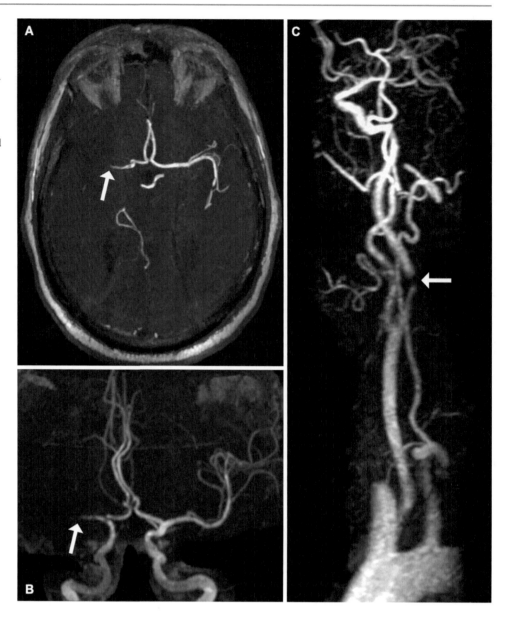

inter-rater reliability, whole brain coverage, is robust against patient motion, and does not require any postprocessing [25].

CT perfusion (CTP) is another popular advanced imaging technique. It can be acquired before or after CTA and requires injection of a second contrast bolus. A slab of 8–16 cm of the brain is continuously scanned again and again over 45–90 s. From these source images, cerebral blood flow (CBF), cerebral blood volume (CBV), mean transit time (MTT) and time-to-maximum of the residue function (Tmax) maps can be calculated. They are typically displayed as color-coded maps (Fig. 7a–d). In theory, ischemic core is characterized by decreased CBV and CBF, and the penumbra shows preserved CBV [26, 27]. Thresholds for ischemic "core" vary (either relative CBV compared to the unaffected hemisphere 0.32–0.34 or absolute CBV of 2 ml/100 g or alternatively

relative CBF compared to the unaffected hemisphere <30% are used as cut-offs), and the variability for penumbra thresholds is even larger [28]. One advantage of CTP is the possibility of automatically obtaining thresholded maps, which are easy to interpret even for physicians with limited experience (Fig. 7e).

Of note, one should be cautious not to over-rely on color-coded perfusion maps, particularly thresholded ones, as they are highly simplistic, and CTP is dependent on complex postprocessing algorithms that are prone to artifacts which can lead to misinterpretation. In a recent study, CTP maps were uninterpretable in 30% of patients [17]. CTP also requires additional time and radiation dose, and we know that CTP-based core and penumbra estimates are often inaccurate [29–31]. MR perfusion relies on the same principles,

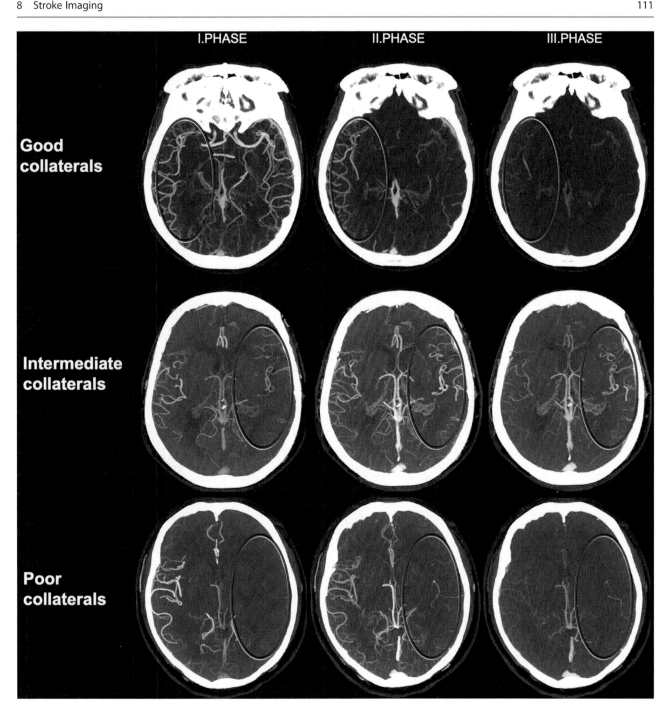

**Fig. 6 Collateral scoring on mCTA**. Top row: Right-sided M1 segment middle cerebral artery occlusion with good collaterals (good backfilling of collaterals in the first phase without significant delay in washout in the third phase). Middle row: Left-sided M1 segment middle cerebral artery occlusion with intermediate collaterals (good backfilling of collaterals in the second, but not in the first phase, slight delay in washout in the third phase). Bottom row: Left-sided M1 segment middle cerebral artery occlusion with poor collaterals (no backfilling of collaterals in the first phase, only very few collaterals visible in the second and third phase)

although image acquisition is more complex than in CTP. The display format of CTP and MR perfusion maps and the thresholds used are similar. Table 1 summarizes the key imaging features along with the clinical patient characteristics that need to be assessed for endovascular treatment decision-making in AIS, and Table 2 provides an overview of the landmark randomized trials on pharmacological and endovascular AIS treatment that formed the basis for current treatment guidelines, including relevant ongoing trials. Of note, no formal evidence exists for patients who were excluded from those trials, but that does not necessarily mean that they do not benefit from treatment.

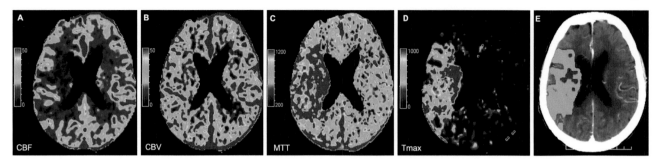

**Fig. 7** CTP imaging in AIS with perfusion abnormality in the right MCA territory in a patient with right-sided M1 segment MCA occlusion. (**a**) CBF map shows a dark blue area on the right side, which is not present on the contralateral hemisphere, indicating decreased CBF. (**b**) CBV map shows no decrease in CBV in the affected territory. (**c**) MTT map shows a red area on the right side, which is not present on the contralateral hemisphere, indicating prolonged MTT. (**d**) Tmax map shows a red and green area on the right side, which is not present on the contralateral hemisphere, indicating an increased Tmax. (**e**) Automatically derived threshold map demonstrating a large estimated ischemic penumbra (green color) and a small area of estimated ischemic core (red color)

**Table 1** Key imaging features and clinical characteristics for endovascular treatment decision-making in AIS [32]

| Suspected acute stroke | | | |
|---|---|---|---|
| NCCT: no hemorrhage, ASPECTS ≥6 | | NCCT: no hemorrhage, ASPECTS <6 | |
| CTA/MRA: LVO and disabling symptoms[a] | CTA/MRA: No LVO and disabling symptoms[a] | CTA/MRA: LVO and disabling symptoms[a] | CTA/MRA: No LVO |
| ≫ Within 6 hours from last-known well: EVT ≫ Beyond 6 hours from last-known well: EVT if advanced imaging shows a target mismatch[c] | ≫ EVT may still be attempted in patients with medium vessel occlusions (MeVOs) | ≫ EVT may still be attempted (EVT for low ASPECTS patients is currently investigated in several ongoing trials) | ≫ EVT may still be attempted, particularly if symptoms are disabling (MeVOs and smaller vessel occlusions usually present with ASPECTS <6 since they supply only a small brain area. EVT for MeVO patients will be investigated in several randomised trials soon) |

In addition, IV alteplase should be administered if indicated, even in the late time window, if mismatch criteria are met[b]. Contraindications for IV alteplase according current guidelines include mainly factors that increase the risk of hemorrhage (e.g., prior hemorrhagic stroke, recent gastrointestinal bleed or malignancy, therapeutic heparinization) [32]
[a]Disabling symptoms defined as NIHSS ≥6. Treatment can also be considered in patients with NIHSS <6 on a case-by-case basis
[b]Diffusion-weighted imaging/fluid attenuation inversion recovery MRI mismatch according to WAKE-UP [33] criteria
[c]Perfusion-based target mismatch according to DAWN or DEFUSE 3 trial criteria [13, 34], although many centers nowadays treat patients beyond 24 hours successfully based on (multiphase) CTA selection criteria

## Hemorrhagic Transformation (HT) in AIS

HT is a frequent complication of AIS, especially after IV thrombolysis therapy and in patient with the history of antiplatelet therapy or oral anticoagulation [44]. HT refers to a spectrum of ischemia-related brain hemorrhage, most commonly affecting the basal ganglia (Fig. 8a). HT can be classified as hemorrhagic infarction or parenchymal hematoma. Hemorrhagic infarction types 1 and 2 represents petechial, punctuate hemorrhages within the infarcted area but with no space-occupying effect. Parenchymal hematoma types 1 and 2 are classified as solid hemorrhage with minor or major mass effect, and especially parenchymal hematoma type 2 is associated with poor outcomes [45].

## Cerebral Venous Infarction

Thrombosis of the dural sinuses and/or cerebral veins is a less frequent type of stroke. It is characterized by venous rather than arterial infarction and accounts for 0.5% to 1% of all

strokes [46]. It predominantly occurs in patients <50 years old and in females. Associated risk factors with the dural sinus/cerebral vein thrombosis are the use of oral contraception, pregnancy, puerperium, recent surgery, trauma, and various prothrombotic states (e.g., coagulation disorders, dehydration, malignancy) [46]. Cerebral venous infarction is caused by fluid extravasation (vasogenic edema development) caused by impaired venous drainage, which results in venous hypertension and eventually leads to cerebral infarction. Venous infarcts are often hemorrhagic, with typical "flame-shaped" hemorrhage (Fig. 8b) [47]. Venous infarcts are located adjacent to venous sinuses and cortical and deep cerebral veins (parasagittal, temporoparietal, deep gray matter). As opposed to arterial infarcts, they frequently cross the borders of arterial vascular territories (Fig. 8b). Although venous infarcts are best seen on a CT or MR venogram, the lack of contrast filling within the affected sinuses/cortical veins can often be seen on CTA (especially in the late phases of mCTA) or CE-MRA as well.

**Table 2** Landmark randomized trials on AIS, including currently ongoing trials

| Trial | Year | Study question | Results |
|---|---|---|---|
| **Pharmacological AIS treatment – thrombolysis** | | | |
| NINDS-tPA [35] | 1995 | Is IV alteplase within 3 hours from symptom onset beneficial in AIS? | IV alteplase improved clinical outcomes despite an increase in symptomatic intracranial hemorrhage |
| ECASS-II [36] | 1998 | Is IV alteplase within 6 hours from symptom onset beneficial in AIS? | IV alteplase did not improve clinical outcomes |
| ECASS-III [37] | 2008 | Is IV alteplase within 3–4.5 hours from symptom onset beneficial in AIS? | IV alteplase improved clinical outcomes despite an increase in symptomatic intracranial hemorrhage |
| IST-3 [38] | 2012 | Is IV alteplase within 6 hours from symptom onset beneficial in AIS? | IV alteplase improved clinical outcomes despite an increase in symptomatic intracranial hemorrhage |
| Effects of IV alteplase for acute stroke on the distribution of functional outcomes: Pooled analysis [39] | 2016 | Meta analysis from nine randomized trials (NINDS-A, NINDS-B, ECASS-I, ECASS-II, ECASS-III, ATLASTIS-A, ATLANTIS-B, EPITHET, IST-3) Is IV alteplase in AIS within 4.5 hours from symptom onset beneficial? | IV alteplase improved clinical outcomes; the earlier that treatment is initiated, the greater the benefit |
| EXTEND-TNK [40] | 2018 | Does IV tenecteplase in addition to EVT within 3–4.5 hours from symptom onset improve outcomes in AIS patients with large vessel occlusion compared to IV alteplase? | IV tenecteplase improved clinical outcomes and reperfusion compared to IV alteplase |
| WAKE-UP [33] | 2018 | Is IV alteplase beneficial in AIS patients with unknown time of onset and mismatch profile on MRI imaging? | IV alteplase improved clinical outcomes |
| **Pharmacological AIS treatment – neuroprotection** | | | |
| ESCAPE-NA1 [41] | 2020 | Is IV nerinetide in addition to EVT within 12 hours from last known well beneficial in AIS patients with large vessel occlusion? | IV nerinetide improved clinical outcomes in those patients who did not receive concurrent IV alteplase (most likely due to a drug-drug interaction that nullified the nerinetide effect in patients with concurrent alteplase treatment) |
| **Endovascular AIS treatment** | | | |
| MR CLEAN [17] | 2015 | Is EVT within 6 hours from symptom onset beneficial compared to medical management in AIS patients with anterior circulation large vessel occlusion? | EVT improved clinical outcomes compared to medical management |
| ESCAPE [15] | 2015 | Is EVT within 12 hours from symptom onset beneficial compared to medical management in AIS patients with anterior circulation large vessel occlusion and moderate to good collaterals? | EVT improved clinical outcomes compared to medical management |
| SWIFT PRIME [42] | 2015 | Is EVT within 6 hours from symptom onset beneficial compared to medical management in AIS patients with anterior circulation large vessel occlusion and absent large ischemic core? | EVT improved clinical outcomes compared to medical management |
| EXTEND-IA [14] | 2015 | Is EVT within 4.5 hours from symptom onset in addition to IV alteplase beneficial in AIS patients with anterior circulation large vessel occlusion and absent large ischemic core? | EVT improved clinical outcomes compared to medical management |
| REVASCAT [18] | 2015 | Is EVT within 8 hours from symptom onset beneficial compared to medical management in AIS patients with anterior circulation large vessel occlusion and absent large ischemic core? | EVT improved clinical outcomes compared to medical management |
| HERMES | 2016 | Meta-analysis of five randomized EVT trials (MR CLEAN, ESCAPE, SWIFT PRIME, EXTEND-IA, REVASCAT) Is EVT beneficial in AIS patients with anterior | EVT improved clinical outcomes compared to medical management |

(continued)

**Table 2** (continued)

| Trial | Year | Study question | Results |
|---|---|---|---|
| | | circulation large vessel occlusion compared to best medical management? | |
| DAWN [34] | 2018 | Is EVT beneficial compared to medical management within 6–24 hours from last known well in AIS patients with anterior circulation large vessel occlusions and a clinical/imaging target mismatch profile on perfusion imaging? | EVT improved clinical outcomes compared to medical management |
| DEFUSE-3 [13] | 2018 | Is EVT beneficial compared to medical management within 6–16 hours from last known well in AIS patients with anterior circulation large vessel occlusions and a clinical/imaging target mismatch profile on perfusion imaging? | EVT improved clinical outcomes compared to medical management |
| DIRECT-MT [43] | 2020 | Is EVT alone within 4.5 hours from symptom onset non-inferior compared to EVT with IV alteplase in AIS patients with anterior circulation large vessel occlusion? | EVT alone was non-inferior compared to EVT with IV alteplase |
| **Ongoing trials – pharmacological AIS treatment** | | | |
| TIMELESS | | Does IV tenecteplase improve outcomes in AIS patients with large vessel occlusion presenting between 4.5 and 24 hours compared to placebo? | |
| AcT | | Does IV tenecteplase improve outcomes in AIS patients who are eligible for IV alteplase compared to IV alteplase? | |
| **Ongoing trials – endovascular AIS treatment** | | | |
| MR CLEAN NO IV, SWIFT-DIRECT | | Is EVT alone within 4.5 hours from symptom onset non-inferior compared to EVT with IV alteplase in AIS patients with anterior circulation large vessel occlusion? | |
| RACECAT | | Does direct transfer to an EVT-capable center compared to transfer to the closest primary stroke center improve outcomes in AIS patients with large vessel occlusion? | |
| TENSION, TESLA, IN EXTREMIS-LASTE | | Is EVT compared to medical management beneficial in AIS patients with large vessel occlusion and large ischemic core at baseline imaging? | |
| IN EXTREMIS-MOSTE, ENDOLOW | | Is EVT compared to medical management beneficial in AIS patients with large vessel occlusion and mild symptom severity? | |
| MR CLEAN LATE | | Is EVT beneficial compared to medical management within 6–24 hours from last known well in AIS patients with large vessel occlusion and moderate to good collaterals? | |

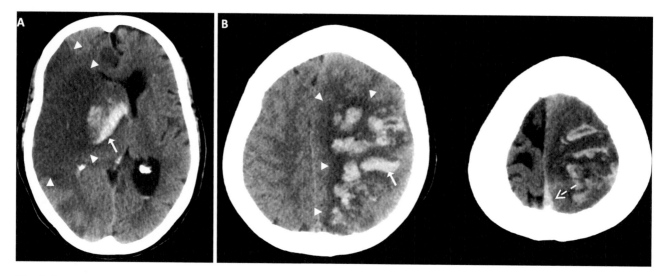

**Fig. 8 Intraparenchymal hemorrhage related to acute ischemic stroke and venous infarction.** (**a**) HT (white arrow) of a large right middle cerebral artery infarct (white arrow heads). (**b**) Hemorrhagic venous infarction in the left frontal and parietal lobe; there are multiple regions of hemorrhage (white arrow) within infarcted tissue (white arrow heads) and a hyperdense superior sagittal sinus (white dashed arrow) representing acute thrombosis of the sinus

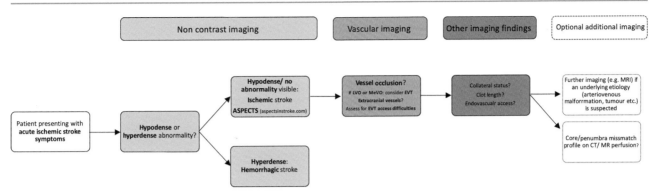

**Fig. 9** Key steps in AIS imaging. Most centers rely on CT imaging in the acute stroke setting; however, the same principles apply to MR imaging-based workflows as well

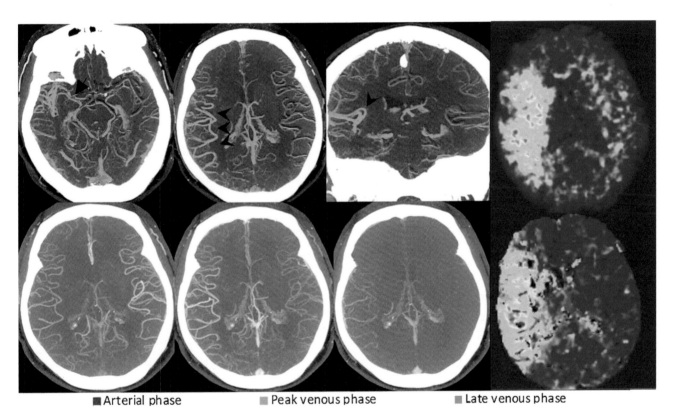

■ Arterial phase          ■ Peak venous phase          ■ Late venous phase

**Fig. 10** Color-coded mCTA maps (three left upper row images) summate all three mCTA phases (shown in the three left bottom row images) in one color-coded map. Vessels with maximum enhancement in the first (arterial) phase are shown in red; those with maximum enhancement in the second (peak-venous) and third (late-venous) phase are shown in green and blue, respectively. This patient presented with a right-sided M1 segment middle cerebral artery occlusion (black arrow); the numerous vessels with predominantly green color that are seen in the color-coded maps (black arrowheads) indicate good collateral backfilling with a one-phase delay. The bottom right image shows the patient's Tmax map that was derived from CTP; the Tmax map that was derived from the mCTA (top right image) looks almost identical

## Summary: Key Concepts in Acute Stroke Imaging

Figure 9 summarizes the key steps in AIS imaging. The first step in a patient presenting with acute stroke symptoms should always consist of non-contrast imaging (CT imaging is preferred in most centers) to distinguish between hemorrhagic stroke, ischemic stroke, and possible stroke mimics. Vascular imaging (mostly CTA) constitutes the second step and is mandatory in AIS patients in order to assess for EVT target occlusions. Additional imaging can be used if necessary, e.g., to evaluate the target mismatch profile in a patient with AIS presenting in the late time window.

# Future Directions in Acute Stroke Management: Simplifying and Automatizing the Imaging Workflow to Allow for Timely Treatment

The numerous different imaging modalities and software solutions that have been developed over the last years and are currently in use in acute stroke imaging have led to lack of standardization and comparability and sometimes even result in misinterpretation of findings. Future efforts should focus on simplification and automatization of AIS imaging. CTP thresholds need to be harmonized throughout different vendors and software packages. Automated ASPECTS scoring based on machine-learning algorithms has been shown to be reasonably reliable [48] and will soon be used routinely in clinical practice. Visual aids, such as color-coded mCTA maps and mCTA-derived CTP-like maps, are promising tools that are obtained within seconds, with very little computational effort, that can help less experienced interpreters and may decrease interpretation time [49, 50] (Fig. 10). Not only imaging-based diagnosis has seen major innovations in over the last years, acute stroke treatment, particularly for AIS, has also made substantial advancements. On the pharmacological side, IV tenecteplase – a genetically modified thrombolytic agent with improved fibrin specificity and longer half-life compared to IV alteplase – has been developed and shown to lead to improved outcomes in AIS patients undergoing EVT in two recent randomized trials, and additional trials are underway. As such, IV tenecteplase could soon replace IV alteplase [40]. Furthermore, the recently published ESCAPE-NA1 trial showed that the neuroprotectant nerinetide is able to improve outcomes in a subset of AIS patients and will hopefully complement pharmacological stroke treatment in the near future [41]. Novel, portable, electroencephalogram, and ultrasound-based large vessel occlusion detection technologies that could be used in the ambulance are under evaluation and might soon allow for faster stroke triage and treatment [51]. Besides these technological innovations, several ongoing randomized trials seek to push the boundaries of EVT indications even further.

In summary, acute stroke treatment options constantly improve, particularly for AIS patients, and so should our imaging tools, because fast and accurate diagnosis is the key to provide the best possible treatment to acute stroke patients.

# References

1. Writing Group M, Mozaffarian D, Benjamin EJ, Go AS, Arnett DK, Blaha MJ, et al. Heart disease and stroke statistics-2016 update: a report from the American Heart Association. Circulation. 2016;133 (4):e38–360.
2. Adams HP Jr, Bendixen BH, Kappelle LJ, Biller J, Love BB, Gordon DL, et al. Classification of subtype of acute ischemic stroke. Definitions for use in a multicenter clinical trial. TOAST. Trial of Org 10172 in Acute Stroke Treatment. Stroke. 1993;24(1):35–41.
3. Kamel H, Navi BB, Merkler AE, Baradaran H, Diaz I, Parikh NS, et al. Reclassification of ischemic stroke etiological subtypes on the basis of high-risk nonstenosing carotid plaque. Stroke. 2019: STROKEAHA119027970.
4. Ospel JM, Singh N, Marko M, Almekhlafi M, Dowlatshahi D, Puig J, et al. Prevalence of ipsilateral nonstenotic carotid plaques on computed tomography angiography in embolic stroke of undetermined source. Stroke. 2020:STROKEAHA120029404.
5. Powers WJ, Rabinstein AA, Ackerson T, Adeoye OM, Bambakidis NC, Becker K, et al. 2018 guidelines for the early management of patients with acute ischemic stroke: a guideline for healthcare professionals from the American Heart Association/American Stroke Association. Stroke. 2018;49(3):e46–e110.
6. Goyal M, Menon BK, van Zwam WH, Dippel DW, Mitchell PJ, Demchuk AM, et al. Endovascular thrombectomy after large-vessel ischaemic stroke: a meta-analysis of individual patient data from five randomised trials. Lancet. 2016;387(10029):1723–31.
7. Saver JL. Time is brain--quantified. Stroke. 2006;37(1):263–6.
8. Olive-Gadea M, Martins N, Boned S, Carvajal J, Moreno MJ, Muchada M, et al. Baseline ASPECTS and e-ASPECTS correlation with infarct volume and functional outcome in patients undergoing mechanical thrombectomy. J Neuroimaging. 2019;29(2):198–202.
9. Bal S, Bhatia R, Menon BK, Shobha N, Puetz V, Dzialowski I, et al. Time dependence of reliability of noncontrast computed tomography in comparison to computed tomography angiography source image in acute ischemic stroke. Int J Stroke. 2015;10(1):55–60.
10. Hagmann P, Jonasson L, Maeder P, Thiran JP, Wedeen VJ, Meuli R. Understanding diffusion MR imaging techniques: from scalar diffusion-weighted imaging to diffusion tensor imaging and beyond. Radiographics. 2006;26 Suppl 1:S205–23.
11. Tortora F, Cirillo M, Ferrara M, Manto A, Briganti F, Cirillo S. DWI reversibility after intra-arterial thrombolysis. A case report and literature review. Neuroradiol J. 2010;23(6):752–62.
12. Edlow BL, Hurwitz S, Edlow JA. Diagnosis of DWI-negative acute ischemic stroke: a meta-analysis. Neurology. 2017;89(3):256–62.
13. Albers GW, Marks MP, Kemp S, Christensen S, Tsai JP, Ortega-Gutierrez S, et al. Thrombectomy for stroke at 6 to 16 hours with selection by perfusion imaging. N Engl J Med. 2018;378(8):708–18.
14. Campbell BC, Mitchell PJ, Kleinig TJ, Dewey HM, Churilov L, Yassi N, et al. Endovascular therapy for ischemic stroke with perfusion-imaging selection. N Engl J Med. 2015;372(11):1009–18.
15. Goyal M, Demchuk AM, Menon BK, Eesa M, Rempel JL, Thornton J, et al. Randomized assessment of rapid endovascular treatment of ischemic stroke. N Engl J Med. 2015;372(11):1019–30.
16. Saver JL, Goyal M, Bonafe A, Diener HC, Levy EI, Pereira VM, et al. Solitaire with the intention for thrombectomy as primary endovascular treatment for acute ischemic stroke (SWIFT PRIME) trial: protocol for a randomized, controlled, multicenter study comparing the Solitaire revascularization device with IV tPA with IV tPA alone in acute ischemic stroke. Int J Stroke. 2015;10 (3):439–48.
17. Berkhemer OA, Fransen PS, Beumer D, van den Berg LA, Lingsma HF, Yoo AJ, et al. A randomized trial of intraarterial treatment for acute ischemic stroke. N Engl J Med. 2015;372(1):11–20.
18. Jovin TG, Chamorro A, Cobo E, de Miquel MA, Molina CA, Rovira A, et al. Thrombectomy within 8 hours after symptom onset in ischemic stroke. N Engl J Med. 2015;372(24):2296–306.
19. Amukotuwa SA, Straka M, Dehkharghani S, Bammer R. Fast automatic detection of large vessel occlusions on CT angiography. Stroke. 2019;50(12):3431–8.
20. Bash S, Villablanca JP, Jahan R, Duckwiler G, Tillis M, Kidwell C, et al. Intracranial vascular stenosis and occlusive disease: evaluation with CT angiography, MR angiography, and digital subtraction angiography. AJNR Am J Neuroradiol. 2005;26(5):1012–21.

21. Hirai T, Korogi Y, Ono K, Nagano M, Maruoka K, Uemura S, et al. Prospective evaluation of suspected stenoocclusive disease of the intracranial artery: combined MR angiography and CT angiography compared with digital subtraction angiography. AJNR Am J Neuroradiol. 2002;23(1):93–101.

22. Demchuk AM, Menon BK, Goyal M. Comparing vessel imaging: noncontrast computed tomography/computed tomographic angiography should be the new minimum standard in acute disabling stroke. Stroke. 2016;47(1):273–81.

23. Jain AR, Jain M, Kanthala AR, Damania D, Stead LG, Wang HZ, et al. Association of CT perfusion parameters with hemorrhagic transformation in acute ischemic stroke. AJNR Am J Neuroradiol. 2013;34(10):1895–900.

24. Roman LS, Menon BK, Blasco J, Hernandez-Perez M, Davalos A, Majoie C, et al. Imaging features and safety and efficacy of endovascular stroke treatment: a meta-analysis of individual patient-level data. Lancet Neurol. 2018;17(10):895–904.

25. Menon BK, d'Esterre CD, Qazi EM, Almekhlafi M, Hahn L, Demchuk AM, et al. Multiphase CT angiography: a new tool for the imaging triage of patients with acute ischemic stroke. Radiology. 2015;275(2):510–20.

26. Allmendinger AM, Tang ER, Lui YW, Spektor V. Imaging of stroke: part 1, perfusion CT--overview of imaging technique, interpretation pearls, and common pitfalls. AJR Am J Roentgenol. 2012;198(1):52–62.

27. Lui YW, Tang ER, Allmendinger AM, Spektor V. Evaluation of CT perfusion in the setting of cerebral ischemia: patterns and pitfalls. AJNR Am J Neuroradiol. 2010;31(9):1552–63.

28. Yu Y, Han Q, Ding X, Chen Q, Ye K, Zhang S, et al. Defining core and penumbra in ischemic stroke: a voxel- and volume-based analysis of whole brain CT perfusion. Sci Rep. 2016;6:20932.

29. McTaggart RA, Ansari SA, Goyal M, Abruzzo TA, Albani B, Arthur AJ, et al. Initial hospital management of patients with emergent large vessel occlusion (ELVO): report of the standards and guidelines committee of the Society of NeuroInterventional Surgery. J Neurointerv Surg. 2017;9(3):316–23.

30. Sheth KN, Terry JB, Nogueira RG, Horev A, Nguyen TN, Fong AK, et al. Advanced modality imaging evaluation in acute ischemic stroke may lead to delayed endovascular reperfusion therapy without improvement in clinical outcomes. J Neurointerv Surg. 2013;5 Suppl 1:i62–5.

31. Schaefer PW, Souza L, Kamalian S, Hirsch JA, Yoo AJ, Kamalian S, et al. Limited reliability of computed tomographic perfusion acute infarct volume measurements compared with diffusion-weighted imaging in anterior circulation stroke. Stroke. 2015;46(2):419–24.

32. Powers WJ, Rabinstein AA, Ackerson T, Adeoye OM, Bambakidis NC, Becker K, et al. Guidelines for the early management of patients with acute ischemic stroke: 2019 update to the 2018 guidelines for the early management of acute ischemic stroke: a guideline for healthcare professionals from the American Heart Association/American Stroke Association. Stroke. 2019;50(12):e344–418.

33. Thomalla G, Simonsen CZ, Boutitie F, Andersen G, Berthezene Y, Cheng B, et al. MRI-guided thrombolysis for stroke with unknown time of onset. N Engl J Med. 2018;379(7):611–22.

34. Nogueira RG, Jadhav AP, Haussen DC, Bonafe A, Budzik RF, Bhuva P, et al. Thrombectomy 6 to 24 hours after stroke with a mismatch between deficit and infarct. N Engl J Med. 2018;378(1):11–21.

35. National Institute of Neurological D, Stroke rt PASSG. Tissue plasminogen activator for acute ischemic stroke. N Engl J Med. 1995;333(24):1581–7.

36. Hacke W, Kaste M, Fieschi C, von Kummer R, Davalos A, Meier D, et al. Randomised double-blind placebo-controlled trial of thrombolytic therapy with intravenous alteplase in acute ischaemic stroke (ECASS II). Second European-Australasian Acute Stroke Study Investigators. Lancet. 1998;352(9136):1245–51.

37. Hacke W, Kaste M, Bluhmki E, Brozman M, Davalos A, Guidetti D, et al. Thrombolysis with alteplase 3 to 4.5 hours after acute ischemic stroke. N Engl J Med. 2008;359(13):1317–29.

38. group ISTc, Sandercock P, Wardlaw JM, Lindley RI, Dennis M, Cohen G, et al. The benefits and harms of intravenous thrombolysis with recombinant tissue plasminogen activator within 6 h of acute ischaemic stroke (the third international stroke trial [IST-3]): a randomised controlled trial. Lancet. 2012;379(9834):2352–63.

39. Lees KR, Emberson J, Blackwell L, Bluhmki E, Davis SM, Donnan GA, et al. Effects of alteplase for acute stroke on the distribution of functional outcomes: a pooled analysis of 9 trials. Stroke. 2016;47(9):2373–9.

40. Campbell BCV, Mitchell PJ, Churilov L, Yassi N, Kleinig TJ, Dowling RJ, et al. Tenecteplase versus alteplase before thrombectomy for ischemic stroke. N Engl J Med. 2018;378(17):1573–82.

41. Hill MD, Goyal M, Menon BK, Nogueira RG, McTaggart RA, Demchuk AM, et al. Efficacy and safety of nerinetide for the treatment of acute ischaemic stroke (ESCAPE-NA1): a multicentre, double-blind, randomised controlled trial. Lancet. 2020;395(10227):878–87.

42. Saver JL, Goyal M, Bonafe A, Diener HC, Levy EI, Pereira VM, et al. Stent-retriever thrombectomy after intravenous t-PA vs. t-PA alone in stroke. N Engl J Med. 2015;372(24):2285–95.

43. Yang P, Zhang Y, Zhang L, Zhang Y, Treurniet KM, Chen W, et al. Endovascular thrombectomy with or without intravenous alteplase in acute stroke. N Engl J Med. 2020;382(21):1981–93.

44. Zhang J, Yang Y, Sun H, Xing Y. Hemorrhagic transformation after cerebral infarction: current concepts and challenges. Ann Transl Med. 2014;2(8):81.

45. Larrue V, von Kummer RR, Muller A, Bluhmki E. Risk factors for severe hemorrhagic transformation in ischemic stroke patients treated with recombinant tissue plasminogen activator: a secondary analysis of the European-Australasian Acute Stroke Study (ECASS II). Stroke. 2001;32(2):438–41.

46. Saposnik G, Barinagarrementeria F, Brown RD Jr, Bushnell CD, Cucchiara B, Cushman M, et al. Diagnosis and management of cerebral venous thrombosis: a statement for healthcare professionals from the American Heart Association/American Stroke Association. Stroke. 2011;42(4):1158–92.

47. Rodallec MH, Krainik A, Feydy A, Helias A, Colombani JM, Julles MC, et al. Cerebral venous thrombosis and multidetector CT angiography: tips and tricks. Radiographics. 2006;26 Suppl 1:S5–18; discussion S42-3.

48. Kuang H, Najm M, Chakraborty D, Maraj N, Sohn SI, Goyal M, et al. Automated ASPECTS on noncontrast CT scans in patients with acute ischemic stroke using machine learning. AJNR Am J Neuroradiol. 2019;40(1):33–8.

49. Byrne D, Walsh JP, Sugrue G, Stanley E, Marnane M, Walsh CD, et al. Subtraction multiphase CT angiography: a new technique for faster detection of intracranial arterial occlusions. Eur Radiol. 2018;28(4):1731–8.

50. Moussady A SA, Al-Sultan A, Maraj N, Najm M, Demchuk A, Goyal M, Menon B. Predicting regional tissue fate in ischemic stroke using color coded mCTA-based collaterals assessment international stroke conference; Hawaii 2019.

51. Forest-Devices. Forest Devices: Alpha Stroke 2020. Available from: https://www.forestdevices.com.

# Imaging of Spontaneous Intracranial Hemorrhage

**9**

Carlos Zamora and Mauricio Castillo

## Contents

**Abstract**

Spontaneous intracranial hemorrhage is a common neurological emergency associated with high morbidity and a case fatality rate between 25% and 48% [1]. Incidence increases with age and is influenced by various factors including hypertension, smoking, and the use of anticoagulation. Hypertensive vasculopathy and cerebral amyloid angiopathy (CAA) represent by far the most common etiologies in the older population. Vascular abnormalities, including ruptured aneurysms and arteriovenous fistulas or malformations, are important causes in younger individuals [2]. In children, arteriovenous malformations are the most common cause of spontaneous intracerebral hemorrhage. Herein, we examine the major conditions that result in nontraumatic intracranial hemorrhage and review the role of imaging in terms of diagnosis and prognostic implications.

C. Zamora · M. Castillo (✉)
Division of Neuroradiology, Department of Radiology, University of North Carolina School of Medicine, Chapel Hill, NC, USA
e-mail: carlos_zamora@med.unc.edu; mauricio_castillo@med.unc.edu

**Keywords**

Intracranial hemorrhage · Intracerebral hemorrhage · Subarachnoid hemorrhage · Hypertensive vasculopathy ·

Cerebral amyloid angiopathy · Arteriovenous fistula · Arteriovenous malformation · Aneurysm

**Key Points**
1. Hypertensive vasculopathy and cerebral amyloid angiopathy are the most common causes of adult spontaneous intracranial hemorrhage.
2. Hypertensive hemorrhages usually involve the deep gray nuclei, brainstem, and cerebellum, while in amyloid angiopathy, hemorrhages are typically peripheral.
3. Vascular abnormalities are an important cause of intracranial hemorrhage in younger patients and require noninvasive and/or invasive imaging for diagnosis.
4. MRI should be used to depict underlying structural abnormalities in patients who are <55 years of age, have no pre-existing hypertension, and present with a lobar hemorrhage.

## Introduction

Spontaneous intracranial hemorrhage is a common neurological emergency associated with high morbidity and a case fatality rate between 25% and 48% [1]. Incidence increases with age and is influenced by various factors including hypertension, smoking, and the use of anticoagulation. Hypertensive vasculopathy and cerebral amyloid angiopathy (CAA) represent by far the most common etiologies in the older population. Vascular abnormalities, including ruptured aneurysms and arteriovenous fistulas or malformations, are important causes in younger individuals [2]. In children, arteriovenous malformations are the most common cause of spontaneous intracerebral hemorrhage. Herein, we examine the major conditions that result in nontraumatic intracranial hemorrhage and review the role of imaging in terms of diagnosis and prognostic implications.

## Role of Imaging in Intracranial Hemorrhage

### Computed Tomography (CT)

Neuroimaging is mandatory in patients with acute neurological symptoms, as the distinction between hemorrhage and ischemia cannot be made on clinical grounds alone. Non-contrast CT is the first-line imaging modality, as it is highly sensitive for the depiction of acute intracranial hemorrhage and allows for rapid assessment of mass effect, herniation, and hydrocephalus. While acute hematomas are hyperdense on CT, freshly extravasated blood has a lower CT attenuation, and therefore areas of hyperacute hemorrhage will appear relatively hypodense. Such areas of low attenuation (including the "swirl sign" and variants) or the presence of two distinct attenuation components (the "blend sign") are independent predictors of hematoma expansion and poor outcomes [3]. The presence of an enhancing focus within a hematoma ("spot sign") on CT angiography (CTA), contrast-enhanced CT (CECT), or MRI is a highly specific predictor of expansion and poor outcomes, although sensitivity decreases after the first 2 h (Fig. 1) [4]. CTA is also highly accurate in the evaluation of underlying vascular anomalies, including aneurysms, arteriovenous malformations (AVMs), and dural arteriovenous fistulas (AFVs).

## Magnetic Resonance Imaging (MRI)

MRI is as sensitive as non-contrast CT for detection of acute intracranial hemorrhage when GRE/SWI sequences are included [5]. Because the CT attenuation of blood decreases over time, MRI is more sensitive for subacute and chronic hemorrhage due to its ability to depict methemoglobin and hemosiderin [6]. The evolution of MRI signal changes over time has been mostly studied with parenchymal hemorrhages. The process is complex and usually begins at the periphery spreading inwards. The MRI appearance is largely determined by the microstructure of the hematoma, as well as the magnetic properties and compartmentalization of the dominant hemoglobin species (i.e., intra- vs. extracellular). Although hematomas have varying degrees of restricted diffusion, this may not be apparent on DWI in the acute and early subacute stages, due to profound T2 effects [7]. Hemosiderin, and to a lesser extent methemoglobin and deoxyhemoglobin, is strongly paramagnetic and appears dark on GRE/SWI, although long T2 relaxation times may affect its appearance in the late subacute stage (Table 1).

Due to its higher contrast resolution, MRI is crucial in patients suspected of having an underlying focal abnormality. A study found a high likelihood of identifying an underlying process on MRI in patients who were younger than 55 years, had no hypertension, or had a lobar hemorrhage [8].

## Cerebral Microbleeds

Cerebral microbleeds (CMBs) are common, with an estimated prevalence between 10% and 25% in aging asymptomatic individuals and up to 68% of patients with spontaneous intracerebral hemorrhage (ICH) [9]. Risk factors include hypertension, CAA, smoking, and decreased serum total cholesterol. Studies also suggest that CMBs may represent an independent risk factor for dementia [10]. Hypertension and CAA are the two most common associated pathologies and show a characteristic spatial distribution which is described below. A small

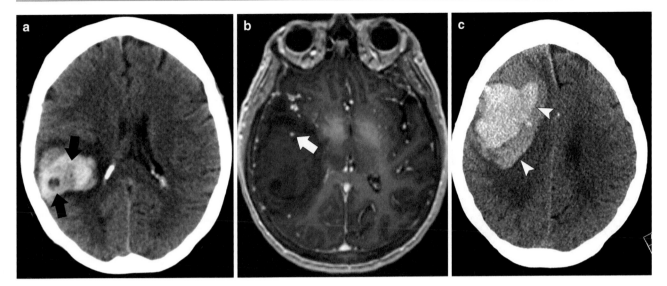

**Fig. 1** Imaging predictors of hematoma expansion. (**a**) Axial non-contrast CT image in a 61-year-old female presenting with lethargy shows a hyperdense hematoma with internal foci of decreased density secondary to active extravasation (black arrows). (**b**) Axial post-contrast 3D T1 MR image obtained several hours later shows that the hematoma has enlarged. There is a small focus of enhancement (white arrow), consistent with a "spot sign." (**c**) Axial non-contrast CT image in an 80-year-old female presenting with left facial droop and dysarthria shows a "blend sign" with distinct areas of attenuation within a hematoma (white arrowheads)

**Table 1** MRI signal intensity changes in ICH over time

|  |  | Dominant Hb species | T1 | T2 | DWI | ADC | GRE/SWI |
|---|---|---|---|---|---|---|---|
| Hyperacute | <12 h | OxyHb | Isointense | ↑ | ↑ | ↓ | ↑ center, ↓ rim[a] |
| Acute | 12 hours–2 days | DeoxyHb | Isointense | ↓ | ↓[b] | ↓[b] | ↓ |
| Early subacute | 2 days–1 week | Intracellular metHb | ↑ | ↓ | ↓[b] | ↓[b] | ↓ |
| Late subacute | 1 week–2 months | Extracellular metHb | ↑ | ↑ | ↑ | ↓ | ↑ center, ↓ rim[c] |
| Chronic | >2 months | Hemosiderin | ↓ | ↓ | ↓ | ↑ | ↓↓↓ |

Note: Hb, hemoglobin; ICH, intracerebral hemorrhage
[a]The dark GRE/SWI rim in hyperacute hemorrhage results from early peripheral conversion to deoxyHb which is paramagnetic. OxyHb is only weakly diamagnetic
[b]Despite the presence of restricted diffusion, DWI is artifactually hypointense due to strong paramagnetic and "T2 blackout" effects. ADC increases in the chronic stage due to facilitated water diffusion
[c]On SWI/GRE, late subacute hemorrhage appears mostly bright centrally due to long T2 relaxation times with a dark rim secondary to early hemosiderin deposition

number of studies suggest an increased risk of intracranial hemorrhage; however, based on current evidence, the presence of CMBs is not a contraindication to intravenous thrombolysis in acute ischemic stroke [11].

## Hypertensive Vasculopathy

Hypertensive vasculopathy is the most common risk factor for spontaneous ICH and frequently affects perforating arteries from the middle cerebral, basilar, and superior cerebellar arteries. These small vessels are thought to be directly susceptible to increased pressures in the parent artery, as they often arise at a nearly 90° angle without gradual tapering [12]. Chronically increased pressures lead to smooth muscle hyperplasia, hyalinization, and fibrinoid necrosis (also called "lipohyalinosis"), which predispose to the formation of microscopic pseudoaneurysms (Charcot Bouchard type) and chronic subclinical leaks, or frank vascular rupture with hemorrhage. Hypertensive hemorrhages favor a central distribution involving the striatocapsular regions (particularly putamen and external capsule), followed by the thalami, brainstem, and deep cerebellar nuclei (Fig. 2, Table 1). Compared to CAA, hypertensive hemorrhage has worse outcomes due to its tendency to involve the brainstem and propensity for an intraventricular extension. The deep hemorrhages seen in hypertension have a lower recurrence rate than the lobar hemorrhages associated with CAA (2.1% vs 15% at 1 year) [13].

**Fig. 2** Hypertensive vasculopathy. (**a**) Axial SWI in a 54-year-old patient with long-standing hypertension demonstrates several microbleeds predominantly in a central distribution (white arrows). (**b**) Axial FLAIR image in a 70-year-old male patient shows a large hemorrhage centered in the right lentiform nucleus (asterisk), with surrounding vasogenic edema and midline shift

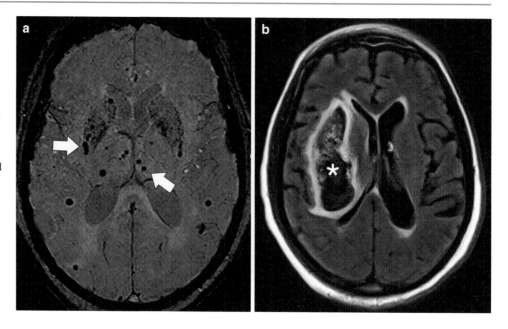

**Fig. 3** Cerebral amyloid angiopathy. (**a**) Axial non-contrast CT image in a 75-year-old male presenting with left-sided weakness and numbness shows a hyperdense acute hematoma in the right parietal lobe (asterisk). (**b**) Axial SWI in the same patient shows profound signal loss within the hematoma due to paramagnetic effects. Additionally, there are numerous microbleeds in a characteristic peripheral distribution (white arrowheads)

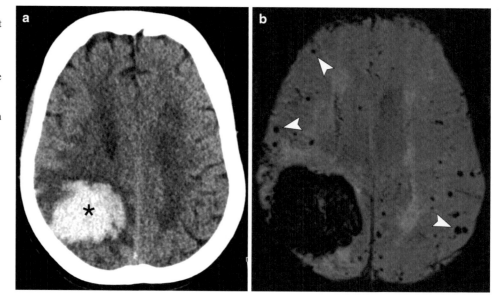

## Cerebral Amyloid Angiopathy

CAA is characterized by the deposition of amyloid-beta peptides preferentially in small capillaries and arterioles along the cerebral cortex and leptomeninges. The amyloid-laden vessel wall degenerates leading to fibrinoid necrosis, microscopic pseudoaneurysms, and subsequent hemorrhage. The disease is strongly age-dependent and, although usually asymptomatic, has been associated with an increased risk of dementia [14]. The widely utilized Boston criteria require a postmortem examination for definite diagnosis; however,

possible or probable CAA can be established based on imaging and clinical grounds [15].

Following the preferential distribution of amyloid-beta peptides, CMBs are typically located along the cortex and most commonly involve the parietal and occipital lobes. Less frequently, they are found in the cerebellum, where they have a superficial distribution along the folia and vermis. In contrast to hypertensive hemorrhage, which has a predilection for deep structures, ICH in CAA occurs in a cortico-subcortical (i.e., lobar) location (Fig. 3). Convexity subarachnoid hemorrhage (SAH) has been increasingly recognized and most commonly occurs along the central sulcus. SAH may occur in isolation and has been associated with an increased risk of recurrent hemorrhage [16]. Superficial siderosis is present in about 40% of patients and is associated with incidental intracranial hemorrhage and poor functional outcomes [17]. The risk for repeat hemorrhages is high, with a cumulative recurrence rate of 21% at 2 years, particularly in patients with a history of previous ICH and a large number of CMBs [18].

## Other Vasculopathies

Intracranial hemorrhage can be a manifestation of a wide range of inflammatory or infectious vasculitides. A study found intracranial hemorrhages in 12% of patients with primary central nervous system vasculitis. These hemorrhages are usually parenchymal but occasionally can be purely subarachnoid [19]. Vasculitis should be suspected as a cause of hemorrhage, in younger patients with small infarcts involving multiple arterial territories, in the absence of other explanations such as embolism. CTA, MRA, and digital subtraction angiography (DSA) may show areas of alternating arterial stenoses and dilatations with a beaded appearance (Fig. 4); however, the sensitivity of this finding is low, and most angiographic examinations are normal. Additionally, reversible cerebral vasoconstriction syndrome (RCVS) can mimic vasculitis on angiography and may present with subarachnoid and less commonly parenchymal hemorrhage. Patients with RCVS classically present with thunderclap headaches,

and their angiographic abnormalities usually resolve spontaneously [20]. Noninflammatory vasculopathy can also be a cause of hemorrhage. In moyamoya disease, this may occur due to rupture of fragile lenticulostriate collaterals or intracranial aneurysms, which have an increased prevalence in this population. Hemorrhage can be intraventricular, intraparenchymal, or rarely subarachnoid [21].

## Hemorrhagic Transformation of Ischemic Infarct

Hemorrhagic transformation can range from minor petechial hemorrhage to frank ICH with mass effect. The reported incidence is highly variable (between 5% and 40%), which reflects study factors including patient selection, time to reperfusion, and accuracy of imaging modalities [22]. Although minor hemorrhages appear to be common with highly sensitive MRI sequences such as SWI, petechial hemorrhages, or small hematomas which occupy <30% of the infarcted territory do not result in worse outcomes. The presence of larger hematomas is a significant predictor of early neurological deterioration and 3-month mortality (Fig. 5) [23]. The most reliable factors that correlate with an increased risk of hemorrhagic transformation are stroke severity (NIHSS ≥22) and large infarct volume on CT or MRI [24]. Areas of hyperattenuation within the infarcted territory are common on non-contrast CT following thrombolysis and usually represent contrast material staining due to

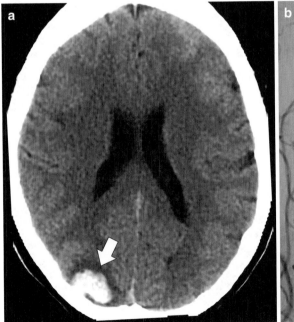
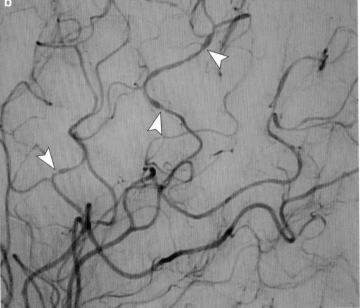

**Fig. 4** Vasculitis. (**a**) Axial non-contrast CT image in a 43-year-old female with severe headaches and seizures shows an acute hematoma in the right parietal lobe (white arrow). (**b**) Lateral view DSA demonstrates alternating stenoses and dilatations (white arrowheads) throughout branches of the middle cerebral artery

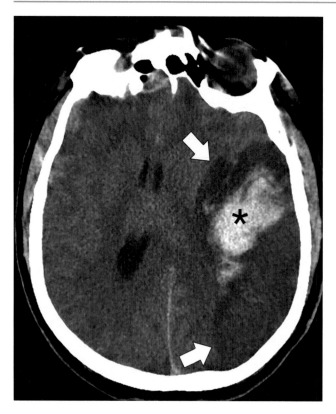

**Fig. 5** Hemorrhagic transformation of ischemic infarct in a 51-year-old male with increasing headaches 1 day after ictus. Axial non-contrast CT image shows an extensive left middle cerebral artery territory infarct (white arrows) with an area of acute hemorrhage (asterisk)

transient disruption of the blood-brain barrier. While differentiating it from hemorrhage may be challenging, contrast staining typically clears on a 24-h follow-up CT. Dual-energy CT has also shown value in this situation, although its availability is currently relatively limited.

## Aneurysmal Subarachnoid Hemorrhage

Aneurysmal rupture is the most common cause of non-traumatic SAH and is a devastating event associated with high mortality and disabling neurological sequelae. It usually presents in patients between 40 to 60 years of age, but children can also be affected. Several complications including vasospasm with delayed cerebral ischemia, intracranial hypertension, hydrocephalus, and seizures contribute to poor outcomes. Thick SAH filling a fissure and cistern and lateral intraventricular hemorrhage are the best predictors of delayed cerebral ischemia due to vasospasm [25]. Patients can rarely present with parenchymal hemorrhage, particularly from middle cerebral and posterior communicating artery aneurysms.

Non-contrast CT can yield sensitivity and specificity of 100% for the depiction of SAH within the first 6 h from headache onset [26]. The sensitivity of MRI is sequence-dependent. Although fluid-attenuated inversion recovery (FLAIR) is sensitive for acute peripheral SAH, its utility is limited in the basal and posterior fossa cisterns due to cerebrospinal fluid pulsation artifacts. However, the combination of FLAIR and SWI sequences is as sensitive as CT [27]. Although initial evaluation for underlying aneurysms can be performed noninvasively with CTA or MRA, DSA is the reference standard and allows for endovascular treatment when indicated (Fig. 6). Up to 20% of patients have no aneurysm on initial angiography, and in up to 17% of them, an aneurysm is found on follow-up angiography which may be performed between several days and 2 weeks after SAH [28]. Most patients with a perimesencephalic pattern of SAH around the brainstem and basal cisterns, without extension into the Sylvian or interhemispheric fissures, do not have aneurysms, and bleeding is thought to be related to venous rupture.

## Vascular Malformations

### Arteriovenous Malformations

An AVM is comprised of anomalous connections between arteries and veins resulting in a vascular nidus, without an intervening capillary bed. The mean age of diagnosis is the fourth decade of life; however, AVMs can present at any age [29]. The majority are single and sporadic, and so the presence of two or more AVMs is highly predictive of hereditary hemorrhagic telangiectasia or RAS mutations [30]. Ten to 20% of AVMs are discovered incidentally, and hemorrhage is the most common complication with an annual rate of 3%, followed by seizures [31]. The most important risk factors associated with rupture are a history of prior hemorrhage, deep location, exclusively deep venous drainage, and associated aneurysms which usually involve feeding arteries [32]. Hemorrhage is most commonly intraparenchymal, but a subarachnoid and intraventricular extension can be present.

Although non-contrast CT is insensitive for the detection of AVMs, the diagnosis may be suspected if the underlying AVM is sufficiently large and accompanied by dilated serpentine vessels which are iso- or hyperattenuating relative to brain parenchyma. Some AVMs may contain hypodense and hyperdense areas of gliosis and dystrophic calcifications, respectively. CTA is highly accurate and demonstrates abnormal feeders and/or draining veins. However, micro-AVMs (those with a nidus <1 cm) which comprise about 10% of surgically treated AVMs may be undetectable without catheter angiography [33]. On MRI, vascular signal voids are best seen on T2-weighted sequences and may indicate the presence of a nidus, feeding arteries, and/or draining veins. MRA is also highly sensitive and specific, and the addition of arterial spin-labeling perfusion and 3D T1-weighted sequences improves the detection of small AVMs [34, 35]. Similar to AFVs, DSA

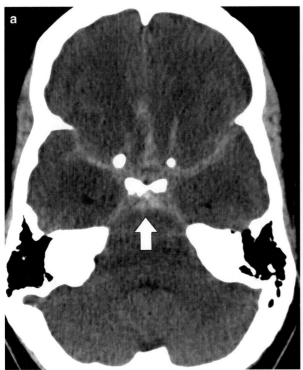 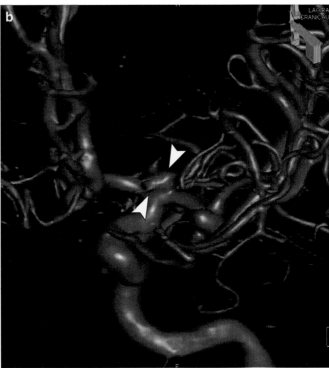

**Fig. 6** Aneurysmal subarachnoid hemorrhage in a 54-year-old female presenting with severe headache, vomiting, and loss of consciousness. Axial non-contrast CT image (**a**) shows extensive hemorrhage centered in the basal cisterns (white arrow) with extension into the sylvian and interhemispheric fissures. (**b**) Frontal 3D reconstruction from DSA demonstrates a multi-lobulated left carotid terminus aneurysm (white arrowheads)

is the reference standard as it allows delineation of the angioarchitecture and flow dynamics and identifies a route for endovascular treatment (Fig. 7; Table 2).

## Arteriovenous Fistulas

Dural AFVs are anomalous connections between dural arteries and dural veins, venous sinuses, or cortical veins without a parenchymal nidus. They are most commonly seen in patients between 50 to 60 years of age and are usually thought to develop secondary to trauma and/or dural sinus thrombosis with the formation of collateral vessels and arteriovenous shunting [36]. The severity of symptoms is determined by AFV location and the pattern of venous drainage. Patients can present with intracranial hemorrhage, seizures, tinnitus, cranial neuropathies, and parkinsonism, among others [37]. Dural AFVs with retrograde flow, or direct drainage into cortical veins, have an aggressive course with an annual hemorrhage rate of up to 8% [38]. Hemorrhage can be intraparenchymal, subarachnoid, and/or intraventricular, and there may be areas of edema from venous congestion or ischemia. CTA or MRA are common initial evaluations and are accurate in demonstrating abnormal clusters of vessels and potential arterial feeders. ASL perfusion is highly sensitive for the depiction of arteriovenous shunting and thus reveals AFVs easily [39]. DSA can determine the presence of cortical venous reflux and identify access for endovascular therapy (Fig. 8). Time-resolved CTA or MRA are alternative noninvasive modalities utilized in some institutions for screening and surveillance.

## Cavernous Malformations

Cavernous malformations (CMs) consist of endothelial-lined, blood-filled sinusoidal spaces without normal intervening brain parenchyma. CMs frequently contain blood at various stages of thrombosis and are surrounded by gliotic tissue and hemosiderin deposits. CMs are more commonly seen in patients with developmental venous anomalies, and their prevalence increases with age suggesting that they may be acquired. After seizures, hemorrhage is the second most common manifestation and occurs at a rate of 2.5% per patient-year; however, up to half of all CMs are discovered incidentally [40]. They are usually located in the hemispheres, followed by the brainstem and cerebellum. The brainstem is the most common symptomatic site and is associated with the highest risk of rebleeding, which tends to occur within the first 2 years [41]. Most CMs are sporadic

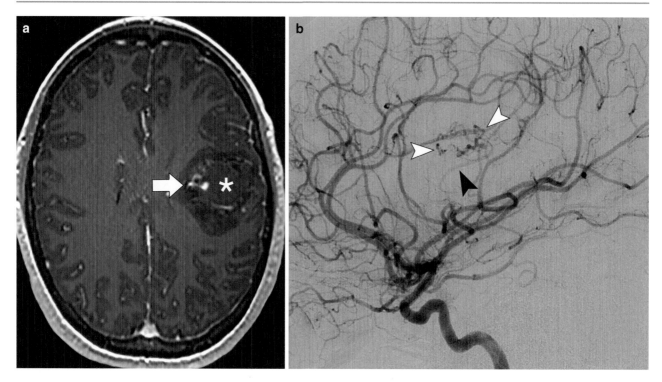

**Fig. 7** Hemorrhagic arteriovenous malformation in an 18-year-old female presenting with aphasia and right hemiplegia. (**a**) Axial post-contrast 3D T1 MR image shows a left frontal hematoma (asterisk) with abnormal vasculature along its medial aspect (white arrow). (**b**) Lateral view DSA shows abnormal vasculature corresponding to the nidus (white arrowheads) and faint early opacification of a draining vein (black arrowhead)

and solitary. Multiple CMs are seen in patients with familial cerebral cavernous malformation syndrome secondary to mutations in the CCM1 (KRIT1, comprising nearly all familial cases among Hispanics), CCM2, and CCM3 (PDCD10) genes. Multiple CMs can also develop following radiation therapy, with a median latency of 12 years [42]. Formation of CMs has also been documented de novo following surgical biopsy and radiosurgery.

CMs may be detected on non-contrast CT if they are sufficiently large or contain areas of thrombosis or calcifications which are common. They show little to no contrast enhancement and are not visible on CTA or DSA due to lack of arterial flow. However, some CMs may be seen on MRA due to the T1 effects of methemoglobin. On MRI, they are frequently lobulated and hyperintense on T2 with a dark hemosiderin rim, resulting in a "popcorn" appearance. Their T1 signal intensity is variable but tends to decrease over time. New T1 hyperintensity, growth, and edema are indicative of rebleeding (Fig. 9).

## Venous Thrombosis

Cerebral venous thrombosis (CVT) most commonly affects individuals younger than 50 years of age. Causes are varied and include transient or chronic hypercoagulable states,

including inherited prothrombotic conditions, pregnancy, dehydration, the use of certain oral contraceptives, infection, and cancer. Most patients present with headaches, which can be complicated by seizures, hydrocephalus, or intracranial hypertension. Hemorrhage occurs in approximately one-third of patients and is the result of increased intracranial pressure leading to venous and capillary rupture. In particular, small juxtacortical hemorrhages (<2 cm) in young patients, in the absence of trauma, are highly characteristic of CVT and are typically secondary to thrombosed cortical veins and superior sagittal sinus thrombosis [43]. Although hemorrhages are usually parenchymal, patients can rarely present with isolated SAH, particularly along the cerebral convexities. Non-contrast CT scan show hyperdense acute thrombus within deep cerebral veins, dural sinuses, or cortical veins with high specificity but only moderate sensitivity [44]. CECT or MRI can show the thrombus as a filling defect (Fig. 10), which may be accompanied by increased collateral vessels. While appropriately timed CECT and MR venography are the modalities of choice, routine non-contrast MRI may reveal the presence of venous thrombosis in the absence of the expected vascular signal void; hyperintense signal on T1, FLAIR, or DWI; or susceptibility effects with blooming artifact on GRE/SWI [45]. DSA is the reference standard but is rarely currently used in the diagnostic workup.

**Table 2** Relevant clinical, epidemiological, and imaging features in various causes of spontaneous ICH

| | Clinical/epidemiological | Imaging |
|---|---|---|
| Hypertensive vasculopathy | Most common risk factor for spontaneous ICH | Central distribution: striatocapsular, thalami, brainstem, and deep cerebellar nuclei |
| Cerebral amyloid angiopathy | Strongly age dependent, usually asymptomatic but associated with dementia | Peripheral distribution: cortex, cortico-subcortical, cerebellar folia and vermis; convexity SAH and superficial siderosis |
| Vasculitis | Younger patients with infarcts in multiple arterial territories | Hemorrhage can be parenchymal or subarachnoid; angiography may show alternating stenoses and dilatations, but sensitivity is low |
| RCVS | Thunderclap headaches | May mimic vasculitis on angiography but findings usually resolve spontaneously |
| Hemorrhagic transformation | Increased risk with NIHSS $\geq$22 and large infarct volumes | Large hematomas (>30%) of infarcted tissue associated with worse outcomes; contrast staining is common after thrombolysis but clears on 24-h follow-up CT |
| Aneurysmal SAH | Most common cause of non-traumatic SAH | Non-contrast CT is highly sensitive for acute SAH; thick SAH filling fissures or cisterns predicts delayed cerebral ischemia; needs angiography to localize aneurysm |
| Perimesencephalic non-aneurysmal SAH | Similar clinical presentation as aneurysmal SAH but often less severe; no vasospasm | Abutting brainstem and basal cisterns without extension to fissures |
| Arteriovenous malformations | Usually sporadic and single; ↑ risk for hemorrhage: deep location, deep venous drainage, and associated aneurysms | MRI with ASL is the most sensitive noninvasive modality; DSA is the reference standard |
| Arteriovenous fistulas | Seizures, tinnitus, cranial neuropathies; AVFs with retrograde flow have aggressive course with ↑ risk for hemorrhage | MRI with ASL is the most sensitive noninvasive modality; DSA is the reference standard |
| Cavernous malformations | Most are sporadic, more common with developmental venous anomalies, multiple abnormalities can be familial or due to radiation | Bright and lobulated on T2 with hemosiderin rim ("popcorn" appearance); new T1 hyperintensity, growth and edema are indicative of rebleeding; not seen on angiography |
| Venous thrombosis | Transient or chronic hypercoagulable states; most patients present with headaches followed by seizures or isolated intracranial hypertension | Typically parenchymal, rarely isolated convexity SAH; CT—increased venous density; CT or MR venogram—filling defect and collateral vessels; MRI—absence of vascular signal void, hyperintense on T1, FLAIR or DWI and blooming on GRE/SWI |
| Neoplasia | Primary (glioblastoma, medulloblastoma, ependymoma) or metastatic (lung, melanoma, breast, renal) | Non-contrast CT—multiple hemorrhages at gray-white interface with greater than expected edema; MRI—contrast enhancement of tumor, mixed signal intensities and delayed evolution of blood products on serial imaging |
| Illicit drug use | Usually cocaine or methamphetamines | Hemorrhage can be parenchymal, subarachnoid, or combined; underlying abnormalities are common |

Note: *ASL* arterial spin labeling, *AVF* arteriovenous fistula, *ICH* intracerebral hemorrhage, *NIHSS* National Institutes of Health Stroke Scale, *RCVS* reversible cerebral vasoconstriction syndrome, *SAH* subarachnoid hemorrhage

## Neoplasia

Intracranial hemorrhage may be the initial presentation of primary or metastatic tumors and is related to factors including angiogenesis, thin and friable vessels, vascular invasion, and tumor necrosis. The most common primary tumor associated with hemorrhage is glioblastoma; however, other malignant and benign neoplasms also have an increased tendency to bleed, including medulloblastoma, ependymoma, pituitary adenoma, and hemangioblastoma, among others [46]. Lung, melanoma, breast, and renal cell carcinoma are the most common tumors leading to hemorrhagic metastases. On non-contrast CT, multiple hemorrhages located at the gray-white matter interface may suggest the diagnosis, particularly

in presence of greater than expected vasogenic edema. Evaluation of underlying neoplasia requires contrast material and MRI is the modality of choice, preferably using 3D T1-weighted sequences. Other features that suggest underlying neoplasia are mixed-signal intensities (a combination of repeated hemorrhages and tumor tissue) and delayed evolution of blood products on serial MRI (Fig. 11).

## Hemorrhage Related to Illicit Drug Use

The two main illicit substances associated with an increased risk of intracranial hemorrhage are cocaine and methamphetamines. Hemorrhage can be parenchymal, subarachnoid, or a combination of both, with or without intraventricular

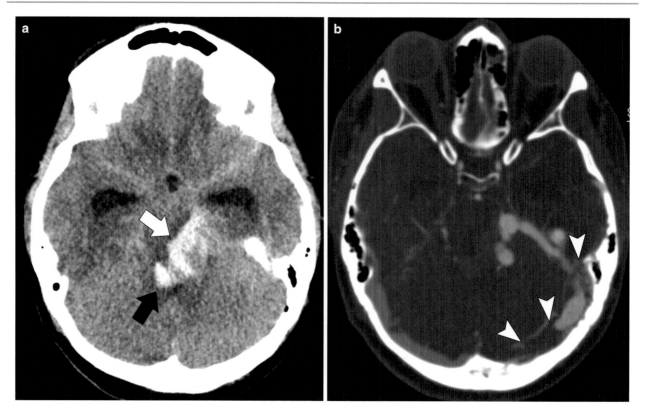

**Fig. 8** Hemorrhagic arteriovenous fistula in a 23-year-old female who was found unresponsive. The patient had a history of dural sinus thrombosis 4 years prior to presentation. (**a**) Axial non-contrast CT image shows a large hematoma centered in the brainstem (white arrow) with intraventricular extension (black arrow). There is obstructive ventriculomegaly.

(**b**) Axial CT venography demonstrates thrombosis of the left transverse sinus (white arrowheads) and a dural fistula at the junction of the left sigmoid and transverse sinuses (white arrow) with drainage into the left petrosal and mesencephalic veins

**Fig. 9** Hemorrhagic cavernous malformation in a 12-year-old presenting with headaches and vomiting. (**a**) Axial T2-weighted MR image shows a hyperintense lobulated focus with a dark hemosiderin rim (white arrow). (**b**) On MRI 2 weeks later, the cavernous malformation has increased in size and shows pronounced surrounding vasogenic edema due to interval hemorrhage

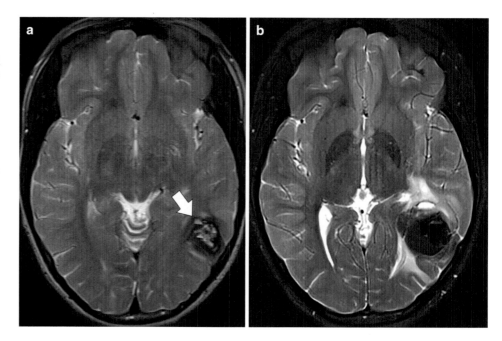

**Fig. 10** Venous thrombosis in a 25-year-old female on oral contraceptives. (**a**) Axial non-contrast CT image shows a large left temporoparietal hemorrhage (white arrows). (**b**) Coronal maximum intensity reconstruction from CT venography shows a lack of enhancement of the left sigmoid-transverse junction (white arrowhead) due to dural sinus thrombosis

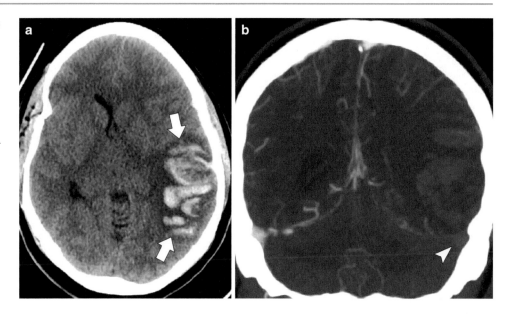

**Fig. 11** Hemorrhagic glioblastoma in a 63-year-old male who was found unresponsive. (**a**) Axial T2-weighted MR image shows a large hemorrhage centered in the right basal ganglia with different signal intensities and marked mass effect (white arrows). There is a midline shift and obstructive ventriculomegaly. (**b**) Axial post-contrast T1-weighted image shows a necrotic enhancing mass along the medial aspect of the hematoma (white arrowheads)

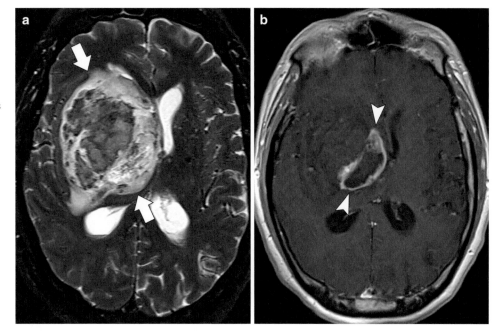

extension. The precise pathologic mechanism is uncertain to our knowledge and is confounded by frequent polysubstance use and the presence of various contaminants that can be found in street drugs. Cocaine is associated with hypoperfusion abnormalities and repeated ischemic episodes which have been proposed as potential mechanisms for hemorrhage. Also, both cocaine and amphetamines are potent sympathomimetics that can lead to abrupt surges in arterial blood pressure and may also induce a vasculitis [47]. Notably, underlying abnormalities are common and have been found in up to 43% of patients with cocaine-related ICH, including

arteriovenous malformations, aneurysms, and neoplasia [48]. A recent large epidemiologic study found that recreational marijuana use was an independent risk factor for aneurysmal SAH [49].

## Conclusion

Spontaneous intracranial hemorrhage can result from several conditions and is associated with high morbidity and mortality. Patient demographics and risk factors are important considerations in the diagnostic workup; however, they are not sufficient to determine the etiology. Neuroimaging plays different roles that vary from assessing acute complications and identifying hemorrhages at risk of expansion to establishing a bleeding source and characterizing underlying abnormalities.

## References

1. Feigin VL, Lawes CM, Bennett DA, Barker-Collo SL, Parag V. Worldwide stroke incidence and early case fatality reported in 56 population-based studies: a systematic review. Lancet Neurol. 2009;8(4):355–69.
2. de Rooij NK, Linn FH, van der Plas JA, Algra A, Rinkel GJ. Incidence of subarachnoid hemorrhage: a systematic review with emphasis on region, age, gender and time trends. J Neurol Neurosurg Psychiatry. 2007;78(12):1365–72.
3. Boulouis G, Morotti A, Brouwers HB, Charidimou A, Jessel MJ, Auriel E, et al. Association between hypodensities detected by computed tomography and hematoma expansion in patients with intracerebral hemorrhage. JAMA Neurol. 2016;73(8):961–8.
4. Dowlatshahi D, Brouwers HB, Demchuk AM, Hill MD, Aviv RI, Ufholz LA, et al. Predicting intracerebral hemorrhage growth with the spot sign: the effect of onset-to-scan time. Stroke. 2016;47(3):695–700.
5. Chalela JA, Kidwell CS, Nentwich LM, Luby M, Butman JA, Demchuk AM, et al. Magnetic resonance imaging and computed tomography in emergency assessment of patients with suspected acute stroke: a prospective comparison. Lancet. 2007;369(9558):293–8.
6. Mitchell P, Wilkinson ID, Hoggard N, Paley MN, Jellinek DA, Powell T, et al. Detection of subarachnoid haemorrhage with magnetic resonance imaging. J Neurol Neurosurg Psychiatry. 2001;70(2):205–11.
7. Shah N, Reichel T, Fleckenstein JL. Diffusion findings in blood clot: the last word? AJNR Am J Neuroradiol. 2004;25(1):157. discussion -8
8. Kamel H, Navi BB, Hemphill JC 3rd. A rule to identify patients who require magnetic resonance imaging after intracerebral hemorrhage. Neurocrit Care. 2013;18(1):59–63.
9. Greenberg SM, Vernooij MW, Cordonnier C, Viswanathan A, Al-Shahi Salman R, Warach S, et al. Cerebral microbleeds: a guide to detection and interpretation. Lancet Neurol. 2009;8(2):165–74.
10. Romero JR, Beiser A, Himali JJ, Shoamanesh A, DeCarli C, Seshadri S. Cerebral microbleeds and risk of incident dementia: the Framingham Heart Study. Neurobiol Aging. 2017;54:94–9.
11. Wang S, Lv Y, Zheng X, Qiu J, Chen HS. The impact of cerebral microbleeds on intracerebral hemorrhage and poor functional outcome of acute ischemic stroke patients treated with intravenous thrombolysis: a systematic review and meta-analysis. J Neurol. 2017;264(7):1309–19.
12. Garcia JH, Ho KL. Pathology of hypertensive arteriopathy. Neurosurg Clin N Am. 1992;3(3):497–507.
13. Hemphill JC 3rd, Greenberg SM, Anderson CS, Becker K, Bendok BR, Cushman M, et al. Guidelines for the management of spontaneous intracerebral hemorrhage: a guideline for healthcare professionals from the American Heart Association/American Stroke Association. Stroke. 2015;46(7):2032–60.
14. Keage HA, Carare RO, Friedland RP, Ince PG, Love S, Nicoll JA, et al. Population studies of sporadic cerebral amyloid angiopathy and dementia: a systematic review. BMC Neurol. 2009;9:3.
15. Greenberg SM, Charidimou A. Diagnosis of cerebral amyloid angiopathy: evolution of the Boston criteria. Stroke. 2018;49(2):491–7.
16. Raposo N, Charidimou A, Roongpiboonsopit D, Onyekaba M, Gurol ME, Rosand J, et al. Convexity subarachnoid hemorrhage in lobar intracerebral hemorrhage: a prognostic marker. Neurology. 2020;94(9):e968–e77.
17. Wollenweber FA, Opherk C, Zedde M, Catak C, Malik R, Duering M, et al. Prognostic relevance of cortical superficial siderosis in cerebral amyloid angiopathy. Neurology. 2019;92(8):e792–801.
18. O'Donnell HC, Rosand J, Knudsen KA, Furie KL, Segal AZ, Chiu RI, et al. Apolipoprotein E genotype and the risk of recurrent lobar intracerebral hemorrhage. N Engl J Med. 2000;342(4):240–5.
19. Salvarani C, Brown RD Jr, Calamia KT, Christianson TJ, Huston J 3rd, Meschia JF, et al. Primary central nervous system vasculitis presenting with intracranial hemorrhage. Arthritis Rheum. 2011;63(11):3598–606.
20. Singhal AB, Hajj-Ali RA, Topcuoglu MA, Fok J, Bena J, Yang D, et al. Reversible cerebral vasoconstriction syndromes: analysis of 139 cases. Arch Neurol. 2011;68(8):1005–12.
21. Liu P, Liu AH, Han C, Chen C, Lv XL, Li DS, et al. Difference in angiographic characteristics between hemorrhagic and non-hemorrhagic hemispheres associated with hemorrhage risk of moyamoya disease in adults: a self-controlled study. World Neurosurg. 2016;95:348–56.
22. Sussman ES, Connolly ES Jr. Hemorrhagic transformation: a review of the rate of hemorrhage in the major clinical trials of acute ischemic stroke. Front Neurol. 2013;4:69.
23. Fiorelli M, Bastianello S, von Kummer R, del Zoppo GJ, Larrue V, Lesaffre E, et al. Hemorrhagic transformation within 36 hours of a cerebral infarct: relationships with early clinical deterioration and 3-month outcome in the European Cooperative Acute Stroke Study I (ECASS I) cohort. Stroke. 1999;30(11):2280–4.
24. Alvarez-Sabin J, Maisterra O, Santamarina E, Kase CS. Factors influencing haemorrhagic transformation in ischaemic stroke. Lancet Neurol. 2013;12(7):689–705.
25. Claassen J, Bernardini GL, Kreiter K, Bates J, Du YE, Copeland D, et al. Effect of cisternal and ventricular blood on risk of delayed cerebral ischemia after subarachnoid hemorrhage: the Fisher scale revisited. Stroke. 2001;32(9):2012–20.
26. Perry JJ, Stiell IG, Sivilotti ML, Bullard MJ, Emond M, Symington C, et al. Sensitivity of computed tomography performed within six hours of onset of headache for diagnosis of subarachnoid haemorrhage: prospective cohort study. BMJ. 2011;343:d4277.
27. Verma RK, Kottke R, Andereggen L, Weisstanner C, Zubler C, Gralla J, et al. Detecting subarachnoid hemorrhage: comparison of combined FLAIR/SWI versus CT. Eur J Radiol. 2013;82(9):1539–45.
28. Jung JY, Kim YB, Lee JW, Huh SK, Lee KC. Spontaneous subarachnoid haemorrhage with negative initial angiography: a review of 143 cases. J Clin Neurosci. 2006;13(10):1011–7.
29. Hofmeister C, Stapf C, Hartmann A, Sciacca RR, Mansmann U, terBrugge K, et al. Demographic, morphological, and clinical characteristics of 1289 patients with brain arteriovenous malformation. Stroke. 2000;31(6):1307–10.
30. Bharatha A, Faughnan ME, Kim H, Pourmohamad T, Krings T, Bayrak-Toydemir P, et al. Brain arteriovenous malformation multiplicity predicts the diagnosis of hereditary hemorrhagic telangiectasia: quantitative assessment. Stroke. 2012;43(1):72–8.
31. Flemming KD, Lanzino G. Management of unruptured intracranial aneurysms and cerebrovascular malformations. Continuum (Minneap Minn). 2017;23(1, Cerebrovascular Disease):181–210.
32. Gross BA, Du R. Natural history of cerebral arteriovenous malformations: a meta-analysis. J Neurosurg. 2013;118(2):437–43.
33. Cellerini M, Mangiafico S, Villa G, Nistri M, Pandolfo C, Noubari H, et al. Cerebral microarteriovenous malformations: diagnostic and therpeutic features in a series of patients. AJNR Am J Neuroradiol. 2002;23(6):945–52.
34. Le TT, Fischbein NJ, Andre JB, Wijman C, Rosenberg J, Zaharchuk G. Identification of venous signal on arterial spin labeling improves

diagnosis of dural arteriovenous fistulas and small arteriovenous malformations. AJNR Am J Neuroradiol. 2012;33(1):61–8.

35. Vella M, Alexander MD, Mabray MC, Cooke DL, Amans MR, Glastonbury CM, et al. Comparison of MRI, MRA, and DSA for detection of cerebral arteriovenous malformations in hereditary hemorrhagic telangiectasia. AJNR Am J Neuroradiol. 2020.

36. Chaichana KL, Coon AL, Tamargo RJ, Huang J. Dural arteriovenous fistulas: epidemiology and clinical presentation. Neurosurg Clin N Am. 2012;23(1):7–13.

37. Gandhi D, Chen J, Pearl M, Huang J, Gemmete JJ, Kathuria S. Intracranial dural arteriovenous fistulas: classification, imaging findings, and treatment. AJNR Am J Neuroradiol. 2012;33(6):1007–13.

38. van Dijk JM, terBrugge KG, Willinsky RA, Wallace MC. Clinical course of cranial dural arteriovenous fistulas with long-term persistent cortical venous reflux. Stroke. 2002;33(5):1233–6.

39. Amukotuwa SA, Marks MP, Zaharchuk G, Calamante F, Bammer R, Fischbein N. Arterial spin-labeling improves detection of intracranial dural arteriovenous fistulas with MRI. AJNR Am J Neuroradiol. 2018;39(4):669–77.

40. Gross BA, Du R. Hemorrhage from cerebral cavernous malformations: a systematic pooled analysis. J Neurosurg. 2017;126(4):1079–87.

41. Taslimi S, Modabbernia A, Amin-Hanjani S, Barker FG 2nd, Macdonald RL. Natural history of cavernous malformation: systematic review and meta-analysis of 25 studies. Neurology. 2016;86(21):1984–91.

42. Cutsforth-Gregory JK, Lanzino G, Link MJ, Brown RD Jr, Flemming KD. Characterization of radiation-induced cavernous malformations and comparison with a nonradiation cavernous malformation cohort. J Neurosurg. 2015;122(5):1214–22.

43. Coutinho JM, van den Berg R, Zuurbier SM, VanBavel E, Troost D, Majoie CB, et al. Small juxtacortical hemorrhages in cerebral venous thrombosis. Ann Neurol. 2014;75(6):908–16.

44. Buyck PJ, Zuurbier SM, Garcia-Esperon C, Barboza MA, Costa P, Escudero I, et al. Diagnostic accuracy of noncontrast CT imaging markers in cerebral venous thrombosis. Neurology. 2019;92(8):e841–e51.

45. Sadigh G, Mullins ME, Saindane AM. Diagnostic performance of MRI sequences for evaluation of dural venous sinus thrombosis. AJR Am J Roentgenol. 2016;206(6):1298–306.

46. Velander AJ, DeAngelis LM, Navi BB. Intracranial hemorrhage in patients with cancer. Curr Atheroscler Rep. 2012;14(4):373–81.

47. Swor DE, Maas MB, Walia SS, Bissig DP, Liotta EM, Naidech AM, et al. Clinical characteristics and outcomes of methamphetamine-associated intracerebral hemorrhage. Neurology. 2019;93(1):e1–7.

48. Tapia JS, J. Case records of the Massachusetts General Hospital. Weekly clinicopathological exercises. Case 27-1993. A 32-year-old man with the sudden onset of a right-sided headache and left hemiplegia and hemianesthesia. N Engl J Med. 1993;329(2):117–124.

49. Rumalla K, Reddy AY, Mittal MK. Association of recreational marijuana use with aneurysmal subarachnoid hemorrhage. J Stroke Cerebrovasc Dis. 2016;25(2):452–60.

# Imaging of Brain Infections

Nader Zakhari, Shivaprakash Hiremath, Paulo Puac, Angela Guarnizo,
Francisco Rivas-Rodriguez, and Carlos Torres

## Contents

**Abstract**

Infections of the central nervous system are potentially treatable emergencies. Imaging plays a central role in the early diagnosis of brain infections and in the detection of related complications, in patients presenting to the ED. While many organisms share non-specific and overlapping manifestations, others have characteristic imaging findings that may allow a prompt confident diagnosis. We describe the manifestations and imaging appearance of the most common acquired acute pyogenic, viral, mycobacterial, fungal, and parasitic infections which may lead to a neurological emergency. Acute opportunistic infections in patients with acquired immunodeficiency syndrome (AIDS) will also be described.

**Keywords**

Abscess · Encephalitis · Bacterial · Viral · Fungal · Parasitic · Mycobacterial

**Key Points**

- Post-contrast FLAIR sequence is the most sensitive sequence for the detection of meningeal inflammation.
- Bilateral asymmetric temporal and frontal signal abnormality is characteristic of HSV encephalitis
- Tuberculoma has different imaging findings depending on its stage with inversely proportional edema to the maturity of the infected focus.
- The eccentric target sign is specific for toxoplasmosis, which is the most common opportunistic infection in HIV/AIDS patients.

N. Zakhari (✉) · S. Hiremath · P. Puac · A. Guarnizo · C. Torres
Department of Radiology, Division of Neuroradiology, University of Ottawa, Ottawa, ON, Canada
e-mail: nzakhari@toh.ca; ppuacpolanco@toh.ca; aguarnizocapera@toh.ca; catorres@toh.ca

F. Rivas-Rodriguez
Department of Radiology, University of Michigan, Ann Arbor, MI, USA
e-mail: frivasro@med.umich.edu

## Imaging of Brain Infections

Infections of the central nervous system (CNS) are potentially treatable emergencies, with the outcome dependent on early diagnosis and treatment. We describe the manifestations and imaging appearance of the most common acquired acute

© Springer Nature Switzerland AG 2022
M. N. Patlas et al. (eds.), *Atlas of Emergency Imaging from Head-to-Toe*,
https://doi.org/10.1007/978-3-030-92111-8_10

pyogenic, viral, mycobacterial, fungal, and parasitic infections which may lead to a neurological emergency. Acute opportunistic infections in patients with acquired immunodeficiency syndrome (AIDS) will also be described.

## Acute Pyogenic Infections

**Acute bacterial meningitis** (ABM): ABM is characterized by meningeal inflammation, typically involving the pia and arachnoid mater. Group B streptococci and coliform bacteria in neonates and *Streptococcus pneumoniae, Neisseria meningitides*, and *Haemophilus influenzae* in children and adults are the most common pathogens. Widespread immunization and immunosuppressed states have led to an increased incidence of *Listeria, Staphylococcus*, and gram-negative bacteria meningitis [1].

Organisms may spread to the CNS hematogenously or by contiguous extension from sinusitis and otitis/mastoiditis or by direct seeding secondary to surgery and trauma [1, 2]. ABM results in proteinaceous exudates and pus accumulation in the cerebrospinal fluid (CSF), blocking CSF resorption leading to communicating hydrocephalus. It can also lead to arteritis and vasospasm, with ensuing infarcts and microhemorrhages. The purulent accumulation in the ventricles results in ventriculitis, ependymitis, and choroid plexitis.

In early ABM, computed tomography (CT) has high false-negative rates especially on routine non-contrast scans in the ED [1–3]. However, with disease progression, more conspicuous leptomeningeal enhancement and hydrocephalus can be seen on contrast-enhanced CT. Magnetic resonance imaging (MRI) is a sensitive modality for the detection of meningeal inflammation with fluid-attenuation inversion recovery (FLAIR) sulcal hyperintensity suggesting proteinaceous and inflammatory exudates and IV contrast-enhanced T1-weighted imaging (T1WI) showing leptomeningeal enhancement. Post-contrast FLAIR is the best sequence for the detection of meningitis compared to magnetization transfer and fat-saturated T1WI [4] (Fig. 1). Diffusion-weighted imaging (DWI) may demonstrate dependent hyperintensities representing purulent fluid, within the ventricles, perivascular spaces, and cortical sulci (Fig. 2).

Communicating hydrocephalus is the most common complication in ABM. Salient early imaging findings include dilatation of the temporal horns of the lateral ventricles,

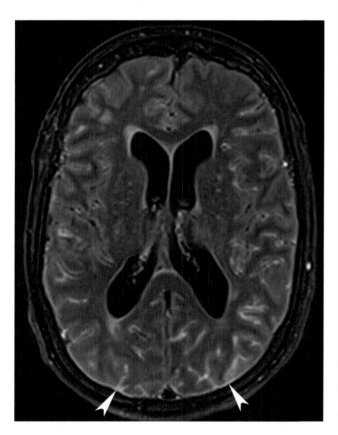

**Fig. 1** *Streptococcus pneumoniae* meningitis in a 42-year-old man. Axial post-contrast FLAIR MR image shows diffuse leptomeningeal enhancement (arrowheads). No definite enhancement was seen on post-contrast T1WI (not shown)

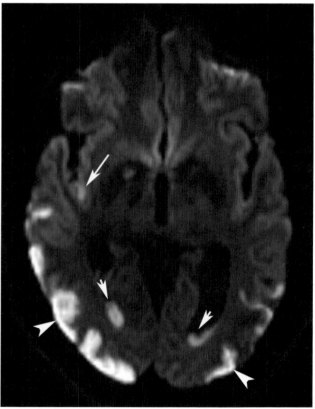

**Fig. 2** *Streptococcus pneumoniae* meningitis complicated with ventriculitis and cortical infarction in a 69-year-old man. Axial DWI image shows restricted diffusion in the right Sylvian fissure (long arrow), as well as within the occipital horns (suggesting ventriculitis, short arrows). Associated bilateral occipitotemporal cortical diffusion restriction (arrowheads) is noted, in keeping with cortical infarcts

with associated transependymal CSF migration in a minority of cases, potentially needing ventricular drainage as the disease progresses [1].

Meningitis may result in vasculitis in 25% of cases [5]. Due to the proclivity to involve the perivascular spaces, infarcts commonly affect the basal ganglia as a complication of meningitis. The involvement of the medium-sized arteries leads to cortical infarctions [1, 5] (Fig. 2). CT and MR angiography may demonstrate narrowing or occlusion of the involved arteries [1].

**Cerebral abscess** is a focal infection of the brain parenchyma, which begins as localized inflammation (cerebritis), and evolves into an encapsulated purulent collection. It is usually caused by a single pathogen, commonly streptococci, staphylococci, and gram-negative bacteria, with polymicrobial infection accounting for ~25% of cases [6].

Cerebral abscess evolves through four stages: early cerebritis (<7 days) with neutrophilic infiltration causing cerebral edema and mass effect; late cerebritis (7–14 days) with blood-brain barrier breakdown and fibroblast accumulation along the margins; and early and late capsule stages (2–4 weeks), when fibroblast induced reticulin matrix evolves to mature collagen, with eventual capsulation and abscess formation [3, 7].

The early and late cerebritis stages demonstrate ill-defined T2 and FLAIR hyperintensity, with irregular, patchy, or nodular enhancement. In the later stages, the capsule is hyperintense on T1WI and hypointense on T2WI owing to free radicals and inflammatory infiltrates, with smooth rim enhancement. The abscess cavity shows restricted diffusion due to the high viscosity of the pus (Fig. 3). Another imaging finding allowing the differentiation of abscess from other ring-enhancing lesions is that the abscess wall is thinner medially due to decreased blood supply, which increases the risk of rupture into the ventricles [1, 3, 7].

The "dual rim sign" seen on susceptibility-weighted imaging (SWI), i.e., a concentric outer hypointense and inner hyperintense rim relative to the intracavitary contents, is typical for a pyogenic abscess [8] (Fig. 3c). Perfusion MRI typically shows low regional cerebral blood volume due to decreased vascularity and mature collagen. MR spectroscopy shows amino acid (valine, leucine, and isoleucine), lipid, and lactate peaks with or without acetate and succinate peaks [7, 9, 10].

**Ventriculitis** may be secondary to rupture of an abscess into the ventricles, or it may occur after the retrograde spread of infection from basal meningitis, hematogenous spread to the subependyma, or choroid plexus, or through direct seeding (e.g., postoperative). Typically, ventriculitis shows layering dependent restricted diffusion and FLAIR hyperintensity in enlarged ventricles strongly suggestive of pus and debris (Fig. 2). Other findings include circumferential T2/FLAIR periventricular white matter hyperintensity, ependymal enhancement, asymmetric enlargement, and enhancement of the choroid plexus [11].

**Extra-axial fluid collections** (EFCs) are either epidural or subdural and develop in up to one-third of patients with meningitis, more commonly in children [1]. EFCs also occur secondary to complicated sinusitis, otitis, and/or mastoiditis [3]. They are generally large, frequently occur in the frontal and temporal regions, and are either sterile or purulent. The sterile effusions follow CSF attenuation and signal

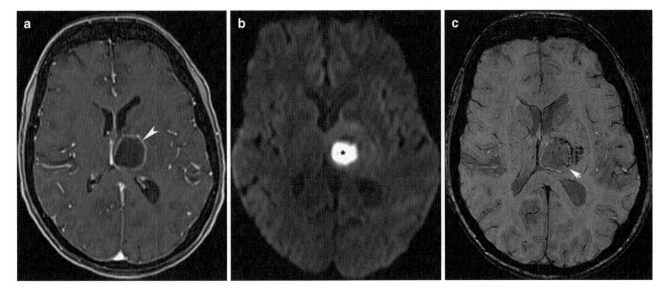

**Fig. 3** *Streptococcus intermedius* cerebral abscess in a 68-year-old woman. Axial post-contrast T1W (**a**), DWI (**b**), and SWI (**c**) MR images show ring-enhancing left thalamic focus (**a**, arrowhead) with central restricted diffusion (**b**, asterisk). SWI image shows the dual rim sign (**c**, arrow) with outer hypointense and inner hyperintense rims

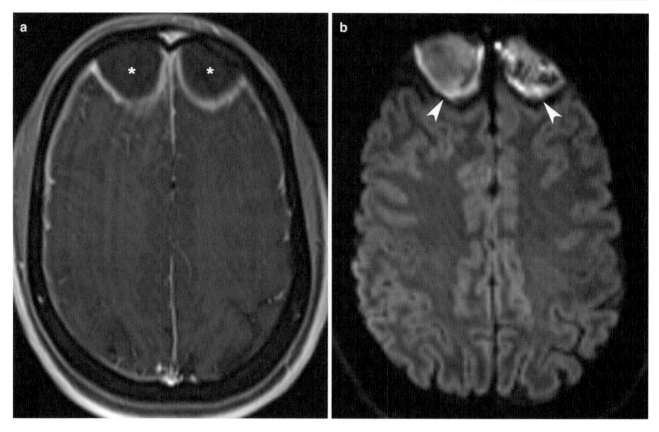

**Fig. 4** Streptococcus bifrontal empyema in a 20-year-old woman. Axial post-contrast T1WI (**a**) and DWI MR (**b**) images show bifrontal rim-enhancing extra-axial collections (**a**, asterisk) with restricted diffusion (**b**, arrowheads)

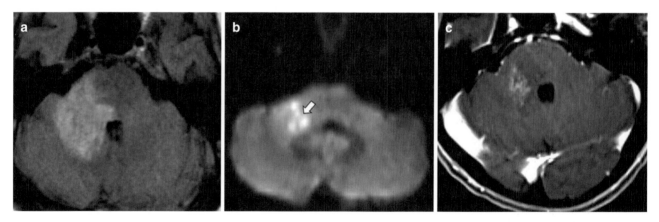

**Fig. 5** Listeria rhombencephalitis in a 52-year-old man. Axial FLAIR (**a**), DWI (**b**), and post-contrast T1WI MR images show mildly expansile FLAIR hyperintensity involving the right pons, middle cerebellar peduncle, and anterior right cerebellar hemisphere (**a**). There are areas of central diffusion restriction within the right middle cerebellar peduncle (**b**, arrows), with heterogeneous enhancement and central non-enhancing components (**c**), in keeping with early abscess formation

characteristics on CT and MRI, respectively. However, they may show a slightly higher signal on FLAIR owing to elevated protein concentration. About 15% of sterile effusions progress to empyemas. Empyemas demonstrate restricted diffusion with a thick rim of enhancement compared with sterile effusions (Fig. 4). Sterile effusions are managed conservatively contrary to empyemas, which require surgical drainage [1, 3].

**Listeria rhombencephalitis:** Listeriosis is caused by the ubiquitous, foodborne, gram-positive bacterium *Listeria monocytogenes*. Listeriosis affects all age groups [12, 13]. In healthy individuals, it usually causes self-limited febrile gastroenteritis. However, patients with impaired immunity may develop invasive listeriosis with sepsis or CNS infections in 60% and 30% of the cases, respectively [12]. CNS infections can present as nonspecific meningitis, meningoencephalitis, rhombencephalitis, or abscess formation. On MRI, rhombencephalitis typically presents as T2 hyperintensity in the brainstem, cerebellar peduncles, and/or cerebellar hemispheres [14] (Fig. 5). Ring enhancement with central diffusion restriction on DWI indicates abscess formation which may be solitary (70%) or multiple (30%) and are located mainly in the pons, thalami, medulla, or subcortical white matter [14] (Fig. 5). The encephalitic form may show findings similar to those of herpes simplex encephalitis (HSE), with involvement of the mesial temporal lobes and insula. This latter presentation can be differentiated from HSE by the additional involvement of the basal ganglia in listeriosis, which is unusual in HSE [14, 15].

## Acute Viral Infections

**Herpes simplex encephalitis (HSE):** HSV-1 and HSV-2 are DNA viruses from the *Herpesviridae* family [16]. HSE is one of the most severe manifestations of these agents with a mortality of 70–90%, if untreated [17]. HSE is caused by HSV-1 in 90% of the cases, with an estimated incidence of 2–4 cases per million population [17]. The virus enters the CNS by retrograde transport from the nasopharyngeal mucosa through the trigeminal nerves [16]. The typical presentation consists of fever (>38°), headache, disorientation,

seizures, and signs of meningitis with a median patient's age of 50 years [15, 17]. The diagnosis is made based on clinical findings, CSF analysis, and MRI.

MRI is more sensitive than CT and enables earlier detection of the disease with abnormality seen on MRI in approximately 75% of patients, as opposed to 40% on CT [17]. On MRI, T2 and FLAIR hyperintensities are typically seen involving the cortex and subcortical white matter of the temporal (70%) and frontal (20%) lobes, followed by the insular and cingulate cortexes [15] (Fig. 6). Bilateral asymmetric distribution is characteristic, but the involvement can be unilateral early in the disease [15, 17]. The lentiform nuclei are typically spared. Isolated signal changes on DWI can be present in the early stage of the disease [17]. Petechial hemorrhage can be seen in 11% of the cases as foci of blooming artifact on gradient-echo sequences [17]. Leptomeningeal and cortical enhancement can also be present [15]. Most advanced cases evolve to liquefactive necrosis and encephalomalacia [15]. Acyclovir is the primary therapy and should be administered as soon as the diagnosis is suspected to reduce potential complications [16].

**West Nile virus (WNV) encephalitis:** WNV is a neurotropic human virus from the *Flaviviridae* family [18]. WNV infection is primarily transmitted to humans by an infected mosquito vector between June and November [18]. The majority of infections are subclinical, with a ratio of asymptomatic/symptomatic illness of 150:1 [19]. In symptomatic patients, WNV causes West Nile fever and encephalitis [18, 19]. The former is the most common presentation (60–80% of cases) and consists of an acute self-limited

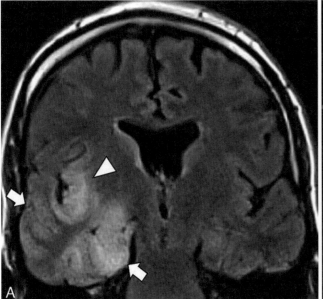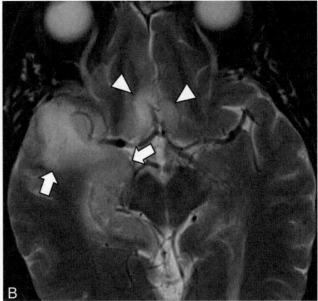

**Fig. 6** Acute HSE in a 65-year-old woman. Coronal FLAIR (**a**) and axial T2WI (**b**) MR images show cortical and subcortical hyperintensity in the mesial and lateral right temporal lobe (**a, b** arrows), insular cortex (**a**, arrowhead), and both inferior cingulate gyri (**b**, arrows). Cortical diffusion restriction was seen in the right temporal lobe (not shown)

flu-like illness. The other subset of symptomatic patients develops neurological deficits in the form of aseptic meningitis, encephalitis, acute flaccid paralysis, or a combination of them [19].

The imaging manifestations in neurological WNV infection are variable, with 30–60% of cases showing no abnormalities [19, 20]. MRI is the imaging method of choice with bilateral asymmetric T2 and FLAIR hyperintensities predominantly involving the thalami and corpus striatum. Other affected areas include the cerebellum, brainstem, and lobar gray/white matter [19, 20]. Signal changes on DWI can precede those on other pulse sequences in half of the patients and are indicative of a good prognosis if they occur in isolation [20]. Patchy T2 signal abnormalities in the spinal cord can also be observed. Leptomeningeal, periventricular, or nerve root enhancement are variably seen [19, 20].

## Mycobacterial Infections

Tuberculosis (TB) remains a prominent cause of morbidity and mortality in developing countries. Increased immigration and the pandemic of acquired immunodeficiency syndrome (AIDS) account for the increase in cases in developed countries as well [21]. Mycobacterium tuberculosis is responsible

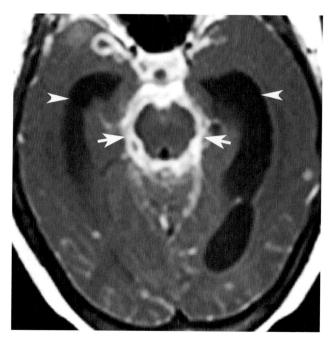

**Fig. 7** Tuberculous meningitis in a 40-year-old patient. Axial post-contrast magnetization transfer (MT) image demonstrates diffuse leptomeningeal enhancement (arrows) around the mid brain and in the suprasellar cistern, with substantial dilatation of the temporal horns of the lateral ventricles, which is consistent with acute communicating hydrocephalus (arrowheads). Evidence of transependymal CSF permeation was seen on T2WI (not shown) (Case courtesy of Dr. Rakesh Gupta, Gurgaon, Haryana, India)

for almost all cases of tubercular CNS infection, which manifests as meningeal and/or parenchymal involvement [21].

*Tuberculous meningitis* can occur by hematogenous spread usually from the lung or by direct extension from mastoids, orbits, or paranasal cavities [21, 22]. Acute tuberculous meningitis occurs when old foci of infection (known as Rich foci) in communication with the meninges rupture, releasing massive numbers of mycobacteria and triggering a significant immune reaction [23].

MRI tends to be normal in the early stages [24]. Post-contrast meningeal enhancement becomes apparent as the disease progresses, characteristically involving the basal meninges (Fig. 7). Communicating hydrocephalus is a known common complication of meningeal TB [24] (Fig. 7). Ischemic brain infarcts resulting from vasculitis of the small- and medium-sized vessels are another potential complication, with preferential involvement of the lenticulostriate arteries and secondary infarcts in the basal ganglia [24] (Fig. 8).

*Parenchymal TB:* Tuberculomas are the most common manifestation of parenchymal TB. Focal cerebritis, tuberculous encephalopathy, and tuberculous brain abscess represent other forms of parenchymal involvement [21, 25]. Most tuberculomas occur at the corticomedullary junction, supporting the pathogenesis of hematogenous spread [21, 26]. They start as a conglomerate of microgranulomata within a region of focal cerebritis, which coalesces to form a mature noncaseating tuberculoma. A solid central caseous necrosis follows, which can subsequently liquefy [21, 27].

Imaging findings will vary depending on the stage of the tuberculoma, and the degree of vasogenic edema tends to be inversely proportional to the maturity of the infected focus [27]. On CT, solid noncaseating tuberculomas are usually isodense to the brain parenchyma and show homogeneous enhancement after contrast administration. On MRI, noncaseating tuberculomas are iso- to hypointense on T1WI and T2WI, with homogeneous post-gadolinium enhancement (Fig. 9). Caseating granulomas are iso- to hypointense on T1WI and T2WI, with a peripheral rim of enhancement on post-contrast images. The solid central T2 hypointense non-enhancing central component of tuberculomas is due to solid caseation, fibrosis, and the presence of free radicals [21, 24, 28].

## Fungal Infection

Fungi can be categorized as yeast (unicellular, e.g., candida and cryptococcus), hyphae (branch-like colonies, e.g., aspergillus and mucormycosis), and dimorphic (e.g., coccidioidomycosis) [29, 30]. Fungal infections of the CNS are rare and depend on the host immune status. Common fungi affecting immunocompromised patients include mucormycosis,

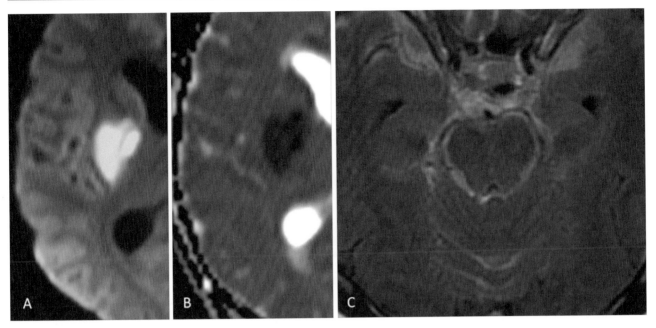

**Fig. 8** Basal ganglia infarct in a 40-year-old patient with tuberculous meningitis. DWI image (**a**) and corresponding ADC map (**b**) show acute infarct of the right lenticulate nucleus. The axial FLAIR sequence (**c**) at the level of the midbrain demonstrates high signal of subarachnoid spaces in the perimesencephalic cisterns, within the sylvian fissures and along the cerebellar folia consistent with TB meningitis

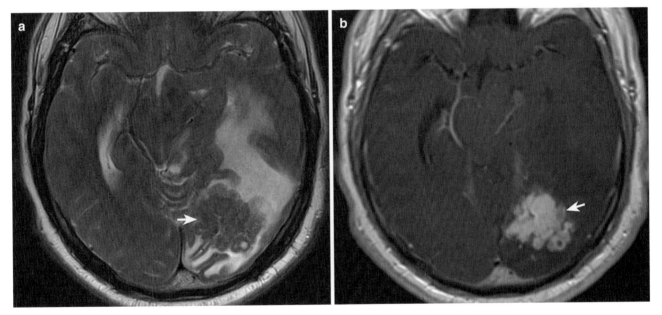

**Fig. 9** Solid noncaseating parenchymal tuberculoma. Axial T2WI (**a**) and post-contrast T1WI MR images show a multi-lobulated T2 hypo-intense left occipital intra-axial focus (arrow **a**), with associated mass effect and surrounding vasogenic edema. The focus shows avid homo-geneous enhancement (arrow **b**) (Case courtesy of Dr. Rakesh Gupta, Gurgaon, Haryana, India)

candida, and cryptococcus. Infection results from hematogenous spread or direct extension from the orbits and paranasal sinuses [30]. Yeast may result in meningeal and parenchymal disease, while hyphae can cause parenchymal and vascular involvement [29].

On MRI, fungal granuloma and cerebritis demonstrate intermediate T2 signal with surrounding edema. Cerebritis may demonstrate variable enhancement and heterogeneous DWI signal. Fungal abscesses are ring-enhancing foci, with hypointense T2 rims and central diffusion restriction (Fig. 10). In immunocompromised patients, fungal abscesses may demonstrate minimal to no enhancement. Crenated margins and diffusion restricting non-enhancing intracavitary projections, seen in some fungal abscesses, help to

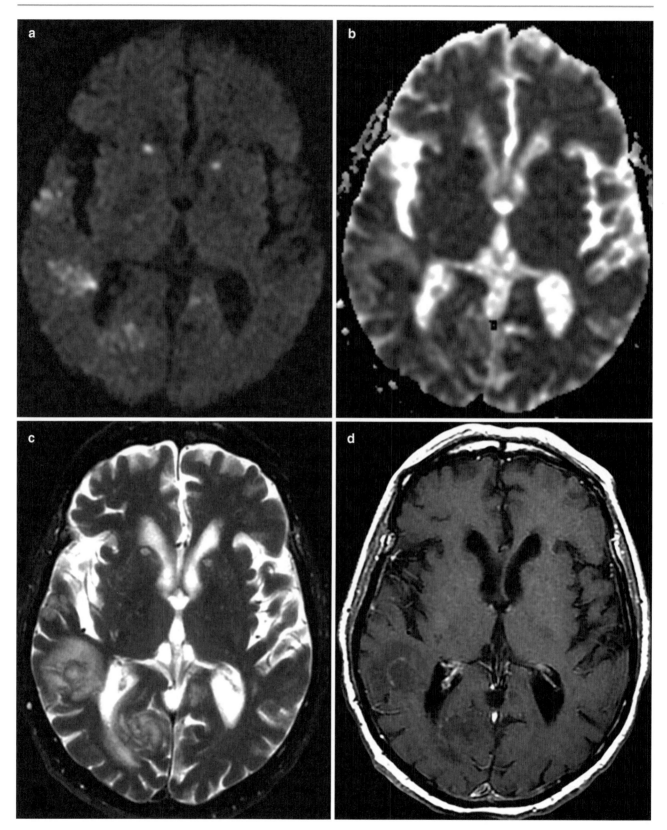

**Fig. 10** Aspergillus abscesses in a 76-year-old patient with lymphoma, altered mental status, sepsis, and respiratory failure. Axial DWI (**a**), ADC (**b**), T2WI (**c**), post-contrast T1WI, (**d**) MR images show multiple parenchymal abscesses in bilateral cerebral hemispheres and bilateral caudate nuclei. Leading temporo-occipital abscesses demonstrate T2 hypointense rim, peripheral enhancement, and central diffusion restriction. *Aspergillus fumigatus* was cultured from blood and alveolar

differentiate them from pyogenic abscesses [9] (Fig. 11). While meningitis remains a clinical diagnosis, MRI may show basal meningeal enhancement and increased leptomeningeal FLAIR signal.

Non-immunocompetent patients have a risk for invasive sinusitis, which rapidly progresses to osteomyelitis, vascular, and parenchymal CNS involvement. Invasive sinusitis demonstrates non-enhancing mucosa with low T1 and T2 signal, related to ferromagnetic material within the hyphae, as well as bone erosions, infiltration of surrounding fat planes, and

extension to the dura, cavernous sinus, and brain parenchyma [31] (Fig. 12).

Aspergillus and mucormycosis have a propensity for angioinvasion of large- and medium-size vessel walls at the skull base. Through the production of elastase, fungi trigger inflammatory vasculitis, in situ thrombosis, and embolization of hyphae, with secondary ischemic brain injury manifesting as low CT attenuation, T2 hyperintensity, and restricted diffusion. Superimposed hemorrhage may be seen. Brain involvement from sino-orbital disease in

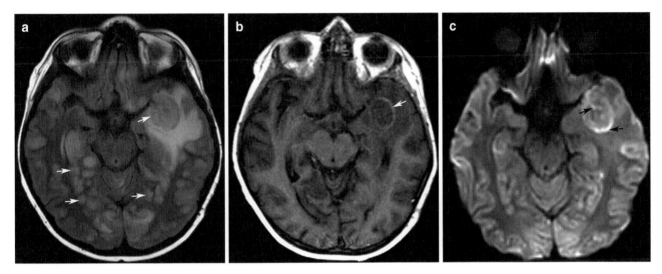

**Fig. 11** Candida abscesses in a 8-year-old patient, history of myelodysplastic syndrome (MDS), hemophagocytic lymphohistiocytosis (HLH), sepsis, and candidemia. Axial FLAIR (**a**), post-contrast T1WI (**b**), and DWI (**c**) MR images show multiple bilateral abscesses (arrows **a**). The largest left temporal abscess demonstrates rim enhancement (arrow **b**) with peripheral restricted diffusion and non-enhancing intracavitary projections that restrict diffusion (black arrows **c**)

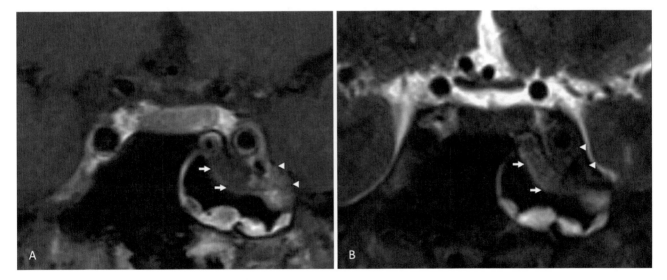

**Fig. 12** Invasive fungal sinusitis in a 61-year-old patient with type 2 DM, progressive headache, photophobia, and diplopia. Coronal post-contrast T1WI (**a**) and T2WI (**b**) show abnormal non-enhancing nodular mucosal thickening with corresponding dark T2 signal at the lateral aspect of left sphenoid sinus roof (arrows **a** and **b**) with abnormal enhancement and comparative thickening of left cavernous sinus (arrowheads **a** and **b**). Frozen biopsy revealed fungal hyphae, surgical specimen culture grew *Rhizopus/Mucormycosis*

mucormycosis predicts a dismal prognosis with a high mortality rate [32].

Vessel wall damage may result in the formation of fusiform aneurysms of intracranial arteries at the base of the brain. Infectious aneurysms account for fewer than 3% of intracranial aneurysms, with aspergillus being the most prevalent cause of fungal aneurysms [33, 34].

## Parasitic Infections

Parasitic infections of the CNS are rare, being more common in developing and tropical countries. However, given the widespread travel and immigration, they are becoming more common globally. Neurocysticercosis is the most common parasitic infection of the CNS and can be found incidentally in 10–20% of the population in endemic countries [35–37].

**Neurocysticercosis** is acquired through feco-oral transmission of *Taenia solium* (pork tapeworm). The primary larvae are released by *Taenia solium* ingested eggs in the intestines and disseminate to the body. The encysted larvae can infect any organ but most commonly affect the CNS, eyes, and muscles [35]. In the CNS, they tend to involve the subarachnoid spaces, brain parenchyma, and ventricles (especially the fourth ventricle) in descending order of frequency [35]. The larval cyst measures between 10 and 20 mm and contains the scolex (larval head) [35, 37].

Neurocysticercosis can present at any age, with a peak incidence from 20 to 50 years of age [37]. The most common clinical presentation includes seizures/epilepsy, followed by headache and focal neurological deficits [37]. On imaging, four stages are identified: *Vesicular*: Viable larvae appear as small (5–20 mm), round, thin-walled non-enhancing cysts, which are isodense/isointense to CSF with an eccentric nodule (scolex 2–4 mm) and no edema. *Colloidal*: Degenerating larvae with inflammatory reaction show avidly enhancing wall, surrounding vasogenic edema, and increased internal density on CT and increased T1/FLAIR signal intensity on MRI,

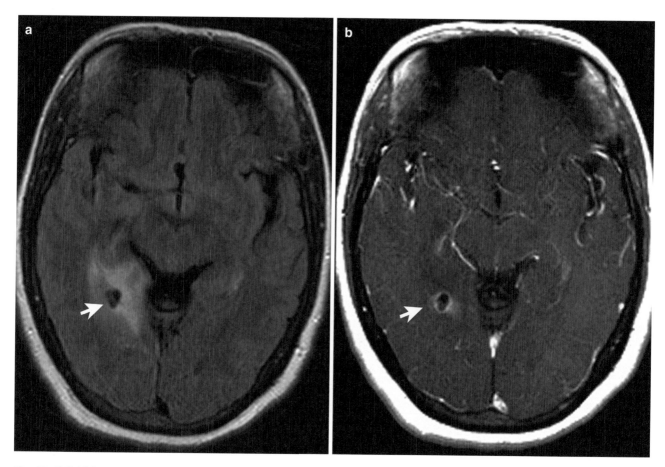

**Fig. 13** Colloidal stage neurocysticercosis in a 42-year-old woman. Axial FLAIR (**a**) and post-contrast T1WI MR (**b**) images show a small cystic focus in the medial aspect of the right temporal lobe (arrow **a**), with rim enhancement (arrow **b**) and surrounding vasogenic edema

compared to CSF, without diffusion restriction (Fig. 13). *Granular nodular*: Retracting cyst shows nodular or retracted faint ring enhancement with mild residual edema. *Nodular calcified*: Calcified nodule seen on CT appears as T1/T2 hypointense non-enhancing nodule on MRI with blooming on T2* GRE or SWI sequences and without edema [35, 36, 38].

*Subarachnoid neurocysticercosis* in the basal cisterns and Sylvian fissures appears as multi-lobular grapelike "Racemose" cystic foci. Associated arachnoiditis can cause basal leptomeningeal enhancement, secondary hydrocephalus, vasculitis, and infarcts [35, 37]. *Intraventricular neurocysticercosis* can be difficult to visualize on CT being isodense to CSF but may be inferred by ventricular distortion and hydrocephalus. It can be better seen on FLAIR, high-resolution T2WI, or cisternography [36, 37]. Treatment consists primarily of albendazole. Steroids may be needed to control inflammatory reaction, and surgical intervention may be necessary for select patients (e.g., shunt for hydrocephalus) [35].

## Acute Opportunistic Infections in Human Immunodeficiency Virus (HIV)/AIDS

Multiple CNS opportunistic infections are associated with HIV infection. Toxoplasmosis, cryptococcosis, cytomegalovirus, and progressive multifocal leukoencephalopathy (PML) are seen with a CD4 cell count below 200 cells/μL, whereas patients with a CD4 count of 200–500 cells/μL are at risk of tuberculous meningitis and PML [39, 40]. Multiple opportunistic infections are present in 15% [40].

**Toxoplasmosis:** Toxoplasmosis is the most common opportunistic CNS infection in HIV patients, caused by *Toxoplasma gondii*, an obligate intracellular parasite [3, 41]. The transmission to humans is by ingestion of cysts in undercooked pork or lamb or food or water contaminated with cat feces [42, 43].

Cerebral toxoplasmosis presents on imaging with multifocal ring-enhancing abscesses in the basal ganglia, thalamus, and at the gray-white matter junction. Solitary foci can occur in one third of the cases [42, 44]. The signal intensity on T2WI varies according to the stage. Central T2 hyperintensity represents liquefactive necrosis, while iso- or hypointense T2 signal is seen in organizing abscesses [43, 45, 46]. Restricted diffusion is seen in the enhancing ring with a central core of low signal on DWI related to necrotic tissue, with low viscosity and absence of purulent material [3, 43]. The eccentric target sign is very specific (95%) [47] for cerebral toxoplasmosis and is seen in 30% of cases. It refers to a small peripheral enhancing nodule along the enhancing margins [3, 42, 48] (Fig. 14). Primary CNS lymphoma which can present with necrotic and hemorrhagic foci in HIV patients is the main differential diagnosis. On perfusion, lymphoma will demonstrate increased cerebral blood volume compared to toxoplasmosis [43]. On MR spectroscopy, lymphoma will show a markedly elevated choline peak, while both will exhibit lactate and lipid peaks, more pronounced in toxoplasmosis [41, 42]. Empirical treatment for 2–3 weeks is indicated if toxoplasmosis is suspected; however, patients may require lifelong maintenance therapy due to the presence of encysted forms [3, 41].

**Cryptococcosis** is the most common fungal infection in HIV patients, found in 5–10%, usually with CD4 count <100 cells/μL [41]. It is caused by *Cryptococcus neoformans*, an encapsulated yeast-like fungus found in soil contaminated by bird excreta [41]. CNS involvement occurs secondary to hematogenous dissemination of a pulmonary focus [41].

Meningitis is the most common presentation affecting 40% of the patients, with a 15–39% mortality rate [49]. In most of the cases, the inflammatory reaction is mild, without meningeal enhancement. Avid meningeal enhancement can be seen in some cases [43] (Fig. 15). The ependymal surfaces are usually involved, and about half of the patients will develop communicating hydrocephalus [48].

Gelatinous pseudocyst results from infection spread to the perivascular spaces, which appear widened and may become confluent with low attenuation on CT and hyperintensity on T2WI without significant enhancement (Fig. 16). The cysts largely suppress on FLAIR with possible hyperintense rim [41, 43]. These foci are usually bilateral and are commonly found in the basal ganglia. The dentate nuclei, thalami, and midbrain can also be involved [43].

Cryptococcomas are granulomas, usually localized in the basal ganglia, thalamus, and cerebellum, and typically hyperintense on T2WI, with a ring or nodular enhancement and surrounding vasogenic edema [41, 43].

## Conclusion

Imaging plays a central role in the early diagnosis of brain infections and in the detection of related complications, in patients presenting to the ED. While many organisms share nonspecific and overlapping manifestations, others have characteristic imaging findings that may allow a prompt confident diagnosis. Knowledge of the patient's immune status and predisposing risk factors, in combination with specific imaging findings, may allow to recognize specific infectious organisms; and therefore targeted therapy may be started.

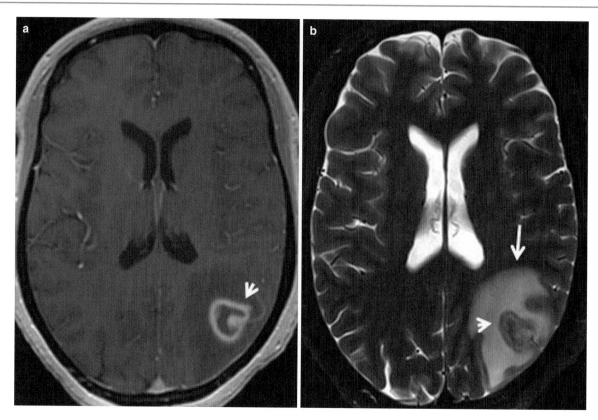

**Fig. 14** Toxoplasmosis in a 43-year-old HIV positive patient. Axial post-contrast T1WI (**a**) and T2WI (**b**) MR images show a left parietal ring-enhancing focus with an eccentric nodule consistent with the eccentric target sign (arrow **a**). The focus is hypointense on T2WI (short arrow **b**), with extensive surrounding vasogenic edema (long arrow **b**)

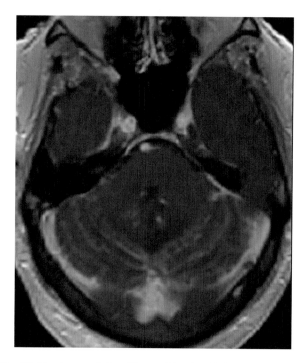

**Fig. 15** Cryptococcosis in a 57-year-old male with fever and headache. Axial post-contrast T1WI image shows prominent leptomeningeal enhancement along the cerebellar folia

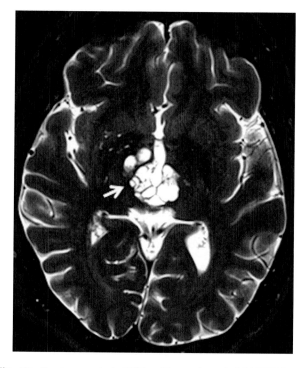

**Fig. 16** Cryptococcosis in HIV-positive patient. Axial T2WI image shows multiple confluent cystic foci in the thalami (arrow) consistent with gelatinous pseudocysts. No significant enhancement was seen with IV contrast administration (not shown)

# References

1. Hughes DC, Raghavan A, Mordekar SR, Griffiths PD, Connolly DJ. Role of imaging in the diagnosis of acute bacterial meningitis and its complications. Postgrad Med J. 2010;86 (1018):478–85.
2. Brouwer MC, Thwaites GE, Tunkel AR, van de Beek D. Dilemmas in the diagnosis of acute community-acquired bacterial meningitis. Lancet. 2012;380(9854):1684–92.
3. Shih RY, Koeller KK. Bacterial, fungal, and parasitic infections of the central nervous system: radiologic-pathologic correlation and historical perspectives. Radiographics. 2015;35(4):1141–69.
4. Azad R, Tayal M, Azad S, Sharma G, Srivastava RK. Qualitative and quantitative comparison of contrast-enhanced fluid-attenuated inversion recovery, magnetization transfer spin echo, and fat-saturation T1-weighted sequences in infectious meningitis. Korean J Radiol. 2017;18(6):973–82.
5. Kanamalla US, Ibarra RA, Jinkins JR. Imaging of cranial meningitis and ventriculitis. Neuroimaging Clin N Am. 2000;10(2): 309–31.
6. Helweg-Larsen J, Astradsson A, Richhall H, Erdal J, Laursen A, Brennum J. Pyogenic brain abscess, a 15 year survey. BMC Infect Dis. 2012;12:332.
7. Rath TJ, Hughes M, Arabi M, Shah GV. Imaging of cerebritis, encephalitis, and brain abscess. Neuroimaging Clin N Am. 2012;22(4):585–607.
8. Toh CH, Wei KC, Chang CN, et al. Differentiation of pyogenic brain abscesses from necrotic glioblastomas with use of susceptibility-weighted imaging. AJNR Am J Neuroradiol. 2012;33(8):1534–8.
9. Luthra G, Parihar A, Nath K, et al. Comparative evaluation of fungal, tubercular, and pyogenic brain abscesses with conventional and diffusion MR imaging and proton MR spectroscopy. AJNR Am J Neuroradiol. 2007;28(7):1332–8.
10. Gupta RK, Jobanputra KJ, Yadav A. MR spectroscopy in brain infections. Neuroimaging Clin N Am. 2013;23(3):475–98.
11. Fujikawa A, Tsuchiya K, Honya K, Nitatori T. Comparison of MRI sequences to detect ventriculitis. AJR Am J Roentgenol. 2006;187 (4):1048–53.
12. de Noordhout CM, Devleesschauwer B, Angulo FJ, et al. The global burden of listeriosis: a systematic review and meta-analysis. Lancet Infect Dis. 2014;14(11):1073–82.
13. Drevets DA, Bronze MS. Listeria monocytogenes: epidemiology, human disease, and mechanisms of brain invasion. FEMS Immunol Med Microbiol. 2008;53(2):151–65.
14. Carmo RLD, Alves Simao AK, Amaral L, et al. Neuroimaging of emergent and reemergent infections. Radiographics. 2019;39(6): 1649–71.
15. Soares BP, Provenzale JM. Imaging of herpesvirus infections of the CNS. AJR Am J Roentgenol. 2016;206(1):39–48.
16. Bradshaw MJ, Venkatesan A. Herpes simplex virus-1 encephalitis in adults: pathophysiology, diagnosis, and management. Neurotherapeutics. 2016;13(3):493–508.
17. Cag Y, Erdem H, Leib S, et al. Managing atypical and typical herpetic central nervous system infections: results of a multinational study. Clin Microbiol Infect. 2016;22(6):568.e569–17.
18. Colpitts TM, Conway MJ, Montgomery RR, Fikrig E. West Nile virus: biology, transmission, and human infection. Clin Microbiol Rev. 2012;25(4):635–48.
19. Tyler KL. West Nile virus infection in the United States. Arch Neurol. 2004;61(8):1190–5.
20. Ali M, Safriel Y, Sohi J, Llave A, Weathers S. West Nile virus infection: MR imaging findings in the nervous system. AJNR Am J Neuroradiol. 2005;26(2):289–97.
21. Torres C, Riascos R, Figueroa R, Gupta RK. Central nervous system tuberculosis. Top Magn Reson Imaging. 2014;23(3):173–89.
22. Dastur DK, Manghani DK, Udani PM. Pathology and pathogenetic mechanisms in neurotuberculosis. Radiol Clin North Am. 1995;33 (4):733–52.
23. Jongeling AC, Pisapia D. Pearls and oy-sters: tuberculous meningitis: not a diagnosis of exclusion. Neurology. 2013;80(4):e36–9.
24. Gupta RK, Kumar S. Central nervous system tuberculosis. Neuroimaging Clin N Am. 2011;21(4):795–814, vii–viii.
25. Helmy A, Antoun N, Hutchinson P. Cerebral tuberculoma and magnetic resonance imaging. J R Soc Med. 2011;104(7): 299–301.
26. Gupta RK, Kohli A, Gaur V, Lal JH, Kishore J. MRI of the brain in patients with miliary pulmonary tuberculosis without symptoms or signs of central nervous system involvement. Neuroradiology. 1997;39(10):699–704.
27. Jinkins JR, Gupta R, Chang KH, Rodriguez-Carbajal J. MR imaging of central nervous system tuberculosis. Radiol Clin North Am. 1995;33(4):771–86.
28. RK G. Tuberculosis and other non-tuberculous bacterial granulomatous infections. In: RK G, RB L, editor. MR imaging and spectroscopy of central nervous system infection. New York: Kluwer Academic/Plenum Publishers; 2001. p. 95–145.
29. Sundaram C, Umabala P, Laxmi V, et al. Pathology of fungal infections of the central nervous system: 17 years' experience from Southern India. Histopathology. 2006;49(4):396–405.
30. Gavito-Higuera J, Mullins CB, Ramos-Duran L, Olivas Chacon CI, Hakim N, Palacios E. Fungal infections of the central nervous system: a pictorial review. J Clin Imag Sci. 2016;6:24.
31. Mathur M, Johnson CE, Sze G. Fungal infections of the central nervous system. Neuroimaging Clin N Am. 2012;22(4):609–32.
32. Yousem DM, Galetta SL, Gusnard DA, Goldberg HI. MR findings in rhinocerebral mucormycosis. J Comput Assist Tomogr. 1989;13 (5):878–82.
33. Keyik B, Edguer T, Hekimoglu B. Conventional and diffusion-weighted MR imaging of cerebral aspergillosis. Diagn Interv Radiol. 2005;11(4):199–201.
34. Hurst RW, Judkins A, Bolger W, Chu A, Loevner LA. Mycotic aneurysm and cerebral infarction resulting from fungal sinusitis: imaging and pathologic correlation. AJNR Am J Neuroradiol. 2001;22(5):858–63.
35. Kimura-Hayama ET, Higuera JA, Corona-Cedillo R, et al. Neurocysticercosis: radiologic-pathologic correlation. RadioGraphics. 2010;30(6):1705–19.
36. Zhao J-L, Lerner A, Shu Z, Gao X-J, Zee C-S. Imaging spectrum of neurocysticercosis. Radiol Infect Dis. 2015;1(2):94–102.
37. Garcia HH, Nash TE, Del Brutto OH. Clinical symptoms, diagnosis, and treatment of neurocysticercosis. Lancet Neurol. 2014;13(12): 1202–15.
38. Lucato LT, Guedes MS, Sato JR, Bacheschi LA, Machado LR, Leite CC. The role of conventional MR imaging sequences in the evaluation of neurocysticercosis: impact on characterization of the scolex and lesion burden. Am J Neuroradiol. 2007;28 (8):1501.
39. Bowen LN, Smith B, Reich D, Quezado M, Nath A. HIV-associated opportunistic CNS infections: pathophysiology, diagnosis and treatment. Nat Rev Neurol. 2016;12(11):662–74.
40. Tan IL, Smith BR, von Geldern G, Mateen FJ, McArthur JC. HIV-associated opportunistic infections of the CNS. Lancet Neurol. 2012;11(7):605–17.
41. Smith AB, Smirniotopoulos JG, Rushing EJ. From the archives of the AFIP: central nervous system infections associated with human immunodeficiency virus infection: radiologic-pathologic correlation. Radiographics. 2008;28(7):2033–58.
42. Akgoz A, Mukundan S, Lee TC. Imaging of rickettsial, spirochetal, and parasitic infections. Neuroimaging Clin N Am. 2012;22(4):633–57.
43. Rumboldt Z, Thurnher MM, Gupta RK. Central nervous system infections. Semin Roentgenol. 2007;42(2):62–91.

44. Swinburne NC, Bansal AG, Aggarwal A, Doshi AH. Neuroimaging in central nervous system infections. Curr Neurol Neurosci Rep. 2017;17(6):49.

45. da Cunha Correia C, Ramos Lacerda H, de Assis Costa VM, Mertens de Queiroz Brainer A. Cerebral toxoplasmosis: unusual MRI findings. Clin Imaging. 2012;36(5):462–5.

46. Brightbill TC, Post MJ, Hensley GT, Ruiz A. MR of Toxoplasma encephalitis: signal characteristics on T2-weighted images and pathologic correlation. J Comput Assist Tomogr. 1996;20(3):417–22.

47. Kumar GG, Mahadevan A, Guruprasad AS, et al. Eccentric target sign in cerebral toxoplasmosis: neuropathological correlate to the imaging feature. J Magn Reson Imaging. 2010;31(6): 1469–72.

48. Vachha B, Moonis G, Holodny A. Infections of the brain and meninges. Semin Roentgenol. 2017;52(1):2–9.

49. Goralska K, Blaszkowska J, Dzikowiec M. Neuroinfections caused by fungi. Infection. 2018;46(4):443–59.

# Imaging of Traumatic Vascular Neck Injuries

## 11

Daniel Furlanetto, Marc Jutras, Nicolas Murray, and Savvas Nicolaou

## Contents

### Abstract

Traumatic injuries of the cervical carotid and vertebral arteries as a result of blunt vascular trauma are identified under the scope of blunt cerebrovascular injuries (BCVI) or blunt vascular neck injuries (BVNI).

The main objective of this chapter is to present the reader the basic as well as the advanced semiology of blunt vascular neck injuries, its most common and less frequently observed patterns, potential pitfalls, and recent imaging techniques that can enhance diagnostic accuracy.

By the end of this chapter, the reader will also have reviewed when to suspect and what patients to screen for BVNI, how to classify the injuries using the most accepted modified Denver/Biffl criteria, and how to guide imaging follow-up and will understand current guidelines for treatment.

D. Furlanetto · M. Jutras · N. Murray · S. Nicolaou (✉)
Department of Radiology, Vancouver General Hospital/University of British Columbia, Vancouver, BC, Canada
e-mail: daniel.furlanetto@vch.ca; marc.jutras@alumni.ubc.ca; nicolas.murray@vch.ca; savvas.nicolaou@vch.ca

### Keywords

Cerebrovascular injury · BCVI · BVNI · Blunt cervical injury · Stroke · Screening

© Springer Nature Switzerland AG 2022
M. N. Patlas et al. (eds.), *Atlas of Emergency Imaging from Head-to-Toe*,
https://doi.org/10.1007/978-3-030-92111-8_11

## Introduction

The term blunt vascular neck injuries (BVNI) encompasses injuries to the extracranial portions of the carotid and vertebral arteries, as a direct cause, or as a sequela of blunt trauma.

Since BVNI was first described in the 1970s [1, 2], there has been progressive understanding of its pathophysiology, importance, and treatment.

Even though these events are relatively rare, their consequences can be tragic. The incidence of BVNI was first believed to be only 0.08% of all blunt cervical traumas and now considered to be between 1% and 3% [1–4].

Taking into consideration both the incidence and potential severity of these injuries, BVNI is a must-know topic for radiologists practicing in the emergency and trauma setting. This chapter will review the most common mechanisms of injury, the natural history, clinical indications for screening, imaging modalities, spectrum of injury, and current classification systems, as well as follow-up and prognostic implications.

## Epidemiology

BVNI was initially considered to be quite a rare entity, with early multicenter studies in the 1990s reporting an incidence of BVNI in approximately 0.1% of all blunt trauma patients in the United States [5]. More recent evidence indicates, however, that BVNI is much more common than originally thought, with a reported incidence of at least 1–3% [1–4, 6]. It is therefore likely that BVNI has been substantially underdiagnosed in trauma patients until recently, given more liberal screening guidelines, advances in technology, and the use of multidetector CT imaging.

The vast majority of BVNI occurs secondary to motor vehicle collisions, with additional etiologies including workplace accidents, falls, and assaults accounting for the remainder of most cases [7–9]. Historically, four fundamental mechanisms of injury have been reported, including direct blunt force, hyperextension with rotation, intraoral trauma, and basilar skull fracture [1]. However, a wider variety of mechanisms is recognized today as being associated with BVNI. In particular, any injury to the head and neck with a strong deceleration component is considered at high risk [8].

Regarding the internal carotid arteries (ICAs), BVNI occurs most frequently within the distal cervical segment, near the base of the skull, with other common sites of injury including the petrous and the cavernous segments [10, 11]. Vertebral artery injuries also tend to occur within the cervical portion, with injuries often associated with fractures of the transverse foramen of the cervical vertebral bodies [11, 12]. Importantly, multivessel injuries are common in trauma patients with BVNI, with a reported incidence of approximately 18–38% [10, 13].

## Screening and Diagnosis

Early studies on the detection and incidence of BVNI [7] utilized invasive digital subtraction angiography (DSA) as the means of diagnosis, which was regarded as the reference standard and indeed was the only true reliable diagnostic method to detect blunt vascular injuries for many years. Less sophisticated CT technology of the 1990s and early 2000s with four or fewer slice multi-detector CT was insensitive for the detection of BVNI [14, 15]. With the advent of modern multi-detector computed tomography (MDCT) techniques (often using 64 or more slices), the use of multi-detector CT angiography (CTA) became an efficient option for diagnosing BVNI [10]. In conjunction with the widespread adoption of rapid whole-body CT imaging for trauma at many institutions [16, 17], the ability to screen for BVNI has expanded substantially over the previous decade, thereby allowing for the detection of many injuries that would previously have gone undiagnosed or diagnosed with delay and its potential severe clinical implications.

Along with advances in MDCT technology that have enabled better screening and detection of BVNI in trauma, screening criteria have also undergone substantial evolution and improvement. The first framework for BVNI screening was published by Biffl et al. in 1999 and has come to be known as the Denver criteria [18]. At that time, screening for BVNI was limited to the use of invasive DSA, and given the resource-intensive nature of this technique, screening recommendations were largely limited to high-risk spinal injury mechanisms, including hyperextension, hyperflexion, and direct blow [18]. In 2010, the Eastern Association for the Surgery of Trauma (EAST) published one of the first comprehensive guidelines on the screening and management of BVNI based on the Denver criteria, the current available evidence, and expert consensus opinion [19].

However, despite the development of standard screening guidelines, some studies found that a sizable proportion of patients who were eventually diagnosed with BVNI were still not being captured by current screening criteria, with a

**Table 1** Denver screening criteria [22, 50]

| Signs/symptoms of BCVI | Risk factors for BCVI |
|---|---|
| Potential arterial hemorrhage from the neck/nose/mouth | High-energy transfer mechanism |
| Cervical bruit in a patient <50 years old | Displaced mid-face fracture (LeFort II or III) |
| Expanding cervical hematoma | Complex skull/basilar skull/occipital condyle fractures |
| Focal neurological deficit: TIA, hemiparesis, vertebrobasilar symptoms, Horner's syndrome | Cervical spine fracture, subluxation, or ligamentous injury at any level |
| Neurological deficit inconsistent with head CT | Near-hanging with anoxic brain injury |
| Stroke on CT or MRI | Clothesline-type injury or seatbelt abrasion with substantial swelling, pain, or altered mental status |
| | TBI with thoracic injuries |
| | Scalp degloving |
| | Thoracic vascular injuries |
| | Blunt cardiac rupture |
| | Upper rib fractures |

*BCVI* blunt cerebrovascular injury, *TIA* transient ischemic attack, *TBI* traumatic brain injury

rate of up to 30% reported at some centers [17, 19]. The original Denver criteria for BVNI screening have therefore undergone many iterations over time, with criteria having been expanded in an effort to promote more liberal screening of all patients who may have BVNI in the appropriate clinical context [21–23]. Notably, the criteria have now been expanded to include any cervical spine injury (whether osseous or ligamentous), at any level [21]. An expanded version of the Denver criteria (Table 1) has been included in an updated practice management guideline for BVNI screening, recently published in 2020 by EAST [24]. A similar, although less comprehensive, screening protocol, known as the Memphis criteria, has also been proposed [25, 26] and is included in the 2020 EAST guidelines as well [24].

Due to the concern of missed BVNI cases in trauma and taking into account the devastating clinical consequences that can result from a delayed diagnosis, some have recently advocated for universal screening of all major blunt trauma patients, with CTA of the head and neck [20]. Of course, the benefit of universal screening for the detection of BVNI must be weighed against the costs of potential overdiagnosis, the associated increased radiation dose delivered, and the risk of iatrogenic patient harm, particularly with respect to bleeding, as many BVNI injuries are ultimately managed with antiplatelets or anticoagulation [20, 24]. Moreover, the situation may be further complicated in complex trauma cases where the iatrogenic risk associated with antiplatelet or anticoagulation therapy may be particularly high due to coexistent injuries, thus necessitating close collaboration between the radiology department and the trauma team when deciding the appropriate diagnostic workup and

when discussing the implications of management that stems from any imaging findings. Currently, at the authors' institution, the decision to add a CTA of the head and neck to the whole-body CT protocol for trauma is made using a combination of major Denver criteria features, injury severity scale (ISS) score, and clinical judgment, in discussion with the acute care and trauma services [27, 28].

## Clinical Features

From a clinical standpoint, the diagnosis of BVNI is often complicated by the fact that most patients do not have neurological symptoms directly attributable to the vascular neck injury itself at the time of presentation [9]. Moreover, many BVNI patients have concurrent substantial polytrauma, which renders the neurological examination difficult due to distracting injuries, as well as the reality of critical care medicine, including the need for intubation and sedation, which further limits the clinical examination.

At the pathophysiologic level, the major risk of BVNI relates to thrombus formation with possible vessel occlusion and/or downstream embolism, leading to cerebral ischemia and infarction. The risk of stroke from BVNI appears to be highest within the first 7 days following injury, with a peak within the first 24 h [9]. With knowledge of this temporal sequence of events, it becomes apparent that there is a window of opportunity in which BVNI can be diagnosed, and appropriate management initiated, before devastating downstream consequences occur. If left untreated, BVNI carries a risk of stroke of up to 40% due to carotid artery

**Table 2** Biffl/Denver scale for BCVI [31]

| Grade I | Vessel wall irregularity, dissection, or IMH with <25% luminal stenosis |
|---|---|
| Grade II | Any raised intimal flap, any intraluminal thrombus, dissection, or IMH with equal to or >25% luminal stenosis |
| Grade III | Arterial pseudoaneurysm |
| Grade IV | Arterial occlusion |
| Grade V | Arterial transection and/or AVF |

*IMH* intramural hematoma, *AVF* arteriovenous fistula

injuries and 15% in the setting of vertebral artery injuries [22, 29, 30]. With appropriate diagnosis and treatment, the stroke rate in BVNI can be reduced to less than 5% [29]. This underscores the importance of having a high index of suspicion and a low threshold for screening any blunt trauma patients who may be at risk for BVNI and justifies the trend toward more liberal screening criteria in recent years [20, 24].

The grading of BVNI (Table 2), discussed further below, is based on the initial work by Biffl et al. [7, 18], and, although originally based on DSA results, the classification has been applied to CTA findings as well. The severity of injury has been shown to correlate with clinical outcomes, and thus, injury grade is an important part of management decisions [10, 30]. For instance, among ICA injuries, research by Biffl and colleagues found a stroke risk of 8% in grade I injuries, 14% in grade II injuries, 26% in grade III injuries, and 50% in grade IV injuries, as well as a high rate of lethality associated with grade V injuries [31]. A direct linear relationship between injury grade and clinical outcome has not been observed for vertebral artery injuries [13], although the same grading scheme has nevertheless been widely adopted in clinical practice for both carotid and vertebral artery BVNI. Most cases of BVNI are ultimately managed with antiplatelet or anticoagulation therapy alone, although higher-grade injuries may require more invasive techniques, including endovascular stenting or coiling for pseudoaneurysms (grade III injuries), or invasive surgical management for transection/extravasation (grade V injuries) [9, 24].

It is important to note that BVNI are not static injuries, but rather are injuries which are dynamic and can frequently evolve, therefore requiring close clinical follow-up. Early work by Biffl and colleagues found that lower-grade injuries on DSA (grades I and II) demonstrated the most heterogeneity in terms of outcome, with several of these injuries progressing to higher-grade injuries on repeat assessment [30]. More recent research examining follow-up CTAs of patients with BVNI diagnosed at the time of initial trauma

assessment produced similar findings, with all cases of worsening BVNI having initially presented as grade I or II injuries [27]. In light of these findings, the Western Trauma Association has recommended early CTA follow-up of BVNI within 7–10 days [21]. For the reasons discussed, this practice may be most important to assess for healing or evolution of lower-grade injuries (grades I or II), whereas early repeat CTA may be unnecessary for higher-grade injuries (grades III–V), which rarely resolve on early follow-up imaging [32]. Depending on the specific injury pattern and management strategy pursued, regular long-term surveillance may also be required. For instance, based on guidelines for stroke management from the American Heart Association (AHA), antithrombotic treatment may be required for several months, or even on a lifelong basis, depending on the specific clinical symptoms and injury pattern in BVNI stroke patients, a situation that would therefore require long-term serial CTA surveillance as well [33].

## Diagnostic Investigations

### Computed Tomography Angiography

Computed tomography angiography (CTA) has become widely accepted as the first screening modality for BVNI, due to its availability, relative low cost, and high diagnostic yield. With CT scanners ranging from 1 to 64 slices, CTA has shown a pooled sensitivity of 66% and a specificity of 97% for the detection of BVNI [34]. Although sensitivity is likely to be higher with scanners ranging from 64 to 256 slices, updated data is still lacking, to our knowledge.

Screening protocols using CTA have shown significantly increased detection and decreased time to diagnosis, mortality, and stroke rates. CTA including the evaluation of the intracranial vasculature can also be used to detect downstream emboli as a consequence of BVNI.

Several advances and new technologies have increased the diagnostic potential of computed tomography. Multiplanar reformation/reconstruction (MPR) and maximum-intensity projections are well known and are broadly utilized post-processing tools to help in the detection and characterization of vascular injuries, as well as in the process of planning any required intervention. MPRs with bone removal have been shown to increase the sensitivity of detection of high-grade carotid stenosis related to calcified atherosclerotic plaques [35]. Multi-energy CT (MECT), with its ability to reveal the composition of specific high-density materials such as iodine and calcium, allows for the creation of multiple material-specific images, including virtual non-calcium (VNCa) images, virtual non-contrast (VNC) images, iodine maps, and virtual monoenergetic (VME) reconstructions, representing additional diagnostic and problem-solving tools. MECT is useful in removing the calcified structures, particularly calcified plaques and osseous structures including the skull base, helping to visualize the lumen of the vessels and the degree of stenosis [36]. VNC images allow for differentiation between acute hemorrhage and iodinated contrast or calcium, while monoenergetic reconstructions can reduce beam-hardening artifacts from dental amalgams or orthopedic hardware [37, 38]. Iodine maps are often used in further evaluating the brain parenchyma and collateral circulation in cases where there is suspected infarction related to the BCVI [39].

## Digital Subtraction Angiography

Digital subtraction angiography (DSA) has traditionally been recognized as the reference standard diagnostic imaging modality for the detection and characterization of BCVI, due to its high sensitivity and collateral pathways evaluation. It is less time-consuming and cost-effective than CTA and, being an invasive procedure, inherently carries a potential complication rate ranging from 1% to 3% [40]. The examination is conceptually a luminogram, defining the luminal abnormalities with high spatial resolution, but often failing to reveal intramural abnormalities, particularly hematomas in the trauma setting.

With the advent of multi-slice scanners and optimized protocols for CTA, the role of DSA has changed from a primary screening tool to a problem-solving tool. It is highly useful in cases where a high pretest probability or strong clinical suspicion of BCVI is accompanied by negative or nondiagnostic findings on CTA. Currently, DSA is mainly used in planning and guiding interventions [40].

## Magnetic Resonance Imaging and Magnetic Resonance Angiography

Magnetic resonance imaging can be used to identify dissections, intramural hematomas, and vascular occlusions. The modality has a safer profile than DSA and CTA, not producing ionizing radiation and with its potential to assess the vascular system without the use of contrast media. Gadolinium, when needed, produces less hypersensitivity reactions. T1-weighted, gradient-echo, and time-of-flight MRA are commonly utilized sequences that do not require IV gadolinium injection. However, IV contrast-enhanced MRA can also be used to diagnose arterial occlusions, stenosis, and pseudoaneurysm formation.

Another major advantage of MR imaging is being able to depict cerebral ischemia while still potentially reversible and to be able to assess for associated cervical spine, ligamentous, and spinal cord abnormalities.

However, MRI has shown to have relatively low accuracy in the diagnosis of BVNI [25], has considerably more contraindications, requires a longer scanning time, and is not as accessible as other modalities in the emergency setting. MRI is therefore not recommended as a primary screening tool, but can be used to further characterize cases where there is suspicion for dissection or intramural hematomas.

## Ultrasound

Duplex sonography of the cervical arteries is not recommended as a screening tool for BCVI. Despite its several strong features in the emergency setting including high specificity, safety, near-universal availability, portability, and the possibility to be used as a bedside tool, it has been shown to have high operator dependency and sensitivity lower than 40% [41].

## Imaging Findings

There is a large range of traumatic vascular injuries that may occur as a result of blunt cervical trauma and may vary greatly depending on the mechanism.

Several classification systems have been proposed to divide this spectral distribution, from mild to severe injuries, and also to guide treatment, prognosis, and follow-up. The most widely accepted severity scale is the modified Denver scale, also known as the Biffl scale (Table 2), as noted above. This grading system comprehensively stratifies vascular injuries from grade I to grade V.

## Grade I Injuries

In this category are included all injuries which produce a mild stenosis of up to 25% of luminal diameter:

- Mild irregularities of the vessel wall: these are the most common injuries and are characterized in CTA and DSA by discrete irregularity of the luminal contour and vessel wall thickening (Fig. 1). These are often

**Fig. 1 Grade I injury.** (a) Sagittal CTA image (a) shows multiple intimal irregularities in the ICA and ECA in keeping with grade I injury. Follow-up scan 72 h after trauma (b) shows complete resolution of the intimal irregularities

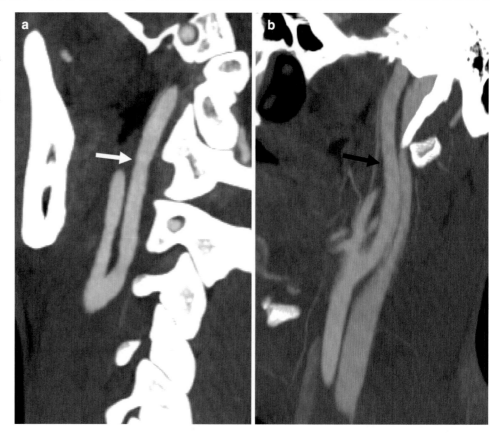

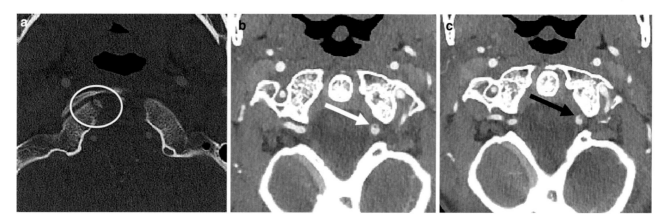

**Fig. 2 Grade I injury.** A 43-year-old man presenting after a motor vehicle collision. Axial CT image with IV contrast image of the craniocervical junction in a bone window (a) demonstrates a type 3 occipital condyle fracture (circle). Axial CT angiogram images (b) and (c) demonstrate a small dissection flap within the proximal V4 segment of the left vertebral artery (white arrow in b), beginning at the junction between the extradural (V3) and intradural (V4) segments (black arrow in c), causing less than 25% luminal narrowing, in keeping with a grade I injury

difficult to distinguish from vasospasm, atherosclerosis, and other diseases including fibromuscular dysplasia [42, 43].

• Intramural hematomas (IMHs): hemorrhage within the vessel wall layers. Pathophysiologically, it is hypothesized to be caused by small intimal tears, rupture of vasa

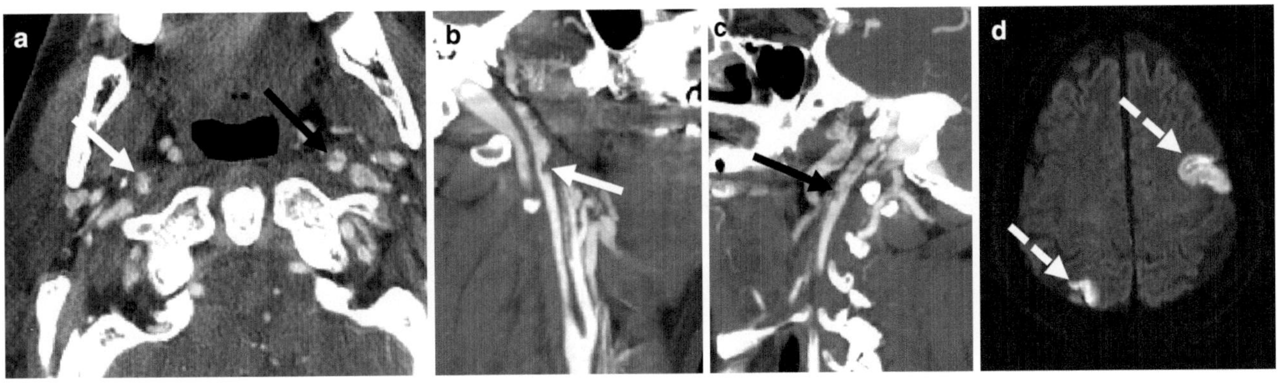

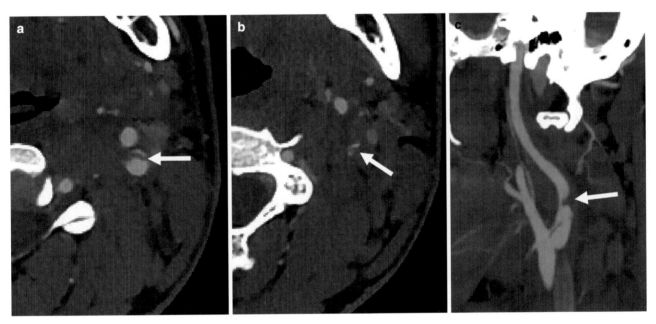

**Fig. 3** **Grade I and II injuries**. A 25-year-old man presenting after a motor vehicle collision. Axial (**a**), sagittal oblique (**b**), and sagittal MIP reformations (**c**) of a CTA of the head and neck show right (white arrows) and left (black arrows) distal cervical ICA injuries, with more than 50% stenosis on the right (grade II) and up to 25% luminal narrowing on the left (grade I). Axial DW image (**d**) of a subsequent MRI of the brain shows bilateral distal MCA territory cortical infarcts (dashed arrows)

**Fig. 4** **Grade II injury**. A 25-year-old man presenting after a police dog bite on the neck. Axial (**a** and **b**) and sagittal (**c**) CTA images demonstrate a focal dissection of the proximal left cervical ICA, with a double-lumen appearance in (**a**) and a raised dissection flap (white arrows), and focal area of narrowing greater than 75% in (**b**) and (**c**), compatible with a grade II injury

vasorum (due to an association between shear stress and different elasticity between each of the vessel layers), or a combination of both. These injuries are seen as focal or segmental wall thickening, with a crescentic, eccentric (Fig. 2), or circumferential appearance on axial imaging. On non-contrast CT, hyperdensity within the wall can be appreciated, despite being a rare finding. On MR imaging, several sequences can be used to study the vessel wall without the use of a contrast agent. The signal intensity on

T1 can help with dating the hematoma, which is more commonly hyperintense on the first 3 days and isointense after 2 weeks [43–45].

## Grade II Injuries

Intramural hematomas, raised dissection flaps, and intraluminal thrombi producing greater than 25% stenosis (Fig. 3):

**Fig. 5 Grade III injury.** Follow-up imaging 24 hours after the presentation for the patient in Fig. 4. CT angiogram with coronal (**a**) and sagittal (**b**) MPRs shows a pseudoaneurysm in the distal right cervical ICA segment (dashed arrows), corresponding to a grade III injury

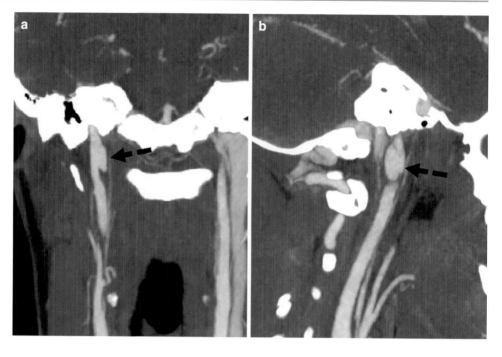

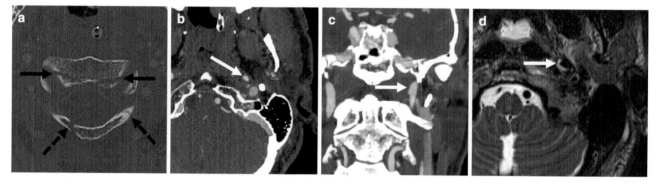

**Fig. 6 Grade III injury.** A 36-year-old man presenting after motor vehicle collision. Axial CT image of the cervical spine in bone window (**a**) demonstrates fractures of the C1 ring (black arrows) and C2 vertebral body (dashed black arrows). Axial (**b**) and coronal (**c**) CTA images show a pseudoaneurysm of the distal left cervical ICA, with partial narrowing of the lumen (white arrows). Axial T2-weighted MR image at the level of the skull base (**d**) shows the pseudoaneurysm and a wall hematoma, corresponding to a grade III injury

- Intramural hematomas: already discussed in the previous section, IMHs are considered grade II injuries whenever they cause more than 25% of luminal stenosis.
- Raised dissection flaps: intimal tears lead to blood flowing between the intima and the middle layers. The most recognized and virtually pathognomonic appearance is that of a vessel with two lumens (double lumen) (Fig. 4).
- Intraluminal thrombus: intimal injury can promote the mixture of blood and thrombogenic factors leading to

thrombus formation. Thrombi are usually observed as nodular or focal filling defects within the vessel lumen [44].

## Grade III Injuries

- Pseudoaneurysm formation: also known as contained rupture, represents a focal or partial vascular wall rupture that is not contained by normal arterial wall components. Potential complications include rupture, distal

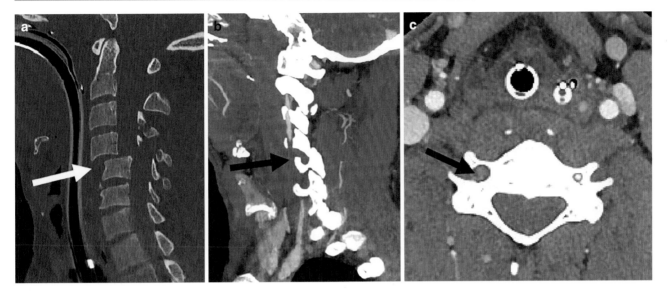

**Fig. 7  Grade IV injury**. A 42-year-old man presenting after semitruck rollover. Sagittal non-contrast CT image (**a**) of the cervical spine in a bone window demonstrates typical findings of bilateral facet dislocation, with greater than 50% traumatic anterolisthesis of C4 on C5 (white arrows). Sagittal (**b**) and axial (**c**) CT angiographic images demonstrate lack of opacification of a short segment of the right vertebral artery at, and proximal to, the cervical spine dislocation (black arrows), corresponding to a grade IV injury

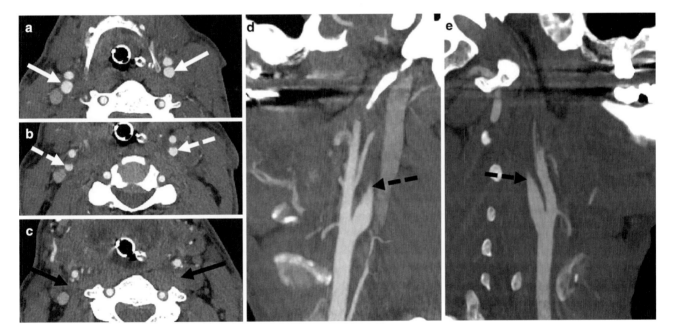

**Fig. 8  Grade IV injuries**. A 56-year-old man presenting to the emergency department after a motor vehicle collision. Axial CT angiogram images from caudal to cranial (**a**–**c**) show normal opacification of the bilateral proximal cervical internal carotid arteries just above the carotid bulbs (white arrows), with progressive tapering of the lumen (dashed white arrows), and then complete occlusion of the vessels (black arrows). Sagittal oblique MPRs (**d**) and (**e**) confirm the classic "rat tail" tapering (dashed black arrows) of the carotid lumen bilaterally, indicating bilateral carotid artery dissection and occlusion, representing a grade IV injury

thromboembolism, and extrinsic compression of the adjacent vessel with luminal stenosis. Radiologically, these are identified as focal saccular or ballooned outpouchings (Figs. 5 and 6) [46, 47].

## Grade IV Injuries

- Arterial occlusion: lack of vessel wall opacification distal to a defined abnormality, including IMHs, thrombi, or

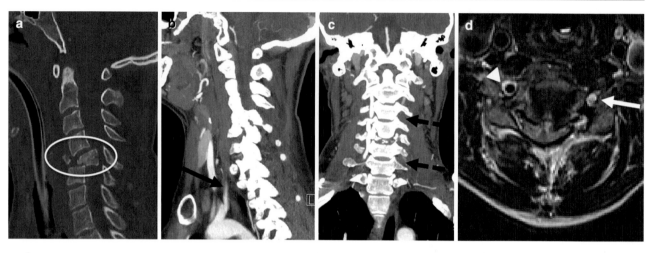

**Fig. 9** **Grade IV injury**. A 30-year-old woman presenting after a ski accident. Sagittal CT image of the cervical spine (**a**) shows a severe flexion teardrop fracture (white circle). Sagittal oblique MIP reformat of a CTA (**b**) demonstrates tapering of the V1 segment of the left vertebral artery with fading of its opacification (black arrow). Coronal CTA image shows lack of opacification of the V2 segment up to the level of the C3 vertebral body (dashed black arrows). Findings are consistent with a vertebral artery dissection and complete occlusion, grade IV injury. MR cervical spine axial T2-weighted image (**d**) at the level of C5 shows loss of the normal flow void in the left vertebral artery (white arrow), which is expected in a patent vessel. Note the normal flow void in the right vertebral artery (white arrowhead), at the same level

dissections. Radiologically, it can be characterized by either progressive narrowing (Fig. 7) or abrupt interruption of the luminal opacification (Figs. 8 and 9). Commonly, the underlying cause (dissection or thrombus) is not identified [47].

## Grade V Injuries

- Arterial transection: extravascular deposition of contrast with associated vessel wall irregularity of the adjacent injured artery. Delayed post-contrast acquisitions are extremely helpful to identify these injuries, as they commonly show pooling of contrast material that increases in size in the interval.
- Arteriovenous fistula formation: when there is concomitant rupture of arterial and venous structures, the arterial flow may find the path of least resistance into the vein's exposed lumen, creating therefore an arteriovenous communication (Figs. 10 and 11). Early opacification of the drainage vein is the hallmark feature of this injury, and, even though this finding is objectively identified on DSA, it may not be that easily appreciated on CTA or MRA. Other than early venous enhancement, CTA and MRA can rely on the comparison with the contralateral side, looking for asymmetry and relative enlargement of the involved sinuses and veins [44, 48].

## Pitfalls and Mimickers

The diagnosis of blunt vascular neck injuries depends not only on the radiologist's awareness of its existence and most common patterns but also on differentiating them from potential imaging mimickers. There are several anatomic variants, nontraumatic vascular entities, and artifacts that can potentially make the diagnostic process more challenging:

- Anatomic variants: which include variations in the origin of the arteries of the circle of Willis, duplications, and fenestrations (Fig. 12), persistent carotid-basilar anastomosis, asymmetry of the pterygoid venous plexuses (Fig. 13), and enhancement of the carotid bodies (Fig. 14).
- Atherosclerosis: more commonly observed in older patients, in the carotid bulbs, and at the origin of the vertebral arteries. The presence of calcifications may be a useful factor for distinction.
- Vasospasm: common finding in early post-trauma imaging and are often indistinguishable from grade I injuries. Short-term follow-up imaging after the first hours to days commonly shows resolution of the abnormality [28, 44].
- Fibromuscular dysplasia: classic "string-of-beads" appearance, due to alternating areas of stenosis and dilatation. Can be encountered in up to 1% of the

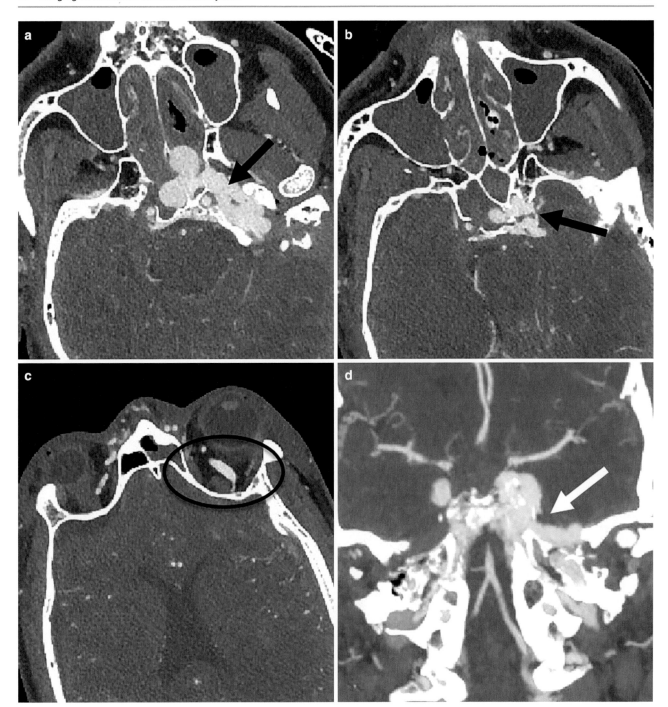

**Fig. 10 Carotid-cavernous fistula (grade V injury).** A 29-year-old man brought to the emergency department after being found down on the side of the road. Axial CTA images (**a–c**) demonstrate a large lobulated pseudoaneurysm of the intracranial segment of the left ICA, extending into the nasopharynx and sphenoid sinuses (black arrows in a and b). In addition, there is early arterial opacification and dilatation of the left superior ophthalmic vein (black circle in **c**). Coronal MIP reformation (**d**) of the CTA shows opacification of the surrounding venous and cavernous sinuses (white arrow). The findings are diagnostic of a carotid-cavernous fistula (grade V injury)

population, most commonly involving the cervical ICAs. Demographic factors (more common in young and middle-aged women), bilaterality, and multi-focality are clues to avoid the pitfall.

- Pseudodissection: faint flow-related linear filling defects (Figs. 15 and 16).
- Carotid webs: linear filling defects usually localized in the posterior wall of the carotid bulbs or proximal ICAs (Fig. 17).

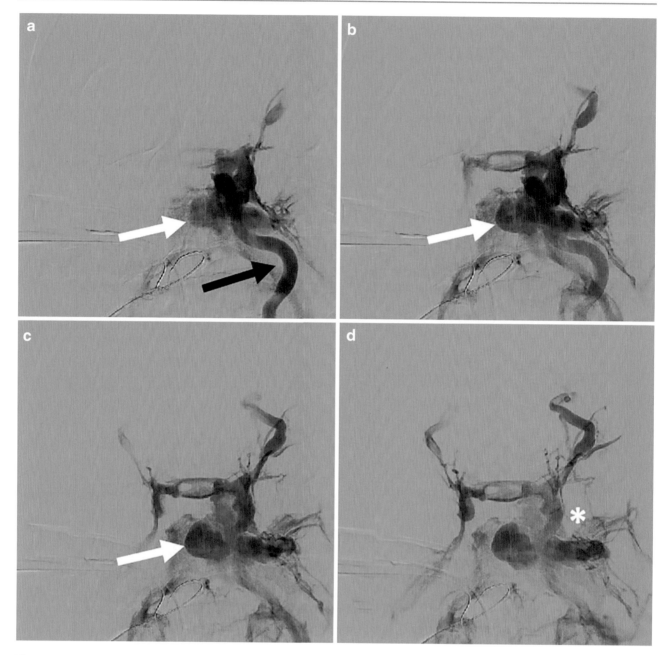

**Fig. 11 Carotid-cavernous fistula (grade V injury)**. The same patient from Fig. 10. Coronal views of the conventional angiogram before interventions (**a–d**) after contrast injection into the left ICA (black arrow) show opacification of a large lobulated pseudoaneurysm of the intracranial segment of the left ICA, with extension into the nasopharynx and sphenoid sinuses (white arrows). Note the early opacification of the adjacent left venous and cavernous sinuses (asterisk), confirming the carotid-cavernous fistula (grade V injury)

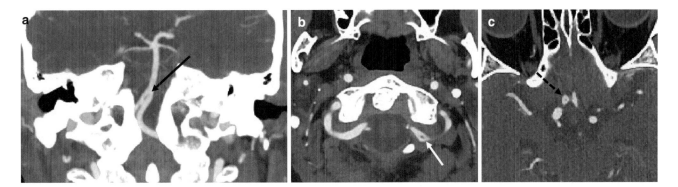

**Fig. 12 Arterial fenestration**. A 32-year-old man following a motor vehicle collision. Coronal MIP image of a post-contrast CTA (**a**) demonstrates a fenestrated proximal basilar artery (black arrow). Axial CTA image (**b**) of a 42-year-old woman after fall from a bicycle shows a fenestrated left vertebral artery involving the V3 segment (white arrow). Axial CTA image (**c**) of another patient centered in the suprasellar region demonstrates a fenestration of the right anterior cerebral artery at the A1–A2 junction (dashed black arrow)

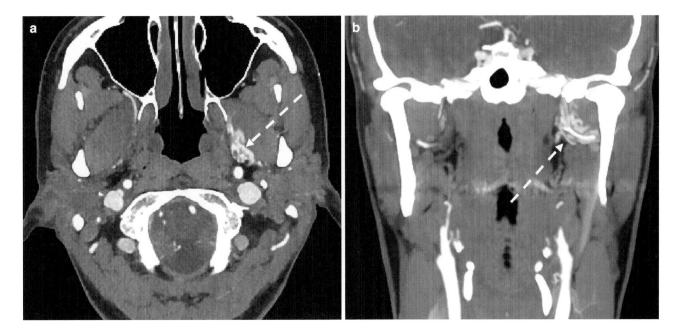

**Fig. 13 Asymmetric pterygoid venous plexus**. A 35-year-old man victim of physical aggression. Axial (**a**) and coronal (**b**) images of a CTA of the head and neck show multiple dilated vascular structures in the left prestyloid parapharyngeal space (dashed white arrows), surrounding the maxillary artery, indicating an asymmetric prominent pterygoid venous plexus, which is a normal variant

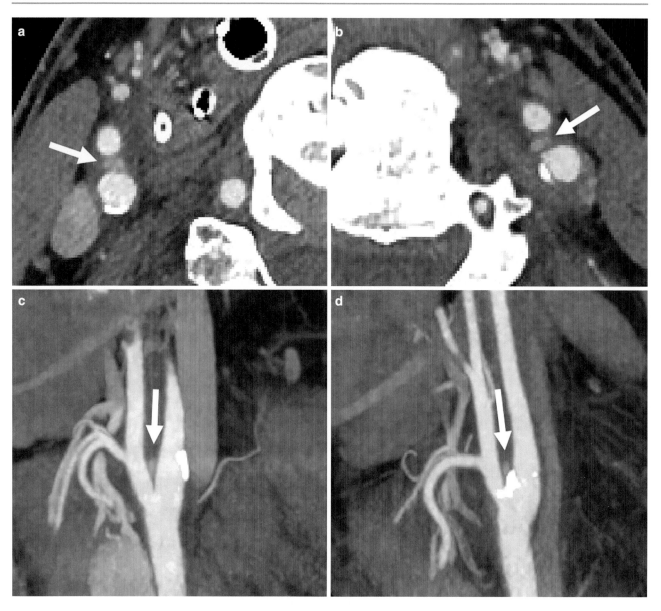

**Fig. 14 Carotid body enhancement**. A 65-year-old man found down with evidence of physical aggression. Axial (**a** and **b**) and sagittal (**c** and **d**) images of a CTA show subtle areas of enhancement between the proximal aspect of the cervical ICAs and ECAs bilaterally, just above the carotid bulbs (white arrows), with less attenuation than the adjacent intravascular contrast. These findings are typical for enhancement of the carotid bodies and should not be mistaken for traumatic injuries

**Fig. 15 Pseudodissection.**
A 40-year-old woman presenting after a ski accident. Sagittal oblique reformats (**a** and **b**) of a CTA show very subtle linear filling defects at the origin of the cervical ICAs (white arrows) representing flow-related abnormality in the absence of atherosclerotic plaques, which is commonly called a pseudodissection

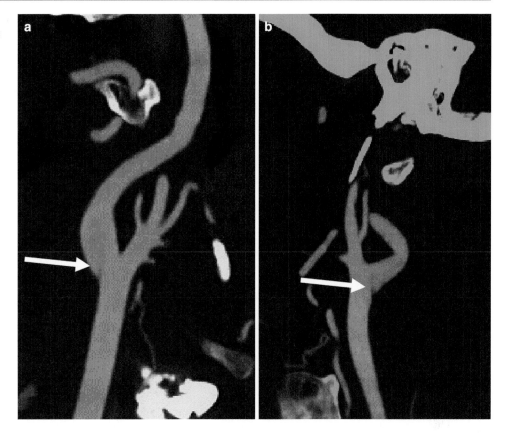

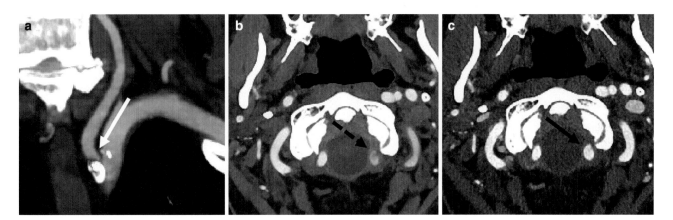

**Fig. 16 Pseudodissection.** A 71-year-old man found down. Coronal CTA image (**a**) shows a severe stenosis at the origin of the left vertebral artery (white arrow), leading to a pseudodissection appearance at the V3–V4 junction on the axial CTA image (**b**) obtained at the level of the skull base (dashed black arrow). Axial follow-up CTA image (**c**) with a slightly more delayed acquisition or multiphasic acquisition can be useful to exclude a vascular injury, as shown in this example (black arrow)

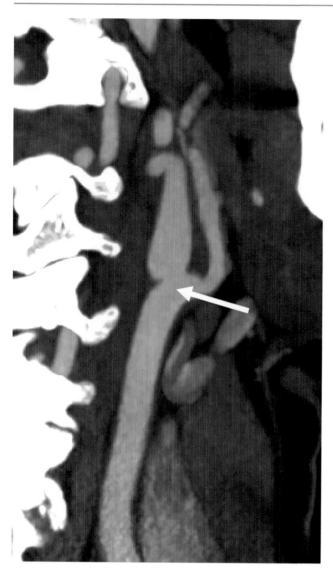

**Fig. 17 Carotid web**. A 52-year-old man brought to the emergency department after motor vehicle collision. There is a linear filling defect localized in the posterior wall of the ICA, at the level of the carotid bifurcation (white arrow)

- Artifacts: motion, step-off, streak, and isocenter artifacts (Fig. 18) are examples of artifacts that may potentially mimic or mask a vascular injury [49].

## Summary

Blunt cerebrovascular injuries (BCVI) are relatively rare injuries with substantial morbidity and mortality rates. Screening protocols for cerebral and cervical vascular injuries are recommended for blunt polytrauma patients. Although DSA is the reference standard for the diagnosis of BVNI, CTA is the universally accepted screening imaging examination. Awareness of the Biffl scale and of the adequate classification of the type of vascular injury is key to determine an affected patient's management and outcome. Recognizing and being familiar with the different pitfalls and mimickers is important for improving the radiologist's individual accuracy and to avoid incorrect diagnoses.

**Fig. 18 Isocenter artifact.** This artifact is attributed to a reconstruction algorithm, more obvious when projecting over a dense tubular object in the isocenter of the gantry following the z-axis (e.g., basilar artery). Initial axial CTA image (**a**) in an asymptomatic 45-year-old female patient, undergoing follow-up for an intracranial aneurysm, shows a target-like concentric hypodense filling defect measuring 3 mm in diameter. On the repeat scan (**b**), obtained with patient's head slightly off the midline, the artifact is no longer identified

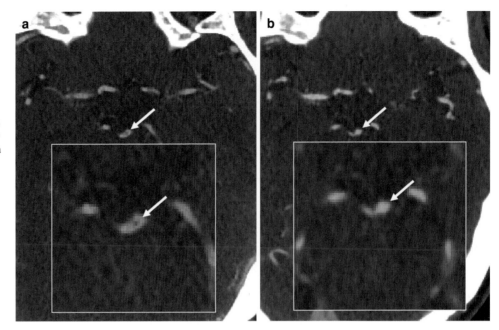

## References

1. Crissey MM, Bernstein EF. Delayed presentation of carotid intimal tear following blunt craniocervical trauma. Surgery. 1974;75:543–9.
2. Fabian TC. Blunt cerebrovascular injuries: anatomic and pathologic heterogeneity create management enigmas. J Am Coll Surg. 2013;216(5):873–85.
3. Davis JW, Holbrook TL, Hoyt DB, et al. Blunt carotid artery dissection: incidence, associated injuries, screening and treatment. J Trauma. 1990;30(12):1514–7.
4. Page P, Josiah D. Traumatic vertebral artery injuries in the geriatric population: a retrospective cohort study. J Neurosurg Spine. 2020:1–4.
5. Cogbill TH, Moore EE, Meissner M, Fischer RP, Hoyt DB, Morris JA, et al. The spectrum of blunt injury to the carotid artery: a multicenter perspective. J Trauma. 1994;37(3):473–9.
6. Grigorian A, Kabutey NK, Schubl S, de Virgilio C, Joe V, Dolich M, et al. Blunt cerebrovascular injury incidence, stroke-rate, and mortality with the expanded Denver criteria. Surgery. 2018;164(3):494–9.
7. Biffl WL, Moore EE, Ryu RK, Offner PJ, Novak Z, Coldwell DM, et al. The unrecognized epidemic of blunt carotid arterial injuries: early diagnosis improves neurologic outcome. Ann Surg. 1998;228(4):462–70.
8. Weber CD, Lefering R, Kobbe P, Horst K, Pishnamaz M, Sellei RM, et al. Blunt cerebrovascular artery injury and stroke in severely injured patients: an international multicenter analysis. World J Surg. 2018;42(7):2043–53.
9. Stone DK, Viswanathan VT, Wilson CA. Management of blunt cerebrovascular injury. Curr Neurol Neurosci Rep. 2018;18(12):98.
10. Sliker CW. Blunt cerebrovascular injuries: imaging with multidetector CT angiography. Radiographics. 2008;28(6):1689–708. discussion 1709–1710
11. Bonatti M, Vezzali N, Ferro F, Manfredi R, Oberhofer N, Bonatti G. Blunt cerebrovascular injury: diagnosis at whole-body MDCT for multi-trauma. Insight Imaging. 2013;4(3):347–55.
12. Torina PJ, Flanders AE, Carrino JA, Burns AS, Friedman DP, Harrop JS, et al. Incidence of vertebral artery thrombosis in cervical spine trauma: correlation with severity of spinal cord injury. AJNR Am J Neuroradiol. 2005;26(10):2645–51.
13. Cothren CC, Moore EE, Biffl WL, Ciesla DJ, Ray CE Jr, Johnson JL, et al. Anticoagulation is the gold standard therapy for blunt carotid injuries to reduce stroke rate. Arch Surg. 2004;139(5):540–5. discussion 545–6
14. Biffl WL, Ray CE Jr, Moore EE, Mestek M, Johnson JL, Burch JM. Noninvasive diagnosis of blunt cerebrovascular injuries: a preliminary report. J Trauma. 2002;53(5):850–6.
15. Berne JD, Norwood SH, McAuley CE, Villareal DH. Helical computed tomographic angiography: an excellent screening test for blunt cerebrovascular injury. J Trauma. 2004;57(1):11–7. discussion 17–9
16. Sedlic A, Chingkoe CM, Tso DK, Galea-Soler S, Nicolaou S. Rapid imaging protocol in trauma: a whole-body dual-source CT scan. Emerg Radiol. 2013;20(5):401–8.
17. Bruns BR, Tesoriero R, Kufera J, Sliker C, Laser A, Scalea TM, et al. Blunt cerebrovascular injury screening guidelines: what are we willing to miss? J Trauma Acute Care Surg. 2014;76(3):691–5.
18. Biffl WL, Moore EE, Offner PJ, Brega KE, Franciose RJ, Elliott JP, et al. Optimizing screening for blunt cerebrovascular injuries. Am J Surg. 1999;178(6):517–22.
19. Bromberg WJ, Collier BC, Diebel LN, Dwyer KM, Holevar MR, Jacobs DG, et al. Blunt cerebrovascular injury practice management guidelines: the Eastern Association for the Surgery of Trauma. J Trauma. 2010;68(2):471–7.
20. Leichtle SW, Banerjee D, Schrader R, Torres B, Jayaraman S, Rodas E, et al. Blunt cerebrovascular injury – the case for universal screening. J Trauma Acute Care Surg. 2020;90(2):224–31.
21. Biffl WL, Cothren CC, Moore EE, Kozar R, Cocanour C, Davis JW, et al. Western Trauma Association critical decisions in trauma: screening for and treatment of blunt cerebrovascular injuries. J Trauma. 2009;67(6):1150–3.
22. Geddes AE, Burlew CC, Wagenaar AE, Biffl WL, Johnson JL, Pieracci FM, et al. Expanded screening criteria for blunt cerebrovascular injury: a bigger impact than anticipated. Am J Surg. 2016;212(6):1167–74.
23. Burlew CC, Biffl WL, Moore EE, Barnett CC, Johnson JL, Bensard DD. Blunt cerebrovascular injuries: redefining screening criteria in

the era of noninvasive diagnosis. J Trauma Acute Care Surg. 2012;72(2):335. discussion 337, quiz 539

24. Kim DY, Biffl W, Bokhari F, Brakenridge S, Chao E, Claridge JA, et al. Evaluation and management of blunt cerebrovascular injury: a practice management guideline from the Eastern Association for the Surgery of Trauma. J Trauma Acute Care Surg. 2020;88(6):875–87.

25. Miller PR, Fabian TC, Croce MA, Cagiannos C, Williams JS, Vang M, et al. Prospective screening for blunt cerebrovascular injuries: analysis of diagnostic modalities and outcomes. Ann Surg. 2002;236(3):386–93. discussion 393–5

26. Ciapetti M, Circelli A, Zagli G, Migliaccio ML, Spina R, Alessi A, et al. Diagnosis of carotid arterial injury in major trauma using a modification of Memphis criteria. Scand J Trauma Resusc Emerg Med. 2010;22(18):61.

27. Elbanna KY, Mohammed MF, Choi JI, Dawe JP, Joos E, Baawain S, et al. What are the expected findings on follow-up computed tomography angiogram in post-traumatic patients with blunt cerebrovascular injury? Can Assoc Radiol J. 2018;69(3):266–76.

28. Abu Mughli R, Wu T, Li J, Moghimi S, Alem Z, Nasir MU, et al. An update in imaging of blunt vascular neck injury. Can Assoc Radiol J. 2020;71(3):281–92.

29. Shahan CP, Croce MA, Fabian TC, Magnotti LJ. Impact of continuous evaluation of technology and therapy: 30 years of research reduces stroke and mortality from blunt cerebrovascular injury. J Am Coll Surg. 2017;224(4):595–9.

30. Biffl WL, Ray CE Jr, Moore EE, Franciose RJ, Aly S, Heyrosa MG, et al. Treatment-related outcomes from blunt cerebrovascular injuries: importance of routine follow-up arteriography. Ann Surg. 2002;235(5):699–706. discussion 706–707

31. Biffl WL, Moore EE, Offner PJ, Brega KE, Franciose RJ, Burch JM. Blunt carotid arterial injuries: implications of a new grading scale. J Trauma. 1999;47(5):845–53.

32. Wagenaar AE, Burlew CC, Biffl WL, Beauchamp KM, Pieracci FM, Stovall RT, et al. Early repeat imaging is not warranted for high-grade blunt cerebrovascular injuries. J Trauma Acute Care Surg. 2014;77(4):540–5. quiz 650

33. Powers WJ, Rabinstein AA, Ackerson T, Adeoye OM, Bambakidis NC, Becker K, et al. 2018 Guidelines for the early management of patients with acute ischemic stroke: a guideline for healthcare professionals from the American Heart Association/American Stroke Association. Stroke. 2018;49(3):e46–e110.

34. Roberts DJ, Chaubey VP, Zygun DA, Lorenzetti D, Faris PD, Ball CG, et al. Diagnostic accuracy of computed tomographic angiography for blunt cerebrovascular injury detection in trauma patients: a systematic review and meta-analysis. Ann Surg. 2013;257(4):621–32.

35. Thomas C, Korn A, Ketelsen D, Danz S, Tsifikas I, Claussen CD, Ernemann U, Heuschmid M. Automatic lumen segmentation in calcified plaques: dual-energy CT versus standard reconstructions

36. Deng K, Liu C, Ma R, et al. Clinical evaluation of dual-energy bone removal in CT angiography of the head and neck: comparison with conventional bone-subtraction CT angiography. Clin Radiol. 2009;64(5):534–41.

37. Shinohara Y, Sakamoto M, Iwata N, et al. Usefulness of monochromatic imaging with metal artifact reduction software for computed tomography angiography after intracranial aneurysm coil embolization. Acta Radiol. 2013;55:1015–23.

38. Srinivasan A, Hoeffner E, Ibrahim M, Shah GV, LaMarca F, Mukherji SK. Utility of dual-energy CT virtual keV monochromatic series for the assessment of spinal transpedicular hardware-bone interface. Am J Roentgenol. 2013;201:878–83.

39. Wiggins WF, Potter CA, Sodickson AD. Dual-energy CT to differentiate small foci of intracranial hemorrhage from calcium. Radiology. 2020;294(1):129–38.

40. Nagpal P, Policeni BA, Bathla G, Khandelwal A, Derdeyn C, Skeete D. Blunt cerebrovascular injuries: advances in screening, imaging, and management trends. AJNR. 2018;39(3):406–14.

41. Liang T, David K, Tso RYW, Chiu NS. Imaging of blunt vascular neck injuries: a review of screening and imaging modalities. Am J Roentgenol. 2013;201(4):884–92.

42. Malhotra AK, Camacho M, Ivatury RR, et al. Computed tomographic angiography for the diagnosis of blunt carotid/vertebral artery injury: a note of caution. Ann Surg. 2007;246(4):632–42.

43. Sliker CW. Blunt cerebrovascular injuries: imaging with multidetector CT angiography. RadioGraphics. 2008;28(6):1689–708.

44. Rutman AM, Vranic JE, Mossa-Basha M. Imaging and management of blunt cerebrovascular injury. Radiographics. 2018;38(2):542–63.

45. Ozdoba C, Sturzenegger M, Schroth G. Internal carotid artery dissection: MR imaging features and clinical-radiologic correlation. Radiology. 1996;199(1):191–8.

46. Núñez DB Jr, Torres-León M, Múnera F. Vascular injuries of the neck and thoracic inlet: helical CT angiographic correlation. RadioGraphics. 2004;24(4):1087–98.

47. Staller B, Múnera F, Sanchez A, Núñez DB Jr. Helical and multislice CTA following penetrating trauma to the subclavian and axillary arteries (pictorial essay). Emerg Radiol. 2005;11(6):336–41.

48. Stallmeyer MJ, Morales RE, Flanders AE. Imaging of traumatic neurovascular injury. Radiol Clin N Am. 2006;44(1):13–39.

49. Borisch I, Boehme T, Butz B, Hamer OW, Feuerbach S, Zorger N. Screening for carotid injury in trauma patients: image quality of 16-detector-row computed tomography angiography. Acta Radiol. 2007;48(7):798–805.

50. Burlew CC, Biffl WL, Moore EE, Barnett CC, Johnson JL, Bensard DD. Blunt cerebrovascular injuries: redefining screening criteria in the era of noninvasive diagnosis. J Trauma Acute Care Surg. 2012;72(2):330–5. discussion 336–337, quiz 539

# Imaging of Neck and Facial Infections

## 12

Prachi Dubey, Amy Juliano, and Gul Moonis

## Contents

P. Dubey (✉)
Houston Methodist Hospital, Houston Radiology Associated, Houston, TX, USA

A. Juliano
Massachusetts Eye and Ear, Harvard Medical School, Boston, USA
e-mail: amy_juliano@meei.harvard.edu

G. Moonis
New York University Langone Health, NYU Grossman School of Medicine, New York, NY, USA
e-mail: gm2640@cumc.columbia.edu

## Abstract

Acute infections in the face and neck can range from minor illnesses to life-threatening surgical emergencies with substantial morbidity and mortality. The cervicofacial soft tissues are compartmentalized in closely approximated spaces such that, despite fascial barriers, there is a high risk for trans-spatial spread with potentially dire consequences. Management relies heavily on understanding not only the anatomic detail but also on the etiopathogenesis and host factors. Delayed or inappropriate management can lead to potentially life-threatening complications. Moreover, the infection can have overlapping features with both neoplasm

© Springer Nature Switzerland AG 2022
M. N. Patlas et al. (eds.), *Atlas of Emergency Imaging from Head-to-Toe*,
https://doi.org/10.1007/978-3-030-92111-8_12

and chronic inflammation in the face and neck. Thus, systematic analysis of structures in the face/neck is critical for accurate and timely diagnosis. Focused attention on three specific elements – anatomic location of the abnormality (source), the region or compartment in which the abnormality dwells (space), and extent of the abnormality (spread) – can aid in the timely diagnosis, detection of complications, and guidance to appropriate management. In this chapter, we present a systematic approach to analyzing commonly encountered face and neck infections with emphasis on the complex interactions between source, space, and pathways of spread.

### Keywords

Head and Neck infections · Spaces · Emergency · Anatomy

### Key Learning Objectives
- Identify imaging features of face and neck infections.
- Characterize the abnormality based on a "source, space, and spread" paradigm.
- Review common case examples highlighting these elements, understanding their role in complications and management.

## Introduction

Acute infections in the face and neck can range from minor illnesses to life-threatening surgical emergencies with substantial morbidity and mortality. The cervicofacial soft tissues are compartmentalized in closely approximated spaces such that, despite fascial barriers, there is a high risk for transspatial spread with potentially dire consequences. The imaging features of common head and neck infections and mimicking conditions have been previously described and are fairly well understood [1, 2]. Management relies heavily on understanding not only the anatomic detail but also on the etiopathogenesis and host factors. Delayed or inappropriate management can lead to potentially life-threatening complications, including necrotizing fasciitis, descending mediastinitis, airway compromise, and sepsis [3–5]. Moreover, the infection can have overlapping features with both neoplasm and chronic inflammation in the face and neck. Thus, systematic analysis of structures in the face/neck is critical for accurate and timely diagnosis. Focused attention on three specific elements – anatomic location of the abnormality (source), the region or compartment in which the abnormality dwells (space), and extent of the abnormality (spread) – can aid in the timely diagnosis, detection of complications, and guidance to appropriate management. In this chapter, we present a systematic approach to analyzing

commonly encountered face and neck infections with emphasis on the complex interactions between source, space, and pathways of spread, as summarized in Table 1.

## Infections from an Odontogenic Source

Odontogenic etiology is common and typically polymicrobial in nature, comprising of anerobic organisms, gram-negative rods, and gram-positive cocci. Odontogenic source infections can originate from dental, alveolar, and/or gingival components and are located in the oral cavity proper. Frequent causes are periapical infections, dental caries or pulpitis, post-extraction infection, and pericoronitis in partially erupted dentition, typically the third molar [6, 7]. These have a tendency to spread into the submandibular/submental, buccal/masticator, and parapharyngeal spaces; more extensive cases can show spread into the floor of mouth (Ludwig angina) and deep cervical spaces. These are prone to additional complications, particularly necrotizing fasciitis and descending mediastinitis. The most common clinical presentation is pain, trismus, and dysphagia. Management strategy depends upon the extent of abnormality and includes antibiotics, tooth extraction, and surgical drainage [7].

### Odontogenic Sinus Disease

Odontogenic sinus disease is one of the common causes of maxillary sinus disease and accounts for 10% to 40% of cases of paranasal sinus disease [8, 9]. Imaging is key in the detection of odontogenic sinus disease, which may be difficult to distinguish from rhinological causes on clinical evaluation. Typically, it involves the maxillary sinuses and is equally prevalent in both immunocompromised and immunocompetent patients [10]. In particular, isolated maxillary sinus disease with periapical lucencies that cause the dentoalveolar unit to breach the Schneiderian membrane is a strong indicator of odontogenic sinus disease [9, 10] (Fig. 1). Other etiologies include post-extraction oroantral fistula, dental implants, and complications related to sinus augmentation ("sinus lift surgery"). Sinus infection from an odontogenic source requires management of the underlying dental condition for a complete response. This is particularly true of unilateral paranasal sinus disease, which in one study was found to be associated with odontogenic infection in 72% of the cases [11]. CT without contrast is the modality of choice for imaging. It may show mucosal thickening, fluid, periapical lucencies, and protrusion of the dentoalveolar unit into the floor of the maxillary sinus, and in complicated cases, an oroantral fistula may be seen. In the setting of medical treatment failure and chronic recurrent episodes of sinusitis, it is therefore essential to evaluate the maxillary dentition for

**Table 1** Face and neck acute soft tissue infections categorized by anatomic source, the space within which the anatomic source resides, and pathways of spread. Commonly encountered clinical entities are also provided for each category

| Source | Space | Spread (extent and destination) | Examples |
|---|---|---|---|
| *Odontogenic* (dentoalveolar unit, gingival mucosa) | Oral cavity (gingivobuccal, retromolar trigone) | Submandibular region Submental space | Odontogenic sinusitis |
| | | Parapharyngeal space | Odontogenic DNSI |
| | | Masticator space | Ludwig angina |
| | | Buccal space | |
| | | Floor of mouth | |
| | | Maxillary sinus | |
| *Salivary* (parotid, submandibular, and sublingual glands) | Parotid region | Floor of mouth | Suppurative or nonsuppurative sialadenitis |
| | Submandibular space | Parapharyngeal space | Ludwig angina |
| | Floor of mouth (sublingual space) | Masticator space | Infected ranula |
| | | Buccal space | |
| *Visceral* (pharynx, hypopharynx, and larynx) | Pharyngeal mucosal space | Parapharyngeal space | Intra-/peritonsillar abscess |
| *Lymphoid* (tonsils, adenoids) | Lymphadenitis (RP, deep neck spaces) | Carotid region | RP necrotizing adenitis |
| | | Retropharyngeal space via danger space to the mediastinum | RP abscess |
| | | | Pharyngitis |
| | | | Lemierre's syndrome |
| *Sinonasal* | Sinonasal[a] | Orbit | Acute rhinosinusitis |
| | | Intracranial compartment | Nasal vestibulitis |
| | | Angioinvasive spread to regions contiguous with the sinonasal cavities | Invasive sinusitis |
| *Otomastoid* | Otomastoid[a] | Parotid space | Coalescent mastoiditis |
| | | Masticator space | Bezold abscess |
| | | Intracranial compartment | Petrous apicitis |
| | | Skull base | Skull base osteomyelitis |
| *Congenital lesions developmental anomalies* (with superimposed infections) | Depends on the anomaly (commonly parotid region, submandibular space, anterior cervical space, and pharyngeal mucosal space) | Retropharyngeal space | Infected branchial cleft cyst, pyriform sinus fistula, infected thyroglossal duct cyst |
| | | Danger space | |
| | | Mediastinum | |
| *Spine* | Prevertebral space | Epidural space | Discitis/osteomyelitis Epidural abscess |
| | Perivertebral space | Prevertebral space | Paraspinal abscess |
| | | Perivertebral space | |

[a]For Sinonasal and Otomastoid categories, the anatomic source and space are equivalent (abbreviation: RP, retropharyngeal; DNSI, deep neck space infection). Please note, it is emphasized that advanced infections can spread into any space; the purpose of this summary is to highlight the early pathways of spread to enable the earliest detection of complications

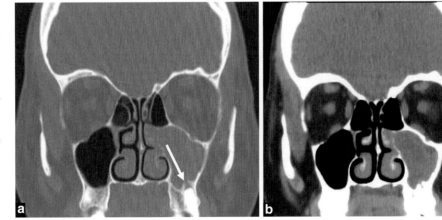

**Fig. 1 Odontogenic sinus disease**. Non-contrast CT image of the sinuses in the coronal plane, in bone (**a**) and soft-tissue (**b**) algorithms, shows complete opacification of the left maxillary sinus and a periapical lucency around the root of a left maxillary molar, which is dehiscent (arrow) into the maxillary sinus antrum. This pattern is due to odontogenic maxillary sinus disease

the presence of an underlying oroantral fistula that may serve as a passage for oral microflora. A recent review on the management of odontogenic sinus disease concluded a need for shared decision-making between patients, dental providers, and otolaryngologists for definitive management [12].

## Ludwig Angina

Ludwig angina is a gangrenous floor of mouth cellulitis with a tendency for the rapid contiguous spread of infection to the submandibular space and sublingual space. It can further extend across the midline, into deep neck spaces across the superficial cervical fascia, platysma muscle, and superficial layer of the deep cervical fascia. This can rapidly lead to substantial oropharyngeal edema and airway compromise [13, 14]. The odontogenic source is one the most common etiologies, most commonly due to a periapical abscess involving the second and third mandibular molars, whose apical processes penetrate the thin lingual cortex of the mandible, below the insertion of the mylohyoid muscle [13, 14] (Fig. 2). Additional sources include suppurative sialadenitis, peritonsillar abscess, foreign body, penetrating trauma, and mandibular osteomyelitis [13]. Early recognition and prompt treatment are critical to avoid complications such as airway obstruction, deep neck abscess, thrombophlebitis, necrotizing fasciitis, mediastinitis, and sepsis. Patients present with pain, fever, dysphagia, and odynophagia. On examination, there is erythema, woody induration, and crepitus. There is no bulky lymphadenopathy due to contiguous soft tissue rather than the lymphatic spread of infection [14]. CT of the neck with IV contrast is the imaging examination of choice and can show soft-tissue edema, inflammatory stranding, abscess formation, and abnormal foci of gas (Fig. 2). Early

airway management is critical. Flexible fiberoptic nasal intubation and elective tracheostomy are preferred due to substantial edema obscuring the oropharyngeal airway, rendering direct laryngoscopic evaluation for oral endotracheal tube placement difficult. Cricothyrotomy can also be challenging due to edema in the neck soft tissues. Intravenous antibiotics are an essential part of management to cover a polymicrobial source of infection. The dental extraction is recommended for odontogenic sources, and surgical management may be needed in severe cases [14].

## Infections from a Sinonasal Source

Sinonasal etiology forms a substantial proportion of face and neck infections. Acute rhinosinusitis in particular accounts for 30 million primary care visits. Although most commonly viral in etiology, it remains a common reason for an antibiotic prescription. In terms of bacterial and fungal etiologies, *Streptococcus pneumoniae*, *Haemophilus influenzae*, *Moraxella catarrhalis*, *Mucor* species, *Rhizopus* species, and *Aspergillus* species are most commonly seen. Patients can present with headache, sinus discharge, fever, and facial congestion [15].

Complicated acute sinus disease entails the spread of infection from the sinus cavities to the surrounding structures. The periorbital and orbital septum act as general physical barriers to prevent the spread of infection to the orbit. However, except at their attachment to the osseous anterior orbital margin, levator aponeurosis, and tarsal plate, they have inherent loose architecture. In addition, these structures contain inherent deficiencies for the passage of neurovascular structures. These lead to potential gaps and spaces for subperiosteal abscess formation and act as a portal of direct entry

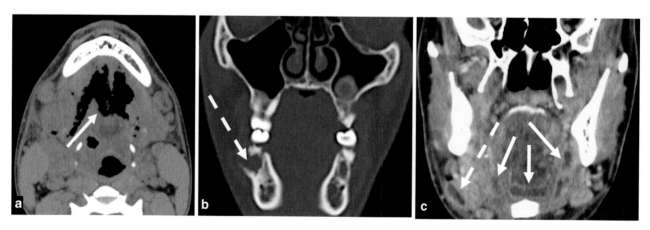

**Fig. 2** **Ludwig angina.** CT images through the floor of the mouth, in the axial (**a**, non-contrast enhanced) and coronal (**b** and **c**, contrast-enhanced) planes. Gas is noted within the soft tissues of the floor of mouth (arrow, **a**) with associated edema in the right submandibular region, and there is abnormal dehiscence/a bone defect surrounding the root of a right mandibular molar (dashed arrow, **b**). Multi-loculated rim-enhancing abscesses are seen in the floor of the mouth (solid arrows, **c**), continuing laterally past the mylohyoid into the right submandibular space (dashed arrow, **c**). Findings are due to Ludwig angina from an odontogenic source

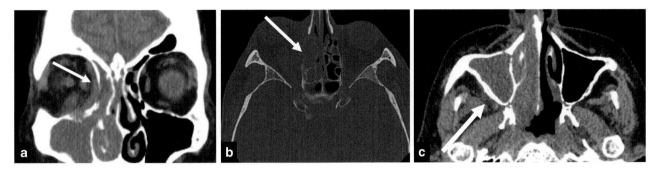

**Fig. 3 Acute invasive fungal sinusitis**. Coronal soft-tissue window (**a**), axial bone window (**b**), and axial soft-tissue window (**c**) images from a non-contrast-enhanced CT of the sinuses show right ethmoid, maxillary, and frontal sinus opacification, with inflammatory soft tissue in the medial aspect of the right orbit (arrow **a**), osseous erosion of the right lamina papyracea, (arrow **B**), and stranding in the right retromaxillary periantral fat (solid arrow **c**). Findings are due to acute invasive fungal sinusitis complicated by right orbital cellulitis

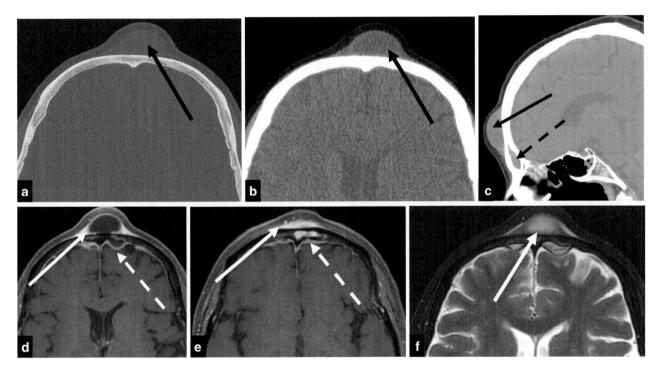

**Fig. 4 Pott puffy tumor**. Non-contrast CT images through the forehead in the axial (**a** in bone window, **b** in soft-tissue window) and sagittal (**c** in soft-tissue window) planes showing a subgaleal low attenuation collection, (arrows **a–c**). MR axial images through the forehead (**d** and **e**, post-contrast T1-weighted images; **f**, T2-weighted image). There is a rim-enhancing subgaleal collection (solid arrows, **d–f**), with associated frontal sinus opacification (dashed black arrow, **c**) and intracranial extension with epidural abscess and dural enhancement (white dashed arrows, **d** and **e**). Findings are diagnostic of Pott Puffy tumor and epidural abscess

for pathogens, including spread via valveless venous channels underneath the inner cancellous bone [16].

Orbital complications from a sinus source commonly originate from disease in the ethmoid or frontal sinuses, with the ethmoid sinus being more common in children [16] (Fig. 3). Imaging of sinus disease is reserved for recurrent cases or patients with suspected complications, particularly for invasive sinusitis with orbital cellulitis (Fig. 3), Pott puffy tumor (Fig. 4), and intracranial involvement including cavernous sinus thrombophlebitis (Fig. 5). Invasive disease is often seen with invasive fungal sinusitis, but it can also be seen in advanced bacterial sinusitis, with a variety of pathogens such as *Pseudomonas aeruginosa* (Fig. 3). CT with intravenous contrast and MRI without and with intravenous contrast are the imaging modalities of choice for invasive sinus disease. On CT, inflammatory extension into the retromaxillary fat pad and skull base, as well as intraorbital extension can be seen. MRI is more sensitive for the depiction of non-enhancing necrotic mucosal lining, cavernous sinus thrombophlebitis or thrombosis, and epidural abscess formation. Purulent cavernous sinus thrombophlebitis and epidural abscess are best detected with the aid of diffusion-weighted imaging with apparent diffusion coefficient mapping, which shows restricted diffusion associated with a peripherally enhancing collection.

## Pott Puffy Tumor

Pott puffy tumor results from frontal sinus disease complicated by frontal bone osteomyelitis and associated subgaleal abscess (Fig. 4). The subgaleal abscess clinically presents as

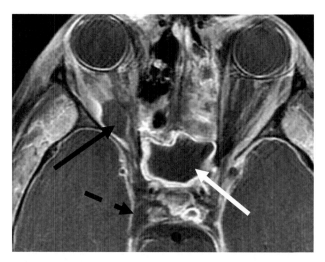

**Fig. 5 Cavernous sinus thrombophlebitis**. Axial contrast-enhanced T1-weighted MR image with fat suppression shows sinus disease, including complete opacification of the sphenoid sinus (white arrow), right cavernous sinus expansion with non-enhancing hypointense material (dashed black arrow), and an expansile collection in the right posterior orbit extending to the orbital apex (solid black arrow). Findings are due to acute sinus disease complicated by cavernous sinus thrombophlebitis, right orbital cellulitis, and intra-orbital abscess

a palpable soft-tissue mass, swelling, and tenderness. The intracranial extension can occur across the calvarium due to osseous erosion, through the valveless diploic space veins or through inherent defects in the inner table of the frontal bone.

## Nasal Vestibulitis

In addition to the sinuses, the nasal cavity can serve as a source of infection with a potential of spread to adjacent soft tissues. Nasal vestibulitis is an example of such a localized infection in the hair-bearing nasal vestibule. It can be seen with minor trauma, such as with nasal hair plucking, and with the use of topical nasal steroids [17] (Fig. 6). It can progress to the development of a nasal septal abscess and can spread into the adjacent soft tissues, resulting in midface cellulitis. Rarely, intracranial complications such as cavernous sinus thrombophlebitis may occur, due to valveless interconnected venous communications between midfacial angular/facial veins with the cavernous sinus and superior ophthalmic vein. CT with intravenous contrast is the imaging modality of choice and may show inflammatory changes including edema, stranding, and enhancement with or without abscess or phlegmon. Methicillin-sensitive *Staphylococcus aureus* is the most common organism causing nasal vestibulitis [17]. Mild cases respond to topical antibiotics, whereas advanced cases such as midface cellulitis require systemic antibiotics.

## Infections from an Otomastoid Source

The temporal bone can be involved by infection, with the external auditory canal, middle ear cavity, mastoid, and petrous apex being potential sites at risk. Acute otitis

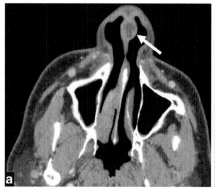 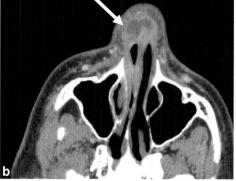 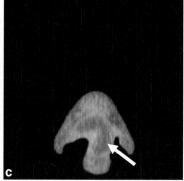

**Fig. 6 Nasal vestibulitis with nasal septal and nasal alar abscess**. IV contrast-enhanced CT images through the nasal septum in the axial (**a** and **b**) and coronal (**c**) planes show a nasal septal abscess (arrows, **a** and **c**), with soft-tissue thickening and fluid collection extending into the nasal alae (arrow **b**). Findings are due to nasal vestibulitis with nasal alar and nasal septal abscess formation

media, otitis externa, petrous apicitis, and acute non-coalescent and acute coalescent mastoiditis are common examples of acute otomastoid source infections [18]. Infection can spread to the suprahyoid neck spaces, including the parotid region, submandibular space, and medially into the masticator and parapharyngeal spaces. Skull base osteomyelitis and intracranial complications including venous sinus thrombosis, meningitis, labyrinthitis, and intracranial abscess may occur as well [19].

## Acute Coalescent Mastoiditis

Acute coalescent mastoiditis is a complicated acute mastoiditis with advanced osteitis and osteoclastic erosion of the mastoid osseous septations. Mastoid pneumatization is incomplete at birth, when there is only an antral air cell and a small opening called the aditus ad antrum, which forms a conduit between the middle ear cavity and mastoid antrum. Subsequent pneumatization in early childhood occurs via

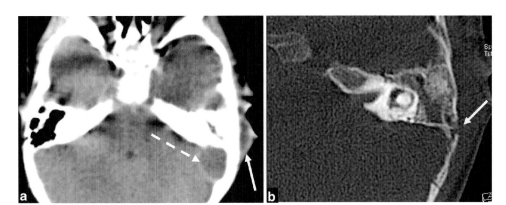

**Fig. 7**  **Coalescent mastoiditis with epidural abscess**. Axial non-contrast CT images in soft-tissue (**a**) and bone (**b**) windows show complete opacification of the left mastoid air cells, along with a retroauricular abscess (solid arrow, **a**), epidural abscess (dashed arrow, **a**), and osseous erosion of the lateral mastoid cortex (arrow, **b**), due to coalescent mastoiditis

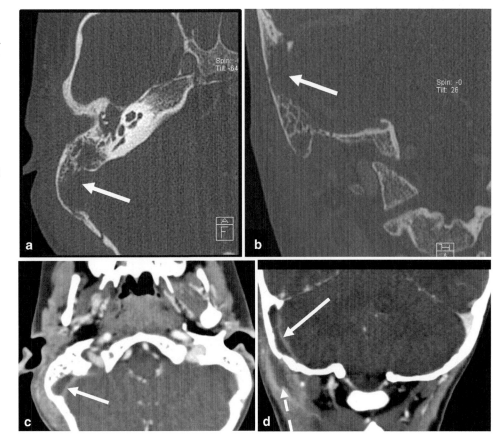

**Fig. 8**  **Coalescent mastoiditis with dural venous sinus thrombosis and Bezold abscess**. IV contrast-enhanced CT images in the axial (**a**, bone window; **c**, soft-tissue window) and coronal (**b**, bone window; **d**, soft-tissue window) planes show right coalescent mastoiditis with osseous erosions (arrows, **a** and **b**), right transverse sinus thrombosis (solid arrows, **c** and **d**), and a Bezold abscess (dashed arrow, **d**)

thinning of the mastoid bone and replacement with air cells, particularly around the tip of the mastoid bone [20]. These mastoid air cells can become obstructed during acute otitis media with trapped purulent secretions. There is subsequent osteitis and osteonecrosis of the bony septations resulting in acute coalescent mastoiditis. Infection can breach the thin mastoid cortex along the digastric ridge, spreading between the digastric and sternocleidomastoid muscles, resulting in a "Bezold" abscess. These changes are best detected on CT of the temporal bones with intravenous contrast. Additional complications can occur intracranially, including epidural abscess (Fig. 7) and dural venous sinus thrombosis (Fig. 8), for which MRI without and with intravenous contrast is the imaging modality of choice. The treatment mainstay involves intravenous antibiotics. Surgical drainage and mastoidectomy may be needed on an individualized basis [20].

## Infections from Salivary Gland Source

There are three paired major salivary glands, namely, parotid, submandibular, and sublingual glands. Infection of the major salivary glands can spread in a contiguous fashion to adjacent structures; depending on the gland of origin, there may be involvement of the floor of the mouth, masticator space, and deep neck spaces. The most common nonneoplastic major salivary gland disorder is post-obstructive sialadenitis, commonly due to sialolithiasis that can be complicated by recurrent bacterial infections [21]. The exact cause of lithogenesis is not entirely known, to our knowledge, but it is thought to be associated with factors such as reduced salivary flow rate, dehydration, altered salivary pH, and impaired crystalloid solubility. The submandibular gland duct is more prone to lithogenesis due to salivary stasis resulting from the angular antigravity course of the duct and also due to the more alkaline and mucoid composition of saliva produced by the submandibular gland, with greater concentrations of calcium and phosphate [21, 22].

Infectious sialadenitis can be bacterial or viral in etiology, including paramyxoviral infection involving the parotids [22, 23]. Host factors such as immunocompromised state, diabetes, and malignancy put patients at an increased risk. A prior study showed a 3% incidence of sialoadenitis in the setting of end-stage cancer, more commonly involving the submandibular gland, followed by the parotid [24]. Acute sialadenitis can be classified as suppurative and nonsuppurative (see below). The most commonly used imaging study in this setting is IV contrast-enhanced CT, which can show glandular enlargement, edema, inflammatory fat stranding, abscess formation, and/or obstructive ductal calculus. Early on in the disease, therapy relies on conservative management with antibiotics, pain relief, and warm compresses. Surgical management with sialolithotomy or sialadenectomy is reserved for advanced or recurrent cases and is dependent upon the location of the stone. Transoral sialolithotomy can be performed in the setting of submandibular duct stones that are within 2 cm from the punctum in the anterior floor of the mouth. Access is more complicated with parotid duct stones, with only the distal-most segment within 1.5 cm from the orifice in the buccal vestibule, opposite the second maxillary molar, being accessible via transoral approach [22]. More recent gland-preserving techniques include sialoendoscopy and extra-corporeal shock-wave lithotripsy [21].

## Acute Nonsuppurative Parotitis

Acute nonsuppurative parotitis is acute inflammation in the parotid gland without phlegmon or abscess formation (Fig. 9). It may be bacterial or viral in etiology. On imaging, there is glandular edema, enhancement, and enlargement without phlegmon, necrosis, or abscess. Pediatric patients may experience recurrent episodes of acute nonsuppurative parotitis due to juvenile recurrent parotitis (JRP). This can persist into adulthood. JRP is the second most common nonobstructive nonsuppurative parotid inflammation with a

**Fig. 9** Acute nonsuppurative parotitis. Axial contrast-enhanced T1-weighted (**a**) and axial T2-weighted (**b**) MR images, both with fat suppression, show left parotid enlargement and enhancement (arrow, **a**) and edema (arrow, **b**). There is no abscess formation and changes are confined to the left parotid

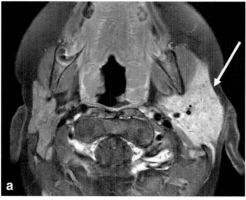 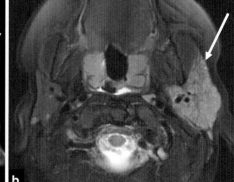

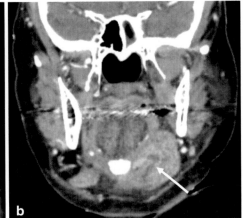

**Fig. 10** Acute suppurative submandibular sialadenitis. Axial (**a**) and coronal (**b**) contrast-enhanced CT images of the upper neck show an enlarged left submandibular gland (arrow, **a**) with intraglandular non-enhancing foci (arrow, **b**), due to acute suppurative submandibular sialadenitis. Note that a portion of the submandibular gland extends into the floor of the mouth, making this a potential source for spread to the floor of mouth that may lead to Ludwig angina or floor of mouth cellulitis

poorly understood etiology. It is usually self-limiting, responding to conservative management but in rare cases requiring a parotidectomy [25].

## Acute Suppurative Submandibular Sialadenitis

On the other hand, acute suppurative submandibular sialadenitis does lead to phlegmon and abscess formation (Fig. 10). This is more often seen in a patient with poor dental hygiene, elderly, and/or debilitated state, severe dehydration resulting in salivary stasis, or in neonates. On imaging, there is edema, glandular enlargement, and intraglandular non-enhancing foci which may reflect focal ductal ectasia or intraglandular abscesses [26].

## Infections from Lymphoid and Visceral Sources

Lymphoid and visceral source infections involve the pharyngeal mucosal space and can originate from lymphoid tissue but also from minor salivary glands or the mucosa itself. As such, patients who have undergone a tonsillectomy, and older patients with atrophied adenoid tissues, remain susceptible to these infections, indicating the role of nonlymphoid sources in such infections. In the following section, we address the lymphoid and visceral source infections separately, but note that they may represent a continuum with substantial overlap in etiology, appearance, and course.

Lymphoid tissues in the pharynx are aggregated in three tonsillar areas: the adenoids, palatine tonsils, and lingual tonsils (collectively termed Waldeyer ring). Alterations in the adenotonsillar microbiome can lead to adenoid

hypertrophy/hyperplasia or tonsillitis; adenoidal enlargement can exert a mass effect on the Eustachian tube opening in the nasopharynx, resulting in obstruction and secondary otitis media (OM). These conditions can often be recurrent and chronic. Common organisms implicated in tonsillar infection are *H. influenzae*, *Neisseria* species, and *S. pneumoniae* [27].

## Peritonsillar Abscess

Peritonsillar abscess (PTA) is one of the most common infections in the head and neck, with an estimated incidence between 19 and 37 per 100,000 persons [28]. PTA is formed due to purulent collection accumulating between the tonsillar capsule and the pharyngeal constrictor muscle (Fig. 11). This is in contradistinction to an intra-tonsillar abscess (ITA), which is seen within tonsillar tissue presumably within the tonsillar crypts, and is relatively rare [29] (Fig. 12). It is important to distinguish ITA from PTA, in order to prevent failed drainage of an ITA by erroneously targeting the peritonsillar space. In addition, unlike for PTA, there is a lack of consensus regarding incision and drainage of an ITA as a management strategy [29].

PTA may develop as a complication of acute tonsillitis. However, PTA has also been described among post-tonsillectomy patients, and therefore minor salivary glands have also been considered a potential source [30]. Patients with PTA can present with a sore throat, fever, trismus, pain, and potential for airway compromise. On physical examination, tonsillar enlargement, exudates, and lymphadenopathy are seen. IV contrast-enhanced neck CT shows tonsil enlargement, phlegmon, or abscess formation in an eccentric location, edema, inflammatory fat stranding in the parapharyngeal spaces, and varying degrees of airway narrowing that may require urgent and close attention.

## Acute Pharyngitis

Acute pharyngitis is one of the most common head and neck infections, accounting for 2% to 5% of outpatient primary care visits. It includes inflammation and infection of the

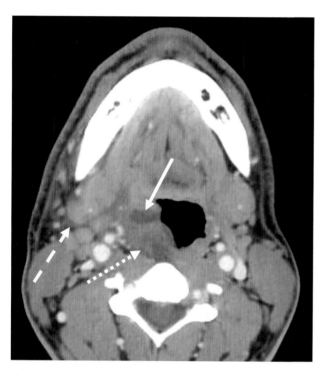

**Fig. 11 Peritonsillar abscess.** Axial IV contrast-enhanced CT image of the upper neck shows a right peritonsillar abscess (solid arrow) with adjacent right parapharyngeal space edema spreading into the right submandibular space (dashed arrow) and a phlegmon in the right retropharyngeal space (dotted arrow)

pharynx and tonsils most often due to viral etiologies (comprising 80% of the cases). The remaining causes are bacterial, by organisms such as *S. pyogenes*, *H. influenzae*, *C. diphtheria*, and rarely fungal. Acute pharyngitis due to viral etiology is typically self-limiting, whereas bacterial and fungal etiologies require prompt treatment and are prone to developing complications. Pharyngeal diphtheriae is now uncommon in the United States due to routine immunization but can be seen among unimmunized and under-immunized groups. This entity is characterized by mucosal necrosis and pseudomembrane formation causing respiratory distress due to airway obstruction. There can be regional spread into deep neck soft tissues, including the parapharyngeal and retropharyngeal spaces. Additional suppurative complications include peritonsillar abscess (which, as noted above, can have lymphoid as well as pharyngeal or minor salivary gland etiology), masticator space abscess (Fig. 13), septic thrombophlebitis/Lemierre's syndrome (Fig. 14), retropharyngeal abscess (Fig. 15), acute necrotizing ulcerative gingivitis (Vincent angina), necrotizing fasciitis, and descending mediastinitis. Clinically, patients present with a sore throat, fever, and odynophagia, with associated pharyngeal and tonsillar erythema. Palatal petechiae and tonsillar exudates may be seen with nonviral etiologies [31]. Imaging may be unrevealing or may show mucosal enhancement. There may be associated tonsillar enlargement and edema in the pharyngeal wall. Severe cases include abscess formation typically in the peritonsillar region, retropharyngeal space, and masticator space. Abnormal foci of gas within soft tissues can be seen with necrotizing infections. Management relies on supportive measures and antimicrobial therapy based on likely source and organism. Surgical incision and drainage may be needed in more advanced cases, when there is abscess formation or necrotizing fasciitis [31].

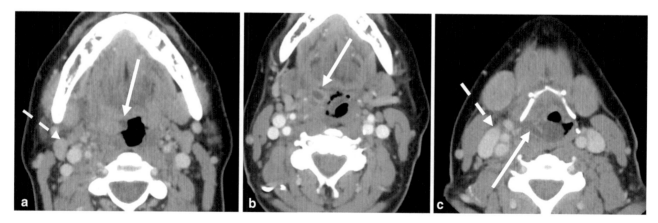

**Fig. 12 Intra-tonsillar and peritonsillar abscesses.** Axial IV contrast-enhanced CT images of the neck in the axial (**a–c**) plane show a small hypodense focus in the medial aspect of the right palatine tonsil (arrow, **a**), indicating an intra-tonsillar abscess (ITA). There is a rim-enhancing right peritonsillar abscess as well (arrow, **b**). There is edema extending around the right carotid sheath (dashed arrow, **a** and **c**) and along the right pharyngeal wall to the right aryepiglottic fold and pyriform sinus (solid arrow **c**)

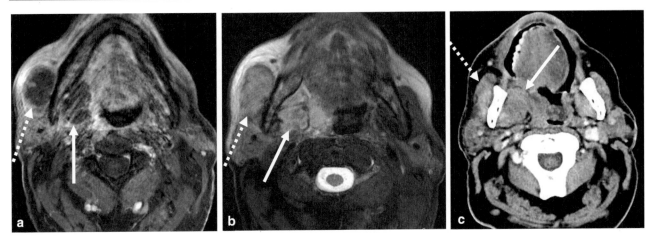

**Fig. 13 Masticator space abscess**. Axial post-contrast T1-weighted (**a**), axial T2-weighted (**b**) MR images, and IV contrast-enhanced axial CT image (**c**) through the face. Rim-enhancing collections are seen in the right masticator space (medial component, white arrows in **a** and **b**; lateral component, dotted white arrows in **a** and **b**), with thickened right masseter muscle (dotted white arrow, **c**) and medial pterygoid muscle (white arrow, **c**). There is an enhancement in the right oropharynx suggesting a visceral/lymphoid source. Odontogenic and salivary sources are other potential sources in this region, and close scrutiny of these structures is warranted

**Fig. 14 Lemierre's syndrome**. Axial (**a**) and coronal (**b**) IV contrast-enhanced CT of the neck shows a right peritonsillar abscess (solid arrow, **a**) and septic thrombophlebitis of the right internal jugular vein (dashed arrow, **a** and **b**). Note inflammatory stranding and edema in the right submandibular region, around the carotid sheath, and in the posterior cervical space

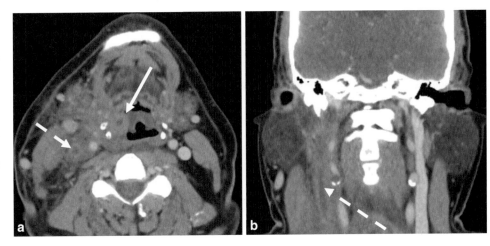

**Fig. 15 Retropharyngeal abscess**. Sagittal (**a**) and axial (**b**) IV contrast-enhanced CT images of the neck show an enhancing retropharyngeal fluid collection (arrow, **a**) with soft-tissue edema (arrow, **b**), due to a retropharyngeal abscess

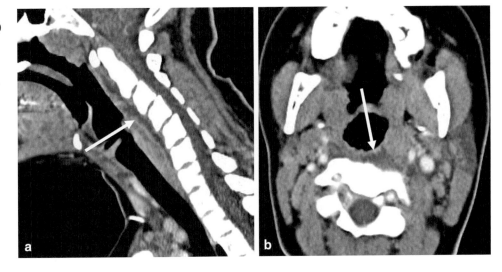

## Lemierre's Syndrome

Lemierre's syndrome is a septic thrombophlebitis commonly resulting from oropharyngeal infections (Fig. 14). It is typically seen in young adults but has been reported in all ages. Predisposing risk factors include diabetes mellitus, head and neck malignancy, and recent procedures, especially dental intervention. Fusobacterium species, specifically *F. necrophorum*, constitute the most common pathogens, but other organisms have also been implicated, with *Streptococcus* species being the second most common. Associated central nervous system (CNS) and pulmonary septic emboli have been reported. Treatment with intravenous antibiotics is the mainstay, with the mean duration of therapy reported to be around 35 days in a recent systematic review. The additional use of anticoagulation therapy and surgical debridement based on the extent of the disease can be considered. It should be noted that the use of anticoagulation is controversial, with a lack of clear guidelines, to our knowledge [32].

## Retropharyngeal Abscess

Retropharyngeal abscess is a common complication of visceral and lymphoid source infections which have spread to the retropharyngeal space (RPS) (Fig. 15). In children, it more commonly results from suppurative necrotizing adenitis that coalesces to form an abscess.

The true RPS extends from the skull base to approximately the T3–T4 level, although it may terminate at as high as the T1 level or extend to as low as the T6 level. It is bound by the alar fascia posteriorly and visceral fascia anteriorly. The inferior extent of the true RPS is variable and depends upon the site where the alar fascia fuses with the visceral fascia [33].

There is a potential space posterior to the alar fascia and anterior to the prevertebral space, which is termed the "danger space." This space extends through the posterior mediastinum down to the level of the diaphragm. However, the danger space or the alar fascia itself cannot be visualized on imaging as separate from the RPS. Pathology is inferred to be located within the danger space, rather than the retropharyngeal space, when it involves locations below the level of T6 down to the level of the diaphragm. Infections can spread from the retropharyngeal space into the danger space in a descending mediastinitis, a potentially life-threatening complication [1, 33]. The mainstay of treatment is antibiotics and surgical drainage based on extent and severity of involvement.

## Necrotizing Fasciitis

Necrotizing fasciitis (NF) is a rapidly progressive destructive soft-tissue infection, with high morbidity and mortality. It is most often reported in the perineum, abdominal wall, inguinal region, and extremities [34]. It is relatively rare in the cranial, cervical, and facial subsites due to the rich vascular supply [35]. NF is more common in immunosuppressed patients and in the setting of comorbidities including diabetes, renal failure, and obesity. On physical examination, skin erythema, cellulitis with purple bluish necrosis, and crepitus due to soft-tissue gas can be seen. It should be noted that the presence of gas is not a requirement for NF and gas is absent in 50% of patients who develop NF. A recent systematic review including 1235 patients found the odontogenic disease to be the commonest cause of NF in the face and neck (47%), followed by visceral and lymphoid inflammation/infection (34%); other rarer causes included salivary infection, iatrogenic/postoperative causes, and trauma (<10%) [36]. NF can spread rapidly across fascial planes due to the destructive nature of this infection, with common complications being descending necrotizing mediastinitis (DNM) and internal jugular vein thrombosis. Other complications include carotid sheath necrosis and hemorrhage [36].

CT neck with IV contrast is the imaging examination of choice due to its superior sensitivity to detection of source and pathways of spread, particularly in the presence of gas, which can obscure detailed assessment on US and MRI. Common imaging findings include cellulitis manifesting as skin thickening and fat stranding, asymmetrical thickening of fascia and muscle, non-enhancing tissues indicating necrosis, fluid collections, and gas crossing tissue planes [37] (Fig. 16). Management relies on antibiotic, surgical debridement, supportive critical care, including early tracheostomy, hyperbaric oxygen, and the potential need for surgical reconstruction [36].

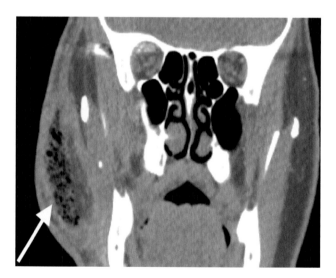

**Fig. 16** **Necrotizing fasciitis**. Coronal IV contrast-enhanced CT image of the face demonstrates skin and soft-tissue thickening, as well as gas formation, in the right face gracilis flap reconstruction, after parotid resection and radiation therapy, due to necrotizing fasciitis

## Infections Superimposed on Congenital/Developmental Anomalies

Congenital or developmental focal abnormalities in the face and neck can become infected, leading to locoregional infection and inflammation. Branchial anomalies, thyroglossal duct cysts and laryngoceles are examples of such processes which can be superinfected (Figs. 17, 18 and 19).

## Infected Branchial Cleft Cyst

Branchial anomalies are hypothesized to arise from incomplete obliteration of branchial apparatus or entrapped cell rests during embryonic development of the neck. These can result in cysts, sinuses, or fistulae. A branchial cleft cyst is completely surrounded by neck soft tissue, and has no internal or external opening. A sinus has an opening on either the inner pharyngeal mucosal surface or the outer skin surface, and a fistula has an opening on both the inner and outer surfaces [38].

Second branchial anomalies are the most common of all types, with 75% of these being cysts, far more common than a sinus or a fistula [39]. The embryologic tract extends from the tonsillar fossa. Bailey classified second branchial cysts into four types, with Type I being the most superficial, lying superficial to the anterior surface of the sternocleidomastoid muscle (SCM), just deep to the platysma. Type II is found at the anterior surface of the SCM, lateral to carotid sheath and posterior to the submandibular gland. Type III is located between the carotid bifurcation and the lateral pharyngeal wall, and type IV is the most medial of all and lies in the pharyngeal mucosal space [40]. There can be displacement of the SCM, submandibular gland, and carotid, depending on the location of the cyst. When superinfected, the cyst can show a thickened enhancing wall and surrounding edema

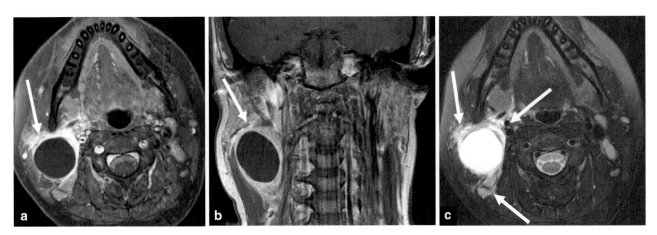

**Fig. 17 Infected second branchial cleft cyst**. Axial (**a**) and coronal (**b**) IV contrast-enhanced fat-suppressed T1-weighted MR images demonstrate a rim-enhancing cystic mass at the level of the angle of the mandible, deep to the right sternocleidomastoid muscle (arrows in **a** and **b**). Surrounding inflammatory stranding and edema can be noted on the axial fat-suppressed T2-weighted MR image (arrows, **c**). This is a second branchial cleft cyst with superimposed infection

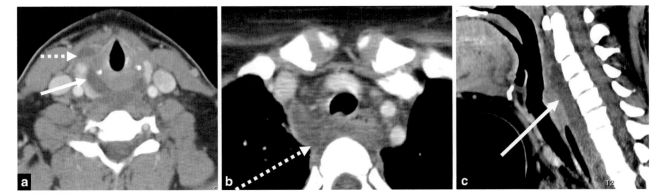

**Fig. 18 Infected fourth branchial anomaly/pyriform sinus fistula**. IV contrast-enhanced CT images in the axial (**a** and **b**) and sagittal (**c**) planes show a fluid collection deep to the right strap muscles (dotted white arrow, **a**) with extension deep to the right thyroid lobe (solid white arrow, **a**) and toward the retropharynx (arrow, **c**). There is fluid continuing inferiorly as descending posterior mediastinitis (dotted arrow, **b**). This is due to the presence of a fourth branchial anomaly and pyriform sinus fistula, leading to neck infection which is often recurrent

**Fig. 19** Infected thyroglossal
duct cyst. IV contrast-enhanced
CT images in the sagittal (**a**) and
axial (**b**) planes show a cystic
mass located just anterior and
inferior to the hyoid bone, with
surrounding fat stranding (arrows,
**a** and **b**) due to an infected
thyroglossal duct cyst

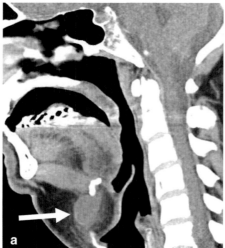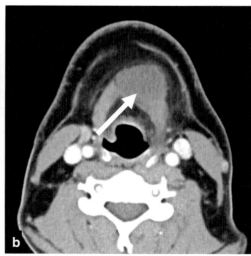

(Fig. 17). Differential diagnosis includes an infected level II node, infected lymphatic malformation or dermoid cyst, and a cystic metastatic node, such as from HPV-associated squamous cell carcinoma of the head and neck or thyroid cancer.

First branchial anomalies are much rarer. These have an association with the external auditory canal (EAC) and are typically located in the upper parotid gland adjacent to the EAC (work type I) or lower in the parotid gland and even down to the angle of the mandible (work type II) [41]. They often become manifest following an episode of otitis externa. Therefore, in a child with a cystic mass in or around the EAC and parotid, a first branchial anomaly should be considered. When infected, thickened enhancing walls and surrounding inflammatory stranding and edema can be seen on imaging. Differential diagnosis includes parotid abscess, infected sialocele, infected lymphatic malformation, nontuberculous mycobacterial infection or adenitis, and even a pilomatrixoma if it closely overlies the parotid.

Third and fourth branchial anomalies are extremely rare, occur lower in the neck than second branchial anomalies, and are more common on the left. A sinus or fistula is much more common than a cyst [38]. Both third and fourth branchial anomalies are related to the pyriform sinus, with the third branchial anomaly tract coursing above the superior laryngeal nerve and the fourth branchial anomaly tract coursing below it [38, 42]. Third and fourth branchial anomalies often become manifest due to the presence of a pyriform sinus fistula which serves as a tract for bacterial seeding from the pharynx (Fig. 18). Another explanation for the pyriform sinus tract is a persistent thymopharyngeal duct, due to failed obliteration of the thymic descent pathway [42]. Both third and fourth branchial anomalies are often associated with infections, with 39% to 42% presenting as neck abscess, and 33% to 45% presenting as acute suppurative thyroiditis [43], and often recurrent in nature. Ultrasound or CT may be used for imaging assessment, which can show inflammatory changes, phlegmon, or abscess in and/or around the thyroid gland. To assess for a sinus or fistula, a fluoroscopic pharyngogram may be performed; however, it is crucial that this be performed following complete resolution of the acute episode of infection, to prevent edema and mass effect from effacing the fistulous tract, by coapting its walls [44, 45]. Definitive treatment is surgical, via complete resection of the tract [43, 46].

## Infected Thyroglossal Duct Cyst

The thyroglossal duct is the embryologic tract through which thyroid primordial cells migrate from the foramen cecum of the tongue, down and around the inferior edge of the hyoid bone, before descending to the final location of the thyroid gland in the lower midline neck. Failure of involution of the thyroglossal duct or entrapped migrating cells within the duct result in a thyroglossal duct cyst and/or ectopic thyroid tissue. Thyroglossal duct cyst is the most common congenital neck mass, suprahyoid in the location in approximately 26% of cases, and intralingual in 2% of cases. The remaining cysts are present at and below the hyoid bone [47]. It is located along the midline in 75% of the cases, and in a paramedian location in 25%, but within 2 cm of the midline, and in close association with the hyoid bone or the strap muscles inferior to the hyoid bone [39]. It commonly presents as a painless midline or paramedian cystic mass; however, it can present as a draining sinus tract in the midline in 25% of the cases [48]. Due to its close association with the oral cavity, it is also prone to infection [48]. An infected thyroglossal duct cyst can demonstrate thickened enhancing walls with surrounding inflammation and edema that can be seen on US, CT, or MRI (Fig. 19). Depending on its location, the spread of infection can lead to the involvement of the visceral space and deep neck soft tissues in advanced cases. Antibiotics are useful for the treatment of the acute infection, while surgical resection via either a classical or modified Sistrunk procedure (includes resection of the center of the hyoid bone), is necessary for complete excision of the cyst and tract, to prevent recurrence [47, 48].

## Conclusion

Infections in the face and neck can have various etiopathogenesis and can potentially lead to life-threatening complications due to rapid trans-spatial spread. A "source, space, and spread" approach provides a systematic framework for defining the source of infection, delineating the anatomic spaces of involvement, and evaluating pathways of spread. This can help facilitate accurate diagnosis and anticipate potential complications, ultimately contributing to better patient care.

## References

1. Rana RS, Moonis G. Head and neck infection and inflammation. Radiol Clin N Am. 2011;49:165–82.
2. Chalifoux JR, Vachha B, Moonis G. Imaging of head and neck infections: diagnostic considerations, potential mimics, and clinical management. Semin Roentgenol. 2017;52:10–6.
3. Osborn TM, Assael LA, Bell RB. Deep space neck infection: principles of surgical management. Oral Maxillofac Surg Clin N Am. 2008;20:353–65.
4. Horváth T, Horváth B, Varga Z, Liktor B Jr, Szabadka H, Csákó L, et al. Severe neck infections that require wide external drainage: clinical analysis of 17 consecutive cases. Eur Arch Otorhinolaryngol. 2015;272:3469–74.
5. Kauffmann P, Cordesmeyer R, Tröltzsch M, Sömmer C, Laskawi R. Deep neck infections: a single-center analysis of 63 cases. Med Oral Patol Oral Cir Bucal. 2017;22:e536–41.
6. Ogle OE. Odontogenic Infections. Dent Clin N Am. 2017;61:235–52.
7. Sánchez R, Mirada E, Arias J, Paño J-R, Burgueño M. Severe odontogenic infections: epidemiological, microbiological and therapeutic factors. Med Oral Patol Oral Cir Bucal. 2011;16:e670–6.
8. Whyte A, Boeddinghaus R. Imaging of odontogenic sinusitis. Clin Radiol. 2019;74:503–16.
9. Simuntis R, Kubilius R, Vaitkus S. Odontogenic maxillary sinusitis: a review. Stomatologija. 2014;16:39–43.
10. McCarty JL, David RM, Lensing SY, Samant RS, Kumar M, Van Hemert RL, et al. Root cause analysis: an examination of odontogenic origins of acute maxillary sinusitis in both immunocompetent & immunocompromised patients. J Comput Assist Tomogr. 2017;41:484–8.
11. Matsumoto Y, Ikeda T, Yokoi H, Kohno N. Association between odontogenic infections and unilateral sinus opacification. Auris Nasus Larynx. 2015;42:288–93.
12. Craig JR, Tataryn RW, Aghaloo TL, Pokorny AT, Gray ST, Mattos JL, et al. Management of odontogenic sinusitis: multidisciplinary consensus statement. Int Forum Allergy Rhinol. 2020; https://doi.org/10.1002/alr.22598.
13. Marple BF. Ludwig angina: a review of current airway management. Arch Otolaryngol Head Neck Surg. 1999;125:596–9.
14. An J, Madeo J, Singhal M. Ludwig Angina. StatPearls. Treasure Island: StatPearls Publishing; 2019.
15. DeBoer DL, Kwon E. Acute Sinusitis. StatPearls. Treasure Island: StatPearls Publishing; 2020.
16. Velayudhan V, Chaudhry ZA, Smoker WRK, Shinder R, Reede DL. Imaging of intracranial and orbital complications of sinusitis and atypical sinus infection: what the radiologist needs to know. Curr Probl Diagn Radiol. 2017;46:441–51.
17. Lipschitz N, Yakirevitch A, Sagiv D, Migirov L, Talmi YP, Wolf M, et al. Nasal vestibulitis: etiology, risk factors, and clinical characteristics: a retrospective study of 118 cases. Diagn Microbiol Infect Dis. 2017;89:131–4.
18. Shekhrajka N, Moonis G. Imaging of nontraumatic temporal bone emergencies. Semin Ultrasound CT M. 2019;40:116–24.
19. Ren Y, Sethi RKV, Stankovic KM. Acute otitis media and associated complications in united states emergency departments. Otol Neurotol. 2018;39:1005–11.
20. Lepore ML, Hogan CJ, Geiger Z. Bezold Abscess. StatPearls. Treasure Island: StatPearls Publishing; 2020.
21. Capaccio P, Torretta S, Ottavian F, Sambataro G, Pignataro L. Modern management of obstructive salivary diseases. Acta Otorhinolaryngol Ital. 2007;27:161–72.
22. Williams MF. Sialolithiasis. Otolaryngol Clin N Am. 1999;32: 819–34.
23. Ogle OE. Salivary gland diseases. Dent Clin N Am. 2020;64:87–104.
24. Watanabe H, Odagiri T, Asai Y. Incidence of acute suppurative sialadenitis in end-stage cancer patients: a retrospective observational study. J Pain Symptom Manag. 2018;55:1546–9.
25. Papadopoulou-Alataki E, Dogantzis P, Chatziavramidis A, Alataki S, Karananou P, Chiona K, et al. Juvenile recurrent parotitis: the role of sialendoscopy. Int J Inflam. 2019;2019:7278907.
26. Abdel Razek AAK, Mukherji S. Imaging of sialadenitis. Neuroradiol J. 2017;30:205–15.
27. Johnston JJ, Douglas R. Adenotonsillar microbiome: an update. Postgrad Med J. 2018;94:398–403.
28. Sunnergren O, Swanberg J, Mölstad S. Incidence, microbiology and clinical history of peritonsillar abscesses. Scand J Infect Dis. 2008;40:752–5.
29. Ali SA, Kovatch KJ, Smith J, Bellile EL, Hanks JE, Truesdale CM, et al. Predictors of intratonsillar versus peritonsillar abscess: a case-control series. Laryngoscope. 2019;129:1354–9.
30. Sanmark E, Wikstén J, Välimaa H, Aaltonen L-M, Ilmarinen T, Blomgren K. Peritonsillar abscess may not always be a complication of acute tonsillitis: a prospective cohort study. PLoS One. 2020;15: e0228122.
31. Sykes EA, Wu V, Beyea MM, Simpson MTW, Beyea JA. Pharyngitis: approach to diagnosis and treatment. Can Fam Physician. 2020;66:251–7.
32. Moretti M, De Geyter D, Goethal L, Allard SD. Lemierre's syndrome in adulthood, a case report and systematic review. Acta Clin Belg. 2020:1–11.
33. Mnatsakanian A, Minutello K, Bordoni B. Anatomy, head and neck, retropharyngeal space. StatPearls. Treasure Island: StatPearls Publishing; 2020.
34. Sepúlveda A, Sastre N. Necrotizing fasciitis of the face and neck. Plast Reconstr Surg. 1998:814–7. https://doi.org/10.1097/00006534-199809030-00028.
35. Lin C, Yeh F-L, Lin J-T, Ma H, Hwang C-H, Shen B-H, et al. Necrotizing fasciitis of the head and neck: an analysis of 47 cases. Plast Reconstr Surg. 2001:1684–93. https://doi.org/10.1097/00006534-200106000-00008.
36. Gunaratne DA, Tseros EA, Hasan Z, Kudpaje AS, Suruliraj A, Smith MC, et al. Cervical necrotizing fasciitis: systematic review and analysis of 1235 reported cases from the literature. Head Neck. 2018;40:2094–102.
37. Zacharias N. Diagnosis of necrotizing soft tissue infections by computed tomography. Arch Surg. 2010:452. https://doi.org/10.1001/archsurg.2010.50.

38. Ibrahim M, Hammoud K, Maheshwari M, Pandya A. Congenital cystic lesions of the head and neck. Neuroimag Clin N Am. 2011;21: 621–39. viii

39. Koeller KK, Alamo L, Adair CF, Smirniotopoulos JG. Congenital cystic masses of the neck: radiologic-pathologic correlation. Radiographics. 1999;19:121–46. quiz 152–3

40. Branchial cysts, and other essays on surgical subjects in the facio-cervical region. By Hamilton Bailey, F.R.C.S., Surgeon to the Dudley Road Hospital, Birmingham, etc. Crown 8vo. Pp. 86 viii, with 50 illustrations. 1929. London: H. K. Lewis & Co. Ltd. 5s. net. Br J Surg. 1929. pp. 362–362. https://doi.org/10.1002/bjs. 1800176648

41. Work WP. Newer concepts of first branchial cleft defects. Laryngoscope. 1972;82:1581–93.

42. Alkire BC, Juliano AF, Hartnick CJ. Neck mass in an adolescent male. Bilateral branchial anomalies of the pyriform sinus. JAMA Otolaryngol Head Neck Surg. 2014;140:275–6.

43. Nicoucar K, Giger R, Pope HG Jr, Jaecklin T, Dulguerov P. Management of congenital fourth branchial arch anomalies: a review and analysis of published cases. J Pediatr Surg. 2009;44:1432–9.

44. Park SW, Han MH, Sung MH, Kim IO, Kim KH, Chang KH, et al. Neck infection associated with pyriform sinus fistula: imaging findings. AJNR Am J Neuroradiol. 2000;21:817–22.

45. Miller D, Hill JL, Sun CC, O'Brien DS, Haller JA Jr. The diagnosis and management of pyriform sinus fistulae in infants and young children. J Pediatr Surg. 1983;18:377–81.

46. Li Y, Lyu K, Wen Y, Xu Y, Wei F, Tang H, et al. Third or fourth branchial pouch sinus lesions: a case series and management algorithm. J Otolaryngol Head Neck Surg. 2019;48:61.

47. Allard RH. The thyroglossal cyst. Head Neck Surg. 1982;5:134–46.

48. Gioacchini FM, Alicandri-Ciufelli M, Kaleci S, Magliulo G, Presutti L, Re M. Clinical presentation and treatment outcomes of thyroglossal duct cysts: a systematic review. Int J Oral Maxillofac Surg. 2015;44:119–26.

# Imaging of Spinal Trauma with MRI: A Practical Guide

## 13

Jason F. Talbott, John F. Burke, Andrew Callen, Vinil Shah, Jared Narvid, and Sanjay S. Dhall

## Contents

J. F. Talbott (✉)
Department of Radiology and Biomedical Imaging, UCSF and Zuckerberg San Francisco General Hospital and Trauma Center, San Francisco, CA, USA

Brain and Spine Injury Center, Zuckerberg San Francisco General Hospital and Trauma Center, San Francisco, CA, USA
e-mail: Jason.talbott@ucsf.edu

J. F. Burke · S. S. Dhall
Brain and Spine Injury Center, Zuckerberg San Francisco General Hospital and Trauma Center, San Francisco, CA, USA

Department of Neurological Surgery, University of California, San Francisco, CA, USA

A. Callen
Department of Radiology, University of Colorado Anschutz Medical Campus, Denver, CO, USA

V. Shah · J. Narvid
Department of Radiology and Biomedical Imaging, UCSF and Zuckerberg San Francisco General Hospital and Trauma Center, San Francisco, CA, USA

© Springer Nature Switzerland AG 2022
M. N. Patlas et al. (eds.), *Atlas of Emergency Imaging from Head-to-Toe*,
https://doi.org/10.1007/978-3-030-92111-8_13

### Abstract

Traumatic spinal injuries are unfortunately common and are clinically important given their potential for severe morbidity and even mortality. Imaging plays a critical role in the evaluation of patients with acute spine trauma. While computed tomography (CT) is well established as the initial imaging modality for evaluating patients with known or suspected spinal trauma, emerging roles for magnetic resonance imaging (MRI) in guiding the emergent management and triage for patients continues to evolve. This review will focus on the added value and limitations of MRI in acute spinal trauma evaluation. Specifically, clinical and imaging indications for MRI will be reviewed. A structured approach to MRI for assessing spinal stability in the context of imaging-based classification systems will also be discussed, with emphasis on the AOSpine cervical subaxial and thoracolumbar classification schemes. MRI assessment of spinal canal contents, with emphasis on the injured spinal cord for both diagnostic and prognostic purposes, will be highlighted. Finally, the added value of MRI for assessing paraspinal soft-tissue injury, specifically for evaluation of whiplash-associated disorder, will be reviewed.

### Keywords

Spinal cord injury · Spinal instability · MRI · Contusion · AOSpine TLICS · Subaxial · BASIC score · Whiplash-associated disorder · Dissection

## Introduction

Spinal traumas comprise a sizable proportion of all musculoskeletal injuries worldwide. Up to 5.9% of polytrauma patients have acute cervical spine injuries, and between approximately 2 and 6% of all blunt trauma patients sustain cervical spine injury [1, 2]. The most frequently reported spinal injury is fracture, with ligamentous and combined injuries comprising a smaller proportion of patients.

A significantly smaller subset of spinal trauma patients has associated spinal cord injury (SCI). The yearly incidence of traumatic SCI is estimated to be 54 cases per one million people in the USA, with approximately 17,700 new injuries each year [3]. Interestingly, the last several decades have witnessed a notable shift in the demographics of SCI patients, with increased prevalence among older patients. For example, the current average age for a SCI patient is 43 years, compared with 29 years in the 1970s [3]. The most frequent injury mechanisms attributed to SCI include motor vehicle crashes and falls, accounting for 38% and 31% of injures, respectively [3]. Although the proportion of spinal trauma patients with SCI is relatively small, the direct financial costs related to SCI are staggering. For example, the lifetime health care and living expense costs for a 25-year-old SCI patient with high cervical tetraplegia averages $4.9M [3]. This figure does not include indirect costs, such as losses in wages and productivity. While these financial tolls are significant, the emotional, physical, and psychological costs on patients and their families are immeasurable.

The reference standard assessment of acute spinal trauma patients, including those with suspected spinal cord injury, remains a comprehensive clinical history and thorough physical examination. Inspection for spinal deformity, midline spinal tenderness, and substantial ecchymosis may be indicative of possible underlying fracture. For SCI, several neurologic and functional assessment tools have been devised to assess patients and to stratify their injury based on injury level and severity. The American Spinal Injury Association (ASIA) has published International Standards for the Neurological Classification of Spinal Cord Injury (ISNCSCI), including a thorough neurologic evaluation updated in 2011, for classification of SCI based on sensory and motor examination findings [4]. The completeness of spinal cord injury can be classified by the ASIA Impairment Scale (AIS), which is a five-point ordinal metric that ranges from complete injury (Grade A) to a normal examination (Grade E). ASIA motor and sensory scores in addition to AIS grade have been validated as predictors of functional recovery at 1 year after injury.

Despite the well-documented value of careful history and physical examination for SCI, there are notable limitations that can hamper early clinical evaluation. Comorbid conditions, including traumatic brain injury, severe pain, endotracheal intubation, sedative medications, and long-bone fractures, among others, all potentially interfere with clinical assessment during the acute phase of injury. Imaging examinations, when appropriately indicated, offer great promise for objective injury assessment, in spite of comorbid conditions that may confound the clinical evaluation.

## Imaging Indications for Blunt Spinal Trauma

There are two well-validated clinical decision rules that are most commonly used to identify patients with blunt trauma, who require screening with imaging for cervical spinal clearance. Both the National Emergency X-Radiography Utilization Study (NEXUS) [5] and the Canadian Cervical Rules (CCR) [6] have high sensitivity for identifying clinically important cervical spine injuries. Although both of these screening tools were originally used to determine patients who should be screened with cervical radiographs, conventional radiography has a very limited role in modern practice, as the initial screening examination for acute blunt spinal trauma. Up to two-thirds of fractures evident on CT are occult on conventional radiographs [7]. As a result, CT has replaced conventional radiography for initial evaluation, given its clear superiority for the depiction and detection of skeletal injuries [8]. Thus, CT is the reference standard initial imaging modality for suspected spinal trauma in patients who meet screening criteria. Although less standardized in clinical practice than NEXUS or the CCR, several criteria have also been suggested to determine if imaging of the thoracolumbar spine is indicated in trauma patients [9].

Appropriate indications for performing MRI, as part of the imaging evaluation in spinal trauma, are less clearly delineated and are more controversial in some cases than indications for CT. Based on literature review and expert opinion, the American College of Radiology (ACR) has published appropriateness criteria for imaging in suspected spinal trauma, with recommendations for MRI as "usually appropriate" in several variant scenarios [10]. This includes patients with confirmed or suspected cervical spinal cord or nerve root injury, independent of CT findings. MRI is also recommended in patients with neurologic abnormalities referable to the thoracolumbar spine. MRI in these cases is valuable for confirming the presence of spinal cord injury and defining the level of potential cord compression [10].

MRI is also recommended as a complementary examination to CT, for patients with mechanically unstable spine injury, for which surgical treatment is planned. MRI is the reference standard for evaluation of discoligamentous spinal injury [9]. As such, MRI is also recommended to further evaluate patients with clinical or imaging findings suggestive of ligamentous injury, independent of imminent surgical planning. Caution is advised by the authors of the ACR criteria, however, as MRI has been shown to overestimate the severity of discoligamentous and other soft-tissue injury. Finally, MRI has been recommended in obtunded patients for which clinical evaluation is not feasible, although literature supporting this recommendation is mixed, to our knowledge [11].

Routine utilization of MRI as the initial imaging examination for blunt spinal trauma is not generally recommended. The value of MRI in patients with initial negative cervical spine CT, whether alert or obtunded, remains questionable. Numerous studies, including those evaluating cost-effectiveness, have concluded that MRI has a low probability of demonstrating soft-tissue injuries requiring surgery that are not apparent on CT, and should not be routinely performed when initial CT is negative [12, 13]. In a meta-analysis examining 23 eligible studies, only 16 unstable injuries were identified with MRI from a pool of 5,286 patients with initial negative CT examinations [14].

In contrast to these data, other recent studies highlight the added value of MRI in select patients with initially negative CT. In a cohort of 259 patients who underwent cervical spine MRI following negative CT and persistent clinical concern for occult trauma-related injury, Onoue et al. [15] detected significant injuries in 31% of patients. This included 15 spinal cord contusions, 9 bone contusions/fractures, 7 spinal canal hemorrhages, and 66 soft-tissue injuries. In the prospective ReCONECT clinical trial, Maung and colleagues [16] reported on MRI findings in 767 patients who underwent MRI, in addition to CT, as part of initial imaging evaluation due to cervicalgia (43%), unevaluable clinical status (44.1%), or both (9.4%). In this select population, MRI revealed injuries occult on CT in 23.6% of patients. Notable abnormalities only identified with MRI included ligamentous injury, soft-tissue swelling, vertebral disc injury, and dural hematomas. The clinical relevance of these abnormalities was not evaluated in that study.

In light of the mixed literature on this topic, MRI utilization relies highly on clinical judgement. Patients with an initially negative CT but persistent neck pain, and patients with mild CT findings, such as prevertebral swelling or stable fractures, may or may not warrant further evaluation with MRI. Future prospective and controlled studies are needed to better inform evidence-based decision-making in these scenarios.

## Structured Approach to MRI for Spinal Trauma

CT and MRI have important and complementary roles in the evaluation of acute blunt spinal trauma, as discussed above. The focus of this section will be on the practical application of MRI in spinal trauma patients. First, the conventional MRI protocol and its individual components will be discussed. Next, a structured approach to MRI evaluation will be described. Specifically, MRI for assessing *i.* spinal stability, *ii.* spinal canal contents, and *iii.* the paraspinal soft tissues will be reviewed.

## Conventional MRI Protocol

The optimal MRI protocol for patients with spine trauma may vary depending on the clinical scenario. For example, if a patient is neurologically unstable or requires emergent surgical intervention, an abbreviated MR examination may be desired to specifically address only emergent surgical questions, such as localizing the level of spinal cord injury and compression with a sagittal survey. With these considerations in mind, the MR examination should be designed so that it may optimally detect emergent spinal cord pathology, including cord compression, extra-axial hemorrhage, and unstable spinal column injuries at a minimum. A standard MRI protocol for blunt spinal trauma is typically comprised of sagittal T1-weighted (T1-W), axial and sagittal T2-W, sagittal fat-suppressed T2-W, and axial T2*-W sequences [9]. Axial or sagittal diffusion-weighted imaging (DWI) sequences are also increasingly incorporated into routine clinical spine trauma protocols, primarily as a supplement to T2-W sequences for spinal cord evaluation. MR angiography (MRA) and fat-suppressed T1-W sequences are optional when evaluation for traumatic vascular injury is indicated.

The conventional MRI examination for spinal trauma is thus heavily weighted toward T2 imaging sequences, each with their own strengths and weaknesses for spinal evaluation. Although not specific with respect to underlying pathophysiologic injury mechanism, T2-W sequences are highly sensitive for intramedullary spinal cord pathology. Axial and sagittal depictions of T2 cord signal abnormality are complimentary with respect to characterization of acute spinal cord injury severity and prognosis [17, 18]. In addition to T2 hyperintense spinal cord edema, T2-W imaging is relatively sensitive for spinal cord blood products, manifesting as hypointense signal in the cord, acutely after injury, due to phase dispersion and accelerated T2 shortening effects of deoxyhemoglobin.

Addition of fat suppression to T2 acquisitions may slightly impair signal-to-noise ratio in the spinal cord and potentially introduce image artifacts, but has the advantage of increasing sensitivity to paraspinal, discoligamentous, and acute bone injury: critical components of the spine MRI evaluation. It is common to obtain sagittal T2-W images with fat suppression with Dixon technique, or short-tau inversion recovery (STIR) technique, to evaluate both the spinal cord and spinal column tissues. Acquiring axial T2-W images can then be performed without fat suppression for optimized spinal cord evaluation.

Increasingly, high spatial resolution sagittal 3D T2-W or balanced steady-state free precession sequences are being incorporated into spine trauma protocols to supplement T1-W images for anatomic delineation of the spine, specifically to aid in assessing the integrity of discoligamentous structures and patency of the CSF spaces [19–21].

T2*-W and susceptibility-weighted imaging (SWI) sequences have increased sensitivity for intramedullary blood products [22]. In the axial plane, T2*-W sequences are less prone to CSF-related flow signal loss than T2-W images, and thus may be useful as a more reliable measure of spinal canal compromise and spinal cord/proximal nerve root compression. It is important to note that T2*-W sequences have enhanced gray-white matter contrast compared to T2-W, with relative intrinsic hyperintensity of the gray matter (GM). Thus, subtle central gray matter hyperintensity as seen with mild SCI may be obscured, or normal hyperintense GM may be misinterpreted as abnormal on this sequence, somewhat limiting its application for diagnosis of mild central cord pathologic edema.

The first set of SCI-specific common data elements (CDEs) was published by a working group of SCI experts in 2015, and these guidelines can be referenced for standardized MRI protocols for SCI evaluation at 1.5 and 3 Tesla [23].

## MRI Evaluation for Spinal Stability

Recognition of the strengths and weaknesses of MRI for discoligamentous assessment, as well as nontraumatic mimics of injury, must be considered in the context of spinal stability evaluation. Studies correlating MRI findings of ligamentous integrity with surgical findings are sparse, to our knowledge [24–26]. Goradia and colleagues showed high sensitivity of MRI for injury to the intervertebral disc (93%), PLL (93%), and interspinous soft tissues (100%), but low to moderate sensitivity for ligamentum flavum (LF) injury (67%). Importantly, agreement between surgical and MRI findings was limited, and the authors concluded that MRI may overestimate the extent of ligamentous disruption. Similarly, Rihn et al. noted relatively low positive predictive value and specificity for MRI in determining posterior ligamentous complex (PLC) integrity, with the authors concluding that MRI may lead to overdiagnosis of PLC injury [27]. Thus, the potential for overdiagnosis should be carefully considered along with the patient's clinical context, particularly when MRI findings are not consistent with clear and unambiguous ligamentous disruption.

Panjabi and White defined spinal stability as "the loss of the ability of the spine under physiologic loads to maintain relationships between vertebrae in such a way that there is neither initial damage nor subsequent irritation to the spinal cord or nerve roots and, in addition, there is no development of incapacitating deformity or pain due to the structural changes." [28] Translating this clinical and biomechanical understanding to an imaging definition of instability for the subaxial cervical and thoracolumbar spine has resulted in dozens of proposed classification systems, a full review of which is beyond the scope of this chapter. Briefly, recent trends in spinal stability classification systems include reliance on morphologic features of injury revealed on imaging, rather than inferred mechanistic-based classifications, and incorporation of clinical data into the injury stratification 29].

The commonly used Denis classification divides the spine into three columns: *i.* anterior column including the anterior two-thirds of the vertebral body and discs; *ii.* middle column, which comprises the posterior third of the vertebral body and discs; and *iii.* posterior column consisting of the spinal posterior elements [30]. Four subtypes of spine injury as defined by Denis include compression, burst, seat-belt-type, and fracture dislocations. While relatively simple to apply in clinical practice, limitations to this classification include unclear identification of ligamentous injury, inability to account for all fracture types, as well as errors in accurately classifying stability and instability based on bony column.

The Arbeitsgemeinschaft für Osteosynthesefragen (AO) classification of thoracolumbar spine injuries builds on the Denis three-column model, and divides injuries based on mechanical forces: type A: compressive vertebral body injury, type B: distraction injuries, and type C: axial torque force-related injuries [31]. Each major injury type is further classified into three divisions, for which each division has an additional three subdivisions, resulting in a highly organized and thorough, but ultimately clinically unwieldy, impractical, and overly complex system.

In 2005 and 2007, the Spine Trauma Study Group introduced the thoracolumbar injury classification (TLICS) [32] and cervical subaxial fracture (SLIC) [33] systems, respectively. Both are based on three injury categories: *i.* injury morphology; *ii.* posterior ligamentous complex (PLC) integrity; and *iii.* involvement of the neuroaxis. Numeric values are assigned to subclassifications of injury within each of these three major groups, from which a comprehensive point total can be derived for guiding surgical management.

Both AO and TLICS/SLIC have been criticized for complexity, low reliability, bias for treatment decision-making based on practice of the original authors, and overdependence on MRI for assessing PLC integrity. To address these limitations and others, the AO established the AOSpine Trauma Knowledge Forum, which was tasked to develop a comprehensive and practical system for the entire spine. The resulting AOSpine TLICS [34] and AOSpine subaxial cervical spine [35] classification systems have become more widely used in recent clinical practice. Similar to TLICS and SLIC, the AOSpine TLICS and subaxial cervical spine systems are imaging based, and consist of three primary injury classifiers: type A compression, type B tension band, and type C translational injury morphologic classifications. Each injury type has several subtypes of injury. AOSpine also incorporates the patient's neurologic status, along with some patient-specific modifiers. For morphologic characterization, the stabilizing structures of the spinal column are divided into

anterior and posterior tension bands. The anterior tension band consists of the vertebral bodies and contiguous interconnecting soft tissues, notably the anterior and posterior longitudinal ligaments, in addition to the intervertebral discs. The posterior tension band includes the posterior elements of each subaxial vertebra, along with the interconnecting ligaments, namely the LF, interspinous ligaments (ISL), supraspinous ligament (SSL), and facet joint capsules. Specific to the subaxial cervical classification, facet injuries have separate descriptors, which can be fully characterized by fracture patterns on CT. Modifiers for indeterminate ligamentous injury and specified comorbidities are also incorporated into the AOSpine classifications.

No classification system for spinal stability has gained universal acceptance for spinal trauma. While the AOSpine TLICS and subaxial cervical spine classifications are among the most current systems, validation of their reliability for morphologic classification, when all subtypes of injury are included, has been mixed [36, 37]. AOSpine TLICS has also been criticized for not clarifying management "greyzones," given there is still heavy reliance on MRI, with its relatively low interobserver reliability for tension band evaluation [38]. Persistent challenges in separating usually stable type A injuries from usually unstable type B injuries are not entirely resolved. Nevertheless, these latest systems are increasingly utilized in clinical practice, and the two-column tension band model establishes a clinically relevant framework for a structured approach to MR evaluation for spinal stability that will provide the foundation for the next section.

## MRI and AOSpine Subaxial Injury Classification

### AOSpine Type A Injuries

Type A injuries of the spine, as defined by the AOSpine TLICS and subaxial cervical spine systems, involve vertebral compression and process fractures, which can be accurately characterized with CT in most cases. A notable exception is the increased sensitivity of MR for vertebral body contusion and mild type A1 compression injury, where fracture only involves a single vertebral endplate [9] (Fig. 1). When there is no associated vertebral height loss, traumatic marrow edema is sometimes referred to as bone contusion or microtrabecular injury. Although diagnosis of these relatively mild injuries may assist in explaining a patient's symptoms, the clinical relevance with respect to urgent and long-term patient management, and thus the added value of MRI, is likely negligible for these CT-occult injuries, where management may be guided primarily by clinical symptoms. For more severe type A compression injuries, MRI adds little to direct characterization of the fracture. However, detection of associated

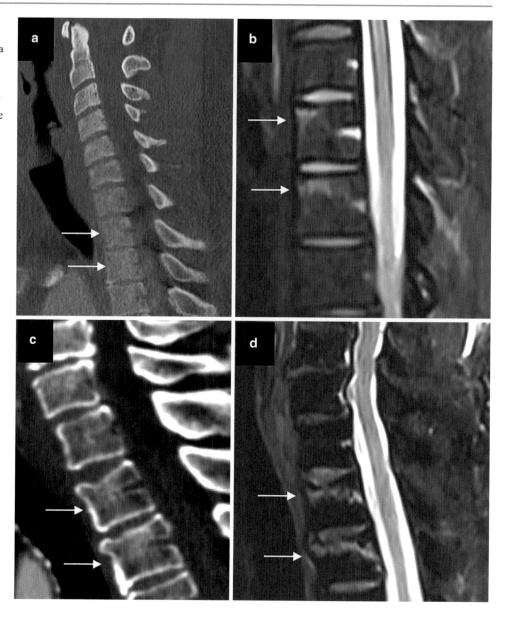

**Fig. 1** MRI is highly sensitive for mild vertebral compression injuries. Sagittal CT image (**a**) in a 34-year-old woman with neck pain following a motor vehicle collision (MVC) did not reveal acute abnormality. Sagittal T2-W FS image (**b**) of the cervical spine shows subchondral marrow edema underlying the superior endplates at T1 and T2, which is consistent with CT-occult mild bone contusions. Sagittal CT image (**c**) in a 62-year-old man with neck pain after fall shows mild superior endplate compression deformities at C6 and C7, which are more conspicuous on same-day sagittal T2-W MRI (**d**). Arrows indicate levels of acute vertebral injury (**a-d**)

CT-occult ligamentous injuries, spinal hematomas, spinal canal compromise, and spinal cord injury often warrants addition of MRI, in patients with higher-grade type A injuries.

## AOSpine Type B Injuries

In the context of AOSpine classification, the major added value of MRI for spinal stability evaluation is for diagnosis of type B injuries. While indications for obtaining MRI to identify type B injuries remain imperfectly defined, some potential clues on CT include facet joint subluxation of more than 2 mm, traumatic spondylolisthesis, and abnormal interspinous or intervertebral space widening [39]. Unfortunately, type B injuries may also be present in the absence of any of these findings on CT (Fig. 2), and other clinical and imaging predictors of unstable discoligamentous injury remain an area of active investigation. When MRI is obtained, evaluation for instability should focus on the integrity of the primary stabilizers for each tension band, as discussed in more detail below.

## Posterior Tension Band Evaluation (B1 and B2 Injury)

Evaluation of the posterior tension band begins with a fluid-sensitive/fat-suppressed T2-W sequence, such as DIXON T2

**Fig. 2** MRI reveals unsuspected posterior ligamentous complex injury in a 48 year old after a fall. Sagittal CT image (**a**) coned in to the mid-thoracic spine shows mild compression and endplate fractures at T5 and T6. (**b**). Sagittal T2-W MRI reveals complete disruption of the ligamentum flavum, interspinous ligament, and supraspinous ligament at T5-T6

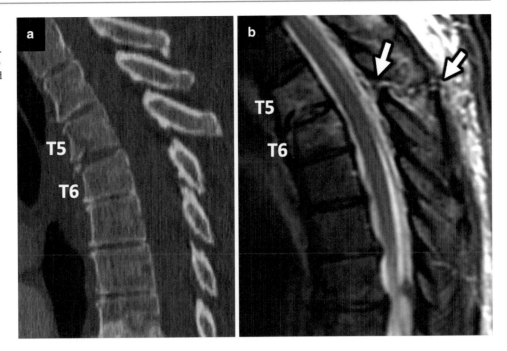

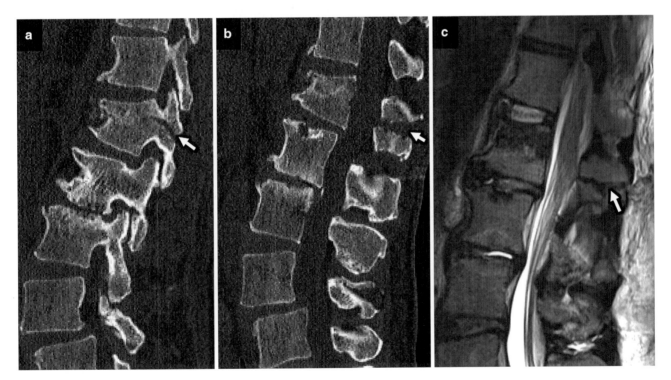

**Fig. 3** AOSpine type B1 injury in a 68-year-old woman after a seatbelt injury. Parasagittal (**a**) and midline sagittal (**b**) CT images at the thoracolumbar junction show a mildly distracted transversely oriented fracture through the posterior elements of the L1 vertebra, which is consistent with AOSpine type B1 injury. Sagittal 3D T2-W SPACE MR image (**c**) in the same patient shows a linear defect corresponding to the posterior tension band bone disruption

or STIR. Type B1 injuries, colloquially referred to as "Chance" fractures, consist of transverse bony disruption of the posterior vertebral elements, a diagnosis readily made with CT. MRI may reveal a thin, linear, T2/STIR hyperintense and T1 hypointense band corresponding to the fracture line (Fig. 3).

MRI plays a more critical role in diagnosis of type B2 injuries, which are defined by unstable, traumatic disruption of the posterior ligamentous complex of the posterior tension band. Relatively low interobserver reliability for type B2 injuries has been reported [37]. As such, familiarity with the normal and abnormal appearance and biomechanical nature of PLC injury should be emphasized, to improve consistency in reporting and diagnosis of these injuries [40].

The major stabilizing ligaments of the PLC are hypointense on all MRI sequences. It is useful to begin evaluation of the PLC with careful examination of the LF on fluid-sensitive/fat-suppressed sequence(s). Because the LF has been shown to be one of the last structures to tear in PLC injury, identification of complete LF disruption is often associated with an unstable B2 injury [40]. Left- and right-sided LF connect the adjacent vertebral lamina. Medially, fibers blend together and laterally, the fibers attach along the facet joint capsules. The LF may not be present at C1-C2. Intrinsic T2 hyperintensity along the course of an otherwise intact LF may suggest partial and/or indeterminate injury (Fig. 4). More definitive evidence of potentially unstable LF disruption, and associated type B2 injury, should include unambiguous focal disruption of the ligament with intervening T2 hyperintensity (Figs. 5, 6, 7, and 8). The injured ligament may also be displaced ventrally into the spinal canal with indentation of the posterior thecal sac [9]. A high spatial resolution sagittal T2-W sequence without fat suppression, such as 3D T2 SPACE, can provide very detailed anatomic delineation of the LF, and can be used to confirm or refute a suspected tear (Figs. 5, 6, 7 and 8).

It is important to recognize that normal occurring spaces or gaps between the left and right LF may be identified with high spatial resolution MRI (Fig. 8) [41]. These naturally occurring gaps may mimic focal traumatic injury. They occur centrally, and are most apparent at the inferior laminar attachment of the LF, with a smooth arc-like morphology and without associated T2 hyperintense edema on a fat-supressed T2-W sequence, as would be expected with a traumatic tear (Fig. 8).

As with the LF, the SSL may be partially injured or completely disrupted. The SSL is an inferior continuation of the nuchal ligament, and usually begins cranially at C6 or C7, and connects adjacent apices of the spinous processes inferiorly, to the level of the sacrum. Focal ligamentous disruption with intervening T2 hyperintensity should be clearly seen for diagnosis of supraspinous disruption as a critical part of a type B2 injury complex (Fig. 6). Initial distracting forces frequently result in avulsion of the SSL at its superior bone attachment, with the vector of ligamentous disruption proceeding inferiorly and ventrally along the contiguous PLC elements [40]. Widening of the interspinous space may also be observed.

In contrast to the LF and SSL, the trilaminar ISL, which connects adjacent spinous processes, is usually not resolved as a discrete, T2-hypointense band on MRI. Injury to this structure is inferred by the presence of abnormal interspinous fluid signal (Figs. 5, 6, 7, and 8). This somewhat complicates distinction of partial and complete ISL disruption. If the SSL and LF remain intact, then distinguishing between partial and complete ISL injury has little clinical relevance, as it is a relatively minor stabilizer of the PLC [40]. Coexisting SSL and LF disruption, however, is sufficient to infer complete ISL disruption, as biomechanical studies have shown that the ISL tears early in the progressive and orderly rupture sequence of the PLC components, always preceding LF disruption [26].

The facet joint capsules are important stabilizers of the posterior tension band. Facet joint fluid and widening are findings suggestive of synovial capsule injury [9, 26]. When these findings are present in the setting of unambiguous SSL, ISL, and LF disruption, type B2 injury is diagnosed.

## Anterior Tension Band Evaluation (B3 Injury)

As with the posterior tension band, evaluation of the anterior tension band on MRI begins with careful examination of the sag T2-W fat-suppressed sequence. The presence of abnormal prevertebral T2 hyperintense fluid and/or hemorrhage is frequently a conspicuous finding which should prompt a detailed search for associated ALL, annular, and/or PLL disruption as part of an unstable type B3 injury complex (Figs. 9, and 10).

The ALL and PLL are normally adherent to the ventral and dorsal aspects of the vertebral body, respectively. Hyperextension injury may entail stripping of the ligament from the annulus and bony vertebral cortex, with or without complete ligamentous disruption. Abnormal intervertebral widening or disc height loss may be associated findings in type B3 injury (Fig. 10). Partial or complete injury to just the ALL or just the PLL should be clearly described, but does not technically qualify as a type B3 injury (Fig. 9). The anterior tension band ligaments may also be traumatically disrupted with severe compression injuries, including A3 and A4 subtypes. However, according to its original description, the B3 injury is defined as anterior tension band distraction-related disruption [34].

## AOSpine Type C Injuries

Type C injuries, with gross translation of spinal elements, are readily diagnosed with CT in most cases. MRI may confirm complete anterior and posterior tension band disruption (Fig. 11), but more importantly help to diagnose associated spinal cord injury, spinal canal hemorrhages, disc herniations, and spinal cord compression.

**Fig. 4** Partial ligamentum flavum injury following a motorcycle collision. Sagittal T2-W FS MR image (**a**) in a 41-year-old man after a fall shows subtle T2 hyperintensity along an otherwise intact LF at the C3-4 level (arrow) on a background of long segment posterior paraspinous and interspinous cervical edema. Sagittal 3D T2-W SPACE image (**b**) in the same patient confirms integrity of the partially injured LF at C3-C4

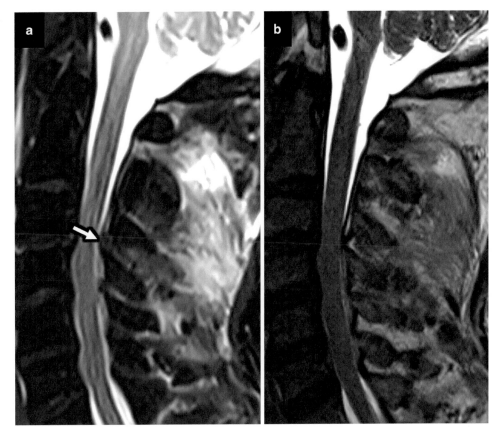

**Fig. 5** AOSpine cervical type B2 injury. Sagittal T2-W FS image (**a**) of the cervical spine of a 29 year old in a motor vehicle collision shows complete disruption of the ligamentum flavum (arrow) and interspinous ligament, which is confirmed on a sagittal 3D T2-W SPACE MR image (**b**) at the same level. Abnormal prevertebral edema and bone marrow edema related to compression fractures at C5, C7, and T1 are also present

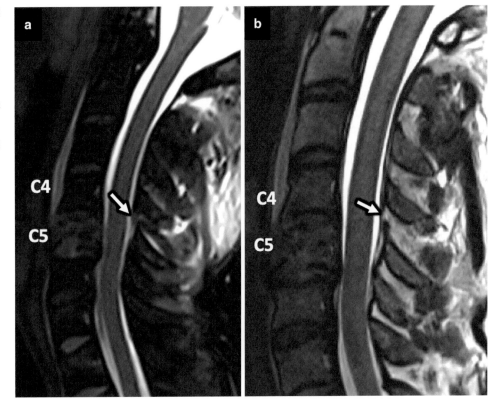

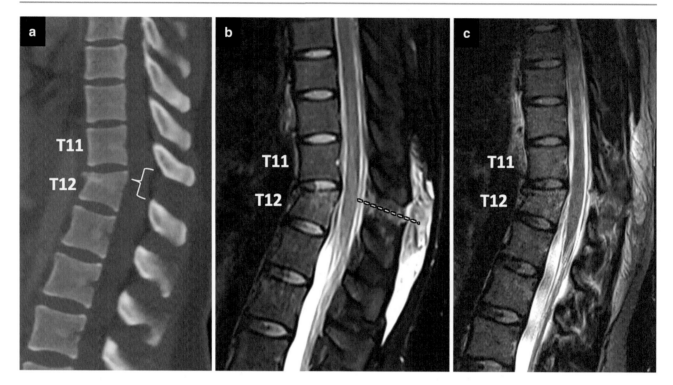

**Fig. 6** AOSpine thoracic type B2 injury in a 31 year old after a fall. Sagittal CT image (**a**) centered at the thoracolumbar junction reveals anterior wedge compression deformity at T12, with focal kyphotic deformity at T11-T12. Associated interspinous widening is seen at this level (bracket). Sagittal T2-W FS MR image (**b**) at the same level shows unambiguous and complete disruption of the ligamentum flavum, interspinous ligament, and supraspinous litament at T11-T12, consistent with type B2 injury

## MRI Evaluation of Spinal Canal Contents

MRI is commonly performed in the setting of blunt spinal trauma, to evaluate the spinal canal for evidence of spinal cord injury, and to identify levels of spinal canal compromise and spinal cord compression. The most common etiologies for traumatic spinal canal compromise include herniated disc, retropulsed bone fragments, traumatic spinal malalignment, and blood in the extra-arachnoid spinal compartments. Preexisting spinal canal narrowing from degenerative spondylosis is common, particularly in the elderly population.

## Acute Traumatic Disc Herniation

Traumatic injury to the intervertebral disc may manifest with asymmetric narrowing or widening of a disc space along with abnormal fluid signal within the disc. Intervertebral disc herniations are commonly seen with flexion-compression and flexion-distraction injuries. Similar to degenerative disc herniations, MRI will frequently show disruption of the disc's outer annulus (Fig. 12), with herniated nucleus pulposus material extruding beyond the expected annular margins. Increased T2 hyperintensity within the extruded disc material is a clue to acuity, along with associated acute traumatic findings at the same or adjacent spinal motion segments (Fig. 12). A combination of axial and sagittal T2-W sequences can be helpful for evaluating the size of the extruded disc material and its associated mass effect on the spinal cord and/or nerve roots (Fig. 12).

In cases of traumatic spinal subluxation, acute disc herniations may be difficult to identify at the subluxed level, and have been defined as extrusion posterior to a vertical line drawn along the posterior cortical margin of the body below the subluxation [42]. Using this definition, identification of acute HNP may be particularly important for patients undergoing closed reduction of spinal dislocations, given the potential for increases in herniation number and size with the reduction procedure. In a study evaluating 11 patients with imaging immediately before and after closed reduction of traumatic spinal dislocations, intervertebral disc herniations were more common after closed reduction [42]. Although neurologic compromise related to worsening of HNPs following closed reduction was not observed in this small study, anatomic progression of HNPs is worrisome, and suggests MRI may be useful in preparation for closed reduction procedures.

**Fig. 7** Three-dimensional T2-W SPACE MR imaging is useful for ligamentum flavum evaluation. Sagittal T2-W FS MR image (**a**) of the cervical spine from a 72 year old who fell down 12 stairs shows traumatic anterolisthesis at C6-C7, long-segment posterior cervical paraspinal and interspinous edema, with indeterminate injury to the LF at C6-C7. Sagittal 3D T2-W SPACE image (**b**) in the same patient confirms complete disruption of LF at C6-C7

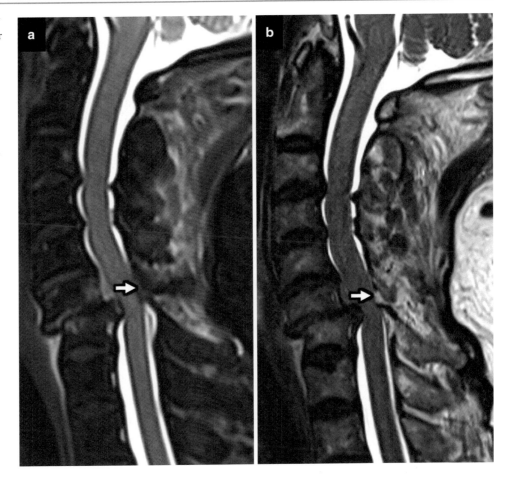

## Traumatic Extra-Arachnoid Collections

Post-traumatic collections contributing to spinal canal compromise include epidural hematomas, subdural hematomas and/or hygromas, and traumatic pseudomeningoceles. Epidural hematomas occur in up to 9% of patients with cervical spinal trauma [43]. In patients with ankylosing spondylitis, the incidence of epidural hematoma is significantly higher. While CT may show epidural hematomas, when they are large, as hyperdense epidural collections, MRI is far more sensitive and the ideal modality for diagnosing this frequent complication of spinal trauma. The stage of blood products and degree of intermixed CSF will primarily dictate the T1 and T2 relaxivity characteristics of the collection(s). Acutely, hemorrhage will be nearly isointense to slightly hyperintense on T1, and hyperintense on T2, when compared to the normal spinal cord (Fig. 13), although variability in T2 signal of acute extra-arachnoid hematomas is common [44]. With time, increasing methemoglobin concentrations will contribute to progressive T1-shortening and associated T1 hyperintensity. Capping of epidural fat along the craniocaudal margins of the hematoma, frequent posterolateral location,

continuity with adjacent bone, and displacement of the dura centrally into the spinal canal are other common imaging features of traumatic epidural hematomas [44]. When ventrally located, especially in the lumbosacral spine, epidural collections may demonstrate the "draped curtain sign," which relates to adherent ventral midline attachment of the meninges to the PLL via Trolard's membrane, with associated uplifting of dura by epidural fluid on either side. When epidural collections more closely match CSF signal on T1 and T2 sequences, they are likely predominantly composed of CSF entering the epidural space via a meningeal defect.

Large, epidural hematomas may contribute to spinal cord compression, necessitating surgical decompression, especially when neurologic symptoms are present. In the absence of referable neurologic deficits, even large epidural hematomas may be treated conservatively, given their propensity for spontaneous resolution and rarity of progression [45].

Subdural hemorrhage and hygromas are less common than epidural hematomas in spine trauma, but may also be identified and characterized using MRI (Fig. 14). Histological analysis suggests "subdural" spinal collections are truly "intradural" in location, and relate to blood and/or CSF

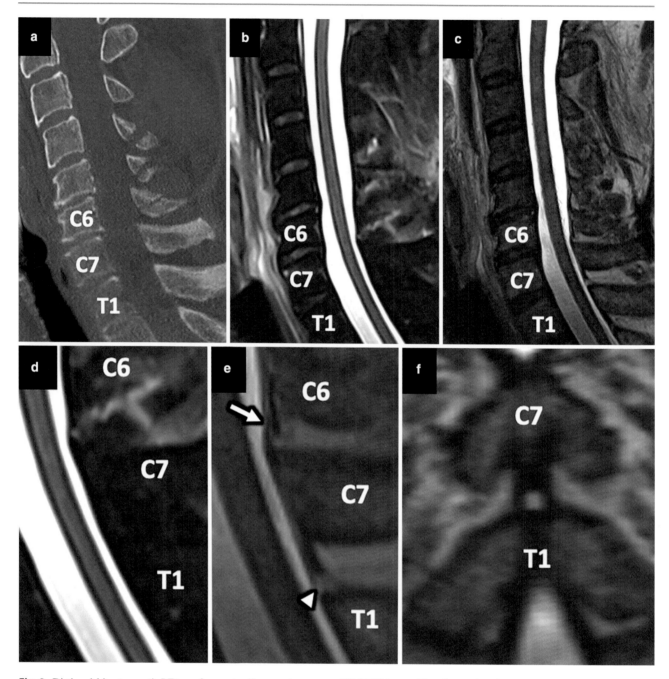

**Fig. 8** Distinguishing traumatic LF tears from naturally occurring gaps. Sagittal CT image (**a**) of the cervical spine, in a 40-year-old man following MVC, shows three-level spinous process fractures at C4, C5, and C6. Sagittal T2-W FS MR image (**b**) in the same patient shows marrow edema related to spinous process fractures, and interspinous edema from C3-C4 through C6-C7 levels. Corresponding sagittal 3D T2-W SPACE image (**c**) shows focal defects at the inferior attachments of LF at C5-C6 and C6-C7. High magnification sagittal T2-W FS image (**d**) at the cervico-thoracic junction shows linear edema extending across the ISL and LF at C6-C7, but no appreciable ISL or LF edema at C7-T1. Sagittal 3D T2-SPACE MR image (**e**) shows disruption and posterior distraction of the LF at C6-C7 (arrow). In contrast, smooth arc-like splaying of LF fibers at C7-T1, and absence of interspinous edema, confirms normal focal gap in image E (white arrowhead) and on a coronal T2-W MR image (**f**)

dissecting between weaker inner and stronger outer dural layers [46]. T1 and T2 signal characteristics are guided by the stage of blood products, as well as by the amount of superimposed CSF fluid. Subdural collections may exert mass effect on the spinal cord or nerve roots; however, a distinct hypointense linear dural margin outlining the hematoma and capping of epidural fat will be absent with subdural collections, often making them more challenging to identify,

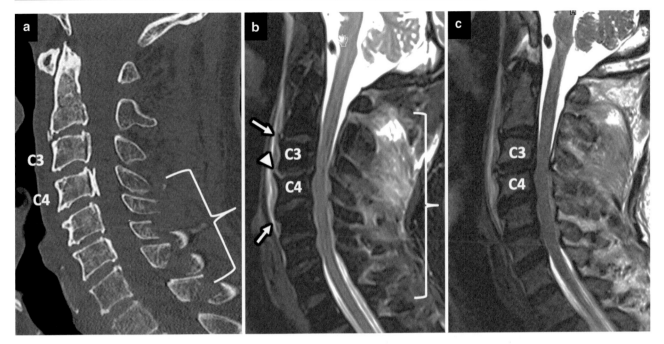

**Fig. 9** Focal disruption of the anterior longitudinal ligament (ALL). Sagittal CT image (**a**) of the cervical spine of a 56-year-old man following a motorcycle collision shows multiple contiguous spinous process fractures (C4-T1). Sagittal T2-W FS (**b**) and 3D T2-W SPACE (**c**) MR images in the same patient show prevertebral swelling and fluid spanning C2-C5 (arrows in **b**), with focal disruption of the ALL and anterior annulus at C3-C4 (arrowhead in **b**)

**Fig. 10** AOSpine type B3 injury in a 72 year old with neck pain after fall. Sagittal CT (**a**) and T2-W FS MR (**b**) images show abnormal intervertebral widening at T10-T11, with traumatic intervertebral fluid signal and complete discoligamentous disruption which is consistent with a type B3 injury

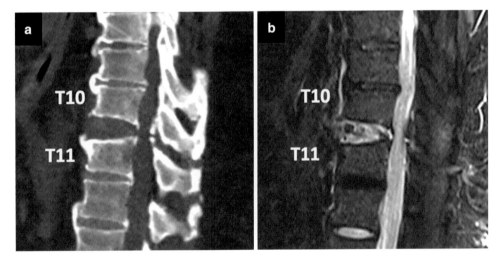

especially when they are predominantly composed of CSF. The curtain sign will also be absent.

Traumatic pseudomeningoceles of the spinal canal are rare, and result from focal dural and arachnoid disruption with progressive contained CSF leakage into the epidural space due to a ball-valve mechanism. When isolated to the spinal canal, traumatic pseudomeningoceles tend to be ventral, with extensive longitudinal spread [47]. More commonly, traumatic pseudomeningoceles will be lateral and extend along one or more neuroforamen, as a harbinger of traumatic nerve root avulsion injury. These collections will follow CSF signal characteristics on all sequences.

## Traumatic Spinal Cord Injury

The best validated and most studied sequence for SC evaluation is simple T2-W imaging, preferably in both the axial and sagittal planes [17, 48]. Sagittal evaluation readily allows for determination of the intramedullary longitudinal length of

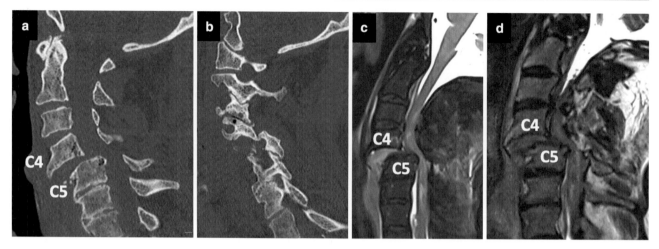

**Fig. 11** AOSpine type C injury following motor vehicle collision. Sagittal (**a**) and parasagittal (**b**) CT images of the cervical spine, in a 72-year-old woman following a MVC, show traumatic anterolisthesis and jumped facet joints at the C4-C5 level. Sagittal T2-W FS (**c**) and sagittal T2 SPACE (D) MR images in the same patient confirm expected complete anterior and posterior tension band discoligamentous disruption at this level

**Fig. 12** Traumatic disc herniation in a pedestrian versus automobile injury. Sagittal (**a**) and axial (**b**) T2-W MR images of the lumbar spine show focal posterior annular disruption at L4-L5, with acute traumatic subligamentous disc extrusion. The herniated disc material combined with acute epidural blood products contribute to severe spinal canal stenosis and cauda equina compression

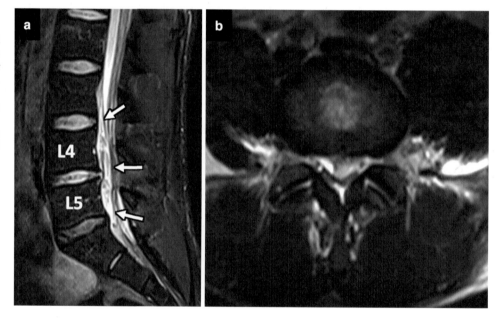

injury (IMLL) and the craniocaudal level of injury, while axial imaging provides important information with respect to transverse extent of contusion and better delineation of relative white and gray matter involvement [49]. As first described by Schaefer et al., the sagittal grade of injury can be determined by assessing the number of vertebral segments the spinal cord injury spans, and for the presence of intramedullary hemorrhage (Fig. 15) [50]. Complete motor and sensory dysfunction was observed in 93% (13/14) of patients with intramedullary cord hemorrhage, designated as type 1 injury. Neurologic deficits were more heterogenous in patients with nonhemorrhagic contusions, reflected by intramedullary T2 hyperintensity spanning more than 1 vertebral segment, classified as type 2 injury. Overall, these patients had more severe deficits than those whose T2-hyperintense contusion was confined to a single vertebral body level (type 3 injury). Patients without evidence for any cord injury on MRI (type 4 injury), not surprisingly, did very well clinically, with none or only mild transient motor and sensory deficits. Numerous subsequent studies have similarly

**Fig. 13** Traumatic epidural hematoma following a high-speed MVC. Sagittal T2-W SPACE (**a**) and T1-W (**b**) MR images show a longitudinally extensive, mildly T2 hyperintense and T1 hypointense epidural hematoma, extending from C1 to T1 (arrows in A), with associated anterior tension band disruption at C6-C7. Dorsal epidural hyperdensity on axial CT (**c**), in the same patient, at the C4 vertebral level, corresponds to hematoma on the axial T2-W MR (D)

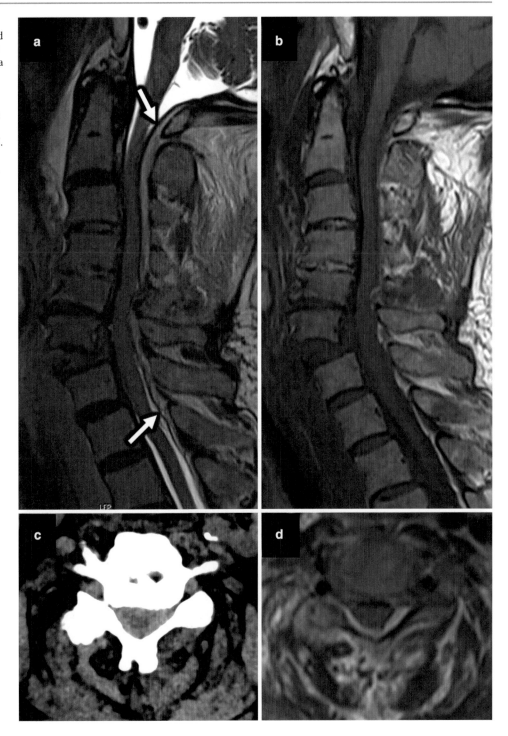

correlated IMLL and cord hemorrhage with clinical measures of injury severity and outcome [48].

It is important to recognize that the timing of MRI can markedly impact the MR imaging appearance of a contusion injury. In one of the earliest longitudinal MRI studies in SCI, Leypold and colleagues showed that edema can expand up to 1 vertebral body segment every 1.2 days between injury and MRI within the first several days after injury [51]. Similar studies have revealed even more rapid injury expansion [52], and these studies highlight the importance of considering time from injury when interpreting MRI findings.

**Fig. 14** Traumatic subdural hygroma. Sagittal T2-W (**a**) image in a patient with mild lumbar compression fractures at L2 and L4 after fall while intoxicated shows central displacement of the cauda equina nerve roots. Axial T2-W (**b**) MR image at the level of L3 in the same patient shows central displacement of the nerve roots by a CSF-isointense collection, without appreciable dural uplifting, which is consistent with intradural/subdural hygroma

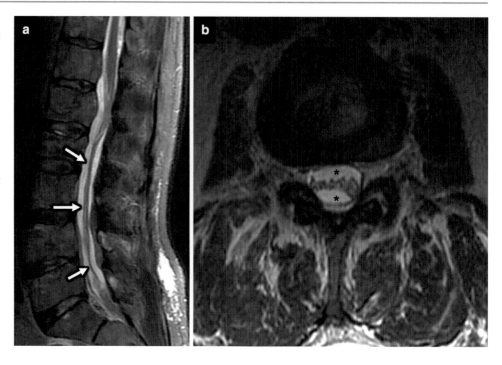

Bozzo and colleagues reviewed the literature spanning more than two decades, between 1988 and 2009, relevant to MRI for short- and long-term SCI prognostication [17]. As part of their meta-analysis, four studies comprising a total of 205 patients were identified, for which MRI findings were correlated with the neurologic examination. In conglomerate, these studies suggest MRI is best used for predicting outcomes in cases where there is very mild (normal cord signal) or very severe (intramedullary hemorrhage) injury. Tremendous variability in outcome, however, was observed when the MRI findings were intermediate in degree. For example, among the 49 patients who demonstrated Schaefer type 2 injury (nonhemorrhagic cord edema spanning greater than 1 vertebral body segment in length), there was a near-equal probability that the neurologic outcome would be ASIA A (26%), ASIA B (22%), ASIA C (24%), or ASIA D (24%). Improved prognostication for patients with this intermediate MRI pattern of injury has been shown, when axial T2 images are used to classify contusion, based on the transverse extent of injury at the contusion epicenter, using the BASIC score (Fig. 16) [49, 53].

Miyanji and colleagues defined standardized methods for determining mid-sagittal mean spinal canal compromise (MCC) and mean spinal cord compression (MSCC) [54]. These measures were prospectively correlated with additional imaging and clinical data in 100 patients [54]. Imaging data included the quantitative measures MCC, MSCC, and longitudinal length of intramedullary cord signal abnormality, in addition to six qualitative dichotomous variables, including the presence or absence of intramedullary hemorrhage, cord swelling, cord edema, soft-tissue injury, disc herniation, and pre-injury stenosis. The authors found that MSCC, cord swelling, and spinal cord hemorrhage were statistically significant predictors of follow-up ASIA motor scores. Importantly, after adjusting for initial ASIA score, only the qualitative variables of cord hemorrhage and cord swelling significantly correlated with outcome.

In a more recent evidence-based SCI guidelines publication, MRI was recommended in the acute stages of SCI, but the quality of evidence and level of recommendation for injury prognostication were rated as "very low" and "weak," respectively [55]. In summarizing the studies included in their meta-analysis, Fehlings et al. concluded that intramedullary hemorrhage was the most substantial prognostic MR biomarker, with moderate evidence associating intramedullary hematoma length with scores of neurologic recovery [56]. Future high-quality prospective longitudinal observation studies are needed to more definitively validate the prognostic significance of conventional MRI biomarkers in acute traumatic SCI.

In summary, the review of axial and sagittal T2-W sequences should focus on the cranio-caudal and transverse extent of SCI, in the context of existing classification systems, such as the Schaefer and BASIC scores (Figs. 17, and 18). The level of injury, along with the presence or absence of hemorrhage, should be documented. Levels of ongoing spinal cord compression may require urgent intervention, and should be emergently communicated given the demonstrated benefits of early surgical decompression.

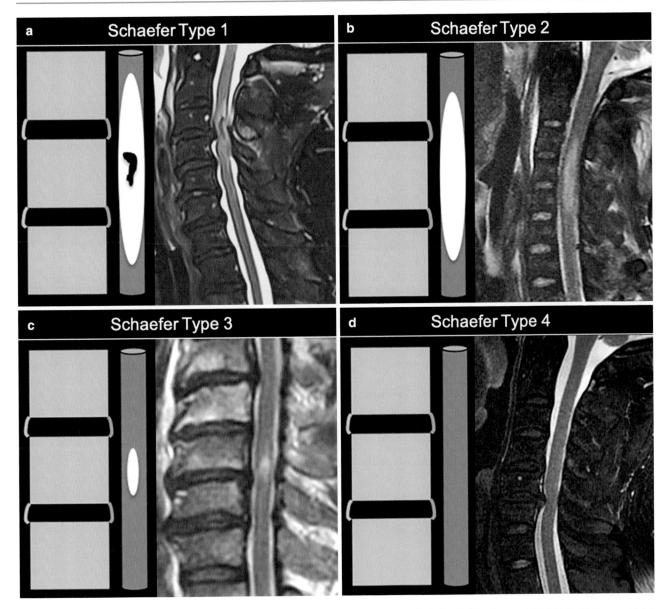

**Fig. 15** Sagittal Schaefer grading scheme for acute traumatic spinal cord injury. Diagram depiction (left) and sagittal T2-W FS MR images (right) for type 1 (**a**), type 2 (**b**), type 3 (**c**), and type 4 (**d**) injuries

## Paraspinous Injury

### Whiplash-Associated Disorder (WAD)

Whiplash-associated disorder (WAD) is the highest reported injury in developed countries. WAD is caused by sudden acceleration-deceleration motion, most commonly resulting from a rear-end motor vehicle collision. A variety of signs and symptoms characterize the WAD, typically developing within days of the initial whiplash injury. Common symptoms include neck pain and stiffness, decreased range of motion in the neck, headaches emanating from the skull base, upper extremity tingling and numbness, fatigue, and dizziness. The highly litigious nature of WAD, and the potential for secondary gain, with amplifications of symptoms, has complicated incidence and severity data.

Diagnosis of WAD is based on clinical evaluation. There are no formal, established, imaging findings that define or confirm the diagnosis of WAD, to our knowledge. However, a number of traumatic findings seen on MRI have been associated with acute WAD. Anderson and colleagues focused on ten cervical spine MRI findings, in a group of

100 patient-control pairs [57]. Overall, the authors found low sensitivity and specificity of these MRI findings for diagnosis of acute WAD. Importantly, although sensitivity was low, identification of occult vertebral fractures or perimuscular fluid was highly specific to findings for WAD, with an odds ratio of greater than 20 when these findings were present. Therefore, close evaluation of the sagittal T2 fat-suppressed sequences for these findings is important for

supporting a clinical diagnosis of WAD, when MRI is performed.

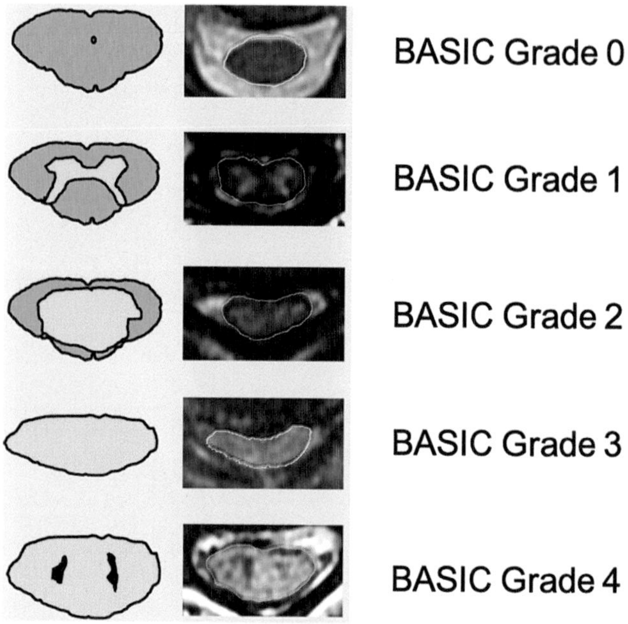

## Conclusion

In summary, MRI is a critically important tool for the evaluation of patients with suspected subaxial spinal trauma, with evolving indications and ever-growing armamentarium of imaging sequences, tailored to improve diagnosis and patient management. Familiarity with the advantages and limitations of MRI for assessing spinal stability, spinal canal contents, and paraspinal injury is vital for those caring for trauma patients with spine injury.

- A structured approach to the MRI examination for spinal stability should include careful evaluation of the anterior and posterior tension band stabilizers.
- Thee-dimensional T2 SPACE or similar high spatial resolution nonfat-suppressed T2-W sequence can be helpful in the evaluation of traumatic spinal injury, particularly for the evaluation of the posterior ligamentous complex.
- Spinal canal evaluation with MRI should focus on traumatic extra-arachnoid collections, canal stenosis, and compression of neural elements, including the spinal cord, the conus, and the cauda equina.
- It is important to recognize the complimentary roles of sagittal and axial characterization of spinal cord contusion, and the prognostic significance of identifying intramedullary hemorrhage.
- Paraspinous muscle edema and vertebral compression injuries are insensitive, but highly specific to findings on

**Fig. 16** BASIC grading scheme for acute traumatic spinal cord injury. Diagram depiction (left) and representative axial T2-W images (right) for BASIC type 0 (top row) through type 4 (bottom row) injuries

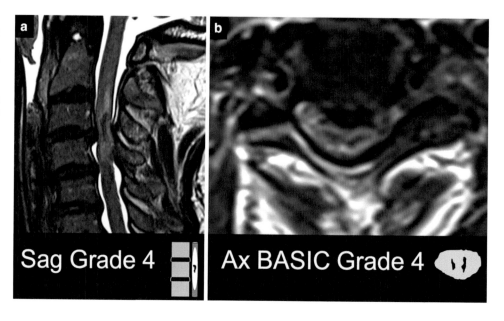

**Fig. 17** Severe acute SCI without recovery. Sagittal (**a**) and axial (**b**) T2-W images of the upper cervical spine in a 72-year-old patient following a MVC shows complete motor and sensory C4 injury, consistent with Schaefer type 1 and BASIC grade 4 injury

**Fig. 18** Acute SCI with significant clinical recovery. Sagittal and axial T2-W images of the upper cervical spine, in a 37-year-old man with initial complete C4 motor and sensory SCI. Sagittal T2-W FS MR (**a**) shows moderate extent of injury consistent with Schaefer type 2, while axial T2-W images (**b**) show central edema primarily confined to the central gray matter, consistent with milder BASIC grade 1 injury. The patient had significant motor and sensory recovery

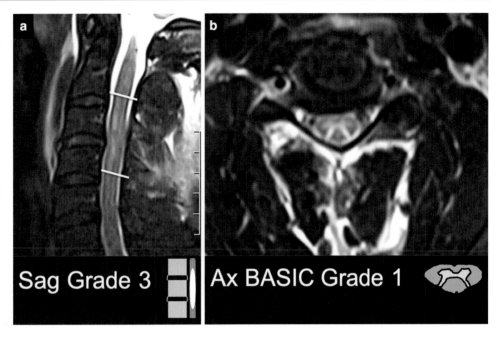

MRI, to support a clinical diagnosis of whiplash-associated disorder.

## References

1. Izzo R, Popolizio T, Balzano RF, Pennelli AM, Simeone A, Muto M. Imaging of cervical spine traumas. Eur J Radiol. 2019;117:75–88.
2. Badhiwala JH, Lai CK, Alhazzani W, Farrokhyar F, Nassiri F, Meade M, et al. Cervical spine clearance in obtunded patients after blunt traumatic injury: a systematic review. Ann Intern Med. 2015;162(6):429–37.
3. National Spinal Cord Injury Statistical Center, Facts and Figures at a Glance. In: Birmingham UoAa, editor. 2017.
4. Kirshblum SC, Burns SP, Biering-Sorensen F, Donovan W, Graves DE, Jha A, et al. International standards for neurological classification of spinal cord injury (revised 2011). J Spinal cord Med. 2011;34(6):535–46.
5. Hoffman JR, Mower WR, Wolfson AB, Todd KH, Zucker MI. Validity of a set of clinical criteria to rule out injury to the cervical spine in patients with blunt trauma. National Emergency X-Radiography Utilization Study Group. N Engl J Med. 2000;343(2):94–9.
6. Stiell IG, Laupacis A, Wells GA, Canadian CTH, Cervical-Spine SG. Indications for computed tomography after minor head injury. Canadian CT Head and Cervical-Spine Study Group. N Engl J Med. 2000;343(21):1570–1.
7. Bailitz J, Starr F, Beecroft M, Bankoff J, Roberts R, Bokhari F, et al. CT should replace three-view radiographs as the initial screening test in patients at high, moderate, and low risk for blunt cervical spine injury: a prospective comparison. J Trauma. 2009;66(6):1605–9.
8. Ghanta MK, Smith LM, Polin RS, Marr AB, Spires WV. An analysis of Eastern Association for the Surgery of Trauma practice guidelines for cervical spine evaluation in a series of patients with multiple imaging techniques. Am Surg. 2002;68(6):563–7. discussion 7-8
9. Shah LM, Ross JS. Imaging of spine trauma. Neurosurgery. 2016;79(5):626–42.
10. Beckmann NM, West OC, Nunez D Jr, et al. ACR appropriateness criteria suspected spine trauma. J Am Coll Radiol: JACR. 2019;16 (5S):S264–85.
11. Daffner RH, Hackney DB. ACR Appropriateness Criteria on suspected spine trauma. J Am Coll Radiol: JACR. 2007;4(11): 762–75.
12. Wu X, Malhotra A, Geng B, Liu R, Abbed K, Forman HP, et al. Cost-effectiveness of magnetic resonance imaging in cervical cpine clearance of neurologically intact patients with blunt trauma. Ann Emerg Med. 2018;71(1):64–73.
13. Wu X, Malhotra A, Geng B, Kalra VB, Abbed K, Forman HP, et al. Cost-effectiveness of magnetic resonance imaging in cervical clearance of obtunded blunt trauma after a normal computed tomographic finding. JAMA Surg. 2018;153(7):625–32.
14. Malhotra A, Wu X, Kalra VB, Nardini HK, Liu R, Abbed KM, et al. Utility of MRI for cervical spine clearance after blunt traumatic injury: a meta-analysis. Eur Radiol. 2017;27(3):1148–60.
15. Onoue K, Farris C, Burley H, Sung E, Clement M, Abdalkader M, et al. Role of cervical spine MRI in the setting of negative cervical spine CT in blunt trauma: critical additional information in the setting of clinical findings suggestive of occult injury. J Neuroradiol Journal de neuroradiologie. 2019;48(3):164–9.
16. Maung AA, Johnson DC, Barre K, Peponis T, Mesar T, Velmahos GC, et al. Cervical spine MRI in patients with negative CT: a prospective, multicenter study of the research consortium of new england centers for trauma (ReCONECT). J Trauma Acute Care Surg. 2017;82(2):263–9.
17. Bozzo A, Marcoux J, Radhakrishna M, Pelletier J, Goulet B. The role of magnetic resonance imaging in the management of acute spinal cord injury. J Neurotrauma. 2011;28(8):1401–11.
18. Haefeli J, Mabray MC, Whetstone WD, Dhall SS, Pan JZ, Upadhyayula P, et al. Multivariate analysis of MRI biomarkers for predicting neurologic impairment in cervical spinal cord injury. AJNR Am J Neuroradiol. 2017;38(3):648–55.
19. Li Z, Chen YA, Chow D, Talbott J, Glastonbury C, Shah V. Practical applications of CISS MRI in spine imaging. Eur J Radiol Open. 2019;6:231–42.
20. Koontz NA, Wiggins RH 3rd, Mills MK, McLaughlin MS, Pigman EC, Anzai Y, et al. Less is more: efficacy of rapid 3D-T2 SPACE in

ED patients with acute atypical low back pain. Acad Radiol. 2017;24(8):988–94.

21. Chokshi FH, Sadigh G, Carpenter W, Allen JW. Diagnostic quality of 3D T2-SPACE compared with T2-FSE in the evaluation of cervical spine MRI anatomy. AJNR Am J Neuroradiol. 2017;38(4):846–50.

22. Wang M, Dai Y, Han Y, Haacke EM, Dai J, Shi D. Susceptibility weighted imaging in detecting hemorrhage in acute cervical spinal cord injury. Magn Reson Imaging. 2011;29(3):365–73.

23. Biering-Sorensen F, Alai S, Anderson K, Charlifue S, Chen Y, DeVivo M, et al. Common data elements for spinal cord injury clinical research: a national institute for neurological disorders and Stroke project. Spinal Cord. 2015;53(4):265–77.

24. Goradia D, Linnau KF, Cohen WA, Mirza S, Hallam DK, Blackmore CC. Correlation of MR imaging findings with intraoperative findings after cervical spine trauma. AJNR Am J Neuroradiol. 2007;28(2):209–15.

25. Rihn JA, Yang N, Fisher C, Saravanja D, Smith H, Morrison WB, et al. Using magnetic resonance imaging to accurately assess injury to the posterior ligamentous complex of the spine: a prospective comparison of the surgeon and radiologist. J Neurosurg Spine. 2010;12(4):391–6.

26. Pizones J, Zuniga L, Sanchez-Mariscal F, Alvarez P, Gomez-Rice A, Izquierdo E. MRI study of post-traumatic incompetence of posterior ligamentous complex: importance of the supraspinous ligament. Prospective study of 74 traumatic fractures. Eur Spine J : Official Publication of the European Spine Society, the European Spinal Deformity Society, and the European Section of the Cervical Spine Research Society. 2012;21(11):2222–31.

27. Rihn JA, Fisher C, Harrop J, Morrison W, Yang N, Vaccaro AR. Assessment of the posterior ligamentous complex following acute cervical spine trauma. J Bone Joint Surg Am. 2010;92(3):583–9.

28. White AA 3rd, Johnson RM, Panjabi MM, Southwick WO. Biomechanical analysis of clinical stability in the cervical spine. Clin Orthop Relat Res. 1975;109:85–96.

29. Chhabra HS, Kaul R, Kanagaraju V. Do we have an ideal classification system for thoracolumbar and subaxial cervical spine injuries: what is the expert's perspective? Spinal Cord. 2015;53(1):42–8.

30. Denis F. Spinal instability as defined by the three-column spine concept in acute spinal trauma. Clin Orthop Relat Res. 1984;189:65–76.

31. Magerl F, Aebi M, Gertzbein SD, Harms J, Nazarian S. A comprehensive classification of thoracic and lumbar injuries. Eur Spine J : Official Publication of the European Spine Society, the European Spinal Deformity Society, and the European Section of the Cervical Spine Research Society. 1994;3(4):184–201.

32. Vaccaro AR, Lehman RA Jr, Hurlbert RJ, Anderson PA, Harris M, Hedlund R, et al. A new classification of thoracolumbar injuries: the importance of injury morphology, the integrity of the posterior ligamentous complex, and neurologic status. Spine. 2005;30(20):2325–33.

33. Vaccaro AR, Hulbert RJ, Patel AA, Fisher C, Dvorak M, Lehman RA Jr, et al. The subaxial cervical spine injury classification system: a novel approach to recognize the importance of morphology, neurology, and integrity of the disco-ligamentous complex. Spine. 2007;32(21):2365–74.

34. Vaccaro AR, Oner C, Kepler CK, Dvorak M, Schnake K, Bellabarba C, et al. AOSpine thoracolumbar spine injury classification system: fracture description, neurological status, and key modifiers. Spine. 2013;38(23):2028–37.

35. Vaccaro AR, Koerner JD, Radcliff KE, Oner FC, Reinhold M, Schnake KJ, et al. AOSpine subaxial cervical spine injury classification system. Eur Spine J: Official Publication of the European Spine Society, the European Spinal Deformity Society, and the

European Section of the Cervical Spine Research Society. 2016;25(7):2173–84.

36. Abedi A, Mokkink LB, Zadegan SA, Paholpak P, Tamai K, Wang JC, et al. Reliability and validity of the AOSpine thoracolumbar injury classification system: a systematic review. Global Spine J. 2019;9(2):231–42.

37. Schnake KJ, Schroeder GD, Vaccaro AR, Oner C. AO spine classification systems (Subaxial, Thoracolumbar). J Orthop Trauma. 2017;31(Suppl 4):S14–23.

38. Pizones J, Izquierdo E, Sanchez-Mariscal F, Alvarez P, Zuniga L. Re: Vaccaro AR, Rihn JA, Saravanja D, et al. Injury of the posterior ligamentous complex of the thoracolumbar spine: a prospective evaluation of the diagnostic accuracy of magnetic resonance imaging. Spine 2009;34:E841-7. Spine. 2010;35(8):929–30. author reply 30

39. Vaccaro AR, Schroeder GD, Kepler CK, Cumhur Oner F, Vialle LR, Kandziora F, et al. The surgical algorithm for the AOSpine thoracolumbar spine injury classification system. Eur Spine J: Official Publication of the European Spine Society, the European Spinal Deformity Society, and the European Section of the Cervical Spine Research Society. 2016;25(4):1087–94.

40. Pizones J, Izquierdo E, Sanchez-Mariscal F, Zuniga L, Alvarez P, Gomez-Rice A. Sequential damage assessment of the different components of the posterior ligamentous complex after magnetic resonance imaging interpretation: prospective study 74 traumatic fractures. Spine. 2012;37(11):E662–7.

41. Reina MA, Lirk P, Puigdellivol-Sanchez A, Mavar M, Prats-Galino A. human lumbar ligamentum flavum anatomy for epidural anesthesia: reviewing a 3D MR-based interactive model and postmortem samples. Anesth Analg. 2016;122(3):903–7.

42. Vaccaro AR, Falatyn SP, Flanders AE, Balderston RA, Northrup BE, Cotler JM. Magnetic resonance evaluation of the intervertebral disc, spinal ligaments, and spinal cord before and after closed traction reduction of cervical spine dislocations. Spine. 1999;24(12):1210–7.

43. Brichko L, Giddey B, Tee J, Niggemeyer L, Fitzgerald M. Cervical spine traumatic epidural haematomas: incidence and characteristics. Emerg Med Australasia : EMA. 2018;30(3):359–65.

44. Sklar EM, Post JM, Falcone S. MRI of acute spinal epidural hematomas. J Comput Assist Tomogr. 1999;23(2):238–43.

45. Lawrence DA, Trotta B, Shen FH, Druzgal JT, Fox MG. Imaging characteristics of cervical spine extra-arachnoid fluid collections managed conservatively. Skelet Radiol. 2016;45(9):1285–9.

46. Haines DE, Harkey HL. al-Mefty O. The "subdural" space: a new look at an outdated concept. Neurosurgery. 1993;32(1):111–20.

47. Horn EM, Bristol RE, Feiz-Erfan I, Beres EJ, Bambakidis NC, Theodore N. Spinal cord compression from traumatic anterior cervical pseudomeningoceles. Report of three cases. J Neurosurg Spine. 2006;5(3):254–8.

48. Talbott JFHJ, Ferguson AR, Bresnahan JC, Beattie M, Dhall SS. Magnetic resonance imaging for assessing injury severity and prognosis in acute traumatic spinal cord injury. Imaging Clin N Am. 2018; In Press

49. Talbott JF, Whetstone WD, Readdy WJ, Ferguson AR, Bresnahan JC, Saigal R, et al. The Brain and Spinal Injury Center score: a novel, simple, and reproducible method for assessing the severity of acute cervical spinal cord injury with axial T2-weighted MRI findings. J Neurosurg Spine. 2015;23(4):495–504.

50. Schaefer DM, Flanders A, Northrup BE, Doan HT, Osterholm JL. Magnetic resonance imaging of acute cervical spine trauma. Correlation with severity of neurologic injury. Spine. 1989;14(10):1090–5.

51. Leypold BG, Flanders AE, Burns AS. The early evolution of spinal cord lesions on MR imaging following traumatic spinal cord injury. AJNR Am J Neuroradiol. 2008;29(5):1012–6.

52. Aarabi B, Simard JM, Kufera JA, Alexander M, Zacherl KM, Mirvis SE, et al. Intramedullary lesion expansion on magnetic resonance

imaging in patients with motor complete cervical spinal cord injury. J Neurosurg Spine. 2012;17(3):243–50.

53. Farhadi HF, Kukreja S, Minnema A, Vatti L, Gopinath M, Prevedello L, et al. Impact of admission imaging findings on neurological outcomes in acute cervical traumatic spinal cord injury. J Neurotrauma. 2018;35(12):1398–406.

54. Miyanji F, Furlan JC, Aarabi B, Arnold PM, Fehlings MG. Acute cervical traumatic spinal cord injury: MR imaging findings correlated with neurologic outcome–prospective study with 100 consecutive patients. Radiology. 2007;243(3):820–7.

55. Kurpad S, Martin AR, Tetreault LA, Fischer DJ, Skelly AC, Mikulis D, et al. Impact of baseline magnetic resonance imaging on neurologic, functional, and safety outcomes in patients with acute traumatic spinal cord injury. Global Spine J. 2017;7 (3 Suppl):151S–74S.

56. Fehlings MG, Martin AR, Tetreault LA, Aarabi B, Anderson P, Arnold PM, et al. A clinical practice guideline for the management of patients with acute spinal cord injury: recommendations on the role of baseline magnetic resonance imaging in clinical decision making and outcome prediction. Global Spine J. 2017;7 (3 Suppl):221S–30S.

57. Anderson SE, Boesch C, Zimmermann H, Busato A, Hodler J, Bingisser R, et al. Are there cervical spine findings at MR imaging that are specific to acute symptomatic whiplash injury? A prospective controlled study with four experienced blinded readers. Radiology. 2012;262(2):567–75.

# Imaging of Nontraumatic Spinal Emergencies

# 14

Shekhar D. Khanpara, F. Eymen Ucisik, and Roy F. Riascos

## Contents

## Abstract

Nontraumatic spinal emergencies (NTSE) present with acute, rapid onset of neurological symptoms without an inciting traumatic event. Pathologies intrinsic and extrinsic to the spinal cord can result in acute neurological deterioration, which generally requires prompt diagnosis, and in some patients requires acute intervention, to sustain function.

## Keywords

Nontraumatic spinal emergencies · Myelopathy · Compressive myelopathy · Non-compressive myelopathy

## Introduction

Myelopathy is a generalized term used to describe conditions affecting the spinal cord resulting in neurological deficit [1]. Several conditions which can present acutely or chronically fall under the umbrella term of myelopathy, which can be divided into two main groups: compressive and non-compressive myelopathy. Trauma, a major cause of compressive myelopathy, will be discussed in detail in ▶ Chap. 10, "Imaging of Brain Infections", we will focus on nontraumatic pathologies that result in acute neurological deterioration requiring immediate intervention to preserve function.

Compressive myelopathy, as the name suggests, is due to extrinsic compression of the spinal cord, which may result in sensory or motor deficits. Patients can present with various

S. D. Khanpara · F. E. Ucisik · R. F. Riascos (✉)
Department of Diagnostic and Interventional Imaging, University of Texas Health Science Center at Houston, Houston, TX, USA
e-mail: shekhar.khanpara@uth.tmc.edu;
fehime.E.UcisikKeser@uth.tmc.edu; roy.f.riascos@uth.tmc.edu

© Springer Nature Switzerland AG 2022
M. N. Patlas et al. (eds.), *Atlas of Emergency Imaging from Head-to-Toe*,
https://doi.org/10.1007/978-3-030-92111-8_14

clinical syndromes depending on the specific tract involved, for example, anterior cord syndrome can occur due to affection of the anterior spinothalamic tracts, while posterior cord syndrome occurs when the fasciculus gracilis and fasciculus cuneatus are affected.

Non-compressive myelopathy is secondary to pathologies arising from the spinal cord that result in alteration in its structure. It may present as acute loss of motor function due to involvement of the anterior horn cells or acute-onset shooting pain due to involvement of the anterior or lateral spinothalamic tracts.

Etiologies for compressive and non-compressive myelopathies can be divided into two groups: neoplastic and non-neoplastic conditions.

Neoplasms can be primary or secondary. Primary tumors can be further divided by location into intradural and extradural tumors; and intradural tumors may be intramedullary or extramedullary. The nonneoplastic category includes ischemic, demyelinating, inflammatory, infectious, and neoplastic conditions (Table 1).

# Epidemiology

Nontraumatic spinal emergencies (NTSE) are more common among the older population, with a female predominance [2]. A true incidence or prevalence of nontraumatic spinal emergencies is not known, to our knowledge, as it includes a constellation of pathologies variably reported across the world. However, differences have been identified regarding the causes of nontraumatic spinal emergencies, between developing and developed countries, mainly due to disparities in demographics and socioeconomic status. Acute spinal cord compression secondary to degenerative changes constitutes the most common etiology for nontraumatic spinal emergencies in developed countries, including North America. On the contrary, in developing countries, infectious conditions including spondylodiscitis and epidural abscess comprise the most common cause of nontraumatic spinal emergencies. Spinal cord compression secondary to tumors or epidural hematoma and myelopathy secondary to vascular causes, demyelinating disorders, or systemic inflammatory diseases constitute other common causes of NTSE in developed countries [3].

**Table 1** Differential diagnoses for nontraumatic spinal emergencies

| Compressive myelopathy | |
|---|---|
| Degenerative | Acute disk herniation |
| | Diffuse idiopathic skeletal hyperostosis (DISH) |
| | Ossification of the posterior longitudinal ligament (OPLL) |
| Infectious | Discitis/osteomyelitis (pyogenic, tuberculous, fungal) |
| | Epidural abscess |
| Neoplastic | Extramedullary intradural tumors – Meningioma, schwannoma, neurofibroma, |
| | Leptomeningeal metastasis, epidermoid cyst |
| | Extradural tumors – Osseous neoplasms, metastasis, multiple myeloma, and lymphoma |
| Vascular | Epidural hematoma |
| **Non-compressive myelopathy** | |
| Ischemic | Spinal cord infarction |
| Demyelinating | Multiple sclerosis (MS) |
| | Neuromyelitis optica (NMO) |
| | Acute demyelinating encephalomyelitis (ADEM) |
| Systemic inflammatory | Sarcoidosis |
| | Systemic lupus erythematosus (SLE) |
| | Behcet's disease |
| Infectious | Acute flaccid myelitis (AFM) |
| | Varicella-zoster myelitis |
| | Poliomyelitis |
| | Parasitic myelitis |
| | Guillain-Barré syndrome |
| Neoplastic | Intramedullary – Hemangioblastoma, lymphoma, paraganglioma |

# Clinical Features

While with trauma the cord injury is generally complete, with nontraumatic injuries the spinal cord abnormality is usually partial, leading to a more variable clinical presentation [4]. Various risk factors, including older age, preexisting degenerative changes, congenital fusion of vertebrae, or spinal canal stenosis due to congenitally short pedicles, predispose patients to nontraumatic spinal emergencies. Other disease-specific risk factors have been described under their respective titles.

In general, nontraumatic spinal emergencies present as acute loss of sensation (touch, pressure, proprioception, or pain sensation), weakness, or complete loss of motor function. Acute compression of the cauda equina may result in saddle anesthesia, loss of bowel and bladder control, sexual dysfunction, and weakness of the lower extremity, which is referred to as cauda equina syndrome (CES).

# Diagnostic Investigations

Imaging plays an essential role in differentiating compressive from non-compressive causes of nontraumatic spinal emergencies. Magnetic resonance imaging (MRI) is the imaging modality of choice in cases of nontraumatic spinal emergencies. Routine imaging includes T2- and T1-weighted sequences performed in the sagittal and axial planes with sagittal STIR sequence. This constitutes a protocol which is usually adequate for diagnosis and management. Post-contrast imaging may be necessary in cases of suspected infection, neoplasm, inflammatory, or vascular conditions. Diffusion-weighted imaging plays a vital role in the diagnosis of spinal cord ischemia and acute demyelinating process. Susceptibility-weighted imaging (SWI) is important for the detection of blood products and calcium, assisting the diagnosis of intramedullary cavernous malformations, hemorrhage within neoplasms, and epidural hematoma.

## Compressive Myelopathy

### Degenerative

Degenerative spondylosis is the most common cause of acute nontraumatic myelopathy in developed countries [3–5]. Degenerative changes are much more common in the cervical and lumbar region than in the thoracic region.

Cervical and lumbar degenerative spondylosis resulting in spinal stenosis is the most common cause of spinal cord dysfunction in the elderly population in North America and is seen more commonly among males at a ratio of approximately 2.7:1 [6]. Compressive myelopathy secondary to degenerative cervical spondylolysis is the result of facet and uncovertebral osteoarthrosis, ligamentum flavum thickening, ligamentous ossification, and disk herniation. An underlying congenitally narrow spinal canal renders the cord more susceptible to compression.

Acute disk herniation superimposed over chronic degenerative changes is an important cause of compressive myelopathy [7] (Fig. 1). Insult to the spinal cord or cauda equina nerve roots occurs from both the primary compression by the disk and by the resulting ischemia [7].

Causes of a rigid spine, including diffuse idiopathic skeletal hyperostosis (DISH) and ossification of the posterior longitudinal ligament (OPLL), render the spine susceptible to relatively minor trauma, resulting in acute spinal cord compression. DISH is an enthesopathy characterized by flowing ossification of the anterior longitudinal ligament with contiguous involvement of at least four vertebral bodies. It is often associated with ossification of the posterior longitudinal ligament and enthesopathy at other sites. Disk spaces are usually well preserved. OPLL is an entity more common in the Asian population, with isolated involvement of the posterior longitudinal ligament and preferential involvement of the cervical spine. However, it can also be associated with DISH and ankylosing spondylitis.

Radiographs are often used for the initial assessment of degenerative conditions. However, MRI is the modality of choice for the evaluation of acute spinal cord compression. Even though it does not provide as much anatomical detail, CT myelography may be performed for the assessment of the thecal sac and its contents, in cases where MRI is contraindicated or MRI artifacts from preexisting spinal hardware substantially interfere with image quality.

## Infection

Infectious conditions of the spine, particularly osteomyelitis and discitis, are the most common cause of nontraumatic compressive myelopathy in developing countries and are one of the leading causes in the developed countries [8]. Certain populations in the developed countries, such as drug abusers, immunocompromised patients, or homeless persons, are considered at high risk.

Spondylodiscitis is a term used to describe a combination of osteomyelitis and discitis. Various pathogens have been implicated as a causative agent. Pyogenic, tuberculous, and fungal spondylodiscitis are the three main broad categories that are commonly encountered. *Staphylococcus aureus* is the most common organism causing pyogenic spondylodiscitis and epidural abscess [9]. *Pseudomonas* and *Salmonella* are other causative agents, relatively more common with intravenous drug use and sickle cell disease, respectively [9, 10]. The pattern of spread can be hematogenous (most common), contiguous, or by direct inoculation due to trauma or surgery. The classic MRI appearance of pyogenic spondylodiscitis includes endplate bone marrow edema (T2 and STIR hyperintensity) on each side of the disk, loss of normal marrow signal, focal enhancement, endplate destruction, and disk space narrowing with associated increased T2 signal of the disk [11] (Fig. 2). While pyogenic spondylodiscitis causes the destruction of both the vertebra and the disk, tuberculosis classically spares the disks at the early stages of the disease [12]. Several other imaging features, including predisposition for the lumbar vertebrae, decreased association with paraspinal abscess, thick and irregular abscess walls, and involvement of more than two vertebral bodies, favor pyogenic over tuberculous spondylodiscitis [13]. Fungal abscesses constitute a rare entity, mostly encountered in

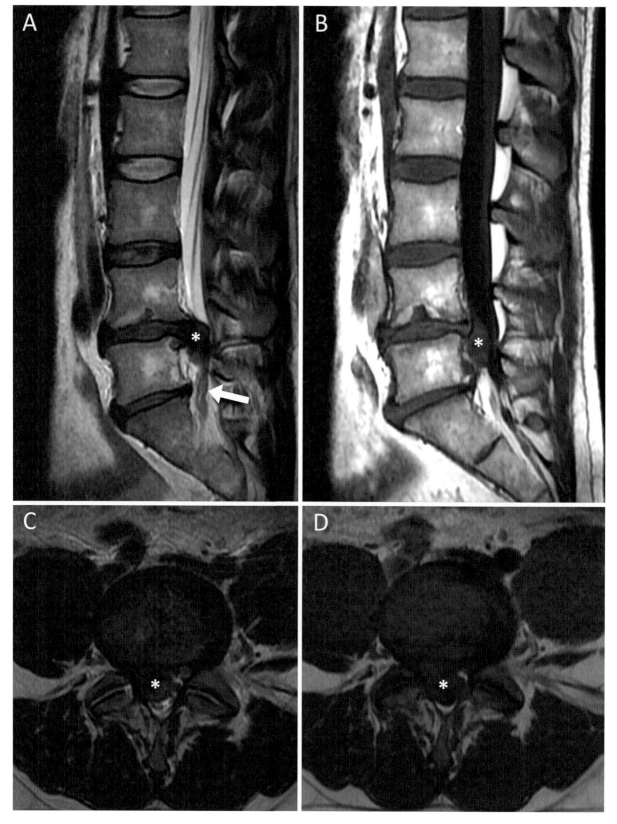

**Fig. 1** Disk extrusion: A 46-year-old man with acute-onset back pain, bilateral lower extremity weakness, and saddle anesthesia. Right parasagittal T2-weighted (**a**) and midline T1-weighted (**b**) MR images demonstrate a large central/right subarticular disk extrusion with inferior migration (asterisk). Axial T2- (**c**) and T1-weighted (**d**) images show moderate to severe stenosis of the spinal canal, with severe compression of the cauda equina nerve roots. Note the clumping of the nerve roots inferior to the disk extrusion (arrow in **a**)

immunocompromised patients. The presence of low signal on T1- and T2-weighted images (relative to muscle) due to the presence of manganese in the fungal hyphae is an important clue to differentiate fungal infection from other etiologies.

An epidural abscess may occur through hematogenous spread or direct extension of spondylodiscitis. Contrast administration helps to differentiate an epidural abscess from noninfectious collections such as a postoperative seroma or a hematoma. An epidural abscess classically has a well-defined wall that shows avid enhancement, while noninfectious collections typically lack these features. Additionally, an epidural abscess classically shows diffusion restriction on MRI due to high cellularity, while seromas do not [11]. An epidural abscess can be preceded by a phlegmon, which will show homogenous enhancement on the post-contrast images with lack of necrosis or pus formation.

## Neoplastic

Neoplastic cord compression is the second most common type of nontraumatic spinal cord injury in developed countries [3, 4]. The tumor is extradural in location about 60% of the time and intradural and extramedullary in 30% of cases and has both intra- and extradural components in 10% [14]. Vertebral metastases are the most common cause of acute compressive myelopathy under this category followed by myeloma and lymphoma. Intradural extramedullary neoplasms including schwannoma, meningioma, and neurofibroma are uncommon causes of acute compressive myelopathy.

Vertebral metastases constitute the vast majority of extradural tumors causing compression of the spinal cord. Five to ten percent of cancer patients develop spinal cord compression, and in 12% to 20% of cancer patients, spinal metastases are the reason for the initial presentation [15, 16]. Breast and lung carcinomas are the most common primary tumors responsible for vertebral metastases. Hematogenous spread to the vertebrae is the most common mechanism, followed by contiguous spread of tumor. Vertebral metastases are often multifocal and are broadly divided into lytic and sclerotic metastases based on the radiographic and CT appearance. MRI is highly sensitive for the depiction of vertebral metastases, which can have variable imaging appearance and different enhancement patterns on MRI. Most often, osteolytic metastases are hyperintense on T2-weighted and hypointense on T1-weighted imaging. Osteoblastic metastases are hypointense on T1-weighted and T2-weighted imaging. Both types of metastatic osseous processes demonstrate heterogenous enhancement on post-contrast images. Associated pathological fractures are a dreaded complication that can result in acute spinal cord compression, more commonly associated with osteolytic metastases. Vertebral metastases often have a soft-tissue component which can occasionally extend beyond the vertebral margins into the epidural space and cause compression of the spinal cord or cauda equina.

Multiple myeloma is the most common primary bone malignancy arising from plasma cells. It primarily affects the red marrow containing axial skeleton in the elderly population (50–70 years of age). Classical clinical presentation includes bone pain, anemia, renal failure, and hypercalcemia. Imaging findings in the spine can range from a normal-appearing vertebral column to diffuse marrow infiltration with a variegated appearance. The tumoral foci have a lytic appearance in majority of the cases, with sclerotic metastases being much less common (approximately 3%) [17]. MRI is the imaging modality of choice in suspected cases of multiple myeloma. The affected vertebrae demonstrate focal or diffuse low T1 signal, with corresponding high T2 signal and heterogenous enhancement after gadolinium administration. Multiple myeloma can present with generalized osteopenia and resultant pathological fracture. CT is less sensitive for depiction of multiple myeloma but is often used to assess the risk of pathological fracture. Extramedullary myeloma is an uncommon form of presentation (7–18% of all newly diagnosed myeloma cases) and most frequently presents as a spinal epidural mass in the absence of skeletal involvement. Spinal cord compression is often present at the time of diagnosis [18, 19].

Primary spinal lymphoma is rare; however, secondary bony involvement occurs in approximately 30% cases of lymphoma [20]. The axial skeleton including the spine (thoracic involvement is most frequent), skull, and pelvis are the most frequently involved sites. It is more common in childhood. Hematogenous spread and direct extension are the two common mechanisms of vertebral involvement. The most common imaging presentation is in the form of a vertebral mass, followed by epidural and intradural deposits. The abnormality is often homogenously hypointense on T1- and T2-weighted imaging due to high cellularity and enhances homogenously after IV gadolinium administration (Fig. 3). The epidural component can result in compression of the spinal cord or nerve roots in approximately 5–10% of systemic lymphoma [21–23].

Schwannoma is the most common intradural extramedullary neoplasm. These are benign tumors of Schwann cell origin that usually arise from the dorsal nerve roots and extend into the neural foramen resulting in a "dumbbell" shape. They show high T2 signal and heterogeneous enhancement and may have central necrosis or hemorrhage

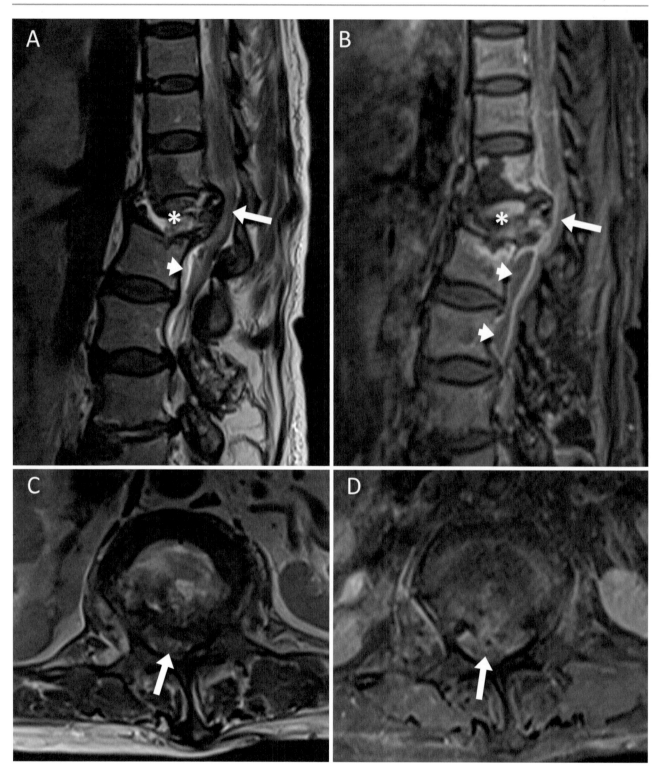

**Fig. 2** Pyogenic spondylodiscitis: An 80-year-old man with bilateral lower extremity weakness and loss of bowel/bladder function and MRSA bacteremia. Sagittal T2-weighted (**a**) and sagittal post-contrast T1-weighted (**b**) MR images show discovertebral destruction at T12-L1, with near-complete collapse of the T12 vertebral body and a fluid-filled cleft along its superior endplate (white asterisk). There is associated retropulsion causing moderate to severe spinal canal stenosis and compression of the conus medullaris (white arrows in **a**–**d**). Axial T2-weighted (**c**) and post-contrast T1-weighted (**d**) MR images confirm these findings. Enhancing marrow edema is seen involving the T11 and L1 vertebral bodies, which is consistent with osteomyelitis. A peripherally enhancing anterior epidural fluid collection is seen extending from T12-L1 to L2-L3 (white arrowheads in **a** and **b**)

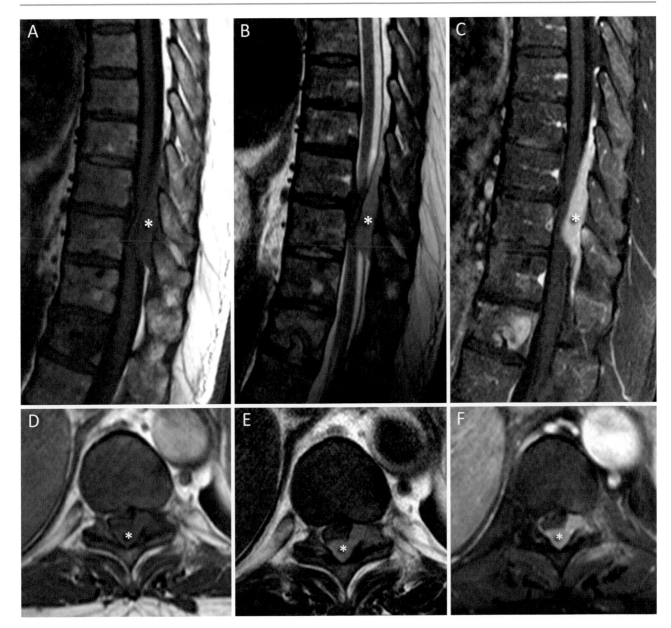

**Fig. 3** Diffuse large B-cell lymphoma: A 63-year-old man with 4 months of back and left flank pain presented with acute onset of altered sensation in the lower extremities. Sagittal T1- (**a**) and T2-weighted (**b**) MR images show a posterior epidural mass (asterisks), hypointense on T1 and of intermediate signal on T2WI, causing compression and anterior displacement of the spinal cord. It demonstrates homogenous enhancement on the post-contrast T1 fat-saturated image (**c**). Corresponding axial T1-, T2-, and post-contrast T1-weighted images (**d**, **e**, **f**) show that the mass is centered along the posterior and left lateral epidural space (asterisks). The patient underwent decompression of the spinal canal with excision of the tumor. The histopathological diagnosis was high-grade diffuse large B-cell lymphoma, germinal center type

[24] (Fig. 4). When multiple, neurofibromatosis type 2 or "schwannomatosis" should be suspected.

Meningioma is the second most common intradural extramedullary neoplasm [25]. They are mostly benign (WHO grade I) but may demonstrate locally invasive behavior (WHO grade II). Approximately 98% of meningiomas are solitary and most commonly involve the thoracic spine. Multiple meningiomas can be seen in association

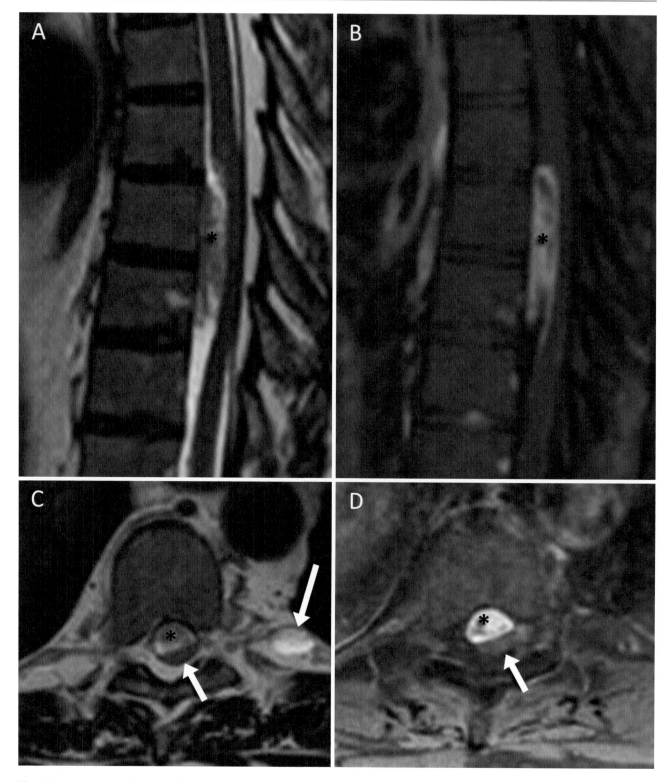

**Fig. 4** Schwannoma: A 57-year-old man with severe back pain radiating to the chest. Midline sagittal T2- (**a**) and T1-weighted MR images with IV contrast (**b**) demonstrate an anterior intradural extramedullary mass (asterisks) with heterogenous signal intensity on T2WI (**a**) and heterogenous enhancement (**b**). Axial T2 (**c**) and post-contrast T1 fat-saturated (**d**) MR images show severe compression and posterior displacement of the spinal cord (short white arrow). Note an oval-shaped cyst within the left intercostal space on image (**c**) (long white arrow), representing a cystic schwannoma along the intercostal nerve

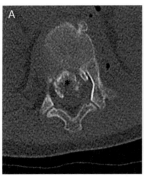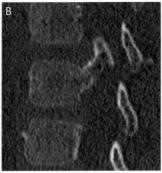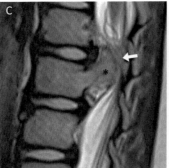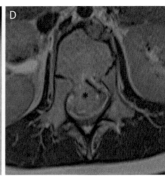

**Fig. 5** Osteochondroma: A 22-year-old woman with worsening of bilateral lower extremity weakness. Non-contrast axial (**a**) and sagittal (**b**) CT images at the thoracolumbar junction demonstrate an exophytic bony mass protruding into the spinal canal, causing moderate to severe spinal canal stenosis (asterisk). Subsequent T2-weighted MR images in the sagittal and axial planes (**c** and **d**) confirmed the exophytic bony origin. The mass (asterisk) is continuous with the posterior wall of the vertebral body, follows similar signal characteristic as the vertebral body on all sequences, and causes severe compression of the thecal sac and cauda equina nerve roots (arrow)

with neurofibromatosis type 2 and meningiomatosis. They follow similar signal characteristics as its intracranial counterpart, with homogenous enhancement and a dural tail [25].

Primary osseous tumors make a small contribution to extradural compressive neoplasms and are rarely responsible for an acute presentation. Common examples include osteoid osteoma, osteoblastoma, aneurysmal bone cyst, giant cell tumor, chordoma, and osteochondroma (Fig. 5).

## Vascular

Causes of hemorrhagic compression include epidural or subdural hemorrhage from arteriovenous malformation (AVM), anticoagulant therapy, bleeding disorders, vascular neoplasms, vasculitis, and iatrogenic trauma during epidural injection or lumbar puncture. While hemorrhage from bleeding disorders or iatrogenic trauma can be seen at any age, epidural or subdural hematoma from an (AVM) most commonly occurs in middle-aged men [26].

AVM-related hemorrhage may result in extradural or intradural cord compression, depending on its anatomical characteristics, and will be discussed in more detail in the non-compressive myelopathy section.

Acute epidural/subdural hematoma is hyperdense on CT, with different degrees in attenuation depending on the age of the hemorrhage. Signal characteristics on MRI are variable and depend on the age of the bleed, as well. With epidural hematoma, the dura is often displaced, and there are effacement of the subarachnoid space and compression of the thecal sac (Fig. 6). Effacement of the epidural fat is an important imaging clue suggestive of epidural hematoma. Subdural hematomas are much less common than epidural hematomas

but may result in more marked compression of the spinal cord [27]. The "inverted Mercedes-Benz" sign can be seen in some subdural hematoma cases [28].

## Non-compressive Myelopathy

### Ischemia

Spinal cord infarction is much less common than its brain counterpart and has a prevalence of approximately 1% [29]. Various risk factors, including arterial hypertension, diabetes mellitus, dyslipidemia, and atrial fibrillation, predispose individuals to spinal cord ischemia. The onset of symptoms is usually within less than 72 h [30]. Clinical presentation includes a range of motor and sensory deficits, ranging from weakness in one limb to tetraparesis, difficulty walking, unexplained radicular pain, or changes in proprioception.

On imaging, spinal cord ischemia can be identified as early as within 24 h of symptom onset. Most common imaging findings include a well-defined linear T2 hyperintensity along the ventral aspect of the cord, in the sagittal plane (pencil-like appearance), and central gray matter T2 signal abnormality with an "H-shaped" appearance on axial images [5]. Restricted diffusion can be seen on DWI in acute cases (Fig. 7). Post-contrast imaging can demonstrate enhancement in the subacute phase like its brain counterpart. Anterior spinal cord infarct involves the anterior 2/3 of the spinal cord. It may present with "owl's eyes" or "snake eyes" appearance, with two T2 hyperintense spots involving the anterior motor horn cells of the spinal cord [30]. A useful adjunct sign to support the diagnosis of spinal cord ischemia is the presence of abnormal T2 signal within the posterior half

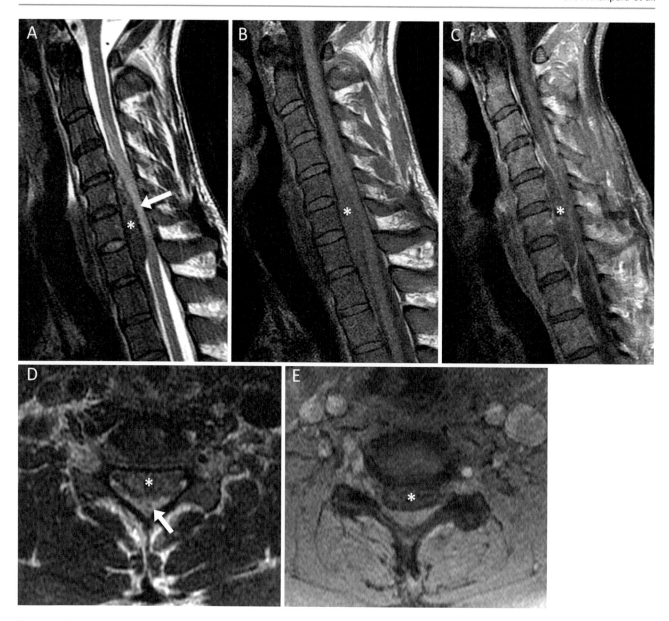

**Fig. 6** Epidural hematoma: A 40-year-old woman on anticoagulants for antiphospholipid syndrome with acute-onset weakness in the upper and lower extremities and radiating pain to the bilateral upper extremities. Sagittal T2- (**a**) and T1-weighted MR images (**b**) demonstrate a large ventral epidural hematoma (asterisk), causing severe spinal canal stenosis, compression of the spinal cord, and increased intramedullary T2 signal (arrow in **a**). The epidural hematoma shows peripheral enhancement in the sagittal T1-weighted fat-saturated MR image following IV contrast (**c**). The axial T2 (**d**) and GRE (**e**) images corroborate the findings. Given the acute presentation, the increased intramedullary signal likely represents spinal cord edema

of the vertebral body at the same level signifying a vertebral body infarct [31]. This has been explained by common blood supply for the anterior spinal cord and the posterior vertebral body.

Fibrocartilaginous disk embolism is a rare cause of spinal cord infarction secondary to retrograde migration of disk material/nucleus pulposus into a spinal artery or vein [32]. Spinal cord infarction, typically in young patients, is secondary to shearing vascular injury from vigorous activities (surfing, gymnastics, falls, etc.) resulting in sudden hyperextension of the spine. This is referred to as surfer's myelopathy, as it was first described in surfers [33].

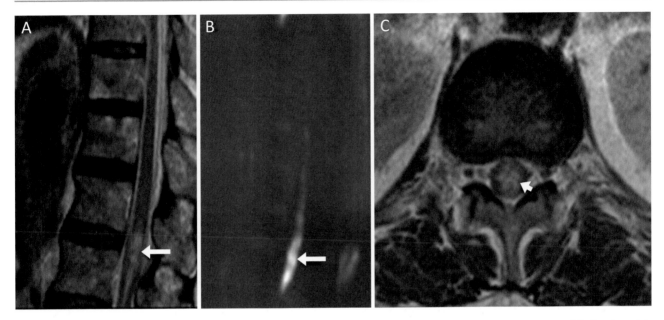

**Fig. 7** Spinal cord infarct: A 75-year-old woman with acute-onset lower extremity weakness following thoracic endovascular aortic repair (TEVAR). Sagittal T2-weighted MR image (**a**) demonstrates a well-defined focal area of hyperintensity within the conus medullaris, with mild associated cord expansion (arrow). Restricted diffusion (arrow) is present on sagittal DWI (**b**). The axial T2-weighted image (**c**) localizes the infarct predominantly within the central gray matter, in an "H-shaped" configuration (arrowhead)

## Demyelinating Disorders

Multiple sclerosis (MS) is the most common demyelinating disease of the central nervous system. Isolated involvement of the spinal cord (more commonly cervical cord) can be seen in 10–20% of the cases. The remainder of the cases have concurrent involvement of the supratentorial or infratentorial brain. Typical onset of the disease is seen from the second to fourth decade, with a female predominance. Caucasians are the most affected ethnicity. Classically, there could be solitary or multiple, asymmetrical T2 hyperintense focal abnormalities involving a short segment (less than two vertebral segments) of the spinal cord. They are peripherally located, and wedge-shaped, with the apex pointing toward the ependymal canal (Fig. 8). There may be associated cord swelling in the acute setting. The presence of enhancement or restricted diffusion might indicate ongoing acute demyelination. Cord edema and restricted diffusion typically resolve within 6–8 weeks.

Neuromyelitis optica (NMO), also known as Devic's disease, is an autoimmune inflammatory condition. It occurs due to autoantibodies directed against the water channel proteins aquaporin-4 (AQP4), which are highly expressed in the optic nerves, spinal cord, periventricular areas, hypothalamus, and area postrema. There is marked female predominance (4:1), with a mean age at presentation between the third and fourth decades. On imaging, it presents as longitudinally extensive myelitis, involving three or more vertebral segments. Longitudinally extensive transverse myelitis (LETM) is less common in children [34]. Spinal cord abnormalities in NMO are hyperintense on T2-weighted images and involve the central spinal cord. The presence of intensely bright T2 hyperintense foci within these abnormalities, known as bright spotty lesions (BSL), is a relatively specific sign for neuromyelitis optica [35] (Fig. 9). Irregular and patchy post-contrast enhancement can be seen in the acute phase. Ring-like enhancement surrounding the bright spotty foci has been described to occur in approximately 1/3 of the patients with NMO and can be used to differentiate NMO from multiple sclerosis. NMO is characterized by long segment and symmetrical T2 hyperintensity of the optic nerves, typically of the posterior aspect (posterior intraorbital, intracanalicular, and intracranial segments of the optic nerves, as well as the optic chiasm), with enhancement after IV gadolinium administration. Concurrent presence of periventricular abnormalities along the third and fourth ventricles and in the area postrema on brain imaging could assist in the diagnosis of NMO. Involvement of the area postrema classically manifests with intractable hiccups, vomiting, and nausea.

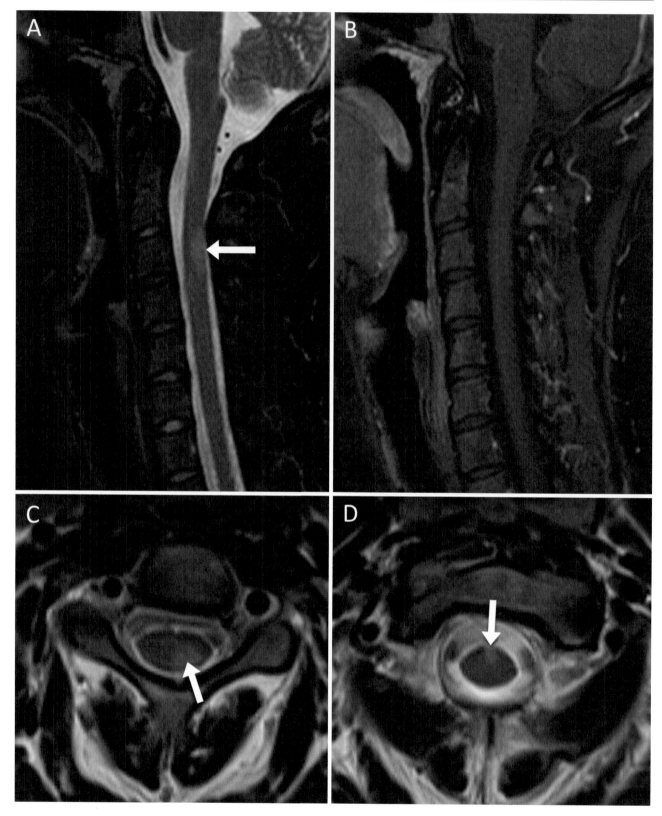

**Fig. 8** Multiple sclerosis: A 17-year-old female with new-onset pain in the left arm. Sagittal T2-weighted fat-saturated MR image (**a**) demonstrates a short-segment hyperintense focal abnormality along the posterior aspect of the spinal cord at the C3 level (arrow) with mild associated cord expansion. There is no enhancement on the sagittal post-contrast T1 fat-saturated MR image (**b**). Axial T2-weighted images (**c** and **d**) at two different levels demonstrate triangular areas of hyperintensity, along the periphery of the spinal cord (arrows)

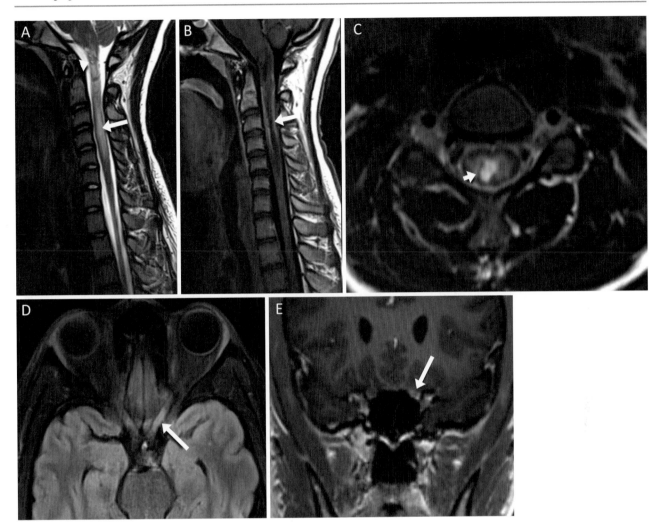

**Fig. 9** Neuromyelitis optica (NMO): A 19-year-old female with new-onset blurring of vision in the left eye and paresthesia in bilateral upper extremities. Sagittal T2-weighted (**a**), sagittal T1-weighted post-contrast (**b**), and axial T2-weighted (**c**) MR images through the cervical spine show long-segment hyperintensity with cord expansion (short white arrow in **a**). There are multiple "bright spots" within the area of abnormal signal (arrowhead in **c**). On the post-contrast T1 image (**b**), there is heterogeneous enhancement (short white arrow in **b**). Axial T2-FLAIR (**d**) and coronal post-contrast T1 fat-saturated (**e**) images demonstrate abnormal hyperintensity within the prechiasmatic segment of the left optic nerve (long white arrow in **d**) with mild homogeneous enhancement (long white arrow in **e**)

Acute disseminated encephalomyelitis (ADEM) is also known as a para−/post-infectious immune-mediated inflammatory disorder of the white matter and is believed to be due to cross-reactivity with myelin basic protein. It is typically seen in children with a recent respiratory or gastrointestinal infection. Monophasic involvement is more commonly seen with complete resolution within few months. Multiphasic involvement occurs in approximately 10% of the cases. ADEM can present as T2 hyperintense abnormality involving the spinal cord, extending for three or more contiguous vertebral segments. The appearance of the is nonspecific and may be indistinguishable from other causes of LETM. Diagnosis of the appearance of ADEM is nonspecific is favored in coexisting involvement of the supratentorial and infratentorial white matter and the basal ganglia (Fig. 10).

## Systemic Inflammatory Diseases

A variety of systemic inflammatory diseases, including sarcoidosis, systemic lupus erythematosus (SLE), Behcet's disease, and Sjogren's syndrome, can present as acute myelopathy. In neurosarcoidosis, there is early involvement of the leptomeninges with centripetal spread to involve the spinal cord as described by Junger et al. [36]. It often presents as longitudinally extensive T2 hyperintense abnormality of the spinal cord, with associated patchy or sheetlike subpial enhancement on post-contrast imaging. It is frequently associated with expansion of the spinal cord (Fig. 11). The presence of pulmonary parenchymal involvement and mediastinal lymphadenopathy on chest CT can serve as an adjunctive imaging marker of sarcoidosis. Imaging in SLE

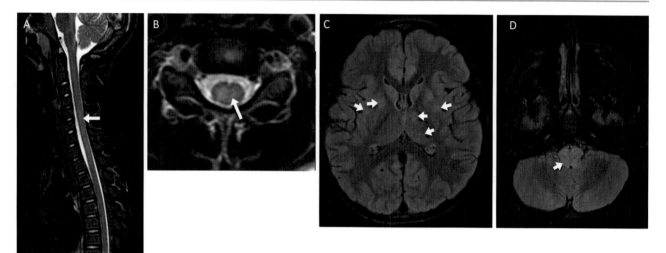

**Fig. 10** ADEM: A 7-year-old boy with acute onset of paresthesia in the upper and lower extremities. Sagittal T2 fat-saturated (**a**) MR image demonstrates abnormal long-segment intramedullary signal (arrow) extending from the lower visible brainstem to the C7 vertebral body level. There is associated mild expansion of the cord. No enhancement was present on the post-contrast images (not shown). Axial T2WI (**b**) demonstrates involvement of the gray and white matter (arrow). Axial T2 FLAIR image through the basal ganglia (**c**) and posterior fossa (**d**) demonstrates multiple focal areas of signal abnormality in the lentiform nuclei, left thalamus, right insula, and medulla (arrowheads). Findings resolved on follow-up imaging 3 months later, with only residual signal abnormality within the cervical spinal cord (not shown)

myelitis or Behcet's disease may be indistinguishable from other causes of LETM.

## Infection

Various bacteria, viruses, and parasites have been associated with infectious myelitis. Viruses are the most common infectious agent, with enteroviruses being the most common among them. Other uncommon infectious agents responsible for acute myelitis include herpes zoster, cytomegalovirus, Epstein-Barr virus, poliovirus, mycobacteria, and parasitic infections including neurocysticercosis and schistosomiasis [37].

Acute flaccid myelitis (AFM) resulting in paralysis of one or multiple extremities is a rare condition related to different viruses. Multiple cases of AFM were recently recorded after an outbreak of enterovirus D68 infection in pediatric patients in the USA, implicating this virus as one of the potential causes [38]. Radiologically, it manifests as non-enhancing T2 signal abnormality within the central gray matter of the spinal cord and, more specifically, along the anterior motor horn cells, as in poliomyelitis (Fig. 12). There may be contiguous involvement of the posterior aspect of the brainstem resulting in the involvement of cranial nuclei. Associated cord expansion can occur in some cases. Enhancement of the cauda equina nerve roots has been described in some cases [39, 40].

Varicella zoster myelitis is a rare condition which presents as asymmetric T2 signal abnormality within the spinal cord, at the level of the involved dermatome. Presence of typical vesicular rash along the involved dermatome, and detection of the varicella zoster IgG in CSF, can confirm the diagnosis. Poliomyelitis, rarely seen in developed countries, predominantly affects the anterior motor horn cells causing flaccid paralysis of the lower extremity. On imaging, T2 hyperintense foci are seen involving the anterior motor horn cells giving a "snake eye" or "owl's eyes" appearance.

Guillain-Barré syndrome (GBS) is a rapidly progressing polyradiculopathy involving the sensory, motor, and autonomic nerves. It is the most common cause of ascending flaccid paralysis. It is believed to be due to autoimmune reaction to anti-GQ1b IgG antigens following a respiratory or gastrointestinal infection. Imaging in these cases is used to rule out other causes of flaccid paralysis. On imaging, presents as thickening and enhancement of the cauda equina nerve roots (Fig. 13). Cranial nerve enhancement can also be seen in some cases, with the seventh nerve being the most commonly involved [41, 42]. Leptomeningeal metastasis and arachnoiditis are in the differential diagnosis and must be excluded before diagnosing GBS.

## Conclusions/Summary

Nontraumatic spinal emergencies may be caused by different neoplastic and nonneoplastic entities. Relevant clinical history and prompt imaging are crucial in the diagnosis of some of these conditions. The use of a compartmental approach might be necessary for appropriate and timely diagnosis and management. Compressive myelopathy

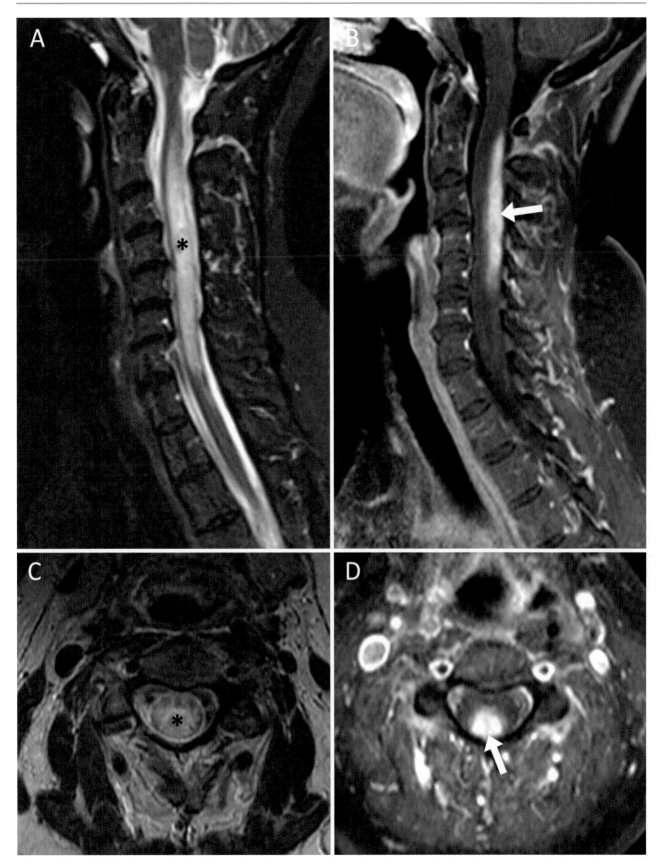

**Fig. 11** Neurosarcoidosis: A 57-year-old woman presents with acute worsening of bilateral upper extremity weakness. Sagittal T2-weighted MR image with fat saturation (**a**) demonstrates a long segment of hyperintensity in the cervical spinal cord with associated cord swelling (black asterisk). On

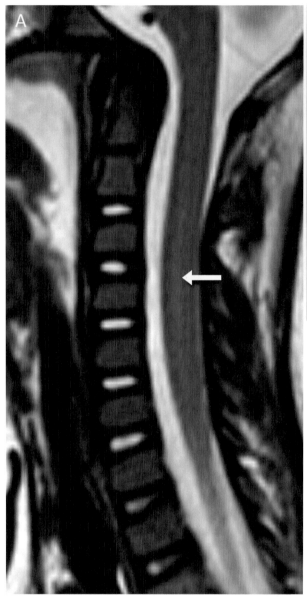

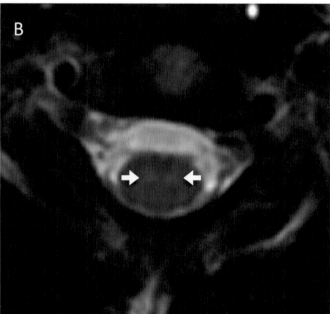

**Fig. 12** Acute flaccid myelitis: A 5-year-old with acute-onset weakness in the upper extremities. Sagittal (**a**) and axial (**b**) T2-weighted MR images demonstrate subtle increased T2 signal within the anterior aspect of the spinal cord at C3 and C4 levels (arrow in **a**). On axial T2-weighted image (**b**), the signal abnormality is centered in the bilateral anterior motor horn cells (arrowheads). No associated enhancement was present on the post-contrast images (not shown). These findings are typical for acute flaccid myelitis

must be initially excluded as it may require urgent neurosurgical attention. Medical management might be appropriate for many of the non-compressive myelopathies, i.e., anticoagulation for spinal cord infarct, glucocorticoids for inflammatory conditions, etc. Adequate knowledge of the common entities and imaging findings of nontraumatic spinal emergencies is pivotal to emergent care.

**Fig. 11** (continued) the post-contrast sagittal T1 fat-saturated MR image (**b**), there is homogeneous sheetlike subpial enhancement along the posterior aspect of the spinal cord (arrow). Corresponding axial T2-weighted (**c**) and IV contrast-enhanced T1-weighted images (**d**) corroborate these findings. The patient was known to have sarcoidosis with mediastinal lymphadenopathy (not shown)

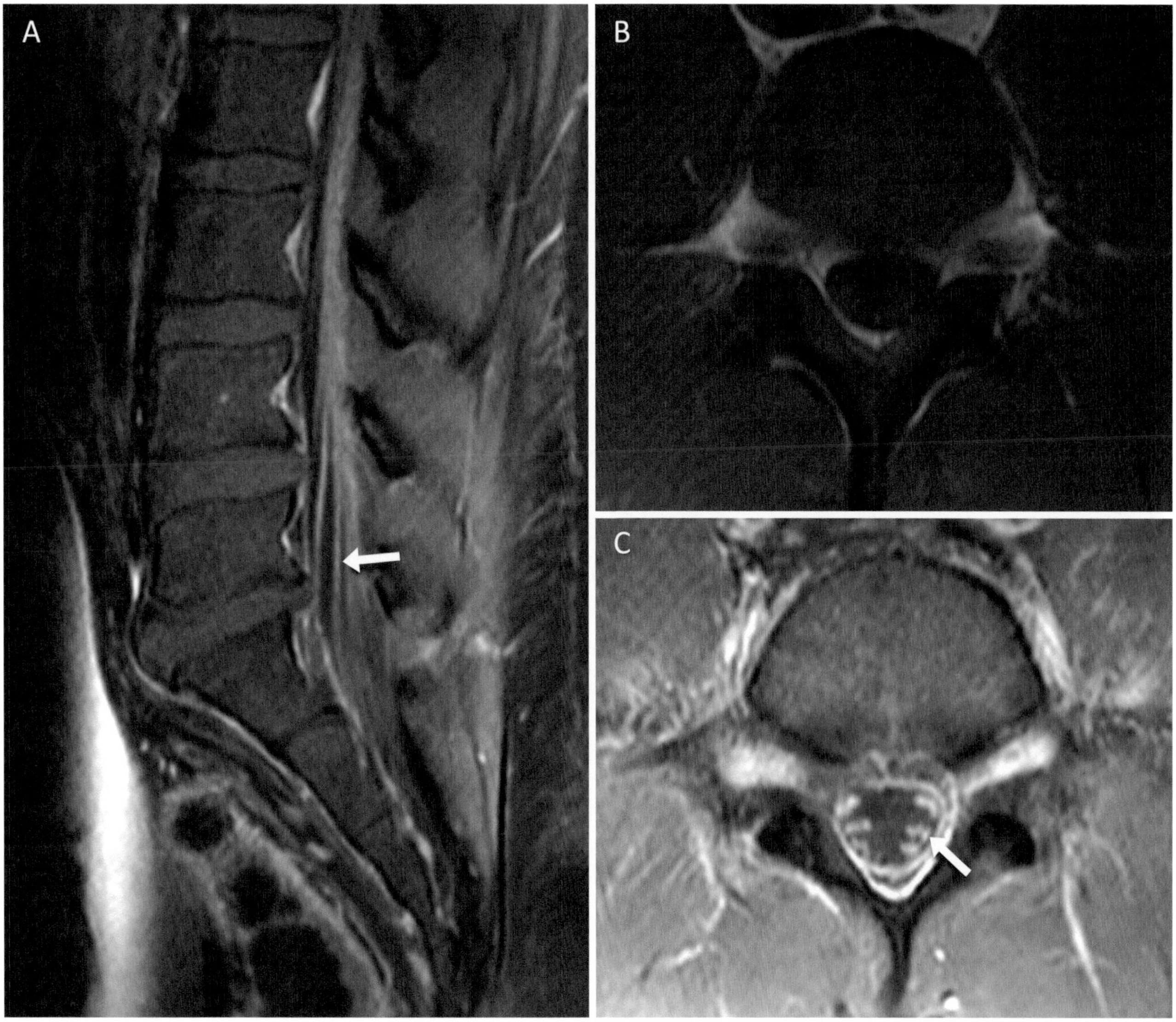

**Fig. 13** Guillain-Barré syndrome: A 33-year-old man with acute onset of weakness and paresthesia in the bilateral upper and lower extremities. Sagittal T1 fat-saturated MR image following IV contrast (**a**) demonstrates smooth, homogeneous enhancement along the cauda equina nerve roots (arrow). Non-contrast axial T1- (**b**) and post-contrast axial T1-weighted (**c**) images allow for an easier visualization of the enhancing nerve roots (arrow in **c**)

# References

1. Seidenwurm DJ. Myelopathy. Am J Neuroradiol. 2008;29(5):1032–4.
2. Harnett A, Bateman A, McIntyre A, Parikh R, Middleton J, Arora M, et al. Spinal cord injury rehabilitation practices. In: Eng JJ, Teasell RW, Miller WC, Wolfe DL, Townson AF, Hsieh JTC, Noonan V, Mehta S, McIntyre A, Queree M, (eds.) Spinal cord injury rehabilitation evidence, version 7.0. 2020;1–100.
3. New PW, Cripps RA, Bonne LB. Global maps of non-traumatic spinal cord injury epidemiology: towards a living data repository. Spinal Cord. 2014;52(2):97–109.
4. McKinley WO, Seel RT, Hardman JT. Nontraumatic spinal cord injury: incidence, epidemiology, and functional outcome. Arch Phys Med Rehabil. 1999;80(6):619–23.
5. Kranz PG, Amrhein TJ. Imaging approach to myelopathy: acute, subacute, and chronic. Radiol Clin. 2019;57(2):257–79.
6. Northover JR, Wild JB, Braybrooke J, Blanco J. The epidemiology of cervical spondylotic myelopathy. Skelet Radiol. 2012;41(12):1543–6.
7. Sabharwal S. Nontraumatic myelopathies. In: Essentials of spinal cord medicine. New York: Demos Medical; 2014. p. 94–182.
8. Nair KPS, Taly AB, Maheshwarappa BM, Kumar J, Murali T, Rao S. Nontraumatic spinal cord lesions: a prospective study of medical complications during in-patient rehabilitation. Spinal Cord. 2005;43(9):558–64.
9. Skaf GS, Domloj NT, Fehlings MG, Bouclaous CH, Sabbagh AS, Kanafani ZA, et al. Pyogenic spondylodiscitis: an overview. J Infect Public Health. 2010;3(1):5–16.
10. Hook EW, Campbell CG, Weens HS, Cooper GR. Salmonella osteomyelitis in patients with sickle-cell anemia. N Engl J Med. 1957;257(9):403–7.

11. Hong SH, Choi J-Y, Lee JW, Kim NR, Choi J-A, Kang HS. MR imaging assessment of the spine: infection or an imitation? Radiographics. 2009;29(2):599–612.

12. Almeida A. Tuberculosis of the spine and spinal cord. Eur J Radiol. 2005;55(2):193–201.

13. Lee KY. Comparison of pyogenic spondylitis and tuberculous spondylitis. Asian Spine J. 2014;8(2):216–23.

14. Traul DE, Shaffrey ME, Schiff D. Part I: spinal-cord neoplasms-intradural neoplasms. Lancet Oncol. 2007;8(1):35–45.

15. Barron KD, Hirano A, Araki S, Terry RD. Experiences with metastatic neoplasms involving the spinal cord. Neurology. 1959;9(2):91–106.

16. Schiff D. Spinal cord compression. Neurol Clin. 2003;21(1):67–86, viii.

17. Filho AG, Carneiro BC, Pastore D, Silva IP, Yamashita SR, Consolo FD, et al. Whole-body imaging of multiple myeloma: diagnostic criteria. Radiographics. 2019;39(4):1077–97.

18. Tirumani SH, Shinagare AB, Jagannathan JP, Krajewski KM, Munshi NC, Ramaiya NH. MRI features of extramedullary myeloma. Am J Roentgenol. 2014;202(4):803–10.

19. Varettoni M, Corso A, Pica G, Mangiacavalli S, Pascutto C, Lazzarino M. Incidence, presenting features and outcome of extramedullary disease in multiple myeloma: a longitudinal study on 1003 consecutive patients. Ann Oncol. 2010;21(2):325–30.

20. O'Neill J, Finlay K, Jurriaans E, Friedman L. Radiological manifestations of skeletal lymphoma. Curr Probl Diagn Radiol. 2009;38(5):228–36.

21. Abdullah BB, Nausheen N, Baksh NK, Keerthi NDT. Non-Hodgkin's lymphoma and spinal cord compression: a diagnostic challenge. Ital J Med. 2015;9(4):380.

22. Cugati G, Singh M, Pande A, Ramamurthi R, Balasubramanyam M, Sethi SK, et al. Primary spinal epidural lymphomas. J Craniovertebr Junction Spine. 2011;2(1):3–11.

23. Thomas AG, Vaidhyanath R, Kirke R, Rajesh A. Extranodal lymphoma from head to toe: part 1, the head and spine. Am J Roentgenol. 2011 Aug;197(2):350–6.

24. Ozawa H, Kokubun S, Aizawa T, Hoshikawa T, Kawahara C. Spinal dumbbell tumors: an analysis of a series of 118 cases. J Neurosurg Spine. 2007;7(6):587–93.

25. Abul-Kasim K, Thurnher MM, McKeever P, Sundgren PC. Intradural spinal tumors: current classification and MRI features. Neuroradiology. 2008;50(4):301–14.

26. Van Dijk JMC, TerBrugge KG, Willinsky RA, Farb RI, Wallace MC. Multidisciplinary management of spinal dural arteriovenous fistulas: clinical presentation and long-term follow-up in 49 patients. Stroke. 2002;33(6):1578–83.

27. Pierce JL, Donahue JH, Nacey NC, Quirk CR, Perry MT, Faulconer N, et al. Spinal hematomas: what a radiologist needs to know. Radiographics. 2018;38(5):1516–35.

28. Grassner L, Marschallinger J, Dünser MW, Novak HF, Zerbs A, Aigner L, et al. Nontraumatic spinal cord injury at the neurological intensive care unit: spectrum, causes of admission and predictors of mortality. Ther Adv Neurol Disord. 2016;9(2):85–94.

29. Sandson TA, Friedman JH. Spinal cord infarction. Report of 8 cases and review of the literature. Medicine (Baltimore). 1989;68(5):282–92.

30. Masson C, Pruvo J, Meder J, Cordonnier C, Touze E, de la Sayette V, et al. Spinal cord infarction: clinical and magnetic resonance imaging findings and short term outcome. J Neurol Neurosurg Psychiatry. 2004;75(10):1431–5.

31. Vargas MI, Gariani J, Sztajzel R, Barnaure-Nachbar I, Delattre BM, Lovblad KO, et al. Spinal cord ischemia: practical imaging tips, pearls, and pitfalls. Am J Neuroradiol. 2015;36(5):825–30.

32. Naiman JL, Donohue WL, Prichard JS. Fatal nucleus pulposus embolism of spinal cord after trauma. Neurology. 1961;11:83–7.

33. Thompson TP, Pearce J, Chang G, Madamba J. Surfer's myelopathy. Spine. 2004;29(16):E353–6.

34. Tenembaum S, Chitnis T, Ness J, Hahn JS. International pediatric MS study group. Acute disseminated encephalomyelitis. Neurology. 2007;68(16 Suppl 2):S23–36.

35. Pekcevik Y, Mitchell CH, Mealy MA, Orman G, Lee IH, Newsome SD, et al. Differentiating neuromyelitis optica from other causes of longitudinally extensive transverse myelitis on spinal magnetic resonance imaging. Mult Scler J [Internet]. 2015. [cited 2020 Jun 13]; https://doi.org/10.1177/1352458515591069.

36. Junger SS, Stern BJ, Levine SR, Sipos E, Marti-Masso JF. Intramedullary spinal sarcoidosis: clinical and magnetic resonance imaging characteristics. Neurology. 1993;43(2):333–7.

37. Jacob A, Weinshenker B. An approach to the diagnosis of acute transverse myelitis. Semin Neurol. 2008;28(1):105–20.

38. Maloney JA, Mirsky DM, Messacar K, Dominguez SR, Schreiner T, Stence NV. MRI findings in children with acute flaccid paralysis and cranial nerve dysfunction occurring during the 2014 enterovirus D68 outbreak. Am J Neuroradiol. 2015;36(2):245–50.

39. Helfferich J, Knoester M, Van Leer-Buter CC, Neuteboom RF, Meiners LC, Niesters HG, et al. Acute flaccid myelitis and enterovirus D68: lessons from the past and present. Eur J Pediatr. 2019;178(9):1305–15.

40. Ertl-Wagner B, Branson H, Shroff M, Bitnun A, Yeh EA. Acute flaccid myelitis in a 10-year-old girl. Radiology. 2018;290(1):31.

41. Fulbright RK, Erdum E, Sze G, Byrne T. Cranial nerve enhancement in the Guillain-Barr√© syndrome. Am J Neuroradiol. 1995;16(4):923–5.

42. Alkan O, Yildirim T, Tokmak N, Tan M. Spinal MRI findings of Guillain-Barré syndrome. J Radiol Case Rep. 2009;3(3):25–8.

# Part III

# Thoracic Emergencies

Kevin Neal and Muhammad Naeem

## Contents

### Abstract

Identification and prompt treatment of nonvascular injuries related to thoracic trauma is critical in the triage and management of trauma patients. Traumatic lung injuries can result in emergent conditions including tension pneumothorax, contusion, and laceration, which can result in substantial respiratory complications. A hemothorax can be a major site of blood loss and result in hemodynamic compromise. Cardiac, tracheal, and esophageal injuries are associated with high morbidity and mortality, and prompt management is critical. Osseous injuries can result in traumatic injuries of the vital mediastinal and lung structures. Rib fractures can impair respiration and if segmental can result in a flail chest. Diaphragmatic injuries can result in both respiratory and abdominal complications, and presentation is often delayed. Correct interpretation of initial radiographs and/or computed tomography in the setting of thoracic trauma requires a thorough and systematic evaluation. In addition to a systematic approach, the radiologist should be aware of common injury patterns, normal variants, and subtle findings which may warrant additional evaluation.

### Keywords

Trauma · Thoracic · Blunt trauma · Penetrating trauma · Lung trauma · Cardiac trauma · Pneumothorax · Diaphragmatic injury

## Introduction

The leading causes of trauma in the United States are accidents, including falls (44%) and motor vehicle collisions (MVCs) (26%). Firearms constitute 4% of trauma but carry a much higher mortality (15%) compared to falls (4%) and

K. Neal (✉)
Mallinckrodt Institute of Radiology, St. Louis, MO, USA
e-mail: kevinaneal@wustl.edu

M. Naeem
Mallinckrodt Institute of Radiology, Washington University School of Medicine, St. Louis, MO, USA
e-mail: mnaeem@wustl.edu

© Springer Nature Switzerland AG 2022
M. N. Patlas et al. (eds.), *Atlas of Emergency Imaging from Head-to-Toe*,
https://doi.org/10.1007/978-3-030-92111-8_15

MVCs (5%). The thorax is the third most injured region after the head and extremities [1]. Radiologists should be comfortable in imaging interpretation related to thoracic trauma to help direct clinical management. Understanding common radiologic findings of nonvascular thoracic trauma and their management is critical for an emergency radiologist.

## Blunt and Penetrating Trauma

Blunt trauma is most commonly the result of motor vehicle collisions, accidents, falls, blast injuries, and assault. Injury patterns are typically multifocal and correspond to forces from blunt impact, acceleration/deceleration, and compression [2].

Penetrating trauma is most commonly related to stab wounds, accidents, and firearms. The injury patterns differ from blunt trauma in that the tissue damage is localized along the tract of the penetrating object. Low-energy objects such as in stabbings have their tissue damage entirely located along the tract. High-energy projectiles such as hunting rifles or military weapons also damage surrounding tissues as they deposit their kinetic energy into the body. Medium-energy projectiles such as from handguns deposit a smaller amount of energy into the body, and the damage is more localized [3].

When assessing stab wounds, determining the depth and trajectory is critical to clinical management. The tract on CT is typically characterized by gas, fat stranding, and blood products. Secondary and direct signs of injury also help to identify the tract. A pneumothorax indicates it extended to the pleural space. A pericardial effusion or thickening indicates that it reached the pericardium and likely the heart [4, 5].

Tracing the path of a projectile is similarly important but is more complicated, as projectiles may follow nonlinear paths in soft tissue and after striking bone. Trajectory interpretation is greatly aided by history and physical examination, placement of entry and exit wound makers, and multi-planar reconstructions [6] (Fig. 1).

## Triage Management and Role of Imaging

In the initial trauma evaluation, an anteroposterior (AP) chest radiograph is primarily used to document and confirm support lines and tubes, but is also useful in guiding resuscitation efforts and for identifying potentially life-threatening injuries, including pneumothorax, hemothorax, large pericardial effusion, foreign bodies, and mediastinal hematoma [7]. Bedside ultrasound or FAST (focused assessment with sonography in trauma) is commonly done in unstable patients. It typically focuses on the presence of fluid in serosal cavities, i.e., the pericardium, pleura, and peritoneum [7].

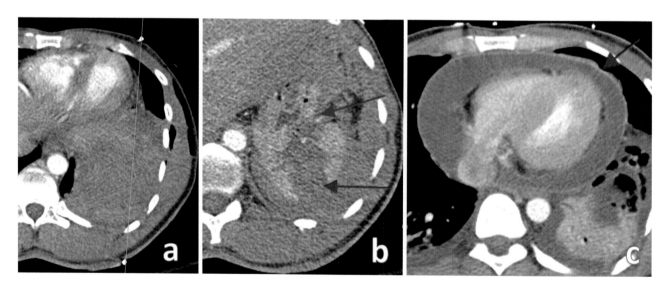

**Fig. 1** "Bullet tract and associated injuries." A 36-year-old man with gunshot to the left anterior chest wall. IV contrast-enhanced computed tomography (CECT) of the chest after multi-planar reconstructions shows the metallic marker at the entry and exit sites with a bullet tract (blue line) in an oblique axial plane (**a**). Notice the bullet tract going through the epicardial fat in close proximity to the heart. The bullet track is shown to cause injury within the left upper quadrant causing a shattered spleen (red arrow in Fig. 1b) and lacerated stomach (blue arrow in Fig. 1b) (even though the tract is shown above the spleen on Figure a). CECT 1 week later in the same patient demonstrates thickened enhancing pericardium (red arrow), which is consistent with post-traumatic pericarditis

Multi-detector computed tomography (MDCT) is the reference standard for imaging major trauma patients who are stable enough to be transported to the scanner. MDCT is far superior to chest radiography for the detection and characterization of both blunt and penetrating thoracic trauma injuries.

## Computed Tomography Protocol

An efficient and uniform protocol for trauma imaging is important not only to provide adequate evaluation of injuries but also to limit unnecessary time-consuming cross-specialty decision-making in patients who may not be stable.

The portal venous phase is most useful in characterizing injuries and soft-tissue differentiation. Injection of 100–125 ml iodinated contrast at a rate of 3 ml/s from a 22-gauge antecubital IV with a delay of 70 s is a standard protocol followed at our institution that may allow continuing the scan through the abdomen and pelvis, if needed. Optional dual- and triple-phase examinations can also be performed if warranted. The arterial phase is useful for detecting subtle vascular injury. In order to optimally assess the vascular and visceral injuries, CT can be performed in both late arterial and portal venous phases. A 5-min delayed phase helps detect pooling of contrast in active bleeding and helps to differentiate a pseudoaneurysm from active bleeding [6].

## Pleural and Extrapleural Injuries

### Pneumothorax

The diagnosis of a pneumothorax is typically made on a chest radiograph. The most common sign of a pneumothorax is a pleural line without lung markings seen distally. This is best seen on an upright radiograph, allowing the air to collect at the lung apices. Chest radiographs in trauma patients, however, are most frequently obtained in the supine position with an anteroposterior acquisition. When supine, air often collects anteroinferiorly and medially rather than at the lung apex, and a pleural line is often not visible. A pneumothorax in the supine position typically manifests as a medial or basilar lucency or deepening of the costophrenic sulcus (Fig. 2). The size of a pneumothorax can be estimated by the distance of the pleural line to the chest wall. A measurement greater than 2 cm indicates a large pneumothorax, with pleural air occupying approximately 50% of the pneumothorax [8].

Skin folds are the most common incorrectly interpreted finding for a pneumothorax, as they can mimic a pleural line. They are differentiated from a pneumothorax by the presence

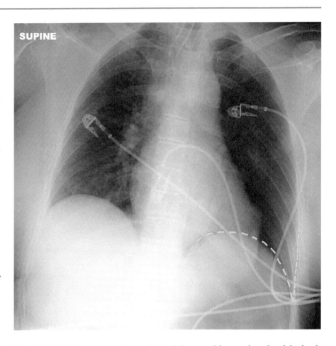

**Fig. 2** "Basilar pneumothorax": A 26-year-old man involved in both penetrating and blunt trauma. On the supine portable radiograph, there is increased lucency in the left hemithorax. Additionally, there is a lucency at the left hemidiaphragm and deepening of the left costophrenic angle (deep sulcus) (yellow dotted line)

of vascular markings beyond the fold, lack of a distinct thin white pleural line (skin folds often have a black edge), and nonanatomic boundaries of the line extending outside the hemithorax (Fig. 3). Bullous disease in the apices can also mimic a pneumothorax. If there is uncertainty, a repeat upright radiograph, opposite lateral decubitus radiograph, or CT can be performed [8].

A tension pneumothorax occurs from a one-way valve mechanism where air progressively enters the pleural space but cannot exit. Radiographically this leads to enlargement of the hemithorax, widening of the intercostal spaces, mediastinal shift to the contralateral side, and flattening of the hemidiaphragm (Fig. 4). While tension physiology is typically a clinical diagnosis, prompt communication of radiographic findings can alert the clinicians to provide lifesaving needle decompression and thoracotomy tube placement [2].

### Thoracostomy Tubes and Persistent Pneumothorax

A pneumothorax despite chest tube placement should raise a suspicion for either thoracostomy tube malfunction or a persistent air leak from a bronchopleural or alveolo-pleural fistula.

Thoracostomy tubes can malfunction from malpositioning or from intrinsic problems including kinking, clogging, or a lack of suction. The tube can be inadvertently placed in the

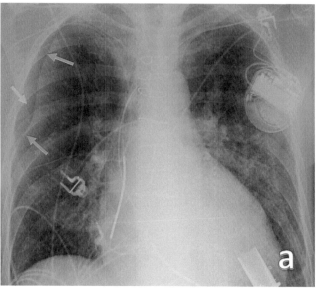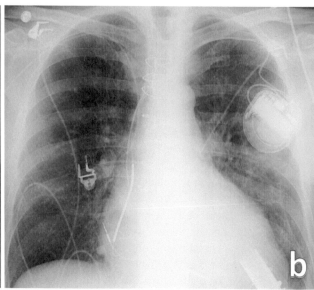

**Fig. 3** "Skin fold": (**a**) Right lateral skin fold (blue arrow) confused for a pleural line in a 70-year-old patient after trauma. Notice the increased density of the line fades to normal density medially rather than representing a sharp thin line. Also notice the pulmonary vessels extending beyond the line (green arrow). (**b**) Second radiograph obtained on the same patient a few hours later showed resolution of the abnormality

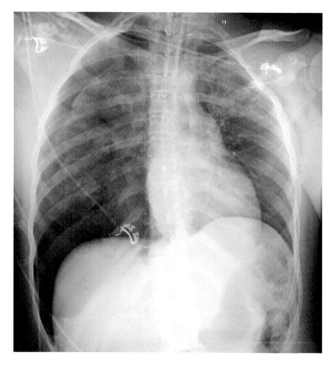

**Fig. 4** "Tension pneumothorax." Large left pneumothorax with flattening of the right hemidiaphragm and leftward mediastinal shift

soft tissues of the back, abdomen, mediastinum, or neck [9]. Placement within the fissure can also provide suboptimal evacuation, but it is often clinically adequate, and the tube only needs to be replaced if it is clinically malfunctioning.

Fissural placement of a thoracostomy tube can be mistaken for intraparenchymal placement. The tube can impress somewhat into the adjacent lung and cause some mild associated atelectasis, but it should remain in the expected course of the fissure with no surrounding hemorrhage. Intraparenchymal thoracostomy tubes cause lung laceration and can cause persistent air leaks. They do not follow the course of the fissure and have consolidation and hemorrhage around them (Fig. 5). Multi-planar CT reconstructions can be helpful to differentiate between the two [10, 11].

## Hemothorax

Bleeding into the pleural space causes a hemothorax. This can be caused by pulmonary laceration, pulmonary vascular injury, mediastinal injury, or intercostal vascular injury.

A pleural effusion on radiograph in a trauma patient is likely a hemothorax in the absence of another plausible explanation. CT can be used to characterize and differentiate a hemothorax from other nontraumatic effusions. Clotted blood has an attenuation between 45 and 65 HU, unclotted blood 35–45, and simple fluid −5–15 HU [2, 12]. In large hemothoraces, clots are common, whereas in smaller or unclotted hemothoraces, high-attenuation material tends to layer dependently within the hemothorax. One should be careful not to confuse streak

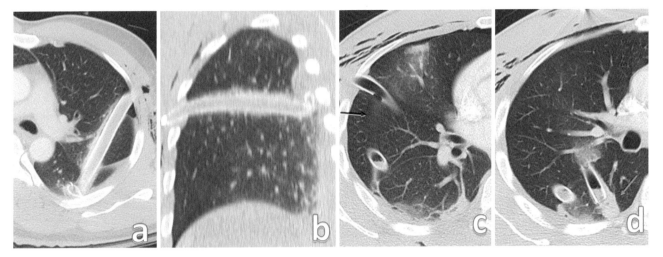

**Fig. 5** "Intraparenchymal and fissural chest tube": A 37-year-old with gunshot thoracic trauma. CECT of the chest (**a** and **b**) on lung windows in the axial and sagittal planes demonstrates laceration and intraparenchymal placement in the left upper lobe. A 29-year-old with gunshot thoracic trauma. CECT of the chest (**c** and **d**) on lung windows in the axial plane demonstrates two thoracostomy tubes positioned within the right minor fissure (red arrow). The more anterior chest tube exits the fissure and takes a short intraparenchymal course in the superior segment of the right lower lobe (green arrow). Notice the adjacent laceration and hemorrhage

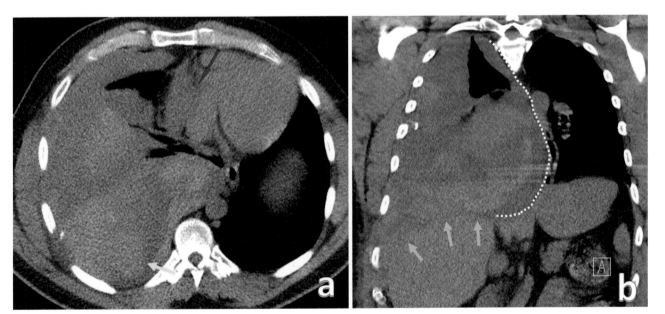

**Fig. 6** "Tension hemothorax": A 20-year-old man presenting with dyspnea 10 days after trauma. Non-contrast CT of the chest in axial (**a**) and sagittal (**b**) planes demonstrates a large hemothorax, with high-density blood products layering posteriorly (yellow arrow). There are signs of tension hemothorax physiology on coronal CT as demonstrated by leftward mediastinal shift (dotted white line) and flattening of the right hemidiaphragm (green arrows). In addition, there is compression/notching of the right atrium by a pericardial hematoma (red arrow) demonstrating early signs of tamponade

artifacts from osseous structures such as the ribs or spine for high-attenuation layering material. MPRs can be helpful in identifying artifacts. As with pneumothoraces, hemothoraces can result in tension physiology requiring emergent drainage [2] (Fig. 6).

## Extrapleural Hematoma

When the chest wall is injured, there is often a disruption of the parietal pleura allowing blood to extend into the pleural space resulting in a hemothorax. An intact parietal pleural and/or the endothoracic fascia can result in blood collection within the extrapleural space causing an extrapleural hematoma. The extrapleural hematoma has a very characteristic imaging appearance of a lenticular high-attenuation fluid collection protruding toward the pleural space, but is separated from the pleural space by a thin layer of fat (Fig. 7). These are managed differently than a hemothorax and are often evacuated by thoracoscopy if large enough. Convex borders of the hematoma are suggestive of an arterial origin of bleeding [13].

## Pulmonary Parenchymal Injuries

Traumatic injury to the lung parenchyma manifests as contusion, laceration, hematoma, and pulmonary vascular injury. Lung contusion is rarely seen in isolation and is commonly seen with pulmonary laceration, rib fractures, pneumothorax, hemothorax, or other injuries. Contusion is important to recognize as it is an independent risk factor for acute respiratory distress syndrome (ARDS), pneumonia, and long-term respiratory distress following trauma [14].

Lung contusion can manifest as minor ground-glass opacity or consolidation on CT immediately after the initial injury, with progressive increase in ground-glass opacity and consolidation over the next 24–48 h [13]. Contusion is often not visible on chest radiography until at least 6 h following the injury, and radiographs often under-reveal the extent of injury [14]. On radiographs, contusion presents as hazy air-space opacities or consolidations which are often peripheral. CT better demonstrates the extent of lung contusions and can

provide prognostic information. One study with 78 patients involved in thoracic trauma found lung involvement of greater than 28% was a predictor of needing ventilator support [15, 16].

The CT and radiographic findings should start to resolve and improve after 48 h (Fig. 8). Lack of improvement after 48 h should prompt consideration that the injury resulted in small lacerations rather than in simply contusion. Worsening after 48 h implies another pathology such as pneumonia or atelectasis.

Lung laceration results from gross parenchymal disruption; the elastic recoil of the lung then pulls apart the lacerated parenchyma and results in a cavity formation which is often surrounded by contusion and hemorrhage (Fig. 9). This cavity when filled with blood is called a hematocele, with air is called a pneumatocele, or when both are present is termed a hemopneumatocele [2].

Contusions and lacerations follow injury patterns related to the mechanism of injury. Chest compression or direct blows often cause peripheral injury. Broken ribs can cause penetrating laceration or contusion. Acceleration/deceleration causes injury at sites of attachment or fixation, such as centrally near the hila or peripherally at pleural adhesions. It also can cause injury adjacent to the spine as the lung moves against spinal osteophytes.

When evaluating an air-space opacity, overlying chest wall injury or rib fracture can indicate traumatic lung injury rather than a nontraumatic process such as aspiration, edema, and pneumonia. Additionally, ground-glass or consolidation

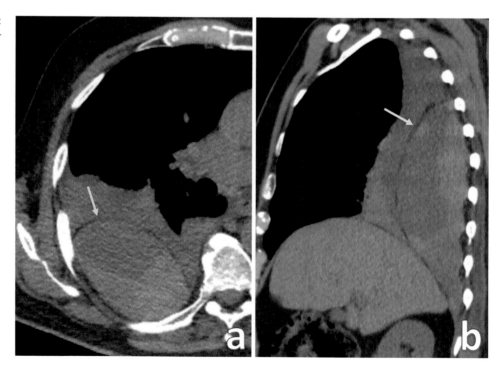

**Fig. 7** "Extrapleural hematoma": After a fall from height, a 36-year-old man presented with both hemothorax and extrapleural hematoma. Non-contrast CT of the chest on axial image (**a**) and sagittal (**b**) reconstruction shows the extrapleural hematoma which is contained under the pleural fat (yellow arrow)

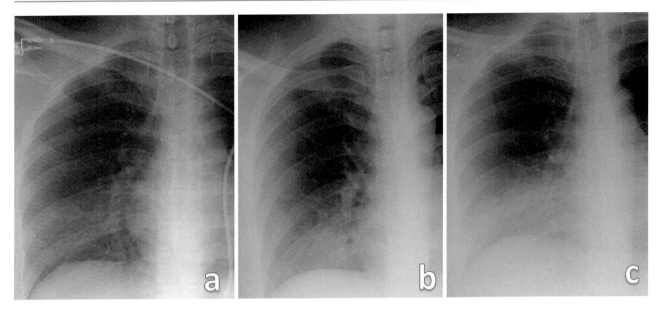

**Fig. 8** "Evolution of contusion at 0, 24, and 48 h": (**a**) Initial radiograph at presentation shows a subtle hazy air-space opacity in the right lung base. (**b**) At 24 h, there is now clear consolidation in the right lung base. (**c**) At 48 h, the consolidation has begun to improve

**Fig. 9** "Lung laceration and hemorrhage": Multiple hemopneumatoceles (yellow arrows) resulting from laceration with surrounding consolidation (green arrows), representing contusion and pulmonary hemorrhage

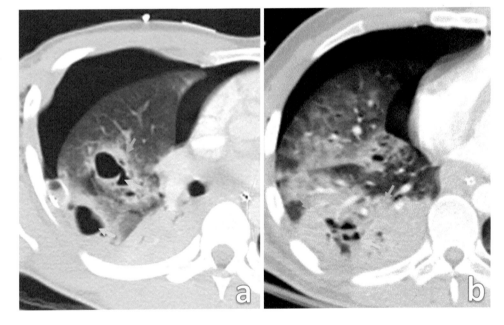

that directly crosses the fissure is typically a finding of traumatic injury rather than another process (Fig. 10).

Aspiration is a common finding in trauma patients, especially those with head injuries or those requiring intubation in the field. Not surprisingly, contusion and aspiration often coexist in trauma, and the appearances can overlap (Fig. 11). In contrast to contusion and laceration, aspiration is often, but not always, dependent and lower lobe predominant with tree-in-bud nodules, peribronchovascular patchy consolidations, and debris in the trachea.

Initially lacerations will often contain both blood products and air but often fill in with fluid after the initial 24–48 h. Development of surrounding pneumonia or filling in of a cavity with fluid and speckled gas locules is suspicious for the development of a secondary pulmonary abscess. In the subsequent months, lacerations may be healed by scarring or a residual pneumatocele [2] (Fig. 12).

Pulmonary vascular injury is rare and typically occurs from penetrating injury. Pulmonary artery pseudoaneurysms on IV contrast-enhanced CT appear as rounded areas of high

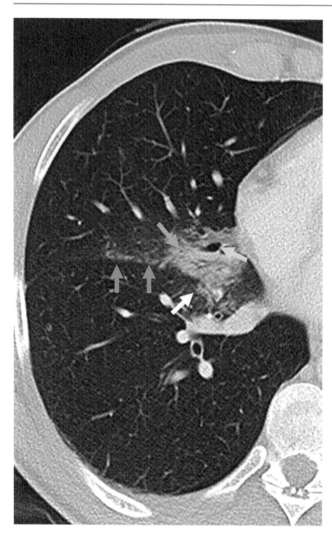

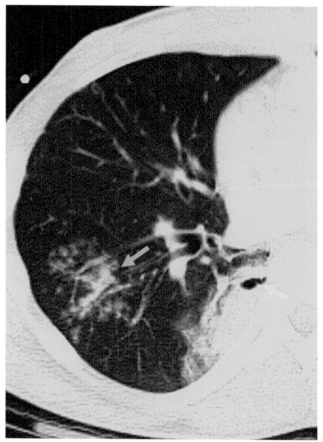

**Fig. 11** "Coexisting aspiration and laceration": A 25-year-old man involved in thoracic trauma. CECT axial image of the chest with a lung window demonstrates a peripheral contusion/laceration seen medially adjacent to the spine with a hemopneumatocele (yellow arrow) from impact with the vertebral body. More laterally, there are tree-in-bud nodules and consolidation in a peribronchovascular distribution from aspiration (green arrow)

**Fig. 10** "Central laceration and contusion": A 20-year-old man involved in rollover motor vehicle collision. CECT of the chest, lung window in the axial plane, demonstrates a right infrahilar contusion and laceration. Small hemopneumatoceles (yellow arrow) are present with surrounding consolidation and ground-glass opacity (green arrow). Notice the contusion crossing the minor fissure (white arrow) and involving the right middle and lower lobes. Also recognize that the contusion crosses the fissure at several locations (white arrow) and not at others (blue arrow)

attenuation arising from a pulmonary artery. This is differentiated from active bleeding which appears as a blush and is less clearly defined. A 5-min delayed acquisition can help differentiate pseudoaneurysms from active bleeding (Fig. 13). Injury to pulmonary veins can also result in a blush of active bleeding, but pseudoaneurysms of the pulmonary veins are rare.

## Fat Emboli Syndrome (FES)

Delayed-onset shortness of breath in a trauma patient who has long bone fractures or recent intramedullary nail placement should raise the suspicion for fat emboli syndrome, which is a clinical syndrome characterized by skin petechiae, altered mental status, and new respiratory distress. It typically occurs 24–72 h after the initial trauma, and respiratory symptoms are often the first manifestation.

Pulmonary parenchymal manifestations are thought to relate to a chemical pneumonitis, with perivascular hemorrhage and edema secondary to the toxic effects of the free fatty acids and glycerol [17].

Radiographically it mimics new pulmonary edema or presents with otherwise relatively nonspecific peripheral air-space opacities. CT findings generally involve new bilateral ground-glass opacities with a peripheral predominance or geographic appearance with associated smooth septal line thickening (Fig. 14). Less frequently, small centrilobular nodules are seen. Filling defects are not

**Fig. 12** "Resolution of laceration over 4 months": A 30-year-old man with gunshot trauma to the chest. CECT axial image of the thorax demonstrates an initial large right lower lobe laceration (green arrow) (**a**), which resolved with small area of scarring at 4-month follow-up (**b**)

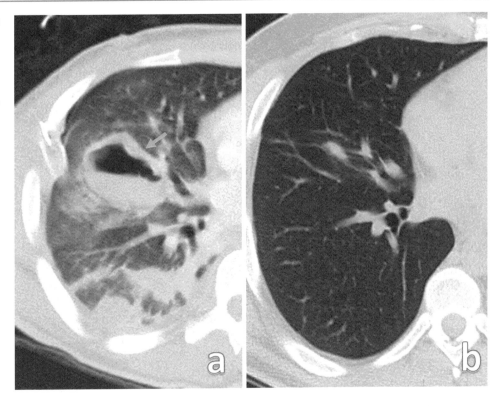

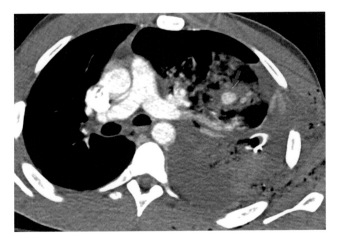

**Fig. 13** "Pulmonary artery pseudoaneurysm": A 19-year-old man with gunshot wound to the chest which caused lung and pulmonary arterial laceration resulting in a pulmonary artery pseudoaneurysm (red arrow)

## Timeline of Lung Opacities

It is useful to have an expected timeline for pulmonary findings and complications in a trauma patient. Initially at presentation and in the first 24 h, contusion, laceration, aspiration, atelectasis, and conditions present prior to the trauma predominate. From 1 to 3 days, consider fat emboli syndrome, evolving aspiration pneumonia, evolving contusion, pulmonary embolism, and pulmonary edema from resuscitation. After 3 days, consider pneumonia, acute respiratory distress syndrome, pulmonary embolism, and pneumonia.

## Pneumomediastinum

Gas within the fascial planes of the mediastinum is pneumomediastinum. There are many radiographic signs of pneumomediastium, including associated findings such as subcutaneous emphysema and pneumopericardium, as well as thin lucencies around the central airways and arteries, thin lucencies outlining the mediastinum, and continuous lucency along the diaphragm.

In blunt trauma pneumomediastium is most often caused by the "Macklin effect," where increased intrathoracic pressure causes rupture of alveoli and gas to enter the pulmonary

seen in the pulmonary arteries except in rare instances. History can be very helpful in differentiating FES from pulmonary edema, which also tends to be more symmetric with peribronchial cuffing and pleural effusions on radiography and on CT [17]. Treatment for FES is typically supportive.

**Fig. 14** "Fat emboli syndrome": A 23-year-old man involved with motor vehicle collision. (**a**) The frontal radiograph of the right tibia and fibula demonstrates midshaft fractures. (**b**) Initial axial CT image of the chest with IV contrast demonstrates no pulmonary parenchymal abnormalities. Follow-up chest CT on coronal (**c**) and axial (**d**) reconstructions demonstrates new peripheral ground-glass opacities which are highly suggestive of fat emboli syndrome in a patient with skin petechiae and altered mental status. Of note, the dependent distribution is somewhat atypical

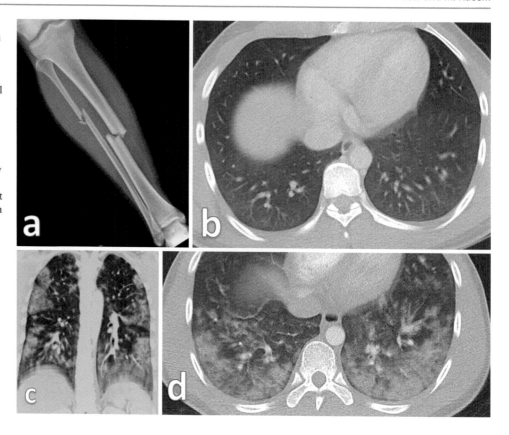

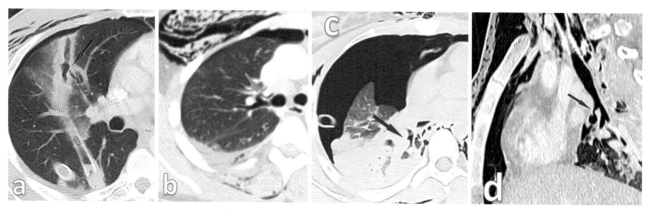

**Fig. 15** "Bronchopleural fistula": (**a**) A 37-year-old man with gunshot trauma to the chest. CT scan of the chest on lung windows demonstrates a peripheral bronchopleural fistula (red arrow). (**b**) A 29-year-old woman after motor vehicle collision with a focal discontinuity of the right upper lobe segmental bronchus resulting in a bronchopleural fistula (green arrow). (**c–d**) A 31-year-old woman with motor vehicle collision. CT chest on axial (**c**) and coronal (**d**) reconstructions demonstrate a laceration of the bronchus intermedius (blue arrow) with associated pneumothorax consistent with bronchopleural fistula

interstitium and travel to the mediastinum. The diagnosis can be made by observing thin air collections around the pulmonary vessels and bronchi on lung windows.

The "Macklin effect" does not affect air exchange, but is a marker of severe blunt trauma, and patients tend to have longer ICU stays because of other injuries [19]. Isolated pneumomediastium related to the "Macklin effect" is typically treated conservatively without requiring further imaging investigation. Pneumomediastinum can also be related to other etiologies including penetrating injury,

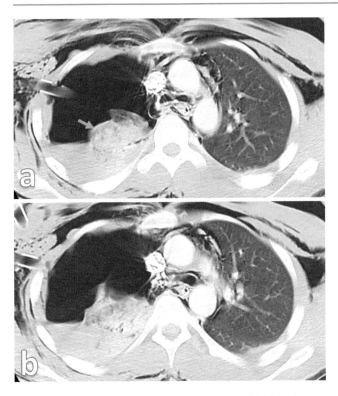

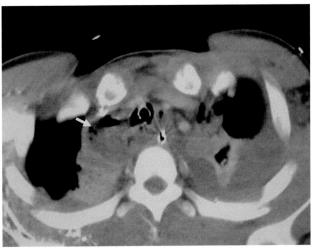

**Fig. 17** "Blunt esophageal injury": A 47-year-old man with blunt thoracic trauma. CT axial image of the chest with IV contrast chest shows a fluid and gas collection surrounding the esophagus (yellow arrow) near the thoracic inlet, which is suspicious for esophageal injury and which was subsequently confirmed surgically

**Fig. 16** "Bronchial avulsion": A 25-year-old man with blunt thoracic trauma. CT scan of the chest on lung windows (**a** and **b**) in the axial plane shows a large right pneumothorax with a "fallen" atelectatic right lung (green arrow). There is discontinuity of the right main stem bronchus consistent with bronchial avulsion (the image a shows the normal bronchus which is not well seen on image **b**)

tracheobronchial injury, esophageal injury, pneumoretroperitoneum, pneumoperitoneum, or cervical subcutaneous emphysema [18].

## Tracheal and Central Bronchial Injuries

Airway injuries often result in secondary signs such as pneumomediastinum or a persistent pneumothorax despite thoracostomy tube placement. However, direct signs such as a defect in the airway are often subtle and frequently missed [9]. These direct signs are best seen on CT lung windows. Multi-planar CT reconstructions can be helpful in confirming communication to the pleural space (Fig. 15). Ultimately, bronchoscopy is the reference standard for the confirmation and evaluation of tracheobronchial injury [9].

A bronchial avulsion results from transection of the bronchus, and discontinuity is usually readily apparent on CT (Fig. 16). The lung or lobe distal to the avulsion will be atelectatic as it is not being ventilated, and it typically falls dependently in the hemithorax. There will be a large air leak, a persistent pneumothorax despite chest tube placement, and extensive pneumomediastinum.

## Esophageal Injury

Traumatic perforation of the esophagus is rare, likely because of its small size and relatively protected position [19]. In blunt trauma, it most often occurs at the thoracic inlet where the esophagus is relatively fixed (Fig. 17), but also at an associated vertebral fracture, or prominent osteophyte. Penetrating injury is more common, and trajectories close to or through the esophagus should prompt endoscopy to prevent mediastinitis and mediastinal abscess, which has a high morbidity and mortality.

The most common finding of esophageal perforation is a gas and fluid collection associated with the esophagus. A perforation can be confirmed with a repeat CT immediately following water-soluble oral contrast administration or possibly with an esophagram (Fig. 18). A dedicated esophagram or endoscopy can be performed after stabilization of the patient to look for more subtle injury if the CT esophagram is negative [19].

In the absence of perforation, injury to the esophagus is often subtle or occult on CT and may only be visible as focal wall thickening, so one should carefully inspect the esophagus near vertebral body fractures, mediastinal hematoma, or large osteophytes.

## Osseous Injuries

### Traumatic Rib Injuries

Rib injuries are common in both penetrating and blunt trauma. When detected on chest radiography, they may alert

**Fig. 18** "Penetrating esophageal Injury": A 29-year-old man with a gunshot injury to the lower neck. CT chest with intravenous contrast (**a**) and oral contrast (**b**) demonstrates a bullet tract (yellow arrow line) traversing through the esophagus, with findings of definitive esophageal injury. There is extraluminal oral contrast surrounding the esophagus and in the neck (red arrow), confirming penetrating esophageal injury. Post-repair fluoroscopy image (**c**) shows an esophageal stent in place

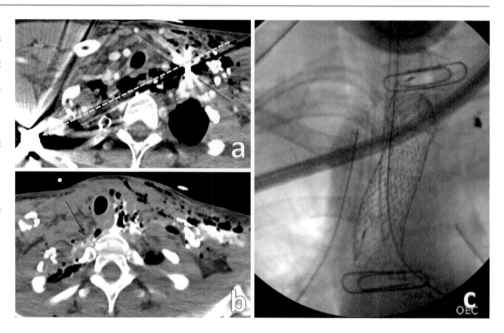

**Fig. 19** "Example of buckle fractures": (**a**) Subtle disruption of the outer cortex with "buckling of the rib" (yellow arrow). (**b**) Displacement of the outer cortex with mild "buckling" (green arrow). In both these examples, the inner cortex (blue arrow) is intact

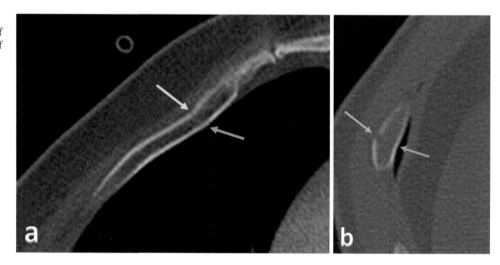

**Fig. 20** "Rib fractures": (**a**) Non-displaced left first rib fracture (yellow arrow). (**b**) Displaced seventh right rib fracture (green arrow) presenting with a delayed massive hemothorax (white star) 10 days after injury

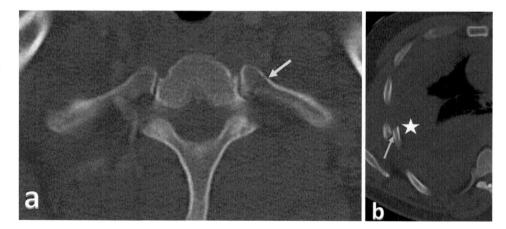

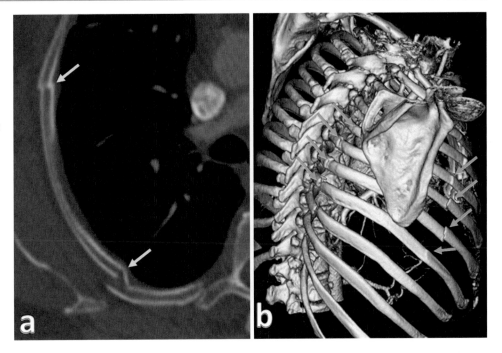

**Fig. 21** "Segmental rib fractures in a 40-year-old man with flail chest": (**a**) MPR reformat of a segmental rib fracture showing posterior and lateral mildly displaced fractures (yellow arrows). (**b**) 3D reconstruction shows multiple contiguous segmental rib fractures in a patient with flail chest (blue arrows)

the clinician to a more severe mechanism of injury and prompt CT evaluation. Radiographs are generally specific but not sensitive for mildly displaced rib fractures. Dedicated rib series slightly increase the sensitivity, but CT is substantially more sensitive for the detection of non-displaced rib fractures [20].

Rib fracture location can help further focus one's search pattern. Ribs 1–3 are associated with high-velocity trauma and often have associated vascular or brachial plexus injuries. Ribs 4–9 are associated with pulmonary contusion or laceration. Ribs 9–12 are associated with liver injury on the right and splenic injury on the left [20].

Rib fractures vary in their severity and ease of detection on CT. Buckle fractures result from disruption of only the inner or the outer cortex with "buckling" the rib. These fractures may be missed at CT. 1 mm reconstructions, bone scintigraphy, ultrasound, or MRI can aid in diagnosis but are rarely clinically necessary (Fig. 19).

Non-displaced rib fractures involving the inner and outer cortices are also commonly missed on CT and are often detected on follow-up when healing callus is seen. Displaced fractures imply both cortical disruption and abnormal alignment. They are associated with intercostal injury, pulmonary contusion, and laceration. Delayed intercostal arterial or lung can occur from displaced rib fractures moving during respiration (Fig. 20).

A segmental rib fracture (Fig. 21) involves complete fractures of a rib in two locations, typically posterior and anterolateral. Three or more contiguous ribs with segmental fractures are associated with flail chest phenomenon.

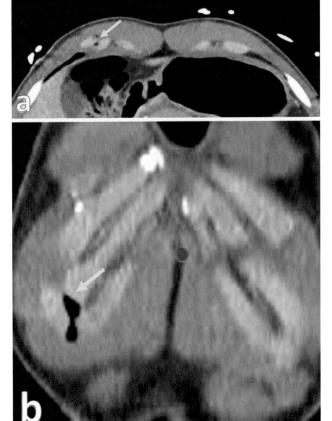

**Fig. 22** "Costochondral fracture": (**a**) Mildly displaced right costochondral fracture with gas between the two fragments. (**b**) The same in coronal reconstruction (yellow arrows)

**Fig. 23** "Sternal fracture": (**a**)
Subtle non-displaced fracture of
the sternum with minimal
surrounding hematoma (blue
arrow). This was a clue that there
was a high-energy trauma and led
to detection of a subtle acute aortic
traumatic injury (red arrow)

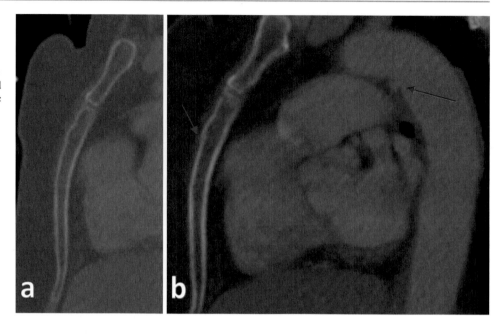

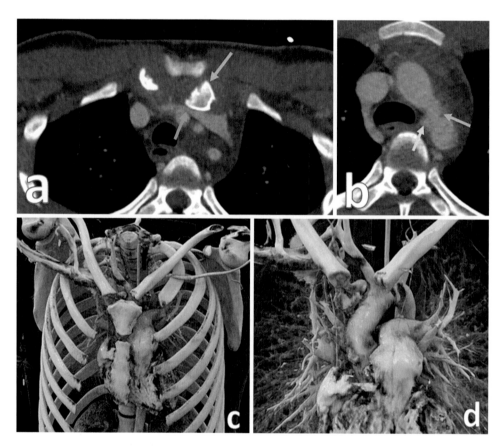

**Fig. 24** "Posterior sternoclavicular dislocation and aortic injury": A
31-year-old man presented after motor vehicle collision. CT of the
chest with intravenous contrast (**a** and **b**) demonstrates posterior
displacement of the left clavicular head (green arrow). It impresses
upon the left brachiocephalic vein (blue arrow) and is in close
proximity to the arch vessels. Associated mediastinal hematoma
and an acute traumatic aortic injury are present with a focal
outpouching (yellow arrow) and a flap (orange arrow). Notice the
clavicular head is no longer in contact with the aorta, but likely
impacted it during the initial trauma and rebounded into a less
displaced position. 3D cinematic rendering of the same patient
(**c** and **d**) showing posteromedial displacement of the proximal
clavicle in relation to the manubrium. Osseous structures removed
to show the aortic injury in figure portion **d**

**Fig. 25** "Thoracic spine fracture and posterior mediastinal hematoma": (**a**) Widening of the left paraspinal line (red arrow) secondary to a thoracic spine fracture in a 36-year-old man involved in motor vehicle collision. The aortic contour is also abnormal secondary to mediastinal hematoma (green arrows). (**b**) Coronal CT reconstruction demonstrating the paravertebral hematoma and severe compression fracture (blue arrow)

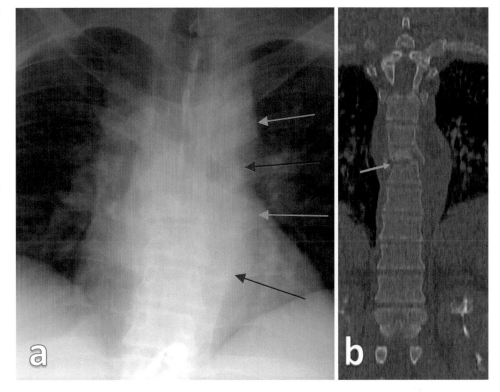

However, this remains a clinical diagnosis [20]. A true flail chest results in paradoxical motion of the segment with respiration. The size of the flail chest segment and the strength of the intercostal muscles play a role in whether it demonstrates clinically substantial paradoxical motion.

Costochondral fractures occur when there is disruption of the rib-cartilage complex. There can be disruption of the cartilage from the sternum, fracture of the cartilage itself, or separation of the costochondral junction. Findings are cartilaginous discontinuity, often with associated locules of gas (Fig. 22).

## Other Osseous Injuries

Sternal fracture is an indication of high-energy trauma and should prompt increased scrutiny of other thoracic structures to evaluate for subtle injuries (Fig. 23). While it can be detected on a lateral radiograph, CT with sagittal reconstruction provides much improved sensitivity and specificity [21]. Evaluation on the axial images alone can make detection difficult.

Sternoclavicular dislocation can result in anterior, superior, or posterior dislocation of the proximal clavicle (Fig. 24). It is a relatively rare injury, seen in only approximately 2–3% of shoulder dislocations [22]. Anterior displacement is more common, more clinically apparent, and associated with less morbidity. Posterior dislocations are associated with potentially life-threatening injuries to the superior mediastinum. Posterior dislocations can result in injury to the lung, superior mediastinal vessels and nerves, trachea, or esophagus. While chest radiography can be used to detect an abnormal position of the clavicle, it lacks sensitivity. CT again is the imaging modality of choice not only for depicting the dislocation but also for characterizing associated injuries. Acute surgical reduction and surgical fixation is often necessary [21, 22].

Thoracic spine fractures are usually best initially characterized using CT. Detection and characterization is best done with dedicated spine reconstructions using thin (1 mm) slices and a sharp bone kernel with axial, sagittal, and coronal reconstructions. Vertebral fractures are a cause of posterior mediastinal hematomas, which can be seen on chest radiography (Fig. 25) and which can occasionally cause or be associated with aortic, esophageal, great vessel, or tracheal injury.

## Chest Wall Soft-Tissue Injury

Contusion or laceration characterized by stranding or hematoma in the chest wall can help detect other more subtle injuries such as rib fractures. Large hematomas should be evaluated for active bleeding. Intramuscular hematomas or muscular tears result in asymmetrical enlargement of the muscle on CT.

## Lung Herniation

When the lung protrudes past the confines of the thoracic chest wall, it constitutes a hernia. Hernias can occur at the thoracic inlet, chest wall, or diaphragm [23].

Traumatic defects in the diaphragm, intercostal space, or supraclavicular space can result in lung herniating beyond the thoracic cavity (Fig. 26). Lung herniation can result in respiratory pain, lung strangulation, or torsion. Symptomatic, diaphragmatic, intercostal, and narrow necked hernias are typically treated surgically [24].

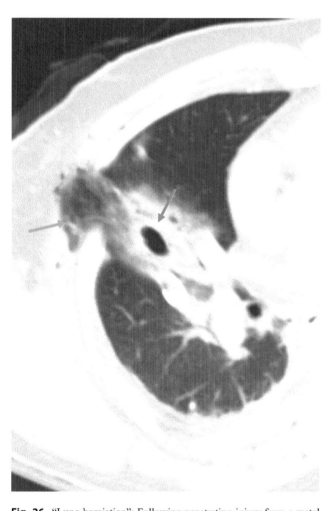

**Fig. 26** "Lung herniation": Following penetrating injury from a metal stake in a 41-year-old man, there is a defect in the chest wall with herniation of a portion of the right upper lobe (green arrow). An associated pulmonary laceration and contusion (blue arrow) is also seen

## Diaphragmatic Injury

Diaphragmatic injury can result in acute or delayed diaphragmatic rupture and herniation of abdominal contents into the thorax. This can cause compression of mediastinal structures, impaired respiration, and bowel obstruction or strangulation. Radiographically rupture can appear as elevation of the hemidiaphragm, air-fluid levels in the thorax, or bowel loops in the thorax (Fig. 27). On CT, rupture is differentiated from eventration or an elevated hemidiaphragm by using several signs (Fig. 28). Discontinuity and thickening of the diaphragm is seen in rupture, but in eventration the diaphragm is thinned but continuous. Abdominal contents falling dependently in the hemithorax or "waisting" of herniated liver with associated hepatic edema at the site of the defect are also signs of rupture [25]. Diaphragmatic rupture and most diaphragmatic injuries are surgically repaired, but some small injuries, particularly on the right where the liver can plug the defect, are treated conservatively [26].

## Cardiac and Pericardial Injuries

### Pericardium

Traumatic pericardial injury is most commonly detected as hemopericardium seen on bedside ultrasound or CT and generally requires surgical exploration to prevent cardiac tamponade [27]. On CT, hemopericardium typically has an attenuation >25 Hounsfield units compared to simple fluid, which is typically <15 Hounsfield units [28]. Pneumopericardium can also result in tamponade and should be differentiated from pneumomediastinum which has a weblike CT appearance (Fig. 29).

The pericardial space can stretch to accommodate a fairly large amount of fluid if it accumulates over the course of many months, but in the acute setting, it is not compliant, and a small amount of fluid can result in cardiac tamponade. CT is not sensitive or specific for tamponade, and echocardiography is the diagnostic modality of choice. Findings of notching of the right atrium or ventricle, or flattening of the interventricular septum or right ventricular free wall, are findings which are occasionally seen on CT. Secondary findings of impaired heart function can frequently be seen as reflux of contrast into the hepatic or renal veins or in severely reduced function layering of contrast in the inferior vena cava [4]. Dependent contrast pooling on CT especially within the right hemi-liver and hepatic veins is a sign of impending cardiac arrest [28].

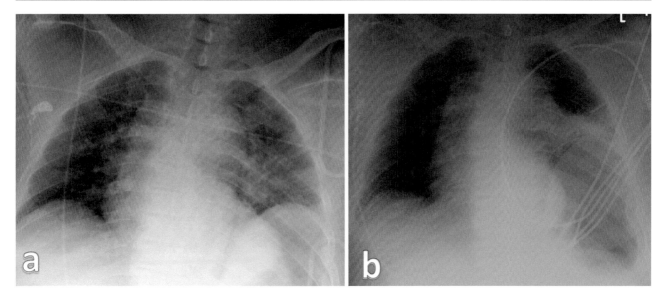

**Fig. 27** "Delayed traumatic diaphragmatic rupture": (**a**) Initial presentation following motor vehicle collision. (**b**) Four hours later there is herniation of the stomach into the left hemithorax

**Fig. 28** "Traumatic diaphragmatic rupture": Different patients with acute diaphragmatic ruptures demonstrating different imaging signs. (**a**) Dependent viscera sign, the stomach protrudes through a left hemidiaphragm rupture and sits posteriorly in the thorax without lung interposed between it and the chest wall. (**b**) Discontinuous diaphragm sign; coronal CT showing abrupt cutoff of the left hemidiaphragm (red arrow) with the stomach extending into the left hemithorax. (**c**) Thickened, retracted, and discontinuous left hemidiaphragm (green arrows). (**d**) "Hump and band sign" – a portion of the liver extends through a right hemidiaphragmatic defect. There is waisting of the herniated liver through the defect (blue arrow)

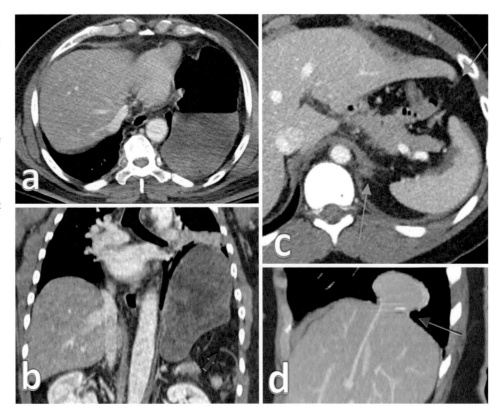

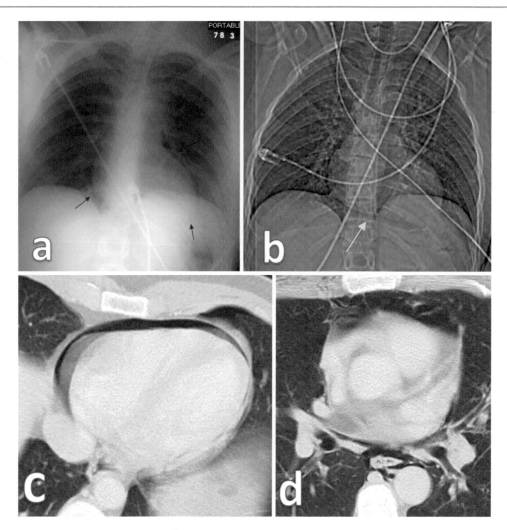

**Fig. 29** "Pneumopericardium vs. pneumomediastium": (**a**) Pneumopericardium on chest radiograph. Lucency outlining the heart (red arrows). (**b**) Topogram with pneumopericardium and a continuous diaphragm sign. (**c**) Pneumopericardium with a single air cavity surrounding the heart. (**d**) Pneumomediastinum with gas surrounding the heart and throughout the mediastinum. Notice the webbing within the mediastinal gas

Rarely, frank disruption of the pericardium with a tear or rupture can cause cardiac herniation and volvulus, or if there is concurrent central diaphragmatic injury, abdominal contents can herniate into the pericardial sac. Both can quickly result in cardiovascular collapse [29].

## Cardiac

Myocardial injury can manifest as concussion, contusion, rupture, or laceration. Concussion and contusion result in decreased myocardial function. Contusion differs in that there are EKG and serum myocardial marker abnormalities from myocardial necrosis. Often only secondary signs are seen on imaging, typically pulmonary edema or transient ventricular enlargement (Fig. 30).

Traumatic disruption of the myocardium can have a variety of manifestations, including subtle free wall laceration with hemopericardium (Fig. 31), septal wall rupture forming a ventriculoseptal defect, papillary muscle rupture with resultant valvular regurgitation, or frank free wall rupture with pseudoaneurysm formation [4, 30].

Traumatic injury to the coronary arteries from penetrating or blunt injury can result in thrombosis, dissection, or transection. Traditional angiography is the diagnostic modality of choice, and typically only secondary CT signs are seen such as pulmonary edema or occasionally subendocardial hypo-enhancement (Fig. 32).

In conclusion, CT plays a pivotal role in the evaluation of penetrating thoracic trauma. Recognition of the common

**Fig. 30** "Cardiac contusion": A 14-year-old following a motor vehicle collision. (**a**) Dependent consolidation and centrally predominant ground-glass opacity, which is consistent with pulmonary edema. (**b**) Mildly dilated left ventricle. (Echocardiography showed markedly decreased ejection fraction.) (**c**) Two days later there is resolving pulmonary edema. (**d**) Left ventricular size has normalized (a subsequent echo showed normal ejection fraction)

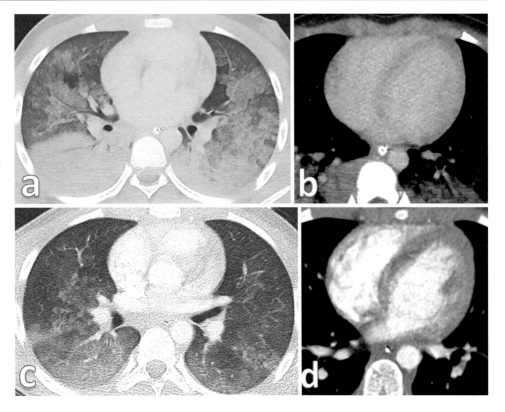

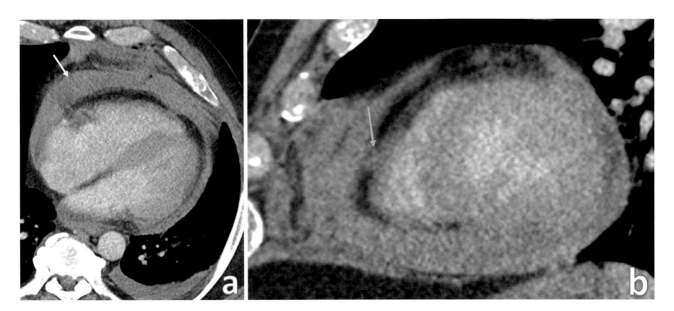

**Fig. 31** "Hemopericardium with RV laceration": (**a**) Following a stab wound to the anterior chest, there was development of hemopericardium (white arrow). (**b**) A small laceration to the right ventricular free wall is seen, accentuated by stranding in the epicardial fat (green arrow)

injury patterns, normal variants, and subtle findings which may warrant additional evaluation are important in the diagnostic evaluation of a penetrating trauma patient and may direct further clinical management.

**Fig. 32** "Coronary dissection": A 15-year-old boy injured playing baseball when another teenager landed on his chest with their knee. He complained of chest pain and then collapsed minutes later. (**a**) Dependent consolidation and ground-glass opacity consistent with pulmonary edema. (**b**) IV contrast-enhanced CT in the portal venous phase showing subtle subendocardial hypoattenuation of the left ventricular myocardium involving the anterior and anteroseptal walls (red arrow) consistent with ischemia. (**c**) Coronary angiogram showing left main coronary dissection (black arrows). (**d**) Post-stenting angiogram showing resolution of the dissection and narrowing

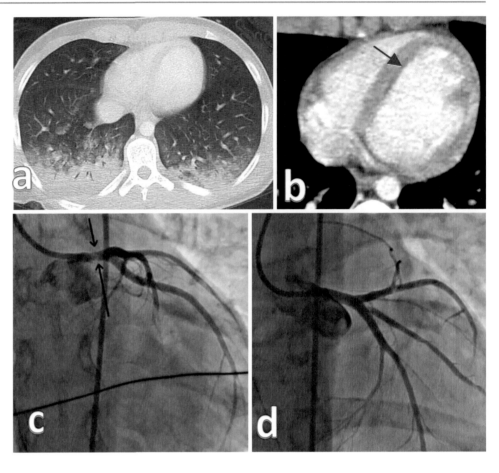

# References

1. NTDB Reports and Publications. In: American College of Surgeons.
2. Sridhar S, Raptis C, Bhalla S. Imaging of blunt thoracic trauma. Semin Roentgenol. 2016;51(3):203–14.
3. Rhee PM, Moore EE, Joseph B, Tang A, Pandit V, Vercruysse G. Gunshot wounds: a review of ballistics, bullets, weapons, and myths. J Trauma Acute Care Surg. 2016;80(6):853–67.
4. Raptis DA, Bhalla S, Raptis CA. Computed tomographic imaging of cardiac trauma. Radiol Clin N Am. 2019;57(1):201–12.
5. Dreizin D, Munera F. Multidetector CT for penetrating torso trauma: state of the art. Radiology. 2015;277(2):338–55.
6. Sodagari F, Katz DS, Menias CO, Moshiri M, Pellerito JS, Mustafa A, et al. Imaging evaluation of abdominopelvic gunshot trauma. Radiographics. 2020;40(6):1766–88.
7. Advanced trauma life support: student course manual. American College of Surgeons; 2018
8. O'Connor A, Morgan W. Radiological review of pneumothorax. BMJ. 2005;330(7506):1493–7.
9. Moser J, Stefanidis K, Vlahos I. Imaging evaluation of tracheobronchial injuries. Radiographics. 2020;40(2):515–28.
10. Gayer G, Rozenman J, Hoffmann C, Apter S, Simansky D, Yellin A, et al. CT diagnosis of malpositioned chest tubes. Br J Radiol. 2000;73(871):786–90.
11. Lim K, Tai S, Chan C, Hsu Y, Hsu W, Lin B, et al. Diagnosis of malpositioned chest tubes after emergency tube thoracostomy: is computed tomography more accurate than chest radiograph? Clin Imaging. 2005;29(6):401–5.

12. Lubner M, Menias C, Rucker C, Bhalla S, Peterson C, Wang L, et al. Blood in the belly: CT findings of hemoperitoneum. Radiographics. 2007;27(1):109–25.
13. Oikonomou A, Prassopoulos P. CT imaging of blunt chest trauma. Insights Imaging. 2011;2(3):281–95.
14. Magret M. Lung trauma. Clin Pulm Med. 2010;17(2):75–81.
15. Cohn S. Pulmonary contusion. J Trauma Inj Infect Crit Care. 1997;42(5):973–9.
16. Wagner RB, Jamieson PM. Pulmonary contusion. Evaluation and classification by computed tomography. Surg Clin North Am. 1989;69(1):31–40.
17. Nucifora G, Hysko F, Vit A, Vasciaveo A. Pulmonary fat embolism. J Comput Assist Tomogr. 2007;31(5):806–7.
18. Zylak C, Standen J, Barnes G, Zylak C. Pneumomediastinum revisited. Radiographics. 2000;20(4):1043–57.
19. Young C, Menias C, Bhalla S, Prasad S. CT features of esophageal emergencies. Radiographics. 2008;28(6):1541–53.
20. Talbot B, Gange C, Chaturvedi A, Klionsky N, Hobbs S, Chaturvedi A. Traumatic rib injury: patterns, imaging pitfalls, complications, and treatment. Radiographics. 2017;37(2):628–51.
21. Restrepo C, Martinez S, Lemos D, Washington L, McAdams H, Vargas D, et al. Imaging appearances of the sternum and sternoclavicular joints. Radiographics. 2009;29(3):839–59.
22. Salgado R, Ghysen D. Post-traumatic posterior sternoclavicular dislocation: case report and review of the literature. Emerg Radiol. 2002;9(6):323–5.
23. Chaturvedi A, Rajiah P, Croake A, Saboo S, Chaturvedi A. Imaging of thoracic hernias: types and complications. Insights Imaging. 2018;9(6):989–1005.

24. Bikhchandani J, Balters M, Sugimoto J. Conservative management of traumatic lung hernia. Ann Thorac Surg. 2012;93(3):992–4.

25. Desir A, Ghaye B. CT of blunt diaphragmatic rupture. Radiographics. 2012;32(2):477–98.

26. Iochum S, Ludig T, Walter F, Sebbag H, Grosdidier G, Blum A. Imaging of diaphragmatic injury: a diagnostic challenge? Radio-Graphics. 2002;22(suppl_1):S103–16.

27. Co S, Yong-Hing C, Galea-Soler S, Ruzsics B, Schoepf U, Ajlan A, et al. Role of imaging in penetrating and blunt traumatic injury to the heart. Radiographics. 2011;31(4):E101–15.

28. Tsai P, Chen J, Huang J, Shen W. Dependent pooling: a contrast-enhanced sign of cardiac arrest during CT. AJR Am J Roentgenol. 2002;178(5):1095–9.

29. Meziane M, Fishman E, Siegelman S. CT diagnosis of hemopericardium in acute dissecting aneurysm of the thoracic aorta. J Comput Assist Tomogr. 1984;8(1):10–4.

30. Restrepo C, Gutierrez F, Marmol-Velez J, Ocazionez D, Martinez-Jimenez S. Imaging patients with cardiac trauma. Radiographics. 2012;32(3):633–49.

# Imaging of Thoracic Vascular Trauma

**16**

Travis S. Henry, Brian M. Haas, and Scott A. Hamlin

## Contents

### Abstract

Injury to the thorax is a common indication for imaging in the emergency setting. Thoracic trauma can be grouped into blunt and penetrating trauma, and vascular injury is a substantial cause of morbidity and mortality in both major types of trauma. Imaging of vascular trauma (including acute traumatic aortic injury and other blunt and penetrating vascular injuries) are discussed in this chapter.

### Keywords

Acute traumatic aortic injury · Minimal aortic injury · Active extravasation · Pseudoaneurysm · Mediastinal hematoma · Aortic rupture · Stab wound · Gunshot wound · Rib fracture

T. S. Henry (✉)
Duke University School of Medicine, Durham, NC, USA
e-mail: travis.henry@duke.edu

B. M. Haas
Zuckerburg San Francisco General Hospital and University of California San Francisco, San Francisco, CA, USA
e-mail: brian.haas@ucsf.edu

S. A. Hamlin
Emory University School of Medicine, Atlanta, GA, USA
e-mail: shamli2@emory.edu

## Introduction

Injury to the thorax is a common cause of morbidity and mortality in trauma patients. Injuries in the chest account for up to 25% of trauma deaths, second only to head injuries, with an overall mortality of approximately 10% [1].

Thoracic trauma can loosely be grouped into blunt injury or penetrating injury. Blunt mechanisms of trauma consist of rapid deceleration from motor vehicle crashes, falls, or blows from a blunt object, while penetrating trauma consists of gunshot wounds, stabbings, or other projectiles. As will be discussed in this chapter, certain mechanisms are associated with different types of injuries identified on imaging. Astute radiologists can use the mechanism or mechanisms of trauma to assist in identifying additional injuries and in categorizing all the injuries present.

## Epidemiology and Clinical Features

### Types of Vascular Injuries

Broadly, traumatic vascular injuries may be classified as contained injuries (e.g., intimal injury, pseudoaneurysm, and traumatic intramural hematoma), frank rupture of an artery or vein resulting in hematoma with or without active extravasation, traumatic arteriovenous fistulae (AVF), transection, or avulsion [2]. The imaging features of each of these types of injury are listed in Table 1. Many of these injuries may be the result of blunt or penetrating trauma, and the rest of this chapter focuses on the approach based on the mechanism(s) of injury.

### Blunt Trauma

Blunt trauma tends to produce somewhat predictable mechanisms of vascular injury. Many patients have other evidence of substantial thoracic trauma (i.e., skeletal fractures, lung contusion/laceration, and diaphragmatic injury), but in some patients, a vascular injury may be present in the absence of substantial additional traumatic findings. Therefore, a high suspicion of vascular injury is paramount in all cases and particularly when assessing the thoracic aorta.

### Penetrating Trauma

Penetrating trauma includes ballistic injury from gunshot wounds (GSW) and piercing injuries including stab wounds (SW). Penetrating trauma generally results in a higher mortality rate than blunt trauma, with GSWs being more likely to cause death than SW [3–5]. In the United States, there are approximately 40,000 firearm-related deaths, over 130,000 nonfatal ballistic injuries, and more than two million piercing injuries, annually [6]. Ballistic trauma in European countries is decidedly less than in the United States, although not insignificant. A retrospective analysis performed of over a 10-year span (1998–2007) in England and Wales from the Trauma Audit and Research Network (TARN) database showed only 0.53% of serious injuries were due to firearms, although this registry does not record prehospital deaths [7]. Another retrospective study analyzing data between 2008 and 2013 from an urban university level 1 trauma center in Western Europe showed 9.3% of injuries were related to penetrating trauma (including stabbings and firearm-related injuries) [8].

## Diagnostic Investigations

Imaging plays an essential role in the evaluation of nearly all trauma patients, regardless of the mechanism(s) of injury. Trauma centers and more generally emergency departments incorporate specific imaging protocols into patient management algorithms [9]. A portable anteroposterior chest radiograph (CXR) is typically the initial examination, as it can be used to quickly screen for life-threatening abnormalities that require immediate intervention, including tension pneumothorax, hemothorax, mediastinal hematoma, or location of a projectile.

In patients stable enough to travel to the radiology department or imaging facility within the emergency department,

**Table 1** CT findings of traumatic vascular injury

| Intimal injury | – Luminal filling defect or flap<br>– Preserved external vessel contour | Blunt (usually high-speed deceleration) |
|---|---|---|
| Traumatic intramural hematoma | – Hyperdense thickening of the vessel wall due to presence of blood in the media | Blunt |
| Pseudoaneurysm | – Focal change in caliber of the vessel with abnormal external contour<br>– Similar enhancement to an adjacent vessel<br>– May be difficult to distinguish from frank rupture | Blunt or penetrating |
| Vessel rupture | – Abrupt change in caliber with full-thickness disruption<br>– High attenuation acute hematoma<br>– Active extravasation – amorphous extraluminal contrast that may be a linear jet or pool | Penetrating or blunt |
| Arteriovenous fistula | Asymmetric, early opacification of a vein of equivalent contrast density to adjacent artery<br>The vein is often enlarged due to increased pressure | Penetrating >> blunt |
| Vessel avulsion or laceration | Abrupt occlusion of a vessel | Penetrating or blunt |

IV contrast-enhanced computed tomography (CT) is unquestionably the current modality of choice for the evaluation of patients with substantial thoracic trauma. Initial radiographs are known to be insensitive, and CT findings change management in at least 20% of patients [1]. Some centers may bypass radiography altogether and screen trauma victims with CT (either focused or whole-body depending upon suspected injuries) [10]. When iodinated contrast is not able to be administered to a patient because of a history of allergic reaction to iodinated contrast or chronic kidney disease, non-contrast CT is the preferred imaging modality for imaging patients with substantial thoracic trauma, although it has some inherent limitations compared with IV contrast-enhanced CT.

Thoracic magnetic resonance imaging (MRI) is generally not the initial imaging modality of choice. However, for patients who cannot receive iodinated contrast and for whom following a non-contrast CT scan, there is a persistent concern for large vessel injury; MRI may be useful to further evaluate for acute aortic syndromes. The use of MRI in the trauma setting is beyond the scope of this chapter.

## CT Parameters

Thoracic CT protocol should include a volumetric, thin-slice acquisition (1–2 mm slice thickness) which can be reformatted in multiple planes. Intravenous contrast should be administered, as noted, if possible, in patients with suspected thoracic trauma to assess for vascular injury. Some institutions perform dual-phase CT with a late arterial phase CT of the chest (or of the full chest/abdomen and/or pelvis), followed by delayed imaging of the abdomen and pelvis. Other institutions obtain a single 70- or 80-s portal venous phase acquisition that enables scanning of the entire body in one pass [2, 11]. Still others utilize a split bolus of contrast, with half of the contrast administered first and timed for the late arterial phase and the second half administered later and timed for the portal venous phase. There is some literature suggesting that dual-phase imaging can better characterize a source of active extravasation [2]. In our experience the benefits of dual-phase imaging are greatest for abdominal and pelvic injuries (and are discussed in more detail in other portions of this book), but either technique is effective for the evaluation of thoracic vascular trauma, especially with modern 64+ detector scanners. A non-contrast series (as may be performed when evaluating for nontraumatic acute aortic syndrome) is generally not necessary.

ECG-gating is unnecessary for a general trauma CT protocol. However, injury to the aortic root or ascending aorta can be subtle and potentially confused for cardiac pulsation on non-gated examinations. Thus, in some instances, ECG gating may be used as a troubleshooting tool in hemodynamically stable patients, as will be discussed later.

## Blunt Aortic Trauma

Traumatic aortic injury is a leading cause of death in blunt trauma and thus warrants considerable discussion. As the body's largest artery responsible for delivering blood from the heart, traumatic aortic injury can be catastrophic with many patients exsanguinating prior to arrival at the hospital. Others are taken immediately to the operating room before imaging can be performed. Whereas penetrating injury to the aorta can occur anywhere and is a direct result of the path of the entering object, blunt trauma tends to produce predictable injury patterns at specific sites.

Blunt thoracic aortic injury (BTAI), also referred to as acute traumatic aortic injury (ATAI), is the second leading cause of death in blunt trauma patients, only behind intracranial hemorrhage [12]. The vast majority of cases of ATAI are due to deceleration from high-speed motor vehicle collisions (MVC), and approximately 70% of patients die at the scene or before they can make it to the hospital [13]. Other less common causes of ATAI include falls from height, crush injuries, and pedestrians who are struck by moving motor vehicles.

Multiple mechanisms of ATAI) have been proposed, and the underlying pathophysiology is likely a combination of multiple factors [14]:

- Rapid deceleration – torsion/shearing forces are applied at locations where the aorta is relatively fixed (aortic annulus, isthmus, and diaphragmatic hiatus).
- Water-hammer effect – forces may result in intravascular pressure exceeding 2000 mmHg in the aorta, which results in pressure bursting the vessel wall.
- Osseous pinch – direct compression of the aorta between the sternum and thoracic spine.

ATAI most often occurs at locations where the aorta is relatively fixed – as noted, the aortic root, the isthmus just distal to the left subclavian artery, and at the diaphragmatic hiatus [15]. The aortic isthmus is by far the most common site of aortic injury for patients that reach the hospital (and CT scanner) alive (>90%). Conversely, injury to the aortic root is often immediately fatal due to hemopericardium (resulting in cardiac tamponade) or coronary artery laceration or dissection [15].

In the past two decades, survival has improved in those with an aortic injury that successfully reach the hospital. The advent of minimally invasive endovascular stent grafts that can be rapidly placed via a percutaneous approach has become the preferred method of repair, with survival rates reaching 80–90% [12, 16].

The clinical presentation of ATAI is variable depending on the severity of the trauma and the co-existence of distracting injuries. If patients are alert, they may complain of pain. Some such patients may be hemodynamically unstable, whereas others may be nearly asymptomatic. As such, a high clinical suspicion and low threshold for CT imaging are necessary. The imager plays an essential role in the evaluation of ATAI patients – first by recognizing the presence of an injury, correctly reporting the location and severity of the injury and providing details which are relevant to the endovascular repair.

## CXR Findings of ATAI

Any patient with suspected ATAI should undergo imaging with CT angiography (which is discussed in more detail below). Based on institutional protocol and level of trauma, some patients may proceed directly to the CT scanner, whereas others may undergo chest radiography (CXR) as an initial method of assessment. CXR is usually performed to evaluate for other suspected life-threatening injuries (e.g., pneumothorax, hemothorax) and/or position of support devices, but the radiologist should be able to recognize salient findings of ATAI on CXR. Findings of ATAI on CXR are listed in detail below (Figs. 1a and 2a).

**Mediastinal widening** – mediastinal widening may represent mediastinal hematoma but lacks specificity as there are many more common causes, including mediastinal bleeding from venous injuries or sternal fractures, increased mediastinal fat/lipomatosis, lymphadenopathy, or poor inspiratory effort and portable CXR technique [11]. Mediastinal widening is defined as >6 cm in width at the level of the left subclavian artery. This finding should not be interpreted in isolation, especially considering that body habitus affects the amount of magnification of the radiograph, and that at least one study has shown it is less sensitive than the radiologist's overall impression of the radiograph when evidence supporting the presence of mediastinal hematoma is taken into consideration [17].

**Obscuration of the aortic arch and loss of aortopulmonary window** – the aortic arch should be clearly visible on CXR as a sharp interface. Mediastinal hematoma from ATAI at the aortic isthmus may result in an abnormal left mediastinal contour with loss of these normal interfaces. These findings have a higher specificity than mediastinal widening seen in isolation.

**Left apical cap** – mediastinal blood may track along the proximal left subclavian artery and result in widening of the left subclavian artery reflection and increased density at the left lung apex.

**Left paratracheal widening; rightward deviation of the trachea and/or nasogastric tube** – hematoma may result in widening of the left paratracheal stripe and/or rightward deviation of the trachea and or esophagus (as indicated by the presence of a nasogastric tube). Deviation of these structures to the right of the T4 spinous process on a properly positioned radiograph is considered abnormal and may be a marker of mass effect from mediastinal hematoma [15].

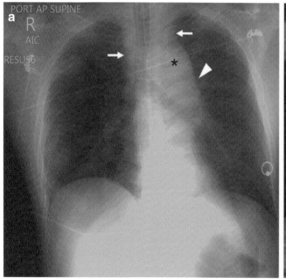 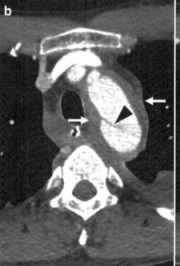 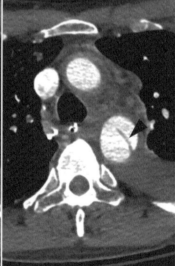

**Fig. 1** Acute traumatic aortic injury (ATAI) in a 40-year-old man from a motor vehicle collision (MVC). (**a**) Portable chest radiograph (CXR) shows multiple findings of mediastinal hematoma, including mediastinal widening with obscuration of the aortic arch (asterisk); loss of the AP window (arrowhead); paratracheal widening (arrows); rightward displacement of the trachea; and depression of the left mainstem bronchus. (**b**) Axial CTA images demonstrate direct and indirect findings of ATAI. Direct findings include intimal flap (arrowheads) and abrupt caliber change of the aorta. Indirect findings include intramural hematoma (arrows) and mediastinal hematoma that effaces the normal fat planes with the aorta

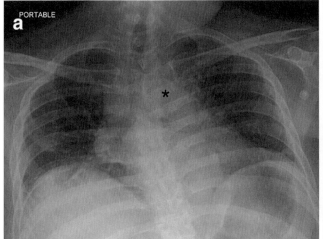

**Fig. 2** Acute traumatic aortic injury in a 35-year-old man from a MVC. (**a**) The chest radiograph shows similar findings to Fig. 1, with mediastinal hematoma including paratracheal widening (arrow), loss of normal aortic contour (asterisk), obscuration of the AP window (white arrowhead), rightward deviation of the trachea (T), and a left apical cap. Widening of the left paravertebral interface is also present (black arrowheads), indicative of hematoma. (**b**) Axial CT images show direct and indirect findings of ATAI. Direct findings include abrupt change of contour of the aorta and intraluminal thrombus (arrowheads). Indirect findings include hematoma in the middle and posterior mediastinum

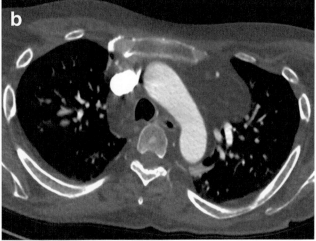

**Fig. 3** Mediastinal fat mimicking mediastinal hematoma in a patient following a fall. (**a**) Portable chest radiograph shows widening of the superior mediastinum and questionable obscuration of the aortic arch (white asterisk), and loss of the AP window that could be representative of mediastinal hematoma. (**b**) Axial CT image with IV contrast shows that the radiographic abnormality represents mediastinal fat (black asterisk). The aorta is normal without direct or indirect findings of traumatic injury

**Depression of the left mainstem bronchus** – mediastinal hematoma may displace the left bronchus into a more horizontal configuration. Historically, a measurement of <40° relative to horizontal has been considered abnormal [15].

**Widening of the paraspinal interface** – a paraspinal width of greater than 5 mm may be indicative of hematoma. This finding is nonspecific for ATAI, as it may be seen with other injuries (e.g., vertebral body fracture) or unrelated to trauma (e.g., mediastinal fat).

Given that the quality of portable chest radiographs can be variable (depending on patient positioning, inspiratory effort, under/over-penetration, overlying support devices) and recognizing that the radiographic findings are not specific, the radiologist should have a low threshold for recommending further imaging evaluation, as the consequences of missing ATAI are potentially fatal. At a minimum, in cases of low clinical suspicion, a repeat upright PA CXR may confirm a normal mediastinal width in 38% of patients where widening was questioned on the portable examination [18]. In all other cases, the patient should proceed to CT for further evaluation (Fig. 3).

IV contrast-enhanced CT approaches 100% sensitivity and specificity for the detection of ATAI for experienced readers and has replaced catheter angiography as the reference standard for the diagnosis. The use of CT has resulted in an increased incidence of ATAI, likely due to the detection of mild injuries that previously went undetected [19]. The choice of CT angiography versus venous phase varies by institution but is essentially equivalent for detection [20]. Regardless of the technique used, the relevant findings of ATAI can be classified as indirect versus direct findings.

## Indirect CT Findings of ATAI

The main indirect finding of ATAI is mediastinal blood *which effaces the fat plane of the aorta (or other injured vessel)*. The location of the hematoma and loss of the fat plane in particular are key findings, as bleeding from other injuries such as injury to small veins or fractures can track through the mediastinum, but should not cause effacement of the fat surrounding the aorta. The hematoma has attenuation typical of blood products (40–70 HU) and displaces and infiltrates normal mediastinal fat (Figs. 1, 2, 4, 6 and 7).

It is important to understand that the presence of mediastinal hematoma in isolation is not a specific finding of ATAI but is thought to arise from injury to the vasa vasorum

or small veins adjacent to the aorta [14]. Any hematoma should prompt scrutiny of the aorta for subtle direct signs of aortic injury and in rare instances intravascular ultrasound (IVUS) or transesophageal echocardiography (TEE) might be appropriate follow-up examinations to evaluate for occult injury. Conversely, mediastinal hematoma does not need to be present to confirm ATAI, particularly for mild injuries limited to the intima or intimo-medial layers (Fig. 5, discussed below).

## Direct CT Findings of ATAI

Direct findings of ATAI encompass specific changes in the morphology of the aorta itself that indicate acute (or chronic) injury. There are many classification schemes and descriptions for the severity of ATAI in the literature, some of which will be discussed below, and the clinical/surgical management of these injuries continues to evolve. In the initial radiologic evaluation, it is essential to assess the aorta on CT with coronal, sagittal, and 3D reformations, as injuries may be subtle and easily overlooked if viewing only axial data sets.

As there is no universally accepted classification scheme, to our knowledge, we believe it is most important to accurately recognize the findings of ATAI and to appropriately describe the location and appearance, which will ultimately guide clinical management. The following are direct findings of ATAI on CT.

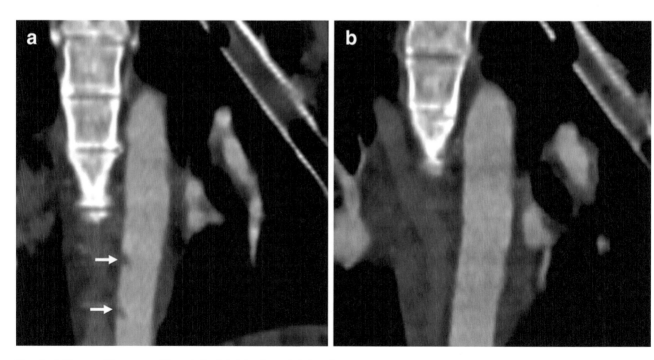

**Fig. 4** A 32-year-old woman with an intimal (minimal) aortic injury from a MVC. (**a**) Coronal CT image shows a subtle intimal flap in the descending aorta (arrows). (**b**) Coronal image from a follow-up CT 2 days later shows that the abnormality resolved with conservative management

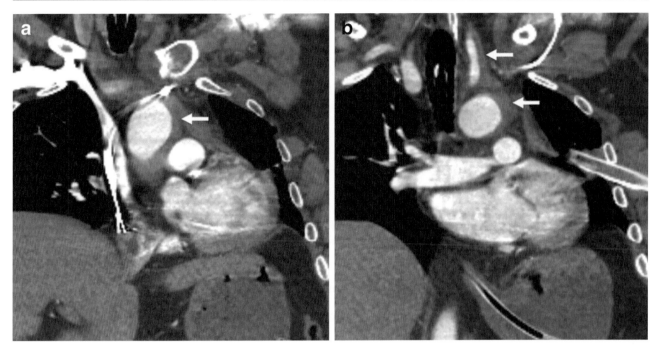

**Fig. 5** ATAI with intramural hematoma in a young male following a MVC. Coronal CT images (**a**, **b**) show wall thickening of the aortic arch and branch vessels, indicative of intramural hematoma (arrows)

## Intimal Injury and Intramural Hematoma

The aorta consists of three primary layers – the intima, media, and adventitia – and injury can be partial thickness or a complete rupture. Partial-thickness injury is often seen only as an intraluminal abnormality, whereas a full thickness injury will result in contour abnormality or change in the caliber of the aorta.

In some cases, ATAI may solely affect the luminal side of the aorta resulting in injury to the intima (or intimo-medial) layer(s). An intimo-medial flap appears as a thin linear structure attached to the internal wall of the aorta, which is visible within the aortic lumen on IV contrast-enhanced CT (Figs. 4 and 8) [21]. An intimo-medial flap is usually smaller than 1 cm and has been described as "minimal aortic injury" (MAI), a concept that will be discussed later [22]. These injuries are most commonly located at the aortic isthmus.

Disruption of the aortic intima may serve as a nidus for thrombus, which is usually a round or triangular-shaped, relatively low attenuation filling defect adherent to the wall of the aorta at the site of injury (Fig. 2) [13]. While thrombus is not a definitive marker of acute intimo-medial injury, any intraluminal filling defect should prompt scrutiny of the surrounding aortic wall for other signs of ATAI.

When traumatic force is significant, the vaso-vasorum (the network of adventitial vessels that supply blood to the wall of the aorta and other elastic arteries) can shear, resulting in the accumulation of blood within the aortic media. The accumulated blood often has a crescentic shape and appears as focal hyperdense wall thickening (Fig. 5). When small and particularly in patients with underlying aortic atherosclerosis, intramural hematomas may be difficult to identify on IV contrast-enhanced CT. In the rare case where intramural hematoma is suspected but not certain on the post-contrast CT, a follow-up non-contrast CT can be confirmatory.

## Full-Thickness Injury

Disruption of the aortic wall is the most straightforward direct finding of ATAI on CT. This can appear as a focal outpouching of the aortic wall containing contrast (Fig. 6), an abrupt change in the contour of the aorta (Figs. 1, 2 and 7), or rarely a wall defect with extravasation of contrast outside of the lumen [11]. The use of the terms "pseudoaneurysm," "contained rupture," or "traumatic dissection" can be confusing and potentially the use of these terms may lead to misunderstanding in terms of underestimating the severity of injury. Thus, the authors discourage using these terms and instead recommend focusing on describing the location and extent of the injury.

As discussed above, injury usually occurs at points of fixation, most commonly the aortic isthmus. Injuries at the diaphragmatic hiatus (Fig. 8) or at the aortic root (Fig. 9) typically result in death prior to the patient reaching the hospital, but on occasion, these injuries may be identified on CT. Careful inspection at the aortic root in particular is important as this region is subject to cardiac pulsation, and a

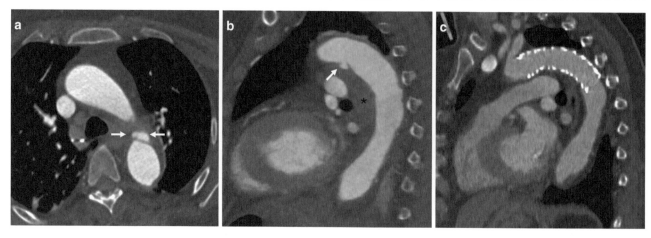

**Fig. 6** A 50-year-old pedestrian hit by a motor vehicle with ATAI. Axial (**a**) and coronal (**b**) CT images show direct findings of aortic injury with a focal contour abnormality (arrows). A small mediastinal hematoma (asterisk) is also visible. Oblique sagittal CT image (**c**) after endovascular repair shows successful treatment of the ATAI

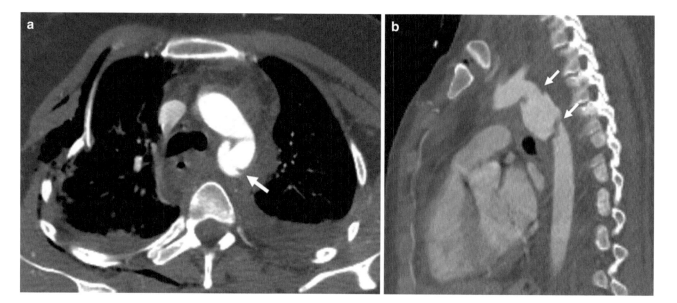

**Fig. 7** Full-thickness ATAI in an MVC patient. Axial (**a**) and sagittal (**b**) contrast-enhanced CT images show a full-thickness injury (rupture) at the aortic isthmus. Note the abrupt caliber change (arrows) that extends for about 3 cm with the normal aorta proximally and distally. Extensive mediastinal hematoma is also present. Several rib fractures are indicative of high-impact trauma

high suspicion for injury in this location should prompt repeat CT with ECG gating (Fig. 9c, d) or echocardiography.

## Classification and Management of ATAI

### Classifying the Severity of ATAI

The increased utilization of CT for diagnosis of ATAI has resulted in increased detection particularly of milder forms of aortic injury in more recent years. ATAI represents a spectrum of abnormalities that range from injuries isolated to the intima, to those that result in disruption of the entire wall.

Many different classification schemes have been proposed to grade the severity of injury and attempt to guide management. Beginning in the early 2000s, some authors have suggested classifying ATAI as either minimal aortic injury (MAI) or as "significant" aortic injury (SAI) [21]. Originally, MAI was defined as a sub-centimeter intimal abnormality (thrombus or flap) without external contour deformity, but many subsequent papers have expanded that definition either to include larger foci (e.g., up to 2 cm intimal flaps). In general, MAI is now considered to be any sub-centimeter intimo-medial abnormality with no external contour deformity of the aorta, which includes small intimal tears and intramural hematomas [21].

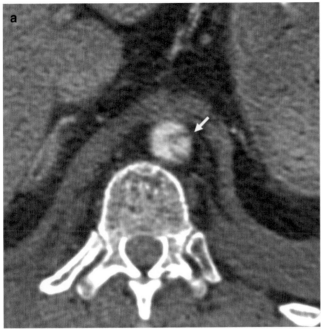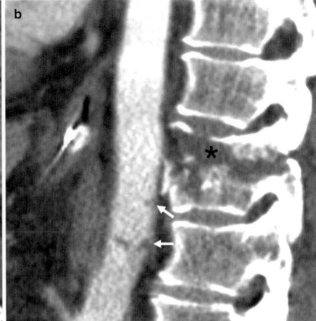

**Fig. 8** ATAI at the diaphragmatic hiatus in a 51-year-old involved in an MVC. Axial (**a**) and sagittal (**b**) CT images show a short segment flap in the descending aorta (arrows) at the diaphragmatic hiatus. The external contour of the aorta is normal. This injury was successfully managed nonoperatively without complication. Adjacent hematoma and pleural effusions attributable to the vertebral body fracture (asterisk, **b**)

Because of the variation of definitions of MAI/SAI, there have been other classification systems put forth. The most widely adopted is the 2011 Society for Vascular Surgery (SVS) severity score, which is now commonly used, and which divides aortic injuries into four categories based on the extent of injury to the aortic wall [12, 23]:

- Grade I – Intimal tear
- Grade II – Intramural hematoma
- Grade III – Pseudoaneurysm
- Grade IV – Rupture

Grade III and IV abnormalities are usually surgically managed (see below). SVS Grade I abnormalities are almost always managed conservatively, whereas grade II represent a "gray zone," with the more recent general trend to conservative management [19]. Regardless of the specific criteria used, injuries confined to the intima (SVS grade I and some grade II) may be managed conservatively, and several studies have shown that most cases resolve within 4–6 weeks, and only a minority of patients (10–15%) progress on follow-up imaging [21].

It may be difficult to precisely classify the SVS severity score based on CT alone, particularly when distinguishing between pseudoaneurysm and rupture (CT may lead to underestimation of grade IV abnormalities in particular). For this reason, and because of the lack of a consensus classification system, we encourage the imager to be thorough in their description of aortic injury, by including details that can help to determine if immediate intervention is needed, rather than simply applying a specific category of injury, as this description will help facilitate the timing and type of repair. Description of any aortic injury should include the following (both pertinent positives and negatives) [11]:

- Location of the injury (i.e., aortic root, isthmus, or descending aorta)
- Length of an intimo-medial flap
- Presence or absence of periaortic hematoma
- Size and length of any focal aortic contour deformity
- Presence or absence of active extravasation of contrast

**Management of ATAI**

Nearly all SVS grade I injuries, and many grade II injuries, are managed conservatively and most resolve on follow-up imaging [19]. Grade III and IV injuries are usually intervened upon if the patient survives and is stable enough for intervention. For patients undergoing treatment, the trend over the past two decades has been towards thoracic endovascular aortic repair (TEVAR), which is now the overwhelmingly favored approach with improved survival and fewer complications (9% vs 16% mortality; 0.8% vs 2.9% spinal cord injury for TEVAR vs. open repair) [19].

Imaging is essential for preoperative TEVAR planning using 3D reconstruction and centerline analysis of the CT (Fig. 10). Endovascular repair requires a 2 cm landing zone

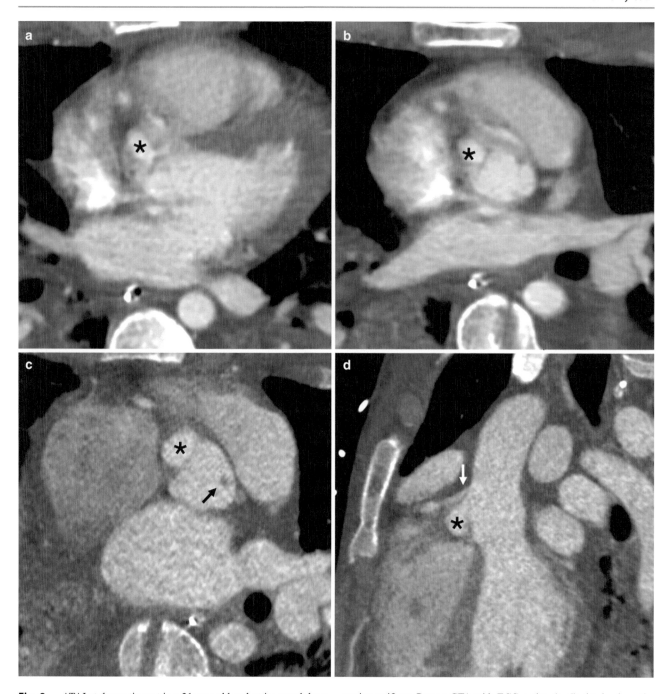

**Fig. 9** – ATAI at the aortic root in a 21-year-old pedestrian struck by a motor vehicle. Axial and 2D MPR images through the aortic root on non-ECG gated CT acquisition show a questionable outpouching (asterisk) at the right coronary sinus, which is incompletely evaluated due to motion artifacts. Repeat CTA with ECG gating (**c**, **d**) clearly show the ATAI involving the aortic root (asterisk, **c**, **d**) just below the right coronary artery (white arrow, **c**). A subtle intimo-medial flap is also visible in the aortic lumen (black arrow, **c**), which was confined at surgery

proximal to the site of injury and about 10 cm of length beyond the injury. Aortic diameter at each of these locations should be reported. Since the most common site of injury is distal to the left subclavian artery, an adequate landing zone may require sacrificing the origin of the left subclavian and placement of carotid to subclavian artery bypass graft. Any arch anomalies (e.g., an aberrant right subclavian artery, a vertebral artery origin directly from the aortic arch) that could be compromised by endovascular repair should also be reported [19].

## Potential Pitfalls and Mimics of ATAI on CT

Understanding pitfalls in the imaging of ATAI is essential to avoiding misdiagnosis due to technical artifacts or anatomic

**Fig. 10** Endovascular treatment of ATAI at the aortic isthmus. Chest CT sagittal MIP with contrast (**a**) shows full-thickness ATAI at the aortic isthmus (asterisk). Curved MPR (**b**) used for stent planning. The proximal landing zone is demarcated by the white lines. The black lines demarcate the length of the injury. LAO fluoroscopic image (**c**) shows a catheter in the aorta prior to stent placement. The aortic injury is visible (asterisk) distal to the left subclavian artery (arrow). Follow-up CT after stent placement (**d**) shows successful treatment of the aortic injury. The proximal stent is at the left subclavian artery (arrow) but does not occlude it

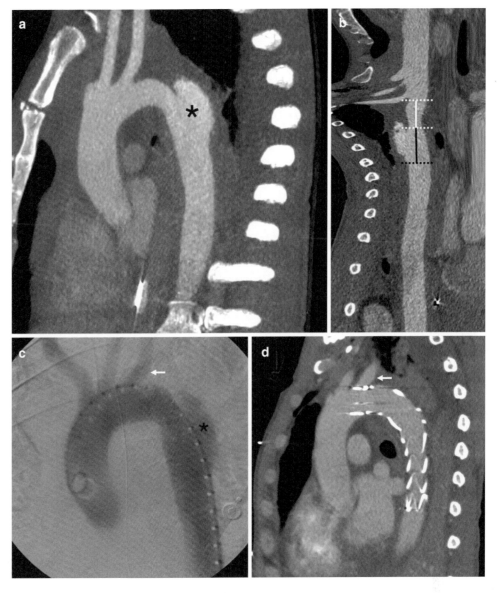

pitfalls/variants. Mediastinal hematoma may be due to other injuries especially when the fat plane surrounding the aorta is preserved (Fig. 11). Technical artifacts include streak artifact from beam hardening/photon starvation, respiratory motion artifact, cardiac pulsation artifact, and contrast/flow-related phenomena. Anatomic variants that can be confused for ATAI include ductus diverticulum, aortic spindle, and infundibula (which will be discussed in more detail below) at the origin of branch vessels. Rarely, the aortic thrombus is encountered in the absence of trauma. If there is any uncertainty as to whether an abnormality represents pathology or artifact, there should be a low threshold to reimage the patient with any necessary adjustment in technical factors (i.e., reposition patient's arms above their head if there is streak artifact, repeat with ECG gating if there is cardiac

pulsation, or re-bolus with delayed imaging if there is flow artifact) [24].

## Streak Artifact

Ideally, patients should be imaged with their arms in the abducted position, but this is not always feasible in trauma patients undergoing CT examinations. If the patient's arms are at their sides, then streak artifact may be substantial (especially in obese patients), which can be confused for hematoma or a flap/filling defect in the aortic lumen. Generally, streak artifact is seen to extend beyond the vessel lumen in a linear fashion, which can help distinguish this entity from true pathology, such as a flap.

Similarly, beam hardening from a dense column of venous contrast can result in linear low attenuation extending across

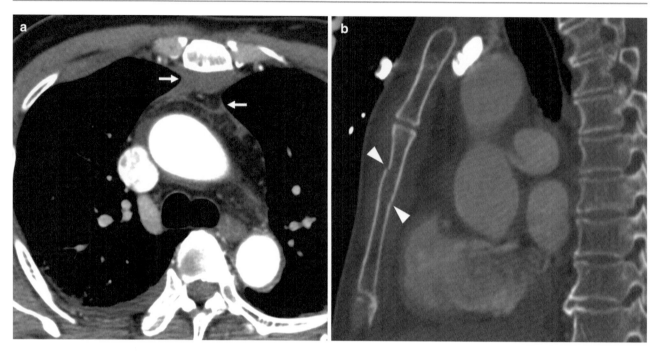

**Fig. 11** A 66-year-old with mediastinal hematoma from a sternal fracture. Axial CT image with contrast (**a**) shows hematoma in the mediastinum (arrows). The fat planes around the aorta are preserved, a clue that this is not due to ATAI. Sagittal reformation with bone windows (**b**) shows a subtle oblique fracture through the sternal body (arrowheads) which accounts for the hematoma

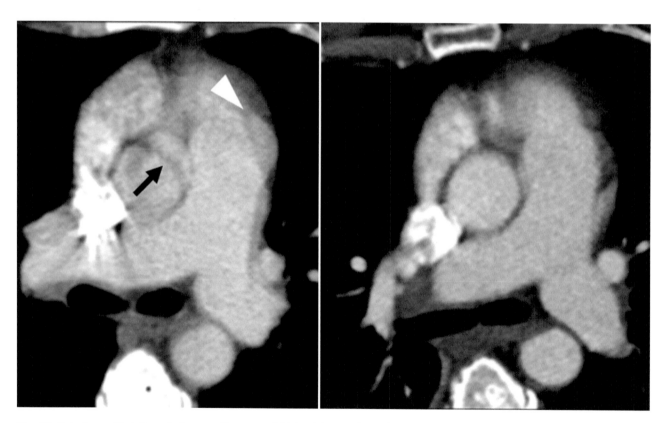

**Fig. 12** Pulsation artifact through the ascending aorta. Initial axial contrast-enhanced CT image (left) shows a curvilinear abnormality in the ascending aorta (arrow) that represents motion and should not be confused for an intimo-medial flap. Motion is also visible in the pulmonary artery (arrowhead). Repeat CT (**b**) confirms that the aorta is normal

the aortic lumen, which can also be confused for pathology (Fig. 12). The use of a saline chaser to flush contrast out of the central veins can be considered in this circumstance but is generally unnecessary [25].

## Respiratory Motion

Trauma patients are often unable to follow commands or hold their breath. Respiratory motion artifact usually manifests as a discontinuity in the aortic wall that is most apparent on sagittal or coronal CT images, in conjunction with similar stepwise discontinuity in other structures at the same level (e.g., the bones, heart, and chest wall), which can help confirm that the finding is artifactual. Similarly, viewing the images on lung windows may be beneficial, where motion artifact can have the appearance of ghosting or a "double vessel" in the adjacent lung parenchyma.

## Cardiac Pulsation

The aortic root and ascending aorta are particularly prone to pulsation artifact that may mimic an aortic contour abnormality or luminal flap. Pulsation artifact is generally curvilinear in configuration and extends beyond the normal expected aortic margins into the adjacent mediastinal fat and/or pulmonary artery (Fig. 12) [11]. Whereas a true flap is a discrete, well-defined abnormality, pulsation is often ill-defined with vague margins. Repeat CT with ECG-gating or further evaluation with echocardiography can be performed if there is any uncertainty.

## Flow Artifact

Flow artifact usually occurs when the scan is obtained before contrast has had time to adequately mix with blood and is usually seen along the lesser curvature of the aortic arch and proximal descending aorta. Flow artifact appears as ill-defined, wispy, smoke-like abnormalities that can be accentuated by narrow window/level settings and can be mistaken for intraluminal flaps (Fig. 13). Flow artifact is especially common when patients are scanned in the arterial phase on fast, modern CT scanners, particularly in patients with reduced cardiac output [26]. A repeat CT examination with delayed imaging can confirm that the flow artifact

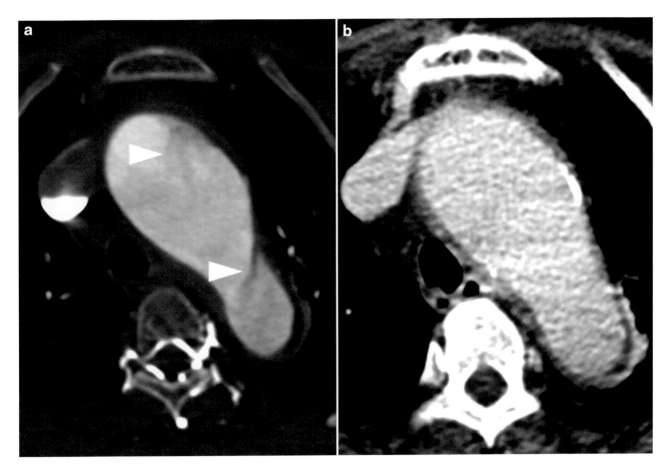

**Fig. 13** Flow artifact mimicking intimal flap in an 82-year-old following a fall. (**a**) Axial CT image in an arterial phase shows several ill-defined apparent filling defects in the aortic arch. (**b**) Venous phase imaging confirms that the abnormality represents flow artifact

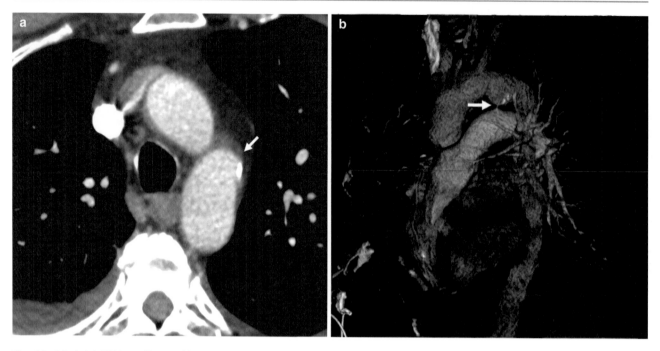

**Fig. 14** (**a**) Axial CT in a 61-year-old man involved in a MVC. A smoothly marginated outpouching along the inferolateral aortic arch (arrow), directed towards the left pulmonary artery, is consistent with a ductus diverticulum. Note the focus of calcification is suggestive of a chronic finding. The absence of indirect findings (e.g., mediastinal hematoma) also supports that this is not ATAI. (**b**) 3D volume-rendered images from CT shows the orientation of the ductus diverticulum towards the left pulmonary artery (arrow), as well as a ligamentum arteriosum

resolves or Hounsfield unit measurements can confirm that the density is too high for thrombus.

## Ductus Diverticulum

A ductus diverticulum (or ductus bump) is a focal bulge along the lesser curvature of the aortic isthmus (just distal to the left subclavian artery origin) at the site of the ductus arteriosus. This normal anatomic variant has a prevalence of approximately 10% and can easily be mistaken for ATAI [27]. A ductus diverticulum usually has smooth margins, forms an obtuse angle with the aortic lumen, and is oriented towards the main pulmonary artery (Fig. 14) [28]. A small calcified or fibrous remnant of the ligamentum arteriosum may be seen extending from the tip of the ductus diverticulum towards the pulmonary artery. ATAI, in contrast, usually forms acute angles relative to the aortic lumen and tends to be more irregular in morphology. Moreover, there should be no other direct or indirect findings of ATAI in the setting of a ductus diverticulum [27].

## Aortic Spindle

An aortic spindle, which is less common than a ductus diverticulum, is a smooth fusiform dilation of the proximal descending aorta just distal to the isthmus [28]. An aortic spindle is thought to represent a remnant of the fetal aorta and may extend over several centimeters. This abnormality is best

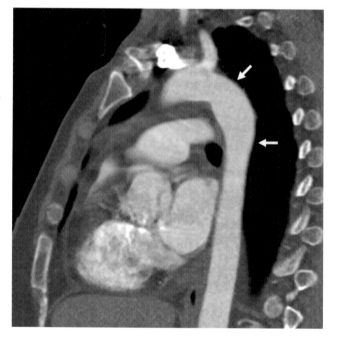

**Fig. 15** Oblique sagittal CT in a middle-aged man following a motor vehicle collision. The proximal descending aorta is focally dilated (arrows). The absence of direct or indirect findings of ATAI support the diagnosis of an aortic spindle, a normal anatomic variant that should not be confused for aortic injury

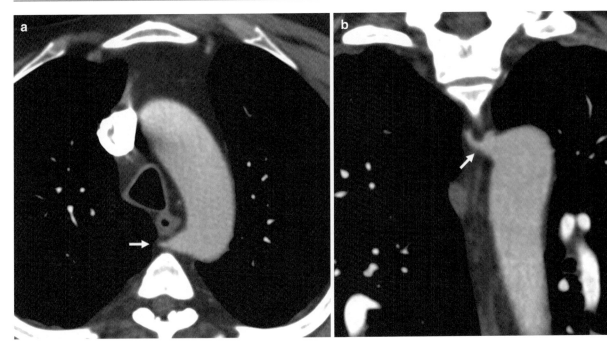

**Fig. 16** A 57-year-old man with a branch vessel infundibulum, which could be confused for ATAI. Axial (**a**) and coronal (**b**) CT images demonstrate a smoothly marginated outpouching from the distal arch with a conical shape and a small vessel arising from the tip of the infundibulum (representing an aberrant right vertebral artery)

confirmed on oblique multi-planar images, and as with other mimics, there should be no other direct or indirect signs of ATAI present (Fig. 15).

## Branch Vessel Infundibula

Branch vessels arising from the aorta may occasionally be dilated at their origins and should not be confused for ATAI. Branch vessel infundibula have a conical shape with smooth margins and a vessel arising from the apex of the outpouching [29]. Infundibula may be seen with the aortic arch vessels, bronchial arteries, intercostal arteries, or rarely, anatomic variants such as a vertebral artery arising directly from the aortic arch (Fig. 16).

## Mobile Aortic Thrombus

Thoracic aortic mobile thrombus is a rare but important mimic of ATAI. Most patients present with distal emboli that can be the cause – rather than the result – of trauma (i.e., a stroke resulting in loss of consciousness or distal limb ischemia resulting in decreased function). Aortic thrombi are discrete low attenuation filling defects in the aorta, may be either sessile or pedunculated, and may span up to several centimeters (usually larger than flaps resulting from aortic trauma) (Fig. 17). Mobile aortic thrombi usually occur along the lesser curve of the aortic arch or proximal descending aorta but can rarely occur in other locations [30]. Patients may have minimal or no underlying

atherosclerotic disease, and the management of these CT findings remains controversial, to our knowledge.

## Acute Traumatic Injury to Aortic Branch Vessels

Injuries to the branches of the thoracic aorta must be evaluated as they can easily be overlooked or obscured by streak artifact from the contrast in adjacent veins on CT. Approximately 30% of patients with branch injury will have a concomitant ATAI, while the rest occur in isolation [31]. The severity of branch artery injury may range from an isolated intimal defect to pseudoaneurysm or rupture (Fig. 18).

On radiography, the findings of branch artery injury are similar to that of ATAI involving the aortic isthmus and result from mediastinal hematoma accumulation. One important exception is an injury that is isolated to the brachiocephalic artery, which may cause right paratracheal widening and/or leftward deviation of the trachea and esophagus [11].

Management of branch artery injuries is less clear, but in our experience these can be managed either surgically or with stent placement in some cases. Failure to recognize branch artery injury may lead to enlargement of a pseudoaneurysm with a delayed presentation due to local mass effect (e.g., SVC syndrome, tracheal compression) or

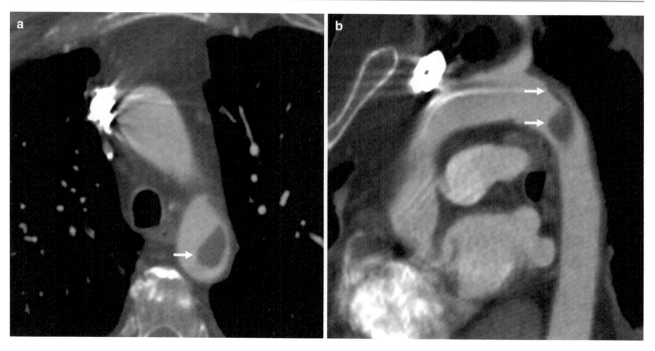

**Fig. 17** Thoracic aorta mobile thrombus in a 68-year-old woman. The patient was "found down" and underwent trauma CT. Axial (**a**) and oblique sagittal (**b**) images show a pedunculated filling defect in the aortic lumen (arrows). There were no other findings of aortic injury. This was confirmed to be a thrombus which had embolized to the brain and caused a stroke

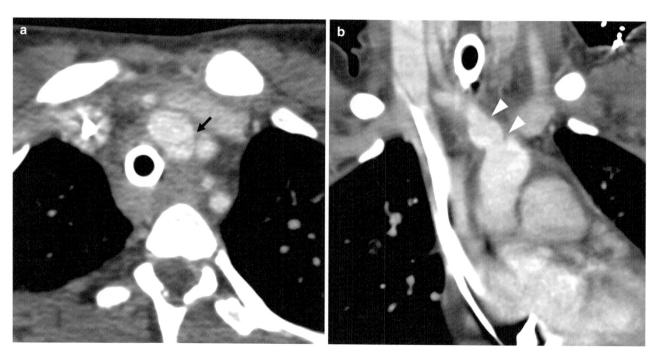

**Fig. 18** Traumatic injury to the brachiocephalic artery in a 17-year-old male involved in a MVC. Axial (**a**) CT image shows focal caliber change of the proximal brachiocephalic artery, a subtle intimal flap (arrow), and surrounding hematoma. The finding is better seen on the coronal image (**b**) as an approximately 1.5-cm-long injury (arrowheads). This was successfully treated with an endovascular stent (not shown)

embolic phenomenon causing stroke or upper extremity ischemia [32, 33].

## Other Blunt Vascular Injuries

Blunt injury to major veins in the thorax is rare and often the result of adjacent fracture/dislocation. There are both direct signs of vessel injury and indirect signs identifiable on imaging. As with arterial injuries, direct signs are more specific and include thrombosis/occlusion, avulsion, rupture with or without active extravasation, and pseudoaneurysm. Fat stranding, hematoma adjacent to a vessel, and vessel wall irregularity are indirect findings that could indicate venous injury but could also be due to bleeding from other sources including arterial injuries, solid organ injury, or fractures [34]. Although any vein can be injured, specific patterns of blunt trauma associated with venous injury include:

**Posterior dislocation of the clavicle with brachiocephalic vein injury:** Direct high-impact force on

the medial aspect of the clavicle may cause posterior dislocation at the sternoclavicular (SC) joint. The posterior movement of the clavicle can cause compression and/or laceration of mediastinal vessels including the brachiocephalic veins [35]. Posterior SC joint dislocation may be difficult to recognize clinically, and the imaging findings including clavicular head malalignment on radiograph and posterior displacement of the clavicular head with surrounding hematoma on CT may be subtle. Hematoma and/or brachiocephalic vein injury should prompt careful examination for posterior SC joint dislocation and vice versa (Fig. 19).

**Vena cava injuries:** Blunt injury to the superior or inferior vena cava is most often due to deceleration, and these injuries are very rare to observe at imaging as patients usually die prior to imaging. As with other vascular injuries, SVC and IVC injuries usually occur at sites of relative fixation near their insertion into the right atrium. Depending on whether or not the injury is intra- or extra-pericardial dictates whether there is hemopericardium or hematoma in the mediastinum/adjacent to the liver. IVC injuries are often associated with severe hepatic parenchymal injuries [34].

**Fig. 19** Posterior dislocation of the left clavicle in a young male with injury to the left subclavian vein. Axial CT images (**a**, **b**) show that the head of the left clavicle is dislocated posteriorly (asterisk) and narrows the left subclavian vein (arrowhead, **b**). A moderate amount of hematoma surrounds the dislocation. Despite the lack of apparent injury, a laceration to the left subclavian vein was found and was repaired at surgery

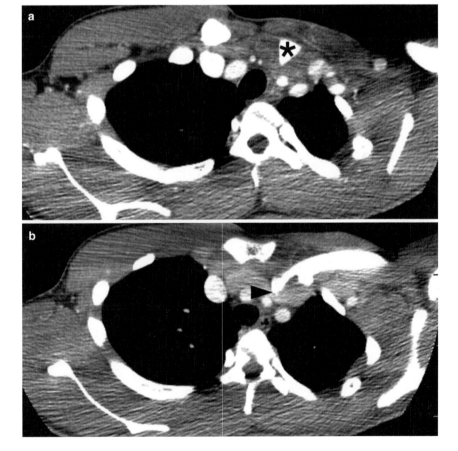

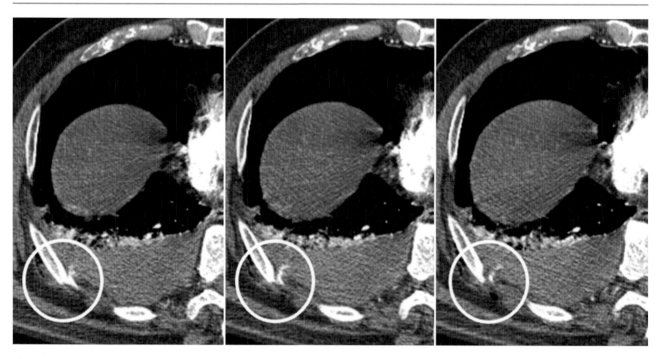

**Fig. 20** A 67-year-old man with intercostal artery injury secondary to blunt trauma/rib fracture. Sequential axial images from a CT show a mildly displaced acute rib fracture (left), with a small jet of arterial contrast flowing into the small right hemothorax (circles)

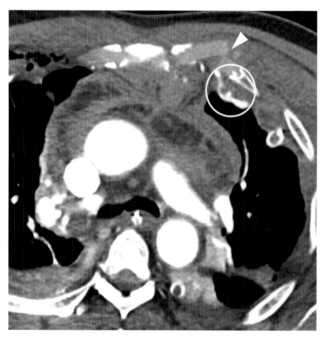

**Fig. 21** Contrast-enhanced axial CT in a 72-year-old man with left internal mammary artery injury from steering wheel impact/MVC. The left second costal cartilage is fractured (arrowhead), with active extravasation in the left extra-pleural space (circle). Extensive mediastinal hematoma is present, although note the preserved fat planes with the pulmonary artery and aorta

**Vessel injury adjacent to fractures:** Any fracture may be associated with adjacent venous injury. Common injuries include intercostal vessel injury secondary to rib fractures (Fig. 20), internal mammary vessel from anterior rib or sternal injury (Fig. 21), and azygos/hemiazygos injury due to spinal fracture [36, 37].

**Extra-pleural hematoma**: Injury to intercostal vessels usually results in hemothorax due to disruption of the parietal pleura. However, hematoma may accumulate in the extra-pleural space if the parietal pleura remains intact. These injuries are frequently misdiagnosed as hemothorax but are important to recognize as they will not be drained by thoracostomy tubes, and may require surgical evacuation if causing respiratory or hemodynamic compromise [38, 39]. Extra-pleural hematoma is most frequently seen in association with rib fractures due to blunt trauma but can rarely be seen in penetrating trauma or aortic rupture.

On CT, the most important imaging finding is a displaced extra-pleural fat sign, where the extra-pleural fat is deviated internally (Fig. 22). Extra-pleural hematomas tend to be lentiform in shape and may show active extravasation from the involved intercostal vessel [38].

## Penetrating Trauma

Most penetrating thoracic trauma is limited to the chest wall and lung parenchyma and therefore may be initially imaged with CXR. Penetrating non-mediastinal trauma in hemodynamically stable patients is often treated conservatively. If hemodynamically stable, patients with evidence of

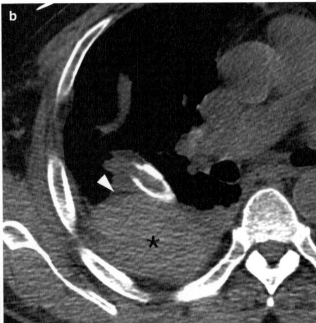

**Fig. 22** A 61-year-old with an extra-pleural hematoma from blunt trauma/rib fracture. (**a**) Axial CT image with IV contrast shows a right pleural effusion is present; however, note the lentiform-shaped high attenuation collection more posteriorly (asterisk) with displaced extra-pleural fat (arrowheads). A minimally displaced posterolateral rib fracture is visible (circle). (**b**) Non-contrast CT after chest tube placement shows that the pleural effusion was successfully drained but does not communicate with the extra-pleural hematoma. The displaced extra-pleural fat is still visible (arrowhead)

substantial mediastinal or vascular injury (such as mediastinal widening on CXR, a large hemothorax, or hemopericardium) may undergo CT [40]. The use of CT has been shown to decrease the number of surgical interventions, reduced length of hospitalizations, and improved outcomes in patients with penetrating trauma [41].

Whereas blunt trauma lends to particular patterns of injury as described above (e.g., at sites of vessel attachment or fixation, adjacent to fractures, etc.), penetrating trauma yields less predictable injury patterns which depend on the type of projectile and the trajectory. Some institutions may place skin markers at sites of entry/exit wounds that can be identified on imaging. It is critical for the imager to identify sites of entry and exit (if applicable), determine the most likely path of the injury (which may not be a straight line with projectiles), and carefully evaluate the entire tract for evidence of injury. Thin-section CT with near-isotropic data sets allows double-oblique reformats to trace the path of penetrating injury (CT trajectory analysis) [42].

The severity of projectile injury will vary with factors beyond the scope of this chapter, including type/velocity of ammunition and distance from the target. GSWs will damage vessels and surrounding tissues by two main mechanisms: (1) laceration from the object traveling through the body and (2) the shockwave of energy transfer along the path perpendicular to the actual projectile (also known as the "temporary cavity"). The temporary cavity may be up to 7 times larger than the size of the projectile and can cause vascular injury not in direct communication to the path of the projectile. Projectiles notoriously travel in a nonlinear fashion as they deflect and ricochet off of bones and other dense tissues (Figs. 23 and 24). Stab wounds may be subtler on imaging but tend to be linear and also tend to be more superficial (Fig. 25) [6]. Distal embolization of bullets and other projectiles is a rare but known phenomenon that can be observed on imaging.

## CT Findings of Penetrating Vascular Injury

The approach to assessing penetrating injury includes:

- Obtain information regarding the type and number of injuries (i.e., GSW vs. SW).
- Determine sites of entry and exit (if applicable).
- Reconstruct the path of the trauma on CT, which may be angular or curved: findings along the path of injury include gas, fragments/debris, bone, and stranding/hematoma.
- Assess every structure along the trajectory and assume that they may have been injured.
- Search for injuries outside of the direct path within the temporary cavity.

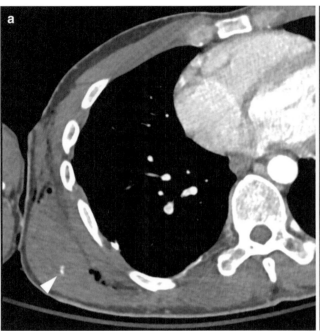

**Fig. 23** A 39-year-old with a gunshot wound to the right chest. Arterial phase (**a**) axial CT image shows a small blush of contrast with a hematoma in the right latissimus dorsi muscle (arrowhead). Venous phase (**b**) axial CT image shows more pooling of extravasated contrast (circle). Injury to a branch of the thoracodorsal artery, which was subsequently confirmed at catheter angiography

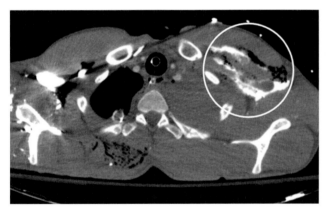

**Fig. 24** Gunshot wound to the left subclavian vein. The entry wound was in the left anterior chest with an exit wound in the right back. Axial contrast-enhanced CT image shows extensive contrast extravasation and soft tissue gas surrounding the left subclavian vessels (circle). Laceration of the left subclavian vein was confirmed at surgery

CT imaging findings of penetrating vascular trauma include direct and indirect findings [6, 40] (Table 2).

Commonly injured vessels include intercostal and internal mammary vessels. Mediastinal vessel injury is less common but potentially more severe. Injury to the aorta or arch vessels results in ~90% mortality, thus only a minority of these patients undergo imaging [6]. Patients with vascular injury may undergo open surgical repair/ligation or percutaneous

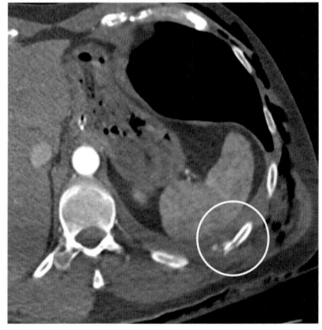

**Fig. 25** Axial contrast-enhanced CT image in a 37-year-old man who was stabbed in the back. A posterior 10th rib fracture is visible with adjacent active extravasation from an intercostal artery (circle). The diaphragm was not injured despite proximity to the injured rib and vessel

treatment with stent grafts or embolization, based on the severity and location of imaging.

**Table 2** CT Findings of Penetrating Vascular Injury

| Direct | Indirect |
| --- | --- |
| Vessel occlusion or abrupt caliber change | Perivascular hematoma |
| Intraluminal filling defect (thrombus or flap) | Perivascular fat stranding |
| Pseudoaneurysm | Projectile resting in proximity to the vessel |
| Active extravasation of contrast | Course of projectile near/through the vessel |
| Arteriovenous malformation | End-organ infarct |

# Conclusion

Thoracic vascular trauma is a substantial cause of morbidity and mortality. The imager must be familiar with the similarities and differences between patterns/mechanisms of injury in blunt and penetrating trauma. CT is the most frequently used modality for diagnosis and treatment planning in vascular trauma. Recognition and thorough description of direct and indirect findings of vascular injury, the vessel(s) involved, and other complications are essential to help guide the appropriate and timely management of trauma patients.

# References

1. Kaewlai R, Avery LL, Asrani AV, Novelline RA. Multidetector CT of blunt thoracic trauma. RadioGraphics. 2008;28:1555–70. https://doi.org/10.1148/rg.286085510.
2. Iacobellis F, Ierardi AM, Mazzei MA, Magenta Biasina A, Carrafiello G, Nicola R, et al. Dual-phase CT for the assessment of acute vascular injuries in high-energy blunt trauma: the imaging findings and management implications. BJR. 2016;89:20150952. https://doi.org/10.1259/bjr.20150952.
3. MMedSci DLC. Emergency operation for penetrating thoracic trauma in a metropolitan surgical service in South Africa n.d.:6.
4. Nummela MT, Thorisdottir S, Oladottir GL, Koskinen SK. Imaging of penetrating thoracic trauma in a large nordic trauma center. Acta Radiol Open. 2019;8. https://doi.org/10.1177/2058460119895485.
5. Clarke DL, Quazi MA, Reddy K, Thomson SR. Emergency operation for penetrating thoracic trauma in a metropolitan surgical service in South Africa. J Thorac Cardiovasc Surg. 2011;142:563–8. https://doi.org/10.1016/j.jtcvs.2011.03.034.
6. Truesdell W, Gore A, Primakov D, Lieberman H, Jankowska D, Joshi G, et al. Ballistic and penetrating injuries of the chest. J Thorac Imaging. 2020;35:W51–9. https://doi.org/10.1097/RTI.0000000000000449.
7. Davies MJ, Wells C, Squires PA, Hodgetts TJ, Lecky FE. Civilian firearm injury and death in England and Wales. Emerg Med J. 2012;29:10–4. https://doi.org/10.1136/emj.2009.085837.
8. Störmann P, Gartner K, Wyen H, Lustenberger T, Marzi I, Wutzler S. Epidemiology and outcome of penetrating injuries in a Western European urban region. Eur J Trauma Emerg Surg. 2016;42:663–9. https://doi.org/10.1007/s00068-016-0630-4.
9. Newbury A, Dorfman JD, Lo HS. Imaging and management of thoracic trauma. Semin Ultrasound CT MRI. 2018;39:347–54. https://doi.org/10.1053/j.sult.2018.03.006.
10. Sierink JC, Treskes K, Edwards MJR, Beuker BJA, den Hartog D, Hohmann J, et al. Immediate total-body CT scanning versus conventional imaging and selective CT scanning in patients with severe trauma (REACT-2): a randomised controlled trial. Lancet. 2016;388:673–83. https://doi.org/10.1016/S0140-6736(16)30932-1.
11. Raptis CA, Hammer MM, Raman KG, Mellnick VM, Bhalla S. Acute traumatic aortic injury: practical considerations for the diagnostic radiologist. J Thorac Imaging. 2015;30:202–13. https://doi.org/10.1097/RTI.0000000000000149.
12. Lee WA, Matsumura JS, Mitchell RS, Farber MA, Greenberg RK, Azizzadeh A, et al. Endovascular repair of traumatic thoracic aortic injury: clinical practice guidelines of the Society for Vascular Surgery. J Vasc Surg. 2011;53:187–92. https://doi.org/10.1016/j.jvs.2010.08.027.
13. Rajput MZ, Raptis DA, Raptis CA, Bhalla S. Imaging of acute traumatic aortic injury. Curr Radiol Rep. 2018;6:19. https://doi.org/10.1007/s40134-018-0278-4.
14. Steenburg SD, Ravenel JG, Ikonomidis JS, Schönholz C, Reeves S. Acute traumatic aortic injury: imaging evaluation and management. Radiology. 2008;248:748–62. https://doi.org/10.1148/radiol.2483071416.
15. Creasy JD, Chiles C, Routh WD, Dyer RB. Overview of traumatic injury of the thoracic aorta. RadioGraphics. 1997;17:27–45. https://doi.org/10.1148/radiographics.17.1.9017797.
16. Demetriades D, Velmahos GC, Scalea TM, Jurkovich GJ, Karmy-Jones R, Teixeira PG, et al. Diagnosis and treatment of blunt thoracic aortic injuries: changing perspectives. J Trauma Inj Infect Crit Care. 2008;64:1415–9. https://doi.org/10.1097/TA.0b013e3181715e32.
17. Ho RT, Blackmore CC, Bloch RD, Hoffer EK, Mann FA, Stern EJ, et al. Can we rely on mediastinal widening on chest radiography to identify subjects with aortic injury? Emerg Radiol. 2002;9:183–7. https://doi.org/10.1007/s10140-002-0219-6.
18. Schwab CW, Lawson RB, Lind JF, Garland LW. Aortic injury: comparison of supine and upright portable chest films to evaluate the widened mediastinum. Ann Emerg Med. 1984;13:896–9. https://doi.org/10.1016/S0196-0644(84)80665-4.
19. Mouawad NJ, Paulisin J, Hofmeister S, Thomas MB. Blunt thoracic aortic injury – concepts and management. J Cardiothorac Surg. 2020;15:1–8. https://doi.org/10.1186/s13019-020-01101-6.
20. Zaw AA, Stewart D, Murry JS, Hoang DM, Sun B, Ashrafian S, et al. CT chest with IV contrast compared with CT angiography after blunt trauma. Am Surg. 2016;82:41–5. https://doi.org/10.1177/000313481608200122.
21. Kapoor H, Lee JT, Orr NT, Nisiewicz MJ, Pawley BK, Zagurovskaya M. Minimal aortic injury: mechanisms, imaging manifestations, natural history, and management. RadioGraphics. 2020;40:1834–47. https://doi.org/10.1148/rg.2020200066.
22. Gunn MLD, Lehnert BE, Lungren RS, Narparla CB, Mitsumori L, Gross JA, et al. Minimal aortic injury of the thoracic aorta: imaging appearances and outcome. Emerg Radiol. 2014;21:227–33. https://doi.org/10.1007/s10140-013-1187-8.
23. Azizzadeh A, Keyhani K, Miller CC, Coogan SM, Safi HJ, Estrera AL. Blunt traumatic aortic injury: initial experience with endovascular repair. J Vasc Surg. 2009;49:1403–8. https://doi.org/10.1016/j.jvs.2009.02.234.
24. Gutschow SE, Walker CM, Martínez-Jiménez S, Rosado-de-Christenson ML, Stowell J, Kunin JR. Emerging concepts in intramural hematoma imaging. RadioGraphics. 2016;36:660–74. https://doi.org/10.1148/rg.2016150094.
25. Kalisz K, Buethe J, Saboo SS, Abbara S, Halliburton S, Rajiah P. Artifacts at cardiac CT: physics and solutions. RadioGraphics. 2016;36:2064–83. https://doi.org/10.1148/rg.2016160079.

26. Henry TS, Hammer MM, Little BP, Jensen LE, Kligerman SJ, Kanne JP, et al. Smoke: how to differentiate flow-related artifacts from pathology on thoracic computed tomographic angiography. J Thorac Imaging. 2019;34:W109. https://doi.org/10.1097/RTI.0000000000000429.

27. Hyung Ann J, Young Kim E, Mi Jeong Y, Ho Kim J, Sik Kim H, Choi H-Y. Morphologic evaluation of ductus diverticulum using multi – detector computed tomography: comparison with traumatic pseudoaneurysm of the aortic isthmus. Iran J Radiol. 2016;13. https://doi.org/10.5812/iranjradiol.38016.

28. Agarwal PP, Chughtai A, Matzinger FRK, Kazerooni EA. Multidetector CT of thoracic aortic aneurysms. RadioGraphics. 2009;29:537–52. https://doi.org/10.1148/rg.292075080.

29. Mirvis SE, Shanmuganathan K. Diagnosis of blunt traumatic aortic injury 2007: still a nemesis. Eur J Radiol. 2007;64:27–40. https://doi.org/10.1016/j.ejrad.2007.02.016.

30. Pagni S, Trivedi J, Ganzel BL, Williams M, Kapoor N, Ross C, et al. Thoracic aortic mobile thrombus: is there a role for early surgical intervention? Ann Thorac Surg. 2011;91:1875–81. https://doi.org/10.1016/j.athoracsur.2011.02.011.

31. Holdgate A, Dunlop S. Review of branch aortic injuries in blunt chest trauma. Emerg Med Australas. 2005;17:49–56. https://doi.org/10.1111/j.1742-6723.2005.00679.x.

32. Kanwar M, Desai D, Joumaa M, Guduguntla V. Traumatic brachiocephalic pseudoaneurysm presenting as stroke in a seventeen-year-old. Clin Cardiol. 2009;32:E43–5. https://doi.org/10.1002/clc.20341.

33. Alamdari NM, Bakhtiyari M. Endovascular treatment of innominate artery pseudoaneurysm. Surg Pract. 2018;22:38–41. https://doi.org/10.1111/1744-1633.12291.

34. Holly BP, Steenburg SD. Multidetector CT of blunt traumatic venous injuries in the chest, abdomen, and pelvis. RadioGraphics. 2011;31:1415–24. https://doi.org/10.1148/rg.315105221.

35. di Mento L, Staletti L, Cavanna M, Mocchi M, Berlusconi M. Posterior sternoclavicular joint dislocation with brachiocephalic vein injury: a case report. Injury. 2015;46:S8–10. https://doi.org/10.1016/S0020-1383(15)30036-X.

36. Endara SA, Davalos GA, Nuñez MF, Manzano JE. Azygous vein laceration secondary to blunt thoraco-abdominal trauma. Interact Cardiovasc Thorac Surg. 2010;11:342–4. https://doi.org/10.1510/icvts.2010.234666.

37. Chen J, Lv J, Ma K, Yan J. Assessment of internal mammary artery injury after blunt chest trauma: a literature review. J Zhejiang Univ Sci B. 2014;15:864–9. https://doi.org/10.1631/jzus.B1400098.

38. Chung JH, Carr RB, Stern EJ. Extrapleural hematomas: imaging appearance, classification, and clinical significance. J Thorac Imaging. 2011;26:218–23. https://doi.org/10.1097/RTI.0b013e3181ebeaba.

39. Choi YS, Kim SJ, Ryu SW, Kang SK. Traumatic extrapleural hematoma mimicking hemothorax. J Trauma Inj. 2017;30:202–5. https://doi.org/10.20408/jti.2017.30.4.202.

40. Durso AM, Caban K, Munera F. Penetrating thoracic injury. Radiol Clin N Am. 2015;53:675–93. https://doi.org/10.1016/j.rcl.2015.02.010.

41. van den Hout WJ, van der Wilden GM, Boot F, Idenburg FJ, Rhemrev SJ, Hoencamp R. Early CT scanning in the emergency department in patients with penetrating injuries: does it affect outcome? Eur J Trauma Emerg Surg. 2018;44:607–14. https://doi.org/10.1007/s00068-017-0831-5.

42. Dreizin D, Munera F. Multidetector CT for penetrating torso trauma: state of the art. Radiology. 2015;277:338–55. https://doi.org/10.1148/radiol.2015142282.

# Acute Aortic Syndrome Imaging

**17**

Kacie L. Steinbrecher, Sanjeev Bhalla, Kaitlin M. Marquis, and Constantine A. Raptis

## Contents

### Abstract

The acute aortic syndrome can be caused by three interrelated conditions involving the aorta with possibility of rupture – aortic dissection, intramural hematoma, and penetrating atherosclerotic ulcer. Diagnostic imaging plays a pivotal role in diagnosis and management, with CT being the most commonly utilized. Although there is significant overlap between these three entities, understanding both the pathophysiology and imaging features is essential for facilitating prompt diagnosis and management.

### Keywords

Aortic Dissection · Intramural Hematoma · Penatrating Atherosclerotic Ulcer · Acute Aortic Syndrome

## Introduction

The acute aortic syndrome is most commonly caused by three interrelated conditions involving the aorta with possibility of rupture – aortic dissection (AD), intramural hematoma (IMH), and penetrating atherosclerotic ulcer (PAU) [1]. These entities can occur as isolated processes or can be found in association to varying degrees and extents. In some cases, these entities can evolve into each other over time, such that what may have originally presented as an IMH may ultimately become an AD. Clinically, these syndromes have similar signs and symptoms. Classically, this includes acute and severe chest pain of a tearing, ripping, migrating, or pulsating nature, but the clinical presentation and physical examination findings may also be vague and variable. All of these pathologies involve disruption of the media layer of the aorta, and can progress to an aneurysm and rupture [2]. As a result, prompt diagnosis and treatment are vital to reduce patient morbidity and mortality [3, 4].

K. L. Steinbrecher (✉) · S. Bhalla · K. M. Marquis · C. A. Raptis
Mallinckrodt Institute of Radiology, St. Louis, MO, USA
e-mail: kacie.steinbrecher@wustl.edu

© Springer Nature Switzerland AG 2022
M. N. Patlas et al. (eds.), *Atlas of Emergency Imaging from Head-to-Toe*,
https://doi.org/10.1007/978-3-030-92111-8_17

## Imaging Considerations

In addition to confirming the diagnosis of acute aortic syndrome, goals of imaging include describing the site and extension of the pathology, identifying complications, and discussing findings relevant to treatment and prognosis. There are three main imaging examinations used to accomplish these goals – computed tomography (CT), transesophageal echocardiography (TEE), and magnetic resonance imaging (MRI) [2]. From a diagnostic standpoint, these tests are equivalent, and have a sensitivity over 98% and specificity over 95% [5–7] in the diagnosis of aortic dissection. Availability, speed, and spatial resolution have made CT the imaging modality of choice, especially in the emergency setting. TEE can be performed at the bedside, and aid in the diagnosis of an unstable patient on the floor or in the operating room. TEE does, however, require an experienced operator, sedation, and intubation. Additionally, TEE is limited in evaluating structures surrounding the aorta, and can have "blind spots" related to the tracheal air column [8]. The main advantages of MR imaging are the lack of ionizing radiation or iodinated contrast. Thus, in the acute setting, MR imaging can also be used as an alternative to CTA in patients with at risk renal function or iodinated contrast allergy. From a diagnostic standpoint, one advantage of MR imaging is the ability to depict dynamic complications including left ventricular dysfunction and valvular regurgitation [9, 10]. Owing to its high-contrast resolution, MR imaging can also be of value in better characterizing or confirming the presence of subtle wall pathology involving the ascending aorta, particularly in the setting of suspected IMH seen on CT.

Given that CT is the most commonly used imaging modality used to evaluate patients with suspected acute aortic syndrome, the remainder of this chapter will focus on CT. At our institution, the CT acute aortic syndrome protocol begins with a noncontrast acquisition of the chest to evaluate for an intramural hematoma, which may become obscured by contrast in the aorta. Additionally, the noncontrast acquisition can help identify blood products in extravascular spaces. The noncontrast portion of the protocol is performed with a slice thickness of 3 mm, reconstruction intervals of 3 mm, and no gap. After the nonenhanced CT, an IV contrast-enhanced CT angiogram is performed with bolus tracking timed off the aorta using an injection rate of 4–5 mL/s. Coverage extends from the thoracic outlet to the femoral heads in order to evaluate the distal extent of pathology, detect potential ischemic pathology in abdominal solid organs and bowel, and to allow for pre-procedure planning if endovascular repair or peripheral bypass is considered. The angiogram portion of the protocol is completed with a slice thickness of 1–2 mm, reconstruction intervals of 1–2 mm, and at least 33% overlap to allow or high-quality 3D and multiplanar reconstructions. Increasingly, multiplanar images are reconstructed directly from the raw data to minimize artifacts.

## Aortic Dissection

Aortic dissection is the most common acute aortic emergency, compromising about 90% of the cases of acute aortic syndrome [6, 9, 11]. AD is characterized by an intimo-medial entry tear that allows blood to enter the medial layer of the aorta, forming a true lumen and false lumen separated by an intimo-medial flap. Hypertension is the most frequent factor predisposing patients to aortic dissection. Connective tissue disorders (Marfan, Turner, Ehlers-Danlos, and Loeys-Dietz syndromes) also are also associated with AD, as is a bicuspid aortic valve, which results in cystic medial necrosis in the ascending aorta [12]. Less common associations include cocaine, anabolic steroids, and autoimmune conditions [13].

## Making the Diagnosis

In most cases, diagnosis of an aortic dissection on CT is straightforward and can be made by identifying an intimo-medial flap separating the true lumen from the false lumen [11, 14]. In a minority of cases involving the ascending aorta, however, a definable intimo-medial flap is not seen or poorly seen; these "flapless type A aortic dissections" have been referred to in the literature as a "localized type A dissection," "limited dissection," or "incomplete dissection." These flapless type A aortic dissections typically involve an intimo-medial tear that causes a contained rupture of the aorta, usually within 2 cm of the aortic valve [7]. On CT, diagnosis of these cases requires recognition of subtle findings, including irregularity along the aortic wall, small focal wall defects or outpouchings, and short strands of intimo-medial tissue extending into the lumen (Fig. 1). If hemopericardium or other findings of ascending aortic rupture are seen without a classic intimo-medial flap, suspicion for a "flapless type A dissection" should be high, prompting close examination of the ascending aortic wall, particularly in the proximal posteromedial aorta near the root where these dissections often occur. In difficult or suspicious cases, CT with EKG gating or ultrahigh pitch may be useful to show these subtle findings in the ascending aorta to advantage.

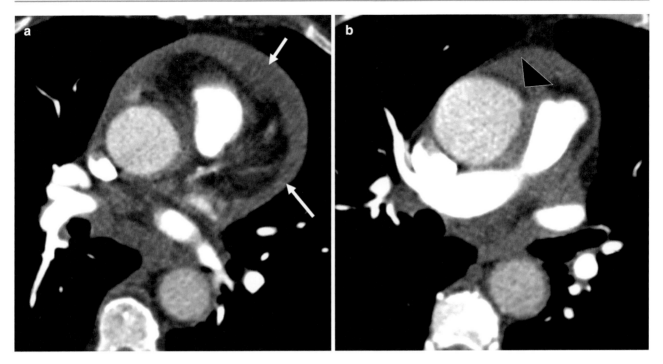

**Fig. 1** Flapless type A dissection (AD) in a patient with chest pain. (**a** and **b**) Two axial CT images from a pulmonary embolism protocol demonstrate high attenuating pericardial fluid consistent with hemopericardium (arrow). Less obvious is a subtle irregularity and bulging contour along the posteromedial ascending aortic wall (arrowhead), indicating the presence of a type A aortic dissection. The patient later expired and an intimo-medial defect along the posteromedial aorta was found at autopsy

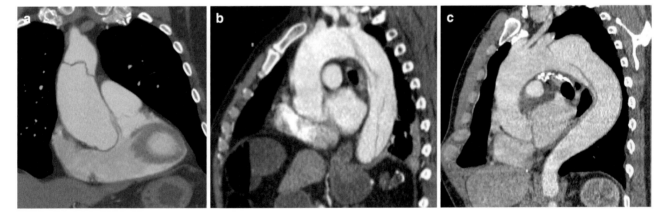

**Fig. 2** Stanford-type classifications of aortic dissections. (**a**) Type A AD in patient with a bicuspid aortic valve; the dissection flap is localized proximal to the brachiocephalic artery. (**b**) Stanford type B AD with arch involvement in a patient with chest pain; the dissection flap is localized distal to the brachiocephalic artery and proximal to the left subclavian artery. (**c**) Stanford type B without arch involvement; the dissection is noted with the dissection flap starting distal to the left subclavian artery

## Describing the Distribution

Classification of AD is based on location and extension of the intimomedial flap. In the emergency radiology setting, the Stanford classification system is preferred due to its implications for management and its relative ease. Stanford type A dissections involve the ascending aorta proximal to the brachiocephalic artery, and are treated surgically. A Stanford type B dissection involves the descending aorta beyond the origin of the brachiocephalic artery. Type B dissections may have aortic arch involvement distal to the brachiocephalic artery and proximal to the left subclavian artery; these are best described as "type B aortic dissection with arch involvement" (Fig. 2). While Stanford type B dissections are often

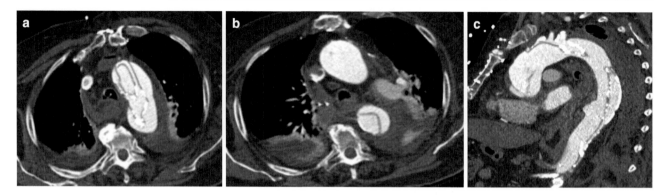

**Fig. 3** Intimo-medial intussusception in a patient with chest pain. Axial (**a** and **b**) and sagittal (**c**) images from a dissection protocol show an easily indefinable intimo-medial flap in the aortic arch (**a**) and proximal descending aorta (**b**). Within the arch (**a**), the flap has an unusual configuration, with invagination of the flap into itself. Extension into the ascending aorta is best viewed on sagittal reconstructions (**c**)

treated conservatively with antihypertensive medication, intervention may be warranted if there are findings of worsening dilatation or rupture, hemodynamic instability, and limb or end-organ compromise [15].

Determining whether the ascending aorta is involved in an AD is often straightforward, but can be difficult in the setting of an intimo-intimal intussusception, which involves a 360-degree tear that causes the intima and inner media to float in the aortic lumen and telescope on itself (Fig. 3). In cases of intimo-intimal intussusception, the intimo-medial tear usually begins in the proximal ascending aorta, but because of the telescoping flap, the proximal extent of the dissection can be difficult to appreciate, particularly on axial images [16, 17]. Thus, when an intimo-intimal intussusception is seen, the interpreting radiologist should closely scrutinize the ascending aorta, particularly on sagittal images, to appreciate the true extent of the dissection.

There are certain circumstances when type A dissections may not be treated surgically. These include iatrogenic aortic dissections (IAD) and spontaneous acute retrograde type A dissections (RTAD) [18]. IAD is a rare care complication of percutaneous coronary interventions, with optimal management being less clear to our knowledge. While initial studies reported a 50% mortality rate following surgical management of IAD, recent registry data suggest that mortality is comparable to that of spontaneous ADs, near 16% [19, 20]. Spontaneous acute retrograde type A dissections have been described in 7–25% of dissections [21]. While most type A dissections begin in the aortic root or ascending aorta with antegrade propagation, RTAD originates from a primary tear in the descending aorta, with the false lumen propagating in a direction that opposes blood flow. These occur spontaneously and as a complication of conventional cardiac surgery or thoracic aortic endovascular repair (TEVAR). A conservative approach for RTAD may be adopted in selected circumstances [18, 22].

Thoracic aortic dissection may also be described according to chronicity, depending on its clinical manifestation. A dissection is considered acute if symptoms last less than two weeks, subacute if symptoms last between 2 weeks and 2 months, and chronic if symptoms persist longer than 2 months [11]. Although a thick flap may suggest a chronic dissection, it can also be seen in acute dissections, and therefore is not a reliable sign in determining chronicity.

Another important factor in describing the distribution of AD is distinguishing between the true lumen and false lumen, which is essential for both surgical and percutaneous intervention. CT features characteristic of the true lumen include direct communication with the aorta tracing back to the valve plane, a smaller centrally located lumen, and greater early enhancement with faster washout. Additionally, intimal calcification generally outlines the true lumen. In contrast, the false lumen is generally larger and demonstrates hypoenhancement in early phase relative to the true lumen with delayed washout due to slower flow. As a result, thrombus is more likely to develop in the false lumen. Early contrast bolus timing may mimic a thrombosed false lumen, and meticulous evaluation is required. Two additional indicators of the false lumen include the "cobweb" sign and the "beak" sign. Slender linear areas of low attenuation, known as the cobweb sign, represent residual medial layers that were sheared during the dissection process (Fig. 4). The beak sign describes the acute angle formed in the false lumen at its interface with the aortic wall and intimo-medial flap [2, 6, 11, 13] (Fig. 5). Table 1 summarizes CT differences that are helpful in distinguishing the true from the false lumen.

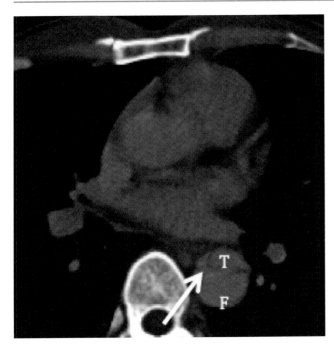

**Fig. 4** "Cobweb" sign. Axial IV contrast-enhanced CT image in a patient with a Stanford type B dissection shows linear areas of low attenuation (arrow) within the false lumen (F). Note the true lumen is smaller than the false lumen

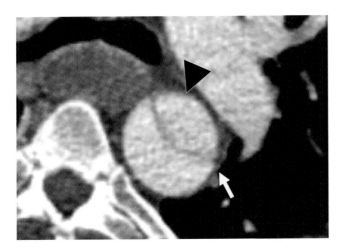

**Fig. 5** "Beak" sign. Axial IV contrast-enhanced CT image in a patient with a Stanford type A dissection shows the acute angle of the false lumen (arrow). Note the true lumen is smaller than the false lumen (arrowhead)

## Identifying Complications

Complications of type A AD can be lethal and must be promptly recognized. Death from AD is usually caused by acute aortic regurgitation, major branch vessel obstruction, tamponade, or aortic rupture. The risk of fatal aortic rupture in patients with untreated proximal aortic dissection is approximately 90% [9, 11]. Signs of aortic rupture include hyperattenuating mediastinal, pericardial, or pleural fluid collections. Rupture of a type A dissection into the pericardial space may result in tamponade – a frequent cause of death (Fig. 6). On CT, patients with cardiac tamponade may demonstrate flattening of the right heart, deviation of the interventricular septum to the left, enlargement of the superior and inferior vena cava and hepatic veins, periportal lymphedema, and reflux of contrast into the azygos vein and other collateral venous pathways [23].

Shared sheath rupture is another complication of type A dissection. The aorta and pulmonary artery have a shared adventitial sheath. If a dissection ruptures within 1 cm of the aortic valve plane, it can gain access into the adventitial sheath, typically via a communication in the posterior wall of the ascending aorta, adjacent to the right pulmonary artery. Blood will track around the periphery of the central pulmonary arterial system, which will appear as high attenuating material that can mimic pulmonary thrombi (Fig. 7). In rare circumstances, the pulmonary artery can be compressed by the blood products leading to acute pulmonary hypertension and potentially death. Thus, when a shared sheath rupture is seen, evaluation for signs of right heart strain is warranted. In addition to its potential clinical manifestations, recognizing shared sheath rupture can be a helpful clue to the presence of a subtle or "flapless" type A AD.

In addition to rupture, dissections involving the ascending aorta may also extend into the aortic valve plane, carotid arteries, or coronary arteries, potentially resulting in aortic regurgitation, stroke, or myocardial infarction, respectively [9, 11]. Aortic regurgitation is a finding best evaluated by TEE or MRI. Carotid and coronary artery extension can be assessed with CT (Fig. 8). While detecting carotid extension is usually straightforward, coronary extension can be difficult to appreciate, especially on

**Table 1**  Common CT findings used to distinguish the true and flase lumen in AD

| CT finding | True lumen | False lumen |
| --- | --- | --- |
| Communication with aorta | Directly communicates with aortic valve plane | No communication with aortic valve plane |
| Lumen size | Smaller than false lumen | Larger than true lumen |
| Enhancement | Early enhancement | Late enhancement |
| Washout | Early washout | Late washout |
| Characteristic signs | Intimal calcification | Cobweb sign |
| | | Birdbeak sign |

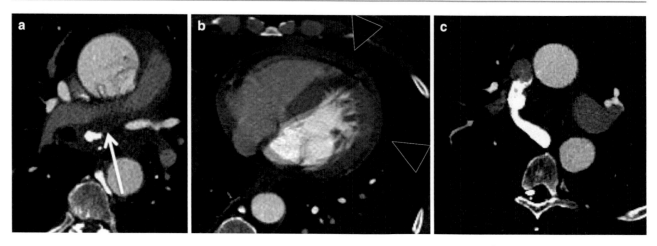

**Fig. 6** Rupture of Stanford type A aortic dissection resulting in cardiac tamponade. (**a–c**) Axial IV contrast-enhanced CT images demonstrate a shared sheath rupture (arrow) and hemopericardium (arrowhead), complications of a ruptured type A AD. The hemopericardium resulted in cardiac tamponade, as evidenced by bowing of the interventricular septum (**b**) and reflux of contrast into the azygos vein (**c**)

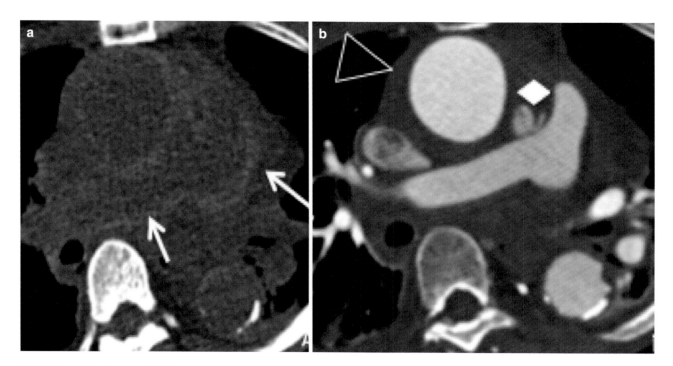

**Fig. 7** Shared sheath rupture in this patient with chest pain. Pre- (**a**) and post-contrast (**b** and **c**) axial CT images demonstrate blood tracking around the main and right pulmonary artery (arrow) in this patient with a not yet filled false lumen (arrowhead). The source of this blood around the pulmonary arterial system is a shared sheath rupture (diamond), which occurs across the shared adventitial sheath between the ascending aorta and the pulmonary artery

CT examinations performed without EKG gating. Thus, when coronary involvement is suspected clinically, EKG gating should be utilized.

Dissections involving the descending aorta can also cause complications via branch vessel involvement. Close interrogation of abdominal solid organs and bowel for signs of ischemia is required in patients with dissections involving the abdominal aorta. Assessment of the aortic branch vessels is also necessary. This involves determining whether vessels arise from the true or false lumen, and whether the intimo-medial flap causes compromise of branch vessels. When there are findings of end-organ or bowel compromise and the intimo-medial flap extends into a branch vessel, this is termed static ischemia. This is in contrast to distal ischemia in the setting of an intimo-medial flap covering a vascular ostium, which is termed dynamic ischemia (Fig. 9). Distinguishing between these causes of ischemia has treatment implications, as static ischemia is typically treated by stenting the branch vessel, while dynamic ischemia is treated by fenestration of the intimo-medial flap in the aorta, or endovascular repair of the aorta itself [6].

## IMH

Intramural hematoma (IMH) accounts for 5–15% of all cases of acute aortic syndrome, with a higher incidence in Asian cohorts. It is defined as acute hemorrhage contained within

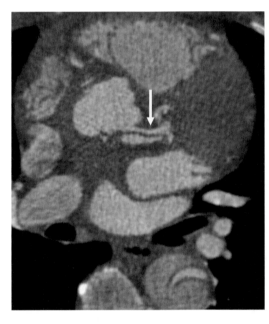

**Fig. 8** Post-contrast early systemic arterial phase image from an EKG-gated CTA demonstrates a dissection flap extending into the left main coronary artery (arrow)

the layers of the aortic wall, thus creating a false lumen [2]. Classically, the mechanism was thought to be rupture of the vasa vasorum within the adventitia. Newer studies suggest that IMH can also arise from microintimal tears, allowing blood to gain access in the media before sealing itself off [24]. IMH may originate spontaneously, or develop as a consequence from a PAU. Resulting aortic wall infarction may be a precursor to evolution into AD [2, 25]. Clinical manifestations, risk factors, classification, complications, and treatment are similar to AD [11]. Compared to patients with AD, patients with IMH are likely to be older, and those with type A IMH are more likely to have a known aortic aneurysm [24].

On nonenhanced CT, a smooth hyperattenuating crescent (typically measuring 40–70 HU), corresponding to a hematoma in the medial layer of the aortic wall, is the imaging hallmark of an IMH (Fig. 10). Intramural hematomas typically do not result in substantial narrowing of the aortic lumen, and should not enhance after contrast administration. The sensitivity of identifying an IMH with both nonenhanced and contrast-enhanced CT has been reported to be as high as 96% [6]. [24]. On some CT examinations, particularly post-contrast acquisitions acquired in an early systemic arterial phase, it can be difficult to distinguish between an IMH and an AD in which the false lumen is not yet filling with contrast. Fortunately, given that IMH and AD are managed similarly, distinguishing these entities is rarely of clinical importance, and they can usually be considered to be equivalent entities [6].

The approach to imaging interpretation of patients with IMH is similar to patients with AD, and consists of making the diagnosis, describing the distribution using the Stanford classification, and evaluating for complications. Complications of IMH are similar to AD, and include rupture, aortic valve disruption, and branch vessel involvement. There are some additional imaging features of IMH which have implications for treatment or prognosis. Total aortic size and IMH thickness should be reported, as total aortic size over 5 cm

**Fig. 9** Mechanisms of end-organ ischemia. In dynamic ischemia, the intimo-medial flap covers a vascular ostium (**a**). In contrast, in cases of static ischemia, the intimo-medial flap extends into a branch vessel (**b**)

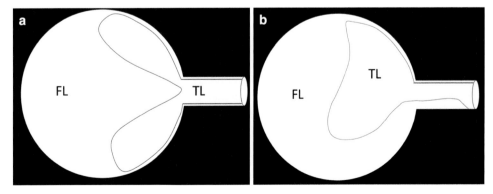

**Fig. 10** Intramural hematoma. (**a** and **b**) Nonenhanced axial CT angiogram shows a hyperdense crescent (arrows) along the anterolateral surface of descending aorta, the hallmark sign of an IMH. Without the noncontrast portion of the CT, an IMH may be difficult to distinguish from a thrombosed false lumen. Contrast-enhanced angiogram (**c** and **d**) does not demonstrate a flow channel or intimo-medial flap, which is characteristic of IMH

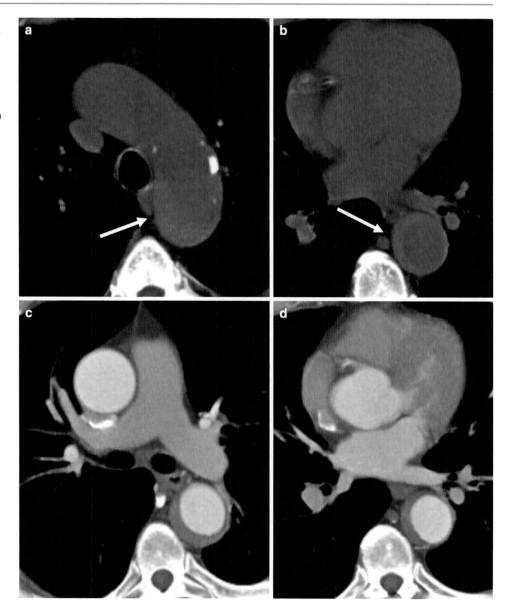

and IMH thickness over 1–1.5 cm have been associated with worse outcomes.

Focal contrast enhancement within the wall of an IMH should also be assessed. Contrast extending into an IMH via a connection from the aortic lumen, which is either broad based or has an opening greater than 3 mm, is best described as an ulcer-like projection (ULP) (Fig. 11). ULPs are the result of an intimo-medial defect which can be atherosclerotic or nonatherosclerotic in origin. While these two underlying causes cannot be reliably distinguished on CT in many cases, this is typically not essential as ULPs are associated with increased risk of complications, and may be targets for endovascular repair. ULPs

may be present in a patient initially presenting with an IMH or can develop on follow-up cross-sectional imaging examinations. Alternatively, a focus of contrast within an IMH that either does not connect to the lumen or connects via a small vessel that passes through it is best described as an intramural blood pool (IBP) (Fig. 12). IBPs are most often due to avulsed branch vessels, and have not been found to be associated with deleterious outcomes. In some instances, IBP can be seen consecutively at multiple levels, a finding called the "Chinese ring sword" sign (Fig. 12).

Treatment strategies for IMH are similar to AD, and depend on whether the IMH is classified as Stanford type A

**Fig. 11** Ulcer-like projection. Axial (**a**) and sagittal (**b**) IV contrast-enhanced CT images demonstrate contrast extending into an IMH via a direct, broad-based connection from the aortic lumen (arrow)

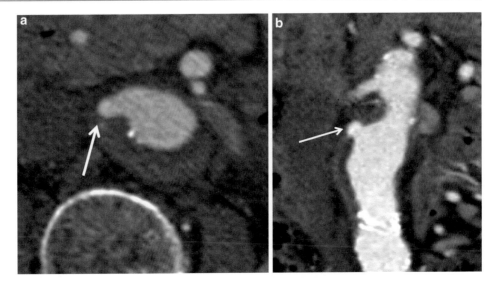

**Fig. 12** Intramural blood pools. (**a**) IV contrast-enhanced CT images demonstrate a focus of contrast within an IMH which does not connect with the aortic lumen (arrow). (**b**) The "Chinese Ring Sword Sign" refers to the appearance of intramural blood pools at multiple levels

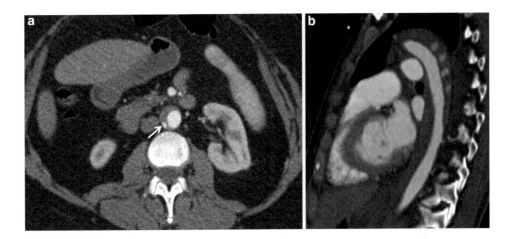

or type B. Most Stanford type A IMH are treated surgically [11]. However, newer data, particularly from Asia, suggests medical treatment with frequent follow-up may be a rational option for uncomplicated type A IMH [26]. In addition, similarly to AD, retrograde-type IMH may not be treated surgically (Fig. 13). Most type B IMH are initially treated medically with antihypertensive medication, with follow-up imaging recommended. While most type B IMH resolves, some can progress to rupture or classic AD. Aneurysm formation is another potential long-term sequela of IMH. As such, short- and long-term imaging follow-up is required for patients with type B IMH, and surgical or endovascular repair can be pursued if complications arise.

## PAU

PAU refers to an atherosclerotic plaque that ulcerates and creates an intimo-medial defect. The incidence of PAU in patients with acute aortic syndrome is estimated to be between 2.3% and 7.6%. Disruption suggests a diseased aortic wall, and therefore PAU generally occurs in elderly patients with atherosclerosis. While PAUs can cause the acute aortic syndrome, the vast majority of PAU are discovered incidentally on CT examinations performed for other reasons [2].

On CT, PAU is diagnosed by demonstrating a focal projection of contrast beyond the intima plus localized

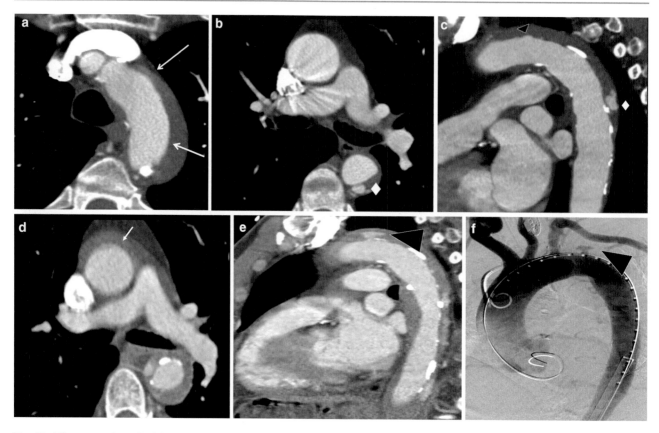

**Fig. 13** IV contrast-enhanced axial and sagittal CT images of a spontaneous acute retrograde type A intramural hematoma in patient with a type B IMH. (**a–c**) At initial presentation, within the type B intramural hematoma (arrow), several intramural blood pools (diamonds) are present as well as a questionable outpouching of contrast from the aortic lumen into the adjacent aortic wall, which is concerning for an ulcer-like projection (arrowhead). The patient was managed with blood pressure control. Less than 48 h later (**d** and **e**), repeat imaging demonstrates extension of the intramural hematoma into the ascending of the aorta (arrow), and enlargement of the ulcer-like projection (arrowhead). The patient was managed with a stent (**f**)

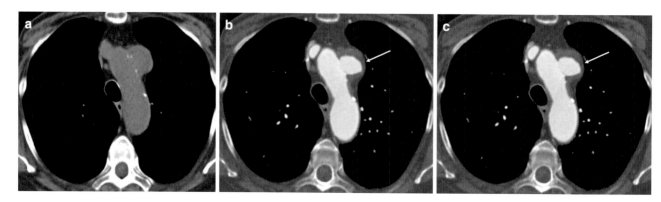

**Fig. 14** Penetrating atherosclerotic ulcer. (**a**) Nonenhanced axial CT image shows atherosclerotic calcification of the aortic wall and medially displaced intimal calcifications. (**b** and **c**) IV contrast-enhanced axial and coronal CT image shows focal saccular outpouching of contrast material outside the aortic lumen (arrow). PAU can be differentiated from other aortic diseases by presence of calcification and lack of compression on the aortic lumen

enlargement of the aorta or saccular pseudoaneurysm (Fig. 14). The outpouching of the outer aortic contour differentiates PAU from ulcerating mural plaque, which is seen within the lumen, central to the wall. PAU may occur anywhere in the aorta, but are most commonly seen in the mid-distal descending thoracic aorta where

**Fig. 15** Ruptured penetrating atherosclerotic ulcer. (**a**) Nonenhanced and enhanced (**b**) axial CT images demonstrate a saccular outpouching of the descending aorta with a "drooped" appearance around the vertebral body. Surrounding high attenuation and inflammatory changes are suggestive of rupture (arrow)

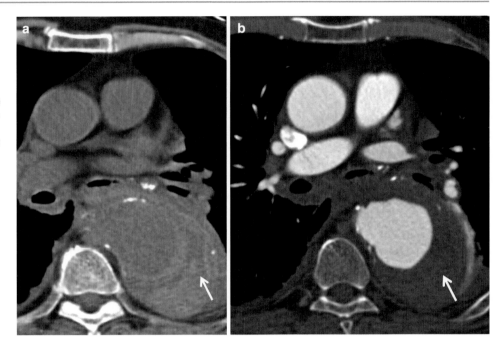

atherosclerosis is more common [6]. PAU can occur as an isolated entity or in association with an IMH; when seen with an IMH, PAU is best described as an ULP as described above.

PAU may resolve, stay stable over time, or progress to an IMH, saccular aneurysm, aortic dissection, or aortic rupture. Prognosis is worse with larger depth (>10 mm) or diameter (>20 mm), when associated with symptoms, or when there is an associated IMH [27]. Surrounding inflammatory fat stranding may suggest an acute or unstable PAU (Fig. 15). Rupture occurs in fewer than 5% of patients, and is higher in patients that present acutely. When a PAU is thought to be the cause of the patient's symptoms, endovascular or surgical repair may be considered.

## Considerations for Endovascular Repair and Treatment Planning

In recent years, thoracic endovascular aortic repair (TEVAR) has been introduced as a less-invasive alternative in patients with complicated type B aortic dissection, type B IMH, and PAU who present with acute or chronic complications. Additionally, TEVAR has been used in repaired type A dissections in cases where the false lumen remains patent. Compared with conventional surgery, repair time and blood loss are

**Table 2** Peritnent CT findings for TEVAR

| Pertinent information for TEVAR |
| --- |
| Location and diameter of primary entry tear |
| Location and diameter of primary exit tear |
| Distance from entry tear to left subclavian artery |
| Relative vertebral artery sizes |
| Coverage length |
| Calcification, tortuosity, and angulation of the aorta |
| Femoral and iliac vessel size |

reduced as TEVAR avoids the need for thoracotomy, bypass, and cross-clamping.

This approach utilizes a stent graft to cover the entry tear, redirect blood flow to the true lumen, and promote false lumen thrombosis. Doing so results in decreased pressure within the false lumen, and thus reduces risk of aneurysm development. Adequate seal zones, meticulous preoperative planning, and appropriate device sizing are all critical to successful results. Specifically, TEVAR requires landing zones of 2 cm in length both proximal and distal to the aortic pathology [28]. On the proximal side, both the site of primary entry tear and its distance to the left subclavian artery should be documented. If coverage of the left subclavian artery is necessary for an adequate proximal seal (within 2 cm from the entry tear), consideration should

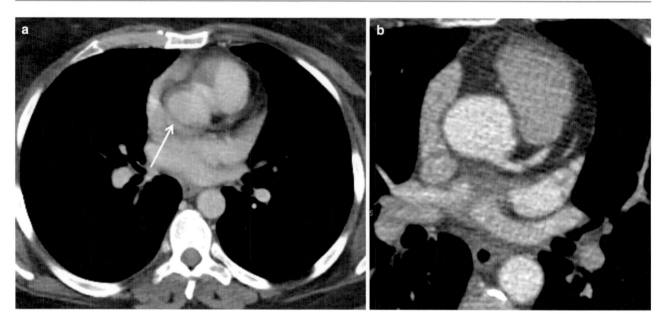

**Fig. 16** Pulsation artifact. (a) Motion of the aorta secondary to the cardiac cycle simulates a dissection flap in this noncardiac gated CT examination. This "flap" is less sharply marginated than an intimo-medial flap, and overlaps with anatomic structures. (b) Cardiac gating in the same patient demonstrates a normal appearing aorta without the presence of a dissection flap

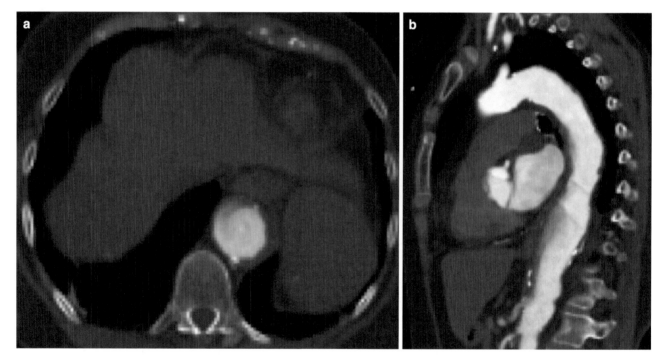

**Fig. 17** Flow artifact. (a) axial and (b) sagittal CT images demonstrate hypodense material along the anterior aspect of the descending aorta. Note the indistinct borders, which sometimes may appear similar to "a cloud of smoke"

be given to preoperative left carotid-subclavian bypass to avoid spinal cord ischemia; as such, relative vertebral artery sizes should be reported as patients with dominant left vertebral arteries are typically treated with bypass. Additionally, information about coverage length, aortic tortuosity, presence of calcification, and angulation should be provided. A vascular stent-graft is sized according to the maximum diameter of the aorta and proximal and distal landing sites, and these values should be reported. It is important to not oversize the graft to avoid stent collapse and intimal tear. Access vessel anatomy is critical, as the thoracic endografts require larger diameter delivery systems, usually 20–26F. Specifically, the femoral and iliac systems need to be evaluated for small diameter or heavy calcification. If there is concern, the subclavian arteries should be assessed, as this alternative approach may need to be considered. Table 2 summarizes pertinent information for TEVAR repair.

## Potential Pitfalls

Several important technical artifacts can affect imaging interpretation in patients with suspected acute aortic syndrome. A commonly encountered technical artifact when evaluating the ascending aorta is pulsation. Pulsation artifact arises due to motion of the aorta secondary to the cardiac cycle, and creates a duplication of the aorta on CT that can simulate a dissection flap. Pulsation can often be distinguished from a true dissection by noting that it is less sharply marginated than an intimo-medial flap and extends outside the confines of the aorta, potentially overlapping with other structures including the central pulmonary arterial system (Fig. 16). In addition, pulsation artifact will not be associated with mediastinal stranding or evidence of aortic rupture that can be seen in the setting of a true dissection. In difficult cases, EKG-gated or ultrafast pitch mode CT can be performed to confirm the artifactual nature of findings suggestive of pulsation.

Another important technical pitfall is flow artifact. Flow artifacts occur due to disruption, mixing, and nonlaminar flow of the contrast column. They are most often seen in patients with decreased cardiac output or in areas of slower flow, particularly along the anterior aspect of the descending aorta (Fig. 17). While flow artifacts can simulate a dissection flap, they are typically thinner, higher attenuating, and will have indistinct borders particularly on multiplanar reconstructions where they may simulate "smoke." Some flow artifacts can extend into branch vessels from the aortic lumen. When flow artifacts are suspected, but not definite, options for definitive characterization include repeat CT in a later phase, MRI, or TEE.

Anatomic and pathologic mimics can also complicate interpretation. On occasion, a large infundibulum, typically from a proximal intercostal artery, can simulate an aortic pseudoaneurysm (Fig. 18). Differentiation can be made by identifying the tiny artery arising from its apex. Pericardial recesses, particularly about the ascending aorta, can simulate a false lumen (Fig. 19). Recognizing that pericardial recesses are fluid attenuation and often have intervening fat between them, the aorta allows for differentiation.

Vasculitis and perivasculitis can also mimic acute aortic pathologies, particularly IMH. Surrounding inflammation, shaggy border, concentric wall thickening, excessively convex configuration, and low attenuation on noncontrast with enhancement help distinguish these entities (Fig. 20). Lastly, infectious pseudoaneurysms have overlapping features with causes of the acute aortic syndrome, particularly PAU. Imaging features characteristic of an infectious pseudoaneurysm include a lack of calcium and a mushroom-shaped or narrow-necked appearance (Fig. 21). On clinical grounds, patients with infectious pseudoaneurysms usually display infectious and constitutional signs and symptoms, which are typically absent in the acute aortic syndrome.

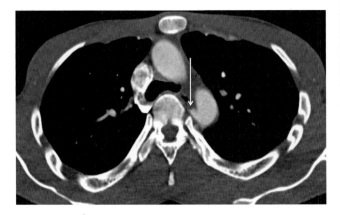

**Fig. 18** Axial IV contrast-enhanced CT image of a branch vessel infundibulum. The superior intercostal artery infundibulum may mimic an ulcer-like projection or pseudoaneurysm. Identifying the tiny artery arising from apex will help differentiate between the two possibilities

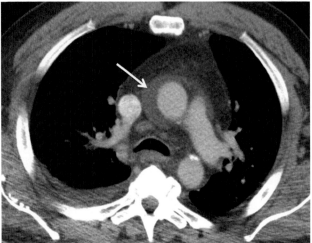

**Fig. 19** IV contrast-enhanced axial CT image of pericardial recesses. Pericardial recesses (arrows) around the ascending aorta may mimic a false lumen. The pericardial recesses are simple fluid attenuation versus false lumens which are higher in attenuation

**Fig. 20** IV contrast-enhanced axial images of vasculitis. Vasculitis and perivasculitis can be differentiated from an intramural hematoma by a shaggy boarder (**a** and **b**), circumferential wall thickening (**b–d**), surrounding inflammatory changes such as lymphadenopathy (**b** and **c**), and contrast enhancement on post-contrast images (**a–d**)

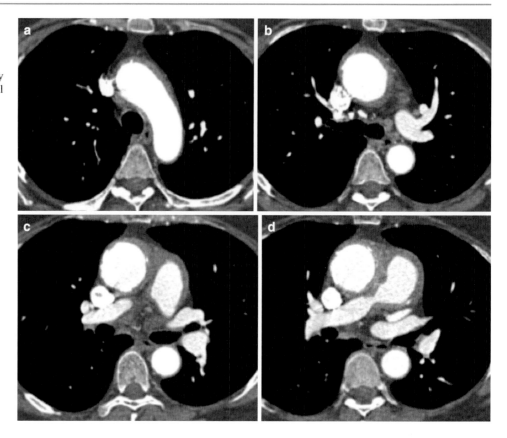

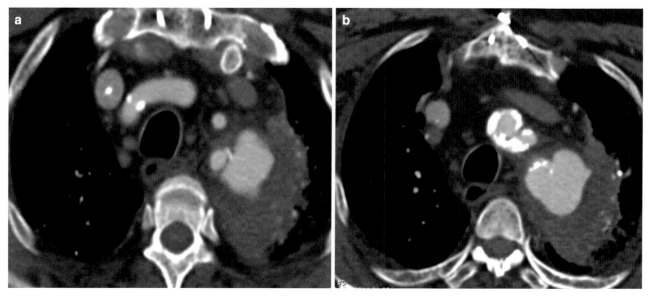

**Fig. 21** IV contrast-enhanced axial images of an infectious pseudo-aneurysm. In addition to rapid growth, infectious pseudoaneurysms can be distinguished from PAU by lack of atherosclerotic calcification (**a** and **b**) and narrow-necked or mushroom-shaped appearance of the saccular aneurysm (**a**)

## Conclusion

The acute aortic syndrome can be caused by three interrelated conditions – aortic dissection, intramural hematoma, and penetrating atherosclerotic ulcer. Diagnostic imaging (TEE, CT, or MR) plays a pivotal role in diagnosis and management, with CT being the most utilized modality in the acute setting. Management depends on location, extent of disease, and complications. Understanding both the pathophysiology and imaging features is essential for facilitating prompt diagnosis and management.

## References

1. Vilacosta I. Acute aortic syndrome. Heart. 2001;85(4):365–8.
2. Maddu KK, Shuaib W, Telleria J, Johnson J-O, Khosa F. Nontraumatic acute aortic emergencies: Part 1, Acute aortic syndrome. Am J Roentgenol [Internet]. 2014; Available from: https://www.ajronline.org/doi/full/10.2214/AJR.13.11437
3. Manriquez M, Srinivas G, Bollepalli S, Britt L, Drachman D. Is computed tomography a reliable diagnostic modality in detecting placental injuries in the setting of acute trauma? Am J Obstet Gynecol. 2010;202(6):611.e1–5.
4. The International Registry of Acute Aortic Dissection (IRAD): New insights into an old disease | Surgery | JAMA | JAMA Network [Internet]. 2020. Available from: https://jamanetwork.com/journals/jama/fullarticle/192401
5. Yoo SM, Lee HY, White CS. MDCT evaluation of acute aortic syndrome. Radiol Clin N Am. 2010;48(1):67–83.
6. Chiu KWH, Lakshminarayan R, Ettles DF. Acute aortic syndrome: CT findings. Clin Radiol. 2013;68(7):741–8.
7. Valente T, Rossi G, Lassandro F, Rea G, Marino M, Muto M, et al. MDCT evaluation of acute aortic syndrome (AAS). Br J Radiol. 2016;89(1061):20150825.
8. Ramanath VS, Oh JK, Sundt TM, Eagle KA. Acute aortic syndromes and thoracic aortic aneurysm. Mayo Clin Proc. 2009;84(5):465–81.
9. Khan IA, Nair CK. Clinical, diagnostic, and management perspectives of aortic dissection. Chest. 2002;122(1):311–28.
10. Hartnell GG. Imaging of aortic aneurysms and dissection: CT and MRI. J Thorac Imaging. 2001 Jan;16(1):35–46.
11. Castañer E, Andreu M, Gallardo X, Mata JM, Cabezuelo MÁ, Pallardó Y. CT in nontraumatic acute thoracic aortic disease: typical and atypical features and complications. RadioGraphics. 2003;23(suppl_1):S93–S110.
12. Bennett CJ, Maleszewski JJ, Araoz PA. CT and MR imaging of the aortic valve: radiologic-pathologic correlation. RadioGraphics. 2012;32(5):1399–420.
13. Larson EW, Edwards WD. Risk factors for aortic dissection: a necropsy study of 161 cases. Am J Cardiol. 1984;53(6):849–55.
14. Rubin GD, Helical CT. Angiography of the thoracic aorta. J Thorac Imaging. 1997;12(2):128–49.
15. Nienaber CA, Eagle KA. Aortic dissection: new frontiers in diagnosis and management: Part I: From etiology to diagnostic strategies. Circulation. 2003;108(5):628–35.
16. Nelsen KM, Spizarny DL, Kastan DJ. Intimointimal intussusception in aortic dissection: CT diagnosis. AJR Am J Roentgenol. 1994;162(4):813–4.
17. Karabulut N, Goodman LR, Olinger GN. CT diagnosis of an unusual aortic dissection with intimointimal intussusception: the wind sock sign. J Comput Assist Tomogr. 1998;22(5):692–3.
18. Tam DY, Mazine A, Cheema AN, Yanagawa B. Conservative management of extensive iatrogenic aortic dissection. Aorta J. 2016;4(6):229–31.
19. Leontyev S, Borger MA, Legare J-F, Merk D, Hahn J, Seeburger J, et al. Iatrogenic type A aortic dissection during cardiac procedures: early and late outcome in 48 patients. Eur J Cardio-Thorac Surg Off J Eur Assoc Cardio-Thorac Surg. 2012;41(3):641–6.
20. Rylski B, Hoffmann I, Beyersdorf F, Suedkamp M, Siepe M, Nitsch B, et al. Iatrogenic acute aortic dissection type A: insight from the German Registry for Acute Aortic Dissection Type A (GERAADA). Eur J Cardio-Thorac Surg Off J Eur Assoc Cardio-Thorac Surg. 2013;44(2):353–9. discussion 359
21. Acute retrograde type A aortic dissection: morphologic analysis and clinical implications | Elsevier Enhanced Reader [Internet]. 2020. Available from: https://reader.elsevier.com/reader/sd/pii/S0022480417300811?token=D887031BB90F8C302E1A295CCE2BB1AD6CB781C6F0F46AA290D1847F4EB124D423364DBCD136456BF94F91577B9C9576
22. Kamohara K, Furukawa K, Koga S, Yunoki J, Morokuma H, Noguchi R, et al. Surgical strategy for retrograde type A aortic dissection based on long-term outcomes. Ann Thorac Surg. 2015;99(5):1610–5.
23. Restrepo CS, Lemos DF, Lemos JA, Velasquez E, Diethelm L, Ovella TA, et al. Imaging findings in cardiac tamponade with emphasis on CT. RadioGraphics. 2007;27(6):1595–610.
24. Gutschow SE, Walker CM, Martínez-Jiménez S, Rosado-de-Christenson ML, Stowell J, Kunin JR. Emerging concepts in intramural hematoma imaging. RadioGraphics. 2016;36(3):660–74.
25. Evangelista A, Mukherjee D, Mehta RH, O'Gara PT, Fattori R, Cooper JV, et al. Acute intramural hematoma of the aorta: a mystery in evolution. Circulation. 2005;111(8):1063–70.
26. Song J-K, Yim JH, Ahn J-M, Kim D-H, Kang J-W, Lee TY, et al. Outcomes of patients with acute type A aortic intramural hematoma. Circulation. 2009;120(21):2046–52.
27. Hayashi H, Matsuoka Y, Sakamoto I, Sueyoshi E, Okimoto T, Hayashi K, et al. Penetrating atherosclerotic ulcer of the aorta: imaging features and disease concept. RadioGraphics. 2000;20(4):995–1005.
28. Saremi F, Hassani C, Lin LM, Lee C, Wilcox AG, Fleischman F, et al. Image predictors of treatment outcome after thoracic aortic dissection repair. RadioGraphics. 2018;38(7):1949–72.

# Imaging of Pulmonary Infections

**18**

Suzanne C. Byrne, Mark M. Hammer, and Richard Thomas

## Contents

### Abstract

Chest radiographs and CT are frequently used in the diagnosis and monitoring of pulmonary infections. The presence and type of immunocompromise influence which infections a patient may be at risk of contracting. Imaging features often overlap among different infections, but some imaging features may help narrow the differential diagnosis. For example, tree-in-bud nodules suggest mycobacterial, atypical bacterial, or viral pneumonias; diffuse ground glass suggests viral or *Pneumocystis* pneumonia; and nodules with ground-glass halos suggest invasive fungal pneumonia in neutropenic patients. Septic emboli present with multiple cavitary nodules, and radiologists should search for a source, such as a valvular vegetation, when they encounter such patients. Radiologists should also be aware of entities which can simulate infection on imaging, including organizing pneumonia and malignancies.

S. C. Byrne · M. M. Hammer (✉)
Division of Thoracic Imaging, Department of Radiology, Brigham and Women's Hospital, Harvard Medical School, Boston, MA, USA
e-mail: scbyrne@bwh.harvard.edu; mmhammer@bwh.harvard.edu

R. Thomas
Department of Radiology, Lahey Hospital & Medical Center, Burlington, MA, USA
e-mail: richard.thomas1@lahey.org

© Springer Nature Switzerland AG 2022
M. N. Patlas et al. (eds.), *Atlas of Emergency Imaging from Head-to-Toe*,
https://doi.org/10.1007/978-3-030-92111-8_18

**Keywords**

Pneumonia · Community-acquired pneumonia ·
Opportunistic infection · Fungal pneumonia · Septic
emboli

## Introduction

Pneumonias are a frequent indication for pulmonary imaging, both with radiographs and CT. Imaging is helpful in making the initial diagnosis of an infection, although identifying a specific microbial etiology is often not possible, as well as monitoring for potential complications, including abscess or empyema. Patients with compromised immune systems are at increased risk of certain infections, depending upon the components of the immune system that are affected. In combination with patient history, certain imaging findings can help to narrow the differential diagnosis. Importantly, radiologists should always consider the potential mimics of infection, such as organizing pneumonia or lung cancer. In this chapter, we will discuss types of immunocompromise, imaging findings of common community-acquired and opportunistic pneumonias, septic emboli, and mimics of infection.

## The Host: Immunocompetent Versus Immunocompromised

The accuracy of radiological diagnosis can be substantially improved if the clinical background of the patient is considered [1]. This includes social history, travel history, and immune status. In particular, immunocompromised patients are at risk of developing opportunistic infections. The type and severity of immunocompromise will determine which infections may occur and their patterns of lung involvement [2, 3].

Immunocompromise can be broadly divided into neutropenia, cellular (B- and T-cell) immunodeficiency, and humoral (antibody) immunodeficiency. Neutropenia, defined as an absolute neutrophil count $<500$ cells/mm$^3$, typically occurs in patients on cytotoxic chemotherapy; the more aggressive regimens seen in the treatment of leukemia produce more severe and long-lasting neutropenia. Neutropenic patients are at risk of severe sepsis from any infection, but they are at particularly increased risk of developing angioinvasive fungal infections, particularly *Aspergillus* and *Mucor*.

Cellular immunodeficiency is best typified in patients with HIV AIDS, in which the virus destroys helper (CD4) T cells. Patients who are solid organ or stem cell transplant recipients also experience cellular immunodeficiency because of their immunosuppressive regimens. These patients are at risk of severe sepsis from any infection; they are also at increased risk of tuberculosis (particularly HIV-infected patients), as well as of *Pneumocystis* and other fungal pneumonias. Humoral immunodeficiency (e.g., in patients with common variable immunodeficiency or other causes of hypogammaglobulinemia) often predisposes to more severe bacterial pneumonias.

Finally, patients on immunosuppressive medications for an autoimmune disease are also at risk of certain opportunistic pathogens, although they do not match exactly to the three categories listed above. In particular, patients on antitumor necrosis factor alpha (TNF-alpha) therapy, which is used for the treatment of inflammatory bowel disease and many connective tissue disorders including rheumatoid arthritis, are at increased risk of tuberculosis. Patients on corticosteroids are at risk of developing *Pneumocystis* pneumonia, among other infections.

Knowing the underlying immune state will help greatly in generating an appropriate differential diagnosis for pulmonary infections. Patient history and medications can also help with differential diagnoses of mimics of infection, which are discussed at the end of this chapter.

## Community-Acquired Pneumonias

Pneumonia is one of the most commonly encountered conditions in emergency radiology. Community-acquired pneumonias (CAP), i.e., those acquired outside of the healthcare setting, may be bacterial or viral in etiology. Common agents include viruses (e.g., rhinovirus, influenza, and human metapneumovirus), as well as bacteria, the most common of which is *Streptococcus pneumoniae* [4]. In most cases, a specific pathogen will not be isolated [4], and therefore the treatment of CAP is typically not targeted to a specific agent [5]. It is important to remember that the most common pneumonia in immunocompromised patients is also CAP, although these patients may experience a more severe course of the disease.

The role of imaging in CAP is to confirm the diagnosis of pneumonia when clinically suspected, to raise the possibility when not clinically suspected, and to look for complications such as empyema. Imaging findings in CAP are generally not specific for a particular infectious agent, although certain findings may suggest bacterial versus viral etiology. It is common to recommend follow-up imaging (chest radiography) in patients with pneumonia to document clearing of the radiographic abnormality after 6–8 weeks and exclude the possibility of malignancy. This recommendation is somewhat controversial, being endorsed by some guidelines but not others given the low yield of these follow-up examinations [5, 6]. However, it is our practice to recommend such follow-up in most patients, at least those of older age.

The initial imaging examination in patients with suspected CAP is the chest radiograph; two-view (PA and lateral)

**Fig. 1** A 42-year-old woman with fever. PA and lateral chest radiographs demonstrate right lower lobe consolidation, which is consistent with lobar pneumonia

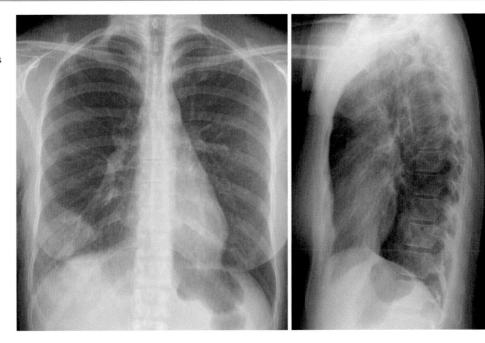

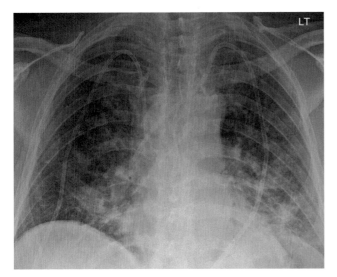

**Fig. 2** A 49-year-old man with fever. AP chest radiograph demonstrates bilateral lower lobe patchy consolidations, which is consistent with bronchopneumonia in this patient with influenza

radiographs are preferable as they can be used to better localize the abnormality. Patients with atypical clinical presentations, unusual imaging findings, or suspected complications may warrant CT. The imaging patterns in CAP may be divided into three major patterns: lobar pneumonia, bronchopneumonia, and "interstitial." Lobar pneumonia refers to a large contiguous area of consolidation, though not always an entire lobe (Fig. 1). This is commonly associated with *S. pneumoniae* and other bacterial pneumonias [7]. It is only rarely present in viral pneumonia. Bronchopneumonia refers to multifocal airway-centered, or peribronchial,

consolidations; it typically has a patchy and mid to lower lung appearance on chest radiography (Fig. 2). Bronchopneumonia may be seen in a large spectrum of infectious agents, including both bacteria and viruses [8]. It is also the typical appearance of aspiration pneumonia. Finally, the "interstitial" pneumonia pattern refers to diffuse reticular or nodular opacities seen radiographically (Fig. 3) [7]. This commonly corresponds to either ground-glass opacities, tree-in-bud nodules, or both on CT (and thus is often not truly interstitial). Interstitial pneumonias are generally associated with viral infections as well as *Mycoplasma*; of note, this is also the radiographic appearance of *Pneumocystis jiroveci* pneumonia.

As noted above, CT is typically only used in CAP in unusual circumstances, such as severe or complicated pneumonias. CT findings, like those of the chest radiograph, are relatively nonspecific. Similar to on chest radiography, lobar pneumonia presents as a large contiguous area of consolidation, often with air bronchograms, and is typically associated with bacterial agents. Bronchopneumonia presents with multifocal peribronchial consolidations, often with associated tree-in-bud nodules (Fig. 4). It may be seen with either bacteria or viruses, as well as aspiration pneumonias [8–10]. Finally, the radiographic "interstitial" pattern is distinguishable as two types of patterns on CT: tree-in-bud nodules, representing bronchiolitis, and patchy or diffuse ground-glass opacities, representing alveolitis (Fig. 5). Both of these patterns are associated with viral pneumonias [8–10]. Tree-in-bud nodules are also a common feature of *Mycoplasma* pneumonia [11]. Finally, while these are discussed elsewhere in this chapter, diffuse ground glass is a feature of *Pneumocystis*

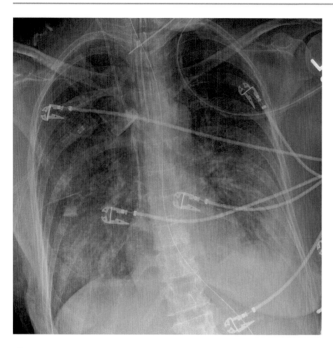

**Fig. 3** A 60-year-old woman with fever. AP chest radiograph demonstrates diffuse interstitial opacities from a viral pneumonia

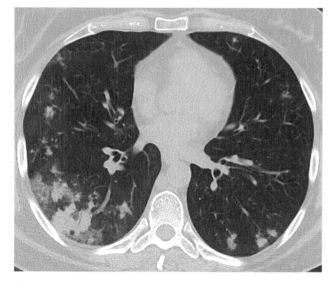

**Fig. 4** A 50-year-old woman with bronchopneumonia from respiratory syncytial virus. Axial CT image of the lungs shows patchy peribronchial consolidations in both lower lobes, as well as tree-in-bud nodules in the right middle lobe

pneumonia, and tree-in-bud nodules are also a major feature of mycobacterial infections.

In summary, the radiologist's role in CAP is primarily to detect an abnormality compatible with pneumonia. While the radiographic pattern may occasionally suggest an infectious agent, it is typically nonspecific, and radiologists should remember that viral pneumonias relatively frequently do cause consolidations.

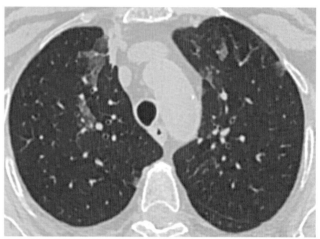

**Fig. 5** A 66-year-old woman with human metapneumovirus. Axial CT image of the lungs shows patchy ground-glass opacities bilaterally

## Mycobacterial Infections

Tuberculosis (TB) and nontuberculous mycobacterial (NTM) infections are important infections in both developed and developing countries. Immunosuppressed patients, particularly those with defects in cellular immunity, are at increased risk for both of these infections. TB may present in primary, postprimary, or miliary forms. NTM may present in *classic* (cavitary) or *non*-classic (bronchiectatic) forms.

## Primary TB

Primary TB refers to a manifestation of infection at the time of the initial infection. This is uncommon in adult patients, in whom the immune system usually controls the initial infection but commonly occurs in children and immunocompromised patients, particularly those with HIV AIDS. The most common radiographic manifestations of primary tuberculosis are mediastinal and hilar lymphadenopathy, which is more apparent on CT [12]. Lobar consolidation is also common and does not have a zonal predominance. Pleural effusions may also be a manifestation of primary tuberculosis [13]. Miliary disease may occur in either primary or postprimary forms and is discussed below.

Lymphadenopathy in tuberculosis typically demonstrates necrosis, i.e., a low-attenuation center with peripheral rim enhancement, on CT. Parenchymal disease most frequently manifests as consolidation, usually without cavitation. Pleural effusions are more common in adults than in the pediatric population. Empyema can also occur and is typically loculated with associated pleural thickening and enhancement on CT. Tuberculous empyema can be complicated by extension into the chest wall, an unusual complication which has been termed *empyema necessitans* [14].

## Postprimary TB

Postprimary TB refers to a pattern of disease that typically occurs in the setting of reactivation of infection. In other words, while the patient has initially controlled the infection, at a later time, often years later, the infection may break free of immune control and develop clinical manifestations. Occasionally, postprimary TB may be a manifestation of initial infection, but this is impossible to distinguish clinically. At imaging, postprimary TB presents with consolidations that are upper lung predominant (involving the upper lobes and superior segments of the lower lobes), often with cavitation [12, 13]. Cavities are typically seen in areas of consolidation

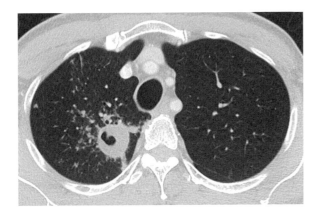

**Fig. 6** A 61-year-old man with post-primary tuberculosis. Axial CT image through the lung apices demonstrates a right upper lobe cavity and adjacent tree-in-bud nodules representing endobronchial spread of tuberculosis

and can be several centimeters in size with thick and irregular walls (Fig. 6) [15]. At CT, tree-in-bud nodules are nearly always present, reflect endobronchial spread of infection (Fig. 6), and are seen in approximately 95% of cases of active TB [12]. TB may also involve the central airways and can lead to bronchial stenoses.

## Miliary TB

Hematogenous dissemination of infection in primary or postprimary tuberculosis leads to miliary TB. This is more common in immunocompromised and pediatric patients. On chest radiographs or CT, miliary disease manifests as diffuse 1–3-mm nodules in a random distribution (Fig. 7). Lymphadenopathy is common as well. Finally, patients with miliary TB may have hematogenous dissemination in other organs, including the spine (Pott's disease), central nervous system, and urogenital system, among others [16].

## Nontuberculous Mycobacteria

Nontuberculous mycobacteria (NTM) are species other than *M. tuberculosis* that infect humans. These mycobacteria are pervasive in the environment, being present in water and soil. In the lungs, the most common agent is the *Mycobacterium avium* complex. Pulmonary NTM disease is a more common cause of mycobacterial infection than tuberculosis in developed countries [17].

NTM manifests in two major forms: cavitary (sometimes known as "classic") and bronchiectatic (sometimes known as "non-classic"), with the latter being far more common [18]. Cavitary NTM infection is characterized by upper lobe

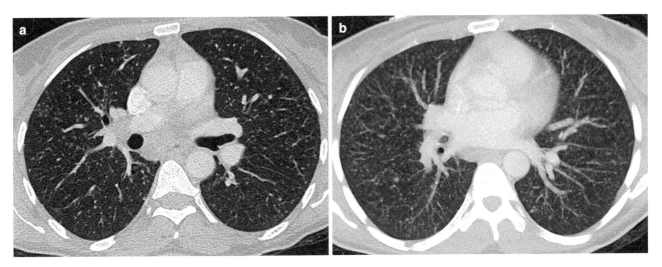

**Fig. 7** A 37-year-old woman with HIV and miliary tuberculosis. (**a**) Axial image and (**b**) axial MIP image of the lungs from a chest CT demonstrate randomly distributed micronodules, as well as mediastinal lymphadenopathy

predominant cavitary consolidations with tree-in-bud nodules, and it is indistinguishable from postprimary tuberculosis. This form typically affects patients with underlying chronic lung disease, e.g., chronic obstructive pulmonary disease. The bronchiectatic form of NTM is far more common and manifests as chronic bronchiectasis and bronchiolitis with a mid-lung predominance. Most characteristically, patients will have bronchiectasis and tree-in-bud nodules (bronchiolitis) in the right middle lobe and lingula (Fig. 8). This form is generally seen in elderly women [19].

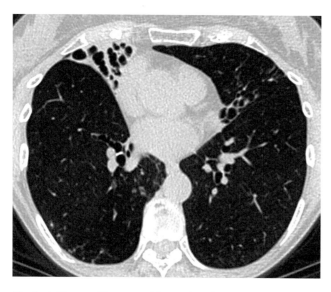

**Fig. 8** A 73-year-old woman with nontuberculous mycobacterial infection. Axial CT image of the mid lungs shows bronchiectasis in the right middle lobe and lingula, as well as scattered tree-in-bud nodules in the right lower lobe

## Septic Pulmonary Emboli

Septic emboli represent infected intravascular thrombi that travel through the bloodstream to obstruct a small vessel and cause an infarct in an organ. While septic emboli are classically associated with endocarditis, they may also be seen in the setting of infected catheters as well as soft-tissue infections (e.g., liver abscess, osteomyelitis) [20–22]. Septic emboli may be asymptomatic, manifest with end-organ damage, or represent a persistently infected site even after treatment of the primary infection. The target organs generally depend on the infectious source: septic thrombophlebitis and right-sided endocarditis are typically associated with septic pulmonary emboli, while left-sided endocarditis may be associated with septic cerebral emboli [23], coronary artery emboli, and splenic infarcts, among other systemic arterial occlusions. It is worthwhile to note that many patients will present with both pulmonary and systemic arterial septic emboli, often because of multiple-valve endocarditis. The presence of one septic embolism should prompt a search for septic emboli in other organs.

Septic pulmonary emboli, which often are a combination of true abscesses and infected pulmonary infarcts, classically present with peripheral nodular or consolidative opacities in the lungs [24–26]. These abnormalities evolve over time, starting as ill-defined consolidative opacities with ground-glass halos (Fig. 9a), later becoming more well-defined and losing the ground-glass halos. Subsequently, they will become more nodular and often develop cavitation (described in 11–34%) (Fig. 9b) [25, 26]. As the patient responds to antibiotics and the immune system clears the infection, the nodules will shrink, and cavities will have decreasing wall thickness. The focus may completely resolve or leave a thin-walled pneumatocele. It is common to see

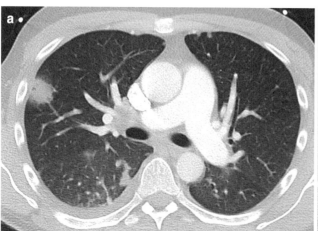
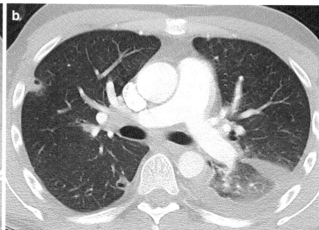

**Fig. 9** A 35-year-old man with endocarditis and septic emboli. (**a**) Axial CT image of the lungs at presentation demonstrates multiple peripheral nodules, particularly in the right lung, with a ground-glass halo in the right upper lobe. (**b**) Axial CT image obtained 10 days later shows that these septic emboli have cavitated

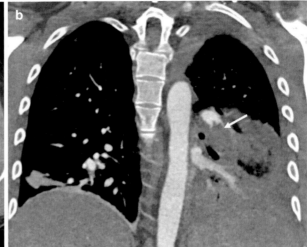

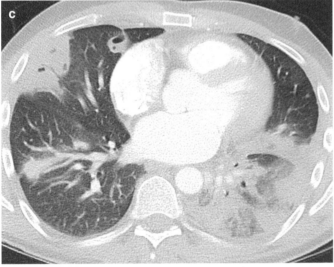

**Fig. 10** A 35-year-old man with endocarditis and septic emboli (same patient as Fig. 9). (**a**) Axial and (**b**) coronal images from a CT pulmonary angiogram demonstrate a pulmonary septic embolus in the left lower lobe artery (arrow) which embolized from a tricuspid valve vegetation (not shown). Note the marked enlargement of the thrombosed vessel, one sign of a macroscopic septic embolus. (**c**) Lung windows show the infarcted left lower lobe with extensive ground-glass and multiple peripheral consolidations

septic emboli in various stages of evolution at a single timepoint, as septic thrombi continue to embolize from their source until adequately treated.

As they are peripheral, septic emboli may secondarily involve the pleura. Rupture into the pleura may cause pneumothorax or, more commonly, empyema. Empyemas generally require drainage for treatment. Typically, septic emboli themselves do not require drainage, although if they form a large enough abscess, drainage may be necessary for adequate infectious source control [20].

In general, the septic embolus itself, i.e., the vascular filling defect, is too small to visualize directly by CT; all the radiologist sees is the distal infarct. However, on occasion, the filling defect is large enough to be directly seen (macroscopic septic emboli). These cases typically result in large, even lobar infarcts (Fig. 10). Pulmonary artery

pseudoaneurysms may result from septic emboli, particularly in the setting of macroscopic septic emboli.

As noted above, when a radiologist encounters pulmonary septic emboli, she or he should look for other embolic sites, to provide the treating physician with a complete picture and alert clinicians to potential drainable collections. He or she should also look for an embolic source, since valvular vegetations may be detected even on noncardiac gated CT examinations and are important to mention if visible.

## *Pneumocystis* Pneumonia

*Pneumocystis jiroveci* is a fungus that causes potentially life-threatening pneumonia in patients with immunocompromised states, including human immunodeficiency virus

(HIV) infection, primary immunodeficiency, transplant recipients, hematological malignancies, steroid therapy, and chemotherapy. Although the incidence of pneumocystis pneumonia (PCP) in HIV-infected patients is decreasing due to prophylaxis and effective antiretroviral treatment, it continues to be one of the most common opportunistic infections [27, 28]. PCP is transmitted by the airborne route, and the initial exposure to PCP occurs early in life. By 4 years of age, two-thirds of healthy humans demonstrate antibodies to *P. jiroveci* [29]. Colonization can be seen in up to 20% of healthy individuals [30].

PCP manifests as gradually progressive fever, cough, dyspnea, and hypoxia. Serum beta-D-glucan is often elevated,

which can be helpful in making the diagnosis. Definitive diagnosis requires identification of the organism in respiratory specimens using stains or polymerase chain reaction (PCR). However, if a definitive diagnosis cannot be made due to the inability to obtain a specimen or a low burden of organisms, a presumptive diagnosis can be made based on typical clinical and radiographic findings and elevated beta-D-glucan [31, 32].

Computed tomography (CT) has higher sensitivity and allows for a more confident diagnosis compared to chest radiography [33]. The most common pattern is bilaterally symmetric and relatively diffuse ground-glass opacities (Fig. 11). The ground glass may at times be subtle and simulate mosaic attenuation [34]. In later stages, ground-glass opacities may be accompanied by septal thickening ("crazy paving," Fig. 12a) and, rarely, consolidation [34, 35]. Lung consolidation is more common in patients without HIV infection, perhaps due to the higher host immune response resulting in more lung damage [36]. Cyst development in PCP is reported in 10–40% of patients; it is more commonly seen in HIV-infected patients and is often seen in more advanced infection [36–38]. Cysts occur mostly in the upper lobes and decrease in size or resolve after treatment [39]. Rupture of subpleural cysts can result in spontaneous pneumothorax which is associated with a high mortality [39]. In fewer than 10% of patients with PCP, nodules may be seen which are solitary or multiple and of varying sizes. These reflect granulomatous reaction and are associated with a better immune status [34, 37, 40]. Some patients may have residual lung parenchymal fibrosis seen as scar-like opacities, with architectural distortion and traction bronchiectasis [37, 41] (Fig. 12b). Pleural effusions are uncommon [42]. Of note, cytomegalovirus pneumonia is in

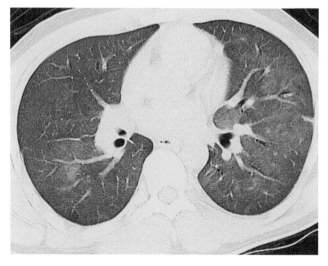

**Fig. 11** A 36-year-old man with HIV and *Pneumocystis* pneumonia. Axial CT image of the lungs shows diffuse ground-glass opacities

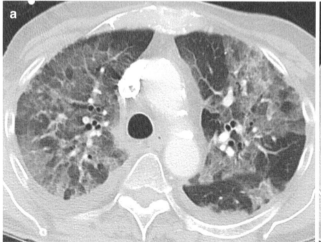
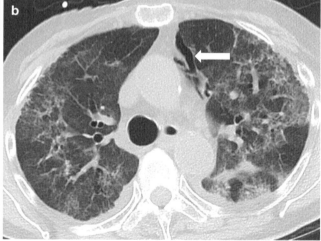

**Fig. 12** An 83-year-old woman with ovarian cancer on chemotherapy, who developed Pneumocystis pneumonia. (a) Axial CT image of the lungs at presentation demonstrates diffuse bilateral ground-glass opacities with interlobular septal thickening ("crazy paving" sign). (b) Follow-up CT image done 6 days later shows the development of architectural distortion and bronchial dilation. Note the small left pneumothorax and pneumomediastinum (arrow)

the differential for PCP. In HIV AIDS patients, it is generally seen only at CD4 less than 50/mm$^3$ [43].

## Invasive Fungal Pneumonias

Fungal pneumonias may be broadly grouped as follows:

1. Endemic includes genera *Histoplasma*, *Coccidioides*, *Blastomyces*, *Paracoccidioides*, *Cryptococcus*, and *Sporothrix*. These can infect both healthy and immunocompromised hosts, occur in certain geographic locations, and are associated with exposure to animal, particularly bird or bat, droppings.
2. Opportunistic includes genera *Aspergillus*, *Mucor*, and *Candida*. These typically occur in immunocompromised patients. Of these, *Aspergillus* and *Mucor* are angioinvasive, i.e., destroying adjacent blood vessels.
3. Hyalohyphomycosis includes fungi that rarely cause pneumonia, such as *Scedosporium* and *Fusarium* [44].

The clinical presentation of fungal pneumonia is nonspecific. In immunocompromised individuals, persistent fever despite antibiotic therapy may indicate a fungal infection. Disseminated fungal infection can present with clinical features reflecting the specific organ involved. In addition, endemic mycosis may present with rheumatologic symptoms [45, 46].

Fungal colonization of the respiratory tract is common [47]. Therefore, invasive fungal disease is considered proven if a biopsy specimen from a normally sterile and clinically or radiologically abnormal tissue, shows evidence of fungal elements on microscopy or culture. In the absence of such evidence, a combination of clinical, laboratory, and radiological data can be used to make a diagnosis [48].

The most characteristic imaging finding of fungal pneumonias is multiple pulmonary nodules (Fig. 13); consolidations may occur as well. Fungal pneumonias, particularly angioinvasive fungi, can manifest as parenchymal nodules or consolidations with surrounding ground-glass opacity, referred to as the "halo sign" (Fig. 14a). The ground-glass opacity generally represents hemorrhage. The halo sign is also seen with several other pathologies, including other fungal pneumonias, viral, bacterial, and mycobacterial pneumonias, septic emboli, and even neoplasms [49]. The "reverse halo sign," characterized by central ground-glass opacity and peripheral consolidation (Fig. 15), represents necrotizing infarction in the setting of angioinvasive fungal pneumonia and was originally thought to help identify mucormycosis. However, in immunocompromised patients, it may be equally common with invasive pulmonary aspergillosis [50]. The reverse halo sign is also nonspecific and may be seen in other conditions such as infectious pneumonias (including COVID-19), organizing pneumonia, lung adenocarcinoma, and granulomatosis with polyangiitis [51]. However, the presence of a reverse halo sign in the appropriate context should prompt radiologists and clinicians to consider mucormycosis; because of its aggressive nature, early diagnosis and treatment are critical. On MRI, pulmonary mucormycosis may show peripheral T2 hypointense signal with central non-enhancement, referred to as the "black-hole" sign [52].

Angioinvasive fungal pneumonias may also be characterized by cavitation and pulmonary infarcts due to vascular involvement [53]. During neutrophil count recovery, separation of necrotic lung parenchyma from adjacent viable tissue by a sickle-shaped gas lucency can give rise to the "air-crescent sign" (Fig. 14b) [54]. Airway-invasive pulmonary aspergillosis is characterized by peribronchial consolidations and centrilobular or tree-in-bud nodules [54].

Endemic fungal pneumonias are often characterized by nodules and consolidations. Travel and exposure history is key to making an accurate diagnosis [53, 55]. Both blastomycosis and histoplasmosis often manifest with pulmonary nodules and mediastinal and hilar lymph nodes (Fig. 16). Calcification is common with healed histoplasmosis. The scarring associated with mediastinal nodal disease may lead to vascular or central airway stenosis – a condition referred to as fibrosing mediastinitis [56]. Pulmonary coccidioidomycosis may present with migratory consolidations, which are referred to as phantom consolidations [57].

## Coronavirus Disease 2019 (COVID-19)

In late 2019, there was an outbreak of a severe viral respiratory illness, determined to be a coronavirus closely related to the severe acute respiratory syndrome (SARS) virus. This virus was named SARS-CoV-2, and the disease named coronavirus disease 2019 (COVID-19). This disease quickly spread across the world, becoming a pandemic that continues at the time of this writing. Patients typically present with cough and fever, although the clinical presentation is quite variable [58]. There is a large spectrum of disease severity, from asymptomatic patients to severely ill patients with acute respiratory distress syndrome (ARDS). The primary target of SARS-CoV-2 is the upper and lower respiratory tracts. Many patients develop pneumonia at imaging, even asymptomatic patients [59]. Some have argued that CT scans may be used as an adjunct in the diagnosis of COVID-19; note that given the large proportion of mild cases without CT manifestations, this strategy will have low sensitivity [60]. The Society of Thoracic Radiology and the American Society of Emergency Radiology issued a joint position statement that CT should not be used as a screening test in patients under investigation for COVID-19 [61]. The reference standard diagnosis of

COVID-19 is through viral nucleic acid detection in naso-pharyngeal swab samples. CT findings typical for COVID-19 in unsuspected patients (e.g., with abdominal complaints) should prompt testing. CT may also be helpful in evaluating patients with suspected complications, including pulmonary embolism or superinfection.

The manifestations of COVID-19 are similar to those of SARS but are different from many other viral and bacterial infections. Manifestations of mild disease mimic organizing pneumonia, with peripheral, basilar predominant ground-glass or consolidative opacities (Fig. 17). The reverse halo sign is not uncommon. A minority of patients progress to diffuse involvement of the lungs, with pathology showing diffuse alveolar damage [62]. As noted, the imaging differential for COVID-19 includes organizing pneumonia; other mimics, depending on the specific appearance, include non-specific interstitial pneumonia, aspiration, pulmonary infarcts, and alveolar hemorrhage [63].

## Mimics of Infection

It is common for pneumonia to persist despite antibiotic therapy due to both host and pathogen-related factors. However, approximately 20% of presumed pneumonia that does not respond to therapy is due to noninfectious causes [64]. Among these, the more common ones are organizing pneumonia, malignancy, and pulmonary infarcts.

## Organizing Pneumonia

Organizing pneumonia (OP) is an inflammatory lung disease that can present with clinical and imaging features similar to an infectious pneumonia. OP can be primary (cryptogenic organizing pneumonia) or secondary, due to drug therapy, connective tissue disorders, malignancies, or infections. A detailed review of the patient's history, medication usage, potential exposures, and underlying systemic disorders is

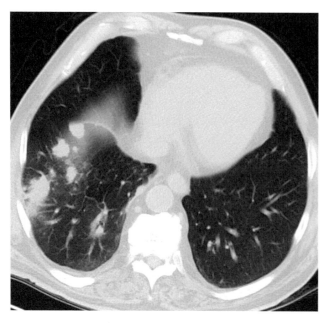

**Fig. 13** A 72-year-old man with Hodgkin's lymphoma, who developed cryptococcal pneumonia. Axial CT image through the lung bases shows multiple pulmonary nodules in the right lower lobe

**Fig. 14** A 47-year-old woman with acute myeloid leukemia and febrile neutropenia, who was found to have *Aspergillus* pneumonia. (**a**) Axial CT image of the right lung at presentation demonstrates a right upper lobe nodule with a subtle ground-glass halo (arrowhead). (**b**) CT performed 17 days later shows the development of an air crescent (arrow)

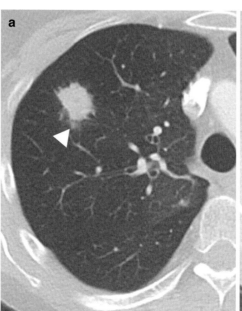
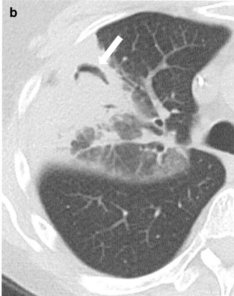

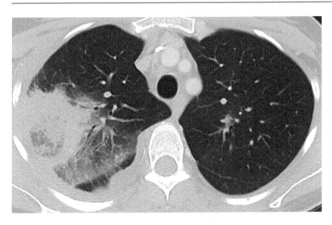

**Fig. 15** A 45-year-old woman with acute lymphocytic leukemia and pulmonary mucormycosis. Axial CT image of the lungs demonstrates a large nodular consolidation in the right upper lobe with central ground glass, representing the "reverse halo" sign. Also note a ground-glass halo surrounding the consolidation

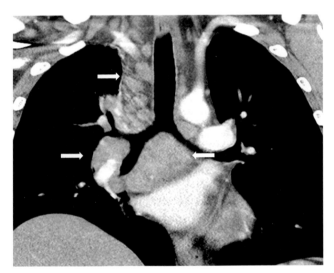

**Fig. 16** A 35-year-old man with histoplasmosis. Coronal CT image of the mediastinum shows extensive mediastinal and hilar lymphadenopathy (arrows)

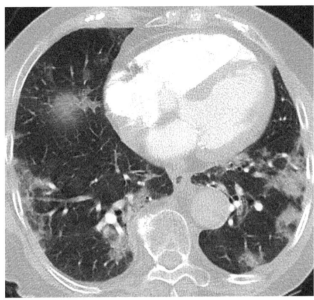

**Fig. 17** An 81-year-old woman with COVID-19 pneumonia. Axial CT of the lungs shows peripheral ground-glass opacities in both lower lobes

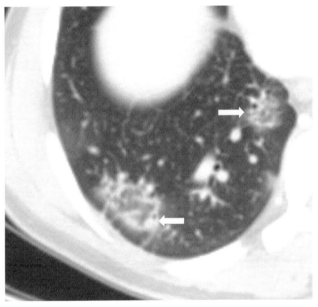

**Fig. 18** A 26-year-old man with Hodgkin's lymphoma on chemotherapy, who developed organizing pneumonia. Axial CT of the right lung demonstrates multiple ground-glass opacities in the right lower lobe with central lucency, indicating the reverse halo sign (arrows)

needed to determine whether OP is primary or secondary [65, 66].

On imaging, the typical appearance of OP is multifocal peripheral or peribronchial consolidative and ground-glass opacities, often with geometric margins or sharp demarcation with adjacent normal lung. Additional findings include reticular opacities, the reverse halo sign (Fig. 18), and bronchial dilatation. Pleural effusion and mediastinal lymphadenopathy are generally not present [67].

Patients with mild symptoms often have spontaneous remission, and therefore they may be managed with observation alone. In patients with moderate or severe disease, glucocorticoid therapy can induce rapid remission [67].

## Malignancies Mimicking Pneumonia

Neoplasms may mimic pneumonia in two forms – postobstructive pneumonia and infiltrative parenchymal neoplasm. In patients with an apparent non-resolving pneumonia, longer duration of symptoms, weight loss, and the absence of fever and leukocytosis can point towards a neoplastic etiology [68].

Endobronchial malignancies (particularly non-small cell lung cancer) may cause post-obstructive pneumonia. About 50% of patients with advanced lung cancer will have post-obstructive pneumonia at some point [69]. Likewise, about 50% of all post-obstructive pneumonias are due to lung cancers [68]. However, malignancies may themselves present as consolidations. These include lung adenocarcinomas

(those formerly known as bronchoalveolar cell carcinoma), as well as primary or secondary pulmonary lymphomas.

Abrupt cut-off of a bronchus (Fig. 19) and differential enhancement of the tumor from adjacent collapsed/consolidated lung are helpful features to distinguish a post-obstructive pneumonia. Primary consolidative malignancies are more difficult to distinguish from infectious or organizing pneumonia. However, persistent or progressive airspace disease over the period of several months should strongly suggest a malignant etiology.

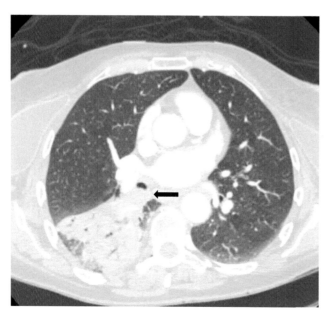

**Fig. 19** A 54-year-old woman with complete occlusion of the right lower lobe bronchus (arrow), with distal atelectasis and consolidation. Transbronchial biopsy revealed primary lung adenocarcinoma

## Pulmonary Infarct

Pulmonary embolism may be complicated by lung infarction. Patients may present with dyspnea, chest pain, and low-grade fever, which can mimic a pneumonia. Thus, infarcts can occasionally be misdiagnosed as pneumonia. A normal D-dimer makes pulmonary embolism (PE) unlikely. However, elevated D-dimer is not specific and can be seen with both PE and pneumonia.

Pulmonary infarcts present as peripheral wedge-shaped ground-glass or consolidation at CT (Fig. 20a). Chest radiographs may demonstrate these subtle opacities at the periphery of the lung, often in the lower lung zones – representing a Hampton's hump. Additional CT imaging features are the reverse halo sign or presence of peripheral consolidation with central ground glass [70]. If these imaging features are present, the radiologist should consider pulmonary infarcts

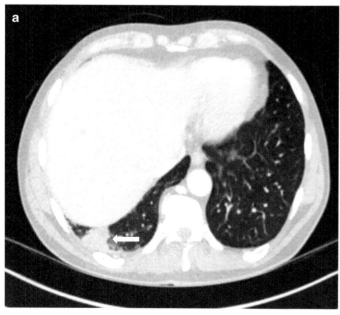
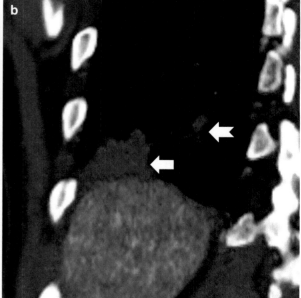
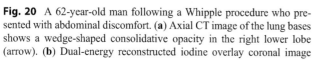

**Fig. 20** A 62-year-old man following a Whipple procedure who presented with abdominal discomfort. (**a**) Axial CT image of the lung bases shows a wedge-shaped consolidative opacity in the right lower lobe (arrow). (**b**) Dual-energy reconstructed iodine overlay coronal image shows the absence of iodine uptake in the opacity (straight arrow) and a filling defect in a right lower lobe subsegmental pulmonary artery branch (notched arrow), indicating acute pulmonary embolism with lung infarction

and should strongly consider recommending CT pulmonary angiography. Dual-energy CT with iodine map overlay can demonstrate the absence of enhancement within the infarct (Fig. 20), although this is a nonspecific finding that may also be seen with pneumonias.

## Conclusion

Pneumonia is a common diagnosis on chest radiography and CT. While some imaging findings can suggest a particular etiologic agent, there is a large degree of overlap in imaging appearance of bacterial, viral, and even fungal pneumonias. Patient immunocompromised state predisposes to particular infections, and this information is critical when providing an accurate differential diagnosis. Equally important to making the diagnosis of pulmonary infection is evaluating for potential alternative diagnoses and mimics that would require different therapies. In this way, radiologists play a key role in evaluating patients with suspected pneumonia.

## References

1. Bajaj SK, Tombach B. Respiratory infections in immunocompromised patients: lung findings using chest computed tomography. Radiol Infect Dis. 2017;4(1):29–37.
2. Peck KR, Kim TJ, Lee MA, Lee KS, Han J. Pneumonia in immunocompromised patients: updates in clinical and imaging features. Precis Future Med. 2018;2(3):95–108.
3. Oh YW, Effmann EL, Godwin JD. Pulmonary infections in immunocompromised hosts: the importance of correlating the conventional radiologic appearance with the clinical setting. Radiology. 2000;217(3):647–56.
4. Jain S, Self WH, Wunderink RG, Fakhran S, Balk R, Bramley AM, et al. Community-acquired pneumonia requiring hospitalization among U.S. adults. N Engl J Med. 2015;373(5):415–27.
5. Metlay JP, Waterer GW, Long AC, Anzueto A, Brozek J, Crothers K, et al. Diagnosis and treatment of adults with community-acquired pneumonia. An official clinical practice guideline of the American Thoracic Society and Infectious Diseases Society of America. Am J Respir Crit Care Med. 2019;200(7):e45–67.
6. Lim WS, Baudouin SV, George RC, Hill AT, Jamieson C, Jeune IL, et al. BTS guidelines for the management of community acquired pneumonia in adults: update 2009. Thorax. 2009;64(Suppl 3):iii1–55.
7. Franquet T. Imaging of pneumonia: trends and algorithms. Eur Respir J. 2001;18(1):196–208.
8. Miller WT, Mickus TJ, Barbosa E, Mullin C, Van Deerlin VM, Shiley KT. CT of viral lower respiratory tract infections in adults: comparison among viral organisms and between viral and bacterial infections. AJR Am J Roentgenol. 2011;197(5):1088–95.
9. Koo HJ, Lim S, Choe J, Choi S-H, Sung H, Do K-H. Radiographic and CT features of viral pneumonia. Radiographics. 2018;38(3):719–39.
10. Kloth C, Forler S, Gatidis S, Beck R, Spira D, Nikolaou K, et al. Comparison of chest-CT findings of influenza virus-associated pneumonia in immunocompetent vs. immunocompromised patients. Eur J Radiol. 2015;84(6):1177–83.
11. Reittner P, Müller NL, Heyneman L, Johkoh T, Park JS, Lee KS, et al. Mycoplasma pneumoniae Pneumonia. Am J Roentgenol. 2000;174(1):37–41.
12. Leung AN. Pulmonary tuberculosis: the essentials. Radiology. 1999;210(2):307–22.
13. Nachiappan AC, Rahbar K, Shi X, Guy ES, Mortani Barbosa EJ, Shroff GS, et al. Pulmonary tuberculosis: role of radiology in diagnosis and management. Radiographics. 2017;37(1):52–72.
14. Choi J-A, Hong KT, Oh Y-W, Chung MH, Seol HY, Kang E-Y. CT manifestations of late sequelae in patients with tuberculous Pleuritis. Am J Roentgenol. 2001;176(2):441–5.
15. Curvo-Semedo L, Teixeira L, Caseiro-Alves F. Tuberculosis of the chest. Eur J Radiol. 2005;55(2):158–72.
16. Rodriguez-Takeuchi SY, Renjifo ME, Medina FJ. Extrapulmonary tuberculosis: pathophysiology and imaging findings. Radiographics. 2019;39(7):2023–37.
17. Prevots DR, Shaw PA, Strickland D, Jackson LA, Raebel MA, Blosky MA, et al. Nontuberculous mycobacterial lung disease prevalence at four integrated health care delivery systems. Am J Respir Crit Care Med. 2010;182(7):970–6.
18. Erasmus JJ, McAdams HP, Farrell MA, Patz EF. Pulmonary nontuberculous mycobacterial infection: radiologic manifestations. Radiographics. 1999;19(6):1487–503.
19. Cassidy PM, Hedberg K, Saulson A, McNelly E, Winthrop KL. Nontuberculous mycobacterial disease prevalence and risk factors: a changing epidemiology. Clin Infect Dis. 2009;49(12):e124–9.
20. Ye R, Zhao L, Wang C, Wu X, Yan H. Clinical characteristics of septic pulmonary embolism in adults: a systematic review. Respir Med. 2014;108(1):1–8.
21. Oh HG, Cha S-I, Shin K-M, Lim J-K, Kim HJ, Yoo S-S, et al. Risk factors for mortality in patients with septic pulmonary embolism. J Infect Chemother. 2016;22(8):553–8.
22. Lin MY, Rezai K, Schwartz DN. Septic pulmonary emboli and Bacteremia associated with deep tissue infections caused by community-acquired methicillin-resistant Staphylococcus aureus. J Clin Microbiol. 2008;46(4):1553–5.
23. Cooper HA, Thompson EC, Laureno R, Fuisz A, Mark AS, Lin M, et al. Subclinical brain embolization in left-sided infective endocarditis: results from the evaluation by MRI of the brains of patients with left-sided intracardiac solid masses (EMBOLISM) pilot study. Circulation. 2009;120(7):585–91.
24. Dodd JD, Souza CA, Müller NL. High-resolution MDCT of pulmonary septic embolism: evaluation of the feeding vessel sign. AJR Am J Roentgenol. 2006;187(3):623–9.
25. Iwasaki Y, Nagata K, Nakanishi M, Natuhara A, Harada H, Kubota Y, et al. Spiral CT findings in septic pulmonary emboli. Eur J Radiol. 2001;37(3):190–4.
26. Kwon WJ, Jeong YJ, Kim K-I, Lee IS, Jeon UB, Lee SH, et al. Computed tomographic features of pulmonary septic emboli: comparison of causative microorganisms. J Comput Assist Tomogr. 2007;31(3):390–4.
27. Sepkowitz KA. Opportunistic infections in patients with and patients without acquired immunodeficiency syndrome. Clin Infect Dis. 2002;34(8):1098–107.
28. Huang L, Cattamanchi A, Davis JL, den Boon S, Kovacs J, Meshnick S, et al. HIV-associated pneumocystis pneumonia. Proc Am Thorac Soc. 2011;8(3):294–300.
29. Pifer LL, Hughes WT, Stagno S, Woods D. Pneumocystis carinii infection: evidence for high prevalence in normal and immunosuppressed children. Pediatrics. 1978;61(1):35–41.
30. Catherinot E, Lanternier F, Bougnoux M-E, Lecuit M, Couderc L-J, Lortholary O. Pneumocystis jirovecii Pneumonia. Infect Dis Clin N Am. 2010;24(1):107–38.
31. Tasaka S, Kobayashi S, Kamata H, Kimizuka Y, Fujiwara H, Funatsu Y, et al. Cytokine profiles of bronchoalveolar lavage fluid in patients with pneumocystis pneumonia. Microbiol Immunol. 2010;54(7):425–33.

32. Tasaka S. Pneumocystis pneumonia in human immunodeficiency virus–infected adults and adolescents: current concepts and future directions. Clin Med Insights Circ Respir Pulm Med. 2015;9 (Suppl 1):19–28.

33. Kang EY, Staples CA, McGuinness G, Primack SL, Müller NL. Detection and differential diagnosis of pulmonary infections and tumors in patients with AIDS: value of chest radiography versus CT. Am J Roentgenol. 1996;166(1):15–9.

34. Fujii T, Nakamura T, Iwamoto A. Pneumocystis pneumonia in patients with HIV infection: clinical manifestations, laboratory findings, and radiological features. J Infect Chemother. 2007;13(1):1–7.

35. Marchiori E, Müller NL, Soares Souza A, Escuissato DL, Gasparetto EL, Franquet T. Pulmonary disease in patients with AIDS: high-resolution CT and pathologic findings. Am J Roentgenol. 2005;184(3):757–64.

36. Tasaka S, Tokuda H, Sakai F, Fujii T, Tateda K, Johkoh T, et al. Comparison of clinical and radiological features of pneumocystis pneumonia between malignancy cases and acquired immunodeficiency syndrome cases: a multicenter study. Intern Med. 2010;49(4): 273–81.

37. Kanne JP, Yandow DR, Meyer CA. Pneumocystis jiroveci pneumonia: high-resolution CT findings in patients with and without HIV infection. Am J Roentgenol. 2012;198(6):W555–61.

38. Boiselle PM, Crans CA, Kaplan MA. The changing face of pneumocystis carinii pneumonia in AIDS patients. Am J Roentgenol. 1999;172(5):1301–9.

39. Chow C, Templeton PA, White CS. Lung cysts associated with pneumocystis carinii pneumonia: radiographic characteristics, natural history, and complications. Am J Roentgenol. 1993;161(3):527–31.

40. Kuhlman JE, Kavuru M, Fishman EK, Siegelman SS. Pneumocystis carinii pneumonia: spectrum of parenchymal CT findings. Radiology. 1990;175(3):711–4.

41. Wassermann K, Pothoff G, Kirn E, Fätkenheuer G, Krueger GR. Chronic Pneumocystis carinii pneumonia in AIDS. Chest. 1993;104(3):667–72.

42. Horowitz ML, Schiff M, Samuels J, Russo R, Schnader J. Pneumocystis carinii pleural effusion. Pathogenesis and pleural fluid analysis. Am Rev Respir Dis. 1993;148(1):232–4.

43. Crowe SM, Carlin JB, Stewart KI, Lucas CR, Hoy JF. Predictive value of CD4 lymphocyte numbers for the development of opportunistic infections and malignancies in HIV-infected persons. J Acquir Immune Defic Syndr. 1991;4(8):770–6.

44. Chen SC-A, Blyth C, Sorrell T, Slavin M. Pneumonia and lung infections due to emerging and unusual fungal pathogens. Semin Respir Crit Care Med. 2011;32(06):703–16.

45. Hage CA, Knox KS, Wheat LJ. Endemic mycoses: overlooked causes of community acquired pneumonia. Respir Med. 2012;106 (6):769–76.

46. Mango ALD, Zanetti G, Penha D, Barreto MM, Marchiori E. Endemic pulmonary fungal diseases in immunocompetent patients: an emphasis on thoracic imaging. Expert Rev Respir Med. 2019;13(3):263–77.

47. Biswas D, Agarwal S, Sindhwani G, Rawat J. Fungal colonization in patients with chronic respiratory diseases from Himalayan region of India. Ann Clin Microbiol Antimicrob. 2010;9:28.

48. De Pauw B, Walsh TJ, Donnelly JP, Stevens DA, Edwards JE, Calandra T, et al. Revised definitions of invasive fungal disease from the European Organization for Research and Treatment of cancer/invasive fungal infections cooperative group and the National Institute of Allergy and Infectious Diseases mycoses study group (EORTC/MSG) consensus group. Clin Infect Dis. 2008;46(12):1813–21.

49. Georgiadou SP, Sipsas NV, Marom EM, Kontoyiannis DP. The diagnostic value of halo and reversed halo signs for invasive mold infections in compromised hosts. Clin Infect Dis. 2011;52(9):1144–55.

50. Thomas R, Madan R, Gooptu M, Hatabu H, Hammer MM. Significance of the reverse halo sign in immunocompromised patients. Am J Roentgenol. 2019;213(3):549–54.

51. Godoy MCB, Viswanathan C, Marchiori E, Truong MT, Benveniste MF, Rossi S, et al. The reversed halo sign: update and differential diagnosis. Br J Radiol. 2012;85(1017):1226–35.

52. Hammer MM, Madan R, Hatabu H. Pulmonary Mucormycosis: radiologic features at presentation and over time. AJR Am J Roentgenol. 2018;210(4):742–7.

53. Orlowski HLP, McWilliams S, Mellnick VM, Bhalla S, Lubner MG, Pickhardt PJ, et al. Imaging Spectrum of invasive fungal and fungal-like infections. Radiographics. 2017;37(4):1119–34.

54. Franquet T, Müller NL, Giménez A, Guembe P, de la Torre J, Bagué S. Spectrum of pulmonary aspergillosis: histologic, clinical, and radiologic findings. Radiographics. 2001;21(4):825–37.

55. Fang W, Washington L, Kumar N. Imaging manifestations of Blastomycosis: a pulmonary infection with potential dissemination. Radiographics. 2007;27(3):641–55.

56. Gurney JW, Conces DJ. Pulmonary histoplasmosis. Radiology. 1996;199(2):297–306.

57. Jude CM, Nayak NB, Patel MK, Deshmukh M, Batra P. Pulmonary Coccidioidomycosis: pictorial review of chest radiographic and CT findings. Radiographics. 2014;34(4):912–25.

58. Huang C, Wang Y, Li X, Ren L, Zhao J, Hu Y, et al. Clinical features of patients infected with 2019 novel coronavirus in Wuhan. China Lancet. 2020;395(10223):497–506.

59. Inui S, Fujikawa A, Jitsu M, Kunishima N, Watanabe S, Suzuki Y, et al. Chest CT findings in cases from the cruise ship "diamond princess" with coronavirus disease 2019 (COVID-19). Radiol Cardiothoracic Imaging. 2020;2(2):e200110.

60. Isikbay M, Hope MD, Raptis CA, Shah A, Bierhals AJ, Bhalla S, et al. CT on the diamond princess: what might this tell us about sensitivity for COVID-19? Radiol Cardiothoracic Imaging. 2020;2(2):e200155.

61. Society of Thoracic Radiology. STR/ASER COVID-19 position statement [Internet]. 2020 [cited 2020 Dec 10]. Available from: https://thoracicrad.org/?page_id=2879

62. Schaefer I-M, Padera RF, Solomon IH, Kanjilal S, Hammer MM, Hornick JL, et al. In situ detection of SARS-CoV-2 in lungs and airways of patients with COVID-19. Mod Pathol. 2020;19:1–11.

63. Simpson S, Kay FU, Abbara S, Bhalla S, Chung JH, Chung M, et al. Radiological Society of North America Expert Consensus Statement on reporting chest CT findings related to COVID-19. Endorsed by the Society of Thoracic Radiology, the American College of Radiology, and RSNA. Radiol Cardiothoracic Imaging. 2020;2(2):e200152.

64. Arancibia F, Ewig S, Martinez JA, Ruiz M, Bauer T, Marcos MA, et al. Antimicrobial treatment failures in patients with community-acquired pneumonia: causes and prognostic implications. Am J Respir Crit Care Med. 2000;162(1):154–60.

65. Cordier J-F. Cryptogenic organising pneumonia. Eur Respir J. 2006;28(2):422–46.

66. Drakopanagiotakis F, Paschalaki K, Abu-Hijleh M, Aswad B, Karagianidis N, Kastanakis E, et al. Cryptogenic and secondary organizing pneumonia: clinical presentation, radiographic findings, treatment response, and prognosis. Chest. 2011;139(4):893–900.

67. Faria IM, Zanetti G, Barreto MM, Rodrigues RS, Araujo-Neto CA, Silva JLP. E, et al. organizing pneumonia: chest HRCT findings. J Bras Pneumol. 2015;41(3):231–7.

68. Abers MS, Sandvall BP, Sampath R, Zuno C, Uy N, Yu VL, et al. Postobstructive pneumonia: an underdescribed syndrome. Clin Infect Dis. 2016;62(8):957–61.

69. Rolston KVI, Nesher L. Post-obstructive pneumonia in patients with cancer: a review. Infect Dis Ther. 2018;7(1):29–38.

70. He H, Stein MW, Zalta B, Haramati LB. Pulmonary infarction: spectrum of findings on multidetector helical CT. J Thorac Imaging. 2006;21(1):1–7.

Mostafa Alabousi, Abdullah Alabousi, Supriya Kulkarni, and Michael N. Patlas

## Contents

### Abstract

A variety of acute breast complaints may present to the emergency department (ED), and it is important for radiologists to be familiar with the important clinical and imaging findings of these pathologies. Although mammography is more commonly utilized for breast imaging, ultrasound (US) is first-line choice of assessment for acute breast complaints in the ED, as it is more readily available and better tolerated by patients. This chapter will review the clinical background and imaging findings of a variety of breast pathologies, which may be seen in the emergency setting, as well as to provide a brief review of management and potential complications. It will cover infectious, inflammatory, traumatic, iatrogenic, pregnancy - or lactation-related, and augmentation- related breast emergencies.

### Keywords

Breast diseases · Breast injuries · Mammography · Ultrasonography, Mammary · Female · Diagnostic imaging · Emergencies

## Introduction

Patients may present to the emergency department (ED) with a variety of breast complaints, which require prompt diagnosis and management [1–3]. It is imperative for radiologists to recognize important clinical and imaging findings for these acute breast conditions, as well as have a good understanding of management and potential complications [1, 3]. In order to do so, radiologists must be familiar with a variety of infectious, inflammatory, traumatic, iatrogenic, pregnancy - or lactation-related, and augmentation-related breast emergencies, which may require urgent intervention [1, 2]. Furthermore, although mammography is more commonly used for breast imaging, breast ultrasound (US) is the workhorse in the ED setting, as it is more readily available, is better tolerated by patients, and provides important information regarding the presence or absence of breast abnormalities

M. Alabousi (✉) · M. N. Patlas
Department of Radiology, McMaster University, Hamilton, ON, Canada
e-mail: mostafa.alabousi@medportal.ca; patlas@hhsc.ca

A. Alabousi
Department of Radiology, McMaster University, St. Joseph's Healthcare Hamilton, Hamilton, ON, Canada
e-mail: abdullah.alabousi@medportal.ca

S. Kulkarni
Department of Medical Imaging, University of Toronto, Princess Margaret Hospital, Toronto, ON, Canada
e-mail: Supriya.Kulkarni@uhn.ca

© Springer Nature Switzerland AG 2022
M. N. Patlas et al. (eds.), *Atlas of Emergency Imaging from Head-to-Toe*,
https://doi.org/10.1007/978-3-030-92111-8_19

[2]. This chapter will review the clinical background and imaging findings of a variety of breast pathologies, which may be seen in the emergency setting, as well as provide a brief review of management and potential complications.

## Clinical Features and Diagnostic Investigations

### Infectious and Inflammatory Disease

#### Infectious Mastitis

Mastitis is defined as inflammation of the breast, which may be related to infectious or noninfectious causes [1]. In infectious mastitis, the most common causative organisms are *Staphylococcus aureus* and *Streptococcus* [2–4]. Classically, mastitis may present with unilateral pain, erythema, and swelling, and it may also result in systemic symptoms, including fever, malaise, and fatigue [1–3, 5]. Mastitis may be complicated by abscess formation, presenting as a painful palpable mass in the breast [5–7]. Infectious mastitis may be acquired spontaneously, or it can be seen in postoperative patients. Additionally, there can be superinfection of a posttraumatic or iatrogenic hematoma [5].

Puerperal mastitis can occur during pregnancy or lactation [6]. It is classically seen in lactating mothers within 3 months of childbirth, affecting 1–9% of nursing mothers [1, 5]. Puerperal mastitis most frequently occurs during the second postpartum week due to milk stasis and resulting retrograde infection [2, 3]. Conservative management strategies consist of analgesia, gentle massage, and warm compresses and ice packs [1]. Continued breastfeeding is suggested, unless the nursing mother is taking an antibiotic which is contraindicated for the newborn [2, 6]. Antibiotic therapy may be administered if symptoms persist; however, the mastitis often resolves without antibiotic therapy [1, 6]. Puerperal mastitis complicated by abscess formation typically responds well to antibiotic therapy and drainage [6].

Non-puerperal mastitis may be classified as peripheral or subareolar [1]. Risk factors include diabetes, smoking, and obesity [6]. Non-puerperal mastitis complicated by central/peri-areolar abscess formation is more commonly seen in younger smokers, while more peripheral abscesses tend to be seen in older women with chronic conditions, such as diabetes, rheumatoid arthritis, or long-term steroid therapy [6]. The main treatment approach is oral antibiotic therapy, as well as aspiration in cases complicated by abscess formation [5]. Success rates for abscess aspiration range from 54% to 100%, and it is most effective in collections <3 cm [1, 5, 6]. There is a higher risk of aspiration failure in larger abscesses and in patients with long-standing symptoms (>6 days) [1]. If aspiration is not successful, drainage catheter placement or ultimately surgical intervention may be

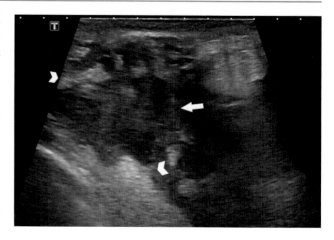

**Fig. 1 Mastitis.** A 35-year-old woman with findings of mastitis on sagittal US images with a heterogeneous appearance of the breast tissue with central hypoechoic changes corresponding to edema (arrow) and peripheral echogenic, inflamed fat (arrowheads)

required for drainage. However, there is a higher recurrence rate in these cases (up to 28%) [1, 5, 6].

Mastitis is often treated empirically without imaging; however, US may be performed if the patient is not completely responding to antibiotics [6, 8–10]. Typical findings on US include dilated lactiferous ducts on a background of heterogeneous echogenic changes in the breast tissue related to inflammatory changes and swelling (Fig. 1) [1]. Abscess formation is characterized by a complex, predominantly centrally hypoechoic collection with a peripheral echogenic rim [1, 2, 5, 6]. Abscesses contain mobile internal debris, posterior acoustic enhancement, and, in some cases, internal septations [1, 2, 5, 6]. They may be variable in shape and size; abscesses are often multilocular [1, 6]. On Doppler assessment, no internal flow is seen, but the periphery is hypervascular, representing hyperemic tissue surrounding the abscess [1, 5, 6].

Mammography may sometimes be considered in women over the age of 30 presenting with clinical signs of mastitis [1]. Delayed mammographic examinations are often recommended, as this improves patient comfort with breast compression, enhancing image quality as a result [1]. Findings on mammography include asymmetric density, as well as skin and trabecular thickening [2, 6]. Associated axillary lymphadenopathy may also be seen [6]. Findings on mammography may be nonspecific, and they should be correlated with the clinical picture and sonographic findings [2]. More importantly, it helps exclude underlying masses and calcifications.

Breast MRI has been proposed to differentiate mastitis from malignancy. However, it is not a first- or second-line imaging option due to higher cost and less ready availability in the emergency setting. Additionally, there can be substantial overlap in imaging findings between malignancy and

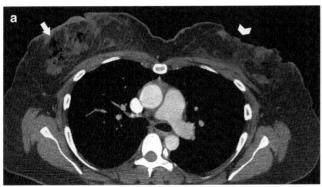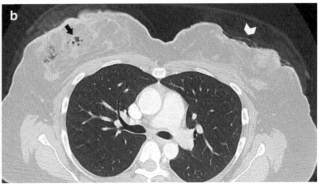

**Fig. 2 Emphysematous mastitis.** A 35-year-old woman with findings of bilateral mastitis on soft tissue (**a**) and lung (**b**) windows axial contrast-enhanced CT images with increased density in the breast tissue, as well as subcutaneous emphysematous changes (arrow) in the right breast. The left breast demonstrates evidence of previous debridement related to prior infection (arrowhead)

infection [1, 5]. An abscess may appear as a rim-enhancing collection on both MRI and CT, but neither of these modalities are first-line options for evaluation of mastitis [5]. In rare cases, emphysematous mastitis may develop as seen in this case on CT (Fig. 2).

## Mondor's Disease

Mondor's disease is a rare, benign, self-limited superficial thrombophlebitis [2, 3]. The classic clinical presentation is a painful, palpable mass or cord-like focus with possible skin discoloration and/or nipple retraction in women of child-bearing age [2, 3, 11]. Many risk factors have been identified, including previous trauma, infection, and breast augmentation [12]. Treatment includes analgesics and warm compresses [2, 3]. Follow-up imaging may be ordered in 4–6 weeks to ensure resolution [2].

Although the diagnosis of Mondor's disease may be made clinically, imaging is often utilized to assist in diagnosing this uncommon entity [2]. On US, a superficial hypoechoic or anechoic noncompressible structure is seen with a beaded appearance, which is the thrombosed vein [2, 3]. A distinct thrombus can occasionally be seen in the vessel. Color Doppler demonstrates a lack of flow in the vein, which is re-established on resolution (Fig. 3) [2, 3]. On mammography, a thick, tubular density can be seen, corresponding to the thrombosed venous segment, which is continuous with a normal-appearing vein [2, 3].

## Hidradenitis Suppurativa

Hidradenitis suppurativa, also known as acne inversa, is an inflammatory condition characterized by recurrent abscesses, nodules, sinus tract formation, and scarring [13, 14]. Although the etiology is unclear to our knowledge, it is favored to be the result of breast follicle occlusion due to follicular hyperkeratosis, ultimately resulting in dilatation and rupture [13, 14]. This leads to spillage of follicular contents into the surrounding dermis, leading to a chemotactic response and

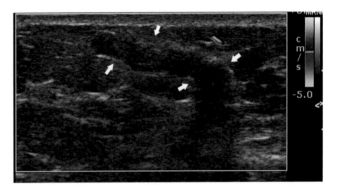

**Fig. 3 Mondor's disease.** A 32-year-old woman with findings of an enlarged, anechoic, tubular structure with no internal vascularity (arrows) on a sagittal US image, which represents an expanded, thrombosed superficial vein (Mondor's disease)

inflammatory reaction [13, 14]. It is more commonly seen in women during puberty, and it generally involves the axilla, inframammary fold, and genitofemoral regions [13, 14]. This condition is chronic and progressive and may require surgical treatment for definitive cure [13, 14].

Findings on US and mammography are fairly nonspecific [13, 14]. Marked skin thickening and induration of the subcutaneous tissue may be seen [13, 14]. Abscess and sinus tract formation are also findings which can be identified in hidradenitis suppurativa (Fig. 4) [13, 14].

## Kikuchi Disease

Kikuchi disease, also known as histiocytic necrotizing lymphadenitis, or Kikuchi-Fujimoto disease, is a rare, benign, self-limited condition characterized by subacute necrotizing lymphadenopathy [15]. It predominantly affects women under the age of 40 [15]. Clinical presentation consists of painful, tender lymphadenopathy, most commonly in the posterior cervical and axillary regions [15]. Patients may develop cutaneous focal abnormalities or rashes, as well as a mild fever or other systemic symptoms [15]. The condition is

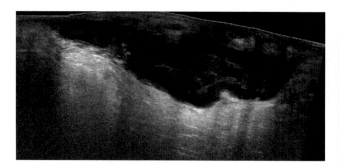

**Fig. 4 Hidradenitis suppurativa.** A 35-year-old woman with hidradenitis suppurativa on a sagittal US image demonstrating a complex hypoechoic collection in the subcutaneous tissue of the axilla with scattered internal septations and debris, as well posterior acoustic enhancement, which represents an abscess secondary to follicular gland obstruction

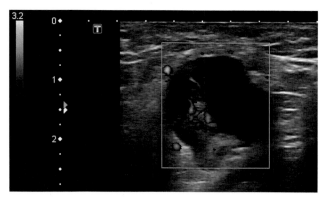

**Fig. 5 Kikuchi disease.** A 29-year-old woman with Kikuchi disease demonstrates findings of axillary lymphadenopathy with an abnormal, enlarged peripherally hypoechoic lymph node with a thickened cortex on an axial US image, which represents abscess formation

self-limited, usually resolving within a few months, with symptomatic treatment [15].

Findings on imaging are relatively nonspecific [16]. They consist of homogenous nodal enlargement, as well as possible perinodal infiltration [16, 17]. Less frequently, central necrotic changes may be seen within the lymph nodes (Fig. 5) [16].

## Traumatic and Iatrogenic Disease

### Hematoma

A breast hematoma may develop secondary to percutaneous biopsy, breast surgery, acute trauma, or, rarely, tumor invasion into a vessel [1]. Following a biopsy, patients usually present within 1–2 days if adequate hemostasis was not achieved, reported to occur in <1% of cases [1, 3, 5, 18]. A motor vehicle collision seat belt injury is the most common cause of traumatic breast hematoma [5, 19]. The clinical presentation consists of a tender, palpable breast mass with

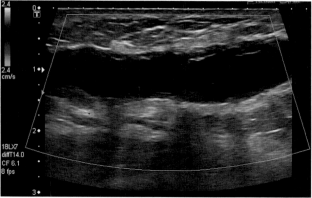

**Fig. 6 Postoperative hematoma.** A 46-year-old woman with findings of a well-defined hypoechoic collection within the breast containing multiple low-level internal echoes, posterior acoustic enhancement, and no internal vascularity on an axial US image, which is a postoperative hematoma

overlying skin bruising, which may extend to the contralateral breast, chest, wall, back, and flanks [1, 5]. Aspirin therapy and anticoagulants are associated with a higher risk of post-biopsy hematoma formation (22% versus 13%), as well as a higher rate of bruising [20, 21]. More severe bleeding complications are thought to occur when a vessel is sliced in the longitudinal plane by the biopsy needle, as opposed to in the cross-sectional plane [1]. Management approaches post-biopsy include a longer period of compression, aggressive vacuum suctioning, or, ultimately, surgical ligation to control the bleeding [21–24]. Management of a post-traumatic hematoma usually involves symptomatic treatment, while significant breast deformity may warrant reconstructive surgery [1]. The most serious post-traumatic complication, breast avulsion, requires emergent surgery due to the accompanying massive hemorrhage [1, 5].

On US, a hematoma is seen as a hypoechoic collection, or a complex collection containing hypoechoic and hyperechoic components, reflecting a mixture of clotted and liquid blood (Figs. 6, 7, and 8) [1, 5]. Scattered areas of hemorrhage on US will appear as hypoechoic foci, for example, seen along the biopsy tract and tissue planes [1]. Superinfection of a breast hematoma often requires correlation with the patient's clinical status (Fig. 9). The mammographic appearance of a hematoma may be an ill-defined or well-circumscribed mass at or near the biopsy site [1, 5]. A gas-fluid level may also be seen on mammography [1]. A focus of hemorrhage may appear as a new focal asymmetry at or near the biopsy site, while hemorrhage may also be seen tracking along the pectoralis major muscle and connective tissue planes [1, 5].

CT is commonly the first-line imaging examination performed in the setting of acute trauma, in which case a hypoattenuating collection may be seen corresponding to a breast hematoma [3, 5]. Findings of contrast blush in or adjacent to the hematoma may represent active extravasation

**Fig. 7 Post-traumatic hematoma.** A 51-year-old woman with findings of an echogenic, irregularly shaped area on axial and sagittal US images in a patient with recent trauma, which is a breast hematoma

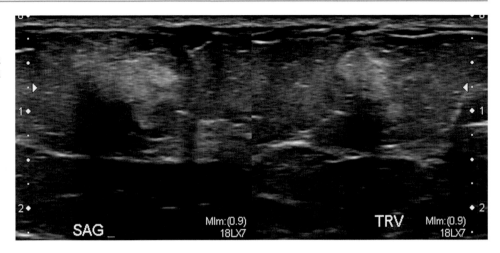

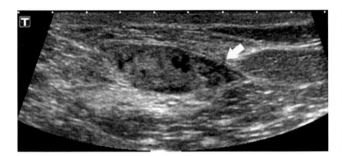

**Fig. 8 Breast hematoma following handlebar injury.** A 22-year-old woman with recent history of bicycle handlebar injury to the right breast demonstrates findings of a superficial, complex, lentiform-shaped collection (arrow) on a sagittal US image, which is a hematoma

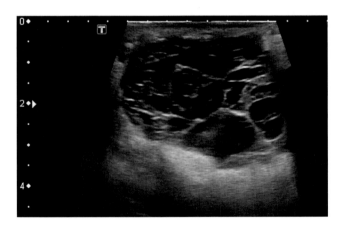

**Fig. 9 Infected postoperative hematoma.** A 74-year-old woman with known postoperative hematoma, now presenting with fever and elevated leukocytes, demonstrates findings of a complex fluid collection with multiple echogenic internal septations, low-level internal echoes, and posterior acoustic enhancement. Findings at the time of drainage confirmed an infected postoperative hematoma

(with delayed pooling) in keeping with active arterial hemorrhage or may represent pseudoaneurysm or both [1, 3, 5]. If only an underlying breast contusion is present, findings of asymmetric breast density and skin thickening may be seen [3, 5].

## Postoperative Seroma

A postoperative seroma is the most common surgical complication, defined as a serous, sterile fluid collection, which does not contain blood contents, that can accumulate in a potential space following surgery [25, 26]. Management of a postoperative seroma, when symptomatic, generally consists of aspiration or surgical drainage [25, 26].

The sonographic appearance of a postoperative seroma consists of an anechoic or hypoechoic fluid-containing mass, which may be round or oval in shape (Figs. 10 and 11) [25, 26]. On mammography, a seroma appears as a soft tissue density or mass [25, 26]. On MRI, a seroma appears hyperintense on T2-weighted imaging and hypointense on T1-weighted imaging [25, 26]. On CT, a round fluid density mass may be seen, corresponding to a postoperative seroma [25, 26]. Early peripheral rim enhancement of a postoperative seroma may be seen on both MRI and CT [25, 26].

## Pseudoaneurysm

A pseudoaneurysm is a hematoma contained by adventitia or surrounding soft tissue that communicates directly with a lumen of an artery [3, 5, 27, 28]. Unlike a true aneurysm, a pseudoaneurysm lacks the normal three layers of a surrounding arterial wall [3, 5, 27, 28]. A pseudoaneurysm most commonly forms secondary to trauma, surgery, or biopsy and is rarely associated with anticoagulation and atherosclerotic disease [1, 5]. Clinically, depending on the size of the pseudoaneurysm, the patient can present with a palpable, pulsatile mass with overlying skin changes, as well as a history of significant bleeding or a large hematoma at the time of biopsy/surgery/trauma [3, 5, 27, 28]. Treatment options consist of manual US-guided compression at the pseudoaneurysm neck as a first-line option, followed by US-guided injection/embolization with thrombin, alcohol,

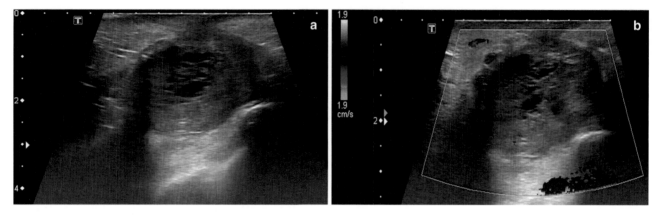

**Fig. 10** **Complex postoperative seroma.** A 53-year-old woman with a history of remote breast surgery demonstrates findings of a complex fluid collection with heterogenous echogenic components and posterior acoustic enhancement (**a**) with no internal vascularity (**b**) on axial US images. Findings at the time of drainage confirmed a complex postoperative seroma

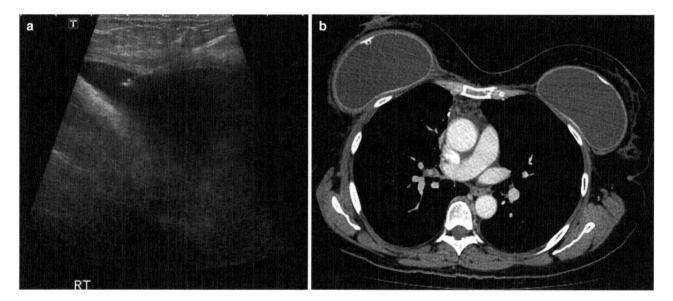

**Fig. 11** **Post-lung biopsy peri-implant collection.** A 56-year-old woman with an US-guided aspiration of the right peri-implant collection (**a**) which developed following biopsy of a lung nodule. Following drainage, axial contrast-enhanced CT shows resolution of the collection with intact breast implants (**b**)

or microcoils, or, in some cases, surgical repair [3, 5, 27, 28]. Treatment of pseudoaneurysms in the breast have lower reported success rates compared to pseudoaneurysms in other parts of the body [1]. Spontaneous pseudoaneurysm resolution has been reported, more commonly in those with a small pseudoaneurysm neck and in patients not on anticoagulation [1, 5].

US is the preferred modality for diagnosis and treatment guidance. It demonstrates an anechoic focal abnormality with an echogenic rim, corresponding to clotting peripheral blood, adjacent to an artery (Fig. 12a) [3, 5, 27, 28]. The pseudoaneurysm neck can sometimes be identified connecting to the culprit artery [1, 5]. Color Doppler imaging will demonstrate flow within the adjacent artery connecting with the pseudoaneurysm via the neck [5]. The "yin-yang" sign may be seen on color

Doppler imaging, demonstrating the classic blood flow pattern within a pseudoaneurysm (Fig. 12b) [1, 3, 5, 28]. Spectral Doppler tracings will demonstrate the "to-and-fro" waveform caused by pressure changes between systole and diastole [1, 3, 5].

On mammography, a pseudoaneurysm may appear as a mass adjacent to and extending from a blood vessel, without any fat density to suggest an intramammary lymph node [1, 5]. A pseudoaneurysm may also be seen on the angiographic phase of CT, which would demonstrate a focal vascular outpouching from a feeding artery [1, 5].

## Localization Wires

Localization wires may be placed for surgical planning of non-palpable masses to guide excision [1]. Potential

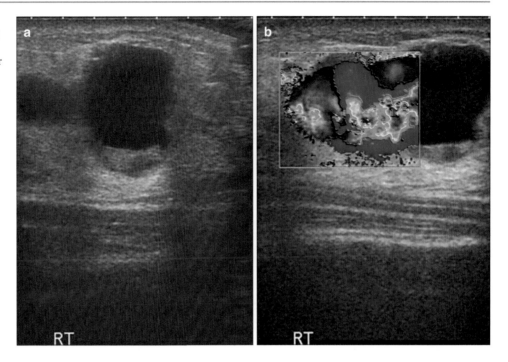

**Fig. 12** Post-biopsy pseudoaneurysm. A 62-year-old woman with US findings of a round anechoic focus in the upper inner quadrant (**a**) which shows classical turbulent flow and yin-yang sign (**b**) on Doppler, which is a pseudoaneurysm following a recent breast biopsy

complications of their placement include wire migration and wire retention following surgery [1, 29–31]. Cases of wire migration into the pericardium, pleural spaces, lung, mediastinum, neck musculature, gluteal regions, axillae, abdominal cavity, and other locations within the breast have been reported [29–32]. Localization wires may migrate at the time of surgery, as well, and they are particularly more prone to migration if they are cut into shorter lengths [29, 32]. Ultimately, migration of localization wires may require significant subsequent surgery for removal [29–31].

Specimen radiography of the excised breast tissue is typically performed during surgery to confirm localization wire presence [1, 32]. If the wire is not easily identified, further imaging with mammography, radiography, CT, or fluoroscopy may be warranted to localize the wire and identify any migration [29–32]. Localization wires will appear hyperdense, and they may be more difficult to localize if they were cut to shorter lengths during surgery [29–32].

### Penetrating Injury

Following penetrating injury, mammography may be used to identify foreign bodies [2, 3]. A bullet may be seen as a high-density foreign body [2]. Smaller bullet fragments may mimic calcifications, but they should appear more dense than typical calcifications [2, 3]. CT may be performed in the acute traumatic setting, which can also identify bullet fragments [2, 3]. A stab wound tract may also be identified with increased tissue density surrounding the tract, as well as subcutaneous emphysema either related to the local injury or secondary to pneumothorax [2, 3].

## Pregnancy and Lactation-Related Disease

### Galactocele

Galactoceles are the most common benign breast "masses" in lactating women, frequently occurring shortly after cessation of breastfeeding as retained milk becomes stagnant. They may also occur in the third trimester of pregnancy [33–35]. Galactoceles are retention cysts containing milk-like fluid with inflammatory or necrotic debris. They form as a result of lactiferous duct obstruction and dilatation [33–35]. The clinical presentation consists of a palpable lump, which may become painful and tender with superimposed infection [34]. Aspiration is both diagnostic and therapeutic, although most will regress spontaneously, and some may recur following aspiration [33, 35]. Antibiotic therapy and pain management may also be used in the setting of superinfection [35].

The imaging appearance of galactoceles varies depending on the proportion of fat and water content, as well as the age of the milk within it [33, 35]. On US, a galactocele with high milk content will appear as a well-defined mass with posterior acoustic enhancement and echogenic internal content [33, 35]. Galactoceles with fresh milk content will demonstrate hyperechoic-hypoechoic fat-fluid levels on US [33, 35]. Meanwhile, mixed contents consisting of old milk and proteinaceous fluid will demonstrate a heterogeneous appearance with mixed low and high internal echogenicity (Fig. 13) [33, 35].

On mammography, a galactocele with high milk and fat content will appear as a completely radiolucent mass

**Fig. 13 Galactocele.** A 40-year-old lactating woman with a palpable breast mass demonstrates sonographic findings of a cystic focus with echogenic fatty internal content, posterior acoustic enhancement, and no internal vascularity, which is highly consistent with a galactocele

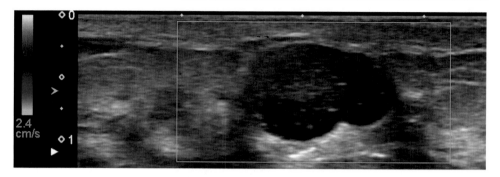

("pseudo-lipoma") [33, 35]. A complex mass with mixed proportions of fresh milk, fat, and water content will appear as a cystic mass with a fat-fluid level [33, 35]. A galactocele consisting of old milk and proteinaceous fluid will demonstrate the "breast-within-breast" appearance resembling a hamartoma ("pseudo-hamartoma") [33, 35].

## Breast Infarction

During pregnancy, typically in the third trimester, bleeding or necrosis may occur in hypertrophic breast tissue or in a preexisting breast abnormality, such as a lactating adenoma [33, 34, 36]. Intravascular thrombosis has been suggested as a possible etiology [33]. The clinical presentation usually involves a poorly defined, painful, palpable breast lump [34]. These infarcts are often biopsied due to their suspicious appearance on imaging; however, fine needle aspiration is not recommended due to the unreliable appearance of ischemic necrosis [34].

On imaging, findings generally consist of a solid-appearing mass, often heterogeneous in appearance, with absent internal vascularity [34]. A surrounding hypoechoic rim or "halo" may be seen, corresponding to regional edema/ischemic changes (Fig. 14). The patient may have associated lymphadenopathy [34]. Correlation with previous imaging may be helpful if there is a previously known breast abnormality in a similar location.

## Milk Fistula

A milk fistula is a tract that forms between a lactiferous duct and the skin, most commonly seen as a complication in lactating women following a biopsy or other surgical procedure [37–39]. Patients often present clinically with milk leakage at the tract of a recent biopsy, and they tend to occur more frequently following biopsies closer to the nipple rather than peripherally [1, 37–39]. Core biopsies pose a higher risk for development of a milk fistula than fine needle aspiration, but they are also more frequently diagnostic [1]. Milk fistulas often resolve spontaneously with supportive management. Some cases require cessation of nursing to stop milk production, allowing the tract to close, although

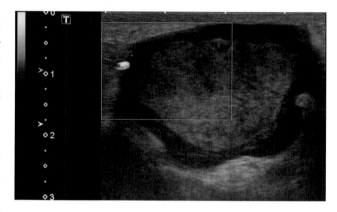

**Fig. 14 Infarcted lactating adenoma.** An 18-year-old woman with sonographic findings of a hypoechoic solid mass, previously showing internal vascularity (not shown), now demonstrating no internal flow, and interval development of a peripheral hypoechoic halo, which represents soft tissue edema/ischemic changes. A biopsy of this process confirmed an infarcted lactating adenoma

severe cases may necessitate bromocriptine therapy to stop milk production [1, 37–39].

Diagnosis is primarily made based on clinical findings and history of recent biopsy [1, 37–39]. However, sonographic findings may include visualization of a lactiferous duct at the site of milk leakage, which may or may not be dilated [39]. Other reported findings include a background of skin thickening and edematous tissue, likely secondary to the recent biopsy [38].

## Breast Augmentation Complications

### Breast Implant Rupture

Implant rupture is often seen in the acute emergency setting following trauma, and it may occur with saline and silicone implants [3]. Saline implant rupture does not require imaging as it can be diagnosed clinically with evidence of a deflated implant on examination [3]. Silicone implant rupture can be intracapsular or extracapsular [40–42]. With intracapsular rupture, the integrity of the implant is breached, but the fibrous capsule remains intact [40–42]. Patients with

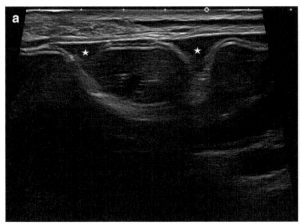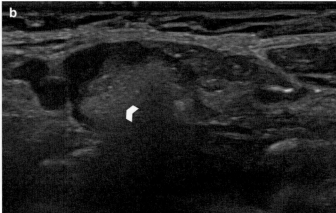

**Fig. 15 Extracapsular breast implant rupture with silicone adenopathy.** A 35-year-old woman with a known silicone implant. Sagittal US images show pericapsular fluid (asterisks) suspected to represent extracapsular silicone (**a**). Sonographic assessment of the axillary region demonstrates a lymph node with increased echogenicity and posterior acoustic shadowing in keeping with a "snowstorm" appearance (arrowhead), which is classic for silicone adenopathy (**b**)

intracapsular rupture are commonly asymptomatic [40–42]. In extracapsular rupture, silicone extends outside the fibrous capsule of the implant [40–42]. Patients usually present with a palpable lump and implant deformity, as well as possible lymphadenopathy due to silicone deposition [40–42]. Treatment for both scenarios involves implant removal, evacuation of free silicone, capsulectomy, and new implant insertion, if desired [3].

On US, intracapsular rupture will demonstrate a "step-ladder sign" with multiple discontinuous, parallel, linear echogenic foci [40–42]. Mammography is limited for assessment of intracapsular rupture. On MRI, a "linguine," "key-hole," or "salad oil" sign may be seen, corresponding to the finding seen on US [41, 42].

Extracapsular rupture will demonstrate a "snowstorm" appearance on US with echogenic noise overlying the region of the implant due to acoustic scattering from silicone debris [40–42]. This appearance may also involve axillary lymph nodes as a result of "silicone adenopathy" (Fig. 15). On mammography, a contour abnormality of the implant can be seen with round- or oval-shaped densities adjacent to the implant corresponding to extracapsular silicone [41, 42]. Similarly, on MRI, extracapsular silicone is seen, as well as possible silicone granuloma formation and adjacent inflammation, in keeping with silicone mastitis [41, 42].

## Conclusion

In the ED, breast US is the imaging workhorse for breast emergencies. Radiologists, including general and emergency radiologists, must be familiar with acute breast pathologies, which may acutely present to the ED, even though their practice scope may not include any other routine breast imaging. Knowledge encompassing infectious, inflammatory, traumatic, iatrogenic, pregnancy- or lactation-related, and augmentation-related breast pathologies can allow radiologists to provide timely diagnoses and facilitate effective management.

**Teaching Points**
- US is the preferred first-line examination for assessment of acute breast complaints in the ED.
- US should be performed in patients with clinical presentation of mastitis and lack of response to antimicrobial therapy to exclude abscess.
- CT is a modality of choice for the demonstration of soft tissue gas in patients with suspicion for emphysematous mastitis.

## References

1. Mahoney MC, Ingram AD. Breast emergencies: types, imaging features, and management. Am J Roentgenol. 2014;202(4):W390–9.
2. Hines N, Leibman AJ, David M. Breast problems presenting in the emergency room. Emerg Radiol. 2007;14(1):23–8.
3. Khadem N, Reddy S, Lee S, Larsen L, Walker D. ED breast cases and other breast emergencies. Emerg Radiol. 2016;23(1):67–77.
4. Givens ML, Luszczak M. Breast disorders: a review for emergency physicians. J Emerg Med. 2002;22(1):59–65.
5. Ingram AD, Mahoney MC. An overview of breast emergencies and guide to management by interventional radiologists. Tech Vasc Interv Radiol. 2014;17(1):55–63.
6. Trop I, Dugas A, David J, El Khoury M, Boileau JF, Larouche N, et al. Breast abscesses: evidence-based algorithms for diagnosis, management, and follow-up. Radiographics. 2011;31(6):1683–99.
7. Spencer JP. Management of mastitis in breastfeeding women. Am Fam Physician. 2008;78(6):727–31.
8. Ozseker B, Ozcan UA, Rasa K, Cizmeli OM. Treatment of breast abscesses with ultrasound-guided aspiration and irrigation in the emergency setting. Emerg Radiol. 2008;15(2):105–8.

9. Ulitzsch D, Nyman MKG, Carlson RA. Breast abscess in lactating women: US-guided treatment. Radiology. 2004;232(3):904–9.

10. Froman J, Landercasper J, Ellis R, De Maiffe B, Theede L. Red breast as a presenting complaint at a breast center: an institutional review. Surgery. 2011;149(6):813–9.

11. Shetty MK, Watson AB. Mondor's disease of the breast: sonographic and mammographic findings. AJR Am J Roentgenol. 2001;177(4):893–6.

12. Yanik B, Conkbayir I, Öner Ö, Hekimoğlu B. Imaging findings in Mondor's disease. J Clin Ultrasound. 2003;31(2):103–7.

13. Lee EY, Alhusayen R, Lansang P, Shear N, Yeung J. What is hidradenitis suppurativa? Can Fam Physician. 2017;63(2):114–20.

14. Kelly AM, Cronin P. MRI features of hidradenitis suppurativa and review of the literature. Am J Roentgenol. 2005;185:1201–4.

15. Perry AM, Choi SM. Kikuchi-Fujimoto disease: a review. Arch Pathol Lab Med. 2018;142(11):1341–6.

16. Kwon SY, Kim TK, Kim YS, Lee KY, Lee NJ, Seol HY. CT findings in Kikuchi disease: analysis of 96 cases. Am J Neuroradiol. 2004;25(6):1099–102.

17. Wallrauch C, Heller T, Dhungel BM, Kayera H, Phiri S, Tomoka TM. Lymphadenopathy due to Kikuchi-Fujimoto disease – a rare differential for a common presentation. Malawi Med J. 2018;30(4):302–4.

18. Parker SH, Burbank F, Jackman RJ, Aucreman CJ, Cardenosa G, Cink TM, et al. Percutaneous large-core breast biopsy: a multi-institutional study. Radiology. 1994;193(2):359–64.

19. DiPiro PJ, Meyer JE, Frenna TH, Denison CM. Seat belt injuries of the breast: findings on mammography and sonography. Am J Roentgenol. 1995;164(2):317–20.

20. Chetlen AL, Kasales C, Mack J, Schetter S, Zhu J. Hematoma formation during breast core needle biopsy in women taking antithrombotic therapy. Am J Roentgenol. 2013;201(1):215–22.

21. Somerville P, Seifert PJ, Destounis SV, Murphy PF, Young W. Anticoagulation and bleeding risk after core needle biopsy. Am J Roentgenol. 2008;191(4):1194–7.

22. Salem C, Sakr R, Chopier J, Antoine M, Uzan S, Daraï E. Pain and complications of directional vacuum-assisted stereotactic biopsy: comparison of the Mammotome and Vacora techniques. Eur J Radiol. 2009;72(2):295–9.

23. Lai JT, Burrowes P, MacGregor JH. Vacuum-assisted large-core breast biopsy: complications and their incidence. Can Assoc Radiol J. 2000;51(4):232–6.

24. Simon JR, Kalbhen CL, Cooper RA, Flisak ME. Accuracy and complication rates of US-guided vacuum-assisted core breast biopsy: initial results. Radiology. 2000;215(3):694–7.

25. Kuroi K, Shimozuma K, Taguchi T, Imai H, Yamashiro H, Ohsumi S, et al. Pathophysiology of seroma in breast cancer. Breast Cancer. 2005;12(4):288–93.

26. Ramirez-Hernandez IE, Hardman RL, Kirkpatrick AD, Sutcliffe J. Post-operative seroma causing spontaneous nipple discharge: diagnosis by Galactography. J Radiol Case Rep. 2013;7(5):16–22.

27. Bitencourt AGV, Cohen MP, Graziano L, Souza JA, Marques EF, Brites MR, et al. Pseudoaneurysm after ultrasound-guided vacuum-assisted core breast biopsy. Breast J. 2012;18(2):177–8.

28. El Khoury M, Mesurolle B, Kao E, Mujoomdar A, Tremblay F. Spontaneous thrombosis of pseudoaneurysm of the breast related to core biopsy. AJR Am J Roentgenol. 2007;189(6):W309–11.

29. Azoury F, Sayad P, Rizk A. Thoracoscopic management of a pericardial migration of a breast biopsy localization wire. Ann Thorac Surg. 2009;87(6):1937–9.

30. Banitalebi H, Skaane P. Migration of the breast biopsy localization wire to the pulmonary hilus. Acta Radiol. 2005;46(1):28–31.

31. Mituś J, Kołodziejski L, Dyczek S, Wysocki WM, Komorowski AL. Localization wire migrating into the hilum of the lung during wire-guided breast biopsy. Breast J. 2004;10(2):165–6.

32. Owen AWMC, Kumar EN. Migration of localizing wires used in guided biopsy of the breast. Clin Radiol. 1991;43(4):251.

33. Sabate JM, Clotet M, Torrubia S, Gomez A, Guerrero R, De Las HP, et al. Radiologic evaluation of breast disorders related to pregnancy and lactation. Radiographics. 2007;27 Suppl 1:S101–24.

34. Langer A, Mohallem M, Berment H, Ferreira F, Gog A, Khalifa D, et al. Breast lumps in pregnant women. Diagn Interv Imaging. 2015;96(10):1077–87.

35. Vashi R, Hooley R, Butler R, Geisel J, Philpotts L. Breast imaging of the pregnant and lactating patient: physiologic changes and common benign entities. Am J Roentgenol. 2013;200(2):329–36.

36. Behrndt VS, Barbakoff D, Askin FB, Brem RF. Infarcted lactating adenoma presenting as a rapidly enlarging breast mass. Am J Roentgenol. 1999;173(4):933–5.

37. Schackmuth EM, Harlow CL, Norton LW. Milk fistula: a complication after core breast biopsy. Am J Roentgenol. 1993;161(5):961–2.

38. Larson KE, Valente SA. Milk fistula: diagnosis, prevention, and treatment. Breast J. 2016;22(1):111–2.

39. Isik A, Karavas E, Firat D. Spontaneous milk fistula from an axillary accessory breast. Breast J. 2019;25(1):154.

40. Ciurea A, Gersak M, Onoe R, Ivan O, Ciortea C. The role of ultrasound in the imaging assessment of the augmented breast. A pictorial review. Med Ultrason. 2014;16(3):256–61.

41. Berg WA, Caskey CI, Hamper UM, Anderson ND, Chang BW, Sheth S, et al. Diagnosing breast implant rupture with MR imaging, US, and mammography. Radiographics. 1993;13(6):1323–36.

42. Caskey CI, Berg WA, Hamper UM, Sheth S, Chang BW, Anderson ND. Imaging spectrum of extracapsular silicone: correlation of US, MR imaging, mammographic, and histopathologic findings. Radiographics. 1999;19(SPEC.ISS):S39–51.

F. Iacobellis, T. J. Fraum, L. Romano, R. Niola, Vincent M. Mellnick, and Mariano Scaglione

## Contents

F. Iacobellis · L. Romano
Department of General and Emergency Radiology, "A. Cardarelli" Hospital, Naples, Italy

T. J. Fraum
Department of Abdominal Imaging and Nuclear Medicine, Mallinckrodt Institute of Radiology, Washington University School of Medicine, Barnes-Jewish Hospital, St. Louis, MO, USA

R. Niola
Department of Diagnostic and Interventional Radiology, "A. Cardarelli" Hospital, Naples, Italy

V. M. Mellnick
Mallinckrodt Institute of Radiology, Washington University School of Medicine, St. Louis, MO, USA

M. Scaglione (✉)
Department of Medical, Surgical and Experimental Sciences, University of Medicine and Surgery, Sassari, Italy

Department of Radiology, James Cook University Hospital, Middlesbrough, UK

Teesside University School of Health and Life Sciences, Middlesbrough, Tees Valley, UK

Department of Radiology, Pineta Grande Hospital, Castel Volturno, Italy

### Abstract

The liver is the second most commonly injured abdominal parenchymal organ in blunt abdominal trauma. Blunt liver trauma may result in different grades of parenchymal, biliary, and vascular injuries, which are variably associated. For correct patient management, it is crucial to promptly and accurately diagnose these conditions. This chapter focuses on the imaging approach in blunt liver trauma patients and on the related management implications of the imaging features, examining parenchymal, vascular, and biliary injuries.

### Keywords

Blunt trauma · Liver parenchymal injuries · Liver vascular injuries · Biliary injuries

## Introduction

The liver is the second most commonly injured abdominal parenchymal organ in blunt abdominal trauma [1], due to direct impact or indirect injury (e.g., from rib fracture). The right hepatic lobe is more commonly injured due to its larger volume and due to its position adjacent to the ribs that may contribute to liver injury when a fracture occurs. Also, the liver surface adjacent to the suspensory ligaments can be more easily injured, due to sudden traction phenomena [2].

Blunt liver trauma may result in different grades of parenchymal, biliary, and vascular injuries, which can manifest in their severity immediately after trauma or in the subsequent days, leading to complications. The reported mortality rate attributable to blunt liver injury ranges from 4.1% to 11.7% [3].

## Parenchymal Liver Trauma

The American Association for the Surgery of Trauma (AAST)liver injury grading scale from 2018 was recently revised and is the most commonly used injury scale for liver injuries [4]. It is based on five grades which refer to the site and extent of injuries, which now incorporates vascular injuries which are identified prospectively on CT. From a management viewpoint, vascular injuries are crucial regardless of the grade of injury, and this incorporation of vascular injuries represents a major revision of the AAST grading scale [1, 4]. Critical points for the radiologist to observe, along with determining the presence and size of hematomas and lacerations, include:

- Capsule breach and hemoperitoneum
- Hepatic vascular injuries
- Hepatic hilar involvement

Accurate injury grading allows for the trauma team to appropriately triage the patient to appropriate treatment. Three different management options are offered to patients with blunt liver trauma:

- Nonoperative management (NOM)
- Interventional radiology (IR)
- Surgery (OM) [1, 5–7]

Clinically, the first points to select the most appropriate treatment include hemodynamic stability or lack of stability and an initial trauma survey. Clinicians also must have knowledge of patients presenting with mechanisms of injury suggesting major trauma. These include sudden deceleration, impact or compression at speeds above 65 km/h in motor vehicle collisions, above 45 km/h in motorcycle collisions, fall from a height of more than 3 m, or crushing between heavy objects.

NOM is strongly suggested for the vast majority of hemodynamically stable patients with liver injuries, even with high-grade injuries, in which CT has been used to exclude arterial vascular injuries (active bleeding, pseudoaneurysm, and AV fistulas), venous vascular injuries, and hepatic capsule breach with hemoperitoneum or injuries affecting the hepatic hilum, regardless the size or extent of parenchymal injuries (Figs. 1 and 2).

Catheter angiography with embolization may be pursued either at initial presentation or when a patient demonstrates ongoing bleeding after a trial of NOM. It is often indicated in stable patients in whom CT has shown hepatic arterial vascular injuries (active bleeding, pseudoaneurysm, or AV fistula) (Figs. 3 and 4).

Surgery is typically viewed as a last option. It is designated in the minority of patients who reach the emergency facility alive but are hemodynamically unstable, with uncontrollable active hemorrhage, in cases of hepatic capsule breach and hemoperitoneum, or with injuries affecting the liver hilum, or with failure of interventional radiology treatment [1, 5–7] (Fig. 4). This may also be the most appropriate course of care in patients with other injuries needing surgical intervention (e.g., bowel or diaphragm injuries). For this reason, it is crucial for radiologists to design protocols and interpret images which allow for accurate injury assessment.

## CT Protocol

Protocols for CT in the setting of major trauma vary widely from institution to institution. There is increasing support for whole-body CT for blunt trauma, however. At our institution, we perform a non-contrast scan of the head, followed by arterial and venous phase scans from the circle of Willis to the symphysis pubis. Iodinated contrast volume is typically 80–130 mL, according to the patient's weight, at a high concentration (370–400 mg I/mL), which is injected at 3.5–5 mL/s, and followed by a 40 mL saline chaser at the same flow rate, to obtain optimal vessel depiction. Automated bolus tracking identifies the arterial phase; a region of interest (ROI) is placed on the aortic arch, and arterial phase scanning begins when an attenuation threshold of 100 Hounsfield units (HU) is reached. The venous phase is performed at a 60- to 70-s delay from the beginning of the injection. Moreover, in selected patients, an additional late phase at 3–5 min may be required to differentiate arterial bleeding from lower-pressure venous bleeding or at 5–20 min to depict urinary extravasation in patients with kidney injuries [8–11].

For accurate vascular and parenchymal evaluation, a slice thickness ranging from 0.5 to 3 mm, and preferably 0.5–1.5 mm, is often useful. Post-processing with three-dimensional (3D) multi-planar reconstructions (MPR) and

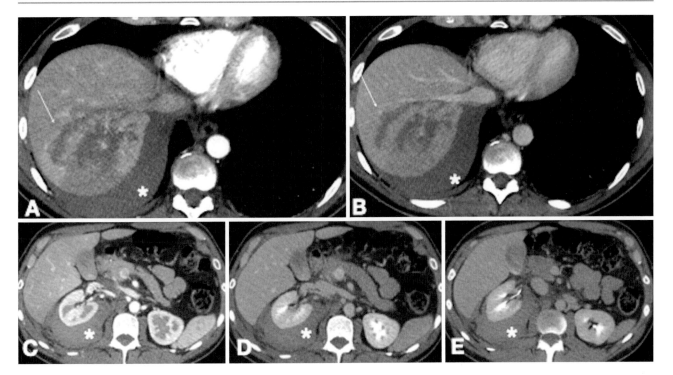

**Fig. 1** IV contrast-enhanced abdominal MDCT images of a 37-year-old-man with multiple injuries due to high-energy blunt trauma (motor vehicle collision). The CT demonstrates hemoperitoneum (**a** and **b**, asterisks), multiple liver lacerations without contained vascular injuries or active bleeding (AAST grade III) (**a**, arterial phase, arrow; **b**, portal venous phase, arrow), and a perirenal hematoma (**c–e**, asterisks). The availability of multiple phases helps exclude the presence of active bleeding or active urine extravasation, thus managing patient conservatively

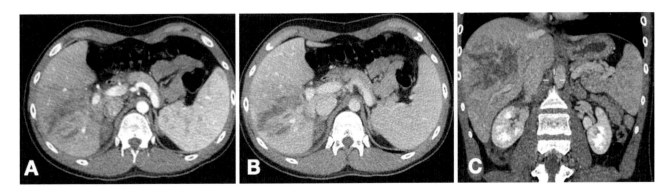

**Fig. 2** IV contrast-enhanced abdominal CT images in arterial (**a**) and venous phases (**b** and **c**) of a 42-year-old patient with high energy blunt trauma. There is an extensive liver laceration in the right lobe (AAST IV). No active bleeding was detected in the arterial (**a**) or the portal venous (**b** and **c**) phases. Non-operative treatment was decided upon, and was successful

volume-rendered reconstructions is helpful for identifying injuries of the vessels and sites of active bleeding, as well as for searching for osseous injuries which can be missed on the axial images [8, 10, 12–14].

## Imaging Findings

The aim of the multiphasic CT examination is to offer to the surgeons a complete patient assessment including not only the description of the parenchymal injuries but also of the presence of vascular injuries, namely, pseudoaneurysms and active contrast extravasation, as these injuries modify patient management (Fig. 5).

Imaging findings of blunt parenchymal injuries are contusions, hematomas, and parenchymal lacerations, as well as avulsion of the hepatic pedicle.

Contusions are ill-defined, hypodense areas detected in the liver parenchyma due to interstitial bleeding. These may be isolated or, more commonly, associated with lacerations. In contrast, liver lacerations are seen as well-defined, irregular linear, or branching low-attenuation areas that are usually parallel to hepatic veins (Fig. 1), whereas hematomas are subcapsular or central blood collections [3].

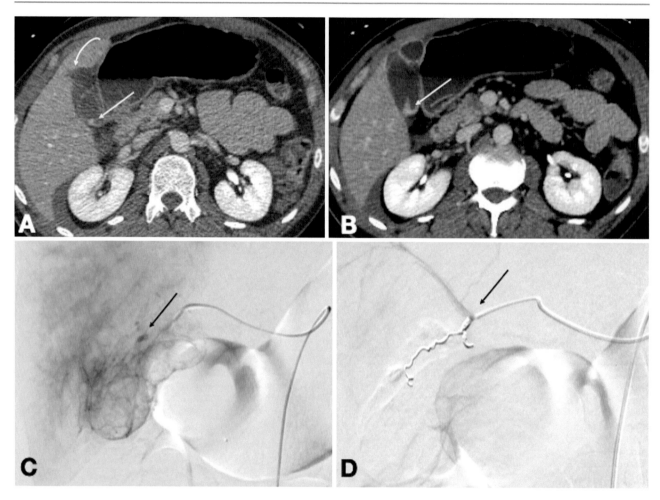

**Fig. 3** IV contrast-enhanced abdominal CT images in the portal venous (**a**) and nephrographic phase (**b**) in a 47-year-old man following major trauma. There is a small liver laceration in the fourth segment-grade II (**a**, curved arrow), hemoperitoneum, and a focus of active bleeding (**a** and **b**, arrow) in the gallbladder lumen. Although the bleeding is best seen in the portal venous phase, it was arterial in origin. The patient underwent angiography, confirming the active bleeding (**c**), followed immediately by successful embolization (**d**)

These injuries may be variably associated with each other depending on the trauma dynamic and specific entity. They are often best seen in the portal venous phase, at which point the normal liver parenchyma is optimally enhancing and most readily differentiated from relatively hypoattenuating lacerations, hematomas, and contusions [1, 2, 8].

To avoid misdiagnosis of liver parenchymal injuries is particularly important to account for upper extremity positioning. When possible, the torso is best imaged with arms up to avoid streak artifact through the liver that may simulate or obscure an injury. Similarly, the removal of all overlying metal lines and devices is ideal, but may not always be possible [8, 15–19].

Among parenchymal injuries, two particularly important observations to make are the presence of capsular breach and extension of the injury into the hepatic hilum.

A capsular breach is at risk of uncontrollable intraperitoneal bleeding. Hepatic hilar involvement also is associated with the risk of major hemorrhage due to the presence of large vessels.

The presence of vascular injuries is important to detect, as their presence is associated with failed NOM and suggests that IR or surgical management should be pursued (Figs. 3, 4, and 5).

Active bleeding is recognized as extraluminal contrast extravasation, increasing and changing its morphology during multiphasic acquisitions. The availability of multiple phases is helpful in the detection and quantification of ongoing bleeding. As blood loss related to hepatic trauma is a major contributor to the morbidity and mortality in patients with abdominal trauma, this is a key observation [1, 15] (Figs. 3 and 4).

In addition to identifying active bleeding, radiologists are also tasked with identifying the bleeding source – generally, arterial, or venous. To do so they must rely on the phase of contrast in which the bleeding first manifests – arterial

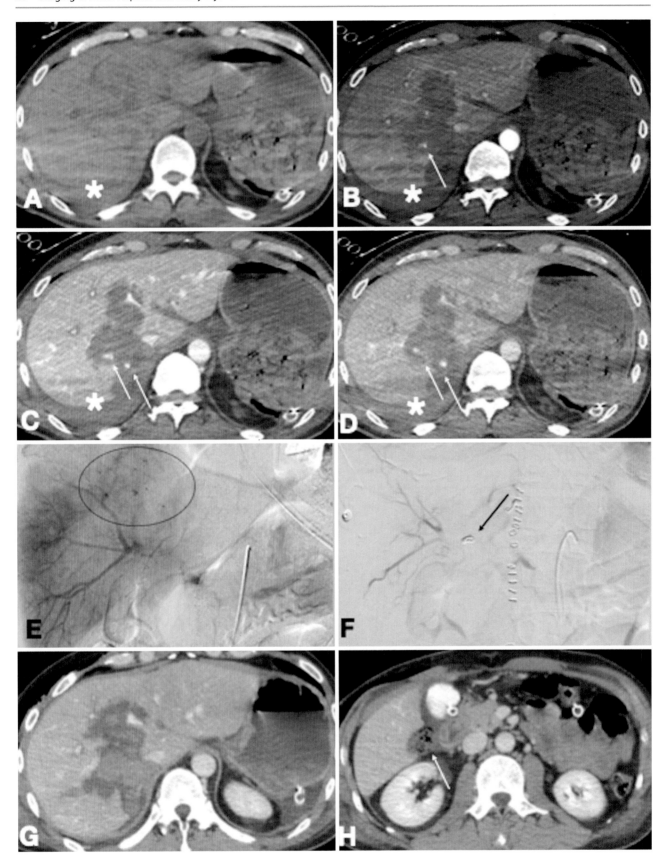

**Fig. 4** Multiphasic IV contrast-enhanced CT images of the abdomen (**a**, non-enhanced scan; **b**, arterial phase; **c**, portal venous phase; **d**, late phase) of a 36-year-old man who sustained high energy blunt trauma (motor vehicle collision). The CT demonstrated hemoperitoneum (**a–d**,

bleeding appearing earlier than with venous sources. However, it should be considered that in patients with hypotension or hypovolemia, arterial bleeding may be first seen in the portal venous phase. In this case, the site and the density and entity of the contrast extravasation, together with the radiologist experience, should suggest the correct diagnosis, even if there are cases in which this may remain undetermined [15]. Regardless, the presence of a contrast "blush" has been used as an indicator for catheter angiography and empiric embolization.

The correct identification of the bleeding origin should lead to correct patient management. When arterial active bleeding is detected, in the majority of cases stable patients may be sent to the interventional radiologist (Figs. 3 and 4), reducing time to treat and invasiveness in comparison with surgery. If the patient is unstable, open surgery remains indicated; however, surgery may be combined with IR intervention in a hybrid operating room for prompt cessation of the arterial bleeding together with the surgical treatment of further associated organ injuries. In most patients, this has saved time and lives, significantly reducing morbidity, death from sepsis and other complications, and financial costs [20].

Contained vascular injuries include pseudoaneurysms and arteriovenous fistulas. Pseudoaneurysms are seen as focal round or oval irregular outpouchings of the outer contour of the arterial vessel wall of equal density to the intra-arterial contrast material, and not changing size over multiple contrast phases. There is often a rim of separation from the vessel lumen [1, 15]. Arteriovenous fistulae consist of a traumatic communications between the arterial and venous systems and are seen as asymmetrical, early contrast opacification of a vein, during the arterial phase [15]. These injuries are best identified and characterized with an adequate multiphasic CT examination. They are relevant clinically, as they can increase in size over time, potentially leading to spontaneous rupture, pseudoaneurysm formation, or circulation overload (Figs. 4 and 5). Once the diagnosis is made at CT, these patients are candidates for IR, with the aim to exclude the vessel injuries with embolization.

## Blunt Biliary Trauma

Biliary tract injury is a rare consequence of blunt abdominal trauma. In a large, single-center study, blunt biliary tract injuries accounted for only 0.1% of all trauma admissions

over a 10-year period [21]. The imaging findings of biliary tract injuries are often subtle or nonspecific. Furthermore, blunt biliary trauma is highly associated with injuries of other abdominal viscera, most frequently the liver (91%), spleen (54%), or duodenum (54%) [22]. Consequently, these biliary injuries are easily overlooked at first presentation. Some biliary injuries are entirely occult on initial imaging, and are not recognized until complications develop and are then seen on subsequent imaging examinations. In this section, we review imaging strategies for the diagnosis of biliary tract injuries in the setting of blunt abdominal trauma.

## Acute Gallbladder Injury

In general, the gallbladder is relatively protected from blunt trauma by overlying hepatic tissue and is very uncommonly injured. Nevertheless, the gallbladder is the most common site of blunt biliary tract injuries. In one single-center study, gallbladder injuries were noted in 2.1% of patients who underwent exploratory laparotomy for blunt abdominal injuries [23]. Gallbladder distension, by means of either physiologic fasting or alcohol-induced sphincter of Oddi spasm, is purported to increase the risk of blunt gallbladder injury [22]. Conversely, the wall thickening associated with chronic cholecystitis has been speculated to be protective [22].

The three original categories of traumatic gallbladder injury included contusion (mural hematoma) (Fig. 6), perforation (also called laceration) (Fig. 7), and avulsion (Fig. 8) [24]. Traumatic cholecystitis, which results from cystic duct obstruction by blood products from traumatic intraluminal hemorrhage, has been subsequently added as a fourth category [25]. In a series of 22 patients with blunt gallbladder trauma at a single center, contusion (45%) and avulsion (45%) were the most frequently observed categories [26]. Similarly, the AAST has published a five-point grading system for the trauma of the gallbladder and extrahepatic bile ducts [27].

By virtue of its speed and availability, computed tomography (CT) for years now has been the primary imaging modality utilized in the setting of blunt abdominal trauma. CT findings of blunt gallbladder injury not specific to any particular category include pericholecystic fluid, an ill-defined gallbladder wall, liver laceration extension into the gallbladder fossa, and high-attenuation material in the gallbladder lumen [28]. It should be noted that biliary sludge and "vicarious" excretion of contrast material are

**Fig. 4** (continued) asterisks), related with an extensive liver laceration with intraparenchymal hematoma and multiple sites of active bleeding (AAST grade IV) (arrows). Angiography confirmed the multiple jets of active bleeding (**e**, circle), and the patient was treated with embolization both with microspheres and coils (**f**, arrow, coil). At surgery, no capsular

laceration was detected, so peritoneal lavage was performed, and absorbable hemostatic agent was placed. (**g** and **h**) The post-surgical follow-up CT performed 3 days after trauma, shows a stable appearance of the large right lobe hematoma and absorbable hemostatic agent (**h**, arrow), but no active bleeding

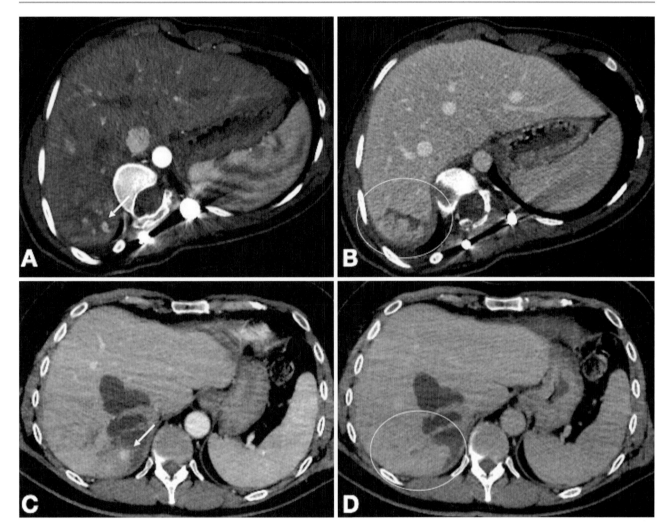

**Fig. 5** IV contrast-enhanced abdominal MDCT images in the arterial (**a**) and venous phases (**b**) in two different patients. Note the presence of contained vascular injuries (**a** and **c**, arrows). These vascular injuries can be only seen on the arterial phase of the CT. In the venous phase (**b** and **d**), contained vascular injuries have an attenuation value similar to those of the surrounding parenchyma and therefore can be easily overlooked

potential mimics of hemorrhage in the gallbladder lumen. A collapsed appearance of the lumen in the setting of gallbladder injury suggests perforation or avulsion with release of bile into the peritoneum. In the setting of avulsion, which can be complete or incomplete, the gallbladder may be physically displaced from its normal anatomic location [29]. Although ultrasound is a mainstay of initial gallbladder imaging in general, its role in the assessment of acute gallbladder trauma is limited, though it may be useful for following known injuries over time.

## Acute Extrahepatic Bile Duct Injury

Injuries to the extrahepatic bile ducts resulting from blunt trauma are exceedingly rare, with only a handful of case reports published in the literature, to our knowledge. These injuries are thought to result from shearing or stretching

mechanisms arising from direct blows to the abdominal wall or sudden decelerations, as from motor vehicle collisions [30]. The most common sites of injury are at points of attachment, specifically the intrapancreatic portion of the common bile duct and the hilar confluence of the right and left intrahepatic bile ducts (Fig. 9) [31].

The findings of extrahepatic bile duct injury on CT, when present, are often subtle, potentially manifesting as nonspecific fluid or stranding along the hepatoduodenal ligament. Direct visualization of a discontinuity is highly unlikely with CT. When not suggested on initial CT, these injuries may be identified on surgical exploration and are managed accordingly to restore continuity of the biliary system. However, extrahepatic bile duct injuries are often made in a delayed fashion, as patients develop jaundice and/or abdominal pain [32]. At this point, repeat imaging (most often CT) often shows new or enlarging fluid collections, raising clinical concern for a biloma, and prompting a

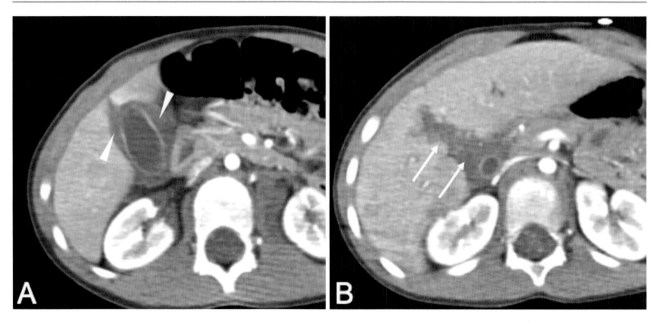

**Fig. 6** Gallbladder contusion following all-terrain vehicle accident. Computed tomography images with contrast from caudal (**a**) to cranial (**b**) with IV contrast of the abdomen show hyperdense thickening of the gallbladder wall (arrowheads), consistent with contusion (mural hematoma). An adjacent liver laceration extending into the gallbladder fossa (arrow) is commonly seen in association with, but is nonspecific for, gallbladder injury

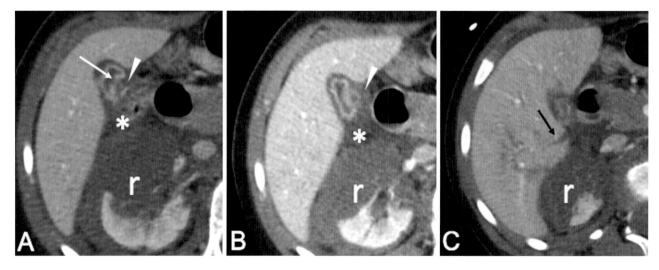

**Fig. 7** Gallbladder perforation in a pedestrian struck by a car. Abdominal computed tomography images with IV contrast from caudal (**a**) to cranial (**c**) show hyperdense thickening of the gallbladder wall (white arrowheads), which is consistent with contusion. A focal discontinuity in the gallbladder mucosa (arrow) with a collapsed lumen suggests superimposed perforation, as was subsequently confirmed by surgery. Hyperdense pericholecystic fluid (asterisks) and an adjacent liver laceration extending into the gallbladder fossa (black arrow) are identified and are commonly associated with gallbladder injuries. Note concurrent right renal laceration (r) with perinephric hematoma

more specific imaging examination for the detection of a bile leak (see section below).

## Acute Intrahepatic Bile Duct Injury

Injuries of the intrahepatic bile ducts occur almost exclusively in the setting of traumatic liver injuries, which are discussed in detail elsewhere in this chapter. In general, longer, deeper, or more centrally located liver lacerations are more likely to disrupt an intrahepatic bile duct in a clinically significant fashion. In the setting of acute trauma, when most patients are imaged with CT, the only suggestion of an intrahepatic bile duct injury may be a laceration traversing a portal tract (Fig. 10). As with acute extrahepatic bile duct injuries, acute intrahepatic bile duct injuries are often suggested only on subsequent imaging examination, when a new or enlarging fluid collection is identified (Fig. 10),

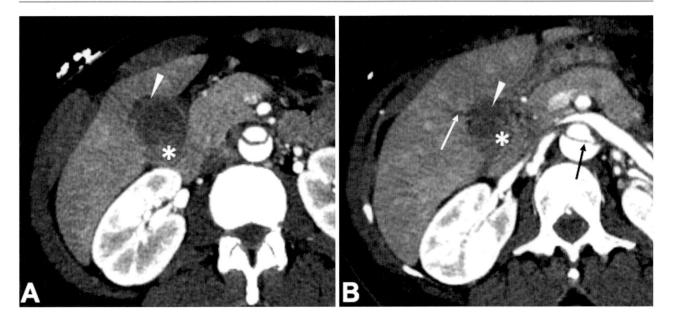

**Fig. 8** Partial gallbladder avulsion in pedestrian struck by a car. Abdominal computed tomography images with IV contrast from caudal (**a**) to cranial (**b**) show hyperdense fluid in the gallbladder lumen (asterisks), likely blood products, with a subtle liver laceration extending into the gallbladder fossa (white arrow). These findings are strongly suggestive of a gallbladder injury. The gallbladder wall is thickened and indistinct (arrowheads), indicating contusion. Surgery showed a partial gallbladder avulsion. The gallbladder may not be displaced from the gallbladder fossa in the setting of a partial avulsion. Note a co-existing traumatic aortic dissection (black arrow)

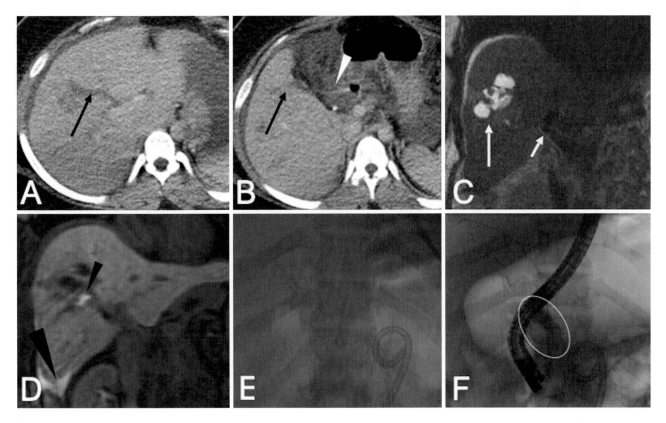

**Fig. 9** Intrahepatic and extrahepatic bile duct injuries in a pedestrian struck by a car. Abdominal computed tomography images with IV contrast from cranial (**a**) to caudal (**b**) show a liver laceration (black arrow) extending into the hepatic hilum, with fluid surrounding the portal structures (white arrowhead). The gallbladder is surgically absent. Due to the subsequent development of bilious ascites, a MRCP examination was performed with a bile leak protocol. Coronal T2-weighted MR images (**c**) show an intrahepatic fluid collection near the hilum, suggestive of a biloma (long white arrow), and a normal-appearing common bile duct (short white arrow). Coronal T1-weighted

raising the possibility of a biloma, and prompting specific imaging for a bile leak (see below).

## Bile Leaks

Any traumatic violation of the biliary tract has the potential to result in a bile leak. Bile leaks arising from the disruption of small intrahepatic bile ducts, such as at the periphery of the liver in the setting of a low-grade liver laceration, may never come to clinical attention or may resolve spontaneously with conservative management. In contrast, bile leaks resulting from disruption of the larger central intrahepatic bile ducts, such as in the setting of high-grade liver laceration, from the extrahepatic bile ducts or from the gallbladder are more likely to become symptomatic and require treatment [31].

In the immediate post-trauma setting, many early bile leaks will be occult or manifested solely by a small amount of free fluid, which is a nonspecific finding in the setting of trauma, especially when accompanied by other abdominal injuries [31]. Importantly, bile is sterile and absorbed by the peritoneum, so bile leaks may not become symptomatic for days or even weeks after an acute injury [33]. However, when collections of bile become superinfected or induce a sterile inflammatory reaction in the peritoneum, patients develop abdominal pain and/or features of sepsis, prompting additional work-up. Rising serum bilirubin levels or jaundice in a patient with recent abdominal trauma should also raise concern for a bile leak, as the conjugated bilirubin that is normally excreted through the gastrointestinal tract is instead resorbed into the bloodstream. Repeat imaging typically reveals a perihepatic or intrahepatic fluid collection that was not present on the initial imaging examination (Figs. 9, 10, and 11). These imaging findings can prompt more specific imaging examinations (see below) or percutaneous drainage procedures, in which case laboratory or even visual analysis of aspirated contents can suffice to make the diagnosis of a biloma.

Whenever a bile leak is suspected, either in the acute setting (on the basis of direct imaging findings or high clinical suspicion) or in the subacute/chronic setting (on the basis of new perihepatic or intrahepatic fluid collections), there are several imaging examinations that can be utilized to make the diagnosis in a highly specific fashion. Hepatobiliary scintigraphy (Figs. 10 and 12),

employing one of the 99mTc-labeled iminodiacetic acid (IDA) derivatives, or magnetic resonance cholangiopancreatography (MRCP) examinations employing delayed imaging with hepatobiliary contrast agents (e.g., gadoxetic acid) (Fig. 9), are options. Both imaging agents are taken up by functional hepatocytes and are excreted into the biliary system, resulting in abnormal sites of intrahepatic or extrahepatic accumulation when a bile leak is present.

To our knowledge, there are no diagnostic accuracy studies comparing these two approaches in a head-to-head fashion. That said, MRCP offers far-superior anatomic detail, potentially allowing identification of the precise site of biliary disruption and directing management appropriately. Hepatobiliary scintigraphy, which can be done as a portable examination and does not have any associated renal function requirements, is a good option for patients with contraindications to MRI or gadolinium-based contrast agents.

Finally, when the above-described noninvasive examinations are nondiagnostic or when a bile leak is diagnosed by other means, endoscopic retrograde cholangiopancreatography (ERCP) can be used to identify the precise site of biliary disruption via the extrabiliary accumulation of iodinated contrast material during injection under fluoroscopy (Figs. 9, 10, and 11). ERCP is also a potential therapeutic procedure, as leaks that are felt to be unlikely to resolve spontaneously can be managed with immediate stenting.

## Bile Leak MRCP Protocol

At our institution, the bile leak MRCP protocol consists of tri-planar thin-slice T2-weighted sequences to delineate the biliary anatomy, as well as standard dynamic pre- and post-contrast T1-weighted images utilizing a double dose of gadoxetic acid (0.05 mmol/kg) as the contrast agent. Diffusion-weighted images are also acquired utilizing $b$ values of 50, 400, and 800 s/mm$^2$. Finally, at 60 min following contrast administration (i.e., a delayed hepatobiliary phase), we acquire tri-planar T1-weighted images of the abdomen to assess for areas of abnormal accumulation of gadoxetic acid, as would be expected for a bile leak or biloma. In many cases, the precise site of bile duct disruption/leakage can be identified and treated accordingly.

---

**Fig. 9** (continued) MR images (**d**) obtained 60 min after intravenous administration of gadoxetic acid show a bile leak originating from the right intrahepatic duct (smaller black arrowhead) and tracking along the inferior liver margin (larger black arrowhead). Because the common bile duct could not be opacified on the MRCP, an ERCP was performed.

Scout (**e**) and postinjection (**f**) images reveal frank extravasation of contrast from the region of the pancreatic head (oval), consistent with a distal common bile duct injury. This case illustrates how difficult the diagnosis of common bile duct injury can be to make using CT or even MRI

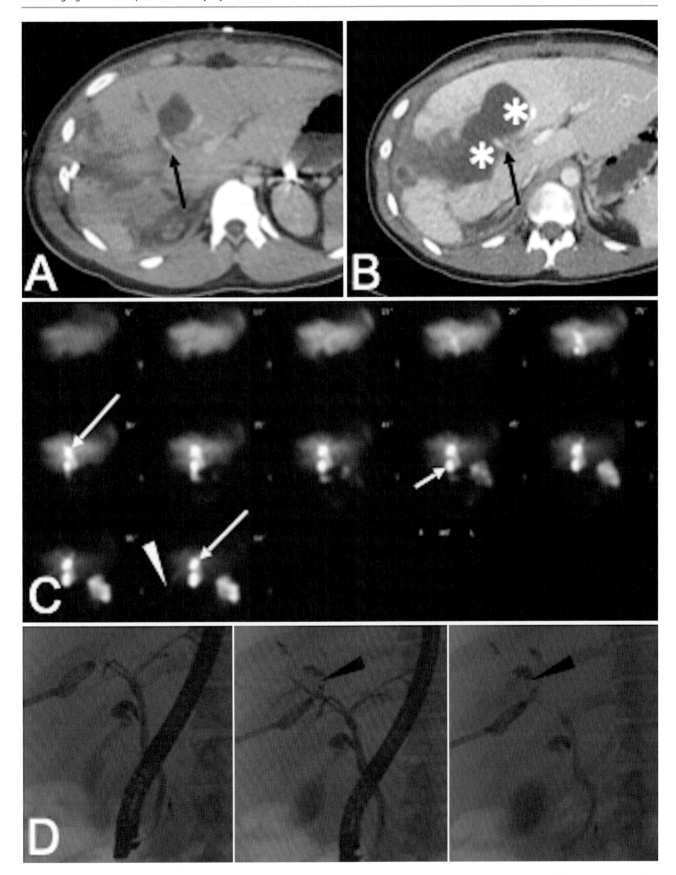

**Fig. 10** Intrahepatic bile duct injury following motor vehicle collision. Abdominal computed tomography images with IV contrast (**a**) acquired immediately after an exploratory laparotomy with hepatic surgery for a high-grade liver injury show a laceration traversing the central right

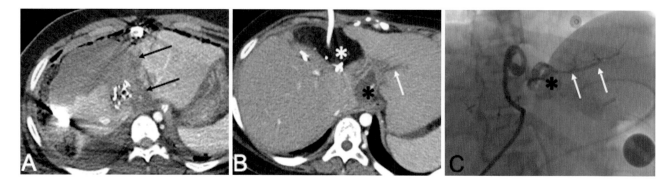

**Fig. 11** Intrahepatic bile duct transection following motor vehicle collision. Abdominal computed tomography (CT) images (**a**) with IV contrast obtained after surgical exploration to control intra-abdominal bleeding show a high-grade liver injury involving a large portion of the right hepatic lobe and completely traversing segment 4 from anterior to posterior (black arrows). A subsequent CT (**b**) with IV contrast after partial segment 4 resection reveals a fluid collection (black asterisk) in the region of the portal structures supplying segment 2/3. The segment 2/3 intrahepatic bile ducts (white arrow) can be seen adjacent to this fluid collection, raising suspicion for a biloma. Note the perihepatic drainage catheter and omental fat packing within the resection cavity (white asterisk). An anterior fluoroscopic image (**c**) from injection of the perihepatic drainage catheter seen in B shows opacification of this fluid collection (black asterisk), with backfilling of a transected segment 2/3 intrahepatic bile duct (white arrows)

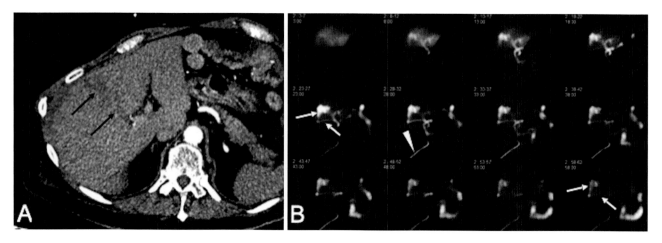

**Fig. 12** Intrahepatic bile duct injury following motor vehicle collision. Abdominal computed tomography images with IV contrast (**a**) show a high-grade liver injury with a laceration extending to the hilum (black arrows). Bilious output from a perihepatic surgical drainage catheter raised suspicion for a bile leak. Sequential anterior images from a hepatobiliary scintigraphy examination (**b**) performed up to 60 min show tracer accumulation in this fluid collection (white arrows), as well as activity in a surgical drainage catheter (white arrowhead), confirming a bile leak

# References

1. Iacobellis F, Scaglione M, Brillantino A, Scuderi MG, Giurazza F, Grassi R, Noschese G, Niola R, Al Zuhir NYS, Romano L. The additional value of the arterial phase in the CT assessment of liver vascular injuries after high-energy blunt trauma. Emerg Radiol. 2019;26(6):647–54. https://doi.org/10.1007/s10140-019-01714-y. Epub 2019 Aug 23

2. Romano L, Giovine S, Guidi G, Tortora G, Cinque T, Romano S. Hepatic trauma: CT findings and considerations based on our experience in emergency diagnostic imaging. Eur J Radiol. 2004;50(1):59–66. https://doi.org/10.1016/j.ejrad.2003.11.015.

3. Yoon W, Jeong YY, Kim JK, Seo JJ, Lim HS, Shin SS, Kim JC, Jeong SW, Park JG, Kang HK. CT in blunt liver trauma.

◄

**Fig. 10** (continued)  portal structures (black arrow). Images from a subsequent CT with IV contrast (**b**) show an enlarging fluid collection (asterisks) straddling the central right portal structures (black arrow), which is suspicious for a biloma. Sequential anterior images from a hepatobiliary scintigraphy examination (**c**) performed up to 60 min show tracer accumulation in this fluid collection (long white arrows), as well as faint activity in a surgical drainage catheter (white arrowhead), confirming a bile leak. Note normal tracer accumulation in the gallbladder (short white arrow). Progressive (earliest on left; latest on right) fluoroscopic ERCP images (**d**) show a bile leak (black arrowheads) originating from the central right intrahepatic duct. This duct was stented to promote healing

Radiographics. 2005;25(1):87–104. https://doi.org/10.1148/rg.251045079.

4. Kozar RA, Crandall M, Shanmuganathan K, Zarzaur BL, Coburn M, Cribari C, Kaups K, Schuster K, Tominaga GT, AAST Patient Assessment Committee. Organ injury scaling 2018 update: spleen, liver, and kidney. J Trauma Acute Care Surg. 2018;85(6):1119–22. https://doi.org/10.1097/TA.0000000000002058. Erratum in: J Trauma Acute Care Surg. 2019;87(2):512

5. Brillantino A, Iacobellis F, Festa P, Mottola A, Acampora C, Corvino F, Del Giudice S, Lanza M, Armellino M, Niola R, Romano L, Castriconi M, De Palma M, Noschese G. Non-operative management of blunt liver trauma: safety, efficacy and complications of a standardized treatment protocol. Bull Emerg Trauma. 2019;7(1):49–54. https://doi.org/10.29252/beat-070107.

6. Matsushima K, Hogen R, Piccinini A, Biswas S, Khor D, Delapena S, Strumwasser A, Inaba K, Demetriades D. Adjunctive use of hepatic angioembolization following hemorrhage control laparotomy. J Trauma Acute Care Surg. 2020;88(5):636–43. https://doi.org/10.1097/TA.0000000000002591.

7. Coccolini F, Catena F, Moore EE, Ivatury R, Biffl W, Peitzman A, Coimbra R, Rizoli S, Kluger Y, Abu-Zidan FM, Ceresoli M, Montori G, Sartelli M, Weber D, Fraga G, Naidoo N, Moore FA, Zanini N, Ansaloni L. WSES classification and guidelines for liver trauma. World J Emerg Surg. 2016;11:50. https://doi.org/10.1186/s13017-016-0105-2.

8. Iacobellis F, Romano L, Rengo A, Danzi R, Scuderi MG, Brillantino A, Scaglione M. CT protocol optimization in trauma imaging: a review of current evidence. Curr Radiol Rep. 2020;8:8. https://doi.org/10.1007/s40134-020-00351-5.

9. Liguori C, Gagliardi N, Saturnino PP, Pinto A, Romano L. Multidetector computed tomography of pharyngo-esophageal perforations. Semin Ultrasound CT MR. 2016;37(1):10–5.

10. West OC, Anderson J, Lee JS, et al. Patterns of diagnostic error in trauma abdominal CT. Emerg Radiol. 2002;9:195–200.

11. Scaglione M, Iaselli F, Sica G, Feragalli B, Nicola R. Errors in imaging of traumatic injuries. Abdom Imaging. 2015;40:2091–8.

12. Monazzam S, Goodell PB, Salcedo ES, Nelson SH, Wolinsky PR. When are CT angiograms indicated for patients with lower extremity fractures? A review of 275 extremities. J Trauma Acute Care Surg. 2017;82(1):133–7.

13. Darling RC III, Byrne J. Diagnosis of vascular trauma. Clin Rev Vasc Trauma. 2014;33:57. https://doi.org/10.1007/978-3-642-39100-2_3.

14. Scaglione M, Laccetti E, Picascia R, Altiero M, Iacobellis F, Elameer M, Grassi R. Errors in imaging of abdominal and pelvic trauma. In: Patlas MN, Katz DS, Scaglione M, editors. Errors in emergency and trauma radiology. New York: Springer; 2019.

15. Iacobellis F, Ierardi AM, Mazzei MA, Biasina AM, Carrafiello G, Nicola R, Scaglione M. Dual-phase CT for the assessment of acute vascular injuries in high-energy blunt trauma: the imaging findings and management implications. Br J Radiol. 2016;89(1061):20150952.

16. Schueller G, Scaglione M, Linsenmaier U, Schueller-Weidekamm C, Andreoli C, De Vargas Macciucca M, Gualdi G. The key role of the radiologist in the management of polytrauma patients: indications for MDCT imaging in emergency radiology. Radiol Med. 2015;120:641–54.

17. Eichler K, Marzi I, Wyen H, Zangos S, Mack MG, Vogl TJ. Multidetector computed tomography (MDCT): simple CT protocol for trauma patient. Clin Imaging. 2015;39(1):110–5.

18. Nguyen D, Platon A, Shanmuganathan K, Mirvis SE, Becker CD, Poletti PA. Evaluation of a single-pass continuous wholebody, 16-MDCT protocol for patients with polytrauma. Am J Roentgenol. 2009;192(1):3–10.

19. Sica G, Guida F, Bocchini G, Codella U, Mainenti PP, Tanga M, Scaglione M. Errors in imaging assessment of polytrauma patients. Semin Ultrasound CT MR. 2012;33(4):337–46.

20. Coccolini F, Montori G, Catena F, et al. Liver trauma: WSES position paper. World J Emerg Surg. 2015;10:39. https://doi.org/10.1186/s13017-015-0030-9.

21. Thomson BN, Nardino B, Gumm K, et al. Management of blunt and penetrating biliary tract trauma. J Trauma Acute Care Surg. 2012;72(6):1620–5. https://doi.org/10.1097/TA.0b013e318248ed65.

22. Gupta A, Stuhlfaut JW, Fleming KW, Lucey BC, Soto JA. Blunt trauma of the pancreas and biliary tract: a multimodality imaging approach to diagnosis. Radiographics. 2004;24(5):1381–95. https://doi.org/10.1148/rg.245045002.

23. Soderstrom CA, Maekawa K, DuPriest RW Jr, Cowley RA. Gallbladder injuries resulting from blunt abdominal trauma: an experience and review. Ann Surg. 1981;193(1):60–6. https://doi.org/10.1097/00000658-198101000-00010.

24. SMITH SW, HASTINGS TN. Traumatic rupture of the gallbladder. Ann Surg. 1954;139(4):517–20. https://doi.org/10.1097/00000658-195404000-00019.

25. Penn I. Injuries of the gall-bladder. Br J Surg. 1962;49:636–41. https://doi.org/10.1002/bjs.18004921816.

26. Sharma O. Blunt gallbladder injuries: presentation of twenty-two cases with review of the literature. J Trauma. 1995;39(3):576–80. https://doi.org/10.1097/00005373-199509000-00029.

27. Moore EE, Jurkovich GJ, Knudson MM, et al. Organ injury scaling. VI: extrahepatic biliary, esophagus, stomach, vulva, vagina, uterus (nonpregnant), uterus (pregnant), fallopian tube, and ovary. J Trauma. 1995;39(6):1069–70. https://doi.org/10.1097/00005373-199512000-00009.

28. Erb RE, Mirvis SE, Shanmuganathan K. Gallbladder injury secondary to blunt trauma: CT findings. J Comput Assist Tomogr. 1994;18(5):778–84.

29. Chen X, Talner LB, Jurkovich GJ. Gallbladder avulsion due to blunt trauma. AJR Am J Roentgenol. 2001;177(4):822. https://doi.org/10.2214/ajr.177.4.1770822.

30. Zago TM, Pereira BM, Calderan TR, Hirano ES, Fraga GP. Extrahepatic duct injury in blunt trauma: two case reports and a literature review. Indian J Surg. 2014;76(4):303–7. https://doi.org/10.1007/s12262-013-0885-5.

31. LeBedis CA, Bates DDB, Soto JA. Iatrogenic, blunt, and penetrating trauma to the biliary tract. Abdom Radiol. 2017;42(1):28–45. https://doi.org/10.1007/s00261-016-0856-y.

32. Gerndt SJ, Seidel SP, Taheri PA, Rodriguez JL. Biliary tract injury following blunt abdominal trauma: case reports. J Trauma. 1995;39(3):612–5. https://doi.org/10.1097/00005373-199509000-00039.

33. Franklin GA, Richardson JD, Brown AL, et al. Prevention of bile peritonitis by laparoscopic evacuation and lavage after nonoperative treatment of liver injuries. Am Surg. 2007;73(6):611–7.

# Imaging of Blunt Pancreatic Injuries

21

Daniel Oppenheimer

## Contents

### Abstract

Blunt pancreatic injuries are uncommon, but they can be life threatening, especially if not recognized promptly. The imaging findings of pancreatic injury may be difficult to identify due to the complex regional anatomy and frequent coexisting injury to adjacent organs and structures. Despite these challenges, the radiologist must be able to recognize the imaging findings of pancreatic injury, and should attempt to characterize the severity of the injury in order to properly guide management decisions. This chapter will review the multimodality imaging findings of blunt injury to the pancreas, describe a commonly used classification system to grade pancreatic injuries, and briefly discuss associated complications.

### Keywords

Pancreatic injury · Pancreatic duct · Abdominal trauma

## Introduction

Injury to the pancreas is relatively rare, occurring in fewer than 2% of cases of blunt abdominal trauma [1]. However, delays in diagnosis of pancreas injuries are associated with increased morbidity and mortality [2]. According to the American College of Radiology Appropriateness Criteria, a radiography trauma series, Focused Assessment with Sonography for Trauma (FAST), and computed tomography (CT) of the whole body are usually appropriate for evaluation of the hemodynamically stable patient following major blunt trauma [3]. In a hemodynamically stable patient, CT is the preferred modality to evaluate a patient who has suffered significant blunt trauma, is faster and less operator dependent than sonography, and readily depicts injuries in multiple body systems simultaneously. Unstable patients may not be suitable for CT, and if the FAST examination is positive, they

D. Oppenheimer (✉)
Abdominal Imaging Division, Department of Imaging Sciences, University of Rochester Medical Center, Rochester, NY, USA
e-mail: daniel_oppenheimer@urmc.rochester.edu

© Springer Nature Switzerland AG 2022
M. N. Patlas et al. (eds.), *Atlas of Emergency Imaging from Head-to-Toe*,
https://doi.org/10.1007/978-3-030-92111-8_21

are generally taken immediately to surgery. However, a negative FAST examination does not exclude the presence of injury in the abdomen [4].

## Anatomy

The pancreas is a "J-shaped" retroperitoneal organ located in the upper abdomen across the midline which measures approximately 15–20 cm in length and weighs 90–100 g. The pancreas secretes hormones and enzymes to maintain euglycemia and assist in digestion. Anatomically, the pancreas is divided into the uncinate process, head, neck, body, and tail. The main pancreatic duct normally measures between 2 and 4 mm diameter within the body and tail, and bifurcates into the dorsal (Santorini) and ventral (Wirsung) ducts in the head, although variations in pancreatic ductal anatomy are common, such as pancreas divisum [5]. The pancreas lies adjacent to the stomach, duodenum, colon, kidneys, liver, and spleen, and is surrounded by several major vascular structures including the aorta, inferior vena cava (IVC), as well as portal, splenic, superior mesenteric, and renal veins, which explains a high association of pancreas trauma with additional injuries.

## Epidemiology

Approximately two-thirds of all pancreatic injuries involve the body. The overall mortality of pancreatic injuries ranges from 9% to 34%, and concomitant injuries to the liver, spleen, stomach, and/or duodenum are present in over 90% of cases [6, 7]. Of those patients who die within 48 h from abdominal trauma, the majority of deaths are secondary to exsanguination from vascular and solid organ injuries. The patients who survive the acute period following trauma may develop complications such as fluid collections, multiorgan failure, and sepsis, which contribute to delayed mortality. This is the subset of patients in whom radiologists have an important role in promptly determining the extent and severity of injuries, because delays in diagnosis and treatment have been shown to adversely affect morbidity and mortality [8, 9]. Therefore, the importance of rapid identification and characterization of pancreatic and additional abdominal injuries cannot be understated.

## Mechanisms of Pancreatic Injury

Despite being relatively protected from trauma by its retroperitoneal location and surrounding fat, the pancreas may be injured secondary to blunt and penetrating trauma. The most common mechanism of pancreatic injury is blunt anteroposterior trauma to the upper abdomen which compresses the pancreas against the spine. This mechanism has been classically associated with handlebar bicycling injury and seat belt motor vehicle injuries, but may also occur with falls, sports-related injury, or in victims of physical assault, including nonaccidental trauma in infants [10]. Blunt trauma to the pancreas is more common in children and young adults, probably because they tend to have less peripancreatic fat compared with older adults [1].

Penetrating injury to the pancreas usually occurs in the setting of gunshot or stab wounds to the upper abdomen. In all cases of penetrating trauma, a careful search along the trajectory of the injury is critical to fully assess the extent of injury. Foci of gas and/or retained foreign material such as bullet fragments are helpful clues to the trajectory of a penetrating wound. Additionally, at our institutions, we place radio-opaque markers on the skin at the entry site(s) to improve our understanding of the trajectory of the trauma and accurately assess the injured structures along the path when interpreting these examinations.

## Clinical and Laboratory Findings

The classic clinical triad of pancreatic trauma is upper abdominal pain, leukocytosis, and elevated serum amylase [11]. However, hyperamylasemia may be absent for up to 48 h after the injury. Furthermore, trauma patients may be sedated, may not be able to provide an accurate history, or may have concomitant or distracting injuries such as long bone fractures.

Hyperamylasemia which rises or remains elevated after blunt traumatic injury to the abdomen is suggestive of pancreatic injury. However, hyperamylasemia may also occur secondary to trauma to the liver or duodenum as well as to the face and neck (due to the salivary production of amylase), and may also be elevated in acute alcohol intoxication. In addition, serum amylase may be normal in up to 40% of patients, even in cases of major pancreatic injury including duct transection. Furthermore, the degree of serum amylase elevation does not correlate with the severity of injury or prognosis [6, 10]. Therefore, while hyperamylasemia may be a sign of pancreatic injury in the appropriate clinical setting, it is nonspecific and does not aid in determining the severity of injury.

## Imaging of Pancreatic Trauma

CT remains a highly effective imaging examination in evaluating the acute trauma patient. The benefits of multidetector CT in the setting of trauma are well known, including a rapid acquisition time, high spatial resolution, and the ability to create multiplanar reformations. The specific CT protocols for trauma vary considerably at different institutions; we perform a single-phase scan through the abdomen and pelvis using a fixed 70 s delay following the intravenous administration of nonionic iodinated contrast material, which is delivered via a power injector into a peripheral IV or central line at a rate of 4–5 cc/s. Oral contrast is generally not administered to acute trauma patients, but water-soluble oral contrast may be considered in follow-up imaging of a trauma patient to evaluate for a leak in the gastrointestinal tract. Follow-up examinations may also be performed with a specific pancreatic protocol, which includes noncontrast CT abdomen followed by scans in the pancreatic parenchymal phase (approximately 30 s after contrast administration) and portal venous phase (70 s).

Previous studies have reported approximately 80% sensitivity and specificity for the detection of pancreatic injury, and less than 50% accuracy for detecting ductal injury on CT [1, 12]. However, because these studies were mostly published before the era of multidetector thin-slice CT, the accuracy of detecting pancreatic ductal injury in particular is believed to be higher [13]. The direct and indirect signs of pancreatic injury are shown in Table 1. Importantly, the pancreas may appear normal in up to 40% of patients imaged within the first 12 h following blunt pancreatic injury [1].

Pancreatic lacerations are an important direct sign of pancreatic injury, and appear on CT and magnetic resonance (MR) as linear or jagged areas of hypoenhancement which may contain small amounts of fluid attenuation/fluid signal material (Fig. 1). T2-weighted fat-suppressed MR images may depict hyperintense fluid signal at the site of laceration, with adjacent milder parenchymal T2 hyperintense edema (Fig. 1d). Pancreatic lacerations are most commonly located in the body and neck region [14]. Some pancreatic lacerations may be difficult to detect acutely (particularly in patients with a paucity of retroperitoneal fat), and may only be apparent on one or two contiguous images if small. In such cases, reviewing multiplanar reconstructions may be helpful in making a diagnosis, particularly if the plane of the laceration is parallel to the transaxial images [15]. If the laceration spans the entire anterior-posterior width of the pancreas, this strongly implies that the pancreatic duct in this segment is transected, whereas if the laceration involves less than 50% of the parenchymal width, injury to the pancreatic duct is unlikely [16]. Injury to the pancreatic duct is an important finding which increases the severity of the injury and impacts treatment decisions. Pancreatic ductal injury is discussed in further detail below.

Other specific signs of pancreatic injury on cross-sectional imaging are pancreatic contusions, pancreatic hematomas, and active hemorrhage from the pancreas. Pancreatic contusions appear as ill-defined area(s) of hypoattenuation on CT, and mildly elevated T2 signal on MR within the pancreatic parenchyma, and may be associated with focal enlargement (Fig. 2). Hematoma within or directly contacting the pancreas is also a direct sign of pancreatic injury, and may result in local mass effect on bowel and vasculature (Fig. 3). Hematomas may be most conspicuous noncontrast-enhanced CT and on T1-weighted fat-suppressed MR images. Active hemorrhage from the pancreatic parenchyma is identified as extravasation of intravenous contrast material, which should increase or change in configuration if multiphasic imaging is performed [6, 17].

Indirect findings of pancreatic injury include hemoretroperitoneum, and peripancreatic fluid and stranding. In one study, fluid specifically located between the splenic vein and pancreas was found in 90% of patients with pancreatic injury (Fig. 4) [18]. However, peripancreatic fluid and stranding in general may be the result of aggressive intravenous hydration, and these nonspecific findings should not be relied upon in isolation to make a diagnosis of pancreatic injury [19].

Potential mimics of pancreatic injury are fatty pancreatic clefts and prominent lobulations of pancreatic tissue, which can be mistaken for superficial pancreatic lacerations (Fig. 5). Conversely, a laceration may be inadvertently dismissed as a normal cleft in the pancreatic contour [1]. In ambiguous cases, the radiologist should attempt to identify additional direct and indirect findings to increase their confidence that a pancreatic injury is actually present.

In the setting of pancreatic trauma, the integrity of the main pancreatic duct is the most important factor which determines the needs for intervention, because major duct injury increases mortality and the likelihood of complications such as fistula and fluid collections [17, 20]. Magnetic resonance cholangio-pancreatography (MRCP) is a highly useful and accurate noninvasive imaging technique which can be used to evaluate the integrity of the pancreatic duct. By utilizing heavily T2-weighted images and three-dimensional reformatting techniques, MRCP reveals the anatomic details of the pancreatic and bile ducts.

**Table 1** Direct and indirect signs of pancreatic injury

| Direct signs of pancreatic injury | Indirect signs of pancreatic injury |
|---|---|
| Pancreatic laceration | Retroperitoneal hemorrhage |
| Pancreatic contusion | Peripancreatic fluid and stranding |
| Pancreatic hematoma | Fluid between the splenic vein and pancreas |
| Active extravasation | Fluid adjacent to the SMA/SMV |
| | Thickening of the left anterior renal fascia |

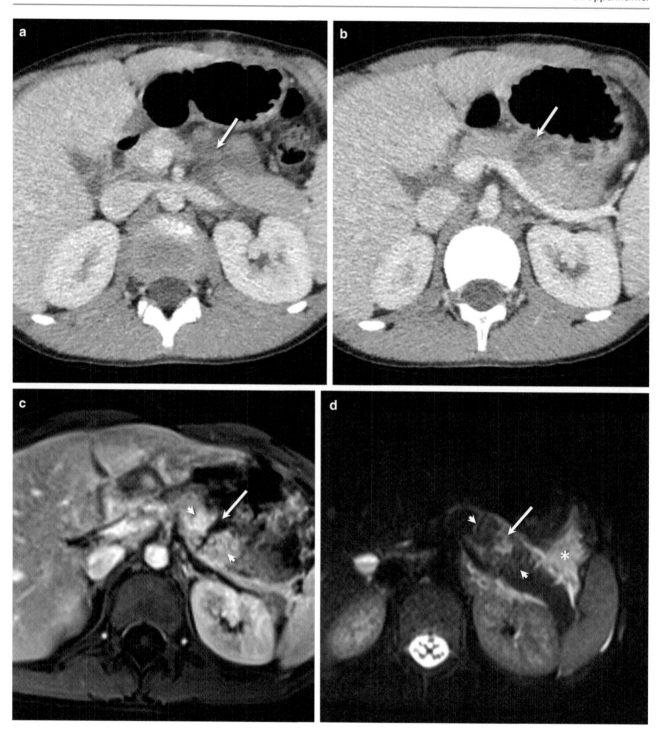

**Fig. 1** A 9-year-old boy with grade 3 pancreatic injury after handlebar bicycle injury. Axial IV contrast-enhanced CT (CECT) (**a** and **b**) images demonstrate a focal area of hypoenhancement involving the entire AP width of the body/tail of the pancreas (arrows) with adjacent edema. Axial T1-weighted fat-suppressed post-gadolinium MR (**c**) image further delineates the area of hypoenhancing laceration (arrow) and adjacent parenchymal hyperemia (arrowhead). Axial T2-weighted fat-suppressed MR (**d**) image demonstrates the high signal laceration extending through the full thickness of the pancreas (arrow), and adjacent parenchymal edema (arrowheads) which shows milder T2 hyperintensity. A small amount of complex peripancreatic fluid is also seen (*)

Discontinuity of the pancreatic duct in the region of pancreatic injury is diagnostic of pancreatic duct disruption (Fig. 6a) [21]. The lack of ionizing radiation with MRCP also makes this technique well suited for follow-up of conservatively managed injuries, particularly in children and younger adult patients [22].

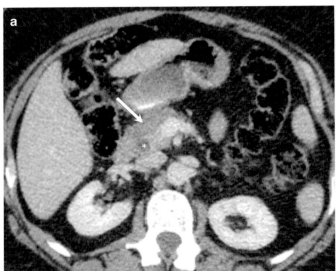
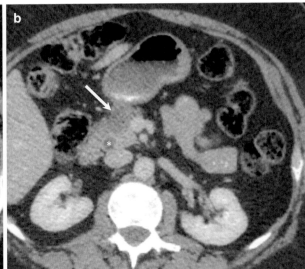

**Fig. 2** A 53-year-old woman with mild pancreatic head contusion (grade 1 injury) after motor vehicle collision. Axial CECT (**a** and **b**) images demonstrate focal hypoenhancement and mild enlargement of the pancreas in the head/neck region (arrows), consistent with a contusion. The patient was treated conservatively, and recovered fully without complication. Asterisk – common bile duct

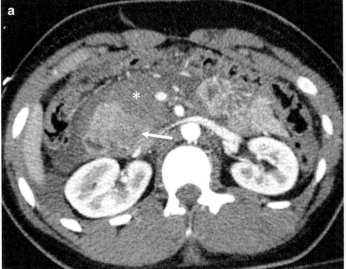
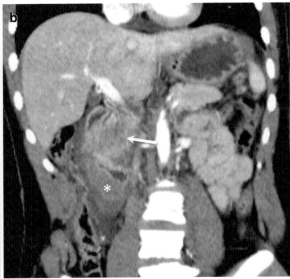

**Fig. 3** A 12-year-old girl with grade 2 pancreatic head and duodenal injury. Axial (**a**) and coronal (**b**) CECT images demonstrate an ill-defined area of hypoenhancement in the pancreatic head (arrow) with large amount of surrounding hematoma (*). At surgery, clot was evacuated, pancreatic and duodenal injuries were repaired without resection, and the patient made a full recovery

MRCP is also useful for preoperative planning prior to endoscopic retrograde cholangio-pancreatography (ERCP) or surgery. In addition to providing a noninvasive assessment of the pancreatic duct integrity in the injured portion of the pancreas, MRCP can also depict ductal anatomic variants, such as pancreas divisum, which may affect cannulation of the pancreatic duct at the time of endoscopic intervention. ERCP can directly confirm ductal injury by demonstrating extravasation of contrast material from the pancreatic duct (Fig. 6b–d), and also permits endoscopic stent placement over the injured segment of duct [23]. ERCP can also determine if the duct is completely transected, or if there remains a portion of the duct distal to the injury which maintains some continuity.

## Grading and Management of Pancreatic Injuries

In the USA, the most frequently used classification system of pancreatic injury is from the American Association for the Surgery of Trauma (AAST), whose systems are also

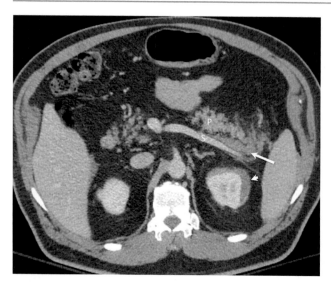

**Fig. 4** A 62-year-old man with grade 1 pancreatic injury after motor vehicle collision with rollover. Axial CECT image demonstrates a small amount of high attenuation hematoma (arrow) located between the splenic vein (S) and tail of the pancreas (P). There was no evidence of pancreatic laceration or contusion. A small left kidney subcapsular hematoma was also present (arrowhead). The patient was treated conservatively and recovered fully without complications

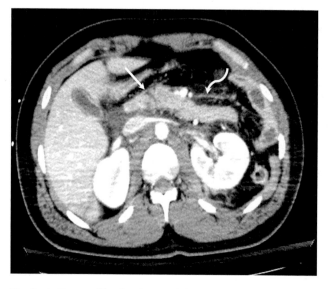

**Fig. 5** A 40-year-old pedestrian struck by an automobile, with a deep pancreatic cleft in the neck mimicking a laceration, and a pancreatic tail injury. Axial CECT image demonstrates a linear area of low attenuation in the pancreatic neck (arrow) which appears to be a laceration, involving approximately 50% of the thickness of the pancreas. There is also mild peripancreatic fat stranding anterior to the tail (squiggly arrow). At surgery, no laceration in the pancreatic neck area was identified, but the patient required distal pancreatectomy for pancreatic tail contusion

commonly used for other organ injuries (Table 2) [24]. The major factors which influence the grade of injury in the AAST system for pancreatic trauma are the location of the

injury and the integrity of the main pancreatic duct. Injuries to the pancreatic head are higher in grade than injuries to the body/tail, and injuries with pancreatic duct involvement are higher in grade than injuries without duct involvement. The most severe type of pancreatic injury is massive disruption of the pancreatic head and duodenum, which is highly associated with hepatobiliary, enteric, and vascular injuries (Fig. 7).

Factors which influence the management of pancreatic trauma include the grade and location of the pancreatic injury, the time elapsed since the injury, and other associated injuries. If duct injury is absent on imaging and the patient does not require surgery for other injuries, a conservative approach is usually undertaken. External drainage of the pancreatic bed can be performed for mild injuries in patients who require laparotomy for other reasons. Omental pancreatorrhaphy may also be performed to repair superficial lacerations to promote healing. If duct involvement is confirmed on imaging, surgery is usually performed. Distal pancreatectomy with or without splenectomy is the treatment of choice for transection of the pancreatic tail (grade 3 injury). In grade 4 or 5 injuries, pancreatoduodenectomy may be necessary, but surgical and/or percutaneous drainage may be performed first as initial damage control in these patients who frequently have additional injuries [25, 26].

## Complications of Pancreatic Trauma

The majority of pancreatic injuries are minor contusions and superficial lacerations, and are treated conservatively [7]. More severe injuries, especially injuries involving the pancreatic duct, are associated with a higher likelihood of complications and death, with approximately 75% of all deaths occurring within the first 72 h [8, 10]. Complications specific to pancreatic trauma include pancreatitis and the development of associated fluid collections. In particular, the development of post-traumatic pseudocysts suggests that pancreatic ductal injury is present, even if not apparent on initial imaging. In these patients, MRCP or ERCP is indicated to further evaluate the integrity of the main pancreatic duct [1, 17]. Fluid collections which develop following pancreatic injury may become infected, fistulize to bowel, or cause mass effect which may require percutaneous or surgical drainage (Fig. 8) [27]. Post-traumatic pancreatitis may also result in pseudoaneurysm formation, which poses risk of rupture and catastrophic hemorrhage. Pancreatic duct stricture(s) may also develop after blunt pancreatic injury, which may predispose to subsequent episodes of pancreatitis.

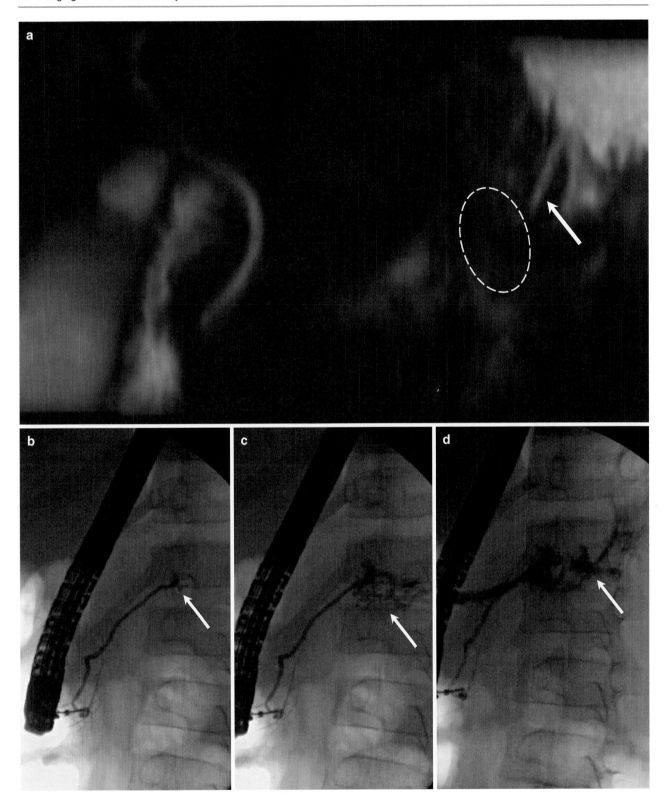

**Fig. 6** A 9-year-old boy with grade 3 pancreatic injury after handlebar bicycle injury (same patient as Fig. 1). (**a**) Coronal MRCP image shows disruption of the pancreatic duct in the distal body (dashed circle), and an adjacent segment of upstream normal caliber pancreatic duct in the tail is visualized (arrow). The pancreatic duct in the head and neck was poorly visualized on MRCP. Sequential images performed during an ERP (**b–d**) show progressive extravasation of contrast (arrows), confirming pancreatic duct disruption in the tail at the site of injury. The patient was treated with distal pancreatectomy, and made a full recovery

**Table 2** AAST pancreatic injury grading

| AAST pancreatic injury grade | Injury | Description |
|---|---|---|
| I | Hematoma | Small contusion, no duct injury |
| I | Laceration | Small laceration, no duct injury |
| II | Hematoma | Major contusion, no duct injury |
| II | Laceration | Major laceration, no duct injury |
| III | Laceration | Laceration in tail with duct injury |
| IV | Laceration | Laceration in head/neck involving ampulla with duct injury |
| V | Laceration | Massive disruption of pancreatic head |

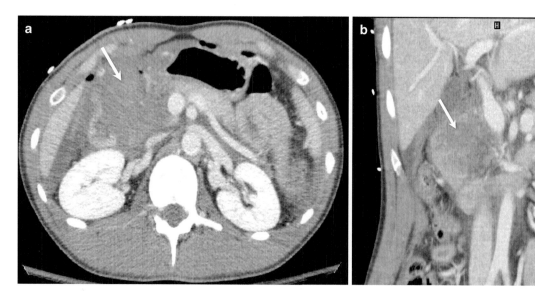

**Fig. 7** A 24-year-old man with grade 5 pancreatic head injury after a fall from height. Axial (**a**) and coronal reformatted (**b**) CECT images demonstrate a large hematoma within and surrounding the pancreatic head (arrows), with mass effect on the adjacent duodenum and portal vein. At surgery, a pancreatic head avulsion was found, which required pancreaticoduodenectomy

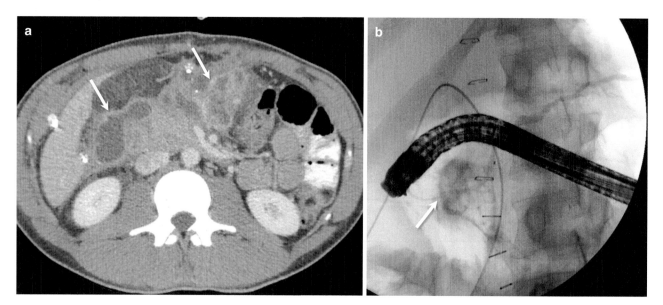

**Fig. 8** A 54-year-old man with multiple solid organ injuries after motor vehicle collision, including pancreatic head injury. (**a**) Several days after exploratory laparotomy, CECT demonstrates multiple rim-enhancing fluid collections adjacent to the pancreas and liver (examples with arrows). Portions of surgical drains are also visible. (**b**) Endoscopic retrograde pancreatography shows extravasation of contrast from the pancreatic head, confirming duct injury (arrow). A pancreatic duct stent was placed, and the fluid collections eventually resolved with percutaneous drainage

## Conclusions

Blunt pancreatic injury is rare but carries substantial morbidity and mortality, and is highly associated with additional injuries in the abdomen. Accurate diagnosis and grading of the injury on initial CT, which may be then followed with MR and possibly other imaging examinations, facilitates appropriate management in these patients. The radiologist should be aware of the spectrum of findings in pancreatic trauma, understand the grading classification, and recognize associated complications if they develop.

## Key Points

- Direct signs of pancreatic injury on IV contrast-enhanced CT include laceration, contusion, active extravasation, and intrapancreatic hematoma.
- Blunt pancreatic injury is commonly associated with injuries to adjacent solid organs, bowel, and vascular structures.
- The presence of injury to the pancreatic duct is an important factor which increases the severity of the injury, and usually requires percutaneous drainage, stent placement, and/or surgery.

## References

1. Cirillo RL Jr, Koniaris LG. Detecting blunt pancreatic injuries. J Gastrointest Surg. 2002;6(4):587–98. https://doi.org/10.1016/s1091-255x(01)00028-2. Review.
2. Smego DR, Richardson JD, Flint LM. Determinants of outcome in pancreatic trauma. J Trauma. 1985;25(8):771–6. https://doi.org/10.1097/00005373-198508000-00007.
3. https://acsearch.acr.org/docs/3102405/Narrative/
4. Laselle BT, Byyny RL, Haukoos JS, et al. False-negative FAST examination: associations with injury characteristics and patient outcomes. Ann Emerg Med. 2012;60:326–34 e3.
5. Quinlan R. Anatomy, embryology, and physiology of the pancreas. In: Shackelford RT, Zuidema GD, editors. Surgery of the alimentary tract. Philadelphia: Saunders; 1983. p. 3–24.
6. Linsenmaier U, Wirth S, Reiser M, Körner M. Diagnosis and classification of pancreatic and duodenal injuries in emergency radiology. Radiographics. 2008;28(6):1591–602. https://doi.org/10.1148/rg.286085524. Review.
7. Bradley EL 3rd, Young PR Jr, Chang MC, et al. Diagnosis and initial management of blunt pancreatic trauma: guidelines from a multi-institutional review. Ann Surg. 1998;227:861–9.
8. Kao LS, Bulger EM, Parks DL, Byrd GF, Jurkovich GJ. Predictors of morbidity after traumatic pancreatic injury. J Trauma. 2003;55: 898–905.
9. Akhrass R, Yaffe MB, Brandt CP, Reigle M, Fallon WF Jr, Malangoni MA. Pancreatic trauma: a ten-year multi-institutional experience. Am Surg. 1997;63:598–604.
10. Venkatesh SK, Wan JM. CT of blunt pancreatic trauma: a pictorial essay. Eur J Radiol. 2007;67:311–20.
11. White PH, Benfield JR. Amylase in the management of pancreatic trauma. Arch Surg. 1972;105:158–63.
12. Wilson RH, Moorehead RJ. Current management of trauma to the pancreas. Br J Surg. 1991;78:1196–202.
13. Teh SH, Sheppard BC, Mullins RJ, Schreiber MA, Mayberry JC. Diagnosis and management of blunt pancreatic ductal injury in the era of high-resolution computed axial tomography. Am J Surg. 2007;193:641–3.
14. Dodds WJ, Taylor AJ, Erickson SJ, Lawson TL. Traumatic fracture of the pancreas: CT characteristics. J Comput Assist Tomogr. 1990;14:375–8.
15. Shanmuganathan K. Multi-detector row CT imaging of blunt abdominal trauma. Semin Ultrasound CT MR. 2004;25:180–204.
16. Wong YC, Wang LJ, Lin BC, Chen CJ, Lim KE, Chen RJ. CT grading of blunt pancreatic injuries: prediction of ductal disruption and surgical correlation. J Comput Assist Tomogr. 1997;21:246–50.
17. Rekhi S, Anderson SW, Rhea JT, Soto JA. Imaging of blunt pancreatic trauma. Emerg Radiol. 2010;17(1):13–9. https://doi.org/10.1007/s10140-009-0811-0. Review.
18. Lane MJ, Mindelzun RE, Sandhu JS, McCormick VD, Jeffrey RB. CT diagnosis of blunt pancreatic trauma: importance of detecting fluid between the pancreas and the splenic vein. AJR Am J Roentgenol. 1994;163:833–5.
19. Chapman VM, Rhea JT, Sacknoff R, Novelline RA. CT of non-traumatic abdominal fluid collections after initial fluid resuscitation of patients with major burns. AJR Am J Roentgenol. 2004;182: 1493–6.
20. Gupta A, Stuhlfaut JW, Fleming KW, Lucey BC, Soto JA. Blunt trauma of the pancreas and biliary tract: a multimodality imaging approach to diagnosis. Radiographics. 2004;24(5):1381–95. https://doi.org/10.1148/rg.245045002. Review.
21. Soto JA, Alvarez O, Munera F, Yepes NL, Sepulveda ME, Perez JM. Traumatic disruption of the pancreatic duct: diagnosis with MR pancreatography. AJR Am J Roentgenol. 2001;176:175–8.
22. Ragozzino A, Manfredi R, Scaglione M, et al. The use of MRCP in detection of pancreatic injuries after blunt trauma. Emerg Radiol. 2003;10:14–8.
23. Kim HS, Lee DK, Kim IW, et al. The role of endoscopic retrograde pancreatography in the treatment of traumatic pancreatic duct injury. Gastrointest Endosc. 2001;54:49–55.
24. Moore EE, Cogbill TH, Malangoni MA, et al. Organ injury scaling. II. Pancreas, duodenum, small bowel, colon, and rectum. J Trauma. 1990;30:1427–9.
25. Subramanian A, Dente CJ, Feliciano DV. The management of pancreatic trauma in the modern era. Surg Clin North Am. 2007;87: 1515–32, x.
26. Wang GF, Li YS, Li JS. Damage control surgery for severe pancreatic trauma. Hepatobiliary Pancreat Dis Int. 2007;6:569–71.
27. Meredith JW, Trunkey DD. CT scanning in acute abdominal injuries. Surg Clin North Am. 1988;68:255–68.

# Imaging of Blunt Splenic Injuries

# 22

Baher R. A. Guirguis, Jennifer F. True, and James T. Lee

## Contents

**Abstract**

This chapter provides a comprehensive review of blunt splenic injury. Beginning with a discussion of the physiologic function of the spleen, historical trends in splenic injury management will then be discussed and then the clinical features of splenic injury.

An in-depth discussion regarding the different types of splenic injury – lacerations, hematomas, and various vascular injuries – and how they are identified on CT, with associated imaging examples, will be presented. CT techniques are reviewed with a discussion of the various phases of contrast, and how different pathologies may be viewed more clearly on certain phases.

A review of the grading and management of the blunt splenic injury is provided. The American Association for the Surgery of Trauma (AAST) organ injury scale of splenic injury is used as a guideline in categorizing various splenic injuries and their subsequent management. A thorough discussion is provided of nonoperative management, surgical management, and selective angiographic embolization, with a brief discussion of potential complications.

Finally, the chapter concludes with a discussion of various pitfalls which a radiologist may encounter with splenic injury imaging, and ways to identify potential splenic injury mimickers.

**Keywords**

Blunt splenic trauma · Blunt splenic injury · AAST splenic injury scale · Splenic vascular injuries · Pseudoaneurysm · AV fistula · Nonoperative management · Selective angiographic embolization

B. R. A. Guirguis · J. F. True · J. T. Lee (✉)
Department of Radiology, University of Kentucky, Lexington, KY, USA
e-mail: b.guirguis@uky.edu; jftrue2@uky.edu; jtlee3@uky.edu

© Springer Nature Switzerland AG 2022
M. N. Patlas et al. (eds.), *Atlas of Emergency Imaging from Head-to-Toe*,
https://doi.org/10.1007/978-3-030-92111-8_22

## Introduction

Though protected by the 9–12th ribs in the left upper quadrant, the spleen is the most commonly injured abdominal organ following blunt trauma – accounting for up to 40% of all abdominal organ injuries [1]. Due to its highly vascular nature (receiving 250–300 mL/min of blood), intraperitoneal location, and relatively thin fibrous capsule, splenic injuries often have a more profound impact on hemodynamic physiology than injury to other abdominal organs (Fig. 1) [2, 3].

Knowledge of the physiologic role of the spleen, and thus subsequent management of splenic injuries, has varied considerably over time. The spleen is composed of red pulp and white pulp. The red pulp is involved in filtering poorly functioning red blood cells and trapping bacteria. White pulp is largely filled with lymphocytes to detect foreign antigens or microorganisms and to help the body in mounting an adequate immune response. The spleen is especially useful in protecting the body against encapsulated bacteria (such as *Streptococcus pneumoniae*, *Neisseria meningitidis*, and *Haemophilus influenzae*) [4].

Even though the spleen is not essential to life, over the past 70 years there has been a significant movement towards spleen-sparing management for blunt traumatic injuries. In the pediatric patient population, for example, close observation and nonoperative management (NOM) have become a standard treatment. Angioembolization is another approach taken with certain types of injury, although the long-term safety and efficacy of this type of management remain under investigation. Finally, despite this more conservative approach, there are cases where aggressive surgical management remains the only life-saving option.

## Historical Context

The function of the spleen has been of interest since ancient Greek times. Plato described the function of the spleen as an organ created "to maintain the liver bright and pure." Other Greek philosophers of that time reinforced this notion by describing the spleen as favoring joviality, a counterbalance to the liver, and even a producer of black bile – one of the four "humors" [5]. What was known, however, was that the spleen was not necessary for life. This helped justify the notion that a diseased or injured spleen was better to be removed.

In more modern times, Dr. Emil Kocher – a pioneering Swiss surgeon and Nobel prize winner – stated "injuries of the spleen demand excision of the gland. No evil effects follow its removal, while the danger of hemorrhage is eventually stopped" [6]. Similarly, William Mayo described how removing the spleen did not produce serious harmful results [5, 7]. Naturally, splenectomies became the standard practice of the time for blunt trauma – up until the 1950s. Interestingly, even though it is now known that asplenic individuals are at increased risk of infection, this pattern was likely not observed due to an overall high incidence of infection in a world without antibiotics [8].

In 1952 King and Schumacker described five cases of fulminant sepsis in asplenic children, arguing that this asplenic state made them more vulnerable to bacterial sepsis [9]. By the 1960s the medical community finally started to have a greater understanding of the function of the spleen – both as an immune and hemofiltration organ. This marked the start of a conservative approach – nonoperative management – to blunt splenic trauma in the modern medical era.

## Epidemiology

Blunt splenic injuries are mostly caused by motor vehicle collisions (MVCs). Other potential etiologies include falls, assaults, and sporting-related injuries. Mortality rates differ depending on the etiology of the splenic trauma – the highest mortality rate is with MVCs compared to other causes [10].

Isolated splenic injuries rarely result in mortality; however, studies have shown that all causes of splenic injury have resulted in mortality rates of up to 10% [11]. Other independent risk factors which have been shown to increase mortality

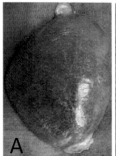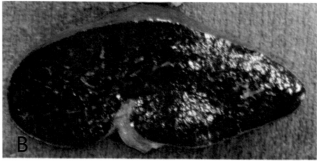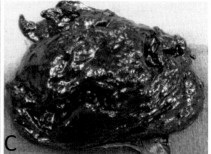

**Fig. 1** Gross pathology picture of the spleen showing (**a**) an intact spleen contained within a thin fibrous capsule; (**b**) cross section showing the thin capsule; (**c**) a different spleen, which has ruptured due to blunt trauma

include concomitant aortic, cardiac, and abdominal injuries and increased age – particularly over 65 [10].

## Clinical Features

For patients involved in MVCs, relevant history, including the location of the patient in the vehicle and the type of impact, are helpful for assessing which patients may be at higher risk for blunt splenic injury. For example, patients in the driver seat in frontal-impact MVCs, and patients in the driver seat or left rear passenger seat in lateral impact MVCs, are at slightly higher risk for splenic injuries. The risk of splenic injury is also increased in unrestrained patients [12].

Surgical and medical history is also important in forming a clinical picture of a critically ill patient. For example, a history of splenectomy will impact management. A history of splenic disease or splenomegaly will also inform a clinician's decision-making. Patients with splenomegaly have a weaker splenic capsule and a less protected and more exposed caudal spleen – due to lack of overlying protective ribs – increasing their risk for splenic injury.

Physical examination can provide useful information when assessing for splenic injury. Localized pain, tenderness, ecchymoses, or abrasions over the left upper quadrant or left chest wall (specifically over left lower ribs) can help quickly identify patients at higher risk of splenic injury [13]. Kehr's sign is also useful in identifying splenic injury. Peritoneal blood following splenic injury is an irritant to the diaphragm. The left hemidiaphragm sensory innervation shares the same cervical roots – C3, C4, C5 – which also innervate the left shoulder. Therefore, on occasion following splenic injury, patients may complain of left shoulder pain.

Of note, the absence of these findings does not exclude splenic injury, and physical examination may be unreliable in patients with altered mental status or other distracting injuries. Finally, there are no sensitive or specific laboratory examinations which are useful in identifying splenic injury. However, it is standard practice to at least obtain a hematocrit and type-and-cross as part of the initial evaluation and resuscitation. A low hematocrit in the setting of the rapid presentation to the hospital following injury, and no prior fluid resuscitation, may point to ongoing hemorrhage.

As is standard, initial evaluation of patients with concern for splenic injury follows the ABCs – airway, breathing, and circulation. When concerned for splenic injury, or after splenic injury has been identified, it is important to assess for other associated injuries including injuries to the gastrointestinal tract, pancreas, and left hemidiaphragm.

## Diagnostic Investigations

### CT Technique

Intravenous contrast-enhanced computed tomography (CECT) is a standard of care for evaluating hemodynamically stable patients who have sustained blunt trauma with suspected intraabdominal injuries. Oral contrast is not needed for the evaluation of blunt splenic trauma [14]. In 2018 the AAST created an imaging criteria column in the splenic trauma grading scale which emulated the CT grading scale initially described and updated by Mirvis et al. [15–17]. The prior version of the AAST grading scaled neglected to account for active bleeding observed by both radiologist and surgeon at imaging and the operating room. The grading system now emphasizes identification of vascular injuries and bleeding on CT, denoting higher-grade injuries as a response to several studies demonstrating that identification of these entities helps select patients for NOM, selective angioembolization (SAE), or splenectomy, and have substantial prognostic and management implications in general [18–21]. Current CT protocols are also tailored to identify these injuries, also resulting from the work by Mirvis and colleagues. Imaging protocol considerations are listed in Table 1. Most major trauma centers currently acquire at least two different time points after the administration of intravenous contrast on CT, if splenic trauma is suspected.

Following IV contrast administration, optimal arterial-phase imaging has complete opacification of the arterial structures in the abdomen, with minimal opacification of the portal venous structures, and no or minimal antegrade contrast in the systemic venous structures. The spleen has a mottled, "tiger stripe" appearance in the arterial phase, which may occasionally mimic (or mask) a splenic laceration (Fig. 2). The portal venous phase allows for maximal homogenous splenic parenchymal enhancement and is ideal to identify lacerations, subcapsular hematomas, and infarcts [22]. A delayed phase may help confirm vascular extravasation [22]. Of note, initial non-enhanced CT of the spleen is not typically performed in the setting of trauma and mainly aids in the detection of splenic calcifications, which would not be expected to alter patient management. Therefore, splenic injury should not be excluded based upon non-enhanced CT (Fig. 3) [22].

### Hemoperitoneum and Splenic Injury

Hemoperitoneum may be the first identified sign of splenic injury [23]. As previously described, hemoperitoneum may accumulate in the hepatorenal fossa, the perisplenic regions, along the paracolic gutters, and in the pelvic cul-de-sac, since these are the most dependent portions of the abdomen and

**Table 1** CT Imaging Protocol

| Imaging protocol considerations | | | Comments |
|---|---|---|---|
| IV access | ≥18G, peripheral | | Central venous and intraosseous access may be used |
| Injection | Volume 100–150 mL, with saline chaser | Rate 2–4 mL/s | Bolus tracking in descending aorta or set time delay after initiation of a contrast bolus |
| Contrast agent | LOCM or IOCM, nonionic | Iodine concentration ≥300 mg/mL | |
| Reconstruction | Axial 1.0–1.5 mm Additional 3–5 mm | Coronal and sagittal 1.5–3 mm at 1.5–2.5 mm intervals | |
| **Phases** | | | |
| Non-enhanced | Not recommended | May aid in the setting of splenic granulomatous disease or calcifications | A virtual non-contrast image may be produced if using DECT |
| Arterial | 25–35 s | Identification of arterial injury, AV fistulas, or arterial pseudoaneurysms | Less parenchymal enhancement, "tiger stripe" spleen |
| Portal venous | 65–120 s | Maximal parenchymal enhancement Venous structures are typically enhanced | Contrast "blush" or extravasation may be arterial or venous |
| Delayed | 3–5 min | Additional time point to help distinguish between non-bleeding and bleeding vascular injuries | "Washed-out" appearance Contrast "blush" or extravasation may be arterial or venous |
| Split-bolus | First bolus inject – No imaging Second bolus imaging in the arterial phase ~25–35 s delay | Decreased radiation exposure Shorter imaging times | Contrast "blush" or extravasation may be arterial or venous May be more susceptible to motion |

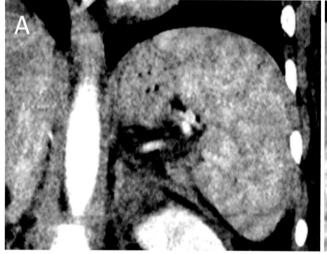 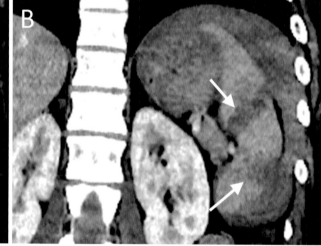

**Fig. 2** Normal "tiger stripe" spleen and splenic lacerations: Coronal CECT examinations show (**a**) a normal "tiger stripe" appearance of the spleen during the arterial phase and (**b**) radially oriented linear regions of the low-attenuation region in the spleen compatible with splenic laceration in a different patient. Care should be made to not mistaken the normal "tiger stripe" appearance with splenic lacerations

pelvis. Splenic hemorrhage more specifically – flowing in a caudal direction in an upright patient – first appears in the perisplenic spaces, and then the left paracolic gutter, before finally reaching the pelvis [24].

CT helps delineate between fluid and blood based on attenuation, making it a highly useful tool for characterizing free intraperitoneal fluid. Blood has a higher attenuation (>25 HU) compared to simple fluid (≤10 HU). Furthermore, the value of the attenuation of blood can also help distinguish between old (clotted) and new (unclotted) blood [24]. The volume of hemoperitoneum – among other clinical factors in the setting of splenic trauma – helps guide patient management. Large volume hemoperitoneum has been implicated in the failure of nonoperative management [19, 25].

When the source of hemoperitoneum is not clearly established, the sentinel clot sign can be used as both as

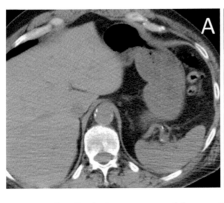
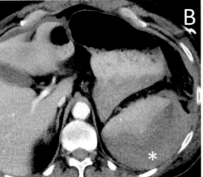
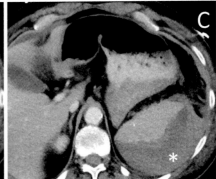

**Fig. 3** Delayed splenic rupture – axial non-enhanced CT image (**a**) following MVC demonstrated no abnormality. Subsequent axial CECT images in the PVP (**b**) and delayed (**c**) phases 1 week later demonstrate

interval development of a large subcapsular hematoma (*). Non-enhanced CT should not be utilized to exclude splenic injury

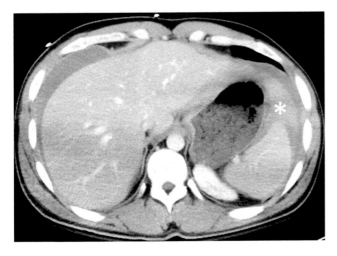

**Fig. 4** Sentinel clot sign – axial CECT image with relatively high attenuation fluid (*) adjacent to the spleen which was injured (not shown). Hemoperitoneum around the liver is also present

sensitive and specific finding on CT. A sentinel clot likely represents a combination of the body's attempt at hemostasis close to the site of an injury with clotted blood attenuating around 45–70 HU and contribution from intravenous contrast into the site of hemorrhage. Therefore, when the hyperattenuating clot is adjacent to the spleen, the splenic injury should be suspected and requires careful examination of the spleen (Fig. 4). Orwig et al. analogized the sentinel clot sign as a diagnostic marker to visceral injury, the way the fat pad sign is a diagnostic marker of elbow trauma on radiographs [23, 24, 26].

It is important to note that there are several variables that may result in different attenuation ranges of hemoperitoneum. First, the concentration of hemoglobin may render blood to appear hyperdense – for example, a diffuse hyperdense appearance of vessels in polycythemia vera, or an isodense/hypodense appearance in the setting of anemia. If patients are anemic, hemoperitoneum may be less than 25 HU. Additionally, current CT radiation dose

modulation techniques may impact the traditional HU cutoff values for the diagnosis of hemoperitoneum, as changing kV alters soft-tissue attenuation [27].

## CT Patterns of Splenic Injury

Following abdominal trauma, CT with intravenous contrast of the abdomen is routinely used as the test of choice to the diagnosis and characterize blunt splenic injury. Injury patterns of blunt splenic trauma include areas of active bleeding, lacerations, hematomas, vascular injuries, and devascularized areas of the spleen, as are described below.

*Splenic lacerations* are linear, low attenuating defects with irregular margins that often extend to the capsular surface. They may be oriented in any direction; however, radially oriented lacerations may have a lower risk for bleeding when compared to those oriented perpendicular to the trabecular vessels of the spleen [28]. Lacerations at times will fill with blood and typically become rounded areas of low attenuation representing an intraparenchymal hematoma with better-defined margins compared to simply lacerations (Fig. 5). It is important not to confuse a splenic parenchymal injury with the normal mottled appearance of the spleen in the arterial phase, which has been referred to as a "tiger stripe" appearance (Fig. 2). Of note, lacerations, intraparenchymal hematomas, and contusion represent an imaging spectrum of parenchymal disruption and may share many CT features. When multiple severe lacerations intersect and result in the complete separation of splenic components, the term "fractured" or "shattered" spleen is often used (Fig. 6) [22, 29, 30].

*Subcapsular hematomas* appear as peripheral, relative low-attenuating, crescent-shaped collections between the enhancing parenchyma of the spleen and the splenic capsule (typically not visible) and that may flatten or deform the adjacent splenic parenchyma (Fig. 7). This mass effect on the spleen may help distinguish subcapsular hematomas from free intraperitoneal blood in the perisplenic spaces. Again, on many occasions, a subcapsular hematoma and free intraperitoneal blood co-exist, and thus are not mutually exclusive.

*Splenic vascular injuries* encompass a large group of injuries that typically diagnosed by CECT or angiography. Being able to identify the location of a hemorrhage associated with the spleen, its acuity, and the suspected type of injury, allows for the identification of cases which require more aggressive surgical or endovascular intervention and thus allow for better and clearer communication to improve management [23, 24, 26]. The term contrast "blush" found throughout the surgical literature is broadly utilized as a CT finding but is a term which has been poorly defined. "Blush" has been applied to active subcapsular or intraperitoneal

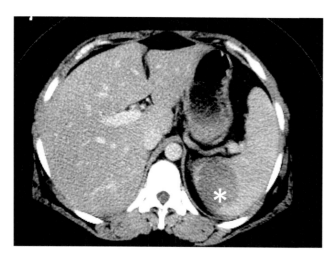

**Fig. 5** Intraparenchymal hematoma – axial CECT image demonstrating a round, low-attenuation nonlinear splenic intraparenchymal hematoma (*)

contrast extravasation, pseudoaneurysm formation, and traumatic AV fistulae. As imaging protocols improve, so does the precision in describing specific splenic vascular injuries, therefore, the preferred term of AACE, active arterial contrast extravasation. Rarely does active venous contrast extravasation occur.

*Active extravasation* is defined as contrast that is actively escaping from injured vasculature. As opposed to free or clotted blood which attenuates between 40 and 90 HU (due to high hemoglobin protein content), active extravasation is highly attenuating ranging from 85 to 350 HU, though usually greater that 100 HU [23, 24, 26]. It has a classic jet-like appearance (Fig. 8) on initial arterial or early PVP imaging and appears as a focal area which increases in size and changes in morphology on subsequent phases of imaging [26, 31].

Similarly, contained vascular foci, i.e., pseudoaneurysms and AV fistulas, appear as well-circumscribed focal areas of extravascular hyperattenuation. The size of these injuries remains similar on different phases of imaging with CT, although the attenuation will typically closely follow that of the blood pool (Fig. 9). Although it is difficult to distinguish between pseudoaneurysms and AV fistulae on CT, they are due to two different processes. Pseudoaneurysms result when the arterial wall is injured, and AV fistulas result when both an artery and adjacent vein are injured, and early filling of splenic veins are observed at conventional as well as CT angiography/arterial phase images. Both have been implicated in delayed splenic hemorrhage [32, 33]. When diagnosing splenic vascular injuries on CT, it is important to remember that these are snapshots in time. For example, contained vascular injuries may subsequently rupture and later cause active contrast extravasation. Conversely, active contrast extravasation can partially thrombose and later become a contained vascular injury.

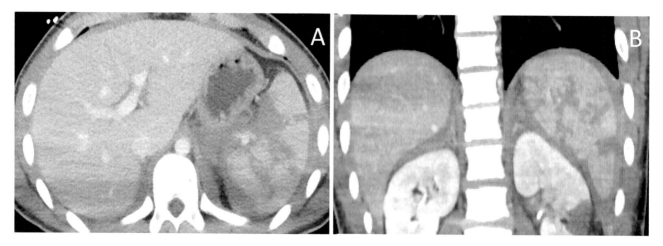

**Fig. 6** Fractured or shattered spleen – axial and coronal CECT images in the PVP shows multiple lacerations completely separating portions of the spleen indicative of a severely fractured or shattered spleen, AAST grade V. Associated perisplenic and perihepatic hemorrhagic fluid is also present

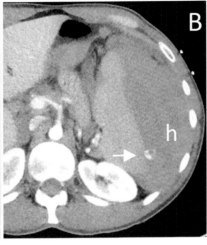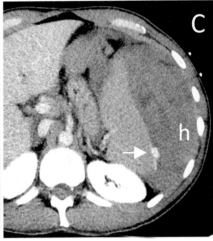

**Fig. 7** Subcapsular hematoma: axial CECT images in the arterial (**a**), PVP (**b**), and delayed (**c**) phases demonstrating a large subcapsular hematoma (h) deforming the contour of the spleen. A subcapsular vascular injury is present along the dorsolateral margin (arrows) and given the presence on arterial phase imaging, active arterial contrast extravasation (AACE) can be diagnosed

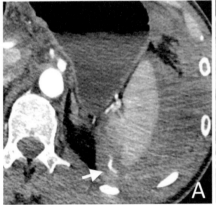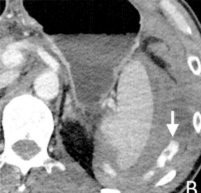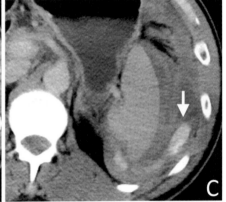

**Fig. 8** Active contrast extravasation – axial CECT images in the arterial (**a**), PVP (**b**), and delayed (**c**) phases demonstrate a jet-like area of high-attenuation contrast extravasating into the peritoneal cavity, changing in attenuation and morphology during arterial, PVP, and delayed phases (arrows). Notice that extravasated contrast remains slightly hyper-attenuating compared to the blood pool

*Splenic infarction* may result from vascular injury and typically appears as a low attenuation wedge-shaped area with the larger portion of the wedge extending away from the splenic hilum (Fig. 10).

*Splenic pedicle injuries* – though very rare – may be fatal complications of blunt splenic injury. They most often occur following severe deceleration injuries and include both intimal dissection of the splenic artery, or avulsion where the spleen gets torn off from its pedicle and may be complete or partial (Fig. 11). The hallmark feature on imaging of this type of injury is poor to no enhancement of the entire spleen or affected portions in the portal venous phase, with or without active intraperitoneal extravasation of contrast. A diagnostic dilemma may arise as the superior pole may maintain some parenchymal enhancement due to collateral circulation from the short gastric arteries [31].

## Grading and Management

A large part of the grading and management of splenic injuries is guided by the Organ Injury Scaling Committee of the American Association for the Surgery of Trauma Association (AAST). The spleen organ injury scale, which provides a grade of injury from grade I to V, was substantially revised in 2018. Firstly, it provided a new column of CT criteria to determine the grade of injury based on these findings (Table 2) [15]. This is in addition to both operative and pathologic grading of injury. Additionally, a significant update was the addition of vascular injury (pseudo-aneurysm, AV fistula) and active bleeding to the organ injury scale. Of note, if more than one grade of injury is present, the highest grade detected should be assigned. If multiple grade I or II injuries are present, grading should be advanced by an additional grade up, to grade III.

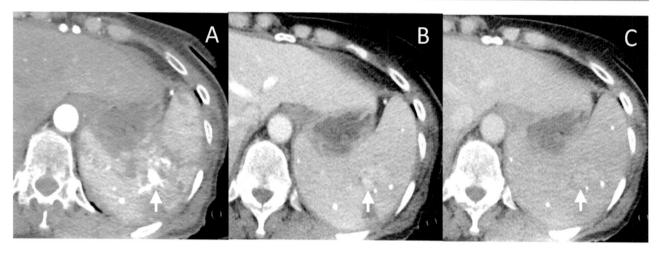

**Fig. 9** Contained Vascular Injury - Axial CECT images in the arterial (**a**), PVP (**b**), and delayed (**c**) phases demonstrate a "blush" that maintains a similar morphology and follows the attenuation of blood pool, and may represent a pseudoaneurysm or arteriovenous fistula (arrows). Splenic granulomas are also present, and do not change in attenuation or morphology

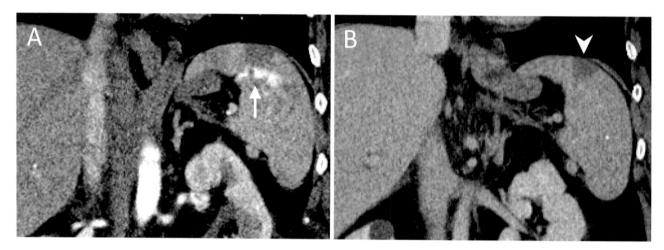

**Fig. 10** Infarct – coronal CECT images in the arterial (**a**) and PVP (**b**) demonstrates a contained vascular injury (arrow) with an associated wedged-shaped region of decreased attenuation extending away from the hilum to the capsule compatible with an infarct (arrowhead)

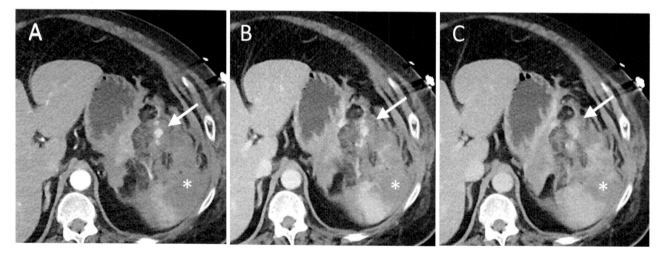

**Fig. 11** Splenic pedicle injury – axial CECT images in the arterial (**a**), PVP (**b**), and delayed (**c**) phases demonstrating an injury to the ventral splenic vascular pedicle with active contrast extravasation (arrows) and with associated devascularization of the ventral spleen (*)

**Table 2** AASST spleen organ injury scale – 2018 revision. (Adapted from Kozar et al. [15])

| AAST grade | Imaging criteria | Operative criteria | Pathologic criteria |
|---|---|---|---|
| I | Subcapsular hematoma <10% surface area<br>Parenchymal laceration <1 cm depth<br>Capsular tear | Subcapsular hematoma <10% surface area<br>Parenchymal laceration <1 cm depth<br>Capsular tear | Subcapsular hematoma <10% surface area<br>Parenchymal laceration <1 cm depth<br>Capsular tear |
| II | Subcapsular hematoma 10–50% surface area;<br>intraparenchymal hematoma <5 cm<br>Parenchymal laceration 1–3 cm | Subcapsular hematoma 10–50% surface area; intraparenchymal hematoma <5 cm<br>Parenchymal laceration 1–3 cm | Subcapsular hematoma 10–50% surface area; intraparenchymal hematoma <5 cm<br>Parenchymal laceration 1–3 cm |
| III | Subcapsular hematoma >50% surface area;<br>ruptured subcapsular or intraparenchymal<br>hematoma ≥5 cm<br>Parenchymal laceration >3 cm depth | Subcapsular hematoma >50% surface area or expanding; ruptured subcapsular or intraparenchymal hematoma ≥5 cm<br>Parenchymal laceration >3 cm depth | Subcapsular hematoma >50% surface area; ruptured subcapsular or intra-parenchymal hematoma ≥5 cm<br>Parenchymal laceration >3 cm depth |
| IV | Any injury in the presence of a splenic vascular injury or active bleeding confined within a splenic capsule<br>Parenchymal laceration involving segmental or hilar vessels producing >25% devascularization | Parenchymal laceration involving segmental or hilar vessels producing >25% devascularization | Parenchymal laceration involving segmental or hilar vessels producing >25% devascularization |
| V | Any injury in the presence of splenic vascular injury with active bleeding extending beyond the spleen into the peritoneum<br>Shattered spleen | Hilar vascular injury which devascularizes the spleen<br>Shattered spleen | Hilar vascular injury which devascularizes the spleen<br>Shattered spleen |

Vascular injury is defined as a pseudoaneurysm or arteriovenous fistula and appears as a focal collection of vascular contrast that decreases in attenuation with delayed imaging. Active bleeding from a vascular injury presents as vascular contrast, focal or diffuse, that increases in size or attenuation in a delayed phase. Vascular thrombosis can lead to organ infarction
Grade based on the highest grade assessment made on imaging, at operation or on pathologic specimen
More than one grade of splenic injury may be present, and should be classified by the higher grade of injury
Advance one grade for multiple injuries, up to a grade III

Management of splenic injury is driven by grade of injury and patient hemodynamics. Blunt splenic traumas are typically managed in one of three ways – nonoperative management, surgical intervention, and selective angiographic embolization (SAE). Most cases of splenic injury currently undergo NOM with low rates of failure, defined as the need for surgical intervention after initial decision towards NOM or SAE [18]. Of note, patients with other injuries requiring operation in the abdomen – mesenteric or bowel injury – may also undergo concurrent operative management of splenic injury.

As previously discussed, there was a turning point in the management of splenic injuries upon the discovery of the immune function of the spleen and the risk of overwhelming post-splenectomy infection (OPSI). In the late 1960s, pediatric surgeons pioneered the concept of NOM for splenic injury in hemodynamically stable children, and this success later served as a guide for adult management [34]. NOM is now the standard of care in most cases of splenic injury.

Grade I (Fig. 12) and II (Fig. 13) injuries include subcapsular hematomas up to 50% of the surface area, parenchymal lacerations up to 3 cm, intraparenchymal hematoma less than 5 cm, and capsular tear, and are specifically outlined in Table 2 [15]. Grade I and II isolated injuries are typically managed nonoperatively.

Grade III (Fig. 14) injuries include subcapsular hematomas which are greater than 50% of the surface area, parenchymal lacerations greater than 3 cm, intraparenchymal hematoma greater than 5 cm, and a ruptured subcapsular hematoma [15]. Furthermore, if there are multiple lower grade injuries, advancing the grade up to but not beyond grade III may be performed (Fig. 15). Depending on patient presentation, other risk factors, and hemodynamic stability, these injuries may be managed nonoperatively, with SAE or with surgery.

Grade IV (Fig. 16) and V (Fig. 17) injuries are often lumped together as "high-grade" and include parenchymal lacerations resulting in greater than 25% devascularization, shattered spleen, evidence of active bleeding confined within the splenic capsule or extending beyond into the peritoneum [15]. Many of these injuries are managed surgically; however, many studies have shown SAE with NOM to be effective alternative to surgery [35–37].

Previously, indications that precluded NOM included grade of injury on CT per AAST guidelines, large volume hemoperitoneum, contrast blush, neurologic status/GCS, age greater than 55, and the presence of other associated injuries. More recent studies, however, have found that these factors do not necessitate surgical intervention, and that a trial of NOM with or without SAE may be attempted [35–37].

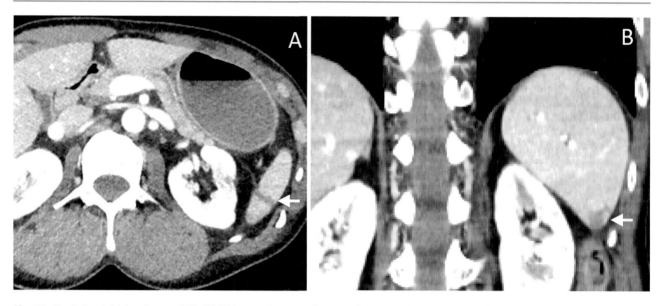

**Fig. 12** Grade I: axial (**a**) and coronal (**b**) CECT images demonstrating a small (<1 cm) laceration at the inferior margin of the spleen (arrows)

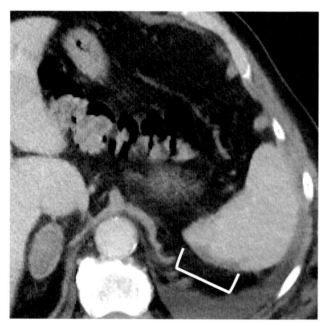

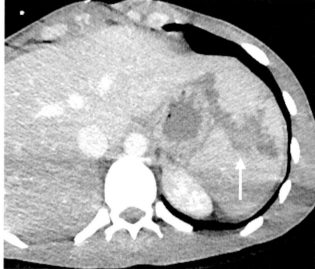

**Fig. 14** Grade III – axial CECT image shows a >3 cm laceration of the spleen (arrow) without associated vascular injury

**Fig. 13** Grade II: Axial CECT image in the PVP phase demonstrates a thin subcapsular hematoma involving between 10% and 50% surface area along the posterior aspect of the spleen (bracket). A small amount of perisplenic hemorrhage (arrowhead), left pleural effusion (*) and right adrenal hematoma (arrow)

Failure of NOM typically results in continued hemorrhage with continuing transfusion requirements or resulting shock and need for surgical intervention with splenectomy [35]. The risk factors for NOM failure include AAST grade of injury, extent of hemoperitoneum, and presence of an AV fistula [38–40]. As a result, grades I–III with no other contraindications are usually given a trial of NOM, whereas grades IV–V are usually more aggressively managed.

There is a growing amount of evidence about the usefulness of angioembolization as an adjunct to NOM. When used as an adjunct, studies have shown that the failure rate has decreased in patients with AAST high-grade injuries, contrast "blush" (active extravasation, pseudoaneurysms), hemoperitoneum, and risk for delayed hemorrhage (Fig. 18) [41–44].

There are absolute contraindications to NOM. Most importantly, patients with diffuse peritonitis or hemodynamic

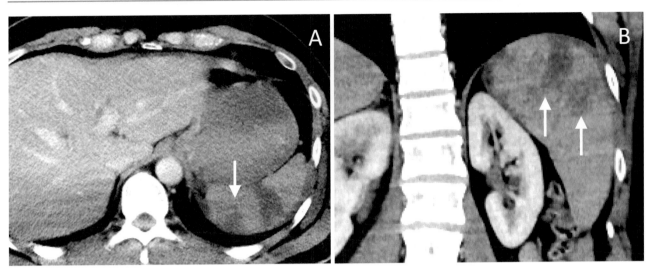

**Fig. 15** Grade III – axial (**a**) and coronal (**b**) CECT images demonstrate two grade II lacerations in one patient (arrows), which now is upgraded to an AAST grade III injury

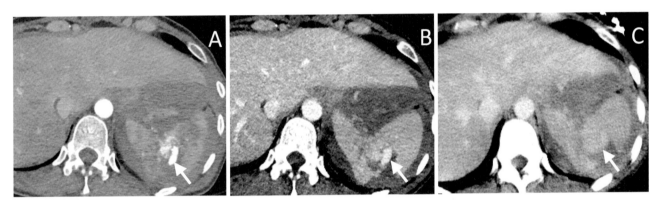

**Fig. 16** Grade IV – axial CECT images in the arterial (**a**), PVP (**b**), and delayed (**c**) phases demonstrate a splenic vascular injury (arrows) without evidence of extracapsular hemorrhage

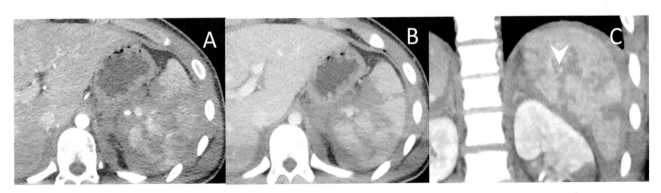

**Fig. 17** Grade V – axial arterial (**a**), axial (**b**), and coronal (**c**) PVP CECT images demonstrate a "shattered" spleen with small splenic vascular injury (arrowhead) within the lacerations

instability not responsive to fluid resuscitation following abdominal trauma are managed operatively [34, 43]. Furthermore, NOM should only be considered in an appropriate setting – a facility that allows for close monitoring, frequent clinical exams, and operating room availability in case emergent intervention is needed.

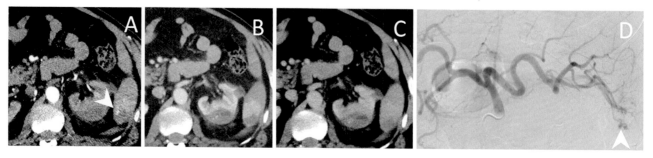

**Fig. 18** Treatment with SAE – axial CECT images in the arterial (**a**), PVP (**b**), and delayed (**c**) phases demonstrate a small non-bleeding splenic vascular injury (arrowhead) at the inferior pole of the spleen, successfully treated by selective splenic artery embolization (**d**)

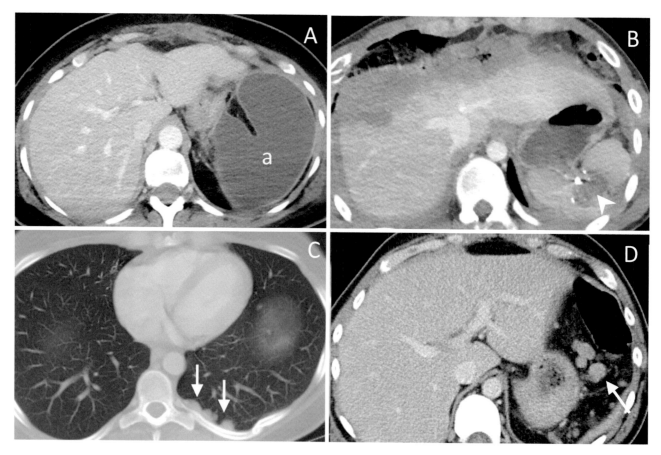

**Fig. 19** Complications – axial CECT images illustrating complications from treatment of blunt splenic trauma. (**a**) Rim-enhancing fluid collection in the splenectomy bed compatible with abscess (a). (**b**) The cystic region in the spleen with the metallic artifact in the hilum compatible pseudocyst (arrowhead) from remote SAE, misdiagnosed as bullet fragments and laceration in the setting of current GSW. (**c** and **d**) Two different patients with remote splenectomy with splenosis in the pleural space and splenectomy bed (arrows), respectively

## Complications

Although splenic trauma has a relatively low mortality rate, recognizing potential complications is important [19]. Delayed splenic rupture describes a clinical scenario in which a patient is managed with NOM for blunt splenic trauma and days to weeks later develops spontaneous hemorrhage from his or her original injury (Fig. 3). The risk for delayed splenic rupture is associated with higher AAST grade and the volume of hemoperitoneum at the time of CT

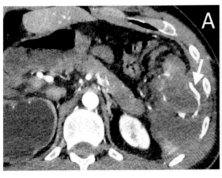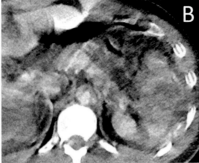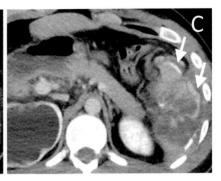

**Fig. 20** Motion artifact – axial CECT in the arterial (**a**), PVP (**b**), and delayed (**c**) phases demonstrates an AAST grade V injury with active bleeding beyond the spleen (arrows) and severe motion artifact making the PVP nondiagnostic (**b**). Multiphasic imaging may help mitigate motion artifact commonly encountered in trauma patients

at presentation. Many point to undiagnosed splenic vascular injuries as the possible etiology [45]. Complications associated with treatment may arise during or after the initial post-procedural or postoperative period. Major complications from SAE include recurrent bleeding, splenic infarction, splenic abscess, and contrast-induced nephropathy [46]. Complications associated with operative management include abscess formation and overwhelming post-splenectomy infection (OPSI). Remote complications from NOM, SAE, and operative management of blunt splenic trauma include pseudocyst formation, OPSI, and splenosis. Current guidelines recommend immediate vaccination for all patients undergoing splenectomy and selective vaccination for those undergoing SAE or splenic salvage surgery (Fig. 19) [19].

## Potential Pitfalls

It is important to avoid common pitfalls in evaluating possible splenic injury on CT; broadly they are artifacts, anatomic variations, and intrinsic abnormalities of the spleen.

Artifacts can degrade image quality – and in worst-case scenarios may render CT nondiagnostic (Fig. 20). Respiratory motion artifacts are common with both the liver and spleen on CT. This artifact appears as a halo that runs parallel to the splenic capsule and should not be confused for a subcapsular hematoma. As previously discussed, the latter is typically distinguishable by the mass effect on the splenic parenchyma [47]. Multiphasic CT protocols may help mitigate respiratory motion artifact. Metallic or beam hardening artifacts are commonly encountered while imaging poly-trauma patients, as arm positioning or overlying life-support artifacts are difficult to completely account for in emergent situations.

Anatomic variations to be aware of include splenic lobules and clefts, and the "sliver of liver" sign. Lobules represent splenic tissues that have persisted from fetal splenic development into adult life. They are frequently seen along the medial aspect of the spleen and may result in contour abnormalities. Clefts, on the other hand, represent the grooves that separated the lobules during fetal splenic development. If they persist into adulthood, they typically have sharp borders and can extend as deep as 2–3 cm into the splenic parenchyma. Although difficult to distinguish from a laceration in the setting of perisplenic hemoperitoneum, clefts will often have smooth, curved margins, and lack adjacent blood [22, 31]. Another anatomic variation, termed the "sliver of liver," is when the left hepatic lobe demonstrates profound extension into the left upper quadrant draping over the spleen. In the setting of trauma, this extended left hepatic lobe may appear as a crescent-shaped mass or complex collection adjacent to or in the spleen, potentially mimicking perisplenic or subcapsular hematoma (Fig. 21) [48, 49]. Diffuse hypoenhancement of the spleen in hypoperfusion complex is a physiologic variation that may be misinterpreted as a splenic pedicle or devascularization injury (Fig. 22).

Intrinsic abnormalities of the patient's spleen can also be a source of diagnostic difficulty. Splenic hamartomas, hemangiomas, and cysts are relatively common and at times can mimic injuries. Furthermore, calcifications within the spleen can make the identification of splenic vascular injuries somewhat difficult (Fig. 23).

## Conclusion

Blunt splenic trauma accounts for approximately a fourth of all intra-abdominal injuries. IV contrast-enhanced computed tomography and radiologists play vital roles in the

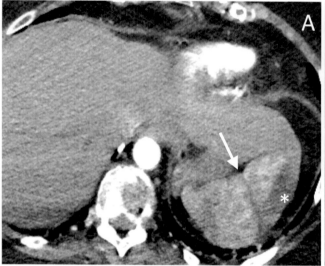
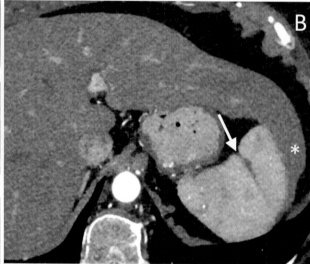

**Fig. 21** Cleft and sliver of liver – axial CECT image (**a**) shows a well-defined linear low attenuation region at the upper pole of the spleen (arrow) with heterogenous low attenuation region (*) along the lateral aspect of the spleen, initially interpreted as an AAST grade II injury; (**b**) however, comparison with a CT examination perform a year prior for preoperative planning for cardiac valvular replacement shows a well-defined splenic cleft (arrow) and a prominent left lobe of the liver (*)

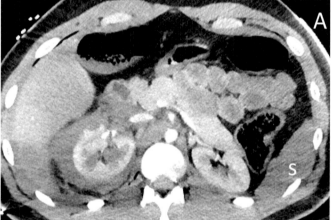
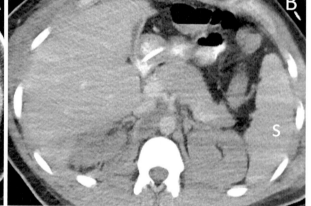

**Fig. 22** Hypoperfusion complex – axial CECT image (**a**) shows diffuse low hypoenhancement of the spleen (s) in the setting of hepatic and right renal injuries and profound hypotension. One week later, axial CECT image (**b**) shows that the spleen (s) enhances normally and is large. The splenic findings on the initial CT (**a**) are compatible with hypoperfusion complex and should not be confused with splenic pedicle injury

evaluation and management of hemodynamically stable patients with splenic trauma. Optimizing imaging protocols, recognizing injury types and patterns, and understanding treatment options and associated complications are vital to caring for these patients. Moreover, the Organ Injury Scaling Committee of the American Association for the Surgery in Trauma recently added a column for computed tomography findings in the most recent update, emphasizing the importance of imaging. Identification of splenic vascular injuries and active bleeding is important as the trend towards a nonoperative management and nonoperative management with selective angioembolization continues to grow.

- Multiphasic IV contrast-enhanced computed tomography plays a vital role in diagnosis, grading, and treatment of patients with suspected splenic trauma
- Identification of splenic vascular injuries with or without active bleeding identifies patients with high-grade injuries
- Management for blunt splenic trauma continues to shift towards a nonoperative management with or without selective splenic artery embolization

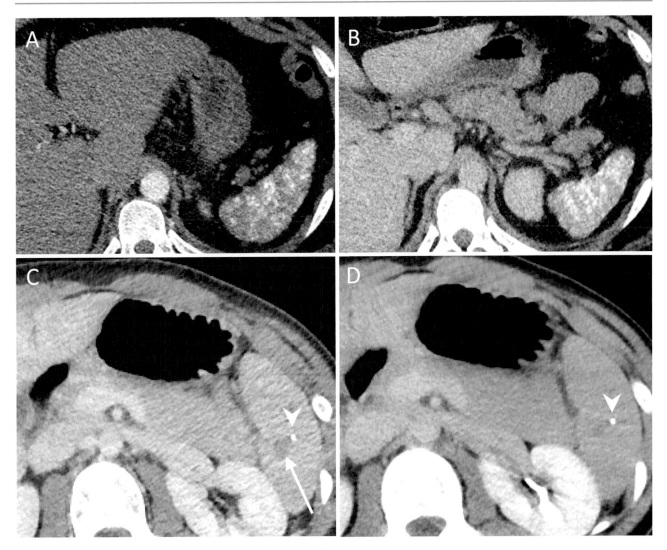

**Fig. 23** Calcifications – axial dual-phase CECT images from two patients. The top row (**a** and **b**) demonstrates splenic calcifications associated with sickle cell anemia, making the diagnosis of splenic vascular injuries extremely challenging. The bottom row (**c** and **d**) shows an AAST grade I splenic hematoma (arrow) with adjacent calcification (arrowhead) mimicking a contained vascular injury

## References

1. Novelline RA, Rhea JT, Bell T. Helical CT of abdominal trauma. Radiol Clin N Am. 1999;37(3):591–612.
2. Brunicardi FC, Andersen DK, Billiar TR, Dunn DL, Hunter JG, Matthews JB, et al. Schwartz's principles of surgery. 10th ed. - New York: McGraw-Hill Education LLC; 2015.
3. Standring S, Adams MA. Gray's anatomy: the anatomical basis of clinical practice. 41st ed. St. Louis: Elsevier; 2016.
4. Petroianu A. Hemostasis of the liver, spleen, and bone achieved by electrocautery greased with lidocaine gel. Surg Today. 2011;41(2):300–2.
5. Dionigi R, Boni L, Rausei S, Rovera F, Dionigi G. History of splenectomy. Int J Surg. 2013;11(1):S42–S3.
6. Kocher T. Text-book of operative surgery. London: Black; 1903/1911.
7. Mayo WJ. Principles underlying surgery of the spleen: with a report of ten splenectomies. JAMA. 1910;LIV(1):14–8.
8. Skattum J, Naess PA, Gaarder C. Non-operative management and immune function after splenic injury. Br J Surg. 2012;99:59–65.
9. King H, Shumacker HB Jr. Splenic studies. I. Susceptibility to infection after splenectomy performed in infancy. Ann Surg. 1952;136(2):239–42.
10. Brady RR, Bandari M, Kerssens JJ, Paterson-Brown S, Parks RW. Splenic trauma in Scotland: demographics and outcomes. World J Surg. 2007;31(11):2111–6.
11. Cadeddu M, Garnett A, Al-Anezi K, Farrokhyar F. Management of spleen injuries in the adult trauma population: a ten-year experience. Can J Surg. 2006;49(6):386–90.
12. Feliciano DV, Mattox KL, Moore EE. Trauma. 8th ed. New York: McGraw-Hill Medical; 2012.
13. Holmes JF, Ngyuen H, Jacoby RC, McGahan JP, Bozorgchami H, Wisner DH. Do all patients with left costal margin injuries require radiographic evaluation for intraabdominal injury? Ann Emerg Med. 2005;46(3):232–6.

14. Stuhlfaut JW, Soto JA, Lucey BC, Ulrich A, Rathlev NK, Burke PA, et al. Blunt abdominal trauma: performance of CT without oral contrast material. Radiology. 2004;233(3):689–94.

15. Kozar RA, Crandall M, Shanmuganathan K, Zarzaur BL, Coburn M, Cribari C, et al. Organ injury scaling 2018 update: spleen, liver, and kidney. J Trauma Acute Care Surg. 2018;85(6):1119–22.

16. Mirvis SE, Whitley NO, Gens DR. Blunt splenic trauma in adults: CT-based classification and correlation with prognosis and treatment. Radiology. 1989;171(1):33–9.

17. Saksobhavivat N, Shanmuganathan K, Chen HH, DuBose JJ, Richard H, Khan MA, et al. Blunt splenic injury: use of a multidetector CT-based splenic injury grading system and clinical parameters for triage of patients at admission. Radiology. 2015;274(3): 702–11.

18. Raza M, Abbas Y, Devi V, Prasad KV, Rizk KN, Nair PP. Non operative management of abdominal trauma – a 10 years review. World J Emerg Surg. 2013;8:14.

19. El-Matbouly M, Jabbour G, El-Menyar A, Peralta R, Abdelrahman H, Zarour A, et al. Blunt splenic trauma: assessment, management and outcomes. Surgeon. 2016;14(1):52–8.

20. Zarzaur BL, Dunn JA, Leininger B, Lauerman M, Shanmuganathan K, Kaups K, et al. Natural history of splenic vascular abnormalities after blunt injury: a Western Trauma Association multicenter trial. J Trauma Acute Care Surg. 2017;83(6):999–1005.

21. Margari S, Garozzo Velloni F, Tonolini M, Colombo E, Artioli D, Allievi NE, et al. Emergency CT for assessment and management of blunt traumatic splenic injuries at a Level 1 Trauma Center: 13-year study. Emerg Radiol. 2018;25(5):489–97.

22. Vancauwenberghe T, Snoeckx A, Vanbeckevoort D, Dymarkowski S, Vanhoenacker FM. Imaging of the spleen: what the clinician needs to know. Singap Med J. 2015;56(3):133–44.

23. Orwig D, Federle MP. Localized clotted blood as evidence of visceral trauma on CT: the sentinel clot sign. AJR Am J Roentgenol. 1989;153(4):747–9.

24. Lubner M, Menias C, Rucker C, Bhalla S, Peterson CM, Wang L, et al. Blood in the belly: CT findings of hemoperitoneum. Radiographics. 2007;27(1):109–25.

25. Coccolini F, Montori G, Catena F, Kluger Y, Biffl W, Moore EE, et al. Splenic trauma: WSES classification and guidelines for adult and pediatric patients. World J Emerg Surg. 2017;12:40.

26. Hamilton JD, Kumaravel M, Censullo ML, Cohen AM, Kievlan DS, West OC. Multidetector CT evaluation of active extravasation in blunt abdominal and pelvic trauma patients. Radiographics. 2008;28(6):1603–16.

27. Hickman D, Zhang J, McQuerry K, Lee J. Should radiologists care about kV? Phantom and clinical study of effects of kV on hemoperitoneum HU in the setting of splenic injuries. Emerg Radiol. 2020;27(2):135–40.

28. Rosenfeld JC. In: Mattox KL, Feliciano DV, Moore EE, editors. Trauma. 4th ed. New York: McGraw-Hill; 2000. p. 1514. 2001, p. 454.

29. Hassan R, Abd Aziz A, Md Ralib AR, Saat A. Computed tomography of blunt spleen injury: a pictorial review. Malays J Med Sci. 2011;18(1):60–7.

30. Herring W. Learning radiology: recognizing the basics. 4th ed. Philadephia: Elsevier; 2019.

31. Pope TL, Harris JH. Harris & Harris' radiology of emergency medicine. 5th ed. Philadelphia: Wolters Kluwer Health/Lippincott Williams & Wilkins; 2013.

32. Clark T, Cardoza S, Kanth N. Splenic trauma: pictorial review of contrast-enhanced CT findings. Emerg Radiol. 2011;18(3):227–34.

33. Saba L, Anzidei M, Lucatelli P, Mallarini G. The multidetector computed tomography angiography (MDCTA) in the diagnosis of splenic artery aneurysm and pseudoaneurysm. Acta Radiol. 2011;52(5):488–98.

34. Stein DM, Scalea TM. Nonoperative management of spleen and liver injuries. J Intensive Care Med. 2006;21(5):296–304.

35. Nix JA, Costanza M, Daley BJ, Powell MA, Enderson BL. Outcome of the current management of splenic injuries. J Trauma. 2001;50(5): 835–42.

36. Haan JM, Biffl W, Knudson MM, Davis KA, Oka T, Majercik S, et al. Splenic embolization revisited: a multicenter review. J Trauma. 2004;56(3):542–7.

37. Myers JG, Dent DL, Stewart RM, Gray GA, Smith DS, Rhodes JE, et al. Blunt splenic injuries: dedicated trauma surgeons can achieve a high rate of nonoperative success in patients of all ages. J Trauma. 2000;48(5):801–5. Discussion 805–6.

38. Haan JM, Bochicchio GV, Kramer N, Scalea TM. Nonoperative management of blunt splenic injury: a 5-year experience. J Trauma. 2005;58(3):492–8.

39. Peitzman AB, Heil B, Rivera L, Federle MB, Harbrecht BG, Clancy KD, et al. Blunt splenic injury in adults: Multi-institutional Study of the Eastern Association for the Surgery of Trauma. J Trauma. 2000;49(2):177–87. Discussion 187–9.

40. Sharma OP, Oswanski MF, Singer D, Raj SS, Daoud YA. Assessment of nonoperative management of blunt spleen and liver trauma. Am Surg. 2005;71(5):379–86.

41. Shanmuganathan K, Mirvis SE, Boyd-Kranis R, Takada T, Scalea TM. Nonsurgical management of blunt splenic injury: use of CT criteria to select patients for splenic arteriography and potential endovascular therapy. Radiology. 2000;217(1):75–82.

42. Dent D, Alsabrook G, Erickson BA, Myers J, Wholey M, Stewart R, et al. Blunt splenic injuries: high nonoperative management rate can be achieved with selective embolization. J Trauma. 2004;56(5):1063–7.

43. Stassen NA, Bhullar I, Cheng JD, Crandall ML, Friese RS, Guillamondegui OD, et al. Selective nonoperative management of blunt splenic injury: an Eastern Association for the Surgery of Trauma practice management guideline. J Trauma. 2012;73(5): S294–300.

44. Liu PP, Lee WC, Cheng YF, Hsieh PM, Hsieh YM, Tan BL, et al. Use of splenic artery embolization as an adjunct to nonsurgical management of blunt splenic injury. J Trauma. 2004;56(4):768–72. Discussion 73.

45. Furlan A, Tublin ME, Rees MA, Nicholas DH, Sperry JL, Alarcon LH. Delayed splenic vascular injury after nonoperative management of blunt splenic trauma. J Surg Res. 2017;211:87–94.

46. Ekeh AP, Khalaf S, Ilyas S, Kauffman S, Walusimbi M, McCarthy MC. Complications arising from splenic artery embolization: a review of an 11-year experience. Am J Surg. 2013;205(3):250–4. Discussion 4.

47. Barrett JF, Keat N. Artifacts in CT: recognition and avoidance. Radiographics. 2004;24(6):1679–91.

48. Cholankeril JV, Zamora BO, Ketyer S. Left lobe of the liver draping around the spleen: a pitfall in computed tomography diagnosis of perisplenic hematoma. J Comput Tomogr. 1984;8(3):261–7.

49. Jones R, Tabbut M, Gramer D. Elongated left lobe of the liver mimicking a subcapsular hematoma of the spleen on the focused assessment with sonography for trauma exam. Am J Emerg Med. 2014;32(7):814.e3–4.

Raffaella Basilico, Andrea Delli Pizzi, Alessio Taraschi, Barbara Seccia, and Roberta Cianci

## Contents

### Abstract

Bowel and mesenteric injuries due to blunt trauma are relatively uncommon; however, a prompt detection of such lesions is vital in order to decrease the mortality and morbidity due to a delayed diagnosis. In addition, since treatment algorithms are conservative oriented, this increases the need to identify bowel and mesenteric trauma early in the treatment process. Multidetector CT (MDCT) is considered the imaging modality of choice for the diagnosis of bowel and mesenteric traumatic injuries, although the detection of these injuries can be challenging because of the presence of multiple simultaneous injuries and subtle imaging findings. Several CT signs of bowel and mesenteric injuries due to blunt trauma have been described in the literature. The major objective in evaluating these signs is to differentiate significant bowel and mesenteric injuries that require surgical treatment from those that can be conservatively treated. Familiarity with direct and indirect CT findings of blunt bowel and mesenteric injuries as well as the recognition of those CT features requiring surgery is crucial to making a timely and accurate diagnosis.

### Keywords

Blunt trauma · Bowel injuries · Mesenteric injuries · MDCT

## Introduction

Bowel and mesenteric injuries are detected in 5% of blunt abdominal trauma patients at laparotomy, and are the third most common type of injury from blunt trauma to the abdominal organs [1]. The incidence of blunt colonic injury

R. Basilico (✉) · A. D. Pizzi · A. Taraschi · B. Seccia · R. Cianci
Department of Neuroscience, Imaging and Clinical Sciences,
G. d'Annunzio University of Chieti, Chieti, Italy

© Springer Nature Switzerland AG 2022
M. N. Patlas et al. (eds.), *Atlas of Emergency Imaging from Head-to-Toe*,
https://doi.org/10.1007/978-3-030-92111-8_23

and blunt small bowel injury is 0.3% and 1.1%, respectively [2]. Although these injuries are relatively rare, prompt diagnosis is crucial because of the substantial morbidity and mortality with a delayed diagnosis, and additionally accurate detection, even with current CT techniques, remains challenging – even for experienced radiologists. A delay in diagnosis as small as five to eight hours may result in peritonitis, worsening hemorrhage, sepsis, bowel ischemia, and necrosis, and potentially death [3–6]. Moreover, due to the increase of conservative treatment of solid organ injuries, the rapid and accurate recognition of surgically important bowel and mesenteric injuries changes the patient's management.

In this scenario, multi-detector CT (MDCT) plays a pivotal role in the diagnosis of blunt bowel and mesenteric injuries, and is the imaging of examination of choice in stable polytrauma patients. Many studies have demonstrated that MDCT has a high negative predictive value; however, the sensitivity and specificity of CT findings of bowel and mesenteric injuries requiring surgery vary in the literature [7]. Radiologist's experience and the number of findings in polytrauma patients are two factors that may contribute to the variability in the CT diagnosis of these injuries [8]. In this chapter, we will review the direct and indirect CT findings of bowel and mesenteric injuries due to blunt trauma, with an emphasis on the importance of focusing on the CT features of injuries requiring surgery.

## Mechanism of Injuries

There are three main mechanisms of blunt traumatic gastrointestinal and mesenteric injuries [9]:

1. A direct force that crushes the gastrointestinal tract or causes its perforation
2. Rapid deceleration that produces shearing force between fixed and mobile portions of the gastrointestinal tract
3. Burst injuries ("blow out") that occur when intraluminal pressure exceeds the tensile strength of intestinal wall

The bowel segments that are most commonly affected by trauma are *the proximal jejunum*, near the ligament of Treitz, and *the distal ileum*, near the ileocecal valve (81%), which is explicable because these segments are more fixed than the rest of small bowel [1]. Moreover, injuries mostly occur on the antimesenteric side than on the mesenteric side [8]. The colon, rectum, duodenum, and stomach may also be injured in blunt trauma, but are even less commonly affected [2]. Bowel and mesenteric injuries usually occur together but also may occur separately, with purely mesenteric avulsions are sometimes seen in the setting of seat-belt-related injuries.

Crush injuries occur as a result of compression of large or small bowel between an external force and the osseous skeleton: frequently, the external force is due to a seat belt across the abdomen, or an impact against steering wheel or dashboard in the context of a high-speed motor vehicle collision. When rapid deceleration occurs, it typically causes stretching and linear shearing at interfaces between fixed and mobile parts of the gastrointestinal tract, thus producing bowel lacerations, mesenteric tears, and interruption of mesenteric vessels. As bowel loops course from their mesenteric attachments, the interruption of the mesenteric blood supply can result in consequent bowel ischemia and infarction [10].

Finally, burst injuries are caused by the increase of intraluminal pressure within loops of bowel, with subsequent perforation. Typically, this kind of mechanism can determine either single perforation or multiple perforations are on the antimesenteric border of the bowel. Ileus, preexisting bowel obstruction, and Crohn's disease are pathologic conditions that can predispose patients to burst injuries. Unlike the blunt bowel and mesenteric injuries due to the crush and shearing mechanism, burst injuries can occur with relatively low-impact trauma and therefore are less likely to be associated with other injuries [11].

## Management and CT Protocol

The main goal in evaluating CT signs of bowel and mesenteric injuries is to recognize and differentiate surgically important bowel and mesenteric injuries from those which can be non-surgically managed. The CT sensitivity and specificity values vary in the literature, ranging between 85–95% and 44–99%, respectively [7, 12]. Moreover, while high false negative rate (12–13%) [3] was reported in the past, with the improved performance of modern CT scanners and optimized protocols, the sensitivity of CT for the diagnosis of surgically significant bowel and mesenteric injuries is near 100%, as reported by some recent studies [13, 14]. However, other authors have demonstrated lower sensitivity values of CT for bowel and mesenteric injuries in blunt trauma, around 58% [15]. In this latter study, the sensitivity was very low mainly due to subtle CT findings of bowel and mesenteric abnormalities retrospectively identified by the two reviewers involved in the study, but nonprospectively diagnosed in the final radiologist's report. In fact, Lawson et al. showed that, except for peripheral musculoskeletal injuries, bowel and mesenteric injuries are the most frequently missed traumatic abnormality on initial CT, especially in patients over 50 year old with an injury severity score (ISS) >14 [16] . Finally, due to the increase of conservative management in polytrauma patients with solid organ injuries, the subtle CT findings are the main reasons why bowel and mesenteric injuries can be missed in blunt trauma [17]. The

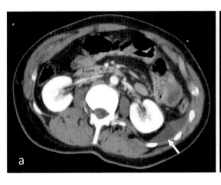
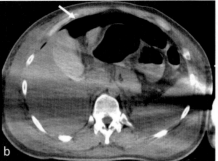
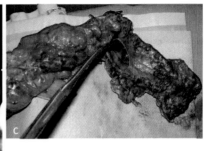

**Fig. 1** A 40-year-old man crushed by a farm tractor. MDCT did not show solid organ injuries, or free air in the abdomen. Fractures of the right hip and the pelvis were present, however. Axial IV contrast-enhanced CT image (**a**) revealed a small quantity of free fluid in the left retroperitoneal space (arrow). The patient was conservatively treated. Four days after the first MDCT examination, the patient became hemodynamically unstable, and a new MDCT examination was performed. A very large amount of free air (arrow in **b**) and free fluid was then present, due to a wide laceration of the left colon which was found at surgery but which was not identified prospectively at CT (**c**), and a colon resection according to Hartmann was performed (Courtesy of Dr M.Cieri, Department of Laparoscopic Surgery, University of Chieti). The only indirect finding of left colon laceration, which could have led retrospectively to a more accurate diagnosis, was the small amount of free fluid in the left retroperitoneal space, not correctly interpreted at the initial CT scan

consequence of missing such findings is delayed diagnosis and surgical intervention (Fig 1).

The diagnostic delay worsens the prognosis and increases the morbidity and mortality. For these reasons, despite several treatment algorithms, the management of patients with these kinds of traumatic injuries is still controversial, to our knowledge. Recently, Lannes et al. demonstrated that an early repeated CT scan, within 48 hours, in initially non-operated patients, improved the sensitivity of CT in the detection of surgically relevant traumatic injuries, as well as the reliability of patient selection for conservative management [18]. However, the exact time to perform repeat CT of the abdomen and pelvis is not definitively established yet, to our knowledge, but there are emerging recommendations, e.g., in a very short-term interval or within a few hours, especially for questionable subtle small bowel/mesenteric injuries – and these scans probably should be performed with water-soluble oral contrast.

Optimization of CT protocols is crucial in the evaluation of trauma patients.

At our institution, trauma protocol consists of whole-body CT from the thoracic inlet to the proximal femora during the arterial phase using bolus tracking, which triggers at 120 HU in the ascending aorta. Then images are obtained from the base of the thorax to the proximal femora during the portal phase. Delayed phase images are acquired in selected cases of renal injuries and pelvic bone fractures. CT examinations are usually performed by using a 64-slice MDCT scanner, preferably located in the emergency department, with a collimation of 64 by 0.6, reconstructed to 3 mm axial slices and 1 mm interval. Subsequently, 1 mm with 0.8 mm overlap coronal and sagittal multiplanar reformatted images are obtained. Oral contrast administration is not routinely used in our institution, especially during the initial CT assessment.

It can be useful in the follow-up of polytrauma patients with the clinical suspicion of bowel injuries. In fact, although leakage of oral contrast is diagnostic of bowel perforation, i.e., has 100% specificity, this finding has a very low sensitivity (12–14%) [19], probably due to a lack of bowel distension during CT or to the subtlety of the leak or to a defect which is "sealed" at the time of imaging but which is still present. Additionally, many blunt bowel injuries are not full thickness and would not cause a luminal disruption to leak enteric contrast. Moreover, an intraperitoneal bladder rupture may be misinterpreted as extraluminal oral contrast material (false positive of bowel perforation). Oral contrast administration has two other downsides: It can cause a potential delay in patient care, and a small yet definite risk of aspiration cannot be excluded. In addition, in a meta-analysis of 32 studies, Lee et al. did not find any difference in the accuracy of CT performed with or without oral contrast agent for the detection of blunt bowel and mesenteric injury [20].

## Bowel Injuries

CT features of **surgically relevant bowel injuries** include: *bowel discontinuity, extraluminal gas, devascularized bowel, large bowel thickening, and abnormal bowel wall enhancement. Isolated small bowel thickening,* which usually indicates bowel wall hematoma or serosal tear, does not always require surgical treatment.

## Bowel Discontinuity

Frank bowel discontinuity appears as a bowel wall defect, and it is an uncommon finding, probably due to the small size of discontinuities which can also be very difficult to detect also at surgical inspection. In fact, in the literature

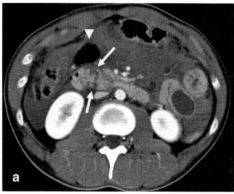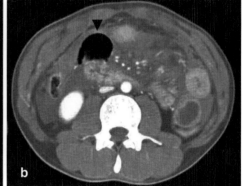

**Fig. 2** Bowel wall discontinuity in a 23-year-old man after a motor vehicle collision. Axial IV contrast-enhanced CT images with soft tissue (**a**) and lung (**b**) window settings show a definitive defect within the wall of the transverse duodenum (white arrows), which is associated with adjacent free extraluminal air (arrowheads in **a** and **b**), and which is diagnostic of bowel perforation

the reported specificity is very high, essentially 100%, but sensitivity has been described very low, ranging from 5–34% [7, 8, 20]. The presence of free air close to bowel discontinuity supports the diagnosis of bowel perforation (Fig 2).

## Extraluminal Air

This sign shows high specificity values up to 95% but very low sensitivity for surgically relevant injuries, 20–30%, as reported by several studies [21–24]. Although extraluminal air is nearly as specific as bowel discontinuity, there are some conditions that may be sources of free air in the abdomen, including intraperitoneal bladder rupture and a Foley catheter in place, diaphragmatic rupture, pneumothorax, mechanical ventilation, and pulmonary barotrauma. In these patients, extraluminal intraperitoneal free air may be considered a false-positive finding. A potential diagnostic pitfall is represented by the so-called "pseudo-pneumoperitoneum," which is described as the presence of air entrapped into the inner layer of the abdominal wall and external to the parietal peritoneum, mimicking true pneumoperitoneum on CT [8].

The location of extraluminal air, as well as free fluid in the abdomen, may be useful in determining the location of bowel injury. The second to fourth portions of the duodenum, the ascending colon, and the descending colon are retroperitoneal. The first portion of the duodenum (duodenal bulb), jejunum, ileum, cecum, transverse colon, sigmoid colon, and upper part of the rectum are intraperitoneal. Retroperitoneal air seems to be more sensitive in the setting of duodenal injury or injury to the ascending and descending colon (Fig 3).

In this context, as a general rule, in all polytrauma patients CT images should be reviewed with lung or bone window settings, in addition to the routine soft-tissue windows, in order to assess even small quantity of free abdominal air and to differentiate fat from air (Fig 4) [25].

## Bowel Wall Thickening and Abnormal Bowel Wall Enhancement

Although focal bowel wall thickening greater than 3–4 mm has been shown to be more sensitive (75%) for bowel wall injury than pneumoperitoneum [26], bowel wall thickening and abnormal bowel wall enhancement are not specific findings to bowel injury because they may be secondary to mesenteric injury, indicating vascular involvement, or to insufficient bowel distension. Moreover, diffuse small bowel wall thickening may represent bowel edema secondary to systemic volume overload or to hypoperfusion complex, the so-called shock bowel. In particular, diffuse bowel wall thickening and mucosal hyper-enhancement in the setting of trauma is usually the result of hypoperfusion rather than the result of trauma injury. In fact, these findings, in combination with other signs of hypoperfusion complex such as inferior vena cava flattening, increased renal and adrenal enhancement, and decreased splenic enhancement, are strong indicators of hypovolemia in trauma patients. Full-thickness bowel wall enhancement is another feature of shock bowel; the proposed explanation is that the increased vascular permeability due to hypoperfusion may result in interstitial leakage of contrast agent [27]. On the other hand, the presence of adjacent hyperenhancing and hypoenhancing segments of small bowel, the so-called "Janus" sign, is highly specific for bowel injury [9] (Fig. 5), as well as areas of decreased or absent contrast enhancement which are indicative of ischemic bowel. Changes in bowel wall enhancement can potentially be better assessed by means of dual- energy CT. The added value of dual-energy CT is that both iodine-selective imaging and virtual monoenergetic imaging highlight the iodine content, which increases the conspicuity of areas of altered bowel wall enhancement [28].

While isolated small bowel thickening without mesenteric infiltration or close free air (which could be from a source

**Fig. 3** A 35-year-old man with free extraluminal air due to trauma from the handlebars of his bicycle. IV axial contrast-enhanced CT images show free intraperitoneal air (arrows in **a**), associated with small free air pockets closely related to the thickened descending colon (arrow in **b**), which is highly consistent with bowel perforation, as was then confirmed at surgery (**c**) (Courtesy of Dr M.Cieri, Department of Laparoscopic Surgery, University of Chieti)

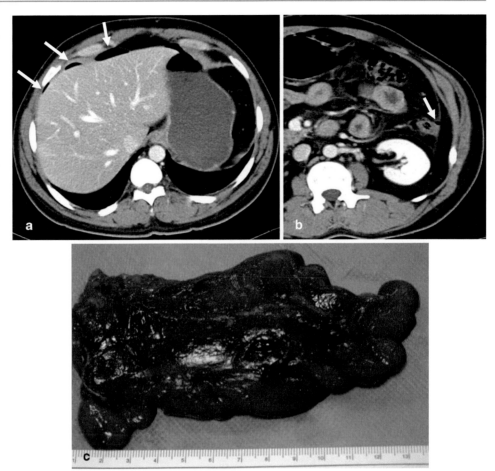

**Fig. 4** A 38-year-old man after a motor vehicle collision. IV contrast-enhanced CT scan revealed a tiny hypodensity (arrow in **a**) in a retroperitoneal fluid collection close to the right psoas muscle, and presumed to be free air from a bowel source. The same image, visualized by using lung window setting, was consistent with fat and not free air (arrow in **b**)

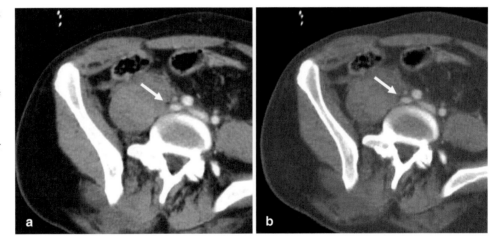

other than the bowel) does not necessarily require surgical treatment, large bowel wall thickening has been found to have high specificity (97%) for bowel injury, and it is considered an "alarming finding" [7]. Moreover, free air close to a thickened bowel loop is a more reliable finding of bowel perforation (Fig 6).

## Mesenteric Injuries

CT features of surgically relevant mesenteric injuries include: *active bleeding within the mesentery, termination of mesenteric vessels, mesenteric vascular beading, mesenteric stranding, or hematoma associated with bowel thickening.*

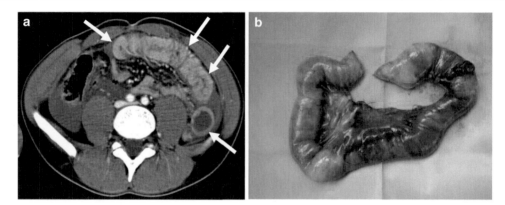

**Fig. 5** Abnormal bowel wall enhancement and focal bowel wall thickening in a 19-year-old man with blunt abdominal trauma. Axial IV contrast-enhanced CT image (**a**) shows thickened jejunal loops, with an inhomogeneous appearance, owing to the presence of interspersed hyperenhancing and hypoenhancing segments (the so-called "Janus" sign, named after the two-headed Roman god representing the "middle ground"), indicative of bowel wall injury with lacerations, as was then confirmed at surgery (**b**) (Courtesy of Dr M.Cieri, Department of Laparoscopic Surgery, University of Chieti)

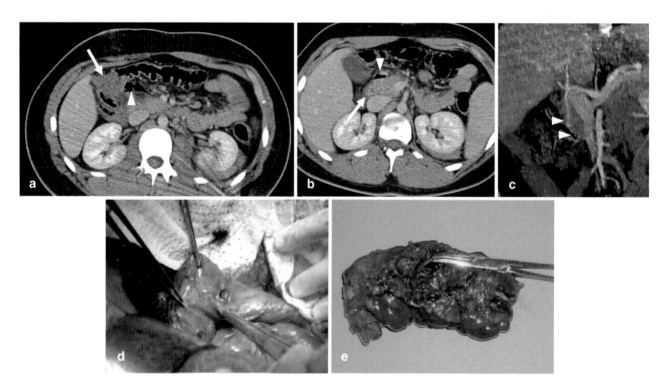

**Fig. 6** A 28-year-old man with trauma from a 4-meter fall. Axial (**a, b**) and MIP (**c**) IV contrast-enhanced CT images show extraluminal air (arrowheads in **a** and **b**) close to a thickened right colon flexure and duodenum (arrows in **a** and **b** respectively), indicating bowel lacerations, as was then confirmed at surgery (**d**: duodenal perforation, **e**: right colon flexure perforation (Courtesy of Dr M. Cieri, Department of LaparoscopicSurgery, University of Chieti)). Vascular beading of the inferior pancreaticoduodenal artery is also evident (arrows in **c**). A left kidney laceration with perirenal hematoma was also present, without associated active bleeding, which recovered after conservative management (**a,b**)

*Focal mesenteric stranding or hematoma without bowel thickening and isolated intraperitoneal fluid* are considered nonsurgical mesenteric injuries [7].

## Active Bleeding Within the Mesentery

Active intravenous contrast extravasation within the mesentery appears as a serpiginous or amorphous high-attenuation

**Fig. 7** Mesenteric hematoma with active bleeding in a 73-year-old man crushed by a farm tractor. Axial arterial-enhanced (**a**), portal venous enhanced (**b**), MIP, (**c**) and cinematic rendering (**d**) CT images demonstrate a large hematoma in the jejunal mesentery (arrowheads), with contrast medium extravasation indicative of active bleeding (arrows) which increases according to the CT phases

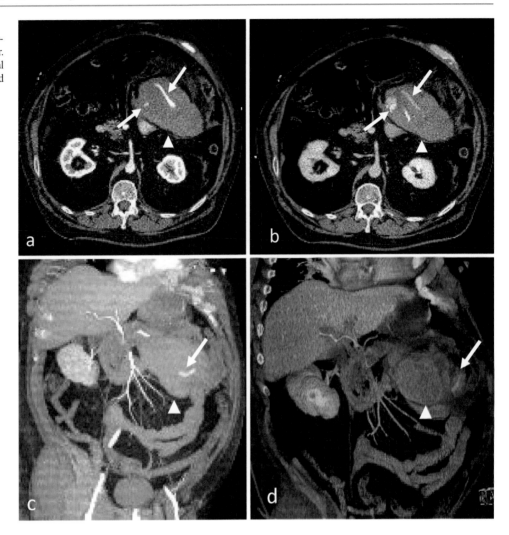

**Table 1** At nonenhanced and enhanced CT, peritoneal fluids show different densities measured by Hounsfield Units (HU). Extravasated IV contrast material consistent with active bleeding shows the highest HU density values compared with ascites/fluid from other etiologies

| Peritoneal fluid | Density (HU) |
| --- | --- |
| Ascites, urine, bile, intestinal contents | 0–10 |
| Unclotted blood (recent bleeding) | 30–45 (< in pts with decreased serum hematocrit level) |
| Clotted blood (within 20 h) | 45–70 |
| Clotted blood (after 72 h) | <30 |
| Extravased contrast material | 85-370 (mean 132) |

area on CT, surrounded by a large hematoma (Fig. 7). The high attenuation of active bleeding can be easily differentiated from other peritoneal fluids (Table 1). This CT sign has high specificity (100%) but low sensitivity (17%) [8]: it is

usually an indication for urgent laparotomy. Mesenteric extravasation is caused by mesenteric laceration with vascular involvement (Fig. 8). When it is associated with bowel injury, other CT features may be present, including bowel thickening and abnormal bowel wall enhancement (decreased or increased) (Fig.9).

## Termination of Mesenteric Vessels and Mesenteric Vascular Beading

Abrupt termination of a mesenteric artery or vein and irregularity (beading) in mesenteric vessels are both indicative of mesenteric vascular injury, and are better visualized on MPR CT images (Fig. 10). Termination of mesenteric vessels has reported to have low sensitivity (35%) [8] but high specificity (97%) [29]. Mesenteric vascular beading was found to be

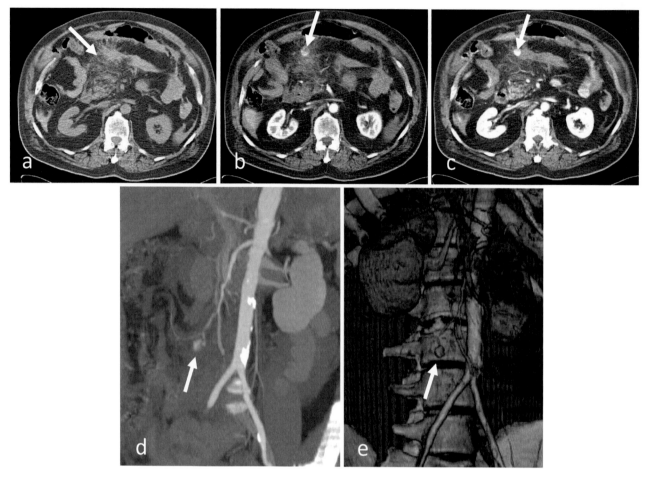

**Fig. 8** Mesenteric laceration with arterial pseudoaneurysm in a 56-year-old man after a motor vehicle collision. Axial nonenhanced (**a**), arterial-enhanced (**b**), portal venous-enhanced (**c**), MIP (**d**), and volumetric rendered CT (**e**) images demonstrate mesenteric stranding (arrow in **a**), with a contained small focus of contrast medium extravasation consistent with a pseudoaneurysm (arrows in **b** and **c**), close to an abrupt termination of the ileocolic artery (arrows in d and e)

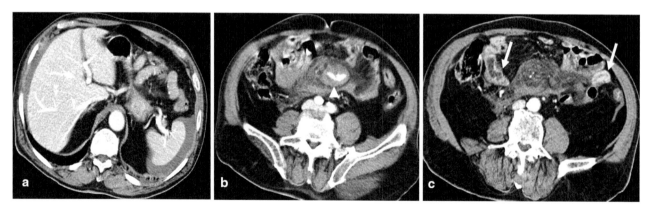

**Fig. 9** A 60-year-old woman after a high-energy car collision. IV contrast-enhanced CT images during the portal phase showed free perihepatic and perisplenic fluid with no evidence for any solid organ injuries (**a**). The free peritoneal fluid was due to a large mesenteric hematoma with contrast extravasation (arrowhead in **b**) associated with abnormal small bowel enhancement (arrows in **c**). At surgery, a wide mesenteric injury with vascular involvement and mucosal hemorrhage of the ileum was demonstrated

**Fig. 10** Same patient with jejunal lacerations illustrated on Fig. 5. MIP CT image (**a**) shows abrupt termination (arrow) and beading (arrowhead) of jejunal arterial vessels due to jejunal lacerations. There was associated extravasation of contrast material, better visualized on delayed contrast-enhanced phase (asterisks in **b**)

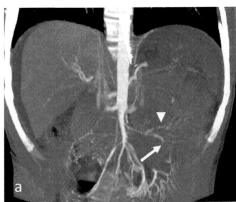
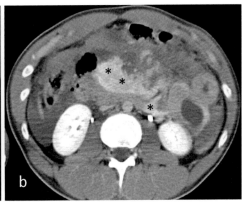

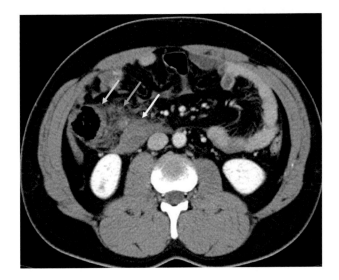

**Fig. 11** A 35-year-old woman after a 3-meter fall. IV contrast-enhanced CT image shows ascending colon wall thickening and decreased enhancement (yellow arrow), mesenteric infiltration (green arrow), and right anterior pararenal hematoma (white arrow). At surgery, an ischemic right colon due to right colic artery injury and associated mesenteric injuries were demonstrated

more frequent than active contrast extravasation in the mesentery as a surgically relevant CT finding [7, 8].

## Mesenteric Stranding or Hematoma Associated with Bowel Thickening

Haziness and fat stranding of the mesentery may indicate mesenteric injury, with a sensitivity of 70–77% and a specificity of 40–90% [30]. If mesenteric infiltration or stranding is associated with bowel thickening (Fig. 11), this finding is highly suggestive of bowel injury requiring surgery with sensitivity and specificity values of 55–75% and 90%, respectively [23]. In contrast, focal mesenteric stranding or hematoma without bowel thickening (Fig. 12) indicates mesenteric injury alone, and may not require surgical repair.

## Common Features in Bowel and Mesenteric Injuries

### Retroperitoneal and Intraperitoneal Fluid

The location of the fluid may indicate the location of the injury. Hemorrhage from the small bowel or the mesentery typically flows into inter-loop spaces with a triangular configuration (Fig. 13), whereas retroperitoneal fluid or hematoma tends to localize at the site of injury. For instance, periduodenal hematoma is a quite specific sign of duodenal injury. Retroperitoneal and intraperitoneal fluid is associated with either bowel and mesenteric injuries in 93% of cases [8], but the specificity of these findings on CT is low for both because of other concomitant injuries. However, hemoperitoneum in the absence of solid organ traumatic injuries, should heighten the possibility of bowel and mesenteric injuries.

### Abdominal Wall Injury

A significant association between abdominal wall traumatic injuries with bowel and mesenteric injuries has been found, such as hematoma or tear or the so-called "seat belt sign," subcutaneous fat haziness along the course of the fastened seat belt. Traumatic lumbar hernias are also strongly associated with bowel and mesenteric injuries.

## Conclusion

Blunt bowel and mesenteric injuries are relatively rare in the setting of blunt abdominal trauma. However, timely and accurate diagnosis is crucial for the appropriate management and for minimizing morbidity, mortality, and hospitalization. It is essential to be aware of the CT findings of bowel and

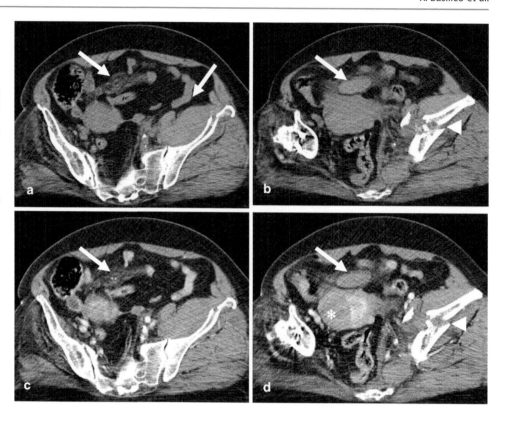

**Fig. 12** Mesenteric injury in a 71-year-old woman following a motor vehicle collision. Axial nonenhanced (**a**, **b**) and IV contrast-enhanced (**c**, **d**) CT images show mesenteric stranding (arrows in **a** and **d**) and a localized mesenteric hematoma (arrows in **b** and **c**), without contrast medium extravasation, pointing to an isolated laceration without active bleeding. Arrowheads in b and d indicate a fracture of the left iliac bone, and asterisk in **d** indicates a uterine fibroid. The patient was conservatively managed with mesenteric healing at follow-up

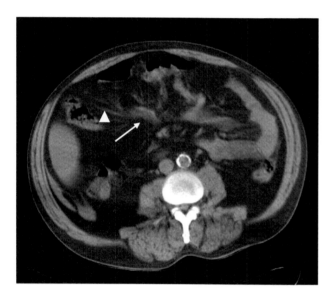

**Fig. 13** Non-enhanced CT scan of a 70-year-old man after a fall from 5 meters. CT image reveals interloop fluid (arrow) and mesenteric stranding (arrowhead) in the absence of bowel wall thickening, findings which are more suggestive of mesenteric injury than of parenchymal organ trauma

mesenteric injuries in order to differentiate those requiring surgical repair from findings/abnormalities which can be conservatively treated. Moreover, due to the fact that these injuries can be easily missed because of factors related to their CT appearance, and even using current equipment and

techniques – and even with experienced radiologists performing the interpretation of such scans – it is necessary to avoid other conditions that can further reduce the diagnostic accuracy of CT. The chaotic trauma setting that may cause findings to be overlooked or misinterpreted, and satisfaction of search error, may also cause mistakes when other injuries are present.

## References

1. Watts DR, Fakhry SM. Incidence of hollow viscus injury in blunt trauma: an analysis from 275.557 trauma admissions from the EAST Multi-Institutional trial. J Trauma. 2003;54:289–94.
2. Williams MD, Watts DR, Fakhry SM. Colon injury after blunt abdominal trauma: results of the EAST multi-institutional hollow viscus injury study. J Trauma. 2003;55(5):906–12.
3. Fakhry SM, Brownstein M, Watts DD, Baker CC, Oller D. Relatively short diagnostic delays (< 8 hours) produce morbidity and mortality in blunt small bowel injury: an analysis of time to operative intervention in 198 patients from a multicenter experience. J Trauma. 2000;48(3):408–14.
4. Malinoski DJ, Patel MS, Yakar DO, Green D, et al. A diagnostic delay of 5 hours increases the risk of death after blunt hollow viscus injury. J Trauma. 2010;69:84–7.
5. Scaglione M, de Lutio di Castelguidone E, Scialpi M, et al. Blunt trauma to the gastrointestinal tract and mesentery: is there a role for helical CT in the decision- making process? Eur J Radiol. 2004;50: 67–73.
6. Hughes TMD, Elton C. The pathophysiology and management of bowel and mesenteric injuries due to a blunt trauma. Injury. 2002;33 (4):295–302.

7. Atri M, Hanson JM, Grinblat L, Brofman N, et al. Surgically important bowel and/or mesenteric injury in blunt trauma: accuracy of multidetector CT for evaluation. Radiology. 2008;249(2):524–33.

8. Brofman N, Atri M, Hanson JM, et al. Evaluation of bowel and mesenteric blunt trauma with multidetector CT. RadioGraphics. 2006;26:1119–31.

9. Khan I, Bew D, Elias DA, et al. Mechanisms of injury and CT findings of bowel and mesenteric trauma. Clin Radiol. 2014;69: 639–47.

10. Hughes TM, Elton C. The pathophysiology and management of bowel and mesenteric injuries due to blunt trauma. Injury. 2002;33:295–302.

11. Bates DDB, Wasserman M, Malek A, Gorantla V, et al. Multi-detector CT of surgically proven blunt bowel and mesenteric injury. Radiographics. 2017;37:313–62.

12. Elton C, Riaz AA, Young N, et al. Accuracy of computed tomography in the detection of blunt bowel and mesenteric injuries. Br J Surg. 2005;92:1024–8.

13. Tan K-K, Liu JZ, Go T-S, et al. Computed tomography has an important role in hollow viscus and mesenteric injuries after blunt abdominal trauma. Injury. 2010;41:475–8.

14. Petrosoniak A, Engels PT, Hamilton P, et al. Detection of significant bowel and mesenteric injuries in blunt abdominal trauma with 64-slice computed tomography. J Trauma Acute Care Surg. 2013;74: 1081–6.

15. Landry BA, Patlas MN, Faidi S, et al. Are we missing bowel and mesenteric injuries? Can Assoc Radiol J. 2016;67(4):420–5.

16. Lawson CM, Daley BJ, Ormsby CB, Enderson B. Missed injuries in the era of the trauma scan. J Trauma. 2011;70:452–8.

17. EurinM HN, Zappa M, et al. Incidence and predictors of missed injuries in trauma patients in the initial hot report of whole-body CT scan. Injury. 2012;43:73–7.

18. Lannes F, Scemama U, Maignan A, et al. Value of early repeated abdominal CTin selective non-operative management for blunt bowel and mesenteric injury. Eur Radiol. 2019;29(11):5932–40.

19. Tsang BD, Panacek EA, Brant WE, et al. Effect of oral contrast administration for abdominal computed tomography in the evaluation of acute blunt trauma. Ann Emerg Med. 1997;30:7–13.

20. Lee CH, Haaland B, Earnest A, Tan CH. Use of positive oral contrast agents inabdominopelvic computed tomography for blunt abdominal injury: meta- analysis and systematic review. Eur Radiol. 2013;23(9):2513–21.

21. Steenburg SD, Petersen MJ, Shen C, et al. Multi-detector CT of blunt mesenteric injuries: usefulness of imaging findings for predicting surgically significant bowel injuries. Abdom Imaging. 2015;40:1026–33.

22. Soto JA, Anderson SW. Multidetector CT of blunt abdominal trauma. Radiology. 2012;265:678–92.

23. Faget C, Taourel P, Charbit J, et al. Value of CT to predict surgically important bowel and/or mesenteric injury in blunt trauma: performance of a preliminary scoring system. Eur Radiol. 2015;25:3620–8.

24. LeBedis CA, Anderson SW, Bates DDB, et al. CT imaging signs of surgically proven bowel trauma. Emerg Radiol. 2016;23:213–9.

25. Pouli S, Kozana A, Papakitsou I. Gastrointestinal perforation: clinical and MDCT clues for identification of aetiology. Insights Imaging. 2020;11:31.

26. Brody JM, Leighton DB, Murphy BL, et al. CT of blunt trauma bowel and mesenteric injury: typical findings and pitfalls in diagnosis. Radiographics. 2000;20:1525–36.

27. Lubner M, Demertzis J, Lee JY, et al. CT evaluation of shock viscera: a pictorial review. Emerg Radiol. 2008;15:1–11.

28. Wortman JR, Uyeda JW, Fulwadhva UP, Sodickson AR. Dual-energy CT for abdominal and pelvic trauma. Radiographics. 2018;38:586–602.

29. Gamanagatti S, Rangarajan K, Kumar A. Blunt abdominal trauma: imaging and intervention. Curr Probl Diagn Radiol. 2015;44:321–36.

30. Alabousi M, Mellnick VM, Al-Ghetaa RK, Patlas MN. Imaging of blunt bowel and mesenteric injuries: current status. Eur J Radiol. 2020;125:108894.

# Imaging of Blunt Genitourinary Trauma

# 24

Gayatri Joshi, Charlotte Y. Chung, and Brittany T. Lewis

## Contents

### Abstract

Genitourinary injury occurs in approximately 10% of abdominal trauma cases, with renal injury being most common, followed by urinary bladder (UB) injury. Most acute traumatic renal injuries (80–90%) are a result of blunt trauma. Though less common, penetrating renal injuries are often more severe. Ureteral injury usually occurs as a result of penetrating trauma, most frequently ballistic insults, and is usually accompanied by other intra-abdominal injuries. UB injuries are relatively uncommon,

most of which are a result blunt trauma (60–85%), as compared to penetrating trauma (15–40%). Pubic rami fractures and diastasis of the pubic symphysis also have a high correlation with UB injury.

Hematuria, though the most common indicator of injury to the genitourinary tract, is not a reliable predictor and is not always present. Additionally, the presence of hematuria does not indicate the site of injury, which may be anywhere along the genitourinary tract. Imaging is routinely used in the diagnosis and grading of genitourinary injuries and may involve a combination of standard trauma protocol CECT, followed by delayed-phase CT imaging, CT cystogram, and/or retrograde urethrography (RUG), depending on the site(s) of suspected injury.

Determination and stratification of injury severity by imaging at initial presentation often directs management

G. Joshi (✉) · C. Y. Chung
Department of Radiology and Imaging Sciences, Emory University School of Medicine, Atlanta, GA, USA
e-mail: gayatri.joshi@emory.edu; charlotte.yuk-yan.chung@emory.edu

B. T. Lewis
Emergency and Trauma Imaging, Emory University School of Medicine, Atlanta, GA, USA
e-mail: brittany.tiana.marie.lewis@emory.edu

© Springer Nature Switzerland AG 2022
M. N. Patlas et al. (eds.), *Atlas of Emergency Imaging from Head-to-Toe*,
https://doi.org/10.1007/978-3-030-92111-8_24

without the need for laparotomy in most patients. Familiarity with commonly used grading systems, including the American Association for the Surgery of Trauma (AAST) grading scales and radiology-based grading scales, is key in relating important findings to clinical providers.

**Keywords**

Genitourinary trauma · Genitourinary injury · GU · Genitourinary · Renal · Kidney · Ureter · Ureteral · Urinary bladder · Trauma · Blunt trauma · Penetrating trauma · Trauma imaging protocol

## Introduction

Diagnosis and grading of genitourinary imaging is primarily performed by computed tomography (CT) at the time of presentation rather than by exploratory laparotomy in most patients. The use of optimized trauma CT protocols has become increasingly pivotal. Management of genitourinary trauma, particularly renal trauma, is shifting toward non-surgical management whenever possible, and accurate grading based on optimal imaging is an important factor in determining which patients can be managed conservatively and which patients require more aggressive intervention. This chapter will discuss not only renal trauma imaging but also ureteral and bladder trauma imaging.

## Renal Trauma

### Epidemiology

Acute traumatic renal injury occurs in approximately 8–10% of patients following blunt or penetrating abdominal trauma, with the majority (80–90%) occurring in the setting of blunt trauma, often secondary to motor vehicle collisions, falls from a height, or direct impact by blunt objects [1–4]. While penetrating renal injuries caused by ballistic or stab injuries are less common (10–20%), they often result in greater injury severity as compared to blunt trauma [3, 5]. High-grade renal injuries are often accompanied by other abdominal injuries; multi-organ injuries occur in approximately 80% of penetrating injuries and 75% of blunt injuries. On the other hand, most isolated renal injuries are low grade [1].

### Diagnostic Investigations

Imaging evaluation of the genitourinary system is generally indicated for trauma patients with (1) gross hematuria,

(2) microscopic hematuria in the setting of hemodynamic instability (systolic blood pressure <90 mm HG) or significant associated injuries, or (3) injury mechanism or examination findings suggestive of renal injury, including rapid deceleration injuries, penetrating flank trauma, penetrating or blunt trauma with concern for retroperitoneal trajectory, rib fractures, or substantial flank hematoma or ecchymosis, even in the absence of hematuria [1, 3, 6, 7].

## IV Contrast-Enhanced Computed Tomography (CECT)

CECT is the imaging modality of choice for acute abdominopelvic trauma and the evaluation of acute renal injuries. Dual-phase trauma CECT protocol involves two separate CT acquisitions after a single IV contrast bolus, with arterial-phase acquisition at approximately 15–25 s delay through the chest and upper abdomen (with some centers including the pelvis) and portal venous-phase acquisition at approximately 70–80 s through the abdomen and pelvis.

The arterial phase allows for optimal detection of vascular injuries, while the portal venous phase (usually corresponding to late corticomedullary or early nephrographic renal enhancement) is used for the detection of parenchymal injuries. Homogeneous enhancement of the renal parenchyma during the nephrographic phase is more ideal for detection of renal parenchymal injuries as compared to the corticomedullary phase when there is suboptimal enhancement of the renal pyramids. However, most centers have standardized trauma CT protocols, and renal enhancement on images acquired during the portal venous phase may vary somewhat between patients, such that optimal nephrographic renal enhancement may not always be obtained. This variation can be due to a variety of factors, including the patient's fluid status and cardiac output. It is important to notice the type of renal enhancement on the portal venous-phase CT images, as this may affect sensitivity for the detection of parenchymal injuries. The portal venous-phase CT images also aid in differentiation of contained vascular injuries from active bleeding, as well as characterization of venous injuries [3].

As an alternative to conventional dual-phase CECT protocol, some centers use the split-bolus trauma CECT protocol. This single-pass CECT protocol consists of a single acquisition through the abdomen following two separate contrast boluses to provide both arterial and portal venous-phase imaging at the same time [8–10]. This technique significantly reduces patient radiation exposure, results in greater renal parenchymal enhancement, and can have overall comparable image quality compared to the dual-phase CT protocol [10]. However, definitive differentiation between arterial and venous injuries can be impaired using this protocol due to simultaneous opacification of arterial and venous structures, although some have suggested that vascular injuries can be characterized based on location, density, and morphology of extravasated contrast [11].

Irrespective of whether the dual-phase or split-bolus trauma protocol is used for the initial trauma CECT evaluation, an additional 5–10 min delayed excretory-phase acquisition should be obtained when there is suspicion for renal collecting system or ureter injury [3, 12]. This delayed phase may also provide increased sensitivity for the detection of venous bleeding.

## Ultrasound

In trauma patients who are unable to undergo CT due to hemodynamic instability and for patients with a documented allergy to intravenous contrast, ultrasound may be considered as an alternative to CT. Focused assessment with sonography in trauma (FAST) scan is well accepted for detection of hemoperitoneum; however, this technique is highly operator and patient body type dependent and has limited sensitivity for the detection of renal parenchymal and vascular injuries. Further, assessment for parenchymal injuries can be limited even when performed by highly experienced sonographers [13]. If large intraperitoneal (IP) fluid is found in a hemodynamically unstable patient, emergent laparotomy may be necessary [1, 13–15].

Intravenous contrast-enhanced ultrasound (CEUS) with the use of microbubble intravenous contrast agents is being employed increasingly in Europe in the setting of trauma after baseline standard ultrasound, although studies regarding the use of CEUS are still ongoing in the United States. Studies thus far show that CEUS has greater sensitivity than standard ultrasound for abdominal solid organ injury. CEUS can be used to identify vascular injuries (including active bleeding), parenchymal infarction, and vascular pedicle avulsion. Active bleeding appears as microbubble contrast extravasation within the IP or retroperitoneal spaces. Vascular pedicle injury appears as absence of organ perfusion. Parenchymal injuries appear as defects within otherwise normally perfused parenchyma. Lacerations may appear as linear or branched hypoechoic defects surrounded by otherwise homogeneous hyperechoic parenchyma following microbubble contrast administration [13]. Still, applications in the trauma patient, particularly pediatric and pregnant patients, are not established to our knowledge, and CEUS has its own logistic and diagnostic limitations. The use of CEUS in the setting of trauma is not widespread in the United States, though this area is being studied at some centers.

## Follow-Up Imaging

Follow-up imaging after renal injury is obtained to evaluate for potential complications, particularly in the setting of expectant management. Persistent urine extravasation (with possible urinoma) is the most common potential early (within 4 weeks) complication [15]. Delayed hemorrhage, shown to occur in up to 25% of grade 3–5 injuries [6], is often related to rupture of contained vascular injuries. Other complications include infected urinoma and perinephric abscess (often seen with concomitant pancreatic or bowel injury), sepsis, and hypertension. Since complications are exceedingly rare following grade 1 and 2 injuries, routine follow-up imaging rarely changes management and is not indicated [5, 14, 16, 17].

For grade 4 and 5 injuries, current guidelines generally recommend repeat CECT with delayed (excretory-phase) images approximately 48 hours after the traumatic event, which can reveal delayed urine extravasation which may have been masked on the initial scan. This unique phenomenon results from urinary urokinase-mediated lysis of the perinephric clot initially plugging the collecting system breech [2, 18]. For patients who are symptomatic with fever, progressive flank pain, ongoing blood loss (as evidenced by labile blood pressures, ongoing transfusion requirement, or down-trending hemoglobin levels), and abdominal distention, follow-up imaging should be obtained earlier. For young patients and pregnant patients in whom judicious use of ionizing radiation is preferred when possible, MRI or CEUS may be utilized instead.

## AAST CT-Based Grading of Kidney Injury

### Overview of AAST Kidney Injury Scale

The AAST OIS is the most widely used grading system for renal trauma [3]. The initial 1989 AAST Renal Injury Scale did not include dedicated imaging criteria and, instead, was clinically based, created to grade kidney injuries at time of laparotomy [2, 19]. Additionally, the 1989 Renal Injury Scale did not fully account for vascular injuries among its criteria. Despite these limitations, the 1989 AAST Renal Injury Scale has been widely used in the United States to grade and stratify severity of traumatic injuries to the kidney by CT without surgical intervention, particularly over the last two decades, as detection of injuries has improved with advances in CT as a diagnostic imaging modality.

The first comprehensive revision of the AAST Renal Injury Scale was published in 2018 as the AAST Kidney Injury Scale and includes dedicated imaging criteria, specifically by CT, as well as separate operative and pathologic criteria [20]. This revision also incorporates renal vascular injury more comprehensively, which are key additions, as vascular injury is now readily detected using CECT, and advances in treatment options have afforded nonsurgical management in a greater portion of renal trauma patients.

The AAST Kidney Injury Scale classifies traumatic injuries to the kidney into five grades, with grade 1 being the least

**Table 1** AAST Renal Injury Scale 2018 revision with newly added CT criteria. Corresponding changes specific to each grade compared to the original injury scale are detailed.

| AAST grade | CT criteria | Specific changes by grade |
|---|---|---|
| 1 | Renal parenchymal contusion (without laceration), subcapsular hematoma, or both | Removed: Clinical descriptors of microscopic or macroscopic hematuria without imaging abnormality<br>Removed: "Non-expanding" as a qualifier for subcapsular hematoma |
| 2 | Renal parenchymal laceration ≤1 cm depth without urinary extravasation<br>Perirenal hematoma confined to Gerota's fascia | Change: Laceration size is now inclusive of 1 cm<br>Removed: "Non-expanding" as a qualifier for perirenal hematoma |
| 3 | Renal parenchymal laceration ≥1 cm depth without urinary extravasation<br>Any injury in the presence of renal vascular injury[a] or active bleeding[b] confined to Gerota's fascia | New definition: Vascular injury includes AVF and pseudoaneurysm<br>Includes active bleeding confined to Gerota's fascia |
| 4 | Renal parenchymal laceration extending into the collecting system<br>Renal pelvis laceration or complete ureteropelvic disruption<br>Segmental renal artery or vein intimal injury/thrombus<br>Segmental or complete renal infarction due to thrombosis in the absence of active bleeding<br>Active bleeding beyond Gerota's fascia | Addition: Renal pelvis laceration and ureteropelvic disruption<br>Addition: Includes active bleeding beyond Gerota's fascia<br>Removed: Laceration/avulsion of main renal vessels, now categorized as grade 5 |
| 5 | Shattered kidney<br>Main renal artery or vein laceration or avulsion from the renal hilum<br>Complete organ devascularization with active bleeding | Addition: The descriptor "laceration" to define main renal vascular injury, in addition to hilar avulsion<br>Addition: Active bleeding in the setting of complete renal infarction |

[a]Vascular injury is defined as pseudoaneurysm or AVF
[b]Active bleeding is defined as vascular contrast either focal or diffuse that increases in size and/or attenuation on delayed imaging (AAST source)
Note: Advance one grade higher for bilateral injuries, up to grade 3 [3, 20]
Note: More than one grade of kidney injury may be present; overall classification should be based on the highest grade [3, 20]

severe and grade 5 the most severe. Each grade is comprised of a set of injury patterns (Table 1). Grade 1 and 2 injuries are considered low grade, are usually treated conservatively, and usually resolve without complications. In contradistinction, grade 4 and 5 injuries are considered high grade with more severe injury patterns and a larger percentage of patients requiring intervention. Grade 3 injuries were previously considered low grade when classified by the 1989 version. However, the 2018 revision categorizes active bleeding confined to Gerota's fascia and vascular injuries such as pseudoaneurysms and arteriovenous fistulas (AVFs) as grade 3. Thus, hemodynamically unstable patients with grade 3 injuries may require intervention [2].

When multiple injuries are present, the grade is determined by the most severe injury. Injury grade should be advanced by one grade for the presence of bilateral injuries, up to grade 3.

## Imaging Findings

Subcapsular hematomas are hemorrhagic fluid collections located between the renal capsule and the renal parenchyma and can have an eccentric, crescentic, or lentiform configuration (Fig. 1). Subcapsular hematomas can vary in attenuation depending on age of the blood products. On NECT imaging, subcapsular hematomas range in attenuation from 30–50 HU (unclotted blood) to 50–70 HU (acute clotted blood) and can appear hyperdense relative to the non-enhanced renal parenchyma [1, 3]. When small, subcapsular hematomas may exert minimal mass effect on the kidney. As they enlarge, however, they tend to take on a biconvex appearance and exert more substantial mass effect on the underlying renal parenchyma, resulting in an indented or flattened renal contour [1, 3]. Unlike subcapsular hematomas, perinephric or perirenal hematomas usually do not exert significant mass effect on the renal contour [4]. Page kidney, a rare complication of persistent or chronic contained subcapsular hematoma, can develop as a result of mass effect, reducing renal blood flow and inducing hyperreninemic hypertension. Page kidney may appear as perirenal soft tissue thickening or a subcapsular collection, as well as with a delayed nephrogram in the affected kidney compared to the contralateral normal kidney. Though secondary hypertension is the most common clinical feature of Page kidney, in settings of diseased contralateral kidney, unilateral kidney, or renal allograft, mass effect by a subcapsular hematoma can manifest as renal insufficiency. Treatment options include percutaneous drainage of a chronic subcapsular hematoma [1].

On the 2018 AAST Kidney Injury Scale, non-expanding subcapsular hematoma has been omitted from the imaging criteria, as it is uncommon to capture hematoma expansion during the short interval between phases on the initial trauma CT [20].

Perirenal hematoma will typically appear as a poorly marginated, hyperattenuating fluid collection (45–90 HU),

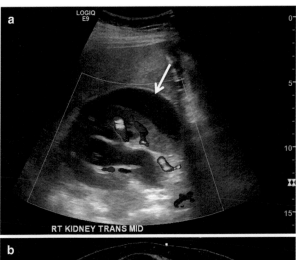

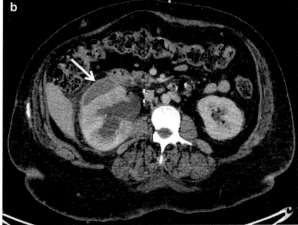

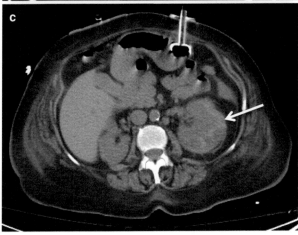

**Fig. 1** **Subcapsular hematoma (AAST grade 1 injury) on ultrasound, contrast-enhanced CT (CECT), and non-enhanced CT (NECT).** (**a**) Transverse color Doppler ultrasound image through the mid-right kidney demonstrates a crescentic hypoechoic subcapsular hematoma (white arrow) along the anterior margin of the kidney. Note concurrent moderate hydronephrosis. (**b**) Subsequent axial portal venous CECT image shows a corresponding hypodense subcapsular hematoma (white arrow). The right kidney is asymmetrically enlarged with moderate hydronephrosis. (**c**) Axial NECT image from a different patient shows a crescentic subcapsular hematoma along the anterolateral aspect of the left kidney, which is heterogeneously hyperdense (white arrow) relative to the unenhanced left renal parenchyma. In all cases, note the associated mass effect with deformation and flattening of the underlying renal contour.

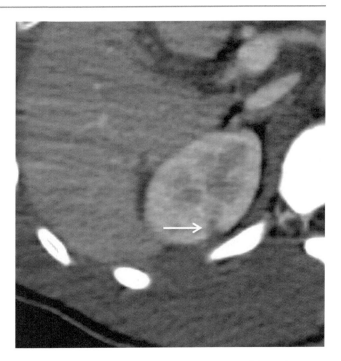

**Fig. 2** **Renal laceration (AAST grade 2 Injury).** Axial portal venous-phase CECT image shows a 0.5 cm linear hypoattenuating laceration (white arrow) in the posterior right renal cortex, which does not extend into the renal collecting system, consistent with a grade 2 injury comprised of a small parenchymal laceration

located between the renal parenchyma and Gerota's fascia [15]. While subcapsular hematomas are often well defined and extend along the contour of the kidney, perirenal hematomas usually have ill-defined margins, implying violation of the renal capsule, and they usually do not exert mass effect on the renal parenchymal contour [2, 3, 15]. Perirenal hematomas may occur in isolation but most often occur alongside renal lacerations and/or vascular injury [3]. Associated findings may include thickening of the lateroconal fascia, mass effect on the adjacent colon, and displacement of the kidney depending on the size and extension of the hematoma [4]. The term "non-expanding" from perirenal hematoma has been removed from the imaging criteria on the 2018 revision of the AAST Kidney Injury Scale, as it is less likely to see hematoma expansion between phases on the initial trauma scan [20].

Deliberate assessment for low attenuation perinephric fluid on the initial trauma CECT is important, as this may indicate urine spillage related to a traumatic collecting system injury, and would therefore constitute a higher-grade injury (at least grade 4). If there is concern for disruption of the renal collecting system, delayed images during the excretory phase can be obtained to assess for spillage of excreted contrast material from the renal collecting system (Fig. 4) [2, 3].

Lacerations typically appear as an irregular, linear, or branching non-enhancing hypoattenuating area (Fig. 2) [2, 3, 15]. In lower-grade injuries, normally enhancing renal parenchyma is typically seen between the deepest margin of the laceration and the renal collecting system. However, if there is ambiguity regarding laceration extension into the renal collecting system, delayed excretory-phase CT images can be obtained to ensure that there is no spillage of excreted contrast material from the collecting system, a finding which would indicate disruption of the collecting system and would correspond with a high-grade renal injury (at least grade 4) [3].

Vascular injuries include pseudoaneurysm and AVF, both of which can appear as a focal collection of vascular contrast material that decreases in attenuation on delayed imaging, without change in morphology between phases of imaging [2, 3, 20]. Pseudoaneurysms are typically well-circumscribed round or ovoid contrast-filled abnormalities that follow arterial blood pool, showing prominent contrast filling on arterial-phase images and diminished contrast on delayed images. AVFs may be associated with early contrast filling and increased diameter of the renal vein. In many cases, however, it can be difficult to differentiate between a pseudoaneurysm and AVF by CT [2, 3]. Moreover, these two entities can coexist in rare occasions [21]. Renal infarctions typically appear as sharply demarcated, wedge-shaped areas of non-enhancing hypoattenuation on delayed images (Fig. 6), whereas contusions are generally less well-defined areas of hypoattenuation and can show enhancement on delayed images [1].

Active bleeding appears as irregular or amorphous extravascular contrast that increases in area and changes morphology with each subsequent phase of imaging. On arterial-phase CT images, active extravasation will appear as a patchy area of extravascular contrast with similar attenuation as the aorta (85–370 HU; mean 132 HU) [1–3, 20]. Active bleeding when contained within Gerota's fascia is classified as a grade 3 injury (Fig. 3), while active bleeding beyond Gerota's fascia is considered a Grade 4 injury (Fig. 5).

Collecting system involvement can be inferred from either a laceration that appears to extend to or through the calyces or renal pelvis or from the presence of low attenuating perirenal fluid centered around the renal hilum on arterial, portal venous, or split-bolus images within the standard trauma CECT protocol; additional delayed (excretory-phase) imaging must be obtained to assess for spillage of excreted contrast material into the perirenal space (Fig. 4) [1, 4, 15].

Isolated renal pelvis injuries are uncommon but, when they occur, can appear as nonspecific low-density fluid adjacent to the renal pelvis with an otherwise normal-appearing kidney on the standard trauma CECT images, highlighting the importance of obtaining delayed (excretory-phase) CT images when free fluid is present adjacent to the ureteropelvic junction (UPJ). On delayed images, normal excretion of contrast within the renal

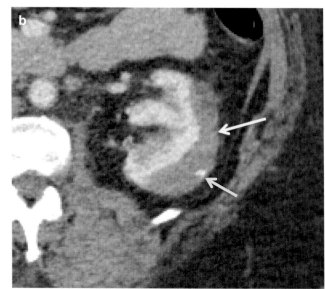

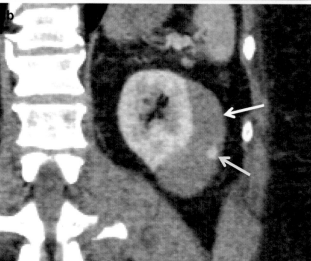

**Fig. 3** **Subcapsular hematoma with active extravasation within Gerota's fascia (AAST grade 3 injury).** Axial (**a**) and coronal (**b**) late arterial-phase CECT images demonstrate a large hypodense left renal subcapsular hematoma (white arrow). A hyperattenuating focus in the lateral aspect of the subcapsular hematoma represents active extravasation (yellow arrow) contained within Gerota's fascia. The presence of active bleeding differentiates this injury from a grade 1 subcapsular hematoma without active bleeding

calyces with spillage of excreted contrast material from the collecting system indicates a UPJ tear or laceration. This spillage characteristically occurs along the medial aspect of the kidney, but circumferential extension of contrast can also be seen. Differentiation between complete and partial UPJ tears is important, as this distinction changes management. Spillage of excreted contrast from the collecting system, with maintained contrast filling of the ipsilateral ureter distal to the site of injury, is diagnostic of a partial tear. Spillage of excreted contrast from the collecting system with failure of the downstream ipsilateral

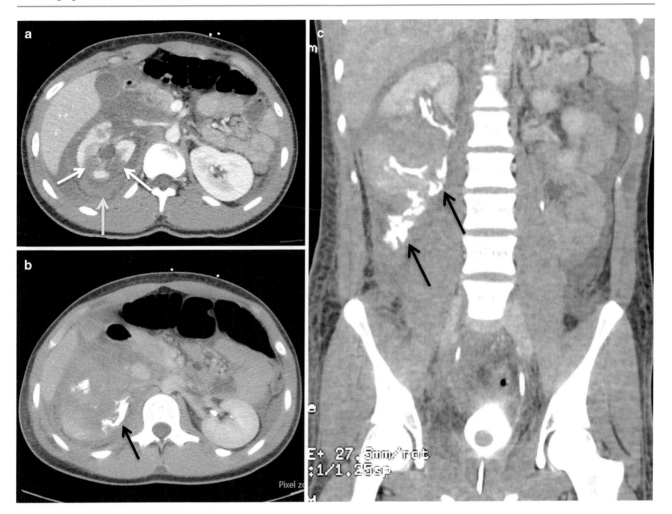

**Fig. 4** Spillage of urine and excreted contrast following traumatic laceration of the renal pelvis (AAST grade 4 injury). (a) Axial arterial-phase CECT image reveals two lacerations extending through the posterior right renal cortex and medulla to the renal pelvis (white arrows), with hyperdense perinephric hematoma posteriorly (yellow arrow), and moderate volume hypoattenuating perinephric fluid surrounding the kidney and extending to both paracolic gutters. Axial (b) and coronal (c) delayed (excretory-phase) CT images show spillage of high-density excreted contrast material into the perirenal space (black arrows), confirming laceration of the renal collecting system

ureter to fill with excreted contrast should raise suspicion for a complete tear. Partial tears can often be treated conservatively with stent placement, while complete tears require surgical repair [2, 4] (Figs. 5 and 6).

Shattered kidney refers to fracturing or fragmentation of the kidney due to severe extensive lacerations, resulting in loss of identifiable parenchymal renal anatomy (Fig. 7) [2, 4]. Distinction between multiple lower-grade lacerations and shattered kidney is subjective, yet the term *shattered kidney* should be reserved for severe tissue destruction that would preclude any meaningful healing and may include devascularized parenchyma, injury to the collecting system, and severe vascular damage with active arterial bleeding [3]. Devitalized regions may not be readily apparent by CT when there is extensive surrounding hematoma [4].

Renal pedicle trauma fortunately is uncommon but is often associated with injuries to other organs [4]. Renal pedicle injury occurs in up to 5% of all renal traumas, although main renal artery injury is even less common, reported in one study by Sangthong et al. to occur in 0.05% of blunt trauma admissions [2–4, 22]. Laceration of the main renal vessels is often associated with large retroperitoneal hematoma and active hemorrhage, warranting emergent surgical intervention [3]. It is important to note, however, that perinephric hematomas are not always large in the setting of renal hilar lacerations [2]. Hematoma located between the aorta and the injured kidney should raise suspicion for renal pedicle injury (Fig. 8) [15]. In patients with large hematomas precluding adequate evaluation of the renal hilar vessels on the initial trauma CECT, further evaluation with CT angiography, CT venography,

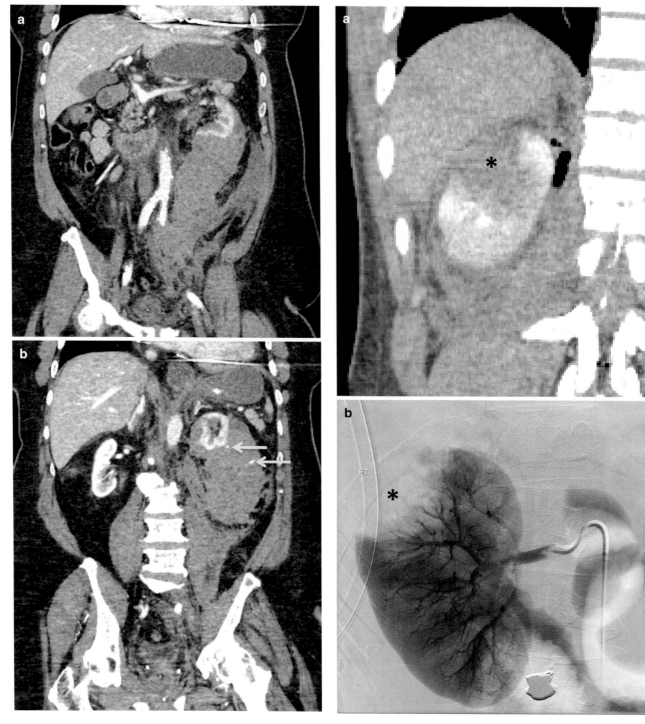

**Fig. 5 Active hemorrhage beyond Gerota's fascia (AAST grade 4 injury).** Coronal arterial-phase CT images show (**a**) a large left perinephric hematoma extending beyond Gerota's fascia into the retroperitoneal space, including the left paracolic gutter and pelvis, and (**b**) at least two high density foci of contrast extravasation within the hematoma representing active bleeding (yellow arrows)

**Fig. 6 Segmental renal infarct without active bleeding status post gunshot wound (AAST grade 4 injury).** (**a**) Coronal CECT image shows a wedge-shaped region of non-enhancing parenchyma in the upper pole of the right kidney (*) and small volume perinephric hemorrhage and stranding. No active extravasation is seen, in keeping with segmental artery injury and thrombosis resulting in segmental infarct. (**b**) Selective right renal artery digital subtraction angiography of the same patient confirms the presence of upper pole infarction without active hemorrhage

or conventional angiography may be considered for diagnosis and management, contingent upon hemodynamic stability [2].

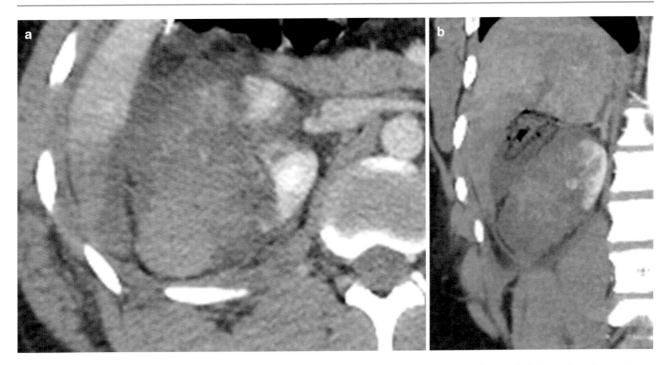

**Fig. 7** **Shattered kidney (AAST grade 5 injury).** (**a**) Axial and (**b**) coronal portal venous-phase CT images show fragmented discontinuous enhancement of the medial renal parenchyma with essentially non-enhancement of the remaining poorly delineated renal parenchyma. A small amount of perinephric and perihepatic fluid is present

In some cases, renal pedicle vascular injury results in devascularization of the entire kidney, although in some cases areas of maintained perfusion may be seen. In contrast to grade 4 devascularization, which results from vascular thrombosis and does not involve active bleeding, traumatic devascularization as a result of pedicular injury with active bleeding constitutes a grade 5 kidney injury [2, 3, 20]. Laceration of the main renal vessels with devascularization of the entire renal parenchyma usually requires emergent nephrectomy, although select rare cases may be amenable to renovascular repair [2, 3, 23].

## Management

Nonoperative management has become the preferred treatment pathway for the majority of blunt renal injuries [5, 7, 14, 24, 25]. This strategy preserves renal function without increasing complication rates [14] and has been reported to be successful in over 80% of cases [26–28], including high-grade injuries in the hemodynamically stable patient. Penetrating renal injuries also are often managed nonoperatively with success [3, 6].

Improved capabilities for close hemodynamic monitoring and advances in diagnostic, endoscopic, and endovascular techniques have made possible the contemporary multidisciplinary management of traumatic renal injuries. Grade 1 and 2 injuries are treated conservatively with observation, bed rest, hydration, serial hematocrit monitoring, and antibiotics. Similarly, expectant management is favored for grade 3 and 4 injuries, while management of grade 5 injuries is more controversial. Importantly, as recommended by the American Urological Association (AUA) guidelines [7], an initial trial of nonoperative management is feasible regardless of injury grade, as long as the patient is hemodynamically stable.

For high-grade injuries involving vascular and/or collecting system injuries, adjunct endovascular and endoscopic management are key to the success of nonoperative management. Angiography with possible selective distal embolization is indicated in stable patients with active extravasation, contained vascular injuries, or nonself-limiting gross hematuria [7, 14, 29]. Additional imaging features, including large (>3.5 cm) or expanding perirenal hematoma, medial parenchymal lacerations, and disruption of Gerota's fascia, may predict the need for angioembolization [7, 30–34]. While repeat intervention may be necessary, angioembolization was shown to eliminate the need for nephrectomy in >75% of high-grade injuries [35, 36]. For renal artery injuries with thrombosis or dissection, endovascular stenting can be attempted promptly after injury, although success rate may be low [24, 29]. Renal

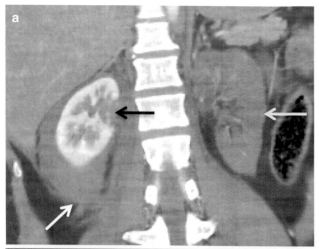

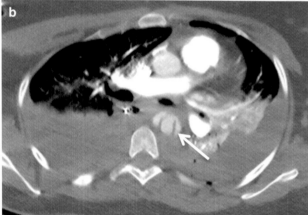

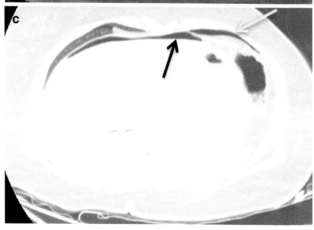

**Fig. 8 Hilar avulsion (AAST grade 5 injury). (a)** Coronal CECT image shows complete devascularization of the left kidney (yellow arrow) due to hilar avulsion. There is no substantial fluid or hematoma around the devascularized left kidney (yellow arrow). Rather, there is a small amount of hematoma between the left kidney and the aorta, which should raise suspicion for a pedicle injury in the setting of a devascularized kidney. Notice the grade 4 type injury of the right kidney with parenchymal laceration (black arrow) and more substantial surrounding hematoma (white arrow) extending beyond Gerota's fascia. High-grade renal injuries, particularly renal pedicle injuries, are associated with polytrauma within the abdomen. **(b)** Axial arterial-phase CECT image shows acute traumatic injury to the descending thoracic aorta (white arrow). **(c)** Axial CECT image in lung window at the thoracoabdominal junction shows a left basilar pneumothorax (yellow arrow) and pneumoperitoneum (black arrow)

vein injuries are usually associated with extensive bleeding and may be better treated surgically.

Surgical exploration aims at early vascular control and renal salvage via renovascular repair, renorrhaphy (primary repair of laceration and/or collecting system injury), or partial nephrectomy [5, 37], although nephrectomy rate still approaches 64% with this approach [25, 35]. Immediate surgical intervention is predominantly indicated for the hemodynamic unstable patient with absent or only transient response to resuscitation. Absolute indications for surgical exploration include persistent potentially life-threatening hemorrhage with renal pedicle avulsion (grade 5 injury), expanding, pulsatile, or uncontained retroperitoneal hematoma, and renal vein injury without self-limiting hemorrhage [5, 14]. Grade 3 and 4 injuries with significant devitalized parenchyma or coexisting pancreatic or bowel injuries [6] may also benefit from open repair, while delayed surgical exploration is indicated for patients who fail nonoperative management or angioembolization, UPJ injury or persistent urinoma not amenable to endoscopic or percutaneous treatment, and patients who develop severe refractory renovascular hypertension.

## Ureteral Trauma

### Epidemiology

Ureteral injury usually occurs as a result of penetrating trauma, most frequently from ballistic trauma. As a result, ureteral injuries often occur with concurrent intra-abdominal injuries. Ureteral injury as a sequela of blunt or external trauma is very uncommon. In the rare setting of blunt ureteral injury, the most common injury site is near the UPJ. It is important to note that hematuria is an unreliable predictor of ureteral injury, highlighting the importance of imaging for identifying this diagnosis [38, 39].

### AAST Ureteral Injury Scale and Imaging Findings

The AAST Ureteral Injury Scale is largely based on operative findings, and while there have been substantial improvements in MDCT, grading of ureteral injuries is still informed by findings at surgery in many cases. According to the AAST Ureteral Injury Scale, injuries are graded from 1 to 5, 1 being the least severe and 5 being the most severe (Table 2) [40].

Stranding or fluid along the course of the ureter without other identifiable injury on the initial trauma CECT, particularly in the setting of hematuria, may indicate a ureteral injury (though notably hematuria does not have to be

**Table 2** AAST ureteral injury scale

| AAST grade | Type of injury | Description of injury |
| --- | --- | --- |
| 1 | Hematoma | Contusion or hematoma without devascularization |
| 2 | Laceration | <50% transection |
| 3 | Laceration | >/=50% transection |
| 4 | Laceration | Complete transection with <2 cm of devascularization |
| 5 | Laceration | Avulsion with >2 cm of devascularization |

Advance one grade for bilateral injuries, up to grade 3
https://www.aast.org/resources-detail/injury-scoring-scale#ureter

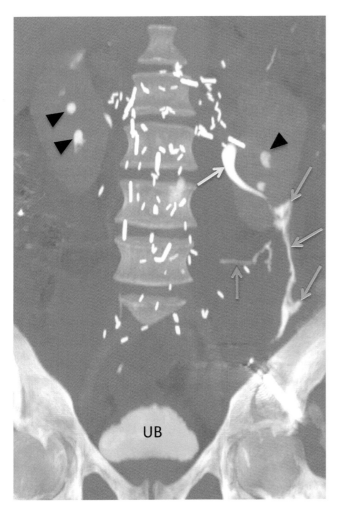

**Fig. 9 Left ureteral laceration.** Coronal delayed-phase MIP image shows excreted contrast material within the renal collecting systems bilaterally (black arrowheads), left ureter (yellow arrow), and urinary bladder (UB). Irregular amorphous contrast is seen extending from the proximal left ureter into the left lateral abdomen (blue arrows), representing contrast leakage secondary to traumatic left ureteral laceration. Notice surgical changes of initial damage-control surgery (DCS) performed prior to CT evaluation, including numerous surgical clips in the central abdomen, and bowel suture material (green arrow) in the left mid abdomen. Ureteral injury was not identified at the time of DCS

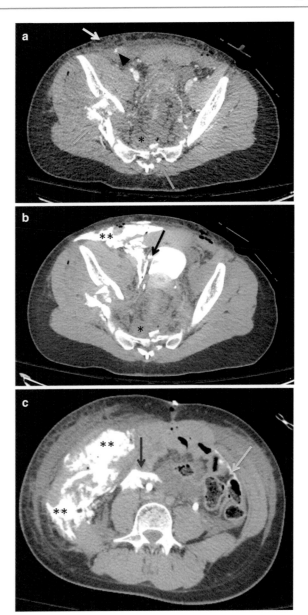

**Fig. 10 UB rupture with combined IP and complex EP components (RCS grade 5 injury). (a)** Axial image from initial trauma CECT shows focal contrast blush within the anterior right pelvic wall (black arrowhead). Overlying subcutaneous fat stranding in the anterior pelvic wall in a seat belt-type configuration (yellow arrow) with acute comminuted fractures of the right iliac bone (blue arrow) and sacrum (green arrow) indicate substantial trauma to the pelvis. Notice concurrent nonspecific fluid in the pelvis, including within the presacral space (*). **(b, c)** Subsequent axial CT cystogram images show leakage of high-density instilled contrast material from a defect in the right lateral aspect of the UB (black arrow) into the EP space and anterior pelvic wall (**), representing complex EP rupture of the UB. This contrast solution extends into the region of active bleeding within the anterior pelvic wall, as seen on initial CECT. If the initial CECT and subsequent CT cystogram had been combined into one examination, the area of active bleeding within the right anterior wall would have been obscured by contrast solution extending from the UB, highlighting the importance of performing separate evaluations. The fluid within the presacral space remains unopacified and represents hematoma (*) related to pelvic fractures. In the upper abdomen, contrast material is seen within the IP space centrally (purple arrow) and along loops of bowel in the left anterior abdomen (orange arrow), indicating concurrent IP rupture of UB

present). In cases of suspected ureteral injury, delayed CT images can be obtained (without administration of additional contrast) from the kidneys though the urinary bladder (UB) to assess for spillage of excreted contrast material (Fig. 9). It is important to note that acquisition of these delayed CT images for the purpose of identifying a ureteral injury should not be combined with dedicated protocols meant for assessing UB injury or bowel injury, both of which also require the use of high-density intraluminal contrast. Combining these protocols can cause diagnostic confusion as to the source of extraluminal free contrast material.

## UB Trauma

## Epidemiology

UB injuries are relatively uncommon though when they occur, the majority are a result of blunt trauma (60–85%), as compared to penetrating trauma (15–40%). The most common mechanisms of injury include motor vehicle collisions and sports-related injuries, although falls, crush injuries, and other types of trauma involving the pelvis can also result in UB injury [41, 42]. Pelvic fractures are present in approximately 80–97% of cases. In particular, fractures of the pubic rami and diastasis of the pubic symphysis have the highest correlation with UB injury, although sacral fractures, iliac fractures, and sacroiliac joint diastasis are also correlated to a lesser degree [41, 43, 44]. Mortality in patients with UB injury can be as high as 44%. However, cause of death usually is attributed to other concurrent injuries rather than the UB injury itself [44, 45]. Still, delays in diagnosis can increase morbidity and mortality as a result of uremia, sepsis, peritonitis, and metabolic imbalances secondary to peritoneal resorption of urine or development of fistulas [41].

Hematuria, the most common indicator of injury to the urinary tract, can be absent in the presence of traumatic injury. Additionally, the presence of hematuria does not indicate site of injury, which may be anywhere along the urinary tract, and, furthermore, multifocal injuries can occur. Consideration of mechanism of injury, the presence of pelvic fractures or diastases, and the presence of gross or substantial microscopic hematuria (>25 RBCs/HPF) should raise suspicion for UB injury, especially in the presence of urinary symptoms including inability to void or suprapubic pain [41]. CT cystogram also can be used to differentiate stranding or indeterminate fluid in the pelvis related to UB injury from other considerations such as fluid tracking from solid organ injuries in the upper abdomen, bowel injury, pelvic hematoma secondary to bony pelvis injuries, vascular injuries,

physiologic fluid as can be seen in premenopausal women, and nontraumatic fluid related to fluid resuscitation.

## Diagnostic Investigations

Dedicated CT cystogram has largely replaced radiography and fluoroscopic cystography in the evaluation for suspected UB injury in the acute setting and can be performed immediately following an initial trauma CECT protocol. It is important to note that CT cystogram should not be combined with the initial CECT, as this may cause diagnostic confusion or missed diagnoses of concurrent injuries (Fig. 10). The presence of pelvic fractures or diastases on initial pelvic radiograph(s) or on initial trauma protocol CECT, hematuria, or suspicious mechanism of injury should prompt performance of a CT cystogram, ideally while the patient is still at the CT scanner following the initial trauma CECT, minimizing movement of a patient with pelvic fractures and expediting diagnosis (Fig. 11).

Prior to performing a CT cystogram, assessment for urethral injury must be performed before Foley catheter placement. Failure to assess for urethral injury may worsen existing partial urethral tears and can transform partial tears (involving a portion of the urethral circumference) into full-thickness tears (complete urethral disruption with laceration across the entire urethral circumference). Partial urethral disruption usually is managed conservatively with a Foley catheter, while complete urethral disruption can involve a suprapubic catheter for 2 months followed by urethral reconstruction and carries increased risk of urethral stricture. Thus, avoidance of this potential complication is rather critical. Blood at the meatus or inability to void may indicate urethral injury [41]. Blood at the meatus is seen in 75% of anterior urethral injuries and in 37–97% of posterior urethral tears [44]. In cases of suspected urethral injury, retrograde urethrography (RUG) may be indicated. Alternatively, in select clinical scenarios, a catheter can be placed across a suspected urethral injury with the guidance of a scope [41].

Once the Foley catheter is in place, the UB must be drained prior to instilling a 3–5% solution of water-soluble contrast in normal saline. Failure to drain the UB reduces sensitivity for the detection of injuries due to poor visualization of wall irregularities along the margin of unopacified urine. Additionally, mixing instilled contrast with urine within an undrained UB results in overall reduced density of intraluminal contents on CT and may cause ambiguity in the origin of free fluid of intermediate density [41].

The contrast solution must be instilled under gravity by placing the saline bag above the patient and allowing the UB to fill, ideally to a volume of at least 350 cc. Contrast solution

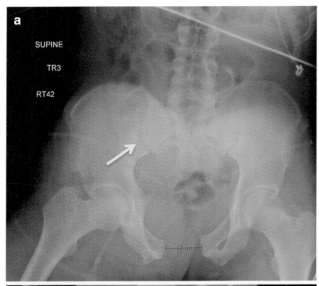

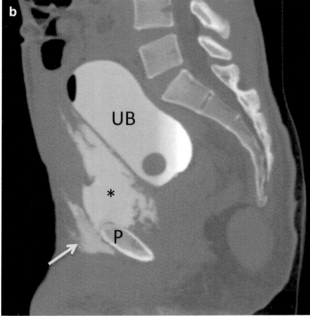

**Fig. 11 Complex EP UB rupture (RCS grade 4b injury).** (a) Initial pelvic radiograph shows 4.7 cm diastasis of the pubic symphysis and asymmetric right sacroiliac joint widening (yellow arrow), which are commonly seen in the setting of UB trauma. (b) Subsequent sagittal CT cystogram image (in bone window and level settings) shows extraluminal contrast material in the prevesical space (*) which extends anterior to the pubis (p) and into the anterior pelvic wall (yellow arrow), representing an RCS grade 4b UB injury

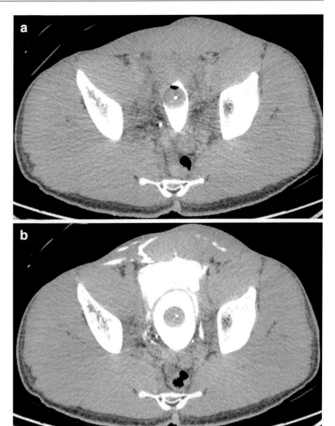

**Fig. 12 Complex EP UB rupture (RCS grade 4b injury).** (a) Axial delayed-phase image, obtained after initial trauma CECT, shows antegrade partial filling of the UB with excreted IV contrast material from the initial CECT. No contrast leakage is elicited due to inadequate UB distension. (b) Subsequent dedicated CT cystogram image at the same level shows greater distension of the UB from retrograde instillation of high-density contrast solution. There is extraluminal leakage into the prevesical space in a "molar tooth" configuration, with further extension into the anterior pelvic wall, representing an RCS grade 4b UB injury, which was not elicited with antegrade filling of the UB

should not be manually pushed through the Foley catheter, as this may cause or worsen an existing injury. If the patient is unable to tolerate 350 cc or reports pain which is worse than the expected discomfort of UB fullness, the drip should be stopped. Infusions greater than 250 cc still have reasonable sensitivity for the detection of UB injuries, but infusions of less than 250 cc are suboptimal, and this limitation should be taken into consideration during image interpretation [41]. Antegrade filling of the UB by excreted IV contrast from the initial trauma CECT must not be used as a replacement for CT cystography, as this will not adequately distend the UB and thus will have inadequate sensitivity for the detection of UB injuries (Fig. 12) [41].

Once the UB is adequately distended, images should be acquired from the iliac crests through the femoral lesser trochanters to include the entire perineum at 0.5–1.0 mm slice thickness. Sagittal and coronal reconstructions can be created at 3–5 mm slice thickness. Thinner reformats can be produced in select cases with ambiguous findings on standard reconstructions. Image width and level settings should be adjusted to optimally visualize the UB wall and

**Table 3** AAST UB injury scale

| Injury grade | Injury type | Description |
|---|---|---|
| 1 | Hematoma<br>Laceration | UB wall thickening related to contusion or intramural hematoma<br>Partial thickness tear |
| 2 | Laceration | EP (<2 cm) UB wall laceration |
| 3 | Laceration | EP (≥2 cm) or IP (<2 cm) UB wall laceration |
| 4 | Laceration | IP (≥2 cm) UB wall laceration |
| 5 | Laceration | IP or EP UB wall laceration extending into the UB neck or ureteral orifice (trigone) |

Adapted from The American Association for the Surgery of Trauma (AAST):
Moore et al. [47]
Note: Advance one grade for multiple injuries up to grade III

**Table 4** RCS for traumatic UB injury

| Injury grade | Injury description | Imaging findings |
|---|---|---|
| 1 | UB contusion | Usually normal CT appearance<br>When detectable, mild focal wall thickening may be seen |
| 2 | IP UB rupture | Contrast leak into the IP space |
| 3 | Interstitial injury | Wall irregularity related to intramural blood and extension of contrast though a defect in the mucosal layer of the UB wall without transmural extension |
| 4 | EP UB rupture | |
| 4a | Simple | Simple: Contrast leakage confined to the EP intrapelvic space |
| 4b | Complex | Complex: Dispersion of extraluminal contrast into the anterior abdominal wall, penis, scrotum, and/or perineum |
| 5 | Combined IP and EP UB rupture | Findings of both type 2 and type 4 injuries |

Adapted from Sandler et al. [46]

its contents. Settings that approach bone window (window width 2000 and window level 300) are especially useful for identifying abnormalities which may be missed on standard soft tissue window settings due to the high density of instilled contrast solution. Post-drainage images are not required in evaluation for suspected traumatic UB injury [41]. In contradistinction, conventional radiographic or fluoroscopic cystography require post-drainage images to elucidate contrast spillage that otherwise may be obscured by the superimposed contrast distended UB.

## AAST UB Injury Scale Versus Radiologic Classification System (RCS)

While trauma surgeons and urologists may use the AAST UB Injury Scale (Table 3) to classify UB injuries, it is important to note that the criteria for each grade are based on surgical or endoscopic findings rather than radiologic findings and include size criteria for lacerations. Due to the spherical shape of the UB, variations in UB distension at CT cystography, and often poor visualization of lacerations themselves, measurement of lacerations is often not

accurate by imaging alone, and most centers utilize the radiologic classification system (RCS) developed by Sandler et al. (Table 4) to grade UB injuries by CT [41, 44, 46, 47].

Though both classification systems grade UB injuries from 1 to 5, it is important to note that grading by the RCS does not translate equivalently to grading by the AAST scale, in that each grade does not indicate the same injuries. Thus, clear communication with the clinical team is paramount, and descriptions of UB injuries should specify which scale is being used (in most cases RCS) and include specific details regarding of the injuries identified, including the site of injury and whether there is IP and/or extraperitoneal (EP) leakage of instilled contrast (Figs. 13, 14, 15, and 16).

## RCS and Imaging Findings

According to the RCS, a grade 1 injury refers to a contusion of the UB wall, which can have a normal appearance on imaging. A grade 2 injury refers to an IP tear or rupture, resulting in spillage of instilled contrast material into the IP space (Figs. 13 and 14). A grade 3 injury is an interstitial injury involving the UB wall without complete

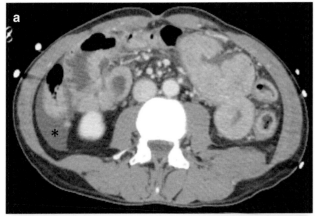

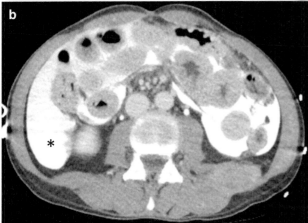

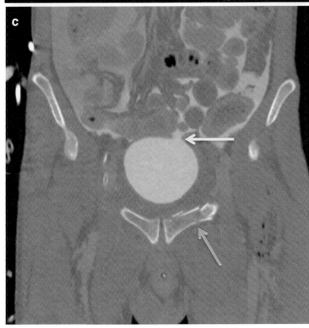

**Fig. 13 IP UB rupture (RCS grade 2 injury). (a)** Axial image through the mid-abdomen from the initial trauma CECT shows nonspecific fluid within the right paracolic gutter (*) and interdigitating between loops of bowel in the IP space. **(b)** Corresponding subsequent axial CT cystogram image at the same level shows new high-density fluid within the right paracolic gutter (*) and throughout the IP space. **(c)** Coronal CT cystogram image shows a defect in the left UB dome, representing the site of laceration (yellow arrow). Notice the fracture of the left superior pubic ramus (blue arrow)

laceration (Fig. 15). A grade 4a injury is a simple EP tear or rupture, in which spilled contrast is confined to the perivesical space (Fig. 16), while a grade 4b injury is a complex EP injury, with contrast extending into the retroperitoneal space, abdominal wall, scrotum, or penis (Fig. 11). A grade 5 injury involves both IP and EP tears.

## Management

Partial thickness injuries (RCS type 1 and 3 injuries) are treated conservatively with urethral Foley catheterization. EP ruptures (RCS type 4 injury) often are treated conservatively with urethral Foley catheterization, although surgical repair may be indicated with large or complex EP lacerations, nonhealing lacerations after a trial of conservative management, and cases complicated by puncture from bone fragments, concurrent rectal or vaginal laceration, or UB neck injury. UB ruptures with an IP component (RCS type 2 and 5 injures) typically require surgical repair of the UB defect with diverting vesicostomy [41]. In cases of EP rupture, it is essential to assess carefully for an IP component, as this would change the RCS grade from grade 4 to grade 5 and also would change management.

## Conclusion

Traumatic injuries to the genitourinary tract are routinely diagnosed using diagnostic imaging, with most centers using CECT as the mainstay for diagnosis but with ultrasound, CEUS, MRI, and cystography as adjunct modalities for initial screening, troubleshooting, and follow-up. These injuries are classified based on location, injury pattern, and severity. Commonly used grading systems allow for efficient communication between radiologists and clinical providers and can inform management decisions without surgical exploration in many patients.

### Key Points
- Approximately 10% of abdominal trauma cases involve genitourinary injuries, with renal injury being the most frequent. Renal and UB injuries are most commonly a result of blunt trauma, whereas ureteral injuries are most commonly the result of penetrating trauma.
- Hematuria, though the most common indicator of injury to the genitourinary tract, is not a reliable predictor and does not indicate site of injury, which may be anywhere along the genitourinary tract. The role of imaging has become standard in the diagnosis and grading of genitourinary injuries and may involve a combination of an initial

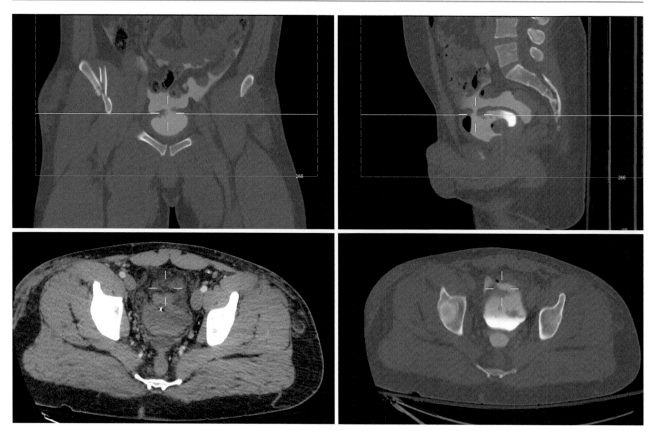

**Fig. 14 UB dome rupture.** Coronal and sagittal reconstructions from CT cystogram (top left and top right) clearly show a defect in the UB dome at midline (yellow crosshairs) through which instilled contrast is leaking into the IP space. This defect is less apparent on an axial CT cystogram image (bottom right), as the laceration is oriented in the axial plane. Irregularities in this region may be confused for debris or clot within the UB, and the defect itself is not definitively apparent. Corresponding axial image from initial trauma CECT (bottom left) shows nonspecific stranding within the pelvis

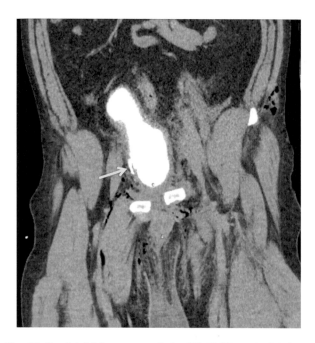

**Fig. 15 Partial-thickness tear of the UB (RCS grade 3 injury).** Coronal reconstruction from CT cystogram shows instilled contrast solution extending into the thickened UB wall (yellow arrow) without extending into the IP or EP spaces, representing a partial-thickness tear with intact serosa

trauma CECT protocol followed by delayed-phase CT imaging, CT cystogram, and/or RUG, depending on the site of suspected injury.

- CECT is the imaging modality of choice in the assessment of acute traumatic injury to the kidney, with most centers using either conventional dual-phase trauma protocol CECT or a single-pass split-bolus technique. Delayed-phase CT imaging can provide additional information regarding injuries to the renal collecting system and ureters. CT cystogram is used to evaluate for suspected UB injury.

- The 2018 revision of the AAST Renal Injury Scale includes dedicated CT criteria for grading kidney injuries and more comprehensively incorporates renal vascular injury. Grade 1 and 2 injuries are low-grade injuries and are usually treated conservatively, while grade 4 and 5 injuries are high grade, with a larger proportion requiring intervention. Grade 3 injuries, previously considered low grade prior to the 2018 revision, now include vascular injuries, which may require intervention in some cases.

- Though the AAST Organ Injury Scale is commonly used to stratify traumatic injuries of many intra-abdominal

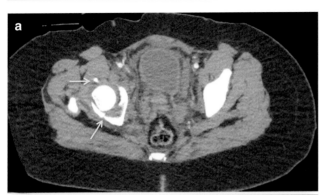

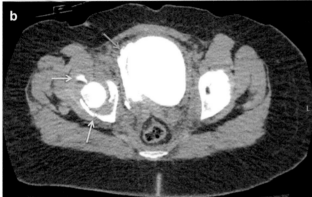

**Fig. 16** **Simple EP UB rupture (RCS grade 4a injury).** (**a**) Axial image from initial CECT shows nonspecific fat stranding and fluid within the pelvis. Notice the right acetabular fracture partially within the field of view (yellow arrows). (**b**) Axial image from subsequent CT cystogram shows leakage of instilled high-density contrast solution into the right perivesical space (blue arrow), creating a partial "molar tooth" configuration. There is no extension of leaked contrast solution beyond the intrapelvic EP space

organs, image-based grading of UB injuries is performed using the RCS. Pelvic fractures are highly correlated with UB injuries.

# References

1. Kawashima A, Sandler CM, Corl FM, et al. Imaging of renal trauma: a comprehensive review. Radiographics. 2001;21(3):557–74. https://doi.org/10.1148/radiographics.21.3.g01ma11557.
2. Hosein M, Paskar D, Kodama R, Ditkofsky N. Coming together: a review of the American Association for the Surgery of Trauma's updated kidney injury scale to facilitate multidisciplinary management. AJR Am J Roentgenol. 2019;213(5):1091–9. https://doi.org/10.2214/AJR.19.21486.
3. Chien LC, Vakil M, Nguyen J, et al. The American Association for the Surgery of Trauma Organ Injury Scale 2018 update for computed tomography-based grading of renal trauma: a primer for the emergency radiologist. Emerg Radiol. 2020;27(1):63–73. https://doi.org/10.1007/s10140-019-01721-z.
4. Alonso RC, Nacenta SB, Martinez PD, Guerrero AS, Fuentes CG. Kidney in danger: CT findings of blunt and penetrating renal trauma. Radiographics. 2009;29(7):2033–53. https://doi.org/10.1148/rg.297095071.
5. Santucci RA, Wessells H, Bartsch G, et al. Evaluation and management of renal injuries: consensus statement of the renal trauma subcommittee. BJU Int. 2004;93(7):937–54. https://doi.org/10.1111/j.1464-4096.2004.04820.x.
6. Chouhan JD, Winer AG, Johnson C, Weiss JP, Hyacinthe LM. Contemporary evaluation and management of renal trauma. Can J Urol. 2016;2016:7.
7. Morey AF, Brandes S, Dugi DD, et al. Urotrauma: AUA guideline. J Urol. 2014;192(2):327–35. https://doi.org/10.1016/j.juro.2014.05.004.
8. Hall FM. Single-pass continuous whole-body CT for polytrauma. Am J Roentgenol. 2009;193(2):594. https://doi.org/10.2214/AJR.09.2328.
9. Ptak T, Rhea JT, Novelline RA. Radiation dose is reduced with a single-pass whole-body multi-detector row CT trauma protocol compared with a conventional segmented method: initial experience. Radiology. 2003;229(3):902–5. https://doi.org/10.1148/radiol.2293021651.
10. Jeavons C, Hacking C, Beenen LF, Gunn ML. A review of split-bolus single-pass CT in the assessment of trauma patients. Emerg Radiol. 2018;25(4):367–74. https://doi.org/10.1007/s10140-018-1591-1.
11. Leung V, Sastry A, Woo TD, Jones HR. Implementation of a split-bolus single-pass CT protocol at a UK major trauma centre to reduce excess radiation dose in trauma pan-CT. Clin Radiol. 2015;70(10):1110–5. https://doi.org/10.1016/j.crad.2015.05.014.
12. Soto JA, Anderson SW. Multidetector CT of blunt abdominal trauma. Radiology. 2012;265(3):678–93. https://doi.org/10.1148/radiol.12120354.
13. Miele V, Piccolo CL, Galluzzo M, Ianniello S, Sessa B, Trinci M. Contrast-enhanced ultrasound (CEUS) in blunt abdominal trauma. Br J Radiol. 2016;89(1061):20150823. https://doi.org/10.1259/bjr.20150823.
14. Panel W-AE, Coccolini F, Moore EE, et al. Kidney and uro-trauma: WSES-AAST guidelines. World J Emerg Surg. 2019;14(1):54. https://doi.org/10.1186/s13017-019-0274-x.
15. Lee YJ, Oh SN, Rha SE, Byun JY. Renal trauma. Radiol Clin N Am. 2007;45(3):581–92, ix. https://doi.org/10.1016/j.rcl.2007.04.004.
16. Breen KJ, Sweeney P, Nicholson PJ, Kiely EA, O'Brien MF. Adult blunt renal trauma: routine follow-up imaging is excessive. Urology. 2014;84(1):62–7. https://doi.org/10.1016/j.urology.2014.03.013.
17. Bukur M, Inaba K, Barmparas G, et al. Routine follow-up imaging of kidney injuries may not be justified. J Trauma. 2011;70(5):1229–33. https://doi.org/10.1097/TA.0b013e3181e5bb8e.
18. Baghdanian AH, Baghdanian AA, Armetta A, et al. Utility of MDCT findings in predicting patient management outcomes in renal trauma. Emerg Radiol. 2017;24(3):263–72. https://doi.org/10.1007/s10140-016-1473-3.
19. Moore EE, Shackford SR, Pachter HL, et al. Organ injury scaling: spleen, liver, and kidney. J Trauma. 1989;29(12):1664–6.
20. AAST Kidney Injury Scale (2018 revision). Accessed 19 July 2020. https://www.aast.org/library/traumatools/injuryscoringscales.aspx#kidney.
21. Benamran D, de Clippele B, Hammer F, Tombal B. Intraparenchymal renal artery pseudoaneurysm and arteriovenous fistula on a solitary kidney occurring 38 years after blunt trauma. Case Rep Urol. 2017;2017:3017501. https://doi.org/10.1155/2017/3017501.
22. Sangthong B, Demetriades D, Martin M, et al. Management and hospital outcomes of blunt renal artery injuries: analysis of 517 patients from the National Trauma Data Bank. J Am Coll Surg. 2006;203(5):612–7. https://doi.org/10.1016/j.jamcollsurg.2006.07.004.
23. Santucci RA, Fisher MB. The literature increasingly supports expectant (conservative) management of renal trauma--a systematic review. J Trauma. 2005;59(2):493–503. https://doi.org/10.1097/01.ta.0000179956.55078.c0.
24. Cimbanassi S, Chiara O, Leppaniemi A, et al. Nonoperative management of abdominal solid-organ injuries following blunt trauma in

adults: results from an International Consensus Conference. J Trauma Acute Care Surg. 2018;84(3):517–31. https://doi.org/10.1097/TA.0000000000001774.

25. Serafetinides E, Kitrey ND, Djakovic N, et al. Review of the current management of upper urinary tract injuries by the EAU Trauma Guidelines Panel. Eur Urol. 2015;67(5):930–6. https://doi.org/10.1016/j.eururo.2014.12.034.

26. van der Wilden GM, Velmahos GC, Joseph DAK, et al. Successful nonoperative management of the most severe blunt renal injuries: a multicenter study of the research consortium of New England Centers for Trauma. JAMA Surg. 2013;148(10):924. https://doi.org/10.1001/jamasurg.2013.2747.

27. McGuire J, Bultitude MF, Davis P, Koukounaras J, Royce PL, Corcoran NM. Predictors of outcome for blunt high grade renal injury treated with conservative intent. J Urol. 2011;185(1):187–91. https://doi.org/10.1016/j.juro.2010.08.085.

28. Lanchon C, Fiard G, Arnoux V, et al. High grade blunt renal trauma: predictors of surgery and long-term outcomes of conservative management. A prospective single center study. J Urol. 2016;195(1):106–11. https://doi.org/10.1016/j.juro.2015.07.100.

29. Martin JG, Shah J, Robinson C, Dariushnia S. Evaluation and management of blunt solid organ trauma. Tech Vasc Interv Radiol. 2017;20(4):230–6. https://doi.org/10.1053/j.tvir.2017.10.001.

30. Dugi DD 3rd, Morey AF, Gupta A, Nuss GR, Sheu GL, Pruitt JH. American Association for the Surgery of Trauma grade 4 renal injury substratification into grades 4a (low risk) and 4b (high risk). J Urol. 2010;183(2):592–7. https://doi.org/10.1016/j.juro.2009.10.015.

31. Hardee MJ, Lowrance W, Brant WO, Presson AP, Stevens MH, Myers JB. High grade renal injuries: application of Parkland Hospital predictors of intervention for renal hemorrhage. J Urol. 2013;189(5):1771–6. https://doi.org/10.1016/j.juro.2012.11.172.

32. Figler BD, Malaeb BS, Voelzke B, Smith T, Wessells H. External validation of a substratification of the American Association for the Surgery of Trauma renal injury scale for grade 4 injuries. J Am Coll Surg. 2013;217(5):924–8. https://doi.org/10.1016/j.jamcollsurg.2013.07.388.

33. Zemp L, Mann U, Rourke KF. Perinephric hematoma size is independently associated with the need for urological intervention in multisystem blunt renal trauma. J Urol. 2018;199(5):1283–8. https://doi.org/10.1016/j.juro.2017.11.135.

34. Fu CY, Wu SC, Chen RJ, et al. Evaluation of need for angioembolization in blunt renal injury: discontinuity of Gerota's fascia has an increased probability of requiring angioembolization. Am J Surg. 2010;199(2):154–9. https://doi.org/10.1016/j.amjsurg.2008.12.023.

35. Kautza B, Zuckerbraun B, Peitzman AB. Management of blunt renal injury: what is new? Eur J Trauma Emerg Surg. 2015;41(3):251–8. https://doi.org/10.1007/s00068-015-0516-x.

36. Hotaling JM, Sorensen MD, Smith TG 3rd, Rivara FP, Wessells H, Voelzke BB. Analysis of diagnostic angiography and angioembolization in the acute management of renal trauma using a national data set. J Urol. 2011;185(4):1316–20. https://doi.org/10.1016/j.juro.2010.12.003.

37. Erlich T, Kitrey ND. Renal trauma: the current best practice. Ther Adv Urol. 2018;10(10):295–303. https://doi.org/10.1177/1756287218785828.

38. Ramchandani P, Buckler PM. Imaging of genitourinary trauma. AJR Am J Roentgenol. 2009;192(6):1514–23. https://doi.org/10.2214/AJR.09.2470.

39. Alabousi A, Patlas MN, Menias CO, et al. Multi-modality imaging of the leaking ureter: why does detection of traumatic and iatrogenic ureteral injuries remain a challenge? Emerg Radiol. 2017;24(4):417–22. https://doi.org/10.1007/s10140-017-1507-5.

40. AAST Ureteral Injury Scale. https://www.aast.org/resources-detail/injury-scoring-scale#ureter.

41. Joshi G, Kim EY, Hanna TN, Siegel CL, Menias CO. CT cystography for suspicion of traumatic urinary bladder injury: indications, technique, findings, and pitfalls in diagnosis: RadioGraphics fundamentals | online presentation. Radiographics. 2018;38(1):92–3. https://doi.org/10.1148/rg.2018170125.

42. Nicola R, Menias CO, Mellnick V, Bhalla S, Raptis C, Siegel C. Sports-related genitourinary trauma in the male athlete. Emerg Radiol. 2015;22(2):157–68. https://doi.org/10.1007/s10140-014-1277-2.

43. Morgan DE, Nallamala LK, Kenney PJ, Mayo MS, Rue LW. CT cystography: radiographic and clinical predictors of bladder rupture. AJR Am J Roentgenol. 2000;174(1):89–95. https://doi.org/10.2214/ajr.174.1.1740089.

44. Kong JP, Bultitude MF, Royce P, Gruen RL, Cato A, Corcoran NM. Lower urinary tract injuries following blunt trauma: a review of contemporary management. Rev Urol. 2011;13(3):119–30.

45. Vaccaro JP, Brody JM. CT cystography in the evaluation of major bladder trauma. Radiographics. 2000;20(5):1373–81. https://doi.org/10.1148/radiographics.20.5.g00se111373.

46. Sandler CM, Hall JT, Rodriguez MB, Corriere JN. Bladder injury in blunt pelvic trauma. Radiology. 1986;158(3):633–8. https://doi.org/10.1148/radiology.158.3.3945731.

47. Moore E, Cogbill T, Malangoni M, Jurkovich G, Champion H. Scaling system for organ specific injuries. PDF. https://www.aast.org/resources-detail/injury-scoring-scale#blatter. Accessed 30 Oct 2020.

# Imaging of Penetrating Abdominal and Pelvic Trauma

# 25

David H. Ballard, Muhammad Naeem, Mark J. Hoegger, Mohamed Z. Rajput, and Vincent M. Mellnick

## Contents

### Abstract

Penetrating abdominal trauma occurs primarily from ballistics and stab wounds. Violation of the peritoneal cavity may cause a substantial number of injuries, often centered along the trajectory of the penetrating agent. Basic ballistic kinematics may be helpful to radiologists in understanding the mechanism of penetrating trauma and are briefly reviewed. CT performed on hemodynamically stable patients without peritonitis is a current near-universal standard, although there are some controversies on preferred CT protocols. Using standard portal venous phase CT imaging, an approach to solid organ, bowel, and vascular trauma is emphasized. Solid organ injuries are rarely isolated, and additional injuries to adjacent structures occur often in a path following the projectile. The direct as well as indirect signs of bowel, mesenteric, and vascular injuries are reviewed. The role of delayed imaging, rectal contrast, CT cystography, and other problem-solving imaging acquisitions performed according to present or suspected injuries is also highlighted. The purpose of this chapter is therefore to review and summarize the imaging of penetrating abdominal trauma.

### Keywords

Penetrating trauma · Abdominal trauma · Computed tomography · Gunshot wound · Penetrating injury

## Introduction

Penetrating abdominal trauma (PAT) involves violation of the abdominal cavity by an impaling object [1]. Though stab wounds are more common than gunshot wounds in one

D. H. Ballard (✉) · M. Naeem · M. J. Hoegger · M. Z. Rajput · V. M. Mellnick
Mallinckrodt Institute of Radiology, Washington University School of Medicine, St. Louis, MO, USA
e-mail: davidballard@wustl.edu; mnaeem@wustl.edu; mhoegger@wustl.edu; mrajput@wustl.edu; mellnickv@wustl.edu

© Springer Nature Switzerland AG 2022
M. N. Patlas et al. (eds.), *Atlas of Emergency Imaging from Head-to-Toe*,
https://doi.org/10.1007/978-3-030-92111-8_25

large series, gunshot wounds remain responsible for 90% of deaths associated with PAT [2]. In contrast, according to the 2016 National Trauma Data Bank report, stab wounds were responsible for 4% of overall trauma, with an associated case fatality rate of only 2% [3]. PAT can result in a lasting impact socially, psychologically, and economically, and by virtue of its predictable pattern, is a public health emergency. Socio-demographic characteristics associated with PAT mortality favor males over females, with the greatest death rate reported among non-Hispanic black males [4, 5].

In the pre-World War I era, penetrating abdominal trauma almost always resulted in death. With the advent of operative management for penetrating injury in World War I soldiers, laparotomy soon became the reference standard for the initial management of penetrating abdominal trauma. Further increase in survival rates was seen with more widespread availability of antibiotics and fluid replacement therapy, along with improved transportation of the wounded [6]. However, in the 1960s, this notion was challenged by a large number of negative laparotomies or laparotomies with no life-threatening organ injuries. As a result, laparotomies performed for penetrating abdominal trauma gradually decreased over time. Since observations by Shaftan [7], nonoperative management for penetrating abdominal trauma has been increasingly recognized and practiced by the trauma surgeons [8].

With the current availability of fast and high-resolution modern scanners, computed tomographic (CT) imaging in the initial evaluation of hemodynamically stable patients with penetrating traumatic injury has become standard practice [9]. Optimizing patient management and outcomes is predicated on prompt recognition of penetrating injuries on CT. To do so, though, requires additional familiarity with appropriate CT imaging protocols for penetrating injury, as well as an understanding of the mechanism and trajectory of the injury itself. This chapter focuses on ballistic mechanics (kinematics), optimal imaging protocols, and salient features of solid and hollow viscus and vascular penetrating abdominal trauma.

## Ballistic Kinematics

Traumatic injuries happen from an interplay between a moving object and the target. In the setting of penetrating trauma, the target is the human body, whereas the moving object is an impaling force. The aim of studying the biophysics behind penetrating trauma is to understand how these injuries occur. In order to do so, one should have a basic understanding of the applicable physics concepts [9–12].

Two basic physics laws define the principles of penetrating traumatic injuries: Joule's first law of thermodynamics, and Newton's first law of motion. Joule's law states that within a closed system, energy can neither be created nor destroyed but can be transformed from one state to another. This law applies in conjunction with Newton's law, which states that an object in motion or rest stays in that state unless acted upon by an external force. When applying these laws to a moving object, such as a bullet in the setting of penetrating trauma, it is understandable that kinetic energy acquired by the bullet will be conserved until it is transformed by an external force (e.g., the human body). The transformation that will happen results in transference of energy attained by a moving bullet into the human body, resulting in alteration of physical form of both the bullet and the organs it interacts with [9–12].

The characteristics of the bullet that dictate the damage within the target are referred to as terminal ballistics. Short, high-velocity bullet yaws are more severe, imparting more kinetic energy to the target from extensive tumbling and rotation as the bullet enters the tissue. Longer and heavier bullets, on the other hand, may not experience much yaw and thus travel over a longer distance, preserving their initial kinetic energy to exit the body. Bullets cause tissue damage in three ways: i) laceration and crushing, ii) cavitation, and iii) shockwaves [9–12].

A bullet passing through tissue creates a crush cavity, characterized by the shape of its nose and penetration depth. A larger wound cavity indicates the true extent of tissue death and is composed of injury from tumbling of the bullet, bullet fragmentation, and temporary cavitation injury. A stretch cavity is also created but is temporary and cannot be seen by imaging. The leading edge of the bullet has a point of maximum pressure and a leading stress wave as it passes through the body [9–12] (Fig. 1). Mass and velocity of the projectile correlate with the maximum wounding potential; however, the resulting injury is also dependent on tissue factors and projectile characteristics.

## Imaging Rationale and Protocols

Appropriate and timely medical imaging can be the difference between life and death in penetrating abdominal trauma. Accordingly, it is critical for the radiologist to promptly identify and report key imaging findings. But an understanding of the best imaging approaches in trauma is also necessary to both improve injury detection and minimizing time wasted in unnecessary radiologic examinations. Central to these imaging approaches are the Advanced Trauma Life Support (ATLS) guidelines [13]. Established by the American College of Surgeons (ACS), the ATLS guidelines provide

**Fig. 1** Injury patterns caused by a bullet traversing through tissue include the primary crush injury and surrounding secondary wound cavity. The outermost stretch cavity is typically not evident on imaging as it collapses

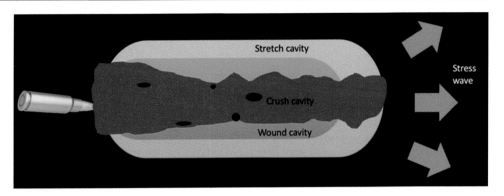

a comprehensive algorithmic and systemic approach for the management of trauma, including penetrating abdominal trauma [13].

After the initial stabilization via the primary survey, patients typically undergo a secondary survey, which is a complete head-to-toe physical examination to further determine injury. In the setting of penetrating trauma, this survey may identify additional entrance and exit wounds. Imaging with ultrasound frequently occurs during the secondary survey. Focused Assessment with Sonography for Trauma (FAST) is a bedside tool often used in blunt and penetrating abdominal trauma, which has largely replaced diagnostic peritoneal lavage to detect intraperitoneal hemorrhage [14]. FAST is used in the ATLS algorithms of most level 1 trauma centers [15]. With FAST, images of the abdominal cavity are typically obtained with a low-frequency (2–5 MHz) curvilinear probe with the patient supine [16]. FAST is aimed at identifying free fluid in several key locations: Morrison's pouch in the right upper quadrant, the left paracolic gutter, the rectovesical space in men, and the rectouterine and vesicouterine pouches in women.

Radiographs and FAST examinations carry the benefit of portability – both can be performed at the patient's bedside and rapidly provide critical information. However, both are inherently technically limited. FAST, for example, has relatively low sensitivity for the detection of fluid volumes less than 200 cc [17] and has even worse sensitivity for the detection of solid organ injury [18]. Moreover, ultrasound can be hampered by suboptimal imaging windows, patient body habitus, and operator-dependent variability. Similarly, radiographs also have poor sensitivity [19]. Thus, given its high sensitivity and specificity, CT is the preferred imaging modality for the detection of penetrating trauma and will be the focus of the remainder of this chapter.

Optimal CT use in penetrating trauma relies on rapid transport to the imaging suite with prompt image acquisition, pathology identification, and reporting. In keeping with this, CT suites are ideally located near – or even

within – the trauma center adjacent to the site of patient drop off by ambulance or airlift. When the patient is imaged, access to life-saving equipment should be available in the event of rapid decompensation. Advances in multidetector CT imaging have allowed for rapid acquisition of high-resolution images with multiplanar reformations. Quickly identifying pathology is also important and is aided by metallic markers placed at the sites of entrance and exit wounds in the skin. To expedite the communication of critical findings, some centers have radiologists review images at the scanner in real time with the trauma team present. With the radiologist present in the control room and reviewing images at the time of acquisition, any necessary additional CT images can be obtained without the patient leaving the table [9].

Obtaining appropriate CT images relies on multiple factors including scan location, patient position, contrast route, and phase of contrast acquisition. Patients with penetrating abdominal trauma typically have a CT performed of the entire torso: the chest, abdomen, and pelvis. This is because in a single penetrating wound, the chest may be involved given the span of the lungs. Also, many patients with penetrating trauma have multiple injury sites [9, 20].

There is some current controversy regarding the optimal imaging protocols in penetrating abdominal trauma, including the use of routine arterial and portal venous phase acquisitions through the upper abdomen to assess for vascular injury. At our institution, we primarily use a single portal venous phase to simplify the protocol and minimize radiation dose.

Some centers also advocate for the routine use of a "triple contrast" regimen, as some studies have indicated that it is more accurate in detecting bowel injuries, relying on the high specificity of an enteric contrast leak (Figs. 2 and 3). At our institution, we do not advocate for routinely administering oral or rectal contrast for penetrating trauma, relying instead on intravenous contrast only. Oral and rectal contrast are primarily reserved as problem-solving tools in our practice, used when necessary to confirm a

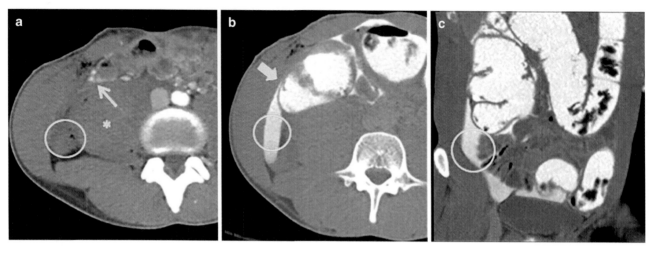

**Fig. 2** Colonic injury with rectal contrast extravasation. Twenty-seven-year-old man following right abdominal gunshot wound. The initial axial CT image (**a**) demonstrates free air within the right retroperitoneum, a right psoas hematoma (*), and mesenteric venous extravasation (thin arrow), along with a tract of low to intermediate attenuation fluid emanating from the cecum (circle). Subsequent administration of rectal contrast (**b** and **c**) shows extracolonic contrast (circles, **b** and **c**, axial and coronal images) emanating from a cecal injury (thick arrow, **b**), which was confirmed surgically

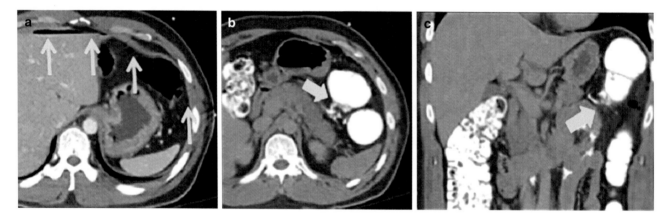

**Fig. 3** Subtle colonic injury confirmed with rectal contrast extravasation. 33-year-old man with a stab wound to the left flank. Initial axial CT image (**a**) demonstrates small foci of gas (thin arrows, **a**) about the left flank stab wound along with generalized pneumoperitoneum (thin arrows, **a**), but no direct evidence of colonic injury. Subsequent administration of rectal contrast shows extracolonic contrast emanating from the distal transverse colon (thick arrows, **b** and **c**, axial and coronal images), which was confirmed surgically

suspected injury [9]. An international survey [21] with majority US respondents revealed that the majority (>65%) of responding centers and radiologists do not routinely employ the triple contrast regimen, with 32% semiroutinely administering rectal contrast, and 26% semiroutinely administering oral contrast. In that survey, the decision to administer oral or rectal contrast is only made by the radiologist in ~50% of cases. In the remaining cases, the treating emergency physician or surgeon makes this decision [21]. A systematic review on penetrating abdominal trauma identified and compared the sensitivity and specificity of studies with and without enteric contrast and found no significant difference in diagnosing bowel injuries with or without enteric contrast [22].

In our experience, administering oral and rectal contrast does not substantially help detect bowel injury and more often delays patient care. In study of 274 patients with penetrating abdominal trauma, CT performed with intravenous contrast, without the use of oral or rectal contrast, demonstrated findings suspicious for bowel injury in 173 cases, and surgery demonstrated bowel injury in 162 cases, with an overall sensitivity of 88% and positive predictive value of 82% [23].

## Imaging Features of Penetrating Trauma

The imaging appearance of a ballistic tract often manifests with small locules of gas, ballistic fragments, contusions, lacerations, and/or abnormal fluid/blood [9, 24]. Retained

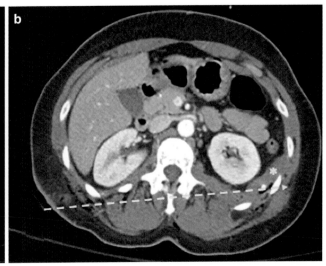

**Fig. 4** Gunshot wound without peritoneal violation. Transverse gunshot wound of the posterior body wall soft tissues and paraspinal muscles (dashed arrows, **a** and **b**, axial CT images with IV contrast), with a bullet lodged in a left posterior intercostal rib space creating a localized extraperitoneal hematoma (*). There are associated lumbar posterior elements and left rib gunshot fractures (not pictured), with accompanying hemorrhage along the bullet trajectory. Otherwise, there is no evidence of peritoneal or retroperitoneal violation

**Fig. 5** Stab wound resulting in penetrating cecal injury. 22-year-old man with a stab wound to the right flank. The entry wound is manifested by a skin discontinuity along with tracking soft tissue contusion (dashed arrow, **a**, axial CT image with IV contrast). Along the tract of the injury, there is focal cecal wall thickening and intramural hemorrhage (dashed box, **a** and **b**, coronal reformation). Despite the absence of free fluid, these findings are highly concerning for cecal injury, which was confirmed and repaired intraoperatively

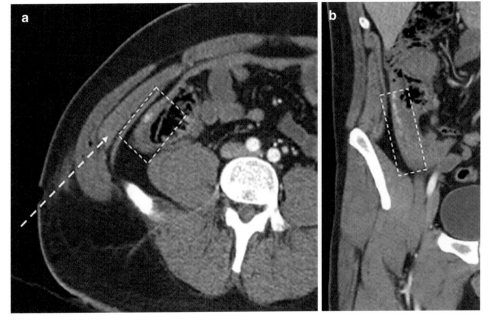

bullets with no exit may lodge anywhere but most frequently do so in bone or large muscle groups. One purpose of imaging and a key point of interpretation is answering if the penetrating injury violated an intraperitoneal or extraperitoneal intraabdominal space (Fig. 4). Knife and other stab wounds often have less contusion and air along their tract due to the lower kinetic injury of these injuries. Resultant intra-abdominal solid or hollow visceral injuries from stab wounds are often less pronounced compared to gunshot trauma. Bowel injury with stab wounds can be particularly subtle, as the depth of injury is not always clear [23] (Fig. 5). Lower caliber bullets, such as shotgun pellets (Fig. 6), may also cause less tissue trauma and will often result in more retained ballistic fragments (Fig. 7).

In penetrating gunshot abdominal trauma, analysis of the ballistic tract (also known as trajectography) can help identify definitive, probable, or possible injuries [9, 24] (Fig. 8). For example, a gas and ballistic tract leading up to a segment of bowel is the most sensitive finding for bowel injury.

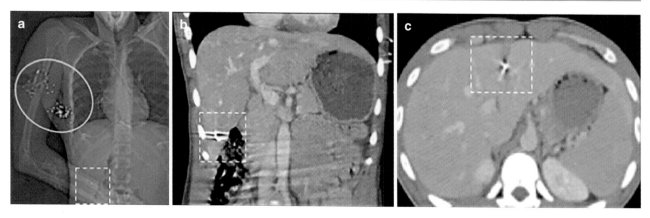

**Fig. 6** Shotgun injuries with pellets acutely lodged in the liver without CT-evident liver injury, highlighting the lower-tissue trauma potential of small caliber rounds. Two patients with upper extremity and right chest wall shotgun injuries. Topogram (**a**) demonstrates the majority of shotgun pellets in the right upper extremity and right chest wall (circle, **a**), with a single metallic focus projecting in the right hemiliver (dashed box, **a**). On CT acquisition, there is a metallic fragment in segment 6 (dashed box, **b**, coronal image with IV contrast). There is dense streak artifact, but the hepatic laceration and tract that lodged the pellet in its position is not evident by imaging. In a different patient (**c**), a metallic fragment lodged in segment 4 (dashed box, **c**, axial image with IV contrast) shows similar findings with surrounding dense streak artifact but no CT-evident liver injury. In both cases, it is not entirely clear how these straight pellets violated the liver as these fragments were away from the trajectory of the primary blast. Liver injury was certainly present, but the low-caliber shotgun pellets did not result in substantial tissue trauma evident on imaging

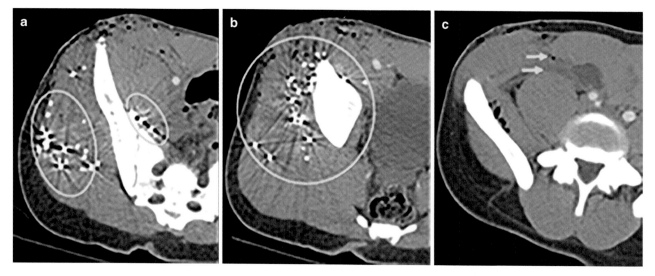

**Fig. 7** Shotgun blast injury. 25-year-old man with a gunshot wound to the pelvis. Axial CT images with IV contrast demonstrate multiple ballistic shot pellets in the right gluteus maximus and right iliopsoas muscles (circles **a** and **b**), with associated intramuscular hematoma. Additionally, there is low-attenuation pelvic free fluid along with locules of pneumoperitoneum (arrows, **c**) which were concerning for bowel injury. These findings were confirmed intraoperatively, where a distal small bowel injury was repaired

Similarly, a trajectory that traverses the hemidiaphragm often implies diaphragmatic injury, as there often will be no definitive disruption of the diaphragm on CT [25, 26]. In the era of modern CT, the use of multiplanar reconstructions is essential and standard practice in the imaging evaluation of trauma at most centers [9]. Delineating the tract in multiple planes to assess for injuries along the ballistic trajectory is a worthwhile endeavor after the radiologist completes her or his search pattern [9, 24]. Some advocate for double obliquing the imaging planes so that the ballistic trajectory is visible in one or few images, using this "tractogram" as a reference for evaluating axial and standard multiplanar image sets. Commercial software also exists for this trajectory analysis. Analysis of stab wound trajectory can also be performed; however, since stab wounds are typically short segment in length, the trajectory is often not a diagnostic dilemma [9, 24]. Stab wound trajectory analysis may be helpful to increase confidence when diagnosing subtle injuries, particularly with obliquely oriented stab wounds. Entry and exit site clinically relevant injuries include traumatic abdominal wall hernias, including lumbar hernias, large abdominal wall hematomas, and gunshot fractures [9, 27, 28] (Fig. 9).

When intraperitoneal injuries are present, they are rarely in isolation [25, 26, 29]. For example, splenic injuries are

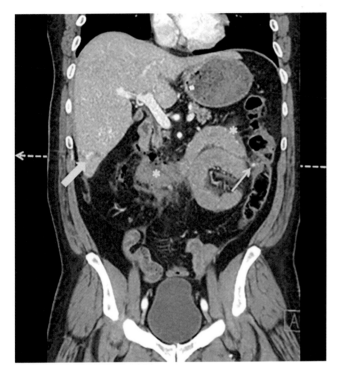

**Fig. 8** Penetrating gunshot wound with multiorgan abdominal injuries identified by trajectory. Coronal CT image with IV contrast reveals multiple injuries along the trajectory of a transversely oriented gunshot wound (dashed arrow). From left to right: descending colonic injury manifested by focally thickened bowel adjacent to a vascular contrast blush (thin arrow); bowel and mesenteric injury with multiple areas of mesenteric hemorrhage and fluid adjacent to thickened jejunal loops (*); and grade 2 segment 6 hepatic laceration (thick arrow)

associated with diaphragmatic injuries in up to 60% of patients [25]. Similarly, although hepatic injuries are the most common isolated organ injury, associated diaphragmatic injury has been reported in up to 40% of cases [26]. Analysis of intra-abdominal gas, fluid, and contusion along the wound tract is often helpful in delineating solid and hollow visceral injuries [23, 30]. Pneumoperitoneum accumulating away from the tract has high specificity (~85%–90%) but low sensitivity (~50%) for the detection of bowel injury [23, 30] (Fig. 10). Free fluid in the setting of penetrating trauma may be due to hemoperitoneum, enteric content, urine, and potentially third spacing from large volume resuscitation. Measurement of attenuation values is helpful to discern simple fluid from blood. Hemoperitoneum is critical to detect and may be due to vascular, solid visceral, mesenteric, or hollow viscus injury. Large-volume simple-attenuating free fluid in the setting of penetrating injury may be due to leaking enteric content or leaking urine [31]. Identifying signs of bowel injury along with the use of delayed excretory phase imaging, and CT cystography, to assess for ureteral and bladder injuries, respectively, will help distinguish between these two entities [9].

## Solid Visceral Injuries

In penetrating abdominal trauma with ballistic peritoneal violation, the liver is the most frequently injured solid organ, followed by the spleen, kidneys, and pancreas. In an older case series published before the advent of modern CT imaging and practice guidelines for trauma patients, the incidence of penetrating liver and pancreatic injuries was reported up to 40% and 6%, respectively [32]. The incidence of renal injuries associated with penetrating trauma is approximately 6% in one more recent series [29]. Splenic penetrating trauma incidence is not well reported, to our knowledge.

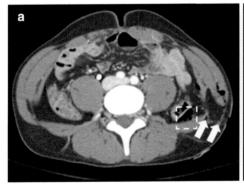
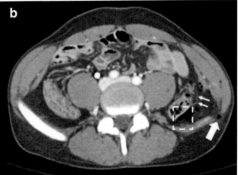

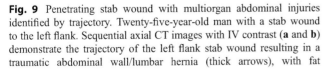

**Fig. 9** Penetrating stab wound with multiorgan abdominal injuries identified by trajectory. Twenty-five-year-old man with a stab wound to the left flank. Sequential axial CT images with IV contrast (**a** and **b**) demonstrate the trajectory of the left flank stab wound resulting in a traumatic abdominal wall/lumbar hernia (thick arrows), with fat interdigitating through the inferior lumbar triangle between the oblique musculature and latissimus dorsi. There is free air adjacent to the descending colon (dashed boxes), with pericolic fluid and fat stranding (thin arrows in **b**), which is suspicious for colonic perforation. These findings were confirmed at exploratory laparotomy

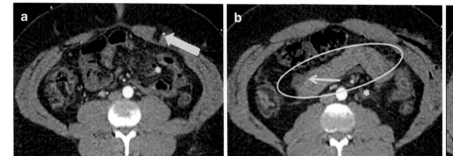

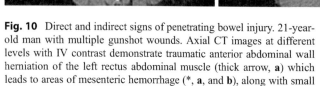

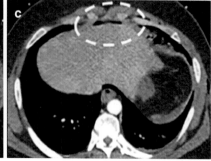

**Fig. 10** Direct and indirect signs of penetrating bowel injury. 21-year-old man with multiple gunshot wounds. Axial CT images at different levels with IV contrast demonstrate traumatic anterior abdominal wall herniation of the left rectus abdominal muscle (thick arrow, **a**) which leads to areas of mesenteric hemorrhage (*, **a**, and **b**), along with small interdigitating locules of air (not shown). A loop of jejunum is thickened (circle, **b**) with apparent wall irregularity and enteric contents spilling out (thin arrow, **b**). Small volume pneumoperitoneum is noted collecting under the diaphragm (dashed circle, **c**)

Penetrating injuries to the liver, spleen, kidneys, and pancreas should be graded with the American Association for the Surgery of Trauma (AAST) grading systems, similar to blunt abdominal trauma, with note of the 2018 AAST organ-grading system update [33].

## Liver and Spleen

The liver and spleen have similar imaging characteristics in the setting of penetrating trauma due to their compact solid parenchyma coupled with the propensity for ballistic injury to cause more damage in denser tissue [24]. On portal venous phase CT, hepatic and splenic parenchymal lacerations will manifest as hypoattenuating linear or geographic tracts disrupting the homogenously enhancing parenchyma. Perihepatic and perisplenic hematomas are visible as high-attenuation fluid around the liver and spleen, which may extend more caudally into the peritoneum and paracolic gutters [25, 26].

When assigning an AAST grade to a hepatic or splenic injury, the radiologist should assess for laceration and hematoma size as well as involvement of the major vessels and the hilar regions (Fig. 11). In addition, one should carefully assess for contrast "blushes" that may be manifestations of active extravasation and/or pseudoaneurysm. In these situations, obtaining a delayed acquisition – either on a case-by-case basis if the initial set of images are reviewed in real time, or as part of a routine protocol on every trauma patient – is valuable in differentiating between the two entities [31].

## Pancreas

Penetrating pancreatic injuries can be devastating with increased morbidity when associated with pancreatic duct injury or need for partial pancreatectomy. In the absence of frank pancreatic parenchymal disruption, confident diagnosis of pancreatic injury on single phase initial trauma CT is often difficult. The radiologist's best guide is often relying on the projectile tract in addition to identifying areas of pancreatic hypoenhancement and assessing peripancreatic fat for blood and/or stranding [34] (Fig. 12). However, assessment of the peripancreatic fat may be confounding if there is an adjacent bowel or solid organ injury, all of which may cause an infiltrative appearance of the peripancreatic fat [31]. In patients with suspected pancreatic injuries, MRI is helpful in assessing pancreatic duct integrity, though it is often obtained several days, if not weeks, after admission and stabilization of other traumatic injuries [34]. As a result, patients with traumatic pancreatic duct injury may present in a delayed fashion, potentially with duct leak and pseudocyst formation. Therefore, it is important for radiologists to suggest these injuries and further workup when seen on the initial examination after trauma.

## Kidneys and Ureters

Isolated renal injuries are rare in penetrating trauma. One study of penetrating trauma at a single center demonstrated a 5.7% (123/2,163 patients) incidence of penetrating renal injuries over a 6-year period [29]. The vast majority (>90%) had associated injuries, most frequently the liver in the setting of right renal injuries and splenic, colonic, and gastric injuries in the setting of left renal injuries [29]. Similar to hepatic and splenic lacerations, renal lacerations will appear as hypoattenuating linear or geographic tracts disrupting the parenchyma [29, 35]. Associated perirenal hematomas may be contained or expand into the retroperitoneum. As with other solid organs, renal injuries should be categorized using the AAST grading system. Most (~80%) are AAST grade III or higher [29].

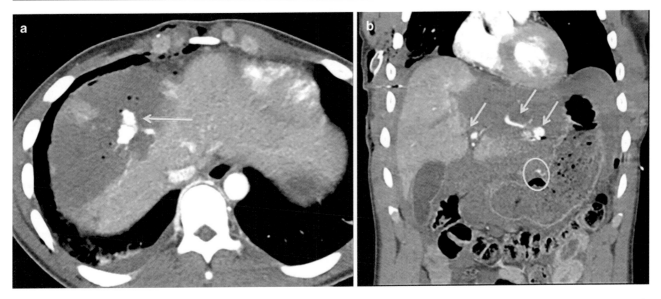

**Fig. 11** High-grade penetrating hepatic injuries in two different patients. (**a**) Grade 4 hepatic injury with a large laceration involving the right hemiliver violating multiple segments with confluent contrast blush in segment 8 indicative of active bleeding or pseudoaneurysm (arrow). (**b**) Grade 5 hepatic injury manifested by near complete laceration/devascularization of the left hepatic lobe with areas of active bleeding/pseudoaneurysm formation in the left lateral section (arrows), and injury to the left hepatic vein (not shown). A left gastric artery injury is also partially profiled (circle) throughout the right and left hemiliver. This grade 5 injury also injured the left hepatic vein (not picture). A left gastric artery injury is also partially profiled

**Fig. 12** Twenty-three-year-old man shot through the upper abdomen. Axial CT images with intravenous contrast show a bullet coursing from the left anterior abdominal wall to the left paraspinal region (**b**, **d**, dashed arrows). Along the bullet track is a left renal hilar injury with a devascularized kidney (**c**, arrows). In the splenic artery territory, there is a rounded blush of contrast (**a**, arrow), consistent with a pseudoaneurysm. A pancreatic tail injury was suspected on the basis of this path of injury and blood surrounding the pancreas. This was confirmed operatively

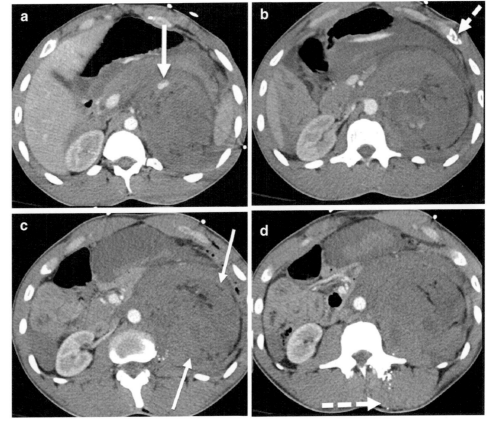

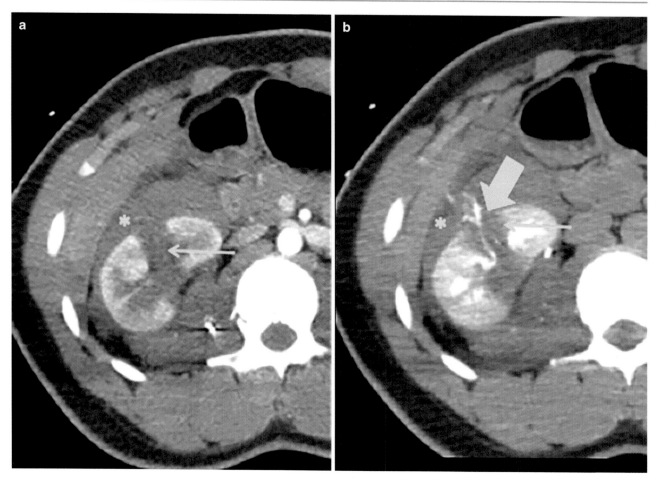

**Fig. 13** High-grade penetrating renal injury. Seventeen-year-old man with gunshot wounds to the right flank. Initial CT axial image (**a**) demonstrates a laceration involving the lower pole of the right kidney (thin arrow), with a perinephric fluid and/or hematoma (*). On the delayed acquisition (**b**), there is extravasation from the collecting system (thick arrow), consistent with a urine leak in the setting of a grade IV injury

Ideally, higher-grade (IV or V) injuries should be assessed in both the portal venous and excretory phases of contrast to evaluate for collecting system injuries [35]. If the collecting system is not adequately opacified at 6–10 min and the patient is stable, a repeat noncontrast scan within several hours can be obtained to assess for collecting system injury while the kidneys continue to excrete contrast. Additionally, an IV contrast-enhanced CT, including excretory phase imaging, several days after admission and/or prior to discharge, is often helpful in identifying urine leaks that are initially obscured by hematoma at the time of presentation (Figs. 13 and 14). Ureteral injuries are assessed in a similar manner to diagnosing collecting system injuries and require a delayed acquisition to show contrast extravasation [35].

Penetrating bladder injuries often present with smaller defects than in blunt trauma. Regardless, it remains imperative to not only identify bladder injuries by the path of the penetrating injury, but also to characterize them as intraperitoneal or extraperitoneal. This distinction is best made by CT cystogram, whereby contrast is instilled into a retrograde fashion into the bladder via a Foley catheter (Fig. 15).

Urethral injures in penetrating trauma are often associated with penile, pelvic, or perineal gunshot wounds. Urethral injuries often require fluoroscopic or radiographic retrograde urethrogram for diagnosis (Fig. 16). In the acute setting, this will show disruption or extravasation of contrast. At follow-up, the sequelae of these injuries may manifest as strictures. Female urethral injuries are extremely rare [36].

With penetrating trauma to the scrotum and penis, CT may be able to reveal, or review of the images may raise suspicion for injury, if these findings are not evident by physical examination. However, the optimal imaging modality to assess the structural and vascular integrity of the testes is ultrasound with Doppler. Testicular rupture is characterized by disruption of

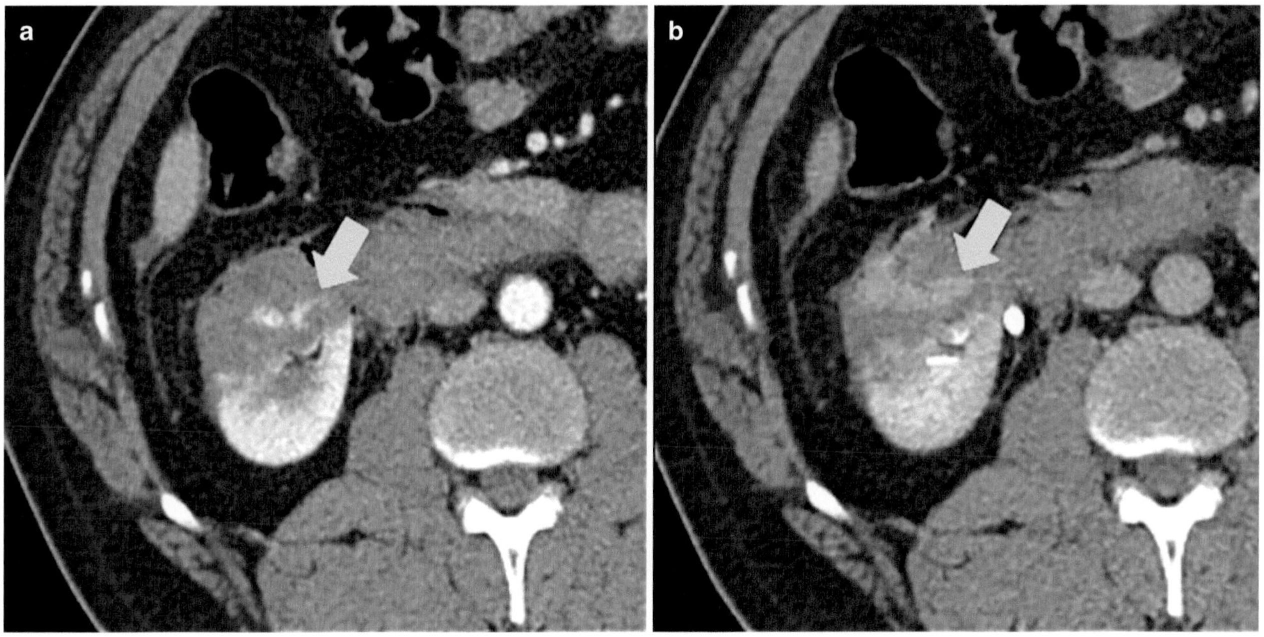

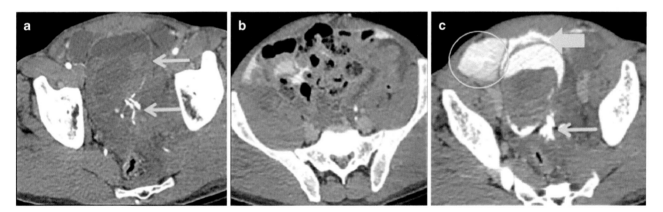

**Fig. 14** Penetrating renal trauma with no collecting system injury. Initial axial CT image (**a**) demonstrates a moderately sized right renal laceration containing small contrast blushes (thick arrow, **a**). To assess for collecting system injury, a delayed CT acquisition (**b**) was acquired 8 min later. The contrast blushes noted in (**a**) have expanded and become overall less dense (thick arrow, **b**), consistent with active intraparenchymal bleeding. No extraluminal high-density contrast to suggest a collecting system injury was seen. These findings are thus compatible with a grade 3 renal injury

**Fig. 15** Penetrating intraperitoneal and extraperitoneal bladder injuries. 47-year-old man with multiple gunshot wounds. The initial CT axial image through the pelvis (**a**) demonstrates extravasated contrast adjacent to the distal left ureter (thin arrow), compatible with ureteral injury, along with low-density fluid surrounding the contour of the bladder (thick arrow), which may represent hemorrhage or urine. Subsequent CT cystogram (**b** and **c**) reveals both intraperitoneal (circle) and extraperitoneal (thick arrow) bladder injuries. Clot is present within the bladder (*)

the tunica albuginea and is demonstrated on ultrasound by loss of the normal elliptical shape, possibly with extruded seminiferous tubules, with or without disrupted flow to the testis on Doppler (Fig. 17). Although both testicles may be injured, testicular trauma is much more often unilateral, so the uninjured testicle can serve as an internal control [36].

## Bowel and Mesentery

In addition to hemodynamic instability and high-grade solid organ injuries, suspected bowel and mesenteric injuries are a common indication for the trauma surgeon to explore patients through laparotomy. These injuries have both indirect and

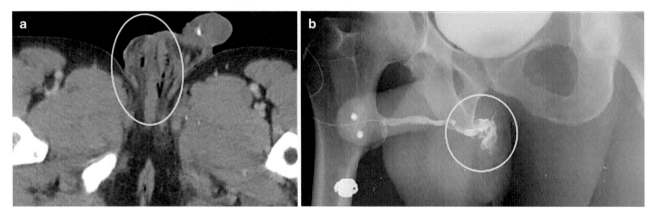

**Fig. 16** Gunshot wound to the penis and perineum with urethral injury. (a) Axial CT image with IV contrast demonstrates a tract of air and contusion throughout the right perineum which tracks toward the base of the penis (circle, **a**). Retrograde urethrogram (**b**) demonstrates a complete injury of the bulbar urethra (Goldman type 5)

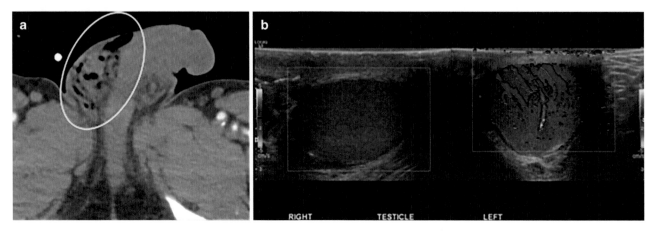

**Fig. 17** Penetrating scrotal injury with compromised blood flow to the testicle. Initial axial CT imaging (**a**) demonstrates a tract of gas and hemorrhage within the right scrotum (circle, **a**) which extends upward toward the inguinal canal (not pictured). (**b**) Doppler ultrasound images profiling both testicles demonstrate absence of flow to the right testicle. These findings were confirmed at exploration

direct signs and may be subtle or equivocal [23, 30]. Direct signs include wound trajectory leading to bowel, which is the most sensitive finding (~90–95%) with moderate specificity (~80%). Disruption of the bowel wall and leakage or oral or rectal contrast are highly specific (>95%) but insensitive findings of penetrating bowel injury [23, 30] (Figs. 8 and 10). Focal wall thickening has moderate sensitivity (~75%) and high specificity (~95%).

Indirect signs of bowel injury include peritoneal or retroperitoneal violation, mesenteric vascular injuries, and hematomas abutting the bowel or mesentery. The mesentery should have near uniform fat attenuation aside from vessels and lymph nodes. Disruption of this normal appearance with fat stranding or higher-attenuating fluid representing contusion/hemorrhage along the path of injury is indicative of mesenteric injury [23, 24, 30]. Mesenteric edema and bowel wall thickening from other causes such as hypoperfusion complex may be potential mimics of bowel injury in penetrating trauma when the path of injury passes near the bowel.

## Diaphragm

Diaphragm injuries in penetrating trauma usually result in small defects that are subtle or occult by CT imaging (Fig. 18). Suspected or implied diaphragm injury is often determined by analyzing the trajectory of the projectile and observing injuries on above and below the diaphragm along with air on both side of the diaphragm with no explanation [37]. There will often be associated thoracic trauma with pneumothorax and pulmonary contusion. In penetrating trauma, diaphragmatic hematomas and herniation of viscera through diaphragmatic defects are uncommon but can occur, particularly with large, shearing injuries.

## Aorta and Vascular

Penetrating abdominal aortic and other major arterial injuries require prompt identification, as a delay in diagnosis

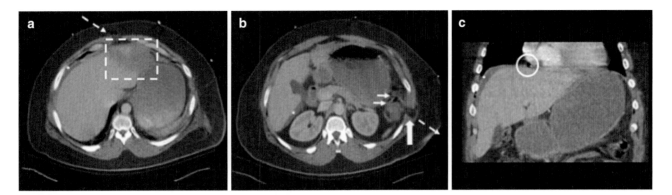

**Fig. 18** Penetrating transdiaphragmatic injury. 30-year-old man with a gunshot wound. Sequential axial IV contrast-enhanced CT images (**a** and **b**) and coronal reconstruction images of the upper abdomen (**c**) demonstrate the trajectory of the gunshot wound (dashed arrows in **a** and **b**), entering though the right anterior chest wall and exiting through the left flank. The entry wound resulted in a small right pneumothorax (not pictured) and injury to the right hemidiaphragm, evidenced by a small laceration surrounding by small locules of gas (circle in **c**). Below the diaphragm, a grade 3 hepatic injury is seen with a laceration involving hepatic segment 2 (dashed box in **a**), and an accompanying small perihepatic hematoma (\*in **a–c**). Within the left upper quadrant, gas is seen adjacent to the thickened splenic flexure (thin arrows in **b**) suspicious for colonic injury, which was subsequently proven intraoperatively. At the exit wound, a traumatic fat-containing left abdominal wall hernia is also noted (thick arrow in **b**)

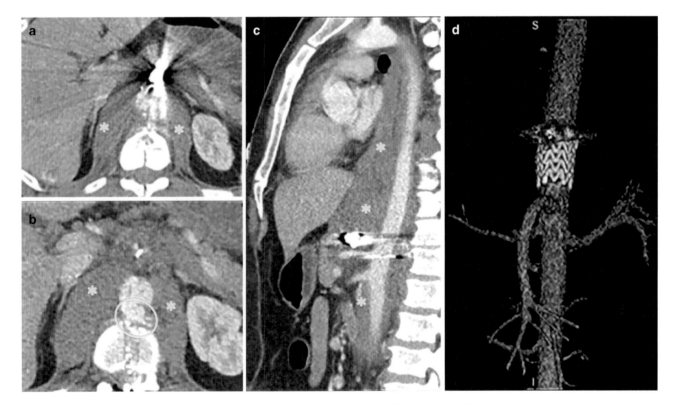

**Fig. 19** Penetrating aortic injury. Posterior gunshot entrance wound results in lumbar vertebral body and posterior element fractures with osseous and ballistic fragments in the spinal canal. A large periaortic hematoma is seen extending from the level of the gunshot wound both cranially and caudally to surround the thoracic and abdominal aorta (\*, **a–c**). There is an area of marked luminal irregularity with a posterior outpouching, compatible with an aortic transection (circle, **b**). This was repaired endovascularly (**d**) requiring stent graft placement covering the celiac axis, at the site where the largest bullet fragment was embedded (dashed box in **a**)

can lead to substantial morbidity. Aortic and other vascular injuries can be assessed with direct and indirect imaging signs. In addition to an injury path through the vessel, direct signs of injury include contour abnormalities of the vessel itself: intramural hematoma, intraluminal thrombus, arteriovenous fistula, and pseudoaneurysm [38]. The primary indirect sign is a hematoma abutting the vessel wall (Fig. 19). As with solid organ vascular injury, small- to moderately sized vascular injuries may manifest as a contrast blush within a hematoma. In these cases, obtaining a

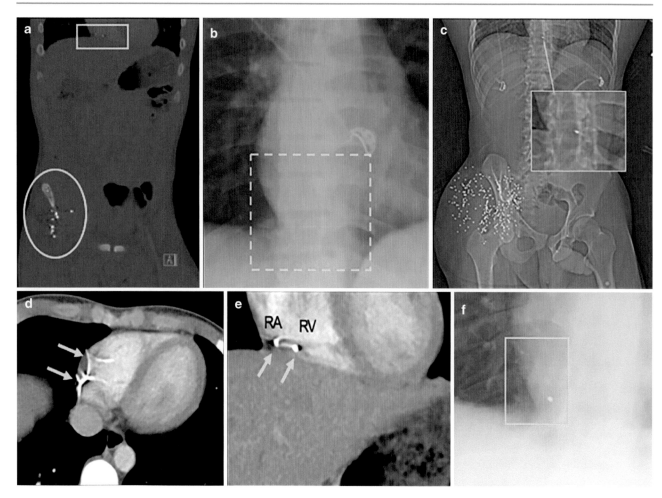

**Fig. 20** Bullet (shotgun pellet) embolism. 25-year-old man with a shotgun injury. (**a**) Coronal CT image demonstrating shotgun blast injury with multiple pellets in the gluteal region and right lower quadrant (**a**, circle). The extent of the intra-abdominal findings is not well profiled on this image and better illustrated in Fig. X (same patient). The subsequently discussed bullet/shotgun pellet emboli are also demonstrated in the right heart (**a**, box). (**b**) Magnified image of the heart and right heart border of the initial trauma bay chest radiograph performed approximately 10 min before subsequent CT examination demonstrates no abnormality and no radiopaque foreign body at the right heart border (dashed box **b**). Topogram (**c**), axial (**d**), and coronal (**d**) CT images demonstrate a radiodensity similar to the check and pellets on the

topogram (**b**), along with two dense metallic foci in the area of the right atrium and right ventricle (yellow arrows, **d** and **e**). When comparing the topogram (**c**) finding to the initial chest radiograph performed minutes earlier (**b**), this opacity and finding are new and are consistent with bullet/shotgun pellet embolism. The patient had an exploratory laparotomy and small bowel resection for management of a small bowel injury, but no intervention directed at the bullet/shotgun pellet embolization. (**f**) Magnified image of the heart and right heart border from chest radiograph performed 4 years later demonstrates similar radiopaque projecting in unchanged positions; follow-up CT examination (not pictured) also demonstrated similar findings. The patient had no cardiac or respiratory sequela

delayed phase is again useful in discriminating between active extravasation, pseudoaneurysms, and potentially clinically insignificant small venous injuries. Rarely, bullet fragments may penetrate the lumen of a large artery or vein and then can embolize to a distant site [39, 40] (Fig. 20). Importantly, vascular injury may present in delayed fashion (Fig. 21). In patients with high suspicion of vascular injury, short interval follow-up imaging may be appropriate.

## Conclusion

Penetrating abdominal trauma requires focused imaging interpretation by radiologists with careful analysis of wound trajectory to help diagnose or raise suspicions of visceral trauma. Knowledge of ballistic kinematics is helpful in the radiologist's understanding of wound trajectories. Solid organ injuries should be graded with AAST

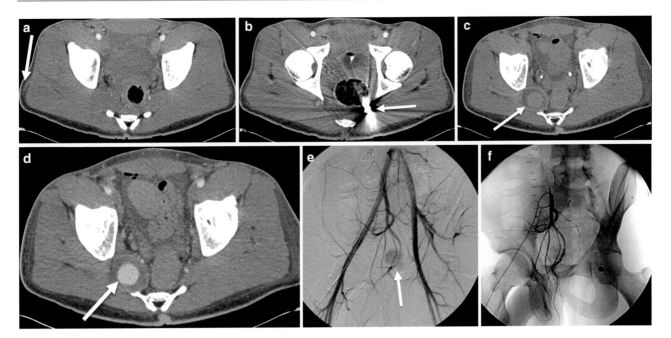

**Fig. 21** Twenty-year-old man shot through the pelvis. Axial CT images with intravenous contrast show bullet entry in the right hip (**a**, arrow), ultimately lodging near the rectum (**b**, arrow). Rectal injury was confirmed operatively. The patient presented with worsening pelvic pain one week later. Axial CT without (**c**) and with (**d**) intravenous contrast demonstrates a new, rounded vascular structure in the territory of the superior gluteal artery compatible with a pseudoaneurysm (arrows). This was confirmed (**e**) and treated (**f**) with angiography and coiling

classifications with careful assessment for associated vascular injuries. High-grade renal injuries warrant delayed acquisitions to assess for collecting system injuries, whereas suspected bladder injuries warrant further assessment with CT cystography. Bowel, mesenteric, and vascular injuries should be identified not only by their position relative to the path of injury, but also by other direct and indirect signs.

## References

1. Dickinson ET, Braslow B. Acute abdominal eviscerations. JEMS. 2006;31(1):70–2, 74, 76–81; quiz 84–85.
2. Zafar SN, Nabeel Zafar S, Rushing A, et al. Outcome of selective non-operative management of penetrating abdominal injuries from the North American National Trauma Database. Br J Surg. 2012;99 (Suppl 1):155–64.
3. Martin MJ, Brown CVR, Shatz DV, et al. Evaluation and management of abdominal stab wounds: a Western trauma association critical decisions algorithm. J Trauma Acute Care Surg. 2018;85(5):1007–15.
4. Nicholas CM, Ward JG, Helmer SD, Haan JM. Incidence of gunshot wounds: before and after implementation of a shall issue conceal carry law. Kans J Med. 2020;13:38–42.
5. Centers for Disease Control and Prevention. Surveillance for violent deaths – national violent death reporting system. Morb Mortal Wkly Rep, 2011. http://www.cdc.gov/mmwr/preview/mmwrhtml/ss6010a1.htm?s_cid=ss6010a1_e. Accessed 15 Aug 2020.
6. Nicholas JM, Rix EP, Easley KA, et al. Changing patterns in the management of penetrating abdominal trauma: the more things change, the more they stay the same. J Trauma. 2003;55(6):1095–108; discussion 1108–1110.
7. Shaftan GW. Selective conservatism in penetrating abdominal trauma. J Trauma. 1969;9(12):1026–8.
8. Como JJ, Bokhari F, Chiu WC, et al. Practice management guidelines for selective nonoperative management of penetrating abdominal trauma. J Trauma. 2010;68(3):721–33.
9. Dreizin D, Munera F. Multidetector CT for penetrating torso trauma: state of the art. Radiology. 2015;277(2):338–55.
10. Jandial R, Reichwage B, Levy M, Duenas V, Sturdivan L. Ballistics for the neurosurgeon. Neurosurgery. 2008;62(2):472–80; discussion 480.
11. Rhee PM, Moore EE, Joseph B, Tang A, Pandit V, Vercruysse G. Gunshot wounds: a review of ballistics, bullets, weapons, and myths. J Trauma Acute Care Surg. 2016;80(6):853–67.
12. Hanna TN, Shuaib W, Han T, Mehta A, Khosa F. Firearms, bullets, and wound ballistics: an imaging primer. Injury. 2015;46(7):1186–96.
13. Henry S. ATLS 10th edition offers new insights into managing trauma patients. J Bull Am Coll Surg. 2018. Available online: http://bulletin.facs.org/2018/06/atls-10th-edition-offers-new-insights-into-managing-trauma-patients/. Accessed 15 Aug 2020.

14. Ollerton JE, Sugrue M, Balogh Z, D'Amours SK, Giles A, Wyllie P. Prospective study to evaluate the influence of FAST on trauma patient management. J Trauma. 2006;60(4):785–91.

15. Scaife ER, Fenton SJ, Hansen KW, Metzger RR. Use of focused abdominal sonography for trauma at pediatric and adult trauma centers: a survey. J Pediatr Surg. 2009;44(9):1746–9.

16. Richards JR, McGahan JP. Focused assessment with sonography in trauma (FAST) in 2017: what radiologists can learn. Radiology. 2017;283(1):30–48.

17. Von Kuenssberg JD, Stiller G, Wagner D. Sensitivity in detecting free intraperitoneal fluid with the pelvic views of the FAST exam. Am J Emerg Med. 2003;21(6):476–8.

18. Poletti PA, Kinkel K, Vermeulen B, Irmay F, Unger P-F, Terrier F. Blunt abdominal trauma: should US be used to detect both free fluid and organ injuries? Radiology. 2003;227(1):95–103.

19. Ziegler K, Feeney JM, Desai C, Sharpio D, Marshall WT, Twohig M. Retrospective review of the use and costs of routine chest x rays in a trauma setting. J Trauma Manag Outcomes. 2013;7(1):2.

20. Brink M, de Lange F, Oostveen LJ, et al. Arm raising at exposure-controlled multidetector trauma CT of thoracoabdominal region: higher image quality, lower radiation dose. Radiology. 2008;249(2):661–70.

21. Ozimok CJ, Mellnick VM, Patlas MN. An international survey to assess use of oral and rectal contrast in CT protocols for penetrating torso trauma. Emerg Radiol. 2019;26(2):117–21.

22. Alabousi M, Zha N, Patlas MN. Use of enteric contrast for abdominopelvic CT in penetrating traumatic injury in adults: comparison of diagnostic accuracy systematic review and meta-analysis. AJR Am J Roentgenol. 2020; https://doi.org/10.2214/AJR.20.24636. Epub ahead of print. PMID: 32997519.

23. Jawad H, Raptis C, Mintz A, Schuerer D, Mellnick V. Single-contrast CT for detecting bowel injuries in penetrating abdominopelvic trauma. AJR Am J Roentgenol. 2018;210(4):761–5.

24. Durso AM, Paes FM, Caban K, et al. Evaluation of penetrating abdominal and pelvic trauma. Eur J Radiol. 2020;130:109187.

25. Berg RJ, Inaba K, Okoye O, et al. The contemporary management of penetrating splenic injury. Injury. 2014;45(9):1394–400.

26. Schnüriger B, Talving P, Barbarino R, Barmparas G, Inaba K, Demetriades D. Current practice and the role of the CT in the management of penetrating liver injuries at a level I trauma center. J Emerg Trauma Shock. 2011;4(1):53–7.

27. Mellnick VM, Raptis C, Lonsford C, Lin M, Schuerer D. Traumatic lumbar hernias: do patient or hernia characteristics predict bowel or mesenteric injury? Emerg Radiol. 2014;21(3):239–43.

28. Ballard DH, Mazaheri P, Oppenheimer DC, et al. Imaging of abdominal wall masses, Masslike lesions, and diffuse processes. Radiographics. 2020;40(3):684–706.

29. Kansas BT, Eddy MJ, Mydlo JH, Uzzo RG. Incidence and management of penetrating renal trauma in patients with multiorgan injury: extended experience at an inner city trauma center. J Urol. 2004;172 (4 Pt 1):1355–60.

30. Saksobhavivat N, Shanmuganathan K, Boscak AR, et al. Diagnostic accuracy of triple-contrast multi-detector computed tomography for detection of penetrating gastrointestinal injury: a prospective study. Eur Radiol. 2016;26(11):4107–20.

31. Lubner M, Menias C, Rucker C, et al. Blood in the belly: CT findings of hemoperitoneum. Radiographics. 2007;27(1):109–25.

32. von Herrmann PF, Nickels DJ, Mansouri M, Singh A. Imaging of blunt and penetrating abdominal trauma. In: Singh A, editor. Emergency radiology. Cham: Springer; 2018. https://doi.org/10.1007/978-3-319-65397-6_9.

33. Kozar RA, Crandall M, Shanmuganathan K, et al. Organ injury scaling 2018 update: spleen, liver, and kidney. J Trauma Acute Care Surg. 2018;85(6):1119–22.

34. Kumar A, Panda A, Gamanagatti S. Blunt pancreatic trauma: a persistent diagnostic conundrum? World J Radiol. 2016;8(2):159–73.

35. Dane B, Baxter AB, Bernstein MP. Imaging genitourinary trauma. Radiol Clin N Am. 2017;55(2):321–35.

36. Bhatt S, Dogra VS. Role of US in testicular and scrotal trauma. Radiographics. 2008;28(6):1617–29.

37. Hammer MM, Raptis DA, Mellnick VM, Bhalla S, Raptis CA. Traumatic injuries of the diaphragm: overview of imaging findings and diagnosis. Abdom Radiol (NY). 2017;42(4):1020–7.

38. Raptis CA, Hammer MM, Raman KG, Mellnick VM, Bhalla S. Acute traumatic aortic injury: practical considerations for the diagnostic radiologist. J Thorac Imaging. 2015;30(3):202–13.

39. Stallings LA, Newell MA, Toschlog EA, Thomas CC, Kypson AP. Right ventricular bullet embolism: diagnostic and therapeutic decisions. Injury Extra. 2013;44(7):64–6.

40. Springer J, Newman W, McGoey R. Intravascular bullet embolism to the right atrium. J Forensic Sci. 2011;56(Suppl 1):S259–62.

# Imaging After Damage Control Surgery

# 26

Armonde Baghdanian, Arthur Baghdanian, Thuy-Huong Pham, and Scott D. Steenburg

## Contents

### Abstract

Abdominopelvic computed tomography (CT) following life-saving damage control surgery (DCS) for trauma is becoming more common in the modern trauma center. Multisystem internal injuries, as well as the postoperative appearance of the peritoneal cavity, organs, bowel, and soft tissues, create a very complex and confusing picture for the interpreting radiologist. Therefore, the knowledge of DCS maneuvers and the process of damage control resuscitation (DCR) in the setting of hypothermia, acidosis, and coagulopathy are important to allow for more accurate and meaningful interpretation. Unexpected injuries are commonly encountered on post-DCS CT, thus rapid diagnosis and communication of these are essential as they may necessitate urgent, unplanned re-intervention. In this chapter, damage control surgery will be described, with special attention to details which are important for the radiologist to know during interpretation. Expected postoperative findings on CT will be reviewed, and special emphasis will be made on frequently encountered unexpected findings on post-DCS CT.

### Keywords

Damage control surgery · Damage control laparotomy · Damage control resuscitation · Coagulopathy · Active bleeding · Solid organ trauma · Bowel trauma

## Introduction

Trauma is the leading cause of death for those age 65 or less, with life years lost greatly exceeding that of malignancy [1]. Computed tomography has been shown to have a high sensitivity and specificity for the diagnosis of acute injuries and can alter patient management [2–7]. While somewhat

A. Baghdanian · A. Baghdanian
Department of Radiology, Keck School of Medicine, University of Southern California, Los Angeles, CA, USA

T.-H. Pham
Department of Surgery, Indiana University School of Medicine, Indianapolis, IN, USA

S. D. Steenburg (✉)
Department of Radiology and Imaging Sciences, Indiana University School of Medicine, Indianapolis, IN, USA
e-mail: ssteenbu@iuhealth.org

© Springer Nature Switzerland AG 2022
M. N. Patlas et al. (eds.), *Atlas of Emergency Imaging from Head-to-Toe*,
https://doi.org/10.1007/978-3-030-92111-8_26

controversial, there is a building body of evidence that whole-body computed tomography (WBCT) in the early evaluation of acute trauma patients can improve survival [2, 5, 8–11]. However, it is relatively common that patients with abdominal and/or pelvic trauma are too unstable to undergo imaging at the time of presentation to the trauma center. It is these patients who are triaged to emergent lifesaving "damage control surgery" (DCS), a series of staged surgical procedures during which life-threatening bleeding is initially identified and controlled. Physiologic resuscitation is then continued in the intensive care unit (ICU) and completed with definitive surgical correction and abdominal wall closure. It is in this patient population that there is emerging evidence that post-DCS abdominopelvic CT can be of substantial clinical use for the diagnosis of clinically occult injuries or injuries not fully explored during laparotomy [12–16]. Unexpected or previously undiagnosed injuries are commonly identified during post-DCS abdominopelvic CT, with many of these injuries necessitating additional intervention [12–16]. In addition,

the imaging features that one would typically be expected to see following DCS are often quite confusing: retained surgical instruments, peritoneal packing material, an open abdominal wall, temporarily altered internal anatomy, and edema due to third spacing resulting in potentially very confusing CT findings, even for the most experienced radiologist [14, 17].

In this chapter, the historical perspective and current state of DCS and damage control resuscitation (DCR) will be detailed, along with descriptions of the major technical features of DCS and how they relate to postoperative imaging appearances. The importance of the "vicious cycle of coagulopathy" will be reviewed, as the physiologic derangements of hemorrhagic shock and volume resuscitation can be manifested on post-DCS abdominopelvic CT. Anticipated imaging findings will be reviewed, as well as the unexpected imaging findings which can lead to operative or nonoperative management. The following chapter is designed to give the radiologist the knowledge and tools needed to approach the interpretation of these challenging examinations (Fig. 1).

**Fig. 1** Imaging findings in the abdomen and pelvis following DCS can be confusing. Multiple expected postoperative findings can be anticipated, including retained surgical instruments, an open abdominal wall, and diffuse edema due to aggressive resuscitation. The radiologist should also look carefully for findings that may not be expected, such as active bleeding and injuries to the unexplored regions, especially the retroperitoneum, spine, and bony pelvis

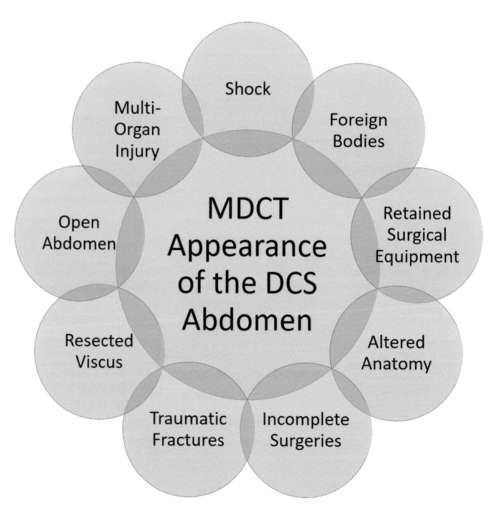

# Damage Control Surgery: The Surgeon's Perspective

As health systems continue to expand and the management and expedition of patients in the field improves, the nature of trauma and its victims has undergone a significant evolution. What were once non-survivable, devastating injuries, have become the trauma activations filling "shock" rooms and operating rooms. Transport times have decreased, standardized evaluations have streamlined initial surveys, and public health endeavors such as the "Stop the Bleed" education movement have resulted in a larger, and arguably sicker, trauma population. As such, the use of damage control laparotomy and a staged resuscitation has become the standard of care in the critically ill operative patient.

The term "damage control surgery" was first coined by Rotundo in 1993 in his landmark paper, demonstrating a sevenfold increase in survivorship with abbreviated laparotomy [18]. However, the concept of expedited hemostasis, resuscitation, and re-evaluation has much further reaching roots. The first open abdomen was described in 1897, wherein septic peritonitis was temporized with the application of gauze to the intestines and a partial skin approximation performed with silkworm gut sutures [19]. William Stewart Halstead thereafter introduced the concept of hepatic packing, detailing a technique wherein rubber sheets were placed directly atop the liver in addition to gauze packing materials as a means of protecting the liver parenchyma. The modern popularization of the abbreviated laparotomy can be attributed to the work of H. Harlan Stone and John Burch. Stone's experience at Grady Memorial Hospital in Atlanta demonstrated increased survivorship with early abortion of laparotomies in the setting of patient instability [20]. Burch similarly demonstrated the utility of temporary abdominal closure and concurrent correction of physiologic derangements [21]. By the early 2000s, DCS would become the accepted standard of care for the unstable trauma patient, as a wealth of research had continued to echo the results of improved mortality in both penetrating and blunt trauma patients.

The process of damage control resuscitation (DCR) follows a natural, intuitive stepwise progression. In Stage 0, the initial evaluation of the patient benefits from a standardized approach, such as the Advanced Trauma Life Support Program (ATLS) from the American College of Surgeons, to establish IV access, initiate balanced volume resuscitation, and to mobilize available resources [22]. In Stage 1, the initial abbreviated laparotomy is performed with the goal of hemostasis and gross control of contamination. After entry into the abdomen, the quadrants are typically widely packed, volume resuscitation continued in concert, and the packing is then sequentially removed in stepwise fashion for evaluation of all abdominal fields. Initial control of vascular hemorrhage can

be achieved with manual compression and suture ligation. Vascular patency can also be maintained through the placement of temporary shunts that would then require formal repair at the time of reoperation [23]. In evaluating the bowel for compromise, perforated and/or marginal segments can be quickly resected and disposed of to control sites of contamination. Owing to the critical status of the patients, the bowel can then be left in temporary discontinuity. Solid-organ injuries can sometimes be temporized by local packing to facilitate tamponade and also by approximation of the visceral defect with methods such as hepatorrhaphy, splenorrhaphy, etc. Upon achievement of adequate hemostasis and source control, a temporary abdominal closure (TAC) is then performed, with the goal of protecting the underlying bowel from desiccation/evisceration, preventing bowel adherence to the abdominal wall, and preventing fascial retraction such that a permanent fascial closure may at some point in the near future be attained. Temporary closure techniques include placement of negative pressure vacuum therapies, skin-only approximation, and, in the setting of the prolonged open abdomen (OA), Wittmann Patches and polypropylene mesh placements [24].

Stage 2 of DCR transitions from the operating room to the intensive care unit and necessitates correction of the vicious cycle of hypothermia, acidosis, and coagulopathy that has manifested since the initial insult. The causes of hypothermia are usually multifactorial, including conductive, radiative, and evaporative heat loss. Additionally, there is a linear and predictable relationship between the volume administered for resuscitation and the heat loss experienced by the patient [25, 26]. The consequences of this hypothermia are profound: decreased cardiac output, decreased glomerular filtration rates, arrhythmias, and exacerbation of ongoing coagulopathy secondary to platelet dysfunction have all been attributed to hypothermia. The effects of acidosis and hypothermia on coagulation are then further compounded by the dilutional effects of an unbalanced resuscitation. The results of this physiologic derangement are often seen on post-DCS CT in these patients, manifested by edema throughout the body (body wall, mesentery, periportal region, Fig. 2), as well as foci of active bleeding near internal injuries or surgical sites (Fig. 3).

As the patient's hypothermia, acidosis, and coagulopathy are mitigated, Stage 3 results in the definitive operative management of the known injuries and temporized repairs and is typically performed 24–48 h after initial DCS. The steps of the initial surgery are reversed. Packs are carefully removed, again in a sequential fashion, and all prior injury sites are re-evaluated. Hemostasis is evaluated and bleeding controlled. Should the patient have undergone a bowel resection without anastomosis, continuity is now restored, whether through anastomosis of proximal and distal limbs or the formation of an ostomy. Gastrostomy tubes and jejunostomy

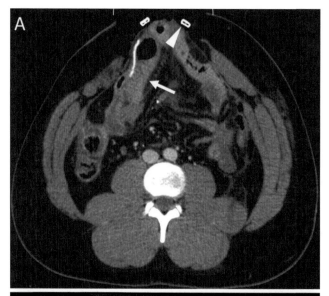

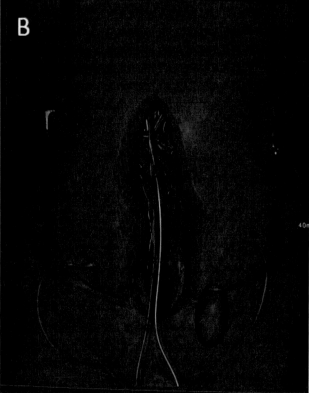

**Fig. 2** Postoperative axial abdominopelvic CT (a) demonstrates bowel wall edema (arrow) with protrusion of bowel through the open abdominal wall (bracket). Overlying vacuum dressing and surgical drains (triangle) are seen. Aggressive IV hydration used to combat shock state increases visceral edema making the approximation of wound edges difficult

tubes can be placed should the patient require prolonged feeding access. The abdomen is then irrigated and pending the degree of contamination, and surgical drains can be placed at this time. Fascia is approximated if possible, and

the skin and subcutaneous tissues are typically left open owing to their frank contamination and concerns for wound healing. Consideration of possible ventral hernia repair, if one should develop, does not typically occur until 6–12 months after initial abdominal wall closure [22].

Successful DCS and DCR require extensive interdisciplinary collaboration. It necessitates an efficient trauma medical system, competent field evaluation, readily available resources, and constant reassessment of the patient's deranged physiology. Should this be achieved, DCS with judicious DCR results in lives saved and resolution of the vicious triad of hypothermia, acidosis, and coagulopathy, as noted, which has plagued their initial clinical presentation. Knowledge of the above surgical strategies and maneuvers by the interpreting radiologist is essential, as the imaging findings seen following DCS can be difficult to interpret (Figs. 4 and 5).

## Utility of CT After Damage Control Surgery

There are a limited number of studies to date which have reviewed/examined the utility of CT imaging solely in patients who have undergone DCS, but in general they present compelling evidence that unsuspected injuries are frequently discovered, often resulting in additional interventions. Haste et al. evaluated at a cohort of 90 patients who underwent diagnostic CT within 48 h of an emergent laparotomy over a 5-year time period. They found that 21% of patients had additional injuries not identified in the initial surgery, and 50% of patients had unsuspected fractures. There were 17 unidentified injuries that were diagnosed on CT, of which 8 were severe enough to warrant immediate surgical or interventional radiology management [13]. Similarly, Matsushima et al. investigated patients who underwent CT within 48 h of receiving emergent neck exploration, thoracotomy, or laparotomy. They found that 59 (66.3%) out of a cohort of 89 patients had new injuries identified. Interestingly, CT imaging in 51 patients (72.8%) necessitated immediate surgical intervention, new consultation from a surgical service, or a higher level of care [16].

Another study by Mendoza et al. investigated 73 penetrating trauma patients who underwent CT following emergent laparotomy. A total of 38 patients (52.0%) had new injuries identified, of which the most frequent were orthopedic or genitourinary injuries. Importantly, 10 patients (13.7%) had injuries that necessitated immediate life-saving repeat surgical intervention. They concluded that CT should be performed after DCS for patients with a high index of suspicion for spine or genitourinary injuries [15].

Weis et al. performed a retrospective 4-year analysis of 124 patients who underwent routine post-laparotomy CT, regardless of postoperative vital signs, laboratory values, or

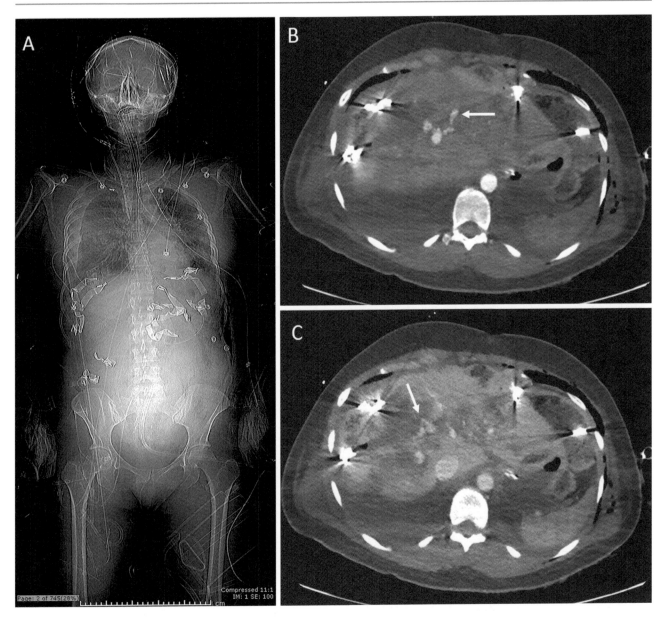

**Fig. 3** A 32-year-old woman with life-threatening thoracic and abdominal injuries after being struck and run over by a car. Scout image (**a**) reveals multiple retained laparotomy pads, as would be expected following DCS. Axial arterial (**b**) and portal venous (**c**) CT images through the upper abdomen demonstrate laparotomy pads in the right upper and left upper quadrants. There is an AAST grade 5 liver injury with continued active bleeding (arrows) despite achieving hemostasis at surgery. Active bleeding is a clinically significant finding that radiologists should actively look for in patients who receive CT following DCS, as it frequently prompts additional intervention such as reoperation or angioembolization

clinical status. They found that 7.3% of patients who had routine CT performed after an exploratory laparotomy had previously unidentified injuries necessitated operative management. This number increased to 10.6% when looking only at patients undergoing damage control surgery. In addition, 29 fractures were identified that may have otherwise been missed as damage control surgery patients typically do not undergo full-body radiographic surveys before being emergently taken to the operating room [12].

## Multidetector CT Imaging Protocol Considerations

The multi-detector CT protocol for damage control surgery patients does not differ substantially from standardized trauma protocols. Optimization is obtained by adhering to standardized CT protocols routinely used for solid organ trauma as a result of blunt or penetrating injury [27]. Damage

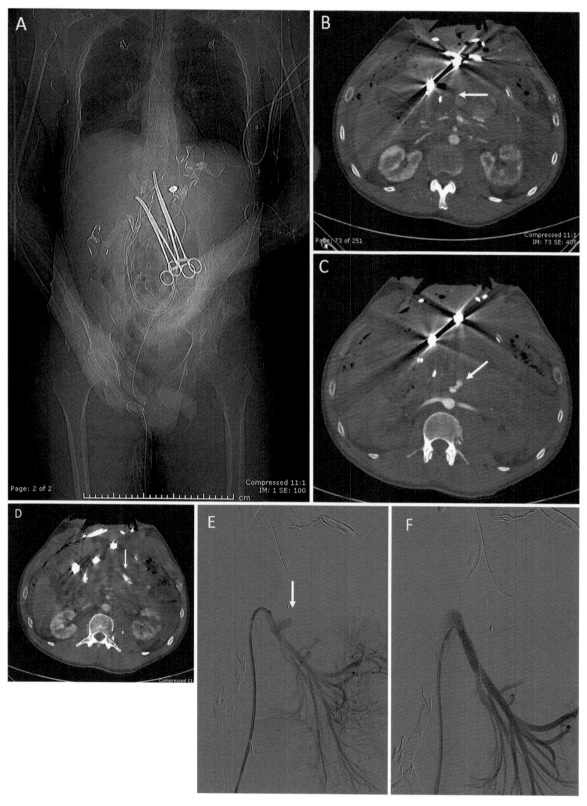

**Fig. 4** A 28-year-old man who was hemodynamically unstable following an abdominal gunshot wound. The patient was taken emergently to the operating room for life-saving damage control laparotomy. Severe injuries to the liver were identified. Hemostasis to the liver injury could not be obtained using hemostatic packing material, so aortic balloon occlusion devices were inserted through the liver injury and secured in place with Kelly clamps. At post-DCS CT, there were numerous retained laparotomy pads and Kelly clamps (**a**). The occlusion balloon could be seen near the portal region (**b**, arrow). There was a pseudo-aneurysm from the SMA (**c**, arrow), and there was active bleeding from a large left abdominal mesenteric injury (**d**, arrow). Selective SMA angiography confirmed the presence of a SMA pseudoaneurysm (arrow) which was treated with a covered stent (E, F). No active bleeding was seen from the SMA branches (not shown)

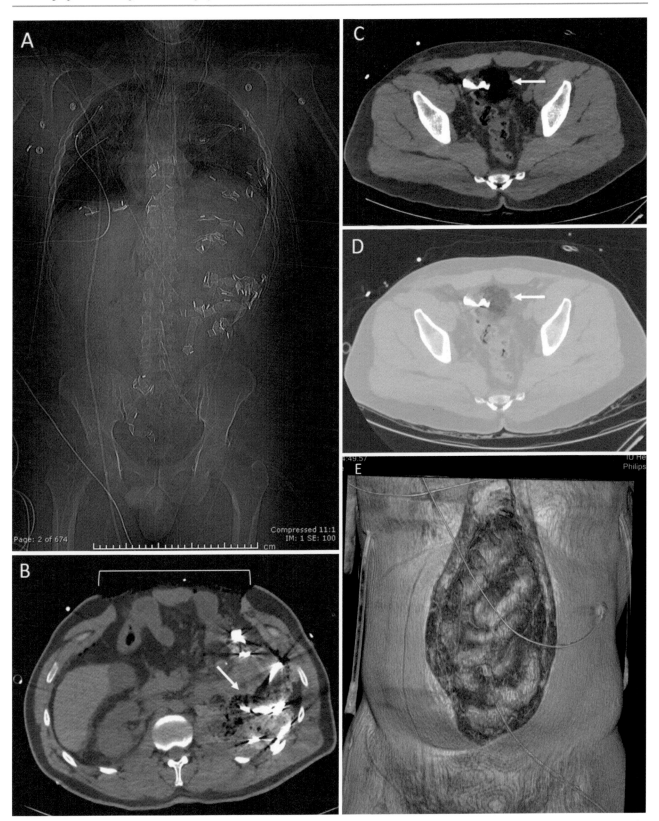

**Fig. 5** A 40-year-old man who sustained life-threatening multisystem trauma following a motorcycle collision. Hemodynamic instability prompted emergency damage control surgery and splenectomy. Postoperative scout image (**a**) reveals numerous retained laparotomy pads in the chest and abdomen. Axial CT through the upper abdomen (**b**) reveals multiple laparotomy pads in the left upper quadrant splenectomy bed (arrow). The patient had an open abdomen (bracket). Axial CT through the pelvis on soft tissue (**c**) and lung windows (**d**) demonstrates laparotomy pad packing material in the pelvis (arrow). The presence of an adjacent metal band is helpful in differentiating lap pads from stool or an abscess. 3D surface-rendered image (**e**) nicely demonstrates the open anterior abdominal wall with protrusion of bowel through the defect

control surgery patients have multiple foreign bodies that include surgical packing material, drains, bone fragments, and possibly metal bullet fragments. Images obtained prior to contrast administration can help differentiate a small focus of contrast extravasation from multiple indwelling foreign bodies. If scanning with a dual-energy CT scanner, virtual non-contrast images may be constructed negating the need to obtain a non-contrast phase [28]. In addition, a dual-energy scanner can be used to reduce beam hardening artifact from metallic foreign bodies such as the radio-opaque markers of surgical packing [29]. However, a notable limitation of this is that institutions differ in their ability to post-process dual-energy images in an expedient manner required for damage control surgery patients.

Multiphase arterial and portal venous phase post-contrast acquisitions are recommended to enhance sensitivity for injury detection. The use of a multiphase examination increases sensitivity for active hemorrhage and for the detection of posttraumatic non-bleeding vascular injuries, such as pseudoaneurysms [30]. Delayed excretory phase imaging may help further increase sensitivity for small foci of active extravasation of contrast. In addition,

excretory phase imaging is useful for the evaluation of the renal collection system and proximal ureters for injuries which may require urinary intervention [31]. If there is concern for bladder trauma, a CT cystogram may then be obtained, as relying solely on delayed phase imaging lacks sensitivity for the detection of bladder injury [31, 32]. As with CT cystograms in the trauma setting, it should be performed after the IV contrast portion of the examination, as bladder contrast leak may obscure active bleeding within the pelvis. Patients undergoing damage control surgery for trauma typically have injuries at more than one site, emphasizing the importance of thorough review and avoiding the pitfall of satisfaction of search [13, 14, 17, 33].

The use of enteric contrast should be made on a case-by-case basis after discussion with the surgical team. CT without the use of enteric contrast has shown to be accurate in the diagnosis of mesenteric and bowel trauma in blunt trauma [34]. The signs of traumatic bowel injury such as bowel wall thickening, free air, free fluid, and mesenteric edema have been described in the literature [35]. However, the imaging features of traumatic bowel injury lack

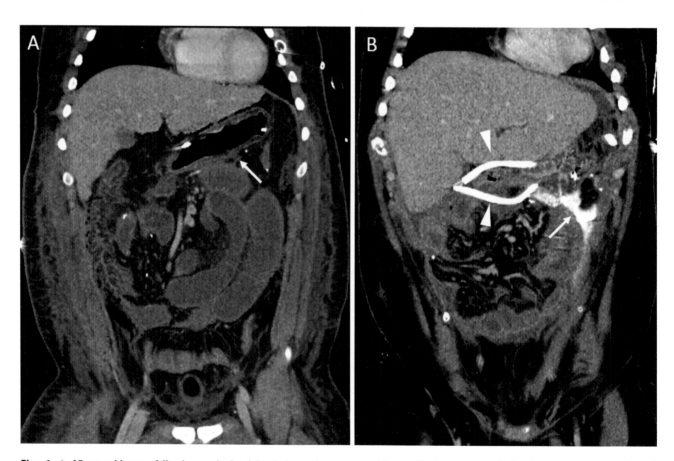

**Fig. 6** A 37-year-old man following a single abdominal gunshot wound. Post-DCS abdominopelvic coronal CT images before (**a**) and after (**b**) enteric contrast administration through the patient's enteric tube. The pre-enteric contrast image (**a**) reveals an irregularity of the wall of the greater curvature of the stomach (arrow). The post-enteric contrast image (**b**) demonstrates a leak of contrast from a gastric wall defect (arrow). There are adjacent subhepatic surgical drains (triangles). Enteric contrast is invaluable for the detection of bowel injury due to the lack of specificity of secondary signs of bowel injury in patients undergoing damage control surgery

specificity in the damage control surgery patients that may already have abnormal bowel imaging features given their postoperative state, shock physiology, and open abdomen. Particularly in patients with penetrating trauma who undergo DCS, the use of enteric contrast should be considered to increase sensitivity for the detection of bowel injury (Fig. 6). The use of enteric contrast can also confirm the stability of surgical repairs of bowel that are performed in an expedited manner [14, 33].

## Expected Imaging Findings Following DCS

Knowledge of the expected postsurgical abdominopelvic CT findings following damage control surgery can help facilitate the expedited and accurate reporting by the radiologist. One of the most striking features of DCS patients is that they have open abdomens with towel clip closures or overlying wound vacuum devices. The aggressive use of intravenous resuscitation and shock state result in a marked visceral edema making wound approximation difficult (Figs. 2, 4, and 5) [36]. In addition, the abdomen is left open for a planned return to the operating room for definitive surgical management. Early closure of the abdomen is associated with wound dehiscence and possible development of an abdominal compartment syndrome [37]. Patients commonly have imaging features of the hypoperfusion complex given the shock state which include pancreatic and peripancreatic edema, renal and adrenal hyperenhancement, a slit-like inferior vena cava, and thickened bowel loops with mucosal edema [38, 39].

Commonly, patients have abdominal surgical packing material in the abdomen that is performed either empirically for hemostasis or placed strategically at sites where there is a concern for persistent injury, such as above and below the liver, spleen, bilateral paracolic gutters, and the pelvis [40–42]. On CT, the radio-opaque band may mimic a bullet or bone fragment, though it can easily be identified on review of the CT scout image (Figs. 3a, 4a, and 5a). The gauze portion of the packing material may mimic the appearance of an abscess, hematoma, feculent material, or a loop of bowel (Figs. 3, 4, and 5). Knowledge of its appearance and typical placement can help avoid these potential pitfalls. The radiologist can also heed closer attention to an area that contains packing as this may be an area of concern for persistent injury. High-grade viscus injuries may be seen that require organ removal as surgical repair is not possible. Patients may be seen with altered anatomy in the form of a full nephrectomy, splenectomy, or hepatic segmentectomy that was performed to control severe hemorrhage [43]. The removed organ fossa will typically be replaced with packing material (Fig. 5b). In the interest of time in these patients at risk of severe coagulopathy, complete bowel repairs such as primary anastomoses and bowel ostomies are usually not performed. Therefore, on CT, end-ligated loops of bowel

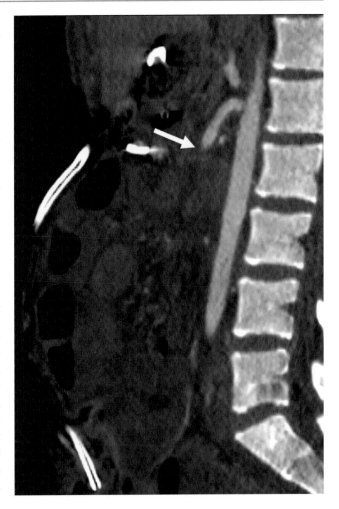

**Fig. 7** A 29-year-old woman with multiple abdominal stab wounds. At surgery, the superior mesenteric artery (SMA) was severely damaged and was subsequently ligated. Sagittal post-DCS CT demonstrates abrupt cutoff of the proximal SMA (arrow) compatible with a history of surgical ligation

without enteric continuity may be seen [43]. In addition, major vessels that are severely damaged may be ligated if there is a limited risk of end-organ ischemia (Fig. 7).

Hemodynamically unstable patients immediately get transported to the operating room upon presentation for life-saving damage control surgery. Consequently, routine trauma imaging protocols, such as whole-body CT and radiographic surveys for the evaluation of fractures, are not performed. Therefore, when interpreting a CT following DCS, close attention should be paid to the spine and pelvis for fractures, as these are often unknown to the surgical team and may require bedside stabilization [15–17]. In addition, patients commonly present with low Glasgow coma scale (GCS) scores and imaging of the head and neck may be obtained. Evaluation for traumatic brain and spine injury is essential as this will have been difficult to evaluate clinically prior to the scan [15–17]. The reporting of the presence of foreign bodies such as bullet fragments and their location should

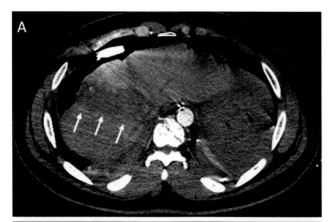

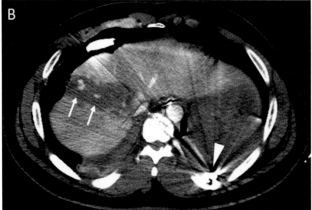

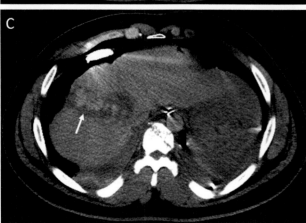

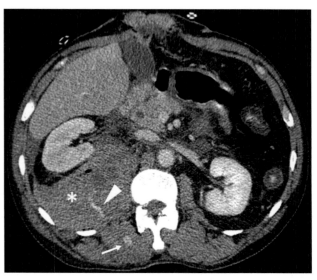

**Fig. 9** A 26-year-old man following an abdominal gunshot wound. Post-DCS axial CT image demonstrates a large posterior pararenal retroperitoneal hematoma (*), with active bleeding in the retroperitoneal hematoma (triangle) and right paraspinal muscles (arrow). The retroperitoneum is not routinely explored during damage control laparotomy, thus emphasizing the importance of postoperative CT in evaluating for suspected injuries in areas that are not fully explored surgically or for unknown injuries outside of the surgical field

## Unexpected Imaging Findings After DCS

Gunshot wounds are a common mechanism of injury that leads to damage control surgery, and thus more than one organ system may be injured [14, 33]. Therefore, it is important to avoid "satisfaction of search" in these patients. In addition, injuries that were treated surgically must be closely evaluated as they may have a persistent injury. This is particularly of concern in hepatic trauma that is notoriously difficult to treat in the coagulopathic patient due to the highly vascularized nature of the hepatic parenchyma and the difficulty in performing a controlled hepatectomy with DCS time constraints [42, 44] (Fig. 8). A multiphasic CT examination can provide confirmation of successful surgical repairs and exclude intraparenchymal injury which is difficult to visualize during expedited open repair [44, 45].

The knowledge of what surgical maneuvers were performed is essential for the diagnosis of clinically unknown injuries, which is especially true for the lesser sac and retroperitoneum (Fig. 9). In the absence of active hemorrhage, an expanding/pulsatile hematoma, or obvious injury, the retroperitoneum may not be surgically explored [13, 43]. Therefore, close attention should be paid to these surgically unexplored areas, as acute injuries may need immediate repair or planned delayed definitive treatment. The evaluation of the kidneys for parenchymal or collecting

**Fig. 8** A 22-year-old man's right upper quadrant gunshot wound. Post-DCS abdominal CT images during arterial (**a**), portal venous (**b**), and 5-min delayed-phase (**c**) images through the upper abdomen demonstrate a transhepatic wound trajectory (**a**, arrows). Portal venous (**b**) and delayed (**c**) images demonstrate active bleeding within the liver along the wound tract, despite attempts at electrocautery for hemostasis during surgery. The bullet traversed the spine, and rested in the posterior left chest wall (**b**, triangle)

be made as these may serve as niduses for infection. They may also preclude the patient from obtaining MRI imaging in the future if they are ferromagnetic and adjacent to vital structures such as the brain parenchyma, globes, spinal cord, or vascular structures [13, 14, 17].

system injury should be made with multiphasic imaging that includes a delayed excretory phase. A urine leak should be excluded as this may necessitate some form of urinary tract diversion. A missed urine leak can lead to sepsis and patient demise [46].

Without CT, a traumatic abdominal aortic injury may be unknown in the absence of retroperitoneal, perivascular, or active hemorrhage in surgery (Fig. 10). Therefore, close evaluation at sites at risk for injury is essential as this will neces-

sitate future repair or follow-up imaging. Evaluation for solid organ posttraumatic injuries such as arteriovenous fistulae or pseudoaneurysms can be diagnosed with multiphase CT examinations. This is essential as these may not have demonstrated active hemorrhage during initial laparotomy but require angiographic embolization due to the risk of future hemorrhage [30, 44, 45]. Close evaluation of the anterior and posterior abdominal wall is also essential as these may be sites of unknown injury with active hemorrhage (Fig. 11).

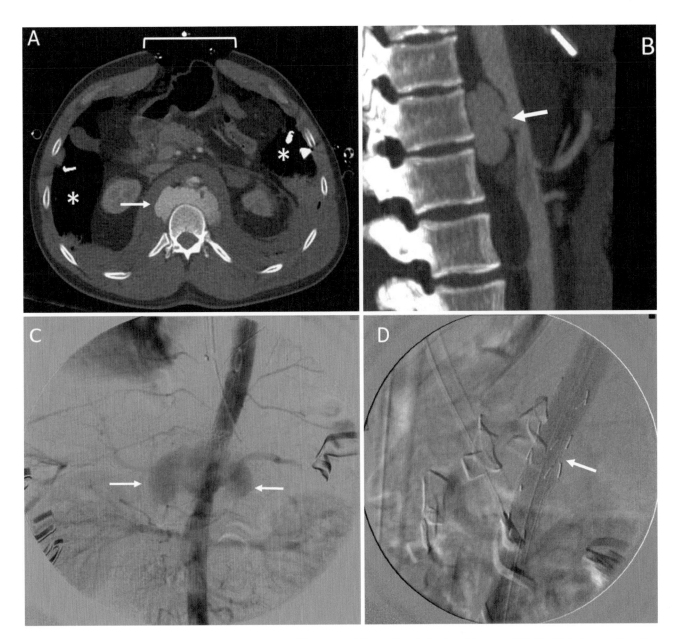

**Fig. 10** Middle-aged man who sustained severe blunt abdominal trauma, who on post-DCS CT was diagnosed with an unsuspected blunt abdominal aortic injury. Axial (**a**) and sagittal (**b**) post-contrast CT images through the abdomen reveal an abdominal aortic rupture with a large contained pseudoaneurysm (arrow). The patient has an open abdomen (bracket) and packing material in the bilateral paracolic gutters (*). The patient underwent catheter angiography (**c**) re-demonstrating the contained rupture (arrows) which was treated with a covered stent (**d**, arrow)

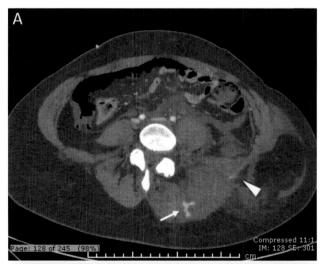

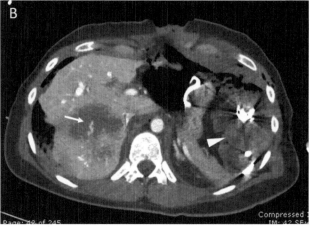

**Fig. 11** A 35-year-old woman who sustained severe multisystem blunt trauma. Axial CT image (**a**) through the lower abdomen demonstrates active bleeding within the left paraspinal muscles (arrow) and an injury to the left abdominal wall and quadratus lumborum (triangle). Axial CT image through the upper abdomen (**b**) demonstrates multiple laparotomy pads in the left upper quadrant (triangle) and a high-grade liver injury with intraparenchymal active bleeding (arrow)

The radiologist should also consider ballistic trajectory in evaluating for unexpected injuries. The integrity of the diaphragm should be evaluated in suspect cases for laceration or elevation as this will require follow-up repair [47, 48]. Portions of the duodenum and pancreas may not be surgically explored; therefore, knowledge of ballistic trajectory can help assess for injuries in these regions. Although injuries to these organs are not common, they are associated with a high mortality and can occur in combination due to close proximity to one another [49]. The bowel should be viewed in association to ballistic trajectory or association with other abdominal injuries in blunt trauma, to evaluate for bowel wall integrity and the potential need for enteric contrast to evaluate for unsuspected injury (Fig. 6).

## Conclusion

CT following life-saving DCS is becoming a common practice in the modern trauma center. Therefore, radiologists who interpret these complex imaging examinations should be familiar with not only the anticipated typical findings but also with unexpected, previously undiagnosed injuries that are routinely identified on CT. The pelvis and spine should be carefully interrogated, as they are typically not imaged preoperatively in these hemodynamically unstable patients. In addition, active bleeding is a common finding on CT following DCS, which is not surprising given the degree of acidosis and coagulopathy as a byproduct of their severe multisystem trauma and shock. Interpretation of post-DCS abdominopelvic CT is challenging; thus, the radiologist should be well informed of the DCS rationale, maneuvers, and postoperative CT findings frequently encountered in this complex patient population.

## Key Points

1. Computed tomography is useful following life-saving damage control surgery (DCS) for trauma.
2. Unsuspected injuries are frequently diagnosed following DCS, especially in the retroperitoneum, spine, and pelvis.
3. Physiologic derangement due to hypothermia and coagulopathy can be seen on post-DCS CT, manifested by third spacing and active bleeding.

## References

1. Years of potential life lost before the age of 65. WISQARS, CDC. 1999–2018. https://webappa.cdc.gov/sasweb/ncipc/ypll.html. Accessed 2 May 2020.
2. Huber-Wagner S, Biberthaler P, Haberle S, et al. Whole-body CT in haemodynamically unstable severely injured patients – a retrospective, multicentre study. PLoS One. 2013;8:e68880.
3. Livingston DH, Lavery RF, Passannante MR, et al. Admission or observation is not necessary after a negative abdominal computed tomographic scan in patients with suspected blunt abdominal trauma: results of a prospective, multi-institutional trial. J Trauma. 1998;44(2):273–80. Discussion 280–2.
4. Salim A, Sangthong B, Martin M, Brown C, Plurad D, Demetriades D. Whole body imaging in blunt multisystem trauma pa-tients without obvious signs of injury: results of a prospective study. Arch Surg. 2006;141(5):468–73. Discussion 473–5.
5. Huber-Wagner S, Lefering R, Qvick L-M, Korner M, Kay MV, Pfeifer K-J, Reiser M, Mutschler W, Kanz K-G. Effect of whole-body CT during trauma resuscitation on survival: a retrospective, multicentre study. Lancet. 2009;373:1455–61.
6. van Vugt R, Kool DR, Deunk J, Edwards MJ. Effects on mortality, treatment, and time management as a result of routine use of total body computed tomography in blunt high-energy trauma patients. J Trauma Acute Care Surg. 2012;72(3):553–9.

7. Wurmb TE, Frühwald P, Hopfner W, et al. Whole-body multislice computed tomography as the first line diagnostic tool in patients with multiple injuries: the focus on time. J Trauma. 2009;66(3):658–65.

8. Caputo ND, Chris S, Lim G, Shah K. Whole-body computed tomographic scanning leads to better survival as opposed to selective scanning in trauma patients: a systematic review and meta-analysis. J Trauma Acute Care Surg. 2014;77(4):534–9.

9. Jiang L, Ma Y, Ye L, Zheng Z, Xu Y, Zhang M. Comparison of WBCT vs selective radiological imaging on outcomes in major trauma patients: a meta-analysis. Scand J Trauma Resusc Emerg Med. 2014;22:54–65.

10. Gordic S, Alkadhi H, Hodel S, Simmen H-P, Brueesch M, Frauenfelder T, Wanner G, Sprengel K. WBCT imaging algorithm for multiple trauma patients: radiation dose and time to diagnosis. Br J Radiol. 2015;88:20140616.

11. Chidambaram S, Goh EL, Khan MA. A meta-analysis of the efficacy of whole-body computed tomography imaging in the management of trauma and injury. Injury. 2017;48:1784–93.

12. Weis JJ, Cunningham KE, Forsythe RM, Billiar TR, Peitzman AB, Sperry JL. The importance of empiric abdominal computed tomography after urgent laparotomy for trauma: do they reveal unexpected injuries? Surgery. 2014;156(4):979–85.

13. Haste AK, Brewer BL, Steenburg SD. Diagnostic yield and clinical utility of abdominopelvic CT following emergent laparotomy for trauma. Radiology. 2016;280(3):735–42.

14. Baghdanian AA, Baghdanian AH, Khalid M, Armetta A, LeBedis CA, Anderson SW, Soto JA. Damage control surgery: use of diagnostic CT after life-saving laparotomy. Emerg Radiol. 2016;23(5):483–95.

15. Mendoza AE, Wybourn CA, Charles AG, Campbell AR, Cairns BA, Knudson MM. Routine computed tomography after recent operative exploration for penetrating trauma: what injuries do we miss? J Trauma Acute Care Surg. 2017;83(4):575–8.

16. Matsushima K, Inaba K, Dollbaum R, Khor D, Jhaveri V, Jimenez O, Strumwasser A, Demetriades D. The role of computed tomography after emergent trauma operation. J Surg Res. 2016;206(2):286–91.

17. Alexander LF, Hanna TN, LeGout JD, Roda MS, Cernigliaro JG, Mittal PK, Harri PA. Multidetector CT findings in the abdomen and pelvis after damage control surgery for acute traumatic injuries. Radiographics. 2019;39:1183–202.

18. Rotondo MF, Schwab CW, McGonigal MD, Phillips GR, Fruchterman TM, Kauder DR, Latenser BA, Angood PA. "Damage control": an approach for improved survival in exsanguinating penetrating abdominal injury. J Trauma. 1993;35:375–82. Discussion 382–3.

19. Leppäniemi A. Who invented damage control surgery? Scand J Surg. 2014;103(3):165–6.

20. Stone HH, Strom PR, Mullins RJ. Management of the major coagulopathy with onset during laparotomy. Ann Surg. 1983;197(5):532–5.

21. Burch JM, Martin RR, Richardson RJ, Muldowny DS, Mattox KL, Jordan GL. Evolution of the treatment of the injured colon in the 1980s. Arch Surg. 1991;126(8):979–84.

22. Waibel BH, Rotondo MM. Damage control surgery: its evolution over the last 20 years. Rev Col Bras Cir. 2012;39:314–21.

23. Hoey BA, Schwab BA. Damage control surgery. Scand J Surg. 2002;91(1):92–103.

24. Dubose JJ, Scalea TM, Holcomb JB, Shrestha B, Okoye O, Inaba K, Bee TK, Fabian TC, Whelan J, Ivatury RR. Open abdominal management after damage-control laparotomy for trauma: a prospective observational American Association for the Surgery of Trauma multicenter study. J Trauma Acute Care Surg. 2013;74:113–20.

25. Schreiber MA. Damage control surgery. Crit Care Clin. 2004;20(1):101–18.

26. Genitello L, Rifley W. Continuous arteriovenous rewarming: report of a new technique for treating hypothermia. J Trauma. 1991;31:1151–4.

27. Shuman WP, et al. Imaging of blunt abdominal trauma. American College of Radiology. ACR Appropriateness Criteria. Radiology. 2000;215(Suppl):143–51.

28. Wortman JR, et al. Dual-energy CT for abdominal and pelvic trauma. Radiographics. 2018;38(2):586–602.

29. Coupal TM, et al. Peering through the glare: using dual-energy CT to overcome the problem of metal artefacts in bone radiology. Skelet Radiol. 2014;43(5):567–75.

30. Uyeda JW, et al. Active hemorrhage and vascular injuries in splenic trauma: utility of the arterial phase in multidetector CT. Radiology. 2014;270(1):99–106.

31. Baghdanian AH, et al. Utility of MDCT findings in predicting patient management outcomes in renal trauma. Emerg Radiol. 2017;24(3):263–72.

32. Haroon SA, et al. Computed tomography (CT) in the evaluation of bladder and ureteral trauma: indications, technique, and diagnosis. Abdom Radiol. 2019;44(12):3962–77.

33. Ahmad ZY, Baghdanian AH, Baghdanian AA. Multidetector computed tomography imaging of damage control surgery patients. Radiol Clin N Am. 2019;57(4):671–87.

34. Stuhlfaut JW, Soto JA, Lucey BC, Ulrich A, Rathlev NK, Burke PA, Hirsh EF. Blunt abdominal trauma: performance of CT without oral contrast material. Radiology. 2004;233(3):689–94.

35. Bates DD, et al. Multidetector CT of surgically proven blunt bowel and mesenteric injury. Radiographics. 2017;37(2):613–25.

36. Shapiro MB, et al. Damage control: collective review. J Trauma. 2000;49(5):969–78.

37. Burch JM, et al. Abbreviated laparotomy and planned reoperation for critically injured patients. Ann Surg. 1992;215(5):476–83. Discussion 483–4.

38. Elst J, et al. Signs of post-traumatic hypovolemia on abdominal CT and their clinical importance: a systematic review. Eur J Radiol. 2020;124:108800.

39. Prasad KR, et al. CT in post-traumatic hypoperfusion complex – a pictorial review. Emerg Radiol. 2011;18(2):139–43.

40. Garrison JR, et al. Predicting the need to pack early for severe intra-abdominal hemorrhage. J Trauma. 1996;40(6):923–7. Discussion 927–9.

41. Gupta M, et al. Abdominal packing for surgically uncontrollable haemorrhage. Trop Gastroenterol. 2010;31(1):61–4.

42. Krige JE, Bornman PC, Terblanche J. Therapeutic perihepatic packing in complex liver trauma. Br J Surg. 1992;79(1):43–6.

43. Germanos S, et al. Damage control surgery in the abdomen: an approach for the management of severe injured patients. Int J Surg. 2008;6(3):246–52.

44. Kutcher ME, et al. The role of computed tomographic scan in ongoing triage of operative hepatic trauma: a Western Trauma Association multicenter retrospective study. J Trauma Acute Care Surg. 2015;79(6):951–6. Discussion 956.

45. Letoublon C, et al. Hepatic arterial embolization in the management of blunt hepatic trauma: indications and complications. J Trauma. 2011;70(5):1032–6. Discussion 1036–7.

46. Smith TG III, Coburn M. Damage control maneuvers for urologic trauma. Urol Clin North Am. 2013;40(3):343–50.

47. Clarke DL, et al. The spectrum of diaphragmatic injury in a busy metropolitan surgical service. Injury. 2009;40(9):932–7.

48. Reber PU, et al. Missed diaphragmatic injuries and their long-term sequelae. J Trauma. 1998;44(1):183–8.

49. Dreizin D, et al. Evaluating blunt pancreatic trauma at whole body CT: current practices and future directions. Emerg Radiol. 2013;20(6):517–27.

# Imaging of Nontraumatic Hepatobiliary Emergencies

**27**

HeiShun Yu and Jennifer W. Uyeda

## Contents

### Abstract

Patients with nontraumatic hepatobiliary emergencies usually present with right upper quadrant abdominal pain, and biliary tract disease is the fifth most common cause of hospital admission. Gallbladder pathologies and other etiologies including infectious, inflammatory, vascular, and postoperative complications can be evaluated on imaging. Being familiar with various imaging appearances of all hepatobiliary disorders is important to provide optimal patient care and equally important is to understand the limitations of each imaging modality.

H. Yu · J. W. Uyeda (✉)
Department of Radiology, Division of Emergency Radiology, Brigham and Women's Hospital/Harvard Medical School, Boston, MA, USA
e-mail: juyeda@bwh.harvard.edu

### Keywords

Hepatobiliary · Emergency · Abdominal pain

## Introduction

Abdominal pain is one of the most common causes of emergency department (ED) visits, and imaging of the hepatobiliary system has an essential role in evaluating patients who present with right upper quadrant pain. Within the 18–44-year-old age group, biliary tract disease is the fifth most common cause of hospital admission [1]. Gallbladder pathologies are common and are the leading cause of hospital admission for gastrointestinal problems, with more than 700,000 cholecystectomies performed annually in the United States [2, 3]. Ethnicity and geography play a role in the prevalence of gallstone disease, as well as the prevalence of the type of gallstone (pigmented or cholesterol), with cholesterol stones being more common in developed countries, while pigmented stones are more common in Asia [4]. Other hepatobiliary emergencies causing right upper quadrant pain include infectious, inflammatory, vascular, and neoplastic diseases, as well as postoperative complications. Imaging plays a crucial role in assessing the hepatobiliary system for acute nontraumatic emergencies, and a variety of imaging modalities are available, including ultrasound (US), computed tomography (CT), hepatobiliary nuclear scintigraphy, and magnetic resonance cholangiopancreatography (MRCP). Dual-energy CT (DECT) is being increasingly utilized in certain clinical practices, with added value in common clinical scenarios including imaging of the hepatobiliary system [6, 7, 8]. In this chapter, we will review various causes of nontraumatic hepatobiliary emergencies and their characteristic imaging features on multiple imaging modalities, and we will review the limitations of each imaging modality.

## Imaging Modalities

### Ultrasound (US)

US is the imaging modality of choice for the initial assessment of known or suspected hepatobiliary disorders. US is sensitive and specific for the detection of gallstones and gallbladder inflammation [9, 10, 11]. Additionally, US can be used to detect biliary ductal dilatation and fluid collections; however, identifying the cause for these imaging findings is somewhat limited with US. Of particular importance in the posttransplant patient is assessing the hepatic vasculature with Doppler US.

### Computed Tomography (CT)

CT is the most common imaging modality used in the evaluation of acute abdominal pain in nonpregnant adults and is commonly used to evaluate acute hepatobiliary disease,

typically after sonography or initially if right upper quadrant abdominal disorders are not specifically identified on initial clinical evaluation. CT with intravenous contrast is preferred and can be used to evaluate the hepatic parenchyma and adjacent organs, including the pancreas, kidneys, and stomach, and can be used to detect identify fluid collections. Harvey et al. [10] found CT to be less sensitive (39%) than US (83%) for the detection of acute biliary disorders, but CT and US have similar specificity, 93% and 95%, respectively (Figs. 1 and 2).

## Nuclear Medicine

The hepatobiliary iminodiacetic acid scan (HIDA) involves the injection of 5 mCi of a technetium-99m iminodiacetic acid analog, which is taken up by hepatic parenchyma within 5 minutes after the injection and is normally excreted into the biliary tract within 10 minutes, and the gallbladder is normally seen within 15 minutes. A HIDA scan can be used to identify cystic duct obstruction in the setting of acute cholecystitis. False-positive results can occur secondary to severe liver disease, sphincterotomy, prolonged fasting, and prior administration of cholecystokinin [11]. A HIDA scan can be helpful in diagnosing a biliary leak in the postoperative setting (Figs. 3 and 4).

## MRCP

MR has high soft tissue characterization and provides superior evaluation of the hepatic parenchyma and adjacent soft tissue organs, in addition to depicting gallstones and choledocholithiasis. The biliary tract is best assessed on MRCP, which relies on heavily T2-weighted images. Hepatobiliary agents, particularly gadoxetate, can be administered in the postcholecystectomy patient to assess the operative anatomy, to depict potential biliary leaks, and to reveal any site of biliary duct injury (Figs. 5 and 6).

## Infection/Inflammation

### Acute Cholecystitis

While gallstones affect people worldwide, cholesterol stones predominate in developed countries with 10–15% of people in the United States having gallstones, affecting more than 20 million American adults [12, 13]. A majority of acute cholecystitis cases, up to 95%, are due to an obstructing calculus at the cystic duct or gallbladder neck, resulting in irritation and inflammation of the gallbladder [14].

**Fig. 1** A 78-year-old woman presented with upper abdominal pain from choledocholithiasis causing acute cholecystitis. IV contrast-enhanced axial CT image (a) demonstrates dependent calculi (arrow) within the gallbladder, with gallbladder wall thickening and pericholecystic fluid. Coronal CT image (b) demonstrates similar gallbladder findings, in addition to a dilated common duct with a calculus in the distal duct (arrowhead), i.e., choledocholithiasis

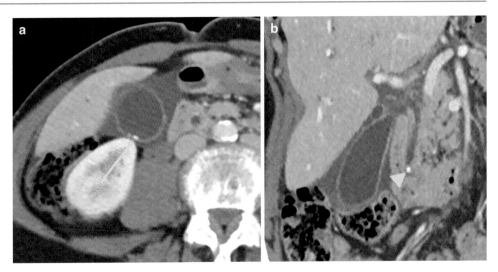

**Fig. 2** A 67-year-old man with 4 days of abdominal pain with perforated acute cholecystitis. IV contrast-enhanced axial (a) and coronal (b) CT images demonstrate a distended gallbladder with numerous dependent tiny calculi, with associated pericholecystic fat stranding and fluid. There is also a defect in the gallbladder wall (arrow), with spillage of gas and calculi into the gallbladder fossa

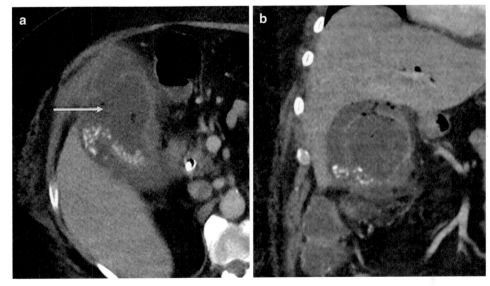

US is the initial imaging modality of choice for the identification of cholelithiasis and cholecystitis but may be limited by patient body habitus. Evaluation for cystic duct obstruction is limited on US, and acute cholecystitis is diagnosed based on secondary signs including cholelithiasis, gallbladder wall thickening greater than 3 mm, pericholecystic fluid, increased mural vascular flow, gallbladder distension >4–5 cm in the transverse plane and >10 cm in the sagittal plane, and a sonographic Murphy's sign [8, 9, 15]. Although US is readily available and does not involve ionizing radiation, the individual sonographic findings of acute cholecystitis are in general relatively nonspecific and can be seen in the setting of other gallbladder diseases (i.e., chronic cholecystitis, cholesterolosis, and malignancy) and in liver, renal, and cardiac diseases [8, 15].

CT is often the first imaging modality used to assess patients who present with otherwise nonspecific acute abdominal pain, and it has been shown to be as sensitive compared to US. A recent study by Wertz et al. showed CT to be statistically significantly more sensitive for the diagnosis of acute cholecystitis than US [16]. However, both imaging modalities are complementary in making the diagnosis and if there remains uncertainty after one imaging modality, the other may be obtained to more conclusively exclude or diagnose acute cholecystitis [16]. CT findings of acute cholecystitis are similar to US, including gallbladder distension, pericholecystic inflammation and fluid, wall thickening, and gallstones. CT is limited for the depiction of many gallstones if the images are not windowed appropriately, particularly for noncalcified stones which are isodense to bile. Using DECT virtual monochromatic imaging can substantially increase the conspicuity of noncalcified gallstones [17, 18, 19]. Cholesterol-filled gallstones have an -energy-dependent X-ray attenuation curve distinct from that of bile, allowing for increased conspicuity and detection

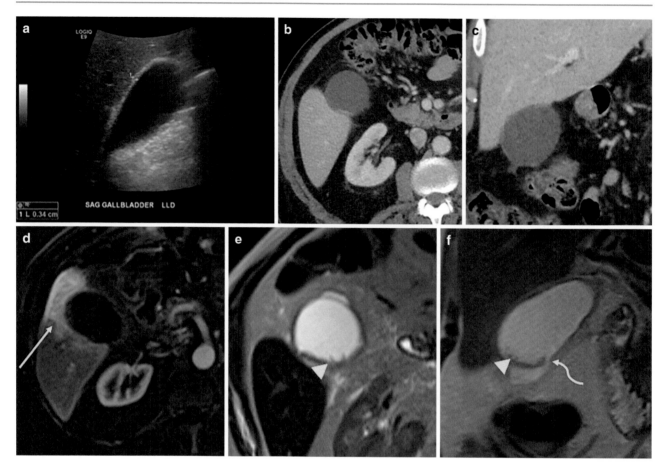

**Fig. 3** A 71-year-old man with nausea and abdominal distention with gangrenous cholecystitis. Long-axis US image (a) demonstrates a distended gallbladder with borderline wall thickening and layering non-shadowing echogenic material, which may represent sludge or tiny calculi. The sonographer reported a positive sonographic Murphy's sign. IV contrast-enhanced axial (b) and coronal (c) CT images demonstrate a distended gallbladder with minimal stranding adjacent to the gallbladder fundus. IV contrast-enhanced T1-weighted fat-saturated axial MR image (d) demonstrates a distended gallbladder with hyperemia in the gallbladder fossa (arrow). Axial (e) and coronal (f) T2-weighted MR images demonstrate irregularity of the gallbladder wall (arrowhead). A wall defect is noted near the fundus (curved arrow)

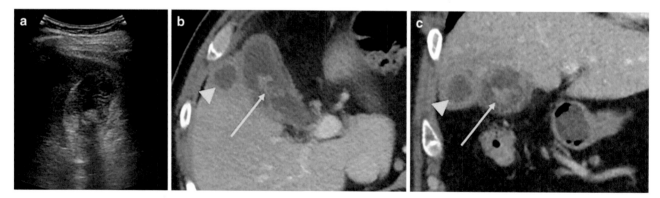

**Fig. 4** A 76-year-old man with fever, elevated white blood count, and abnormal liver function tests, with gangrenous cholecystitis and pericholecystic abscess. Long-axis US image (a) demonstrates a distended gallbladder with wall thickening and edema, as well as a dependent calculus. IV contrast-enhanced axial (b) and coronal (c) CT images demonstrate a distended gallbladder with irregular gallbladder wall thickening and edema and minimal pericholecystic stranding. Intraluminal membranes/debris is noted (arrow). Additionally, there is an organized collection in the gallbladder fossa which is highly consistent with a pericholecystic abscess (arrowhead)

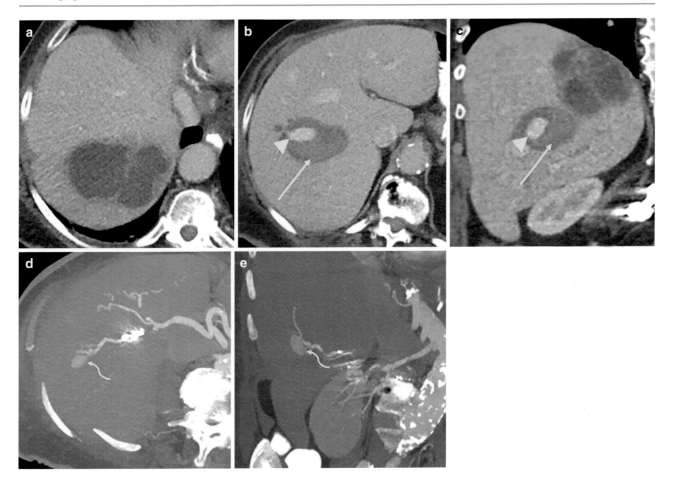

**Fig. 5** A 68-year-old woman following cholecystectomy 3 months ago, with a postoperative course complicated by sepsis and intra-abdominal hemorrhage requiring coil embolization in the region of the porta hepatis, currently presenting with 1 week of abdominal pain. IV contrast-enhanced axial CT image (a) demonstrates a thick-walled intrahepatic collection with thick septations, which is highly consistent with an abscess. Additional axial CT image at a lower level (b) demonstrates a second predominantly hypoattenuating collection with dependent faintly hyperdense material (arrow). Also within this collection is a hyperattenuating ovoid focus (arrowhead). Sagittal oblique IV contrast-enhanced CT image (c) demonstrates the relationship of the two collections. Follow-up CT angiogram of the abdomen was performed with axial (d) and coronal (e) maximum intensity projection images, demonstrating a hepatic artery pseudoaneurysm (curved arrow) corresponding to the ovoid focus seen on the prior scan

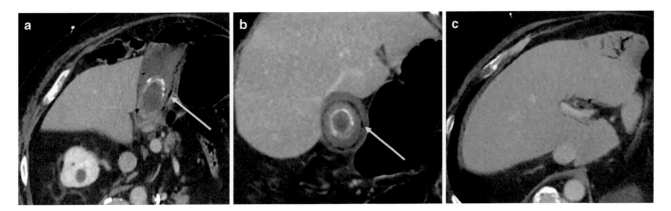

**Fig. 6** A 77-year-old man with a past medical history of diabetes presented with 2 days of altered mental status and was found to have emphysematous cholecystitis. IV contrast-enhanced axial (a) and coronal (b) CT images demonstrate a distended gallbladder with a large calculus in the gallbladder neck and intraluminal gas. There are also numerous tiny foci of gas within the gallbladder wall (arrow). Additional axial CT image at the level of the porta hepatis (c) demonstrates portal venous gas

[17, 18, 19]. MR/MRCP show similar findings of acute cholecystitis as CT, with the added benefit of T2-weighted MRCP images for the identification of gallstones and choledocholithiasis. Additionally, diffusion-weighted images can be used to differentiate acute from chronic cholecystitis with restricted diffusion seen in cases of acute cholecystitis, and multiphasic post-gadolinium images show increased transient pericholecystic hepatic parenchymal enhancement on the arterial phase and increased enhancement of the gallbladder wall [20, 21, 22].

Equivocal cases can be assessed with a HIDA scan, where cystic duct obstruction in acute cholecystitis is shown as radiotracer excretion into the small bowel without accumulation in the gallbladder [8, 23].

## Acute Acalculous Cholecystitis

Acute acalculous cholecystitis is often seen in critically ill patients, particularly those who have had surgery, trauma, burn injury, and cardiac arrest. Other associations include diabetes, vasculitis, and congestive heart failure [24]. Acute acalculous cholecystitis is characterized by gallbladder inflammation without cystic duct obstruction. Early imaging is critical, as these patients have a worse prognosis, with 30–50% mortality given their increased propensity to develop complications of cholecystitis [25]. Imaging findings are similar to those seen in acute calculous cholecystitis.

## Complications of Acute Cholecystitis

Imaging plays an important role for the detection of complications of acute cholecystitis, which include gangrenous cholecystitis, emphysematous cholecystitis, hemorrhagic cholecystitis, gallbladder perforation, and pericholecystic abscess formation. Secondary infection of an inflamed gallbladder can lead to emphysematous cholecystitis and gangrenous cholecystitis. Gangrenous cholecystitis is the most common complication and is associated with increased morbidity and mortality. It is characterized by intramural hemorrhage, necrosis, micro-abscesses, and intraluminal purulent debris, and sloughed membranes are characteristic of gangrenous cholecystitis [26, 27, 28]. Perforated cholecystitis is commonly seen in association with gangrenous cholecystitis and typically occurs at the gallbladder fundus. On imaging, a focal discontinuity of the gallbladder wall with pericholecystic fluid and inflammation are seen, and extraluminal gallstones may also be identified [29]. Superinfection by gas-forming organisms can result in emphysematous cholecystitis, which more commonly affects diabetics, men, and patients between the ages of 40 and 60 [26, 29].

## Xanthogranulomatous Cholecystitis (XGC)

XGC is a chronic form of cholecystitis with focal or diffuse destructive inflammation resulting in perforation, abscess formation, fistula, and invasion of adjacent structures, which can closely mimic gallbladder carcinoma [30]. Intramural accumulation of lipid-laden foamy macrophages occurs and results in scarring and proliferative fibrosis. On imaging, XGC manifests as focal or diffuse gallbladder wall thickening with hypoattenuating intramural nodules on CT, heterogeneously enhancing gallbladder wall, and infiltration of adjacent hepatic parenchyma and pericholecystic fat [28, 30]. These hypoattenuating intramural nodules on CT and T2 hyperintense intramural nodules on MR are very helpful in discriminating XGC from gallbladder carcinoma (Figs. 7 and 8).

## Acute Ascending Cholangitis

Ascending cholangitis most commonly occurs from choledocholithiasis, resulting in biliary obstruction; however, other causes including malignant obstruction or biliary manipulation can also result in acute cholangitis. Acute cholangitis is usually a clinical diagnosis and can be seen in the presence of the Charcot triad of fever, jaundice, and right upper quadrant

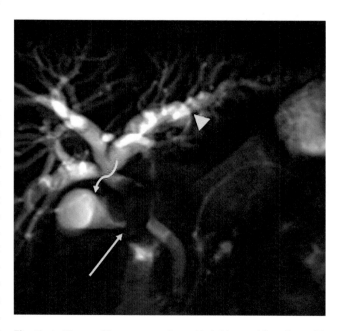

**Fig. 7** A 68-year-old man presenting with itching and jaundice, with Mirizzi syndrome. Heavily T2-weighted coronal maximum intensity projection MRCP image demonstrates a large filling defect in the cystic duct (arrow), which is a calculus and which is causing compression of the adjacent common hepatic duct. There is associated dilatation of the intrahepatic ducts (arrowhead) as well as of the gallbladder (curved arrow)

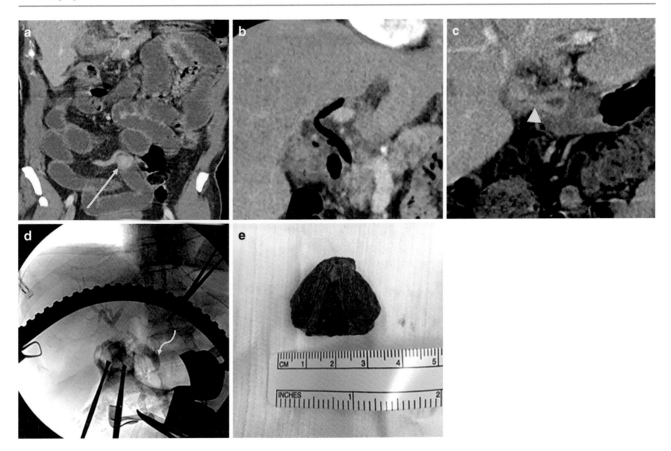

**Fig. 8** A 55-year-old man presenting with colicky abdominal pain, nausea, and vomiting, with gallstone ileus. IV contrast-enhanced coronal CT image (a) demonstrates diffusely distended small bowel loops to the level of an obstructing intraluminal gallstone (arrow), i.e., gallstone ileus. Coronal CT image through the porta hepatis (b) demonstrates pneumobilia. Coronal oblique CT image through the gallbladder (c) demonstrates a cholecystoduodenal fistula (arrowhead). Intraoperative cholangiogram (d) demonstrates the corresponding cholecystoduodenal fistula (arrowhead), as well as filling of the common duct (curved arrow)

pain. US can show biliary ductal dilatation, and findings on CT and MR include choledocholithiasis, periductal inflammation, ductal wall thickening, and mural enhancement [31]. MR/MRCP can also show parenchymal changes of wedge-shaped or peribiliary regions of T2 hyperintense signal and parenchymal enhancement [31, 32]. Choledocholithiasis can be seen on CT and MR/MRCP, although MRCP has a higher sensitivity for the detection of calculi, and CT can be used to readily differentiate pneumobilia from choledocholithiasis [8] (Figs. 9 and 10).

## Mirizzi Syndrome

Common hepatic duct obstruction can occur from extrinsic compression by a gallstone in the gallbladder infundibulum or cystic duct in Mirizzi syndrome. Anatomically the cystic and common hepatic ducts are oriented in a parallel configuration to a long and low-inserting cystic duct, which

predisposes individuals to this syndrome [33, 34]. US may reveal an ectatic common hepatic duct. On CT, periportal inflammation can be seen. MRCP can best depict the biliary duct anatomy, and MRCP sequences will show the calculus impacted in the cystic duct, resulting in compression of the dilated common hepatic duct, with dilation proximal to the calculus and normal caliber distal to it.

## Gallstone Ileus

Gallstone ileus is characterized by mechanical obstruction of the gastrointestinal tract due to an impacted gallstone, usually involving large stones >2 cm. The gallstone erodes through the gallbladder wall into an adjacent loop of small bowel, usually the duodenum, and then lodges typically at anatomical sites – and occasionally of pathologic sites – of narrowing, resulting in obstruction of loops of small bowel proximal to the level of obstruction (and occasionally of the

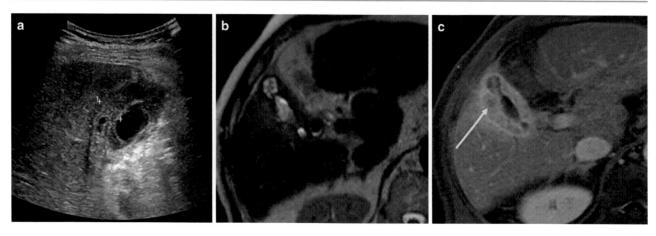

**Fig. 9** A 83-year-old man with right upper quadrant pain found to have XGC. Sagittal US image through the liver (a) demonstrates incidental asymmetric gallbladder wall thickening. Axial T2-weighted (b) and T1-weighted fat-saturated IV contrast-enhanced (c) MR images through the gallbladder demonstrate irregular wall thickening with intramural nodules (arrow) and intact mucosa

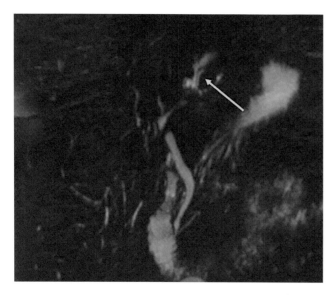

**Fig. 10** A 37-year-old woman with a history of PSC. Heavily T2-weighted coronal maximum intensity projection MRCP image demonstrates irregular, beaded intrahepatic ducts with an area of focal dilatation in the left hepatic lobe (arrow)

stomach as well), with decreased luminal diameter, with the transition zone with the lodged calculus most commonly at the terminal ileum and ileocecal valve. Bouveret syndrome can rarely occur, where the gallstone migrates proximally, resulting in gastric outlet obstruction. On CT, gallstone ileus is diagnosed when there are dilated bowel loops, an ectopic gallstone, and pneumobilia [28, 35].

## Primary sclerosing cholangitis (PSC)

PSC is a result of chronic inflammation and fibrosis of the intrahepatic and extrahepatic bile ducts and is commonly seen in association with inflammatory bowel disease, specifically ulcerative colitis. Patients with PSC are at increased risk of cholangiocarcinoma [32, 36]. Patients typically present with abdominal pain, pruritus, and jaundice, and recurrent bouts of cholangitis are common. MR/MRCP is the best imaging modality to assess PSC, and the resultant multifocal beading of the biliary tract with associated areas of ductal dilatation is the typical imaging feature [26, 37].

## Recurrent Pyogenic Cholangitis (RPC)

RPC has been associated with infection and infestation with parasitic disease, including *Clonorchis sinensis*, *Ascaris lumbricoides*, and *Opisthorchis viverrini*, and is characterized by repeated bouts of cholangitis. Patients are predisposed to repeated bouts of bacterial cholangitis. Presenting symptoms include abdominal pain, fever, and jaundice. Potential complications include abscess, portal vein thrombus, and biliary strictures [26, 32]. On imaging, portal vein thrombus and abscess can be seen on CT and MR. Biliary strictures are best visualized on MRCP.

Parasitic Infection

Parasitic infections can affect the biliary tract, most commonly *Echinococcus granulosus*. Patients have presenting symptoms similar to those seen with ascending cholangitis. Echinococcal infections occur in stages and if left untreated can lead to cholangitis due to fistulization into the biliary ducts. Early (active) stage of infection can be seen as a simple- appearing cyst on US and CT but may also present as a multivesicular cyst with multiple daughter cysts. The cyst enters a transitional stage as the parasite dies, and an endocyst can detach from the pericyst which is seen as a floating membrane. Multiple membranes can appear with progression of the disease, which is known as the "water lily" sign. As the disease progresses into the

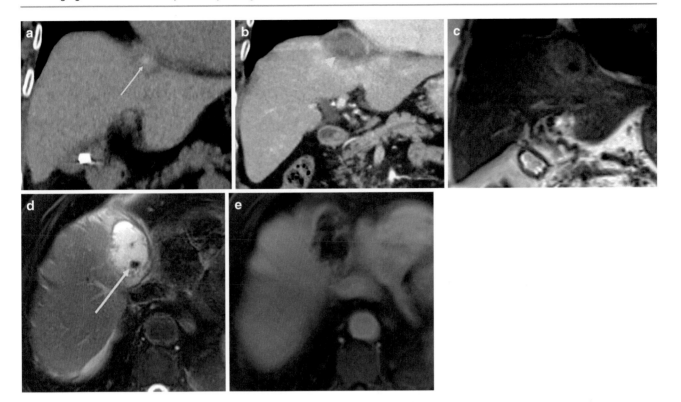

**Fig. 11** A 91-year-old man following cholecystectomy 3 months ago, with a dropped gallstone. Non-contrast coronal CT image (a) demonstrates an ill-defined hyperdensity over the hepatic dome with surrounding inflammatory changes, representing a dropped gallstone (arrow). Coronal image from a subsequent IV contrast-enhanced CT (b) demonstrates interval development of an organized collection (arrowhead) in the region of previously identified hyperdensity. Corresponding T2-weighted coronal (c) and T2-weighted fat-saturated axial (d) MR images demonstrate a fluid collection with surrounding inflammation and a hypointense filling defect (arrow), corresponding to the dropped gallstone seen on initial non-contrast CT. IV contrast-enhanced T1-weighted fat-saturated MR image (e) demonstrates irregular wall enhancement

inactive stage, the cyst becomes more solid and may calcify. Intrahepatic ductal dilatation, cystobiliary fistulae, and extension of daughter cysts or hydatid membranes into the biliary tract can be seen on imaging [26] (Figs. 11 and 12).

## Immunocompromised Patients

Immunocompromised patients are predisposed to opportunistic infections of the biliary tract. Human immunodeficiency virus (HIV) patients are predisposed to biliary tract infections when CD4 counts fall below 100/mm3, and biliary disease in this patient population includes a spectrum of disease which is called acquired immunodeficiency syndrome (AIDS) cholangiopathy. This includes acute acalculous cholecystitis, sclerosing cholangitis, lymphoma, and Kaposi's sarcoma [38]. Hepatic, biliary, and pancreatic parenchymal abnormalities can be seen in AIDS cholangiopathy, where US and CT may show hepatomegaly, periportal lymphadenopathy, and acalculous cholecystitis. CT and MR findings include patchy arterial enhancement in hepatitis. Biliary abnormalities are best assessed on MR/MRCP, and the imaging findings are similar to those of PSC, with intrahepatic and extrahepatic stenoses and ductal dilatation, commonly with long-segment extrahepatic strictures [26, 38].

## Acute Hepatitis

There are acute and chronic forms of viral hepatitis, which can be caused by hepatitis A, hepatitis B, hepatitis C, HBV-associated delta agent/hepatitis D, or hepatitis E viruses and sometimes by more than one of these viruses in the same patient. Inflammation and necrosis occur in chronic hepatitis, and complications can include varices, bleeding, ascites, encephalopathy, and hepatocellular carcinoma [39]. On US, hepatomegaly with increased echogenicity of the portal trial, the so-called "starry night" pattern, can be seen [39]. On CT and MR, hepatomegaly is seen, and periportal edema appears as periportal low attenuation around the portal triads on CT and as T2 hyperintense periportal regions on MR. Of note, a normal-appearing liver on imaging does not exclude this diagnosis.

**Fig. 12** A 50-year-old woman with history of hepatocellular carcinoma resulting in Budd-Chiari syndrome. IV contrast-enhanced axial CT images through the liver (a, b) demonstrate a large heterogeneous mass within the left hepatic lobe (arrow). The remaining hepatic parenchyma demonstrates heterogeneous enhancement, representing congestion. Note the absence of hepatic venous enhancement. Axial CT images through the level of the heart (c) demonstrate a filling defect within the right atrium. Corresponding image from an echocardiogram (d) confirms the presence of a tumoral thrombus within the right atrium

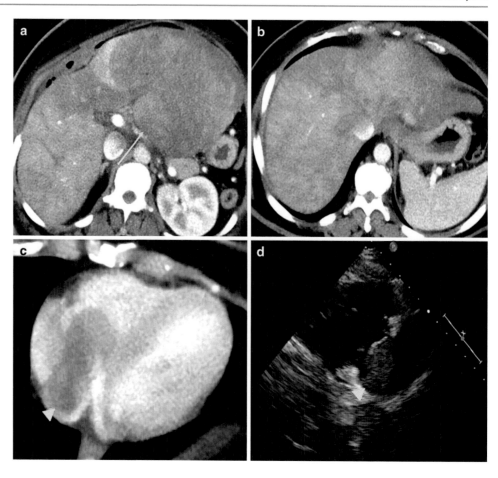

## Vascular

### Budd-Chiari Syndrome

Several disorders compromise Budd-Chiari syndrome and involve venous outflow obstruction of the liver. The most common cause is a clotting disorder; however, malignant causes, particularly hepatocellular carcinoma, can also be the underlying etiology, which typically involves invasion and partial or complete obstruction of the hepatic veins, inferior vena cava, and/or right atrium. The obstruction may lead to portal hypertension, hepatic congestion, and reduced perfusion [40]. Doppler US can show a lack of flow in the obstructed hepatic veins or reversal of flow, while gray-scale US may show changes in echotexture of the hepatic parenchyma [40]. CT may show hepatomegaly in the setting of congestion and decreased attenuation as a result of edema, while hypoattenuating thrombus can be seen in the hepatic veins. With MR, loss of signal on T1-weighted images with associated T2 hyperintense signal can be seen in the liver, particularly in the periphery reflecting edema. After the administration of IV gadolinium, decreased peripheral enhancement with preserved central enhancement can be seen, particularly where edema and vascular congestion is most severe. There may be compensatory hypertrophy and caudate lobe enhancement due to preservation of the IVC, which directly drains the caudate lobe.

### Portal Vein Thrombosis

Portal vein thrombus can be seen in cirrhosis or may be secondary to an ascending infection originating from a gastrointestinal infection, including diverticulitis, appendicitis, inflammatory bowel disease, and pancreatitis, and may be due to hypercoagulability and reduced portal venous flow [41, 42]. While patients with portal vein thrombus can be asymptomatic, presenting symptoms include abdominal pain, vomiting, diarrhea, nausea, gastrointestinal bleeding, and fever. Portal vein thrombophlebitis has a mortality rate up to 50% due to the associated complications of bowel ischemia, hepatic abscess formation, and sepsis [42]. CT and MR show the portal vein thrombus as well as hepatic abscess(es), if present.

On US, thrombus in the portal vein can be seen, and, with Doppler, absence of flow is seen. The thrombus can be identified on IV contrast-enhanced CT or MR and can provide the added benefit of evaluating for bowel ischemia in the setting of superior mesenteric venous thrombus [41, 42]. The thrombus may exclusively occur in the main portal vein or can extend into the superior mesenteric and/or splenic veins.

## Postoperative/Post-procedural Complications

### Cholecystectomy

A laparoscopic or open approach can be performed for cholecystectomy, with an increase in complication rate with an open approach. Potential complications of cholecystectomies include bile leak, dropped gallstones, retained gallstones, bleeding, and abscess formation [43]. Various imaging modalities can be used to depict cholecystectomy complications, and the diagnosis may require a multi-modality approach. US and CT can be used to identify fluid collections and to detect biliary dilatation; however, neither modality can be used to definitely identify a bile leak, although a large amount of surrounding low-density fluid without any other explanation is highly suspicious for a bile leak. CT can be used to detect vascular injury, as well as to reveal a dropped calcified gallstone(s). MR/MRCP can be used to depict fluid collections, vascular injuries, and dropped gallstones and has the added benefit of revealing and localizing bile leaks with the use of a hepatobiliary agent and for the detection of calculi in the biliary tract [44].

### Trans-arterial Chemoembolization (TACE)

TACE utilizes chemotherapeutic agents and thrombogenic material which are injected into hepatic artery branches which supply tumors [45]. Due to the peribiliary capillary plexus arising from the hepatic artery branches and the sole vascular supply to the biliary tract, ischemia of the biliary tract is a potential complication of TACE. Pathophysiologically, ischemia of the biliary tract leads to necrosis, potentially leading to biliary leaks and biloma formation. Bilomas are the most common complication after TACE and can become superinfected to form abscesses, which can readily be detected on CT or MR. Another potential complication of TACE leading to ischemia is the formation of strictures [45]. The larger bile ducts are typically affected, and this can be assessed with MR/MRCP.

### Transplant

Liver transplants are the treatment for end-stage liver disease as well as for major post-liver transplant complications,

including organ rejection, vascular, and biliary complications.

Imaging can be used to detect vascular and biliary complications, although organ rejection is a clinical diagnosis. US should be the initial imaging modality to assess postoperative complications. Doppler US should be performed to evaluate the hepatic vasculature given that hepatic artery thrombosis is the most common posttransplant vascular complication, accounting for more than half of such vascular complications [46, 47]. Hepatic artery stenosis and pseudoaneurysm formation are other arterial complications, and pseudoaneurysms may rupture and result in fistula formation with the portal vein and/or biliary tract. Venous complications involving the portal and hepatic veins and IVC include stenosis and thrombosis [46, 47], which can be detected on US, CT, and MR.

Potential biliary complications after a liver transplant include biliary obstruction and bile leak. US will show biliary duct dilatation, obstruction, or the presence of a fluid collection. MR is the best imaging modality to assess biliary obstruction, which may be secondary to an anastomotic or non-anastomotic stricture or choledocholithiasis.

## Conclusion

Hepatobiliary emergencies typically cause right upper quadrant pain, and a number of underlying disorders can be identified on imaging, including infectious, inflammatory, vascular, and postoperative complications. Other clinical considerations to consider include immunocompromised status or recent procedures and surgery. A multi-modality approach is usually required to make a definitive diagnosis including one or more of the following imaging examinations: US, CT, MR/MRCP, and HIDA scan. It is important to be familiar with the imaging appearances of all hepatobiliary disorders and equally important to be familiar with the limitations of each imaging modality.

## References

1. Weiss AJ, Wier LM, Stocks C, et al. Overview of emergency department visits in the United States, 2011. HCUP Statistical Brief #174. Agency Healthc Res Qual. 2014:1–13.
2. Russo MW, Wei JT, Thiny MT, et al. Digestive and liver diseases statistics, 2004. Gastroenterology. 2004;126(5):1448–53.
3. Shaffer EA. Gallstone disease: epidemiology of gallbladder stone disease. Best Pract Res Clin Gastroenterol. 2006;20(6):981–96.
4. Stinton LM, Shaffer EA. Epidemiology of gallbladder disease: cholelithiasis and cancer. Gut Liver. 2012;6(2):172–87. https://doi.org/10.5009/gnl.2012.6.2.172.
5. Sodickson AD, Keraliya A, Czakowski B, et al. Dual energy CT in clinical routine: how it work sand how it adds value. Emerg Radiol. 2020. [Online ahead of print].
6. Marin D, Boll DT, Mileto A, Nelson RC. State of the art: dual-energy CT of the abdomen. Radiology. 2014;271(2):327–42.

7. Bauer RW, Fischer S. Dual-energy CT: applications in abdominal imaging. Curr Radiol Rep. 2015;3:9.
8. O'Connor OJ, O'Neill S, Maher MM. Imaging of biliary tract disease. Am. J. Roentgenol. 2011;197:W551–8.
9. Gore RM, Thakrar KH, Newmark GM, Mehta UK, Berlin JW. Gallbladder imaging. Gastroenterol Clin North Am. 2010;39(2):265–87. ix. 9
10. Harvey RT, Miller WT Jr. Acute biliary disease: initial CT and follow-up US versus initial US and follow-up CT. Radiology. 1999;213(3):831–6.
11. Moparty B, Carr-Locke DL. Biliary emergencies. In: Tham T, Collins J, Soetikno, editors. Gastrointestinal emergencies. 2nd ed. Blackwell Publishing; 2009. p. 134–40.
12. Wilkins T, Agabin E, Varghese J, et al. Gallbladder dysfunction: cholecystitis, choledocholithiasis, cholangitis, and biliary dyskinesia. Prim Care. 2017;44:575–97.
13. Everhart JE, Khare M, Hill M, Maurer KR. Prevalence and ethnic differences in gallbladder disease in the United States. Gastroenterology. 1999;117(3):632–9.
14. Gurusamy K. Gallstones. Br Med J. 2014;348:1–6.
15. Ralls PW, Colletti PM, Lapin SA, et al. Real-time sonography in suspected acute cholecystitis. Prospective evaluation of primary and secondary signs. Radiology. 1985;155(3):767–71.
16. Wertz JR, Lopez JM, Olson D, Thompson WM. Comparing the diagnostic accuracy of ultrasound and CT in evaluating acute cholecystitis. Am. J. Roentgenol. 2018;211:W92–7.
17. Chen A, Liu A, Wang S, et al. Detection of gallbladder stones by dual-energy spectral computed tomography imaging. World J Gastroenterol. 2015;21:9993–8.
18. Uyeda JW, Richardson IJ, Sodickson AD. Making the invisible visible: improving conspicuity of noncalcified gallstones using dual-energy CT. Abdom Radiol. 2017;42(12):2933–9.
19. Yang CB, Zhang S, Jia YJ, et al. Clinical application of dual-energy spectral computed tomography in detecting cholesterol gallstones from surrounding bile. Acad Radiol. 2017;24(4):478–82.
20. Altun E, Semelka RC, Elias J Jr, et al. Acute cholecystitis: MR findings and differentiation from chronic cholecystitis. Radiology. 2007;244(1):174–83.
21. Gupta A, LeBedis CA, Uyeda J, et al. Diffusion-weighted imaging of the pericholecystic hepatic parenchyma for distinguishing acute and chronic cholecystitis. Emerg Radiol. 2018;25:7–11.
22. Wang A, Shanbhogue AK, Dunst D, et al. Utility of diffusion-weighted MRI for differentiating acute from chronic cholecystitis. J Magn Reson Imaging. 2016;44:89–97.
23. Chamarthy M, Freeman LM. Hepatobiliary scan findings in chronic cholecystitis. Clin Nucl Med. 2010;35:244–51.
24. Barie PS, Eachempati SR. Acute calculous cholecystitis. Gastroenterol Clin North Am. 2010;39:343–57.
25. Jones MW, Ferguson T. Acalculous cholecystitis. [Updated 2021 Feb 8]. In: StatPearls [Internet]. Treasure Island (FL): StatPearls Publishing; 2021 Jan-. Available from: https://www.ncbi.nlm.nih.gov/books/NBK459182/
26. Catalano OA, Sahani DV, Kalva SP, et al. MR imaging of the gallbladder: a pictorial essay. RadioGraphics. 2008;28(1):135–55.
27. Jeffrey R, Laing F, Wong W, et al. Gangrenous cholecystitis: diagnosis by ultrasound. Radiology. 1983;148:219–21.
28. Ratanaprasatporn L, Uyeda JW, Wortman JR, et al. Multimodality imaging, including dual-energy CT, in the evaluation of gallbladder disease. Radiographics. 2018;38:75–89.
29. Shakespear JS, Shaaban AM, Rezvani M. CT findings of acute cholecystitis and its complications. AJR Am J Roentgenol. 2010;194(6):1523–9.
30. Kang T, Kim S, Park H, et al. Differentiating xanthogranulomatous cholecystitis from wall-thickening type of gallbladder cancer: added value of diffusion-weighted MRI. Clin Radiol. 2013;68:992–1001.
31. Yeh BM, Liu PS, Soto JA, et al. MR imaging and CT of the biliary tract. RadioGraphics. 2009;29:1669–88.
32. Walshe TM, Bao MBB, Rcsi FFR, et al. Infection, inflammation and infiltration. Appl Radiol. 2016;4:20–6.
33. Yu HS, Gupta A, Soto JA, et al. Emergency abdominal MRI: current uses and trends. Br J Radiol. 2016;89:20150804.
34. Chen H, Siwo E, Khu M, et al. Current trends in the management of Mirizzi syndrome. Medicine (Baltimore). 2018;97:1–7.
35. Chung AYA, Duke MC. Acute biliary disease. Surg Clin North Am. 2018;98:877–94.
36. Silveira MG, Lindor KD. Primary sclerosing cholangitis. Can J Gastroenterol. 2008;22:689–98.
37. Bali MA, Pezzullo M, Pace E, et al. Benign biliary diseases. Eur J Radiol. 2017;93:217–28.
38. Bilgin M, Balci NC, Erdogan A, et al. Hepatobiliary and pancreatic MRI and MRCP findings in patients with HIV infection. Am J Roentgenol. 2008;191:228–32.
39. Mortele KJ, Segatto E, Ros PR. The infected liver: radiologic-pathologic correlation. Radiographics. 2004;24:937–55.
40. Brancatelli G, Vilgrain V, Federle MP, et al. Budd-Chiari syndrome: spectrum of imaging findings. Am J Roentgenol. 2007;188:168–76.
41. Von Kockritz L, De Gottardi A, Trebicka J, et al. Portal vein thrombosis in patients with cirrhosis. Gastroenterol Rep (Oxf). 2017;5:148–56.
42. Jha RC, Khera SS, Kalaria AD. Portal vein thrombosis: imaging the spectrum of disease with an emphasis on MRI features. Am J Roentgenol. 2018;211:14–24.
43. Vollmer C, Callery M. Biliary injury following laparoscopic cholecystectomy: why still a problem? Gastroenterology. 2007;133:1039–45.
44. Thompson CM, Saad NE, Quazi RR, et al. Management of iatrogenic bile duct injuries: role of the interventional radiologist. Radiographics. 2013;33:117–34.
45. Sueyoshi E, Hayashida T, Sakamoto I, Uetani M. Vascular complications of hepatic artery after transcatheter arterial chemoembolization in patients with hepatocellular carcinoma. AJR Am J Roentgenol. 2010 Jul;195(1):245–51.
46. Singh AK, Nachiappan AC, Verma HA, et al. Postoperative imaging in liver transplantation: what radiologists should know. Radiographics. 2010;30:339–51.
47. Caiado A, Blasbalg R, Marcelino A, et al. Complications of liver transplantation: multimodality imaging approach. Radiographics. 2007;27:1401–17.

# Imaging of Nontraumatic Splenic Emergencies

Maria Zulfiqar and Vincent M. Mellnick

## Contents

## Abstract

Acute abnormalities in the spleen are frequently traumatic but also include nontraumatic entities which can be potentially life-threatening if not recognized and managed in a timely manner. In the nontraumatic setting, emergent splenic pathology can be identified diagnosed on cross-sectional imaging obtained for left upper quadrant or otherwise nonspecific abdominal pain, as history and physical examination are often inconclusive. A wide spectrum of nontraumatic splenic pathology can be seen, ranging from vascular conditions to infections and inflammatory processes. Given the potential for high morbidity and mortality associated with most of these entities, radiologists must be familiar with the imaging features to circumvent delayed or missed diagnosis.

## Keywords

Nontraumatic splenic emergencies · Splenic rupture · Splenic abscess · Splenic aneurysm

## Introduction

The spleen is a part of the reticuloendothelial system and represents the largest lymphoid organ in the human body, constituting approximately 25% of the total body lymphocytes stored in the white pulp. In addition, the spleen functions as a blood filter and carries a reserve of approximately 250 mL of blood volume. The blood flow through the spleen is also very high and is estimated to be between 5% and 10% of the cardiac output in the resting state [1]. Therefore, any insult to the spleen, traumatic or nontraumatic, carries high risk for bleeding. Diagnosing nontraumatic splenic emergencies can be problematic on physical examination due to the high location of the spleen in the left upper quadrant between the stomach and the diaphragm. The spleen can be evaluated by various imaging modalities, including ultrasound, computed tomography (CT), magnetic resonance imaging (MRI), and, in the

M. Zulfiqar (✉) · V. M. Mellnick
Mallinckrodt Institute of Radiology, Washington University School of Medicine, St. Louis, MO, USA
e-mail: mariazulfiqar@wustl.edu

traumatic setting in particular, conventional angiography. As is the case for many acute settings, CT is the workhorse and first-line imaging modality to identify splenic pathology due to fast acquisition times and excellent soft tissue detail.

***Splenic Size*** Enlargement of the spleen (splenomegaly) is the most common sign of splenic pathology and may be present as the only finding on imaging pointing toward splenic involvement by congestion, hematological disorders, or infiltration by infectious or neoplastic processes. Although splenic volume is considered the best measure for splenic size, with a normal volume considered between 236 + and - 78 mL [2], in the fast-paced environment of the ED, a maximum splenic length or two-dimensional coefficient obtained on CT by multiplying the maximal splenic length with vertical height has also been shown to correlate with splenic area, with a cutoff of normal in the average-sized adult at 115 cm$^2$ [3].

The length of the spleen measured vertically from the splenic dome to the level of the inferior splenic margin is considered enlarged when it exceeds 13 cm, as defined by the Lugano classification for evaluation of lymphoma published in 2014 (Fig. 1) [4].

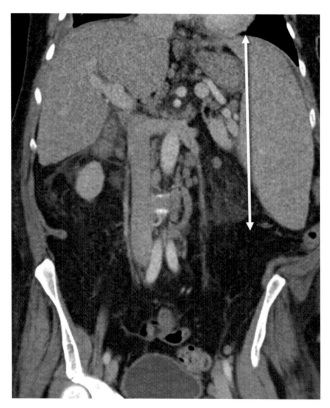

**Fig. 1** Splenic length measurement for the assessment of splenomegaly. Coronal CT image of the abdomen and pelvis with intravenous contrast shows a vertical line drawn from the splenic dome to the level of the inferior splenic margin, which correlates well with splenic volume in adults, with a measurement above 13 cm indicative of an enlarged spleen

***Normal Splenic Parenchyma*** Histologically, the spleen is composed of lymphoid tissue (white pulp) and sinusoidal spaces containing blood (red pulp). This architecture imparts the splenic parenchyma with a characteristic "tiger striped" pattern of enhancement, which is transient and lasts for the first 60 seconds of contrast injection, thought to be due to differential rates of blood flow through the cords of red and white pulp. Although it has its advantages in the detection of traumatic splenic hemorrhage and contained vascular injuries [5], imaging the spleen in the arterial phase (on CT and also on MRI) for nontraumatic pathology may not be always beneficial due to decreased conspicuity of certain focal abnormalities including infarcts, small abscesses, and infiltrative malignancies on this phase of contrast when compared to the portal venous phase, where the splenic parenchyma demonstrates a uniformly homogenous pattern of enhancement [6].

***Splenic Vasculature*** A high incidence of splenic arterial and/or venous involvement by ongoing disease process and an increasing trend toward managing most splenic emergencies through minimally invasive interventional approaches warrant the radiologist to have good understanding of the splenic blood supply. Arising from the celiac trunk, the splenic artery takes an inherently tortuous retroperitoneal course and travels anterior and superior to the splenic vein along the superior margin of the pancreas. Both vessels traverse the splenorenal ligament into the splenic hilum. One should keep in mind that the branches of the main artery to the spleen are noncommunicating end arteries, the blockage of which will lead to varying degrees of splenic infarction [7].

## Atraumatic Splenic Rupture

***Epidemiology*** Atraumatic splenic rupture is a rare but potentially life-threatening complication, with an estimated mortality rate of approximately 12%. Multiple predisposing conditions have been identified as detailed in Table 1 but broadly include coagulopathy, infection, inflammatory disorders, and neoplasms [8].

***Clinical Features*** Due to the location of the spleen in the left upper quadrant immediately below the left hemidiaphragm, blood products from the rupture can irritate the diaphragmatic lining, leading to left chest wall or left shoulder pain (Kehr's sign) which can be misleading [9]. If the bleeding is substantial, the pain is often accompanied by refractory hypotension. Rarely, the spleen can rupture in an iatrogenic setting following optical colonoscopy or colonic surgery secondary to significant tension on the splenocolic ligament during the procedure and resultant avulsion of the spleen [10].

**Table 1** Various causes of atraumatic splenic rupture

| Coagulopathy | • Therapeutic anticoagulation<br>• Platelet and factor VIII deficiency<br>• Idiopathic thrombocytopenic purpura<br>• Uremia-hemodialysis |
|---|---|
| Infections | • Infectious mononucleosis (Epstein-Barr virus infection)<br>• Endocarditis<br>• HIV<br>• Cytomegalovirus (CMV)<br>• Typhoid fever<br>• Malaria<br>• Babesiosis<br>• Dengue fever |
| Inflammatory disorders | • Systemic lupus erythematosus (SLE)<br>• Polyarteritis nodosa<br>• Pancreatitis<br>• Amyloidosis |
| Neoplastic conditions | • Lymphoma<br>• Leukemia<br>• Waldenstrom macroglobulinemia<br>• Splenic metastases<br>• Splenic angiosarcoma |
| Other | • Pregnancy<br>• Ruptured benign splenic focal masses, including cyst, infarction, hamartoma, hemangioma, and peliosis |

*Imaging Findings* On non-contrast CT, in the hyperacute phase, the blood attenuation measures between 35 and 50 Hounsfield units (HU). As clotting ensues, the hematoma becomes denser and measures 60–80 HU in the acute phase. The focus of highest attenuation (sentinel clot) within the hematoma is often located near the site of the splenic bleeding (Fig. 2). At times, the bleeding may be slow or intermittent, and the only finding on CT will be hemoperitoneum in the paracolic gutters or pelvic cul-de-sac in association with splenomegaly. Following contrast administration, pseudoaneurysms, arteriovenous fistulas, frank contrast extravasation, or some combination of these may be present [11].

## Splenic Infarction

*Epidemiology* Splenic infarcts can occur due to either deficient arterial supply or obstructed venous drainage. Common causes of splenic infarction include thromboembolic phenomenon – usually from a cardiac source, hypercoagulable conditions such as hemoglobinopathies, lymphoproliferative disorders, portal hypertension, inflammation such as from acute pancreatitis, infections including mononucleosis and malaria, or rarely splenic torsion [12].

*Clinical Features* Clinical presentation depends on the degree of splenic infarction and complications. Approximately 30–50% of patients are asymptomatic, which is likely

due to segmental nature of infarction, often detected incidentally on imaging subsequently obtained for other purposes. Multifocal or global large-volume splenic infarcts can present with left upper quadrant or diffuse abdominal pain or even constitutional symptoms of fever and chills with or without leukocytosis [13]. There is high incidence of complications in the setting of thromboembolic splenic infarction, including abscess, liquefaction, rupture, and hemorrhage.

*Imaging Findings* In the acute setting, CT demonstrates a well-defined hypoattenuating area of perfusion abnormality within the splenic parenchyma, which is wedge-shaped, with the tip of the wedge pointing toward the splenic hilum. With time, the subacute infarcted parenchyma becomes almost fluid in attenuation appearing cyst-like and decreases in size. Chronic infarcts heal with fibrosis and atrophy with or without focal calcification [14]. Infarcts can be multiple and at times involve the entire spleen (Fig. 3). Development of internal gas, progressive expansion, or liquefaction of the affected splenic parenchyma can be seen with superinfection and at times herald splenic rupture [15].

## Splenic Artery Aneurysm (SAA) and Pseudoaneurysm

*Epidemiology* After the abdominal aorta and iliac arteries, the splenic artery is the third most common site of intraabdominal aneurysms, with an estimated incidence up to 10.4% [16]. SAAs are four times more common in women but are three times more likely to rupture in men, with an overall rupture incidence of 4.6% [17]. A true aneurysm wall comprises of three layers of intima, media, and adventitia. In contrast, the wall of a pseudoaneurysm (PSA) is weaker due to presence of only intima and media. Nontraumatic splenic PSAs are less common and usually occur secondary to pancreatitis or infection [16].

*Clinical Features* Of patients, 97.5% are asymptomatic, and SAAs are often discovered incidentally on cross-sectional imaging performed for other indications. The risk of SAA rupture has been well documented in association with pregnancy, hypertension, cirrhosis, and portal hypertension, as well as aneurysm size greater than 2 cm [17, 18]. Splenic pseudoaneurysms are commonly symptomatic, as they have a higher risk of rupture nearing 37%. Sudden-onset abdominal pain, gastrointestinal (GI) bleeding, oozing of blood through the ampulla of Vater seen on endoscopy (hemosuccus pancreaticus), and hemodynamic instability indicate SAA or PSA rupture that carries a mortality rate of almost 90% if left untreated [19]. Occasionally, the rupture occurs into the lesser omental sac instead of the retroperitoneum, leading to transient tamponade in the small space, and the patient

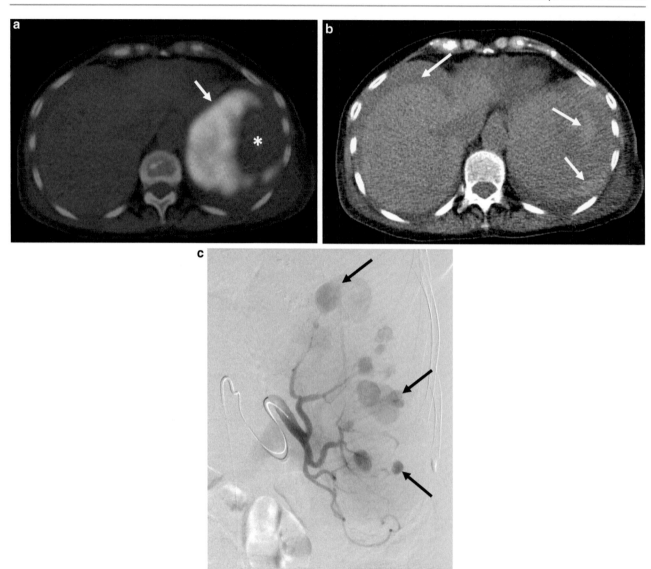

**Fig. 2** Spontaneous splenic rupture and hemorrhage. Composite axial PET-CT image (**a**) of a 74-year-old woman with diffuse large B-cell lymphoma shows an enlarged hypermetabolic spleen (arrow) representing lymphomatous involvement. There is an eccentric area of absent FDG tracer activity within the spleen (asterisk). Axial CT image of the abdomen without contrast (**b**) shows high attenuation blood products within and around the spleen, as well as anterior to the liver (arrows) compatible with splenic rupture. Digital subtraction angiography was performed (**c**) showing multiple pseudoaneurysms in the spleen (arrows); this was then followed by embolization of the splenic artery

remains hemodynamically stable during this time. However, if there is persistent bleeding, spillage of hemorrhage into the greater omental sac via the foramen of Winslow may lead to sudden hemorrhagic shock and collapse of the patient, a manifestation termed as the "double-rupture" phenomenon. Intraperitoneal bleeding from SAA or PSA rupture can also occur along the gastrosplenic ligament. Less commonly, rupture can occur into a hollow viscus such as the stomach or the pancreatic duct or into the splenic vein forming an arteriovenous fistula [17].

***Imaging Findings*** SAA can be solitary or multiple, with a predilection for the distal splenic arterial segment. Around 80% of SAAs demonstrate atherosclerotic changes including peripheral calcifications and mural thrombi [20]. Lack of calcification, an irregular aneurysmal margin, and surrounding inflammatory changes, such as from pancreatitis or infection, favor the diagnosis of a PSA. It is recommended that the CT protocol for evaluating SSAs and splenic PSAs should include both an arterial and portal venous phase, to distinguish between active bleeding and splenic PSA. A PSA remains unchanged in size and follows the intensity of the aorta on arterial and delayed images (Fig. 4). Increased area of contrast pooling on the delayed images is consistent with non-contained hemorrhage [11]. [17]. In addition, when an SAA is large, turbulent flow may lead to lag in the

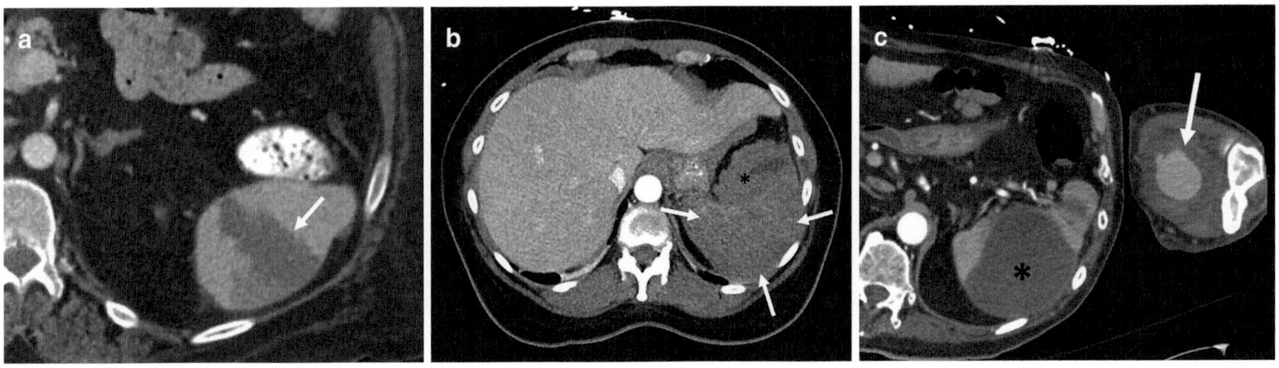

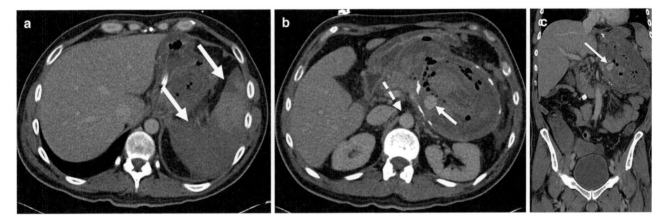

**Fig. 3** Splenic infarction in three different patients. Axial CT image of the abdomen with intravenous contrast (**a**) in a 45-year-old man shows a wedge-shaped area of non-perfusion in the spleen (arrows), which is highly consistent with an infarct. Axial image CT of the abdomen (**b**) performed for generalized abdominal pain in a 57-year-old man with amyloidosis shows complete lack of enhancement in the spleen (arrows). There is small- to moderate-volume hemorrhage anterior to the spleen in the left upper quadrant (asterisk), indicating splenic rupture. Axial CT image of the abdomen and left upper extremity with intravenous contrast (**c**) of a 37-year-old man with intravenous drug abuse and infective endocarditis shows a wedge-shaped area of cystic attenuation in the spleen with a mild contour bulge representing an evolving subacute splenic infarct, which is likely infected due to bacteremia (asterisk). Also noted is a left brachial artery infectious pseudoaneurysm (arrow)

**Fig. 4** Splenic pseudoaneurysm in a 67-year-old man with necrotizing pancreatitis. Axial CT image of the abdomen with IV contrast demonstrates splenic infarcts (**a**, arrows). Within the pancreatic tail, there is a hemorrhagic postnecrotic collection with internal foci of gas. There is a focal area of contrast pooling within the hemorrhage (**b, c**, arrows) along the expected course of the splenic artery representing a splenic artery pseudoaneurysm, which enhances with similar attenuation as the aorta (**b**, dashed arrow)

enhancement of the aneurysm, so it can appear less dense compared to the aorta (Fig. 5a). In this situation or when the patient cannot receive intravenous contrast, ultrasound can be used where it shows the classic "yin-yang" appearance of the pseudoaneurysm on color Doppler (Fig. 5b). Ultrasound may also be useful endoscopically: Due to the intimate course of the splenic artery along the pancreas, PSAs can sometimes be confused with a hyperenhancing pancreatic neuroendocrine tumor by the radiologist, and this can lead to erroneous biopsy with detrimental patient outcome. This pitfall can also be avoided by carefully examining the abnormality on multi-planar reformats to confirm communication with the splenic artery, as well as scrutinizing the contrast enhancement to be similar to the aorta on angiography, contrast US, multiphasic CT, or MRI (Fig. 5c-f) [16]. More recently, minimally invasive transcatheter embolization of SAA and

PSAs is gaining favor over surgery due to low procedural morbidity and mortality, with the added benefit of conserving splenic tissue. Symptomatic SAAs or those with size greater than 2 cm especially in high-risk individuals are treated. Invariantly, all splenic PSAs are embolized due to the high risk of rupture [16, 19].

## Splenic Venous Thrombosis (SVT)

*Epidemiology* SVT is much more common than arterial thrombosis and commonly occurs in the setting of acute or chronic pancreatitis or pancreatic neoplasms. Other causes include extension of portal venous clot, septic thrombophlebitis, and hypercoagulable states [21].

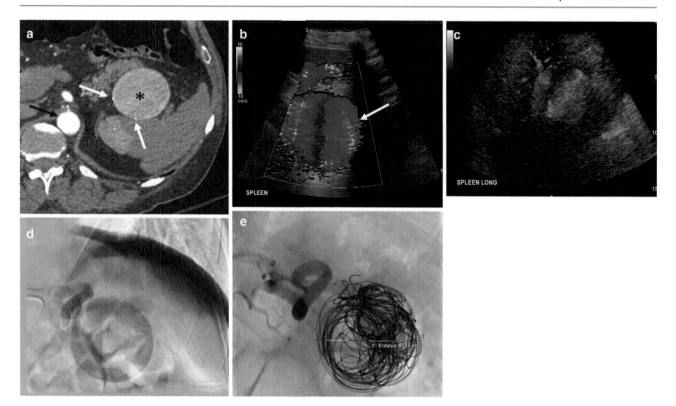

**Fig. 5** SAA . Axial CT image of the abdomen with IV contrast in the arterial phase (**a**) of a 71-year-old man with back pain shows a 5-cm round abnormality near the splenic hilum (asterisk) that communicates with the splenic artery (not shown) but which enhances less compared to the aorta (black arrow). Also noted are specks of peripheral calcifications along its wall (white arrows). Follow-up ultrasound with color Doppler (**b**) shows the characteristic "yin-yang" pattern of color (arrow) due to swirling blood flow in the large SAA. Contrast-enhanced ultrasound (**c**) shows uniform enhancement, compatible with a vascular structure. Digital subtraction angiography (**d**) pre- and (**e**) post-coiling confirms a treated SAA

***Clinical Features*** SVT is often clinically silent or may be masked by abdominal pain related to pancreatic pathology. In about 22% of patients, chronic SVT can present with upper GI bleeding from submucosal gastric varices that form secondary to increased splenic venous pressure, which is referred to as sinistral or left-sided portal hypertension. In this setting, the venous drainage of the spleen is achieved by collateral flow via short and posterior gastric veins into the coronary veins and gastroepiploic veins into the superior mesenteric vein (SMV) [22, 23].

***Imaging Findings*** On ultrasound, the splenic vein is seen distended with echogenic intraluminal thrombus and no color flow on Doppler imaging. However, this may be difficult to image with ultrasound given its location posterior to the stomach. Portal venous phase CT and MRI are both excellent for evaluating SVT and also can delineate the cause, such as pancreatic pseudocysts or parenchymal changes of acute or chronic pancreatitis. In acute to subacute SVT, there is lack of enhancement of the vein, which can be focal or complete (Fig. 6). In cases of thrombophlebitis, surrounding fat stranding is often present. Chronic SVT is characterized by fibrosis and obliteration of the vein, potentially with calcification, with dilated collaterals especially in the gastric, peripancreatic, and gastroepiploic regions [24].

## Splenic Torsion

***Epidemiology*** With an incidence of 0.2%, splenic torsion is a rare entity and occurs due to splenic hypermobility (also known as wandering or meandering spleen) allowing the spleen to migrate from the left upper quadrant into an ectopic location and twist around an abnormally long and lax vascular pedicle, potentially leading to splenic infarction. Congenital causes include absent or underdeveloped splenic support ligaments and can be associated with intestinal malrotation. Pregnancy, prior splenic surgery, splenomegaly, and prior splenic trauma are some causes of acquired splenic hypermobility [25].

***Clinical Features*** The clinical presentation of splenic torsion is variable depending on the degree of torsion, similar to other organs which can torse in the abdomen and pelvis. Patients usually present with severe sudden-onset abdominal pain with complete torsion or with recurrent episodic

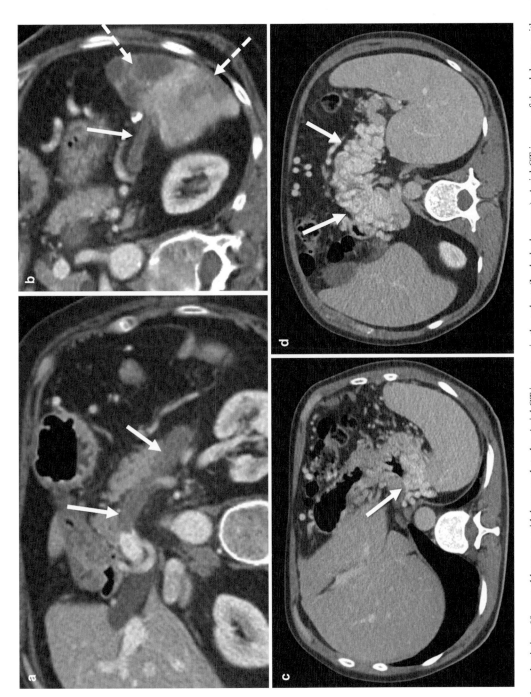

**Fig. 6** Splenic vein thrombosis in a 60-year-old woman with lupus and stroke. Axial CT image of the abdomen with IV contrast (**a**) shows non-opacification of the splenic vein, which is slightly distended with bland thrombus (arrow). In addition, there are multiple segmental infarcts in the spleen (**b**, dashed arrows). Axial CT images of the abdomen with contrast in a different patient (**c**, **d**) with chronic splenic vein thrombosis shows multiple dilated submucosal gastric varices and intrapancreatic collateral vessels (arrows)

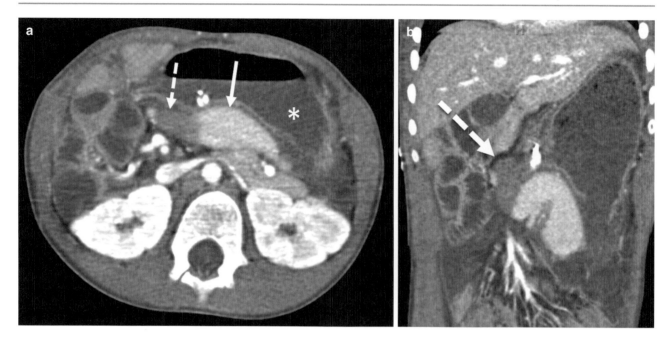

**Fig. 7** Wandering spleen with torsion in an 8-year-old girl. Axial and coronal CT images of the abdomen with IV contrast show ectopic location of the spleen in the mid-abdomen (**a**, arrow) anterior to the pancreas. There is a wedge-shaped area of splenic parenchymal hypoenhancement (**a**, **b**, dashed arrows) representing an infarct due to vascular twisting. The patient also has gastric distention (asterisk) from concomitant gastric volvulus and findings of intestinal malrotation (not shown).

abdominal pain when the torsion is incomplete or intermittent. Initial workup may show fever, leukocytosis, and a palpable abdominal mass that confuses the clinical picture [26].

*Imaging Findings* US is useful to confirm ectopic malpositioning of the wandering spleen. If the splenic vascular pedicle is torsed, Doppler flow will be reduced or absent in the spleen, and on gray scale, the parenchymal echotexture will be heterogeneous. Elevated resistive indices with decreased or even reversed diastolic splenic arterial flow can be detected [27]. On CT, an enlarged malpositioned spleen is present with an ovoid- or comma-shaped contour without or without surrounding fat stranding, fluid, or hemorrhage (Fig. 7a,b). Depending on the degree of vascular compromise, segmental or global splenic infarction may be seen. A "whirled" appearance of the splenic hilum has been reported as a specific sign of splenic torsion [28]. When infarcted from torsion, spleen is typically surgically removed. However, a viable spleen can be managed with manual detorsion followed by splenopexy [29].

## Splenic Sequestration Crisis

*Epidemiology* Sudden pooling of blood occurs within the splenic red pulp commonly in hemoglobinopathies such as sickle cell anemia, hemolytic anemias, or beta thalassemia. Sequestration crisis is commonly seen in the pediatric population due to increased distensibility of the spleen and accounts for 50% mortality in children with sickle cell disease under 2 years of age. Rarely, sequestration can be seen in young adults [30]. Splenic sequestration should not be confused with hypersplenism, which refers to rapid and premature destruction of blood cells in an overactive chronically enlarged spleen leading to mono-lineage or multi-lineage cytopenias, commonly seen in chronic liver diseases including cirrhosis, leukemias and lymphomas, and infection including infectious mononucleosis or malaria [31].

*Clinical Features* The abnormally shaped sickled red blood cells occlude the splenic capillaries and venules, leading to sudden massive splenic enlargement, acute drop in hemoglobin more than 2 g/dl, and thrombocytopenia. Patients often present with acute-onset abdominal pain, fever, lethargy, tachycardia, and tachypnea. Severe splenic sequestration can lead to hypovolemic shock and death [32]. The diagnosis of acute splenic sequestration is primarily clinical one, with imaging reserved to evaluate for complications such as splenic rupture and hemorrhage.

*Imaging Findings* Worsening splenomegaly may be the only finding on imaging with splenic size often greater than 15 cm. On US, the splenic echogenicity may be heterogeneous due to areas of infarction and hemorrhage in the presence of a patent splenic artery and vein (Fig. 8). Of note, flow in the splenic vein in this setting is retrograde from the portal vein. On CT, two distinct splenic patterns of

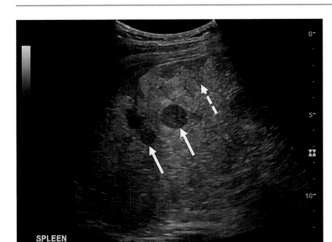

**Fig. 8** Splenic sequestration in a 30-year-old man with sickle cell disease and acute drop in hemoglobin with abdominal pain. Left upper quadrant sonogram transverse view shows an enlarged spleen with multiple round areas of decreased echogenicity within the parenchyma (arrows) representing foci of evolving hemorrhage. In addition, there are peripheral areas of wedge-shaped hypoechogenicity representing infarcts (dashed arrow)

enhancement have been identified: multiple small non-enhancing low-density parenchymal foci in a predominant peripheral location or larger, more diffuse areas of low density. The presence of perisplenic fat stranding or fluid implies impending rupture [33]. Mild episodes are treated conservatively with blood transfusions only. Severe or complicated cases may require splenectomy.

## Splenic Infections and Abscess

*Epidemiology* Splenic infection is most commonly caused by disseminated bacterial or fungal organisms, with a high propensity in immunocompromised patients such as with neutropenia or human immunodeficiency virus (HIV), uncontrolled diabetes, and intravenous drug abuse. Phillips et al. [34] reported an incidence of splenic abscess between 0.14% and 0.7% in patients with HIV and intravenous drug abuse. Hematological seeding of the spleen from septic emboli, superinfection of a large splenic infarct, and contiguous spread from adjacent organs such as stomach or colon are some of the common routes of spread [35]. Rarely, parasitic infections such as echinococcosis can involve the spleen, commonly in conjunction with the liver and peritoneum, accounting for up to 8% of cases of abdominal hydatid cysts [36].

*Clinical Features* Patients often present with fever, left abdominal, chest wall, or referred left shoulder pain. Signs of peritonitis when present often indicate abscess or splenic

rupture. Splenic hydatid cysts usually become symptomatic when large and can reach more than 10 cm in size.

*Imaging Findings* Bacterial abscesses are typically large, can be parenchymal or subcapsular, and are often solitary. On US, a splenic abscess can be predominantly cystic or appear as a complex hypoechoic mass. Internal echogenic debris can be seen with foci of gas associated with "dirty" posterior acoustic shadowing [37]. On CT and MRI, similar features are present, but rim enhancement and diffusion restriction may also be helpful features to distinguish from other cystic processes, including lymphangiomas (Fig. 9a). Perisplenic fat stranding and fluid and a reactive left pleural effusion may be present. Neutropenic patients are prone to developing fungal microabscesses that commonly involve both spleen and liver, appearing as multifocal hypo-attenuating subcentimeter foci (Fig. 9b,c) [38]. A splenic hydatid cyst appears as a unilocular cyst without internal architecture in the early stages. Multiple daughter cysts within a single large cyst are seen in the intermediate stage (Fig. 9d-f). End-stage disease shows complete calcification of the cyst, which indicates death of the parasite. Gray-scale ultrasound delineates a thick bilayered wall and multiple internal mobile echogenic foci (hydatid sand) that are pathognomonic of hydatid cyst [39]. On T2-weighted MR sequences, a low-signal-intensity outer rim is seen representing the dense fibrous pericyst. The signal intensity of maternal and daughter cysts may differ depending on the matrix contents. When detached, the inner wall of the maternal cyst can be seen as floating membranes. These cysts also restrict diffusion [36].

## Conclusions/Summary

Nontraumatic emergent splenic pathology can be seen in patients with acute abdominal pain and/or hypotension and is equally important to diagnose, as delay in management can be potentially fatal. Efforts to conserve immunocompetence have encouraged preservation of splenic tissue, with imaging playing a vital role in helping to diagnose as well as illustrate the severity of these acute abnormalities, which help in decisions regarding conservative, interventional, or surgical management.

### Key Points
- Splenic hemorrhage can occur without trauma due to spontaneous parenchymal rupture or rupture of an SAA or pseudoaneurysm.
- Vascular compromise (artery, vein, or sequestration) may result in splenic infarction.
- Imaging findings of splenic infections can be variable and depend on the pathogen. Bacterial abscesses are often

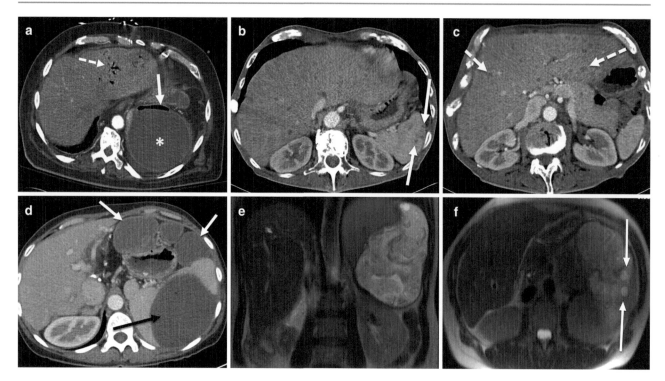

**Fig. 9** Splenic infections in three different patients. Axial CT image of the abdomen with IV contrast of a 30-year-old man with fever and intravenous drug abuse (**a**) shows a rim-enhancing fluid collection replacing almost the entire spleen (asterisk), representing an abscess. There is nondependent gas within the collection (white arrow), as well as portal venous gas in the liver (black arrow). Axial CT image of the abdomen with IV contrast of a 42-year-old woman with chronic myelogenous leukemia and neutropenic fever (**b**) demonstrates innumerable subcentimeter hypoattenuating foci in the spleen (**b**, arrows), as well as within the liver (**c**, dashed arrows), representing hepatosplenic candidiasis. Axial CT image of the abdomen with IV contrast of a 42-year-old woman with prior echinococcal cyst resection from the left liver (**d**) shows a large dominant cyst in the spleen (black arrow) as well as multiple peritoneal cysts (arrows). MRI (**e**, **f**) subsequently shows T2 hyperintense, swirled appearance of the lesions with daughter cysts (**f**, arrow) noted as well

large and few in number. Fungal infections commonly lead to microabscesses. Both may be associated with mycotic pseudoaneurysms.

# References

1. Barnhart MI, Lusher JM. Structural physiology of the human spleen. Am J Pediatr Hematol Oncol. 1979;1(4):311–30.
2. Linguraru MG, Sandberg JK, Jones EC, Summers RM. Assessing splenomegaly: automated volumetric analysis of the spleen. Acad Radiol. 2013;20(6):675–84.
3. Kucybała I, Ciuk S, Tęczar J. Spleen enlargement assessment using computed tomography: which coefficient correlates the strongest with the real volume of the spleen? Abdom Radiol. 2018;43(9):2455–61.
4. Cheson BD, Fisher RI, Barrington SF, Cavalli F, Schwartz LH, Zucca E, et al. Recommendations for initial evaluation, staging, and response assessment of Hodgkin and non-Hodgkin lymphoma: the Lugano classification. J Clin Oncol. 2014;32(27):3059–68.
5. Uyeda JW, LeBedis CA, Penn DR, Soto JA, Anderson SW. Active hemorrhage and vascular injuries in splenic trauma: utility of the arterial phase in multidetector CT. Radiology. 2014;270(1):99–106.
6. Karlo CA, Stolzmann P, Do RK, Alkadhi H. Computed tomography of the spleen: how to interpret the hypodense lesion. Insights Imaging. 2013;4(1):65–76.
7. Emery KH. Splenic emergencies. Radiol Clin N Am. 1997;35(4):831–43.
8. Renzulli P, Hostettler A, Schoepfer AM, Gloor B, Candinas D. Systematic review of atraumatic splenic rupture. Br J Surg. 2009;96(10):1114–21.
9. Rutkow IM. Rupture of the spleen in infectious mononucleosis: a critical review. Arch Surg. 1978;113(6):718–20.
10. Levenson RB, Troy KM, Lee KS. Acute abdominal pain following optical colonoscopy: CT findings and clinical considerations. Am J Roentgenol. 2016;207(3):W33–40.
11. Alabousi A, Patlas MN, Scaglione M, Romano L, Soto JA. Cross-sectional imaging of nontraumatic emergencies of the spleen. Curr Probl Diagn Radiol. 2014;43(5):254–67.
12. Tonolini M, Bianco R. Nontraumatic splenic emergencies: cross-sectional imaging findings and triage. Emerg Radiol. 2013;20(4):323–32.
13. Nores M, Phillips EH, Morgenstern L, Hiatt JR. The clinical spectrum of splenic infarction. Am Surg. 1998;64(2):182–8.
14. Balcar I, Seltzer SE, Davis S, Geller S. CT patterns of splenic infarction: a clinical and experimental study. Radiology. 1984;151(3):723–9.
15. Stuart E, Murvis WSK, Shanmuganathan K, Soto JA, Yu JS. Nontraumatic abdominal emergencies. In: Patlas MS MN, Romano L, Soto JA, editors. Problem solving in emergency radiology. 1st ed. Philadelphia: Elsevier; 2015. p. 368–458.
16. Agrawal GA, Johnson PT, Fishman EK. Splenic artery aneurysms and pseudoaneurysms: clinical distinctions and CT appearances. Am J Roentgenol. 2007;188(4):992–9.
17. Abbas MA, Stone WM, Fowl RJ, Gloviczki P, Oldenburg WA, Pairolero PC, et al. Splenic artery aneurysms: two decades experience at Mayo clinic. Ann Vasc Surg. 2002;16(4):442–9.

18. Lakin RO, Bena JF, Sarac TP, Shah S, Krajewski LP, Srivastava SD, et al. The contemporary management of splenic artery aneurysms. J Vasc Surg. 2011;53(4):958–65.
19. Tessier DJ, Stone WM, Fowl RJ, Abbas MA, Andrews JC, Bower TC, et al. Clinical features and management of splenic artery pseudoaneurysm: case series and cumulative review of literature. J Vasc Surg. 2003;38(5):969–74.
20. Dave SP, Reis ED, Hossain A, Taub PJ, Kerstein MD, Hollier LH. Splenic artery aneurysm in the 1990s. Ann Vasc Surg. 2000;14(3):223–9.
21. Uy PPD, Francisco DM, Trivedi A, O'Loughlin M, Wu GY. Vascular diseases of the spleen: a review. J Clin Transl Hepatol. 2017;5(2):152–64.
22. Butler JR, Eckert GJ, Zyromski NJ, Leonardi MJ, Lillemoe KD, Howard TJ. Natural history of pancreatitis-induced splenic vein thrombosis: a systematic review and meta-analysis of its incidence and rate of gastrointestinal bleeding. HPB (Oxford). 2011;13(12): 839–45.
23. Marn CS, Glazer GM, Williams DM, Francis IR. CT-angiographic correlation of collateral venous pathways in isolated splenic vein occlusion: new observations. Radiology. 1990;175(2):375–80.
24. Marn CS, Edgar KA, Francis IR. CT diagnosis of splenic vein occlusion: imaging features, etiology, and clinical manifestations. Abdom Imaging. 1995;20(1):78–81.
25. Herman TE, Siegel MJ. CT of acute splenic torsion in children with wandering spleen. Am J Roentgenol. 1991;156(1):151–3.
26. Chawla S, Boal DKB, Dillon PW, Grenko RT. Best cases from the AFIP. Radiographics. 2003;23(2):305–8.
27. Nemcek AA Jr, Miller FH, Fitzgerald SW. Acute torsion of a wandering spleen: diagnosis by CT and duplex Doppler and color flow sonography. AJR Am J Roentgenol. 1991;157(2):307–9.
28. Swischuk LE, Williams JB, John SD. Torsion of wandering spleen: the whorled appearance of the splenic pedicle on CT. Pediatr Radiol. 1993;23(6):476–7.
29. Lubner MG, Simard ML, Peterson CM, Bhalla S, Pickhardt PJ, Menias CO. Emergent and nonemergent nonbowel torsion: spectrum of imaging and clinical findings. Radiographics. 2013;33(1): 155–73.
30. Roshkow JE, Sanders LM. Acute splenic sequestration crisis in two adults with sickle cell disease: US, CT, and MR imaging findings. Radiology. 1990;177(3):723–5.
31. Caro J, Nagalla S. Hypersplenism and hyposplenism. In: Kaushansky K, Lichtman MA, Prchal JT, Levi MM, Press OW, Burns LJ, et al., editors. Williams Hematology, 9e. New York, NY: McGraw-Hill Education; 2015.
32. Powell RW, Levine GL, Yang YM, Mankad VN. Acute splenic sequestration crisis in sickle cell disease: early detection and treatment. J Pediatr Surg. 1992;27(2):215–8.
33. Sheth S, Ruzal-Shapiro C, Piomelli S, Berdon WE. CT imaging of splenic sequestration in sickle cell disease. Pediatr Radiol. 2000;30(12):830–3.
34. Phillips GS, Radosevich MD, Lipsett PA. Splenic abscess: another look at an old disease. Arch Surg. 1997;132(12):1331–6.
35. Chang K-C, Chuah S-K, Changchien C-S, Tsai T-L, Lu S-N, Chiu Y-C, et al. Clinical characteristics and prognostic factors of splenic abscess: a review of 67 cases in a single medical center of Taiwan. World J Gastroenterol. 2006;12(3):460–4.
36. Pedrosa I, Saíz A, Arrazola J, Ferreirós J, Pedrosa CS. Hydatid disease: radiologic and pathologic features and complications. Radiographics. 2000;20(3):795–817.
37. Ralls PW, Quinn MF, Colletti P, Lapin SA, Halls J. Sonography of pyogenic splenic abscess. Am J Roentgenol. 1982;138(3):523–5.
38. Orlowski HLP, McWilliams S, Mellnick VM, Bhalla S, Lubner MG, Pickhardt PJ, et al. Imaging spectrum of invasive fungal and fungal-like infections. Radiographics. 2017;37(4):1119–34.
39. Turgut AT, Ödev K, Kabaalioğlu A, Bhatt S, Dogra VS. Multitechnique evaluation of renal hydatid disease. Am J Roentgenol. 2009;192(2):462–7.

# Imaging of Nontraumatic Gastrointestinal Emergencies

Varun Razdan and Meghan Lubner

## Contents

V. Razdan · M. Lubner (✉)
University of Wisconsin School of Medicine and Public Health,
Madison, WI, USA
e-mail: Vrazdan@uwhealth.org; mlubner@uwhealth.org

## Abstract

Acute abdominal pain is a very common presentation of patients in the emergency department. The spectrum of pathologies range from benign and self-limiting to high morbidity and potentially life-threatening. Although clinical history, physical examination, and laboratory tests are critical

© Springer Nature Switzerland AG 2022
M. N. Patlas et al. (eds.), *Atlas of Emergency Imaging from Head-to-Toe*,
https://doi.org/10.1007/978-3-030-92111-8_29

for evaluation, imaging plays a key role in many clinical scenarios. Imaging can help clinicians' diagnostic confidence, as many acute abdominal pathologies present with nonspecific symptoms. Furthermore, imaging can evaluate for complications, some of which can be life-threatening. Lastly, imaging can help guide management, especially with regard to whether the patient needs urgent surgery.

In this chapter, we review common causes of acute abdominal pain: appendicitis, small bowel obstruction, diverticulitis, colitis, mesenteric ischemia, and acute gastrointestinal bleeding. In each section, we start with a brief discussion of epidemiology and clinical features. Next, we compare different imaging modalities, with specific recommendations from the American College of Radiology appropriateness criteria. The specific imaging techniques are detailed. Lastly, we discuss common imaging findings, as well as important associated complications.

## Keywords

Appendicitis · Small bowel obstruction · Diverticulitis · Colitis · Mesenteric ischemia · Acute gastrointestinal bleed

## Imaging Techniques

Computed tomography (CT) for acute abdominal pain typically involves thin section (≤5 mm) multiplanar imaging of the entire abdomen and pelvis. The use of intravenous (IV) and oral contrast material will be discussed with each specific pathology.

Magnetic resonance imaging (MRI) protocols for acute abdominal pain are varied, but a sample protocol [1] is as follows: multiplanar T2-weighted single-shot fast spin-echo imaging without and with fat saturation; non-enhanced and IV contrast-enhanced 3D spoiled gradient-echo T1-weighted imaging at 40 s, 90 s, and 3 min; and axial diffusion-weighted imaging. Gadolinium-based contrast agents should not be used in pregnant patients.

## Acute Appendicitis

### Epidemiology

The annual rate of acute appendicitis (AA) was 9.4/10,000 in 2008, which had increased from 7.6/10,000 in 1993 [2]. The most commonly affected age group is between 10 and 19 years old, although the incidence of AA in adults has increased since 1993, partially attributed to changing national demographics [2]. Males are more frequently diagnosed than females (56.6% versus 43.4%), although the gap has narrowed over time [2].

## Clinical Features

The classic presentation of AA is acute onset of periumbilical abdominal pain, which migrates to the right lower quadrant. However, many patients present with atypical symptoms, such as indigestion, flatulence, bowel irregularity, diarrhea, and generalized malaise [3]. Commonly described physical examination signs include maximal tenderness in the right lower quadrant at McBurney's point, pain in the right lower quadrant with palpation of the left lower quadrant (Rovsing's sign), and right lower quadrant pain with passive right hip extension (Psoas sign).

Common appendicitis mimics include epiploic appendagitis, mesenteric adenitis, omental infarct, terminal ileitis, cecal diverticulitis, cecal and appendiceal carcinoma, and appendiceal mucocele [4].

## Diagnostic Investigations

### Imaging Modalities

Computed tomography (CT) remains the most commonly used and recommended modality for nonpregnant adults with suspected AA [5]. CT has the highest accuracy, with reported sensitivities of 88–100%, specificities of 91–99%, negative predictive values of 95–100%, and accuracies of 94–98% [4]. Furthermore, CT can evaluate the complications of AA and can be used to determine other causes of acute abdominal pain. The major disadvantages of CT are ionizing radiation and the risk of an IV contrast reaction.

Ultrasound (US) is the favored modality for pediatric [6] and pregnant patients [5], due to the lack of ionizing radiation (Fig. 1). Although US can be used in adults, there are common situations where it can be difficult to accurately diagnose AA: obesity, overlying bowel gas, and a retrocecal appendix. Furthermore, US is highly operator dependent and has lower sensitivity and specificity when compared to CT [4].

Magnetic resonance imaging (MRI) is also used for diagnosing AA, especially in pediatric and pregnant patients (Fig. 2). Improvements in MRI technique and technology have led to high sensitivity (96.6%) and specificity (95.9%), similar to CT [7]. MRI can better evaluate other causes of abdominal pain when compared to US. The major disadvantages of MRI include the length of the examination (typically 15–20 min) and limited access to MRI in the emergency setting.

### Technique

The use of oral and/or IV contrast in diagnosing AA is still somewhat controversial. Many studies have shown similar diagnostic accuracy with versus without oral and IV contrast [8–10]. Furthermore, oral contrast delays the examination, and IV contrast has the potential to cause adverse reactions. Proponents of oral contrast claim improved diagnostic

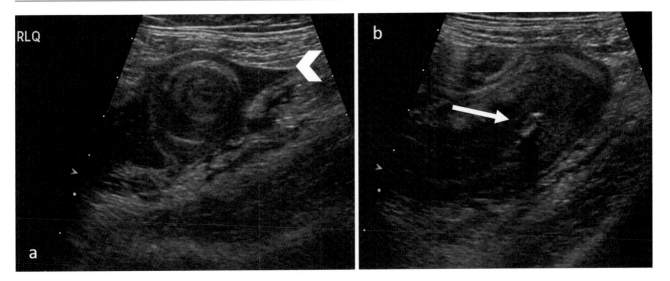

**Fig. 1** A 35-year-old pregnant woman with right lower quadrant (RLQ) pain and appendicitis on US. Transverse (**a**) and longitudinal (**b**) gray-scale ultrasound images demonstrate a dilated, non-compressible blind ending appendix with surrounding free fluid (arrowhead, **a**). Note the calcified appendicoliths with shadowing (arrow, **b**)

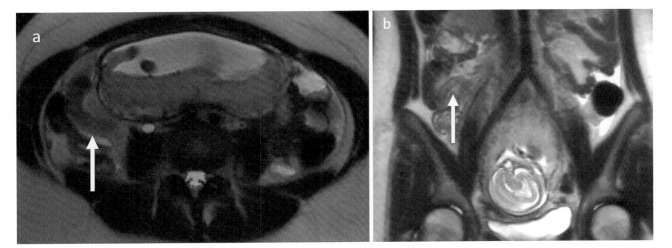

**Fig. 2** A 19-year-old 20-week pregnant patient with right lower quadrant pain. Axial (**a**) and coronal (**b**) T2 weighted images demonstrate free fluid in the RLQ and a dilated fluid-filled appendix (arrows) consistent with appendicitis

confidence [11]. If oral contrast is given, approximately 1000 ml of Iohexol 300 over 1 h may opacify the distal small bowel and cecum.

## Imaging Findings

The classic imaging findings of AA include appendiceal dilation with some degree of periappendiceal inflammatory changes. Appendiceal dilation is defined as a transverse diameter greater than 6 mm, when measured between each outer wall. Importantly, the normal appendix measures greater than 6 mm in up to 42% of asymptomatic patients [12]. Some authors classify an appendiceal diameter of 6–10 mm as indeterminate [4]. Therefore, the diagnosis of AA should be interpreted in the context of other imaging and clinical findings and not just based on size measurement alone.

Appendiceal wall thickening ≥3 mm and wall hyper-enhancement are also seen with AA. Appendicolith(s) can be seen in approximately one third of patients with AA. Appendicoliths are an important prognostic factor, as it increases the risk for appendiceal perforation (Fig. 3) [13].

Focal cecal apex thickening is commonly seen with AA. The arrowhead sign is described as enteric/rectal contrast in the thickened cecal apex "pointing" to the abnormal appendix. The cecal bar sign is described as inflammatory soft tissue at the base of the appendix that separates the appendix from the contrast-filled cecum [4].

Periappendiceal inflammatory changes are common, such as fat stranding, thickening of the lateroconal fascia and mesoappendix, and inflammation of adjacent structures (e.g., bowel, bladder).

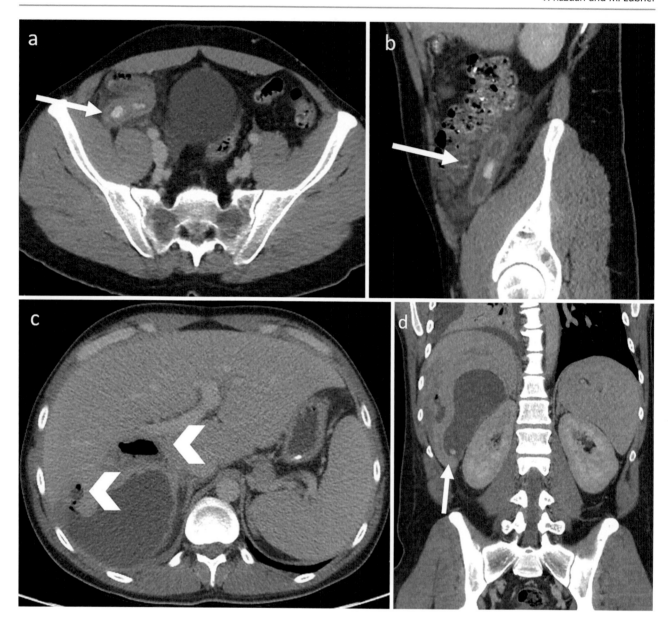

**Fig. 3** A 29-year-old man with right lower quadrant pain. Axial (**a**) and sagittal (**b**) IV contrast-enhanced CT images demonstrate a dilated, thick-walled appendix containing appendicoliths (arrows, **a** and **b**), measuring up to 2 cm, with exuberant surrounding inflammatory change and complex fluid. Axial (**c**) and coronal (**d**) CT images in the same patient 2–3 weeks later demonstrate a rim-enhancing hepatic fluid collection with internal appendicoliths (arrow, **d**) and gas (arrowheads, **c**), compatible with hepatic abscess, which was subsequently drained

MR findings of AA are similar to CT, such as appendiceal dilation, wall thickening, and hyperenhancement. MR-specific findings include increased T2 signal in the appendiceal wall and diffusion restriction of the appendix [1].

## Complications

The most frequent complication of AA is abscess formation (Fig. 3). The classic imaging findings are a loculated rim-enhancing fluid collection, which can sometimes contain an appendicolith. Large abscesses are typically treated with percutaneous drainage, followed by delayed appendectomy.

AA can lead to ischemia and necrosis of the appendiceal wall, leading to perforation. The most sensitive findings include a focal defect in enhancing the appendiceal wall (64%), phlegmon (46%), abscess (36%), extraluminal air (26%), and extraluminal appendicolith (21%). These findings have a specificity between 95% and 100% [14].

Early appendiceal rupture can lead to bacterial peritonitis, characterized by enhancing and thickened peritoneal reflections with associated free fluid, mesenteric vessel engorgement, and bowel hyperemia [4].

Bowel obstruction as an immediate complication of AA is uncommon. Bowel obstruction more commonly occurs postoperatively due to adhesions, in pediatric and elderly patients, and in patients with atypical presentations.

## Conclusion/Summary/Key Points

- Acute appendicitis is a common cause of acute abdominal pain, especially in children and young adults.
- CT with or without oral and enteric contrast is the initial study of choice in adults with suspected AA. US and MRI are typically reserved for pediatric or pregnant patients.
- Common CT findings include appendiceal dilation and wall thickening, focal cecal thickening, and periappendiceal inflammatory changes.
- Potential complications include abscess, perforation, bacterial peritonitis, and bowel obstruction.

## Small Bowel Obstruction

### Epidemiology

Small bowel obstruction (SBO) accounts for 12–16% of hospital admissions for abdominal pain [15]. The mortality rate ranges from 2% to 8% but can be as high as 25% with delay in surgical management. There are numerous causes of SBO, with adhesions accounting for up to 74% [16]. Other causes include inflammatory bowel disease, hernias, intussusception, volvulus, gallstones, foreign bodies, bezoars, and trauma [16].

### Clinical Features

The classic symptoms for SBO include diffuse abdominal pain, abdominal distention, and vomiting. Symptoms and laboratory findings have limited sensitivity and specificity for diagnosing SBO [17].

### Diagnostic Investigations

#### Modality
Abdominal radiography is frequently the first imaging examination obtained for a patient with acute abdominal pain. The reported accuracy of radiography is 50–86% [15]. Both dependent and nondependent views should be obtained. An oral contrast challenge (detailed in Sect. 3.3.2) with interval radiography helps to predict if conservative measures (e.g., NG tube placement) will be successful (Fig. 4).

CT is the recommended modality for the evaluation of suspected SBO as its reported diagnostic accuracy is greater than 90% [17]. Furthermore, CT can help determine the SBO

etiology and the site of obstruction, evaluate for complications, and identify alternative causes for abdominal pain.

Both MRI and US are not frequently used or recommended for SBO evaluation in the emergency setting, except in pregnant patients.

#### Technique
Patients with suspected high-grade SBO should not receive oral contrast as it may lead to aspiration. Furthermore, non-opacified fluid in the bowel provides intrinsic contrast [17].

The oral contrast challenge can be started with oral or enteric tube administration of 100 ml of hyperosmolar iodinated contrast agent mixed with 50 ml of water. Subsequently, radiographs are obtained at 8 and 24 h to determine if oral contrast reaches the colon.

#### Imaging Findings
The classic imaging finding on radiography is dilated (>3 cm) gas or fluid-filled small bowel. Other important findings include two or more air-fluid levels, which are wider than 2.5 cm and differ more than 2 cm in height in the same bowel loop (Fig. 4) [18]. The absence of rectal gas and a distended stomach can also be seen. The key imaging finding on CT is dilated small bowel (>2.5 cm outer wall to outer wall), with normal or collapsed bowel distally.

SBO lies on a spectrum from low-grade partial obstruction, to high-grade partial obstruction, to high-grade complete obstruction. Low-grade partial obstruction demonstrates flow of contrast through the level of obstruction. High-grade partial obstruction demonstrates delayed passage of contrast with minimal contrast past the obstruction. There is no contrast flow through a high-grade complete obstruction. The small bowel "feces sign" can also be seen with a complete obstruction.

The etiology of SBO can often be determined by evaluating the area adjacent to the transition point. Intrinsic causes of SBO include Crohn disease, neoplasia, intussusception, radiation enteritis, small bowel hematoma, and vascular occlusion [18]. Extrinsic causes include adhesions, hernias, and endometriosis (Fig. 5). Intraluminal causes include gallstone ileus, bezoar, DIOS, and foreign body ingestion [18].

#### Complications
Closed-loop physiology is defined as the occlusion of a bowel segment at two adjacent points. The obstructed bowel segment will be enlarged and is fluid-filled, classically with a C- or U-shaped configuration (Figs. 5 and 6). When a long segment of bowel is involved, this has been described as resembling balloons on a string or a bag of bowel. Closed-loop physiology is highly specific (0.95) for the need for surgery [19].

Bowel obstruction can eventually lead to strangulation and bowel ischemia. Common findings include bowel wall thickening, mesenteric edema with engorged vessels, pneumatosis, and abnormal bowel wall enhancement (Figs. 5 and 6).

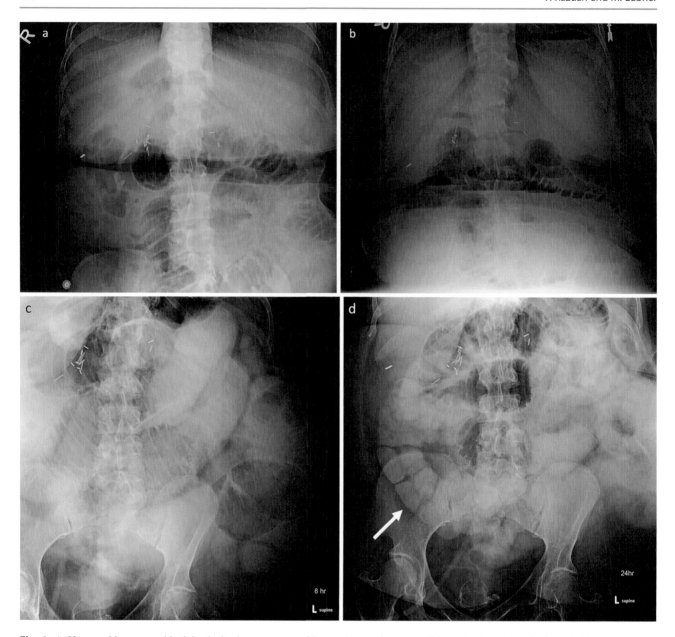

**Fig. 4** A 52-year-old woman with abdominal pain, nausea, vomiting, and history of prior surgery. Supine (**a**) and upright (**b**) radiographs demonstrated dilated gas-filled loops of small bowel measuring up to 5 cm, with multiple air-fluid levels on upright radiographs. A small amount of colonic gas is seen, but the small bowel is dilated out of proportion to the colon and CT (not shown) demonstrated small bowel obstruction due to ventral/incisional hernia. Additional radiographic images from a small bowel oral contrast challenge in the same patient. For this challenge, 100 mL of oral contrast (iohexol 300) was administered, and radiographs were obtained 8 h (**c**) and 24 h (**d**) after the administration of contrast. At 8 h, the small bowel loops are dilated, and no contrast has advanced to the colon, but after 24 h, contrast is seen in the right colon (arrow, **d**). If the contrast has not reached the colon by 24 h, this suggests that the patient may need surgical intervention

## Conclusions/Summary

- Small bowel obstruction is a common cause of abdominal pain in the emergency setting and can have high mortality if surgical management is delayed.
- CT with IV contrast is the recommended imaging examination to evaluate for SBO and for its complications.

- Key imaging findings include dilated small bowel with normal or collapsed bowel distally. Although there are many causes for SBO, the etiology can often be determined by evaluating the site of obstruction on CT.
- Complications include closed-loop obstruction and strangulation/bowel ischemia.

**Fig. 5** An 81-year-old woman with abdominal pain, nausea, and vomiting. Axial and coronal CT images demonstrate dilated small bowel loops with a transition at the level of the incarcerated left femoral hernia (arrows). Note the decreased enhancement of the small bowel loop in the hernia sac, concerning for developing ischemia. At surgery, an incarcerated femoral hernia was found with necrotic small bowel and associated purulence

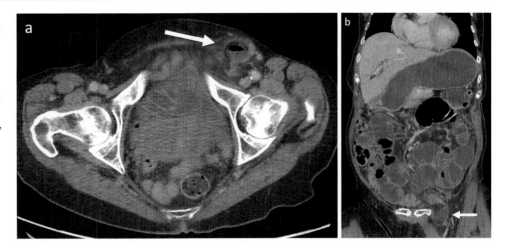

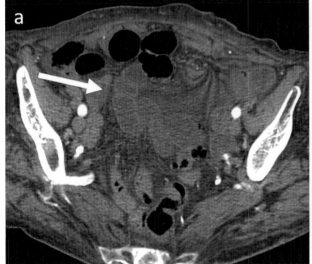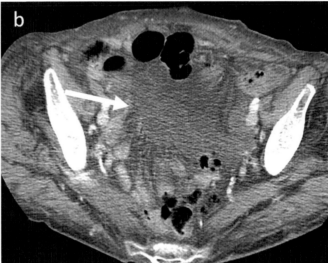

**Fig. 6** An 86-year-old woman with abdominal pain. Axial CT images from mesenteric ischemia protocol CT (arterial phase **a**, portal venous phase **b**) demonstrate loops in a radial configuration, resembling balloons on a string (arrows) with a decreased enhancement of the bowel wall seen on **b**. This was concerning for closed-loop obstruction with developing ischemia, and at surgery infarcted small bowel was found to be torsed around or herniated under the left round ligament and an associated dense adhesive band

## Acute Diverticulitis

### Epidemiology

Diverticulosis is a term used to describe the presence of uninflamed diverticula, which can occur throughout the GI tract but are seen most commonly in the descending or sigmoid colon. The frequency of diverticulosis increases with age, affecting 5–10% of the US population over the age 45 and nearly 80% over age 85 [20]. The frequency is similar in male and females.

Acute diverticulitis (AD) refers to acute inflammation of diverticula. It is estimated that 20% of patients with diverticulosis will develop acute diverticulitis. Although 80% of patients who present with AD are 50 years or older [21], there has been a significant increase in hospitalizations for AD in patients below age 45, attributed to increasing rates of obesity [22].

The pathophysiology of diverticulosis in the colon is related to increased intracolonic pressures leading to outpouchings of the colonic wall. These outpouchings can become obstructed, leading to bacterial overgrowth and inflammation. There is an association between diverticulosis and low-fiber diets [21].

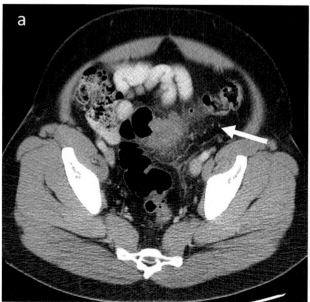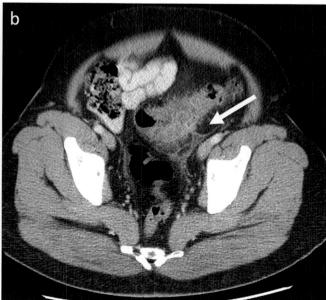

**Fig. 7** A 71-year-old woman with left lower quadrant abdominal pain. Axial CT images (**a** and **b**) demonstrate multiple inflamed sigmoid colonic diverticula with associated colonic wall thickening, adjacent inflammatory stranding, fascial thickening, and free fluid (arrows) consistent with acute uncomplicated diverticulitis

## Clinical Features

The classic presentation of AD is left lower quadrant abdominal pain. Changes in bowel habits, lower GI bleeding, and dysuria are common symptoms. Common mimics of AD include inflammatory bowel disease, pelvic inflammatory disease, cystitis, colon cancer, and infectious colitis [21].

## Diagnostic Investigations

### Imaging Modalities

CT is the modality of choice for the evaluation of suspected AD [23]. Furthermore, CT can better evaluate complications of AD and alternative diagnoses [24]. US can be used for evaluating AD, and studies have shown similar diagnostic accuracy to CT [24], although US evaluation is operator dependent and limited in obese patients. MRI can also be used for evaluating AD, although the modality is typically reserved for pregnant women and children, demographics that have a very low incidence of AD.

### Technique

IV contrast is typically used to better evaluate potential complications of AD. The use of oral contrast is controversial (see Sect. "Acute Appendicitis" for further discussion).

### Imaging Findings and Complications

The classic CT findings of AD are inflammation surrounding a diverticulum with adjacent bowel wall thickening and fat stranding. Highly specific and sensitive (90–96%) imaging findings include bowel wall thickening and fat stranding. Highly specific (97–100%) but less frequent signs include fascial thickening (50%), free fluid (45%), and inflamed diverticula (43%) (Fig. 7) [25].

Uncommon presentations of diverticulosis and AD include giant colonic diverticula and small bowel diverticula. Giant colonic diverticula are large, mass-like collections typically arising from the sigmoid colon. Inflammatory giant colonic diverticula is the most common subtype, which contains dense fibrous tissue, inflammatory cells, and foreign body giant cells [26]. Giant colonic diverticula can perforate and form abscesses. Resection is the definitive treatment. Small bowel diverticula are most commonly identified in the duodenum. They are usually incidentally found but rarely present with AD.

The most common complication of AD is abscess formation, found in approximately 15% of patients, typically adjacent to the inflammatory process [27] (Fig. 8). These can potentially be treated with percutaneous drain placement. More serious complications include distant intraperitoneal abscess (e.g., hepatic abscess), colovesical fistula, pylephlebitis or septic thrombophlebitis of the portal vein, and peritonitis (Fig. 9).

## Conclusion/Summary/Key Points

- AD presents with left lower quadrant abdominal pain.
- CT with IV contrast is the imaging modality of choice for evaluating AD.

- Classic imaging findings of AD are inflammation surrounding a diverticulum with adjacent bowel wall thickening and fat stranding.
- Complications include abscess formation, colovesical fistula, pylephlebitis, and peritonitis.

## Colitis

### Epidemiology/Clinical Features

Colitis is a nonspecific term referring to inflammation of the colon, which typically is related to an infectious etiology, inflammatory disease, or underlying ischemia. Clinical

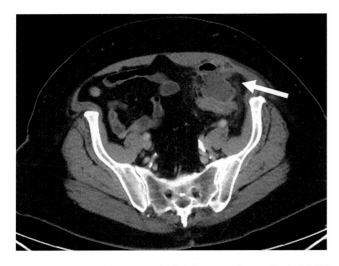

**Fig. 8** A 60-year-old woman with left lower quadrant pain. Axial CT image demonstrates a rim-enhancing fluid collection with associated gas in the left lower quadrant (arrow) adjacent to an inflamed sigmoid colon, compatible with perforated diverticular abscess

history plays a key role in helping the radiologist determine the etiology of colitis. Acute nonlocalized abdominal pain is the most common overlapping clinical symptom. Elevated white blood cell count is the most common laboratory finding. Definitive diagnosis can be obtained with colonoscopy and biopsy.

Infectious colitis is caused by bacterial, viral, fungal, and parasitic organisms. For example, pseudomembranous colitis is caused by *Clostridium difficile*, which is typically preceded by recent antibiotic use. Diarrhea is a common clinical symptom. Inflammatory colitis is related to two common inflammatory bowel diseases: Crohn disease and ulcerative colitis. These are typically seen in younger patients presenting with crampy abdominal pain, tenesmus, and rectal bleeding. Ischemic colitis is typically seen with older patients and is related to "low flow states," for example, hypovolemic shock or arrhythmias.

There are other, less common, causes of colitis. Neutropenic colitis (also known as typhlitis) is seen with immunocompromised patients. Immune-mediated colitis is associated with immunotherapy, first described with Ipilimumab. Stercoral colitis is related to chronic constipation or fecal impaction, which can lead to ischemic pressure necrosis of the colonic wall.

### Diagnostic Investigations

#### Imaging Modalities and Technique
CT is the first-line imaging modality for acute nonlocalized abdominal pain [28]. Both IV and oral contrast is typically used to better evaluate bowel pathology and to evaluate for complications.

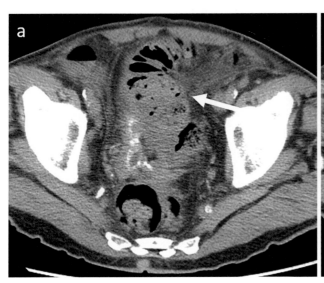
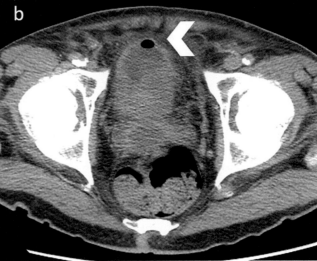

**Fig. 9** Axial CT images (**a** and **b**) demonstrated a thickened, inflamed sigmoid colon due to diverticulitis (arrow, **a**), with an associated thick-walled bladder containing gas (arrowhead, **b**), indicating a colovesical fistula

CT and MRI enterography is a specialized protocol, often used for Crohn disease. It involves the use of negative oral contrast (e.g., Volumen, 0.1%, or Breeza), which aids in the evaluation of mucosal enhancement and mesenteric vasculature.

## Imaging Findings and Complications

Key overlapping CT and MR imaging findings in colitis include bowel wall thickening, pericolonic stranding, and ascites. As mentioned before, clinical history plays a key role in narrowing the wide range of etiologies.

Infectious colitis is classically seen with a pan-colonic distribution, with associated mesenteric edema and ascites. Uncommon infectious causes can favor more specific colonic distributions. For example, there is a favored right colon distribution of salmonella, yersina, tuberculosis, and amebiasis, and there is a favored left colon distribution of schistosomiasis, shigellosis, herpes, gonorrhea, syphilis, and lymphogranuloma venereum [29]. Pseudomembranous colitis almost always involved the rectosigmoid colon.

Ulcerative colitis demonstrates symmetric continuous wall thickening, almost always involving the rectum, and can extend to the left colon or involve the entire colon. Crohn disease demonstrates asymmetric segmental wall thickening, commonly involving the right colon and terminal ileum, and typically sparing the rectum.

Ischemic colitis classically affects the watershed areas (i.e., the splenic flexure and rectosigmoid colon) and typically spares the rectum (Fig. 10). With profound hypotension, CT hypoperfusion complex can occur. Bowel imaging findings of hypoperfusion complex include thickened small bowel loops with hyperdense walls on non-contrast imaging and hyperenhancing walls on IV contrast-enhanced imaging.

## Complications

Common complications of colitis include abscess, toxic megacolon, and perforation. Abscess formation is commonly seen with Crohn disease and is identified as a fluid collection with enhancing borders (Fig. 11). Toxic megacolon is seen with inflammatory bowel disease and in infectious colitis. The classic imaging features are enlarged ahaustral colon, with thinned walls, which eventually leads to perforation.

## Conclusion/Summary/Key Points

- Colitis has numerous etiologies, most commonly infectious, inflammatory, or ischemic. Clinical history plays a key role in helping the radiologist narrow the differential diagnosis.
- CT with IV contrast is the recommended imaging modality for acute nonlocalized abdominal pain and suspected colitis.

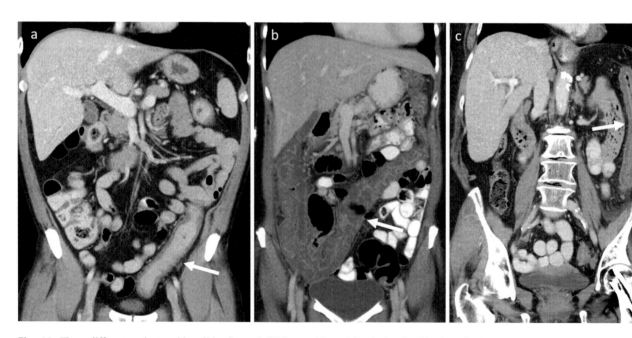

**Fig. 10** Three different patients with colitis. Coronal CT image (**a**) from a 46-year-old man with bloody diarrhea, with symmetric moderate wall thickening of the left colon (arrow, **a**) contiguous from the rectum (not shown). Colonoscopy showed pancolitis with biopsy compatible with ulcerative colitis. Coronal CT image (**b**) demonstrates exuberate colonic wall thickening and edema in a pancolonic distribution (arrow, **b**) with rectal sparing (not shown) in a 63-year-old woman with abdominal pain, bloating diarrhea, and fevers. Stool studies demonstrated enterohemorrhagic *E. coli*, compatible with infectious colitis. Coronal CT image (**c**) in a 61-year-old woman demonstrates homogeneous wall thickening of the left colon spanning the splenic flexure with minimal surrounding inflammatory stranding (arrow, **c**) following an episode of abdominal pain and a bloody bowel movement, compatible with ischemic colitis

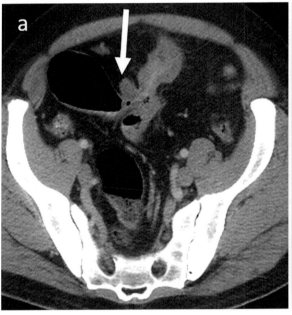
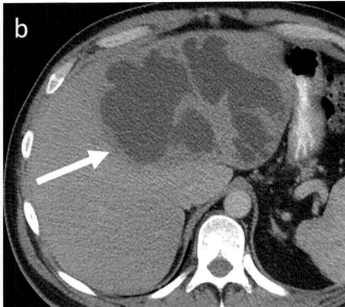

**Fig. 11** A 46-year-old man presenting with right lower quadrant pain and fevers. Axial CT images demonstrate an inflamed terminal ileum and sigmoid colon with a coloenteric fistula (arrow, **a**), with a rim-enhancing complex collection in the liver (arrow, **b**) compatible with hepatic abscess. This was the patient's first presentation of complicated Crohn disease

- Key overlapping imaging findings in colitis include wall thickening, pericolonic stranding, and ascites. The distribution of wall thickening can help to narrow the differential diagnosis.
- Complications of colitis include toxic megacolon, perforation, phlegmon/abscess formation, stricture, and fistula.

## Acute Mesenteric Ischemia

### Epidemiology

Acute mesenteric ischemia (AMI) is a rare but deadly disease process. Approximately 1% of patients presenting with acute abdominal symptoms are diagnosed with AMI [30]. Clinical diagnosis can be challenging, and treatment is frequently delayed, leading to a mortality rate estimated over 50% [31]. Early detection by imaging can lead to a significant decrease in mortality, less than 10% with immediate management [30].

Arterial embolization, typically from a cardiac origin, is the most frequent etiology of AMI (40–50%). Less frequent causes include arterial thrombosis (20–30%), nonocclusive processes (25%), or venous thrombosis (5–15%) [32]. The lack of mesenteric blood flow to the bowel can lead to a cascade from ischemia to necrosis to perforation and peritonitis. The risk factors for AMI include atrial fibrillation, coronary artery disease, and peripheral arterial occlusive disease [30].

## Clinical Features

Clinical symptoms are nonspecific; classically the patient presents with sudden onset of severe abdominal pain out of proportion to the clinical examination. Frequently, there is a pain-free interval (3–6 h) after the initial symptoms. Elevated lactate and d-dimer levels can be seen, but are nonspecific for AMI.

## Diagnostic Investigations

### Modalities

CT angiography with IV contrast is the recommended test of choice in adults with suspected acute mesenteric ischemia [32]. Dual-energy CT is an emerging modality which may help to identify subtle bowel wall enhancement differences. MR angiography has high sensitivity and specificity for diagnosing AMI but is typically not used in the emergency setting due to availability and length of examination. Furthermore, MRA has limited value in evaluating bowel ischemia. Conventional angiography has a high sensitivity and specificity but is more invasive than CTA and may lead to a delay in surgery.

### Technique

CTA involves thin section (at least 5 mm, but frequently 1–2 mm) arterial phase imaging of the entire abdomen and pelvis. Often, the portal venous phase is also performed through the entire abdomen and pelvis. Typically, negative oral contrast (e.g., barium sulfate or water) is given to distend the bowel, which can help evaluate for bowel wall pathology [32]. 3D reconstructions of the vasculature is performed which can help aid in diagnostic confidence. Concurrent non-contrast CT is performed at most institutions and is recommended by some authors [32], but may not always be necessary for accurate diagnosis [33]. Dual-energy CT is performed with high- and low-energy x-ray spectra concurrently, with post-processing techniques allowing iodine selective imaging.

## Imaging Findings

Classic and specific CT findings for occlusive AMI include a filling defect in the mesenteric arteries, with associated hypoenhancing or non-enhancing bowel wall (Fig. 12). The most frequent occlusion location is the superior mesenteric artery, near the middle colic artery. Non-contrast imaging can demonstrate high attenuation vascular filling defects (i.e., clot)

and hyperattenuating bowel wall, indicative of hemorrhagic infarction. Nonspecific CT findings include mesenteric congestion, ascites, and bowel wall thickening. These findings are more commonly seen after arterial reperfusion.

Thrombotic AMI imaging findings can be similar to embolic AMI. Typically, there are also extensive atherosclerotic calcifications, especially at the origin of the mesenteric arteries. With venous occlusion, imaging findings include filling defects in the mesenteric and portal veins, with associated mesenteric congestion and bowel wall thickening with a halo/target appearance.

Of note, nonocclusive ischemia, as could be seen with low flow states and ischemic colitis, is further discussed in the Sect. "Colitis".

Complications of AMI include bowel infarction, which leads to perforation. Classic imaging findings of infarcted bowel include thinning of the bowel wall with pneumatosis and/or portal venous gas (Fig. 12). Gross pneumoperitoneum indicates bowel perforation.

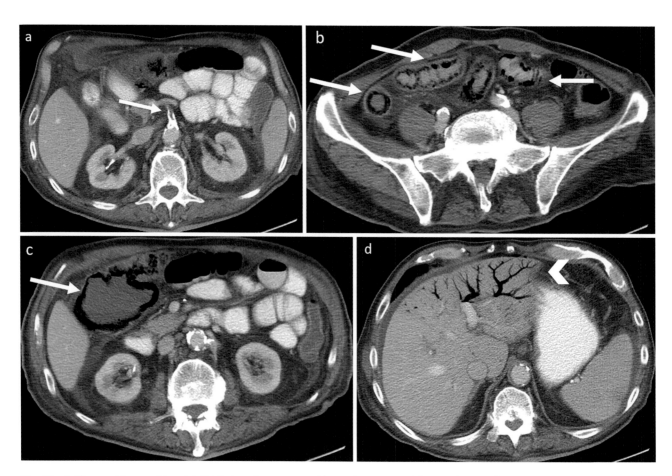

**Fig. 12** A 72-year-old man with atrial fibrillation who presents with abdominal pain and bloody diarrhea. Axial CT images demonstrate severe atherosclerotic disease with probable occlusion at the origin of the SMA (arrow, **a**), with distal small bowel wall thickening, mesenteric edema and pneumatosis (arrows, **b**) and decreased right colonic enhancement with extensive mural pneumatosis (arrow, **c**) and associated portal venous gas (arrowhead, **d**). The patient was taken emergently to the operating room, where necrotic small bowel and cecum/ascending colon were resected

## Conclusions/Summary/Key Points

- AMI is a rare but deadly cause of acute abdominal pain, and early detection with imaging can lead to a significant decrease in mortality.
- CTA is the first-line imaging modality for evaluating AMI.
- Classic CT findings for embolic AMI include a filling defect in the mesenteric arteries with non-enhancing bowel.
- AMI can lead to necrosis and perforation; the imaging findings include bowel wall thinning, pneumatosis, portal venous gas, and pneumoperitoneum.

## Acute GI Bleeding

### Epidemiology

Acute gastrointestinal bleeding is a common pathology, accounting for 1–2% of all hospital admissions in the United States [34]. The ligament of Treitz is the anatomic location separating upper gastrointestinal bleeding (UGIB) from lower gastrointestinal bleeding (LGIB). Although GIB can resolve spontaneously, massive bleeds can lead to mortality rates up to 40% [35].

### Clinical Features

Although imaging can be used for evaluating UGIB, upper endoscopy has a higher sensitivity and specificity in diagnosing the cause for UGIB. Furthermore, upper endoscopy can be used for treating UGIB. Imaging is typically used when upper endoscopy is inconclusive or cannot be used (e.g., post-upper GI surgery).

The rest of this section will focus on imaging in acute LGIB. The most common etiologies for LGIB include diverticulosis/diverticulitis, ischemic colitis, hemorrhoids, neoplasm, angioectasia, and IBD [36].

Patients with LGIB present with hematochezia or melena. If the blood loss is greater than 500 ml, hypotension and hypovolemic shock may occur. There are multiple clinical scenarios for patients presenting with LGIB, each with its own specific imaging recommendations. This includes hemodynamically stable patients, unstable patients, recurrent bleeding after colonoscopy treatment, or intermittent bleeding with negative colonoscopy [37].

### Diagnostic Investigations

### Imaging Modalities

Colonoscopy assessment for LGIB is the preferred assessment but can be challenging, as patients must undergo colon preparation which can be difficult and time-consuming in the emergency setting. Therefore, imaging can play a critical role in determining the cause and location of LGIB.

Conventional angiography is recommended in hemodynamically unstable patients and patients with recurrent bleeding after colonoscopy. Conventional angiography can be used to accurately diagnose LGIB and to also perform therapeutic interventions at the same setting (e.g., embolization). The bleeding rate detection is up to 0.5–1 ml/min.

CTA is recommended in hemodynamically stable patients and patients with intermittent or obscure nonlocalized recurrent bleeding after negative colonoscopy, such as an occult small bowel bleed [35].

Tagged red blood cell scintigraphy has a high sensitivity for the detection of UGIB, with a bleeding rate detection as low as 0.1 ml/min. On the other hand, scintigraphy has high false-negative rates and poor positive predictive value in determining the site of the bleeding, and is not easily available in the emergency setting [37]. This modality is better used for detecting slow intermittent bleeding.

### Technique

CTA technique for GI bleeding can involve up to three phases of imaging: non-contrast, arterial, and portal venous. No oral contrast should be given as it can obscure luminal blood. Dual-energy CT can be used and is performed with high- and low-energy x-ray spectra concurrently, with post-processing techniques allowing iodine selective imaging.

### Imaging Findings

Classic CTA findings for GI bleeding are intraluminal extravasation of contrast, with a blush in the arterial phase and subsequent variable change in morphology during the portal venous phase (Fig. 13) [33]. Importantly, the non-contrast imaging should confirm that there is no hyperattenuating intraluminal material in this location. Non-contrast imaging can show clotted blood as hyperattenuating material, indicating a recent bleed.

Frequently, the etiology of LGIB can be determined by imaging. As discussed above, the most common etiologies of LGIB include diverticulosis/diverticulitis, ischemic colitis, hemorrhoids, neoplasm, angioectasia, and IBD [36]. A diverticulum may be the site of active extravasation of contrast. Ischemic colitis is characterized by bowel wall thickening in the watershed areas (see Sect. "Colitis" for further details). Hemorrhoids are characterized by large veins near the anus or rectum, best seen on portal venous phase imaging [36]. The neoplasm may present as a focal segment of bowel wall thickening and luminal obstruction. Angioectasia can be characterized by a nidus of enhancement, often only visible during the enteric phase of contrast [36]. Inflammatory bowel disease has variable bowel wall thickening (see Sect. "Colitis" for further details).

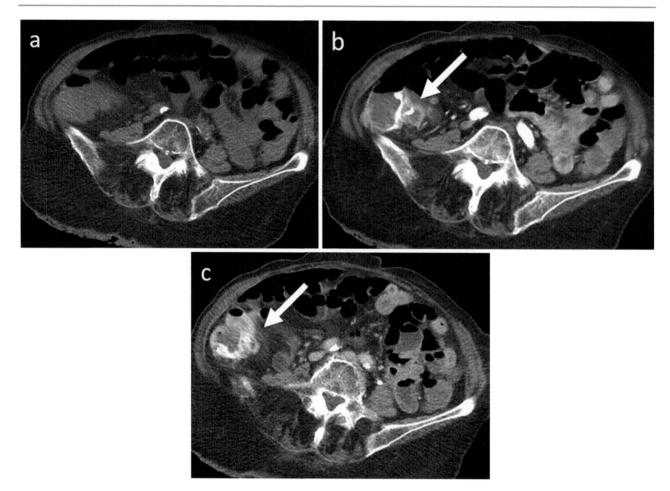

**Fig. 13** A 93-year-old woman who presented to the ED with lower GI bleeding. Axial CT images from a GI bleeding protocol including non-contrast (**a**), arterial phase (**b**), and a 3-min delay image (**c**) demonstrate serpiginous high attenuation material in a cecal diverticulum (arrow, **b**) not seen on pre-contrast images at this location that accumulates on a 3-min delay (arrow, **c**), indicating active bleeding from a right-sided colonic diverticulum

## Conclusions/Summary/Key Points

- Acute LGIB is a common pathology with many different etiologies, including diverticulosis/diverticulitis, ischemic colitis, hemorrhoids, neoplasm, angioectasia, and IBD.
- Colonoscopy is an excellent way to evaluate and treat LGIB but can be challenging during the emergency setting. CTA is the recommended non-invasive modality to evaluate LGIB.
- Classic imaging findings include intraluminal contrast blush on the arterial phase, with increase in accumulated contrast in the portal venous phase.

## References

1. Pickhardt PJ, Reeder SB. Contrast-enhanced abdominal MRI for suspected appendicitis: how we do it. AJR Am J Roentgenol. 2016; https://doi.org/10.2214/AJR.15.15948.

2. Buckius MT, McGrath B, Monk J, Grim R, Bell T, Ahuja V. Changing epidemiology of acute appendicitis in the United States: study period 1993–2008. J Surg Res. 2012;175(2):185–90.

3. Martin RF. Acute appendicitis in adults: Clinical manifestations and differential diagnosis. In: Post TW, ed. UpToDate. Waltham, MA: UpToDate. https://www.uptodate.com/contents/acute-appendicitis-in-adults-clinicalmanifestations-and-differential-diagnosis#H5346248. Last updated: February 4, 2016. Accessed: June, 2020.

4. Pinto Leite N, Pereira JM, Cunha R, Pinto P, Sirlin C. CT evaluation of appendicitis and its complications: imaging techniques and key diagnostic findings. AJR Am J Roentgenol. 2005;185(2):406–17.

5. Garcia EM, Camacho MA, Karolyi DR, Kim DH, Cash BD, Chang KJ, et al. ACR Appropriateness Criteria® right lower quadrant pain-suspected appendicitis. J Am Coll Radiol. 2018;15(11):S373–87.

6. Koberlein GC, Trout AT, Rigsby CK, Iyer RS, Alazraki AL, Anupindi SA, et al. ACR Appropriateness Criteria® suspected appendicitis-child. J Am Coll Radiol. 2019;16(5 Suppl):S252–63.

7. Repplinger MD, Levy JF, Peethumnongsin E, Gussick ME, Svenson JE, Golden SK, et al. Systematic review and meta-analysis of the accuracy of MRI to diagnose appendicitis in the general population. J Magn Reson Imaging. 2016;43(6):1346–54.

8. Keyzer C, Cullus P, Tack D, De Maertelaer V, Bohy P, Gevenois PA. MDCT for suspected acute appendicitis in adults: impact of oral

and IV contrast media at standard-dose and simulated low-dose techniques. AJR Am J Roentgenol. 2009;193(5):1272–81.

9. Anderson SW, Soto JA, Lucey BC, Ozonoff A, Jordan JD, Ratevosian J, et al. Abdominal 64-MDCT for suspected appendicitis: the use of oral and IV contrast material versus IV contrast material only. AJR Am J Roentgenol. 2009;193(5):1282–8.

10. Lane MJ, Liu DM, Huynh MD, Jeffrey RB Jr, Mindelzun RE, Katz DS. Suspected acute appendicitis: nonenhanced helical CT in 300 consecutive patients. Radiology. 1999;213(2):341–6.

11. Pickhardt PJ. Positive oral contrast material for abdominal CT: current clinical indications and areas of controversy. AJR Am J Roentgenol. 2020;8:1–10.

12. Brown MA, Tamburrini S, Furtado CD, Nanigan D, Sirlin CB, Casola G. Prospective evaluation of normal appendiceal diameter on CT. In: 103rd annual meeting of the American Roentgen Ray Society, San Diego. 2003.

13. Kaiser S, Frenckner B, Jorulf HK. Suspected appendicitis in children: US and CT – a prospective randomized study. Radiology. 2002;223(3):633–8.

14. Horrow MM, White DS, Shurman A. Differentiation of perforated and non-perforated appendicitis by CT. Radiology. 2003;227:46–51.

15. Paulson EK, Thompson WM. Review of small-bowel obstruction: the diagnosis and when to worry. Radiology. 2015;275(2):332–42.

16. Miller G, Boman J, Shrier I, Gordon PH. Etiology of small bowel obstruction. Am J Surg. 2000;180(1):33–6.

17. Chang KJ, Marin D, Kim DH, Fowler KJ, Camacho MA, Cash BD, et al. ACR Appropriateness Criteria® suspected small-bowel obstruction. J Am Coll Radiol. 2020;17:S305–14. https://doi.org/10.1016/j.jacr.2020.01.025.

18. Silva AC, Pimenta M, Guimarães LS. Small bowel obstruction: what to look for. Radiographics. 2009;29(2):423–39.

19. Scrima A, Lubner MG, King S, Pankratz J, Kennedy G, Pickhardt PJ. Value of MDCT and clinical and laboratory data for predicting the need for surgical intervention in suspected small-bowel obstruction. AJR Am J Roentgenol. 2017;208:785–93. https://doi.org/10.2214/ajr.16.16946.

20. Ferzoco LB, Raptopoulos V, Silen W. Acute diverticulitis. N Engl J Med. 1998;338(21):1521–6.

21. Jacobs DO. Diverticulitis. N Engl J Med. 2007;357(20):2057–66.

22. Nguyen GC, Sam J, Anand N. Epidemiological trends and geographic variation in hospital admissions for diverticulitis in the United States. World J Gastroenterol. 2011;17(12):1600.

23. Galgano SJ, McNamara MM, Peterson CM, Kim DH, Fowler KJ, Camacho MA, et al. ACR Appropriateness Criteria® left lower quadrant pain-suspected diverticulitis. J Am Coll Radiol. 2019;16 (5 Suppl):S141–9.

24. Laméris W, van Randen A, Bipat S, Bossuyt PMM, Boermeester MA, Stoker J. Graded compression ultrasonography and computed tomography in acute colonic diverticulitis: meta-analysis of test accuracy. Eur Radiol. 2008;18(11):2498–511.

25. Kircher MF, Rhea JT, Kihiczak D, Novelline RA. Frequency, sensitivity, and specificity of individual signs of diverticulitis on thin-section helical CT with colonic contrast material: experience with 312 cases. AJR Am J Roentgenol. 2002;178(6):1313–8.

26. Thomas S, Peel RL, Evans LE, Haarer KA. Best cases from the AFIP: giant colonic diverticulum. Radiographics. 2006;26(6): 1869–72.

27. Stoker J, van Randen A, Laméris W, Boermeester MA. Imaging patients with acute abdominal pain. Radiology. 2009;253(1):31–46.

28. Scheirey CD, Fowler KJ, Therrien JA, Kim DH, Al-Refaie WB, Camacho MA, et al. ACR Appropriateness Criteria® acute non-localized abdominal pain. J Am Coll Radiol. 2018;15(11):S217–31.

29. Thoeni RF, Cello JP. CT imaging of colitis. Radiology. 2006;240(3): 623–38.

30. Klar E, Rahmanian PB, Bücker A, Hauenstein K, Jauch K-W, Luther B. Acute mesenteric ischemia: a vascular emergency. Dtsch Arztebl Int. 2012; https://doi.org/10.3238/arztebl.2012.0249.

31. Adaba F, Askari A, Dastur J, Patel A, Gabe SM, Vaizey CJ, et al. Mortality after acute primary mesenteric infarction: a systematic review and meta-analysis of observational studies. Color Dis. 2015;17(7):566–77.

32. Furukawa A, Kanasaki S, Kono N, Wakamiya M, Tanaka T, Takahashi M, Murata K. CT diagnosis of acute mesenteric ischemia from various causes. Am J Roentgenol. 2009;192(2):408–16.

33. Ginsburg M, Obara P, Lambert DL, Hanley M, Steigner ML, Camacho MA, et al. ACR Appropriateness Criteria® imaging of mesenteric ischemia. J Am Coll Radiol. 2018;15:S332–40. https://doi.org/10.1016/j.jacr.2018.09.018.

34. Artigas JM, Martí M, Soto JA, Esteban H, Pinilla I, Guillén E. Multidetector CT angiography for acute gastrointestinal bleeding: technique and findings. Radiographics. 2013;33(5):1453–70.

35. Darcy MD, Ray CE Jr, Lorenz JM. ACR Appropriateness Criteria® radiologic management of lower gastrointestinal tract bleeding. Reston: American College of Radiology; 2011.

36. Wells ML, Hansel SL, Bruining DH, Fletcher JG, Froemming AT, Barlow JM, et al. CT for evaluation of acute gastrointestinal bleeding. Radiographics. 2018;38:1089–107. https://doi.org/10.1148/rg.2018170138.

37. Singh-Bhinder N, Kim DH, Holly BP, Johnson PT, Hanley M, Carucci LR, et al. ACR Appropriateness Criteria® nonvariceal upper gastrointestinal bleeding. J Am Coll Radiol. 2017;14: S177–88. https://doi.org/10.1016/j.jacr.2017.02.038.

# Non-traumatic Emergent Genitourinary Conditions

Victoria Chernyak

## Contents

### Abstract

Nontraumatic emergent genitourinary conditions require timely diagnosis to ensure timely treatment and an improved clinical outcome. This chapter summarizes the multimodality imaging findings in nontraumatic emergent genitourinary conditions, such as urolithiasis, infections of the GU tract, renal and adrenal infarction, renal and adrenal hemorrhage.

### Keywords

Non-traumatic emergencies · Upper GU track

## Urolithiasis

Urolithiasis is a common condition, affecting approximately 1.2 million Americans annually, with a prevalence of up to 9% [1, 2]. The prevalence of urolithiasis is 11% in men and 7% in women, with the lifetime risk of urolithiasis of up to 14% in men and 6% in women [1–3]. Computed tomography (CT) is the modality of choice for assessment of urolithiasis due to its exceptional sensitivity of 95–98%, specificity of 98%, and 96–97% accuracy [4, 5]. Ultrasound (US) is inferior to CT in assessment of urolithiasis, with only 40% of calculi identified on CT also detected on US [6]. Discrepancy between US and CT is more pronounced with smaller calculi and with calculi in ureteral locations [6]. US has a sensitivity, specificity, and accuracy of 40%, 84%, and 53% for the detection of urolithiasis, respectively [6]. Low-radiation-dose CT, aimed at decreasing radiation dose, has a sensitivity of 94%, a specificity of 100%, and an accuracy of 95% for the detection of urolithiasis [7].

Acute flank pain is the most common acute symptom in patients with urolithiasis, with marked relief of symptoms once the calculus passes [8]. Up to 81% of ureteral calculi pass spontaneously, while approximately 19% require intervention [9]. Calculi impacted at the ureteropelvic junction mainly result in flank pain, whereas those lodged in the proximal ureter above the iliac vessels cause flank pain radiating to the genitals, and calculi lodged at the ureterovesical junction (UVJ) result in voiding urgency and suprapubic discomfort, as well as radiation of pain to the inguinal region [8]. Associated signs and symptoms include hematuria (either gross or microscopic), nausea, and vomiting.

V. Chernyak (✉)
Beth Israel Deaconess Medical Center, Boston, MA, USA
e-mail: vchernya@bidmc.harvard.edu

© Springer Nature Switzerland AG 2022
M. N. Patlas et al. (eds.), *Atlas of Emergency Imaging from Head-to-Toe*,
https://doi.org/10.1007/978-3-030-92111-8_30

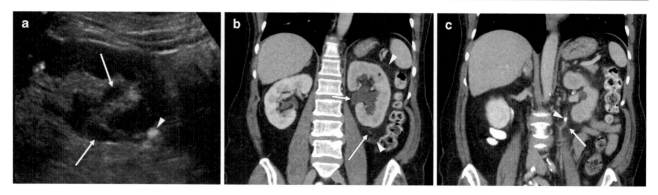

**Fig. 1** Obstructing urolithiasis in a 68-year-old man with acute back pain. Gray-scale US in sagittal plane (**a**) demonstrates mild left hydronephrosis and proximal hydroureter (arrows) to the level of hyperechoic calculus (arrowhead) in the proximal ureter. Coronal IV contrast-enhanced CT performed on the following day (**b** and **c**) shows left hydronephrosis (short arrow, **b**) and a 6-mm left ureteral calculus (arrowhead, **b**), similar to US. Note that perinephric stranding (long arrow, **b**), periureteral stranding (arrow, **c**), and thickening of perirenal fascia (arrowheads, **b**) are evident on CT only. The left renal parenchyma (\*) demonstrates slightly diminished enhancement as compared to the non-obstructed right kidney

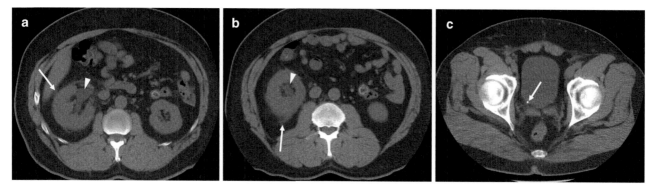

**Fig. 2** Obstructing urolithiasis in a 34-year-old man with acute right flank pain. Axial non-contrast CT images demonstrate mild right hydronephrosis (arrowheads, **a** and **b**) and asymmetric perinephric stranding (arrows, **a** and **b**). The findings are caused by a 3-mm calculus (arrow, **c**), which is lodged at the right ureterovesical junction

The acute flank pain in patients with urolithiasis is usually due to obstruction of the urinary tract by a lodged calculus. While US may be a good screening imaging examination to exclude hydronephrosis, it has a limited ability to visualize and follow the ureter. In patients presenting with renal colic, US can be used to detect approximately 76% of the calculi seen on CT (Fig. 1) [10]. Negative predictive value of US is 86% for all calculi and 98% for calculi > 5 mm [10].

Acute obstruction of the urinary tract is seen as dilatation of calyces, renal pelvis, and ureter to the level of the calculus (Fig. 2). CT demonstrates hydroureter in up to 83% of patients with acute renal colic, hydronephrosis in 80%, periureteric edema in 59%, and unilateral renal enlargement in 57% [9]. Mild asymmetric perinephric and periureteral stranding as well as thickening of perirenal fascia may be seen (Figs. 1 and 2). When obstructing urolithiasis is suspected, intravenous (IV) contrast is not administered for CT, as the contrast can obscure visualization of small calculi [11]. When the clinical presentation is unclear or suggests other etiologies, patients may undergo CT with IV contrast. Contrast-enhanced CT is 99% sensitive for calculi ≥3 mm [11]. The obstructed kidney often shows diminished enhancement and delayed transit of IV contrast (Figs. 1 and 3).

Renal calyceal rupture is due to perirenal urinary extravasation associated with ureteral obstruction. While the majority (74%) of cases with calyceal rupture are due an obstructing ureteral calculus, other benign and malignant causes of ureteric obstruction need to be excluded [12]. Approximately 58% of calculi associated with calyceal rupture are lodged at the ureterovesical junction [12]. The diagnosis of renal calyceal rupture is suggested when an obstructed collecting system is accompanied by an irregularity of a single renal calyx, infiltration of renal sinus fat, asymmetric perinephric stranding, or a discreet perinephric fluid collection (Fig. 3) [12]. Urinary tract infection can also present with asymmetric perinephric fluid, and the distinction between the two entities may be difficult. No evidence of infection on urinalysis and lack of fever can help distinguish between the two.

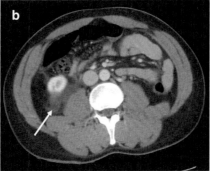
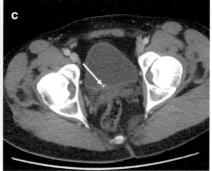

**Fig. 3** Calyceal rupture in a 47-year-old man with acute right abdominal pain and vomiting. Axial post-contrast CT images demonstrate mild right hydronephrosis (arrowhead, **a**) due to a 3-mm calculus (arrow, **c**) at the right ureterovesical junction. Asymmetric ill-defined fluid collection around the right kidney (arrows, **a** and **b**) represents calyceal rupture. Note that the right kidney is in the corticomedullary phase, whereas the left kidney is in the nephrographic phase, indicating delayed function of the right kidney (**a**)

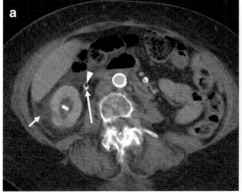
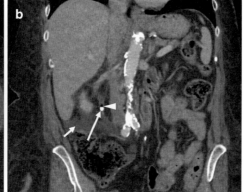

**Fig. 4** Pyonephrosis in a 66-year-old woman with fever and abdominal pain. Axial (**a**) and coronal (**b**) post-contrast CT images demonstrate a 6-mm calculus (long arrow) lodged in the proximal right ureter. Focus of air superior to the calculus (arrowhead) confirms superimposed infection (pyonephrosis). Asymmetric fluid around the right kidney (short arrow) may be a result of calyceal rupture or inflammatory changes related to infection

Superimposed infection can complicate obstructive urolithiasis, resulting in pyonephrosis, uroseptic shock, and acute kidney injury (AKI) [13]. In hospitalized patients with urinary tract infection, urolithiasis is associated with nearly twofold increased risk of uroseptic shock, AKI, and bacteremia [13]. As discussed above, infection may be difficult to distinguish from calyceal rupture; the presence of gas in the obstructed collecting system helps establishing the diagnosis of pyonephrosis (Fig. 4).

## Infection

Urinary tract infection is reported to affect 150 million patients annually worldwide [14]. In most uncomplicated cases, the diagnosis is made based on clinical symptoms and urinalysis, with no need for imaging. Diagnostic imaging plays an important role in the evaluation of complications, indicated clinically by lack of response to antibiotic treatment. Imaging can also identify structural abnormalities of the urinary tract, which can guide management.

## Pyelonephritis

Acute pyelonephritis is a multifocal infection of the kidneys, which can result from either hematogenous spread or from ascending infection from the bladder. Imaging is not necessary to establish the diagnosis but is important in detecting complications in patients who failed to improve with treatment. When imaging is warranted, CT is the modality of choice [15]. Non-enhanced CT may be useful for identifying urinary tract calculi, gas, hemorrhage, renal enlargement, and obstruction [15]. In the absence of these abnormalities, the CT may appear normal.

On IV contrast-enhanced CT, acute pyelonephritis appears as areas of decreased parenchymal enhancement, reflecting areas with diminished function due to vasospasm, tubular

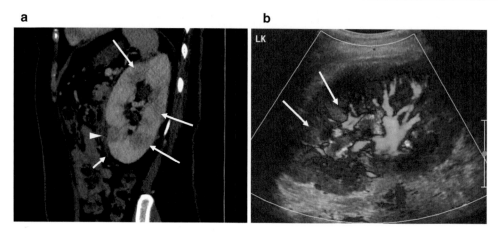

**Fig. 5** Acute pyelonephritis in a 47-year-old man with fever and flank pain. Sagittal post-contrast CT image (**a**) demonstrates geographic areas of decreased enhancement in the left kidney (long arrows). There are inflammatory changes in the perirenal fat (arrowhead) and thickening of the Gerota fascia (short arrow). Color Doppler US image of the left kidney (**b**) demonstrates geographic areas of decreased perfusion (arrows), equivalent to hypoenhancing areas seen on the CT

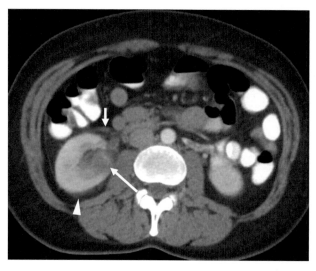

**Fig. 6** Acute pyelonephritis in a 39-year-old woman with history of IV drug use, presenting with sepsis. Axial post-contrast CT image demonstrates a rounded ill-defined area of decreased enhancement in the right kidney (the long arrow), with associated perinephric stranding (arrowhead) and thickening of Gerota fascia (short arrow). The history suggests hematogenous spread as the cause of acute pyelonephritis. The rounded appearance should not be mistaken for a neoplasm

obstruction, obstruction by inflammatory debris, or interstitial edema (Fig. 5) [14, 16]. The affected areas often alternate with areas of normal enhancement, resulting in a striated nephrogram [17]. Typically, the affected areas are wedge-shaped; however, hematogenous seeding of infection can result in rounded appearance of the affected areas, mimicking focal masses (Fig. 6) [15]. The corticomedullary phase is the most sensitive in detecting of acute pyelonephritis [16, 17]. Inflammatory changes result in thickening of the Gerota fascia, as well as in thickening and hyperenhancement of the urothelium of the renal sinuses (Fig. 5) [16].

US may appear normal in 75–80% of patients with acute pyelonephritis [15]. Positive findings of pyelonephritis on gray-scale US include renal enlargement, loss of renal sinus fat due to edema, heterogeneity of the parenchyma with decreased echogenicity due to edema, or increased echogenicity due to hemorrhage, loss of corticomedullary differentiation, and abscess formation [15]. Doppler interrogation demonstrates areas of hypoperfusion (Fig. 5) [15].

On MRI, parenchymal edema in acute pyelonephritis manifests as ill-defined areas of increased signal intensity on T2-weighted images, with or without decreased signal intensity on T1-weighted images. Decreased conspicuity of corticomedullary differentiation may be present [18]. The distribution of inflammatory foci is typically patchy with wedge-shaped areas radiating from the papilla to the cortical surface, with the renal parenchyma demonstrating a typical striated appearance due to interspersed areas of parenchyma spared, equivalent to the striated nephrogram sign. Similar to CT, areas of decreased enhancement can be seen on post-contrast T1-weighted images, reflecting parenchyma with diminished function (Fig. 7) [16]. Perirenal inflammatory changes on MRI manifest as streaks of increased signal on T2-weighted sequences and are most conspicuous with the application of fat saturation [16].

On diffusion-weighted imaging (DWI), the affected areas appear hyperintense, with the corresponding hypointensity on the apparent diffusion coefficient (ADC) map (Fig. 7) [19]. DWI is more sensitive for detection of acute pyelonephritis as compared to post-contrast imaging [19]. The use of DWI offers an accurate means of diagnosing acute pyelonephritis while avoiding the use of contrast media and radiation exposure [20, 21].

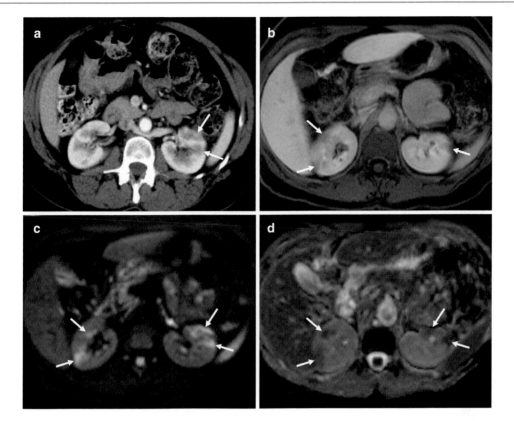

**Fig. 7** Acute pyelonephritis in a 63-year-old man presenting with fever and abdominal pain. Axial post-contrast CT image (**a**) demonstrates wedge-shaped areas of decreased enhancement extending to the cortex in the left kidney (arrows), consistent with acute pyelonephritis. MRI performed on the next day for evaluation of an incidental liver mass (not shown) demonstrates wedge-shaped areas of decreased enhancement in the kidneys bilaterally on the post-contrast T1-weighted sequence (arrows, **b**), similar to the CT. The affected areas demonstrate high signal intensity on diffusion-weighted image (DWI) (arrows, **c**), with corresponding hypointensity on the apparent diffusion coefficient (ADC) map (arrows, **d**). Note that the affected areas are most conspicuous on DWI and ADC map

## Renal Abscess

Renal abscess is a complication of acute pyelonephritis and should be suspected when appropriate therapy does not lead to clinical improvement. Patients with diabetes mellitus are predisposed to abscess formation, with approximately 75% of all renal abscesses occurring in this patient population [15]. Normal urine culture does not exclude a renal abscess, and normal urine culture is seen in 15–20% of patients with renal abscesses [15]. On CT, renal abscesses appear as rounded low-attenuation collections with a peripheral enhancing rim of variable thicknesses (Fig. 8). A halo of diminished enhancement may be seen around the abscess during the nephrographic phase, reflecting parenchymal edema (Fig. 8) [15].

On US, the typical abscess appears as a hypoechoic mass with an increased through transmission, internal debris, and lack of internal flow on color Doppler flow images (Fig. 9) [15].

On MRI, the signal intensity of the abscess cavity on T1- and T2-weighted sequences is variable, depending on the amount of internal debris and protein, but most commonly demonstrates low and high signal intensity, respectively [16]. The abscess cavity is usually surrounded by thick peripheral enhancing rim, and the surrounding parenchyma may be edematous (Fig. 9). Renal abscess often demonstrates restricted diffusion and should not be misinterpreted as malignancy [22].

## Emphysematous Cystitis and Pyelonephritis

Emphysematous pyelonephritis (EPN) is a severe necrotizing renal infection with mortality rates of 40–50% [23]. EPN is more common in women, and diabetes mellitus is a major risk factor, seen in 75–96% [24, 25]. EPN can also occur in the setting of urinary tract obstruction with superimposed infection [24, 25]. *Escherichia coli* and *Klebsiella pneumoniae* are the most common pathogens, although urine culture may be negative in about 20–35% [24, 25]. Patients present with fever, flank or abdominal pain, nausea, vomiting, change in mental status, and septic

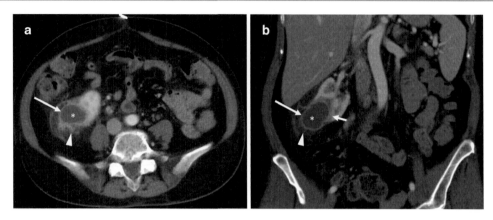

**Fig. 8** Renal abscess in a 68-year-old woman with history of pyelonephritis and persistent fever, despite antibiotics. Axial (**a**) and coronal (**b**) post-contrast CT images demonstrate a low-attenuation collection in the right kidney (*), with thick peripheral enhancing rim (long arrow) and perinephric inflammatory changes (arrowhead). Note a halo of diminished enhancement in the adjacent parenchyma (**b**, short arrow), reflecting parenchymal edema

**Fig. 9** Renal abscess in a 41-year-old man with bacteremia following heart transplant. Grayscale (**a**) and color Doppler (**b**) transverse US images demonstrate a mass in the left kidney (arrow) with heterogeneous echotexture, increased through transmission (arrowhead, **a**), and no internal flow (**b**). Axial post-contrast T1-weighted (**c**) and T2-weighted (**d**) images demonstrate a non-enhancing T-hyperintense abscess cavity (white arrowhead, **c** and **d**). The peripheral rim of the abscess (long arrow) enhances avidly (**c**) and demonstrates low signal intensity on the T2-weighted image (**d**). Note increased signal intensity in the adjacent parenchyma on T2-weighted image (black arrowhead, **d**) due to edema, as well as perinephric stranding (short arrow, **d**)

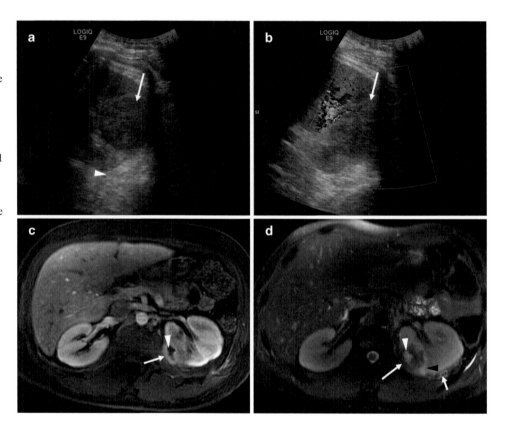

shock [24, 25]. CT has become the reference standard for diagnosis of EPN, and the classification system proposed by Huang and Tseng is commonly used for assessment of disease severity. According to this classification system, class 1 is characterized by the presence of gas in the collecting system only (emphysematous pyelitis) (Fig. 10); class 2 is characterized by gas in the renal parenchyma without extension to extrarenal space; class 3A is characterized by extension of gas or abscess to perinephric space; class 3B is characterized extension of gas or abscess to pararenal space; and class 4 is characterized by bilateral EPN or a solitary kidney with EPN (Fig. 11) [24]. Prognosis is the best for patients with class 1 EPN, where antibiotics and relief of obstruction, if present, may suffice [24]. Prognosis in patients with class 2 EPN is similar to class 1, but management requires percutaneous drainage along with antibiotics; nephrectomy is seldomly necessary [24]. Percutaneous drainage and antibiotics are successful in about 60% of class

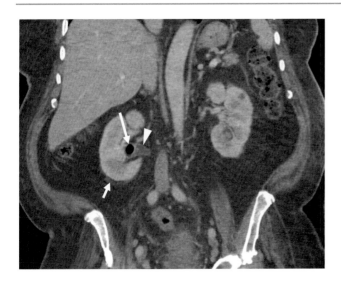

**Fig. 10** Class 1 EPN in a 76-year-old man with fever and back pain. Coronal post-contrast CT image demonstrates air within the collecting system (long arrow) without extension into the renal parenchyma, corresponding to class 1 EPN. Note hyperemia of the urothelium in the renal pelvis (arrowhead) and asymmetric perinephric stranding (short arrow)

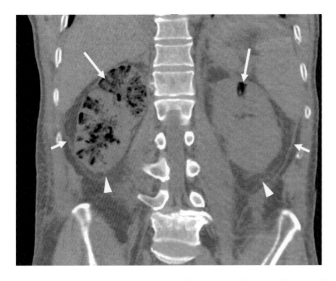

**Fig. 11** Class 4 EPN in a 60-year-old man with fever and signs of septic shock. Coronal non-contrast CT image demonstrates air (long arrows) in the renal parenchyma bilaterally, right greater than left, corresponding to class 4 EPN. Note bilateral perinephric stranding (arrowheads) and thickening of the lateral conal fascia (short arrows)

3 EPN; nephrectomy is required in a third of patients with class 3A EPN and in all patients with class 3B and 4 EPN [24, 25].

Emphysematous cystitis is analogous to EPN in that it is a urinary tract infection formed by gas-forming organisms. Contrary to EPN, emphysematous cystitis has a much better prognosis, with the mortality rate of 7%, where 90% of patients with emphysematous cystitis are successfully treated with antibiotics [26]. Prompt diagnosis and treatment is

necessary to prevent the potential morbidity and mortality [26]. Diabetes mellitus is the most common predisposing condition, seen in 67% of patients with emphysematous cystitis [26]. Clinically, emphysematous cystitis presents similar to uncomplicated cystitis, with symptoms of dysuria, hematuria, pelvic pain, and urinary urgency and frequency [27]. Pneumaturia can be a distinguishing symptom of emphysematous cystitis [27]. Concomitant emphysematous cystitis and pyelonephritis are rare [28].

On CT, emphysematous cystitis is diagnosed by the presence of foci of gas in the bladder wall, with or without the presence of intraluminal gas (Fig. 12). On US, hyperechoic foci with "dirty" shadowing are evident (Fig. 12).

## Renal Infarction

Patients with renal infarction present with acute flank pain, with or without hematuria [29]. Renal infarcts are typically caused by an embolic event, aortic dissection, trauma, or venous thrombosis [29]. Careful scrutiny of the renal vasculature is warranted to identify the area of vascular compromise (Fig. 13).

On CT, renal infarcts appear as focal wedge-shaped areas of decreased enhancement that involve both the cortex and medulla and extend to the capsular surface (Fig. 13) [29]. Occlusion of the main renal artery causes global infarction, where the entire kidney is nonperfused. Preserved capsular enhancement via collateral flow creates a peripheral rim of enhancement, known as the cortical rim sign, and may be seen in approximately half of the cases (Fig. 13) [29, 30].

While CT is usually the modality of choice when renal infarction is suspected, US may be performed in cases with indeterminate clinical presentation. On US, acute infarction appears as an absence of perfusion on color Doppler examination, patchy if segmental arteries are involved, or complete when infarction is global (Fig. 13). Doppler imaging may also reveal the absence of flow in the renal vasculature. IV contrast-enhanced ultrasound (CEUS) may be particularly useful for assessment of renal infarction. On CEUS, infarcts appear as wedge-shaped regions of nonperfusion.

MRI is not usually performed for the diagnosis of renal infarction. The findings on post-contrast T1-weighted sequences are similar to those of post-contrast CT (Fig. 13). The infarcted areas typically demonstrate high signal intensity on T2-weighted sequences due to parenchymal edema.

## Renal Hematoma

Renal hematomas may be intrarenal, subcapsular, or perirenal and are usually a result of a trauma or iatrogenic injury [31]. Spontaneous renal hematomas in the absence of trauma

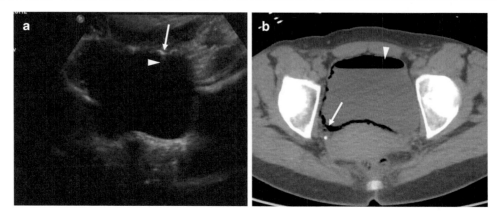

**Fig. 12** Emphysematous cystitis in a 56-year-old woman with a history of diabetes, presenting with abdominal pain and vomiting. Gray-scale US transverse image through the bladder (**a**) demonstrates hyperechoic foci in the bladder wall (arrow) with posterior urinary shadowing (arrowhead), consistent with foci of gas. Axial non-contrast CT (**b**) image demonstrates gas within the bladder wall (arrow) and in the lumen (arrowhead)

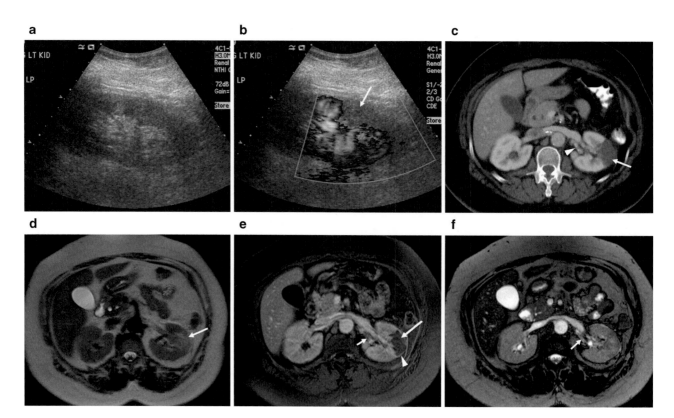

**Fig. 13** Acute renal infarct in a 69-year-old woman presenting with back pain and vomiting. Gray-scale sagittal US image through the left kidney (**a**) demonstrates no abnormalities. Color Doppler US image (**b**) demonstrates a wedge-shaped area of hypoperfusion (arrow). Axial post-contrast CT image (**c**) demonstrates a large wedge-shaped area of decreased enhancement (arrow) in the left kidney. The visualized branch of the left renal artery (arrowhead) demonstrates calcifications; the luminal patency is difficult to assess. The area of infarct demonstrates increased signal intensity on a T2-weighted MR image (arrow, **d**) due to parenchymal edema. On a post-contrast T1-weighted MR image (**e**), the area of infarct demonstrates no enhancement (long arrow). Note the preserved enhancement of the overlying renal capsule (arrowhead, **e**), resulting in a cortical rim sign. There is lack of enhancement in the left renal arterial branch (short arrow, **e**) with a corresponding signal void on balanced gradient echo image (arrow, **f**), confirming arterial occlusion

are rare. Renal tumors, benign or malignant, are the most common cause of spontaneous renal hemorrhage, accounting for 50–65% [32, 33]. Following renal masses, vascular disease is the next most common cause of spontaneous perirenal hemorrhage, accounting for approximately 17% of cases, with the polyarteritis nodosa being the most frequent etiology [33]. Spontaneous renal hematomas may present with acute flank pain, tenderness, and symptoms of internal bleeding

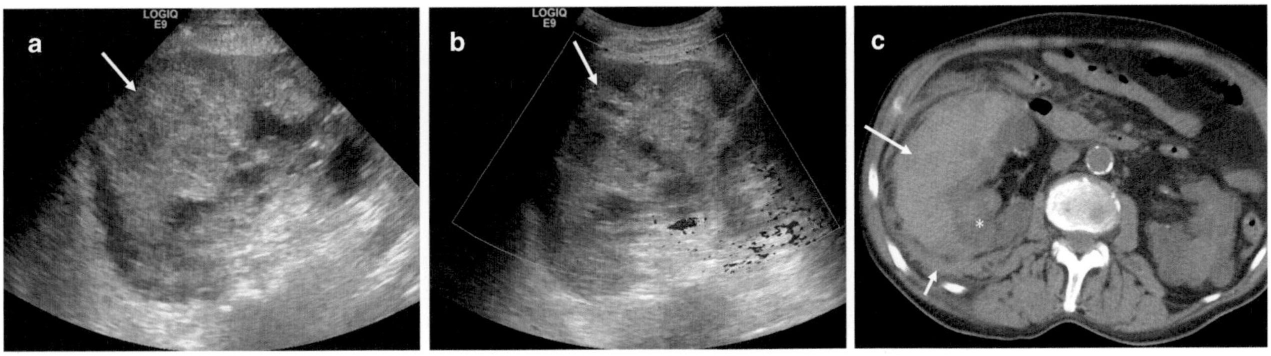

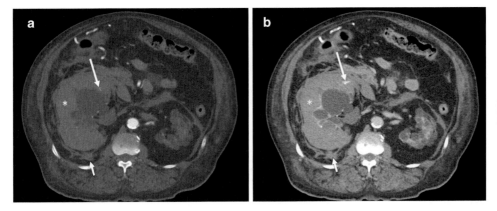

**Fig. 14** Subcapsular renal hematoma in a 78-year-old man with end-stage renal disease, presenting with hypovolemic shock. Grayscale US image through the right kidney (**a**) demonstrates a large heterogeneous hyperechoic subcapsular collection (arrow) with no internal flow on color Doppler US (**b**). Axial non-contrast CT image (**c**) demonstrates a uniformly hyperdense subcapsular hematoma (long arrow), exerting mass effect on the right kidney (*). Hyperdense streaks are seen in the perirenal space (short arrow), consistent with perirenal component of hematoma

**Fig. 15** Subcapsular renal hematoma with active bleeding in a 60-year-old woman presenting with abdominal pain and distention. Axial CT images in the arterial phase (**a**) and portal venous phase (**b**) demonstrate a large right subcapsular hematoma (*) and small amount of hemorrhage in the perirenal space (short arrow). There is contrast extravasation in the hematoma (long arrow), which changes shape and becomes larger on the portal venous phase

("Lenk's triad"), but the symptoms may be nonspecific and may mimic other acute intra-abdominal conditions [34].

Subcapsular hematoma appears as a crescentic collection along the renal border, often with mass effect on the adjacent parenchyma (Fig. 14). On US, hemorrhage appears as heterogeneous collection of variable echogenicity (Fig. 14). On CT, hyperacute hemorrhage has attenuation values of 30–45 Hounsfield units (HU), and the attenuation increases to 70–80 HU in the acute state due to the high concentration of hemoglobin [35]. Perirenal hematoma appears as streaks and/or collections in perirenal space, with imaging characteristics of hemorrhage. If IV contrast is administered, images should be scrutinized to identify areas of active bleeding (Fig. 15). On MRI, the signal intensity on T1- and T2-weighted sequences is variable, depending on the stage of the hemorrhage. Increased signal intensity on T1-weighted sequences indicates subacute blood. Following administration of IV contrast on either CT or MRI, areas of hemorrhage demonstrate no enhancement. In cases with increased signal intensity on pre-contrast T1-weighted images, subtraction images are required to assess the presence of enhancement (Fig. 16).

Since an underlying renal mass is the most common cause of spontaneous renal and perirenal hemorrhage, imaging is crucial for assessment of the underlying cause. While both US and CT are nearly 100% sensitive for detection of hematoma, sensitivity and specificity for determining the underlying cause on CT are 57% and 82%, respectively, and 11% and 33% on US, respectively [33]. MRI may offer an advantage for detecting a small underlying mass [34].

## Adrenal Hemorrhage

Adrenal hemorrhage is most commonly caused by non-traumatic causes, as the deep location of the adrenals is protective against damage in trauma [36]. Nontraumatic adrenal hemorrhage can be caused by stress, bleeding disorders,

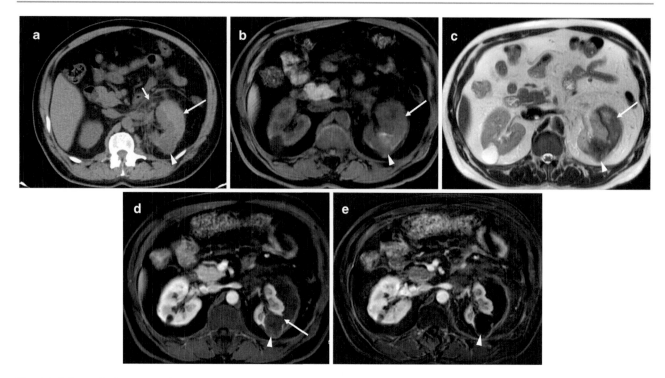

**Fig. 16** Subcapsular hematoma due to a ruptured hemorrhagic renal cyst in a 52-year-old man presenting with acute flank pain. Axial non-contrast CT images (**a**) demonstrate a uniformly hyperdense subcapsular hematoma (long arrow), a small amount of perirenal hemorrhage (short arrow), and an indeterminant contour-deforming mass (arrowhead). Axial pre-contrast T1-weighted (**b**) and T2-weighted (**c**) MR images demonstrate the subcapsular hematoma to have intermediate (arrow, **b**) and low (arrow, **c**) signal intensity, respectively, consistent with acute blood products. The left renal mass (arrowhead) demonstrates intermediate to high signal intensity on the pre-contrast T1-weighted MR image (**b**) and low signal intensity on T2-weighted MR image (**c**), indicating internal acute and subacute blood products. Disruption of the left lateral wall (arrow, **d**) is evident on post-contrast T1-weighted image (**d**). A subtraction image (**e**) confirms lack of internal enhancement within this hemorrhagic cyst

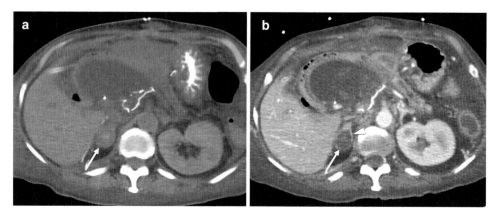

**Fig. 17** Adrenal hemorrhage in the 59-year-old woman with postoperative hypovolemic shock. Axial non-contrast CT image (**a**) demonstrates an oval mass in the right adrenal (arrow) with heterogeneously high attenuation, consistent with an adrenal hemorrhage. Axial post-contrast CT image (**b**) demonstrates no enhancement in the hematoma (arrow) and enhancement in the preserved peripheral adrenal tissue (arrowhead)

iatrogenic causes, or an underlying mass [37]. Patients present with acute abdominal or flank pain, fever, nausea, vomiting, and mental status changes [37]. Because these signs and symptoms are nonspecific, adrenal hemorrhage is often not suspected clinically and is discovered on an imaging examination performed for another indication [37].

On US, an acute adrenal hematoma may appear solid, heterogeneous, and of variable echogenicity [35]. As the hematoma evolves and liquefies, heterogeneity increases [35].

On CT, adrenal hemorrhage appears as a round or oval mass (Fig. 17), often associated with periadrenal fat stranding

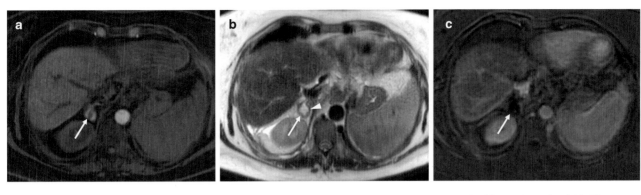

**Fig. 18** Hemorrhagic adrenal infarction in a 53-year-old woman following orthotopic liver transplant. Axial T1-weighted (**a**) and T2-weighted (**b**) MR images demonstrate a rounded process (arrow) in the right adrenal with high signal intensity on both sequences, with a low signal intensity rim on T2-weighted image (arrowhead, **b**). The process is new from pretransplant imaging (not shown). Subtraction image (**c**) shows no enhancement (arrow), confirming diagnosis of a hemorrhagic infarction

**Fig. 19** Nonhemorrhagic adrenal infarcts in an 84-year-old man presenting with sepsis. Axial post-contrast CT image (**a**) demonstrates enlarged hypoenhancing adrenals (arrows) with surrounding stranding (arrowheads). The findings are new from CT 3 months prior (**b**), at which point the adrenals were not enlarged (arrows), and there was no adjacent fat infiltration

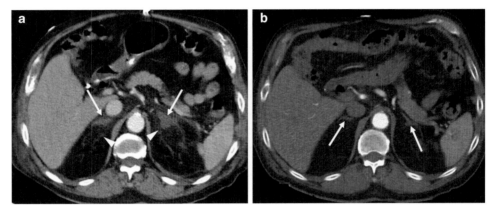

and poorly defined adrenal margins [38]. On non-contrast CT, hyperacute hemorrhage has attenuation similar to the blood pool; as blood evolves to acute stage, the attenuation increases, both of the hemorrhage itself and of the periadrenal fat stranding [35, 39]. On IV contrast-enhanced CT, peripheral enhancement may be seen due to preserved normal adrenal tissue (Fig. 17) [39].

## Adrenal Infarction

Patients with adrenal infarction may present with acute chest, back, and upper abdominal pain and signs of adrenal insufficiency, including hypoglycemia, hyponatremia, and hyperkalemia [40, 41]. Prompt diagnosis of adrenal infarction is essential for preservation of adrenal vitality and function [41]. Hemorrhagic adrenal infarctions can be life-threatening due to acute primary adrenal insufficiency [36]. Hemorrhagic infarction in the right adrenal is a known complication of orthotopic liver transplantation and should not be mistaken for an adrenal metastasis or a postoperative abscess (Fig. 18)

[42]. Right adrenal infarction is a result of the ligation and division of the right adrenal vein during recipient hepatectomy [43].

Nonhemorrhagic adrenal infarction is less common than hemorrhagic infarction. In approximately 70% of patients, nonhemorrhagic adrenal infarction is associated with thrombosis of the adrenal vein, leading to ischemia and parenchymal necrosis [44]. Thrombotic conditions predispose the patient to develop microvascular thrombosis, which then leads to ischemia of the adrenal parenchyma [40]. Additionally, nonhemorrhagic adrenal infarctions can occur in patients with shock, terminal hypotension, disseminated intravascular coagulation, and pregnancy [40, 44].

On CT, a hemorrhagic adrenal infarction has a typical appearance of blood. A nonhemorrhagic adrenal infarct appears as a diffusely enlarged and hypoenhancing adrenal, with associated stranding and fluid (Fig. 19) [40, 41]. A high index of suspicion is needed, based on appropriate provided history to suggest this diagnosis. A "capsular sign," defined as a subtle peripheral line of hyperenhancement around a hypoenhancing adrenal, can be seen in 83% [41].

## Adrenal Infections

Adrenal infections rarely lead to insufficiency, as more than 90% of the gland must be affected for the insufficiency to ensue [45, 46]. Infection of the adrenals is relatively uncommon, but adrenals may be involved in the setting of the disseminated viral infection, so-called adrenalitis. On cross-sectional imaging, adrenal infection is seen as a thickened adrenal with surrounding edema [46]. However, the appearance on cross-sectional imaging is not specific.

Fungal infections of the adrenals typically present with bilateral adrenal thickening. However, the symptoms and imaging findings are nonspecific, and definitive diagnosis requires biopsy [46]. *Histoplasma capsulatum* (histoplasmosis) can affect the adrenals and can be seen in immunocompromised patients, in organ transplant recipients, and in the elderly [46].

Pyogenic infections and bacterial sepsis may lead to Waterhouse–Friderichsen syndrome: bilateral adrenal hemorrhage with subsequent acute adrenal insufficiency [47]. Adrenal abscesses are very uncommon in adults [48].

The adrenals are among the most common extrapulmonary sites *of Mycobacterium tuberculosis* (TB) infection. Up to 6% of patients with active TB have adrenal involvement on pathology, and in some the adrenal may be the only site of infection [45]. On cross-sectional imaging, active TB infection appears as diffuse enlargement of the affected gland.

## References

1. Uyeda JW, Gans BS, Sodickson A. Imaging of acute and emergent genitourinary conditions: what the radiologist needs to know. AJR Am J Roentgenol. 2015;204(6):W631–9.
2. Scales CD Jr, Smith AC, Hanley JM, Saigal CS. Prevalence of kidney stones in the United States. Eur Urol. 2012;62(1):160–5.
3. Soucie JM, Thun MJ, Coates RJ, McClellan W, Austin H. Demographic and geographic variability of kidney stones in the United States. Kidney Int. 1994;46(3):893–9.
4. Dalrymple NC, Verga M, Anderson KR, Bove P, Covey AM, Rosenfield AT, et al. The value of unenhanced helical computerized tomography in the management of acute flank pain. J Urol. 1998;159(3):735–40.
5. Vieweg J, Teh C, Freed K, Leder RA, Smith RH, Nelson RH, et al. Unenhanced helical computerized tomography for the evaluation of patients with acute flank pain. J Urol. 1998;160(3 Pt 1):679–84.
6. Viprakasit DP, Sawyer MD, Herrell SD, Miller NL. Limitations of ultrasonography in the evaluation of urolithiasis: a correlation with computed tomography. J Endourol. 2012;26(3):209–13.
7. Weinrich JM, Bannas P, Regier M, Keller S, Kluth L, Adam G, et al. Low-dose CT for evaluation of suspected urolithiasis: diagnostic yield for assessment of alternative diagnoses. AJR Am J Roentgenol. 2018;210(3):557–63.
8. Kambadakone AR, Eisner BH, Catalano OA, Sahani DV. New and evolving concepts in the imaging and management of urolithiasis: urologists' perspective. Radiographics. 2010;30(3):603–23.
9. Ege G, Akman H, Kuzucu K, Yildiz S. Acute ureterolithiasis: incidence of secondary signs on unenhanced helical CT and influence on patient management. Clin Radiol. 2003;58(12):990–4.
10. Moak JH, Lyons MS, Lindsell CJ. Bedside renal ultrasound in the evaluation of suspected ureterolithiasis. Am J Emerg Med. 2012;30(1):218–21.
11. Dym RJ, Duncan DR, Spektor M, Cohen HW, Scheinfeld MH. Renal stones on portal venous phase contrast-enhanced CT: does intravenous contrast interfere with detection? Abdom Imaging. 2014;39(3):526–32.
12. Gershman B, Kulkarni N, Sahani DV, Eisner BH. Causes of renal forniceal rupture. BJU Int. 2011;108(11):1909–11. discussion 12
13. Hsiao CY, Chen TH, Lee YC, Hsiao MC, Hung PH, Chen YY, et al. Urolithiasis is a risk factor for urosepstic shock and acute kidney injury in patients with urinary tract infection. Front Med. 2019;6:288.
14. Nicola R, Menias CO. Urinary obstruction, stone disease, and infection. In: Hodler J, Kubik-Huch RA, von Schulthess GK, editors. Diseases of the abdomen and pelvis 2018–2021: Diagnostic imaging – IDKD Book. Cham: Springer; 2018. p. 223–8.
15. Craig WD, Wagner BJ, Travis MD. Pyelonephritis: radiologic-pathologic review. Radiographics. 2008;28(1):255–77. quiz 327-8
16. Cruz J, Figueiredo F, Matos AP, Duarte S, Guerra A, Ramalho M. Infectious and inflammatory diseases of the urinary tract: role of MR imaging. Magn Resonance Imaging Clin N Am. 2019;27(1):59–75.
17. Kawashima A, Sandler CM, Goldman SM, Raval BK, Fishman EK. CT of renal inflammatory disease. Radiographics. 1997;17(4):851–66. discussion 67-8
18. Martina MC, Campanino PP, Caraffo F, Marcuccio C, Gunetti F, Colla L, et al. Dynamic magnetic resonance imaging in acute pyelonephritis. La Radiologia Medica. 2010;115(2):287–300.
19. Faletti R, Cassinis MC, Fonio P, Grasso A, Battisti G, Bergamasco L, et al. Diffusion-weighted imaging and apparent diffusion coefficient values versus contrast-enhanced MR imaging in the identification and characterisation of acute pyelonephritis. Eur Radiol. 2013;23(12):3501–8.
20. Bosakova A, Salounova D, Havelka J, Kraft O, Sirucek P, Kocvara R, et al. Diffusion-weighted magnetic resonance imaging is more sensitive than dimercaptosuccinic acid scintigraphy in detecting parenchymal lesions in children with acute pyelonephritis: a prospective study. J Pediatr Urol. 2018;14(3) 269.e1-.e7
21. Aoyagi J, Kanai T, Odaka J, Ito T, Saito T, Betsui H, et al. Non-enhanced magnetic resonance imaging versus renal scintigraphy in acute pyelonephritis. Pediatr Int. 2018;60(2):200–3.
22. Goyal A, Sharma R, Bhalla AS, Gamanagatti S, Seth A. Diffusion-weighted MRI in inflammatory renal lesions: all that glitters is not RCC! Eur Radiol. 2013;23(1):272–9.
23. Dutta P, Bhansali A, Singh SK, Gupta KL, Bhat MH, Masoodi SR, et al. Presentation and outcome of emphysematous renal tract disease in patients with diabetes mellitus. Urol Int. 2007;78(1):13–22.
24. Huang JJ, Tseng CC. Emphysematous pyelonephritis: clinicoradiological classification, management, prognosis, and pathogenesis. Arch Intern Med. 2000;160(6):797–805.
25. Elawdy MM, Osman Y, Abouelkheir RT, El-Halwagy S, Awad B, El-Mekresh M. Emphysematous pyelonephritis treatment strategies in correlation to the CT classification: have the current experience and prognosis changed? Int Urol Nephrol. 2019;51(10):1709–13.
26. Thomas AA, Lane BR, Thomas AZ, Remer EM, Campbell SC, Shoskes DA. Emphysematous cystitis: a review of 135 cases. BJU Int. 2007;100(1):17–20.
27. Eken A, Alma E. Emphysematous cystitis: the role of CT imaging and appropriate treatment. Can Urol Assoc J. 2013;7(11–12):E754–6.
28. Li S, Wang J, Hu J, He L, Wang C. Emphysematous pyelonephritis and cystitis: a case report and literature review. J Int Med Res. 2018;46(7):2954–60.
29. Urban BA, Fishman EK. Tailored helical CT evaluation of acute abdomen. Radiographics. 2000;20(3):725–49.

30. Kawashima A, Sandler CM, Ernst RD, Tamm EP, Goldman SM, Fishman EK. CT evaluation of renovascular disease. Radiographics. 2000;20(5):1321–40.

31. Schaner EG, Balow JE, Doppman JL. Computed tomography in the diagnosis of subcapsular and perirenal hematoma. AJR Am J Roentgenol. 1977;129(1):83–8.

32. Bosniak MA. Spontaneous subcapsular and perirenal hematomas. Radiology. 1989;172(3):601–2.

33. Zhang JQ, Fielding JR, Zou KH. Etiology of spontaneous perirenal hemorrhage: a meta-analysis. J Urol. 2002;167(4):1593–6.

34. Baishya RK, Dhawan DR, Sabnis RB, Desai MR. Spontaneous subcapsular renal hematoma: a case report and review of literature. Urol Ann. 2011;3(1):44–6.

35. Hammond NA, Lostumbo A, Adam SZ, Remer EM, Nikolaidis P, Yaghmai V, et al. Imaging of adrenal and renal hemorrhage. Abdom Imaging. 2015;

36. Chernyak V, Patlas MN, Menias CO, Soto JA, Kielar AZ, Rozenblit AM, et al. Traumatic and non-traumatic adrenal emergencies. Emerg Radiol. 2015;22(6):697–704.

37. Simon DR, Palese MA. Clinical update on the management of adrenal hemorrhage. Curr Urol Rep. 2009;10(1):78–83.

38. Burks DW, Mirvis SE, Shanmuganathan K. Acute adrenal injury after blunt abdominal trauma: CT findings. AJR Am J Roentgenol. 1992;158(3):503–7.

39. Jordan E, Poder L, Courtier J, Sai V, Jung A, Coakley FV. Imaging of nontraumatic adrenal hemorrhage. AJR Am J Roentgenol. 2012;199(1):W91–8.

40. Michiels JJ, Berneman Z, Schroyens W, Krestin GP. Bilateral adrenal swelling as a cause of chest, back, and upper abdominal pain in essential thrombocythemia and polycythemia vera is due to microvascular ischemic thrombosis rather than to hemorrhage. Ann Hematol. 2002;81(12):691–4.

41. Moschetta M, Telegrafo M, Pignatelli A, Stabile Ianora AA, Angelelli G. Value of the CT "capsular sign" as a potential indicator of acute adrenal ischemia. Emerg Radiol. 2015;

42. Boraschi P, Donati F. Complications of orthotopic liver transplantation: imaging findings. Abdom Imag. 2004;29(2):189–202.

43. Bowen AD, Keslar PJ, Newman B, Hashida Y. Adrenal hemorrhage after liver transplantation. Radiology. 1990;176(1):85–8.

44. Fox B. Venous infarction of the adrenal glands. J Pathol. 1976;119(2):65–89.

45. Lam KY, Lo CY. A critical examination of adrenal tuberculosis and a 28-year autopsy experience of active tuberculosis. Clin Endocrinol. 2001;54(5):633–9.

46. Upadhyay J, Sudhindra P, Abraham G, Trivedi N. Tuberculosis of the adrenal gland: a case report and review of the literature of infections of the adrenal gland. Int J Endocrinol. 2014;2014:876037.

47. Tormos LM, Schandl CA. The significance of adrenal hemorrhage: undiagnosed Waterhouse-Friderichsen syndrome, a case series. J Forensic Sci. 2013;58(4):1071–4.

48. Joshi P, Lele V. FDG PET/CT findings in a case of nontuberculous abscess of adrenal gland. Clin Nucl Med. 2014;39(1):57–8.

# Imaging of Pelvic Emergencies

Victoria Chernyak

## Contents

### Abstract

Various nontraumatic emergent conditions occur in the pelvis. As with acute conditions in other organs, timely and accurate diagnosis helps to ensure prompt and optimized treatment and contributes to optimal clinical outcome. This chapter summarizes the imaging findings on US, CT, and MRI in various emergent conditions in the pelvis, including those affecting men, women, and pregnant women specifically.

### Keywords

Non-traumatic pelvic emergencies · Non-traumatic emergencies of lower male GU track · Non-traumatic emergencies of lower female GU track

V. Chernyak (✉)
Beth Israel Deaconess Medical Center, Boston, MA, USA
e-mail: vchernya@bidmc.harvard.edu

## Pregnancy-Related Emergent Conditions

### Ectopic Pregnancy

Ectopic pregnancy, defined as an implantation of a fertilized ovum outside of the endometrial cavity, occurs in 1–2% of all pregnancies [1]. The incidence of ectopic pregnancy is increasing due to an increasing prevalence of assisted reproductive technology [1]. The fallopian tube is the most common site, accounting for at least 95% of all ectopic pregnancies [2, 3].

Transvaginal ultrasonography (US) is the imaging modality of choice for the diagnosis of ectopic pregnancy. In the setting of a positive hCG and acute pelvic pain and/or vaginal bleeding, transvaginal US has a sensitivity of 87%, a specificity of 94%, and a positive predictive value of 92% for the diagnosis of ectopic pregnancy [4].

In patients with an inconclusive US, MRI can be a valuable problem-solving tool, as it can accurately localize the extrauterine gestational sac in 93–100% [5]. Accurate detection of the sac location can help to guide management in surgical candidates, as well as in candidates for conservative treatment [2, 6]. Due to its longer acquisition time and relatively limited availability, MRI is reserved only for hemodynamically stable patients.

CT is not usually employed in the assessment of ectopic pregnancy due to use of ionizing radiation, particularly since US and MRI offer accurate radiation-free diagnostic options. However, CT may be inadvertently performed in a symptomatic pregnant patient if the screening was not performed.

## Hemoperitoneum

Isolated hemoperitoneum in a patient with positive hCG has an 86–93% positive predictive value for the diagnosis of ectopic pregnancy [2]. Hemoperitoneum is not pathognomonic for ectopic pregnancy, as it can be seen in patients with placenta accreta, rupture of a hemorrhagic cyst, or a spontaneous abortion [7]. On US, hemoperitoneum appears as complex pelvic fluid with internal echoes (Fig. 1). On CT, acute hemoperitoneum demonstrates attenuation values of 50–80 HU (Fig. 2). On MRI, the signal intensity of hemoperitoneum is variable, depending on the stage of blood. Hyperacute blood, occurring within hours of bleeding, appears as intermediate signal intensity on T1-weighted sequences and high signal intensity on T2-weighted sequences [8]. Acute blood, hours to 3 days after the initial event, appears as intermediate signal intensity on T1-weighted sequences and low signal intensity on T2-weighted sequences [8]. High signal intensity on T1-weighted sequences is the hallmark of subacute blood; in early subacute stage (3–7 days), the signal intensity on T2-weighted sequences is low, and it progresses to high signal intensity in the late subacute stage (1 week–months) [8].

A pseudogestational sac, which appears as thickened decidua with an irregular fluid collection within the endometrial cavity on sonography or MRI, may be present in about 20% of ectopic pregnancies. A pseudogestational sac should be distinguished from a normal gestational sac, which is typically round, eccentric in location, and may contain a visible embryo [9, 10]. Since a yolk sack is not routinely seen on MRI, its absence cannot be used to differentiate between a pseudogestational sac and a true gestational sac [9].

## Tubal Ectopic

As stated above, the fallopian tube is the most common site of ectopic implantation, and in the vast majority, the ampulla is involved [3]. When a fertilized egg implants in a fallopian tube, trophoblasts invade the wall of the fallopian tube, leading to formation of hematosalpinx. In the setting of positive hCG without an intrauterine gestation, unilateral hematosalpinx is concerning for an ectopic pregnancy, even when an extrauterine gestation sac is not demonstrated [7]. Hematosalpinx appears as a distended tubular structure with imaging characteristic of hemorrhage on all modalities [11].

A non-cystic adnexal mass with a peripheral hyperechoic rim and a "ring of fire" appearance on Doppler sonography has a sensitivity of 84%, specificity of 99%, and a positive predictive value of 96% for the diagnosis of tubal ectopic on US [3]. Applying external pressure over the ovary and observing the adnexal mass moving separately from the ovary ensures that the observed abnormality is distinct from the ovary and therefore is not a corpus luteum. When the ectopic gestational sac is detected, its dimensions, the

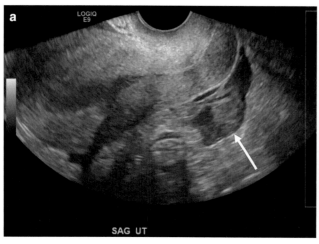
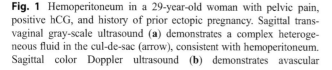
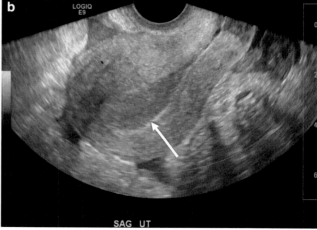

**Fig. 1** Hemoperitoneum in a 29-year-old woman with pelvic pain, positive hCG, and history of prior ectopic pregnancy. Sagittal transvaginal gray-scale ultrasound (**a**) demonstrates a complex heterogeneous fluid in the cul-de-sac (arrow), consistent with hemoperitoneum. Sagittal color Doppler ultrasound (**b**) demonstrates avascular heterogeneous material in the endometrial cavity (arrow), compatible with blood products, without an intrauterine gestational sac. No ectopic gestational sac was discerned elsewhere. Left tubal ectopic pregnancy was confirmed by pathology

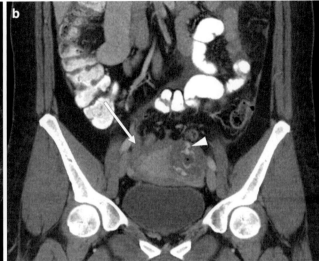

**Fig. 2** Ruptured interstitial ectopic pregnancy in a 34-year-old woman with severe pelvic pain. Axial (**a**) and coronal (**b**) post-contrast CT images demonstrate an eccentrically located gestational sac, centered at the interstitial portion of the left fallopian tube (*). There is disruption of the wall of the gestational sac (short arrow), with areas of active contrast extravasation (arrowhead). A hyperdense lobulated collection in the pelvis (long arrow) represents hemoperitoneum

presence of an embryo, and the presence of an embryonic heartbeat should be described, as these factors affect selection for conservative management with methotrexate (Fig. 3) [3].

## Ovarian Ectopic

Ovarian ectopic pregnancy is rare, constituting approximately 3% of all ectopic pregnancies. On imaging, an ovarian ectopic is seen as a gestational saclike structure within the ovary, often with internal blood products [2]. Since other hemorrhagic ovarian cysts/masses, such as corpus luteal cyst or endometrioma, are much more common than an ovarian ectopic, establishing the diagnosis may be challenging [2]. Visualization of a clear yolk sac or an embryo within the ovary improves the confidence of the diagnosis prospectively, but the definitive diagnosis can only be established by surgery [2, 12].

## Cervical Ectopic

A cervical ectopic is a result of a pregnancy implantation inferior to the internal cervical os [2]. Cervical ectopic pregnancies are rare, occurring in 1 in 4500 pregnancies [13]. The imaging characteristic is an hourglass shape of the uterus with an empty endometrial cavity superiorly and expansion of the cervix by the gestational sac (Fig. 4) [13]. Cervical ectopic appears as a poorly defined cervical mass with internal hemorrhagic contents [14]. If contrast is administered for CT or MRI, the mass typically demonstrates avid irregular enhancement peripherally, often with enhancing papillary solid components [14].

US can be used to distinguish between a cervical ectopic pregnancy and an incomplete abortion – during the real-time US assessment, progression of the gestational sac through the cervical canal can be observed in the latter. An accurate distinction between these two entities is important for appropriate management, since dilatation and curettage, a standard treatment for an incomplete abortion, may lead to severe and potentially life-threatening hemorrhage if performed in a patient with cervical ectopic [6]. MRI can help in assessment of inconclusive cases and can accurately evaluate for complications of cervical ectopic, including the presence and the extent of placental invasion beyond the cervix and involvement of the bladder wall [6, 15].

## Cesarean Section Scar Ectopic

Cesarean section scar ectopic occurs in <0.1% of all pregnancies [16]. The risk of cesarean ectopic is approximately 6% in patients with prior cesarean delivery [17]. A diagnosis of cesarean section scar pregnancy is made when a gestational sac is located in the lower uterine segment, anterior to the endometrial stripe, with <5 mm of overlying myometrium [18]. MRI is the preferred imaging modality for detailed assessment of cesarean section scar ectopic due to its superior soft-tissue resolution. MRI reveals a cesarean scar defect in 86% of cases and shows the associated protrusion of a low-lying gestational sac through the defect [19]. MRI can accurately depict the thickness of the myometrium between the gestational sac and the bladder, which helps determine eligibility for conservative treatment with methotrexate, where the myometrial thickness <2 mm between the gestational sac and the bladder is an indication for methotrexate therapy [20]. Additionally, conservative medical treatment is appropriate for hemodynamically stable patients with a gestational sac of l < 8 weeks of gestation and no evidence of a rupture [20].

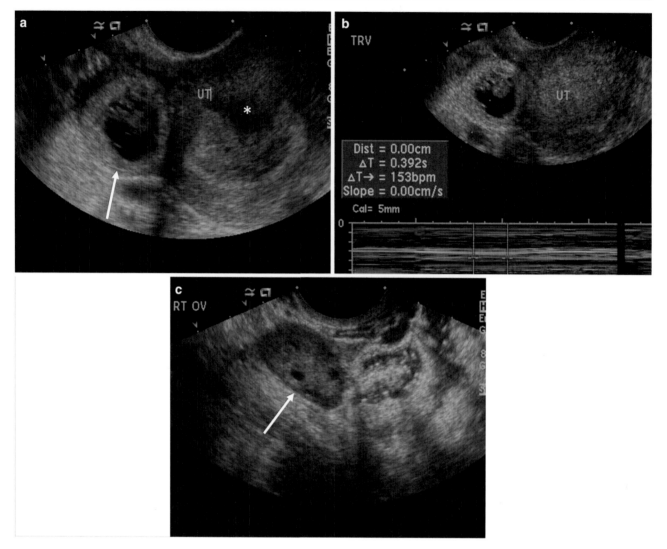

**Fig. 3** Live tubal ectopic pregnancy in a 29-year-old woman presenting with cramps and vaginal bleeding. Transverse gray-scale ultrasound (**a**) demonstrates a gestational sac (arrow) to the right of the uterus (*). No intrauterine gestation sac is seen. A fetal heart rate is detected (**b**). The right ovary (arrow, **c**) is seen separately

## Interstitial Ectopic

Interstitial pregnancy, defined as an implantation of the gestational sac in the intramyometrial segment of the fallopian tube, accounts for 2%–4% of all ectopic pregnancies [21]. Due to relatively high distensibility of this segment of the fallopian tube, interstitial pregnancies may be seen as late as the 16th week of gestation [21]. Due to proximity of the uterine artery to the fallopian tube, rupture of an interstitial pregnancy can result in life-threatening hemorrhage [21].

On imaging, an interstitial pregnancy is seen an eccentrically located gestational sac with the overlying myometrial layer measuring <5 mm (Fig. 5) [21]. On US, the presence of an interstitial line sign, defined as a hyperechoic line between the endometrium of the uterine horn and the eccentrically located gestational sac, is 80% sensitive and 98% specific for the diagnosis of an interstitial pregnancy [22].

## Retained Products of Conception

Retained products of conception (RPOC) are defined as the presence of any fetal or placental tissue within the endometrial cavity after miscarriage, termination of pregnancy, or preterm/term delivery. Patients with RPOC typically present with bleeding and pelvic pain following one of the above scenarios.

On US, an echogenic or heterogeneous process within the endometrium is the most sensitive sign of RPOC, seen in nearly 80% of patients (Fig. 6) [23]. Complex endometrial fluid can be seen in almost 30%, and endometrial thickening >10 mm is seen in 7% [23]. Lack of any of the aforementioned findings has a negative predictive value of 100% for RPOC [23].

On CT, RPOC appear as diffuse thickening of the endometrium (Fig. 6). On MRI, RPOC are seen as an endometrial

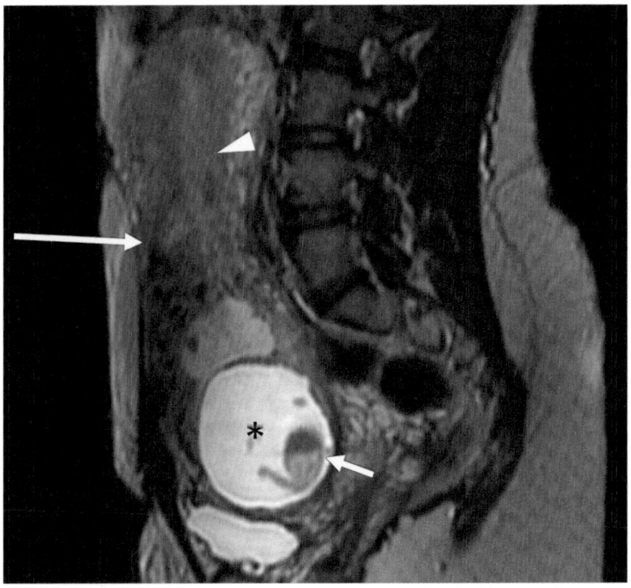

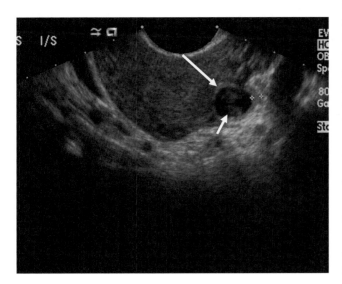

**Fig. 4** Cervical ectopic pregnancy in a 27-year-old woman. Sagittal T2-weighted MR image demonstrates a gestational sac in the cervix (*). There is an embryo (short arrow) in the sac. Note an hourglass shape of the uterus (long arrow) with an empty endometrium superiorly (arrowhead). MRI was performed prior to surgical planning

**Fig. 5** Interstitial ectopic pregnancy in a 29-year-old woman with pelvic pain and vaginal bleeding. Transverse gray-scale ultrasound image demonstrates an eccentrically located gestational sac (long arrow) with an internal embryo (short arrow). The overlying myometrium measures 3 mm (calipers)

mass with heterogeneous signal intensity on both T1-weighted and T2-weighted sequences, with variable degree of heterogeneous enhancement (Fig. 7) [24, 25].

Imaging characteristics of the gestational trophoblastic disease and RPOC overlap, making the distinction potentially difficult. However, accurate differentiation between RPOC and gestational trophoblastic disease is important, as these entities require different management options [25]. One distinguishing feature is the location of the abnormality: while gestational trophoblastic disease is predominantly intramural in location, RPOC are confined to the endometrial cavity [26].

## Uterine Scar Dehiscence and Rupture

Approximately one-third of live births in the United States are delivered via cesarean section, with an overall postoperative complication rate of 36% [27, 28]. Although rare, uterine scar dehiscence and rupture are well-documented complications, with an estimate rate of occurrence of 0.2 to 4.3%, with prior cesarean section being the greatest risk factor [29]. Cesarean scar dehiscence is defined as disruption of the endometrium and myometrium with an intact overlying serosal layer. In the cesarean scar rupture, there is complete disruption of all three uterine layers, including the serosa. Symptoms are nonspecific and can include dysmenorrhea, dyspareunia, or abdominal pain [30].

IV contrast-enhanced CT is not accurate for diagnosing cesarean scar dehiscence and rupture due to overlap in appearance with the normal postoperative appearance of the uterus on CT, where fluid within the scar or edema of the adjacent myometrium can mimic discontinuity of the myometrium on CT (Fig. 8) [31]. MRI is more accurate for the identification of areas of discontinuity in the endometrium, myometrium, and serosa (Fig. 9) [30]. In cases of partial dehiscence, the minimum wall thickness at the site of the dehiscence helps to determine management, as a minimum wall thickness of less than 2.5 mm requires surgical repair [32].

## Emergent Pelvic Conditions in Nonpregnant Women

### Ovarian Torsion

Ovarian torsion, a result of the ovarian vascular pedicle twisting, is associated with a lead-point mass in 50–90% of cases [33–35]. Torsion of the vascular pedicle results in circulatory compromise, which initially affects the venous outflow and later affects the arterial inflow. Vascular compromise leads to early parenchymal edema and, as arterial inflow diminishes, to gangrenous and hemorrhagic necrosis. If untreated, hemorrhagic ovarian infarction may be complicated by infection, peritonitis, and, occasionally, death [36]. In patients with partial or intermittent torsion with spontaneous untwisting, symptoms may be recurrent, improving and then worsening within hours, days, or weeks [36].

Timely and accurate diagnosis of ovarian torsion is essential to prevent the detrimental outcome of ovarian infarction. Establishing the diagnosis of ovarian torsion based on clinical

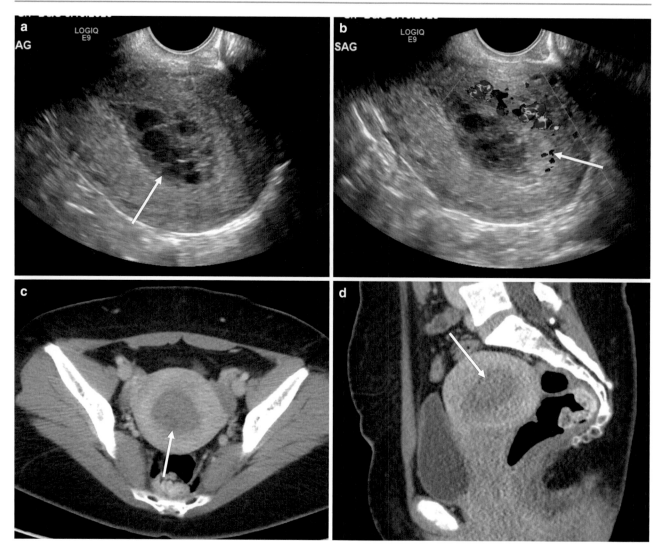

**Fig. 6** Retained products of conception in a 34-year-old woman with pelvic pain 7 days after dilation and curettage. Sagittal gray-scale (**a**) and color Doppler (**b**) US demonstrates thickened heterogeneous endometrium (arrow, **a**) with internal vascularity (arrow, **b**). Axial (**c**) and sagittal (**d**) post-contrast CT images demonstrate thickening and slight heterogeneity of the endometrium (arrow)

evaluation alone can be challenging, as the clinical presentation can be nonspecific and can overlap with other acute gastrointestinal or urinary disorders. Symptoms of ovarian torsion include acute onset of unilateral lower abdominal pain and can be associated with nausea, vomiting, and fever [33].

Regardless of the modality, imaging of patients with ovarian torsion demonstrates an enlarged ovary >4 cm, peripherally displaced follicles, and often a lead-point ovarian mass (Fig. 10) [35]. Corpus luteum or physiologic follicles are the most common lead-point masses, and dermoid is the most commonly associated tumor, seen in approximately 17% of cases of ovarian torsion [35]. Pelvic US is the initial imaging modality in both pregnant and nonpregnant patients presenting with acute-onset pelvic pain. Twisting of the vascular pedicle is visible on US in approximately 87% of patients with ovarian

torsion [37]. Both arterial and venous flow can be preserved in more than half of patients with a visible twisted pedicle, and the presence of flow in the twisted pedicle is associated with preserved ovarian viability at surgery [37].

Twisting of the vascular pedicle is pathognomonic for ovarian torsion and therefore is the most specific finding on cross-sectional imaging [35]. However, presence of a twisted pedicle is seen in fewer than a third of patients [35]. On MRI, a twisted vascular pedicle is seen as a swirling configuration in an enlarged adnexal mass. Since the twisted pedicle may be discerned only in one of the three orthogonal planes, multi-planar acquisition on MRI or multi-planar reconstruction on CT improves detection [35].

Several other findings of ovarian torsion can also be identified on CT and MRI. Asymmetric thickening of the fallopian

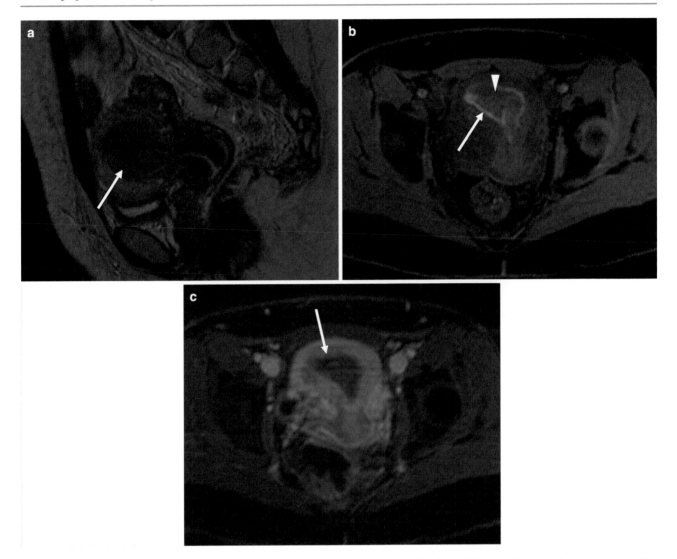

**Fig. 7** Retained products of conception in a 26-year-old woman with pelvic pain and bleeding 3 days after dilation and curettage. Sagittal T2-weighted MR image (**a**) demonstrates an endometrial cavity distended with hypointense material (arrow). Axial T1-weighted pre-contrast (**b**) image demonstrates central intermediate signal intensity (arrowhead) and peripheral high signal intensity (arrow), corresponding to acute and early subacute blood products, respectively. Axial T1-weighted post-contrast image (**c**) demonstrates a small peripheral irregular enhancing area (arrow)

tube ipsilateral to the torsed ovary is seen in almost 85% of cases [36]. A thickened fallopian tube is seen as an amorphous or target-like structure adjacent to an adnexal mass [36]. Since the thickened fallopian tube may be best apparent on only one plane, multi-planar imaging can improve assessment [36]. Twisting of the vascular pedicle results in its foreshortening; consequently, the uterus may deviate toward the affected side in 35% of cases [36]. Although nonspecific, ascites is present in approximately 65% of cases [36].

While decreased ovarian enhancement strongly suggests torsion, the opposite is not true: preserved ovarian enhancement does not exclude ovarian torsion, as dual-blood supply to an ovary helps preserve a near-normal enhancement [35]. Additionally, partial torsion may be associated with near-normal enhancement [35].

The above features are common to all three modalities. However, the superior tissue contrast resolution MRI provides an advantage over CT and US in assessment of ovarian torsion. Edema of the affected ovary is an early sign of ovarian torsion, preceding infarction, and it is best demonstrated on T2-weighted sequences as parenchymal increase in signal (Fig. 11) [34]. On CT, a solid enlarged ovary with abnormal enhancement can be difficult to distinguish from a non-enhancing cyst, yet this distinction is easily made on MRI due to characteristic high signal intensity of cysts on T2-weighted sequences [35].

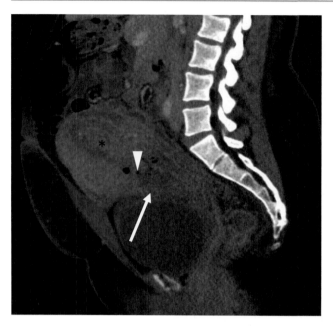

**Fig. 8** Postoperative dehiscence of the cesarean section scar in a 31-year-old woman with fever and pain on postoperative day #3 after cesarean section. Sagittal post-contrast CT image demonstrates low attenuation of the myometrium in the lower uterine segment (arrow) with associated foci of air (arrowhead), indicating cesarean section scar dehiscence. Note that CT cannot accurately reveal whether the overlying serosa is intact

## Ruptured Ovarian Cyst

Rupture of an ovarian cyst, either hemorrhagic or simple, may be spontaneous or can be the result of trauma or pregnancy. Right-sided ovarian cysts are more predisposed to rupture, and the sigmoid colon may provide a protective barrier to the left ovary in the setting of a direct trauma [38]. Although a rupture of an ovarian cyst may result in massive hemoperitoneum, conservative supportive treatment is indicated in patients who are hemodynamically stable [38].

Appearance of hemoperitoneum on various modalities was described earlier. The ruptured cyst may have an irregular shape, and discontinuity of the wall may be observed. A blood clot can be seen adjacent to the ruptured cyst on any of the modalities (Fig. 12). CT or MRI can demonstrate discontinuity of the cyst wall. Occasionally, active bleeding can be seen, if IV contrast was administered.

## Pelvic Inflammatory Disease

Pelvic inflammatory disease (PID) refers to a spectrum of diseases affecting female genital tract, which result from ascending infection, most commonly *Chlamydia trachomatis* and *Neisseria gonorrhea* [39, 40]. In early stages, the patients present with cervicitis, endometritis, and salpingitis, which can progress to pyosalpinx and tubo-ovarian abscesses (TOA). US has a sensitivity of 81%, a specificity of 78%, and an accuracy of 80% for detection of laparoscopically proven PID; MRI performs better, with a sensitivity of 95%, specificity of 89%, and accuracy of 93% [41]. CT may not provide enough anatomic detail to establish a definitive diagnosis of PID, even at the later stages [42]. General findings of PID on CT include thickening of the uterosacral ligaments, obliteration of fascial planes, pelvic fat haziness, reactive lymphadenopathy, and signs of peritonitis [43].

Cervicitis is often occult on US and CT. Endometritis manifests on CT as an enlarged uterus, expansion of the endometrial canal by fluid, and endometrial hyperemia [43]. On MRI, cervicitis and endometritis result in increased signal intensity on T2-weighted sequences and avid enhancement of the cervix and endometrium and thickening of the uterosacral ligaments [39].

The findings of salpingitis are often subtle on US, resulting in tubal tortuosity, mural hyperemia, and tubal thickening >5 mm [43]. Since normal fallopian tubes are not typically discernable on CT, tubal thickening >5 mm is highly specific for salpingitis [43].

Pyosalpinx manifests on US as a dilated tube with internal debris, with associated mural thickening and hyperemia (Fig. 13) [43]. On CT, pyosalpinx is seen either as a tortuous tubular structure with internal debris and a thick enhancing wall or as a complex cystic mass (Fig. 13) [43]. Surrounding fat infiltration and reactive lymphadenopathy are often seen.

MRI can be helpful in distinguishing between pyosalpinx and hydrosalpinx. Similar to hydrosalpinx, pyosalpinx appears as a fluid-filled serpentine structure; mural thickening and hyperenhancement, as well as the signal intensity that is higher on T1-weighted images and lower on T2-weighted sequences, when compared with those of simple fluid, help to establish the diagnosis of pyosalpinx [39, 44]. Since high viscosity of pus may result in restricted diffusion, it should not be misinterpreted as a malignant process [39, 44].

Establishing a diagnosis of TOA is important for management guidance, as TOA necessitates intravenous antibiotics, and possible drainage, as opposed to oral antibiotics required for management of less complex PID cases [39]. CT may not be able to accurately reveal the presence of ovarian involvement, particularly when the degree of tubal dilation is severe [42, 43]. On all imaging modalities, TOA appear as complex cystic mass, with multiple septations and internal debris, and destruction of normal ovarian tissue [43]. CT and MRI also depict adjacent inflammation and peritoneal enhancement [39]. Since TOA can be difficult to differentiate from an ovarian neoplasm on all imaging modalities, patient history is required to make the appropriate diagnosis [8].

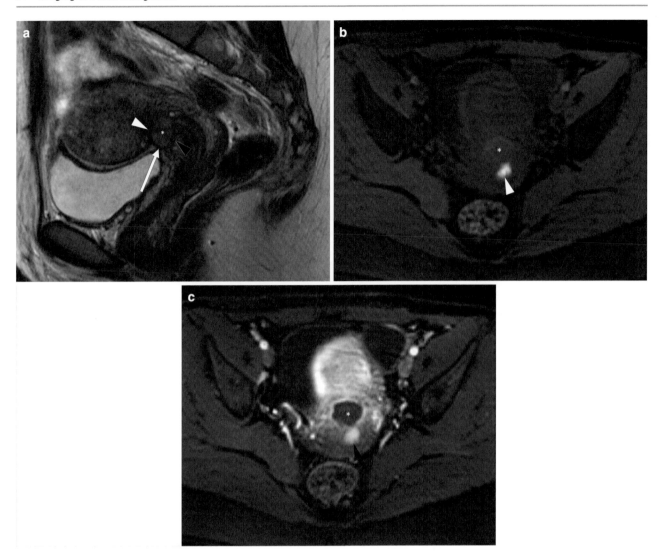

**Fig. 9** Cesarean scar dehiscence in a 28-year-old woman with pelvic pain. Sagittal T2-weighted (**a**), axial pre-contrast T1-weighted (**b**), and axial T1-weighted post-contrast (**c**) MR images demonstrate a defect (*) at the site of the cesarean section scar, between the myometrium in the lower uterine segment (white arrowhead, **a**) and the anterior cervical wall (black arrowhead, **a**). The defect is filled with material which is hypointense on T2-weighted sequence and mildly hyperintense on the T1-weighted sequence and demonstrates no enhancement, consistent with early subacute blood. The thin T2-hypointense line overlying the defect (arrow, **a**) represents intact serosa, distinguishing the dehiscence from rupture. Note subacute blood products distending the endocervical canal (arrowhead, **b** and **c**)

## Emergent Condition in Men

### Testicular Torsion

Testicular torsion is a surgical emergency, and testicular viability is related to the duration of ischemia [45, 46]. Testicular viability can be salvaged in 97% of patients presenting within 6 hours of onset of symptoms, in 50% of patients presenting after 12 h, and in only 10% of patients presenting after 24 h [45]. Patients usually present with acute unilateral testicular pain, which may radiate to the lower abdomen and may be accompanied by nausea and vomiting.

Lack of detectable blood flow in the testis on color Doppler US is diagnostic of torsion (Fig. 14). On gray-scale US, the torsed testicle may have a normal appearance in early stages. As ischemia progresses, the torsed testicle becomes enlarged and heterogeneous. Heterogeneity on preoperative US is predictive of testicular necrosis and the need for orchiectomy in almost all patients [45, 46]. Conversely, almost 90% of testes with homogeneous echotexture and iso-echogenicity to the contralateral testicle are viable at exploration [45]. While immediate emergent surgical exploration is a standard of care, with the goal of salvaging testicular viability, it is suggested that patients with a nonviable torsed testicle can be offered delayed orchiectomy electively,

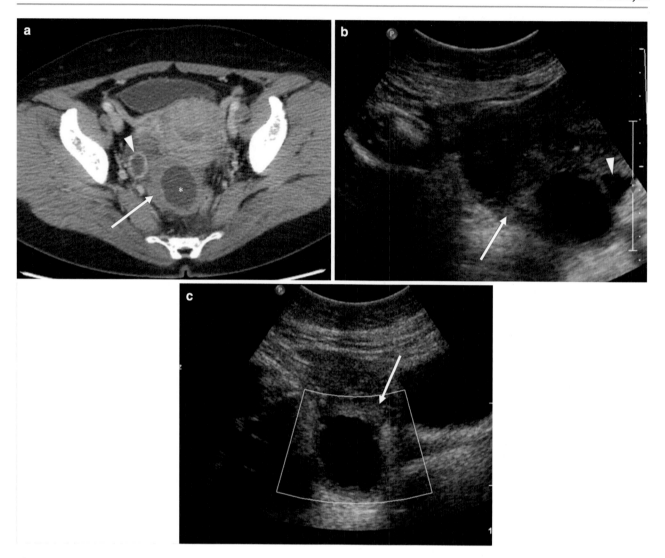

**Fig. 10** Ovarian torsion in a 31-year-old woman with right acute lower quadrant pain. Axial post-contrast CT image (**a**) demonstrates an enlarged edematous poorly enhancing right ovary (arrow) with a dominant cyst (*) and a corpus luteum (arrowhead). Transverse gray-scale ultrasound image of the right ovary (**b**) demonstrates an enlarged right ovary (arrow), with small amount of adjacent fluid (arrowhead). Color Doppler ultrasound image (**c**) demonstrates no flow in the right ovary (arrow)

particularly if the patient has risks for general anesthesia, such as recent oral intake [45, 46]. As heterogeneous echotexture of the parenchyma is highly predictive of a nonviable testicle, description of homogeneity vs heterogeneity in the clinical report can guide the appropriate management [45, 46].

## Epididymitis and Epididymo-orchitis

Epididymitis and epididymo-orchitis are caused by retrograde spread of urethral pathogens via the ejaculatory ducts and the vas deferens. *Neisseria gonorrhoeae* and *Chlamydia trachomatis* are the most common pathogens in sexually active men, and *Escherichia coli* is the most common pathogen in children and older men

[47]. Patients typically present with painful scrotal swelling [48].

Due to retrograde spread of infection, the epididymal tail is usually involved before the body and head; as a result, evaluation of the entire epididymis, especially the tail, is necessary to detect early epididymitis. On gray-scale US, epididymitis manifests as an enlarged heterogeneous epididymis [47]. The echogenicity is often diminished due to associated edema. Color Doppler US reveals asymmetric hyperemia and may be the only finding of early acute epididymitis [47]. Epididymal abscess, a rare complication of epididymitis, can form if the treatment is delayed [48].

In 20–40% of patients with epididymitis, infection progresses to the testicular parenchyma, forming epididymo-orchitis [47]. On US, the affected testicle appears heterogeneous, with increased flow on Doppler US (Fig. 15).

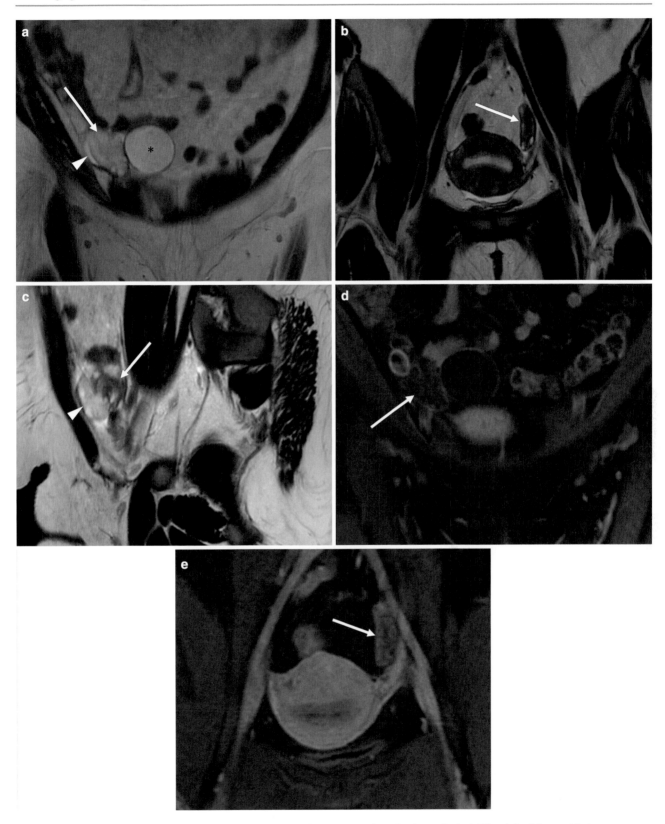

**Fig. 11** Ovarian torsion in a 23-year-old woman with pelvic pain. Coronal T2-weighted MR images (**a** and **b**) demonstrate an enlarged right ovary (arrow, **a**) with an exophytic cyst (*) and adjacent fluid (arrowhead). The right ovary demonstrates increased signal intensity in the parenchyma compared to the left ovary (arrow, **b**), indicating parenchymal edema. Sagittal T2-weighted image (**c**) demonstrates a swirling structure (arrow) adjacent to the right ovary (arrowhead), representing a twisted vascular pedicle. Coronal post-contrast T1-weighted images (**d** and **e**) demonstrate diminished enhancement in the right ovary (arrow, **d**) as compared to the left (arrow, **e**)

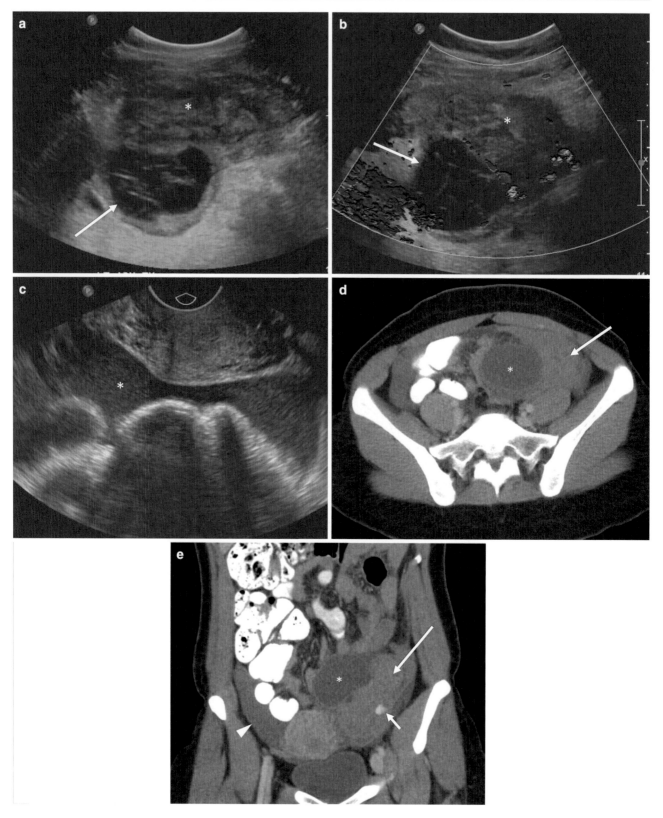

**Fig. 12** Ruptured ovarian cyst in a 26-year-old woman with severe pelvic pain. Gray-scale (**a**) and color Doppler (**b**) ultrasound images of the right ovary demonstrate a hemorrhagic cyst in the right ovary (arrow), with adjacent heterogeneous hyperechoic avascular process (*), consistent with a hematoma. Gray-scale ultrasound image (**c**) of the cul-de-sac demonstrates pelvic fluid with low-level internal echoes (*), consistent with hemoperitoneum. Axial (**d**) and coronal (**e**) post-contrast CT images demonstrate a large left adnexal cyst (*) with an adjacent lobulated hyperdense blood clot (long arrow). An ill-defined collection of contrast within the blood clot (short arrow, **e**) represents an area of active bleeding. Hyperdense ascites (arrowhead, **e**) represents hemoperitoneum

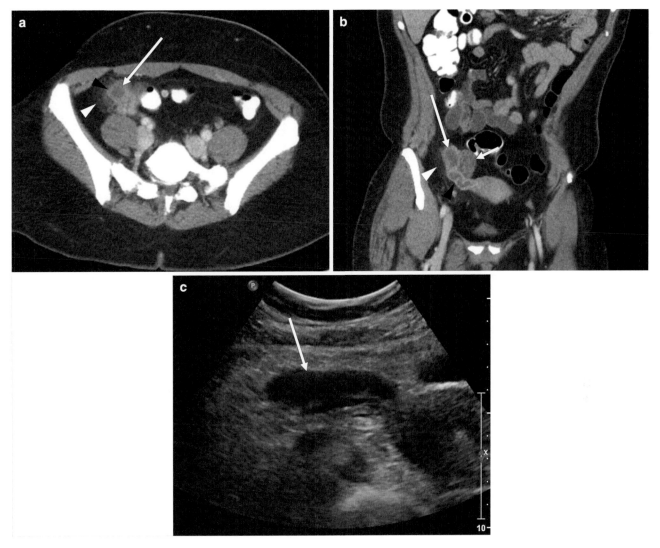

**Fig. 13** Pyosalpinx in a 29-year-old woman with pelvic pain and fever. Axial (**a**) and coronal (**b**) post-contrast CT images demonstrate a dilated fluid-filled right fallopian tube (long arrow) with a thick hyperenhancing wall (black arrowhead) and infiltration of the adjacent fat (white arrowhead). A normal right ovary is seen distinct from the pyosalpinx (short arrow, **b**). Gray-scale ultrasound view of the right adnexa (**c**) demonstrates a dilated right fallopian tube (arrow), filled with debris

While cross-sectional examinations are not typically performed for the diagnosis of epididymo-orchitis, asymmetric hyperenhancement of the affected testicle and epididymis may be evident (Fig. 15). Scrotal edema may be seen as well.

Severe testicular edema may limit testicular venous outflow, leading to parenchymal necrosis. Late or failed treatment of epididymo-orchitis may result in a pyocele or formation of a testicular abscess (Fig. 16) [49]. Pyocele manifests as a complex fluid with internal echoes and septations around the affected testicle (Fig. 15). An abscess appears as a central hypoechoic area on gray-scale US with no associated flow on Doppler US (Fig. 16) [47].

## Prostatic Abscess

Prostatic abscesses are uncommon complications of acute bacterial prostatitis, with the pathogen extending through reflux of infected urine into prostatic ducts [50]. Elderly patients with diabetes, patients with chronic liver failure, and those with immunocompromised states are at the highest risk, and *Escherichia coli* is the most common pathogen [50]. Differentiation between uncomplicated prostatitis and an abscess is difficult based on clinical examination alone, as the symptoms often overlap and include dysuria, urinary urgency, frequency, the sensation of incomplete voiding, and suprapubic or perineal pain [50]. Fever, malaise, and

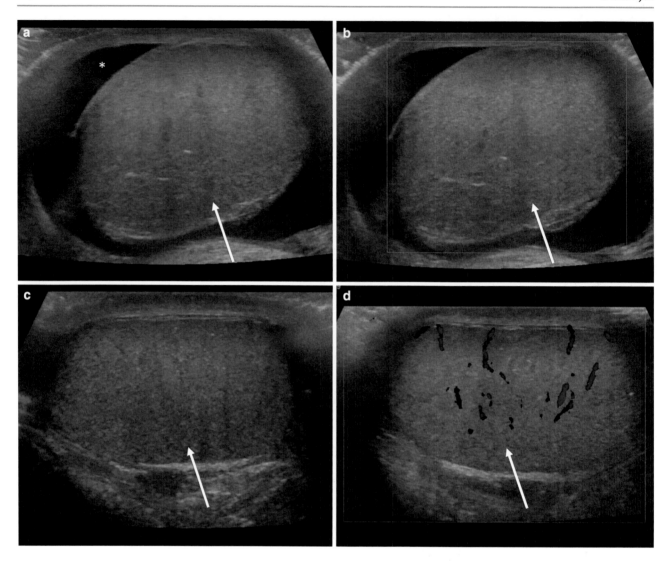

**Fig. 14** Testicular torsion in a 17-year-old man with scrotal pain and swelling. Gray-scale (**a**) and color Doppler (**b**) images demonstrate oblique rotation of the right testicle (arrow) with no detectable flow (**b**). In contrast, the left testicle demonstrates a normal rotation on a gray-scale ultrasound image (arrow, **c**) and preserved flow on the color Doppler image (**d**). Note a simple hydrocele on the right (*, **a**)

sepsis may be the presenting symptoms in approximately one-third of patients [50]. Imaging plays an important role, as the presence of an abscess necessitates drainage in addition to antibiotics.

On US, prostatic abscesses appear as focal hypoechoic or anechoic avascular foci with thick wall and internal septations (Fig. 17) [51]. CT findings are similar to US, and abscesses appear as low attenuation foci with enhancing wall and internal septations (Fig. 17) [52]. In addition, CT can identify extraprostatic spread, show reactive lymphadenopathy, and potentially depict other sites of infection, when hematogenous spread is suspected [50]. Intravenous contrast should be administered, as the abscess cavity may be difficult to discern from the background parenchyma on a non-contrast CT, particularly if the abscess is small or is lacking internal foci of air.

MRI may be helpful for detecting an early abscess when US is inconclusive [50]. On MRI, the abscess cavity usually has low signal intensity on T1-weighted sequences and high signal intensity on T2-weighted sequences, although the signal may be variable depending on the degree of internal debris [50]. If contrast is administered, the abscess wall and septations enhance.

## Fournier Gangrene

Fournier gangrene is a necrotizing infection involving both superficial and deep fascial planes of perineal, perianal, and genital regions. The condition has a strong male predominance, with over 90% of cases occurring in men [47]. Fournier gangrene is a urologic emergency with high mortality rates,

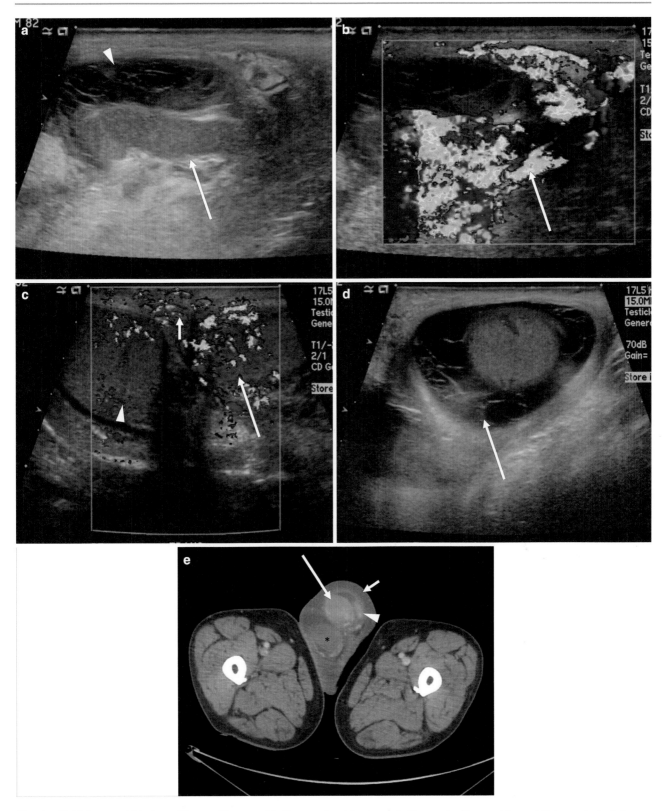

**Fig. 15** Epididymo-orchitis in a 47-year-old man with fever and scrotal pain. Gray-scale (**a**) and color Doppler (**b**) images demonstrate thickened left epididymis (arrow) measuring up to 0.9 cm, with marked internal flow (**b**). Color Doppler ultrasound image through the testes (**c**) demonstrates asymmetrically increased vascularity in the left testicle (long arrow) as compared to the right testicle (arrowhead). Note thickening and hyperemia of the overlying scrotal wall (short arrow). Gray-scale ultrasound image (**d**) demonstrates left scrotal fluid with internal echoes and debris, consistent with a pyocele. Axial post-contrast CT image (**e**) demonstrates asymmetrically increased enhancement of the left testicle (long arrow), thickened and hyperemic left epididymis (arrowhead), and scrotal edema (short arrow). The right testicle (*) has a normal appearance

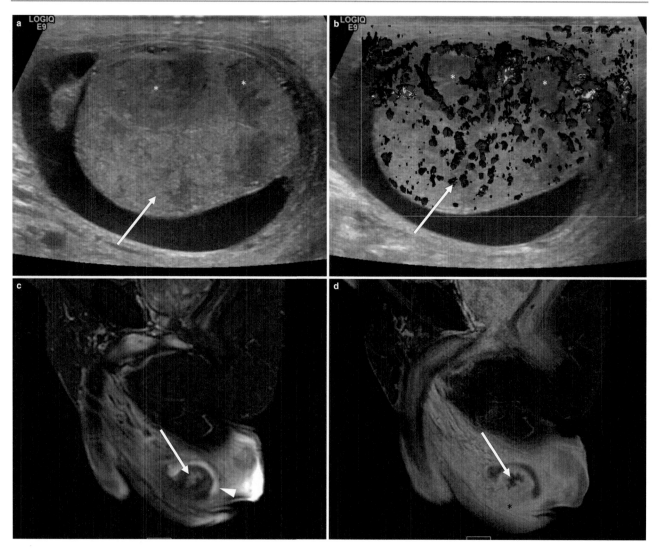

**Fig. 16** Testicular abscess in this 72-year-old man with history of orchitis and persistent symptoms despite antibiotics. Gray-scale (**a**) and color Doppler (**b**) ultrasound views of the right testicle (arrow) demonstrate heterogeneous echotexture with increased vascularity, consistent with known orchitis. Two distinct areas of decreased echogenicity (*) are associated with lack of internal vascularity and peripheral rim of enhancement, concerning for abscesses. Sagittal T2-weighted (**c**) and post-contrast T1-weighted (**d**) MR images demonstrate an irregular T2-hyperintense non-enhancing collection (arrow), confirming a small abscess. Note a small hydrocele (arrowhead) and thickening and hyperemia of the scrotal wall (**d**, *)

ranging from 15% to 50% [53]. Diabetes mellitus is the most common predisposing condition and can be found in 40–60% of patients with Fournier gangrene [53]. Other important predisposing factors include alcohol abuse, immunocompromised states such as steroid use, chemotherapy, radiation therapy, human immunodeficiency virus, indwelling catheters, localized trauma, malignancy, and prolonged hospitalization [53]. Most Fournier gangrene infections are polymicrobial, including both aerobic and anaerobic organisms, but the source of infection may be occult in 6–45% of patients [47]. Patients with Fournier gangrene present with scrotal swelling, fever, pain, and hyperemia [53]. On physical examination, crepitus is detected in 20–64% of patients [53].

Although the diagnosis of Fournier gangrene can be made based on clinical examination, CT is valuable for evaluation of the extent of disease, as it has greater specificity than physical examination or US [53]. CT accurately reveals the extent of the gangrene, anatomic pathways of spread of the infection and subcutaneous gas, and the presence of fluid collection or abscesses (Fig. 18) [53]. While the epicenter of Fournier's gangrene is the perineum, CT coverage should include the abdomen in addition to the pelvis, in order to detect intra-abdominal sources of infection and to accurately evaluate the extent of involvement [47].

On CT, Fournier gangrene is seen as soft-tissue thickening, fat infiltration, and subcutaneous emphysema.

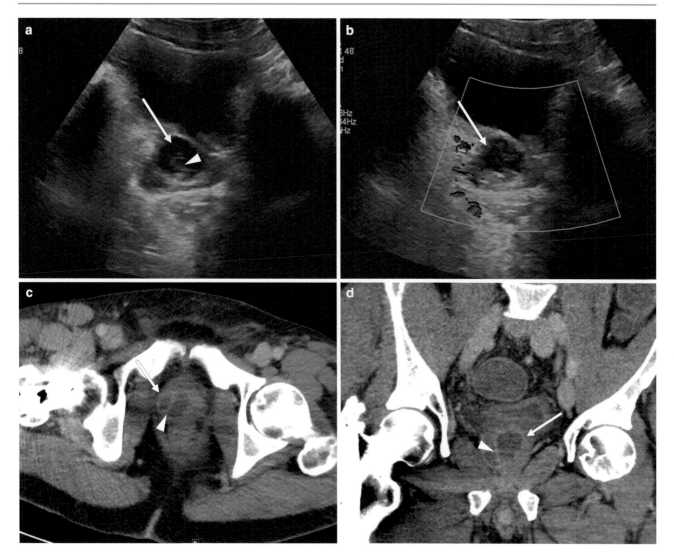

**Fig. 17** Prostate abscess in a 54-year-old man with history of HIV, hepatitis C, cirrhosis, and persistent *E. coli* bacteremia despite antibiotics. Gray-scale (**a**) and color Doppler (**b**) ultrasound images demonstrate a complex avascular fluid collection (arrow) in the prostate, with internal septations/debris (arrowhead, **a**). Axial (**c**) and coronal (**d**) post-contrast CT images demonstrate a fluid collection in the prostate with peripheral rim enhancement (long arrow) and internal enhancing septation (arrowhead)

The subcutaneous emphysema dissects along the fascial planes and can involve the soft tissues of the scrotum, perineum, inguinal regions, retroperitoneum, abdominal wall, and thighs [53]. Concomitant abscesses appear as organized fluid collections with peripheral enhancing wall.

US is usually not a modality of choice for the assessment of Fournier's gangrene, since the direct pressure on the perineum from the transducer is not well tolerated. Additionally, US is limited in the assessment of the deep extent of disease (Fig. 18) [47]. However, US may be useful in patients who cannot leave the emergency department or intensive care unit and may depict fluid and gas in the subcutaneous tissues [47]. On US, Fournier's gangrene is seen as a thickened, edematous perineal and scrotal wall [54]. Foci of air appear as hyperechoic foci with ring-down artifact and "dirty" acoustic shadowing (Fig. 18) [54].

Due to the long acquisition time and potential lack of added value over CT, MRI is not the primary imaging modality for the diagnosis of Fournier gangrene. While not a first-line modality, MRI can be a useful tool for problem-solving, particularly when US or CT findings are equivocal or suboptimal. On MRI, Fournier gangrene manifests as increased signal intensity in the perineal region on T2-weighted sequences, indicating inflammation, fascial thickening, soft-tissue gas, and collections, or fistulas [54]. Foci of gas on MRI appear as foci of signal void and susceptibility artifacts, best appreciated on gradient-echo sequences.

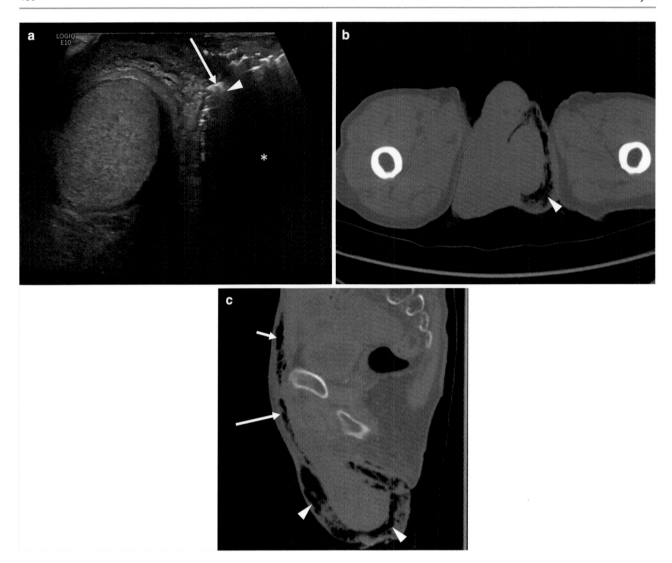

**Fig. 18** Fournier gangrene in an 82-year-old man with scrotal pain and skin ulceration. Transverse gray-scale ultrasound (**a**) of the scrotum demonstrates multiple echogenic foci in the left scrotal wall (arrow) with dirty shadowing (arrowhead), consistent with foci of air. Note that the air obscures visualization of the left testicle (*). Axial (**b**) and sagittal (**c**) non-contrast CT images also demonstrate air in the scrotal wall (arrowheads). CT also allows visualization of the extension of air superiorly through the left inguinal canal (long arrow, **c**) into the soft tissues of lower anterior abdominal wall (short arrow, **c**)

## Priapism

Priapism, a prolonged painful penile erection not associated with sexual arousal, is classified as low flow (ischemic) or high flow (arterial or nonischemic). Low-flow priapism is more common and is caused by obstruction of penile venous outflow resulting from a variety of conditions, such as malignancy, hypercoagulable states, sickle cell disease, and medications. Low-flow priapism is a true emergency since prolonged high cavernous pressures may lead to irreversible ischemic changes and permanent erectile dysfunction. High-flow priapism is due to unregulated penile arterial inflow, usually as a result of arterial injury in the setting of genitoperineal trauma. High-flow priapism is usually painless, is less common, and does not constitute an emergency since permanent erectile dysfunction is unusual.

The distinction between the two types of priapism is usually based on clinical evaluation: the low-flow priapism is acute, painful, and rigid, whereas high-flow priapism is painless and has a more prolonged manifestation after a trauma, and the erection is incomplete. On US, low-flow priapism manifests as thrombosis of the corpora cavernosa or corpus spongiosum and decreased or absent color flow or spectral Doppler in the cavernosal arteries (Fig. 19). Flow in the superficial penile vein may be preserved. In high-flow priapism, US may demonstrate an arteriovenous fistula, with normal (>25 cm/s) or elevated velocity in the penile arteries.

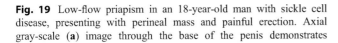

**Fig. 19** Low-flow priapism in an 18-year-old man with sickle cell disease, presenting with perineal mass and painful erection. Axial gray-scale (**a**) image through the base of the penis demonstrates enlargement of the left crus (arrow) with dilated anechoic vascular channels (arrowhead). No flow in the left crus (arrow) is seen on the color Doppler image (**b**)

# References

1. Sivalingam VN, Duncan WC, Kirk E, Shephard LA, Horne AW. Diagnosis and management of ectopic pregnancy. J Fam Plann Reprod Health Care. 2011;37(4):231–40.
2. Srisajjakul S, Prapaisilp P, Bangchokdee S. Magnetic resonance imaging in tubal and non-tubal ectopic pregnancy. Eur J Radiol. 2017;93:76–89.
3. Condous G, Okaro E, Bourne T. The conservative management of early pregnancy complications: a review of the literature. Ultrasound Obstet Gynecol. 2003;22(4):420–30.
4. Shalev E, Yarom I, Bustan M, Weiner E, Ben-Shlomo I. Transvaginal sonography as the ultimate diagnostic tool for the management of ectopic pregnancy: experience with 840 cases. Fertil Steril. 1998;69(1):62–5.
5. Masselli G, Derme M, Piccioni MG, Spina V, Laghi F, Gualdi G, et al. To evaluate the feasibility of magnetic resonance imaging in predicting unusual site ectopic pregnancy: a retrospective cohort study. Eur Radiol. 2018;28(6):2444–54.
6. Ramanathan S, Raghu V, Ladumor SB, Nagadi AN, Palaniappan Y, Dogra V, et al. Magnetic resonance imaging of common, uncommon, and rare implantation sites in ectopic pregnancy. Abdom Radiol (NY). 2018;43(12):3425–35.
7. Parker RA 3rd, Yano M, Tai AW, Friedman M, Narra VR, Menias CO. MR imaging findings of ectopic pregnancy: a pictorial review. Radiographics. 2012;32(5):1445–60. discussion 60–2.
8. Somberg Gunther M, Kanmaniraja D, Kobi M, Chernyak V. MRI of acute gynecologic conditions. J Magn Reson Imaging. 2020;51(5):1291–309.
9. Viets ZJ, Raptis CA, Fowler KJ, Hildebolt CF, Yano M. Magnetic resonance imaging of first trimester pregnancy: expected intrauterine contents in relation to gestational age. Abdom Radiol (NY). 2017;42(9):2334–9.
10. Shin DS, Poder L, Courtier J, Naeger DM, Westphalen AC, Coakley FV. CT and MRI of early intrauterine pregnancy. AJR Am J Roentgenol. 2011;196(2):325–30.
11. Si MJ, Gui S, Fan Q, Han HX, Zhao QQ, Li ZX, et al. Role of MRI in the early diagnosis of tubal ectopic pregnancy. Eur Radiol. 2016;26(7):1971–80.
12. Raziel A, Schachter M, Mordechai E, Friedler S, Panski M, Ron-El R. Ovarian pregnancy-a 12-year experience of 19 cases in one institution. Eur J Obstet Gynecol Reprod Biol. 2004;114(1):92–6.
13. Kung FT, Lin H, Hsu TY, Chang CY, Huang HW, Huang LY, et al. Differential diagnosis of suspected cervical pregnancy and conservative treatment with the combination of laparoscopy-assisted uterine artery ligation and hysteroscopic endocervical resection. Fertil Steril. 2004;81(6):1642–9.
14. Jung SE, Byun JY, Lee JM, Choi BG, Hahn ST. Characteristic MR findings of cervical pregnancy. J Magn Reson Imaging. 2001;13(6):918–22.
15. Kao LY, Scheinfeld MH, Chernyak V, Rozenblit AM, Oh S, Dym RJ. Beyond ultrasound: CT and MRI of ectopic pregnancy. AJR Am J Roentgenol. 2014;202(4):904–11.
16. Jurkovic D, Hillaby K, Woelfer B, Lawrence A, Salim R, Elson CJ. First-trimester diagnosis and management of pregnancies implanted into the lower uterine segment Cesarean section scar. Ultrasound Obstet Gynecol. 2003;21(3):220–7.
17. Seow KM, Huang LW, Lin YH, Lin MY, Tsai YL, Hwang JL. Cesarean scar pregnancy: issues in management. Ultrasound Obstet Gynecol. 2004;23(3):247–53.
18. Rheinboldt M, Osborn D, Delproposto Z. Cesarean section scar ectopic pregnancy: a clinical case series. J Ultrasound. 2015;18(2):191–5.
19. Peng KW, Lei Z, Xiao TH, Jia FG, Zhong WX, Gao Y, et al. First trimester caesarean scar ectopic pregnancy evaluation using MRI. Clin Radiol. 2014;69(2):123–9.
20. Ash A, Smith A, Maxwell D. Caesarean scar pregnancy. BJOG. 2007;114(3):253–63.
21. Lin EP, Bhatt S, Dogra VS. Diagnostic clues to ectopic pregnancy. Radiographics. 2008;28(6):1661–71.
22. Ackerman TE, Levi CS, Dashefsky SM, Holt SC, Lindsay DJ. Interstitial line: sonographic finding in interstitial (cornual) ectopic pregnancy. Radiology. 1993;189(1):83–7.
23. Durfee SM, Frates MC, Luong A, Benson CB. The sonographic and color Doppler features of retained products of conception. J Ultrasound Med. 2005;24(9):1181–6. quiz 8–9.
24. Zuckerman J, Levine D, McNicholas MM, Konopka S, Goldstein A, Edelman RR, et al. Imaging of pelvic postpartum complications. AJR Am J Roentgenol. 1997;168(3):663–8.

25. Noonan JB, Coakley FV, Qayyum A, Yeh BM, Wu L, Chen LM. MR imaging of retained products of conception. AJR Am J Roentgenol. 2003;181(2):435–9.

26. Brandt KR, Coakley KJ. MR appearance of placental site trophoblastic tumor: a report of three cases. AJR Am J Roentgenol. 1998;170(2):485–7.

27. Dresang LT, Leeman L. Cesarean delivery. Prim Care. 2012;39(1):145–65.

28. van Ham MA, van Dongen PW, Mulder J. Maternal consequences of caesarean section. A retrospective study of intra-operative and postoperative maternal complications of caesarean section during a 10-year period. Eur J Obstet Gynecol Reprod Biol. 1997;74(1):1–6.

29. Sawada M, Matsuzaki S, Nakae R, Iwamiya T, Kakigano A, Kumasawa K, et al. Treatment and repair of uterine scar dehiscence during cesarean section. Clin Case Rep. 2017;5(2):145–9.

30. Alamo L, Vial Y, Denys A, Andreisek G, Meuwly JY, Schmidt S. MRI findings of complications related to previous uterine scars. Eur J Radiol Open. 2018;5:6–15.

31. Twickler DM, Setiawan AT, Harrell RS, Brown CE. CT appearance of the pelvis after cesarean section. AJR Am J Roentgenol. 1991;156(3):523–6.

32. Moshiri M, Osman S, Bhargava P, Maximin S, Robinson TJ, Katz DS. Imaging evaluation of maternal complications associated with repeat cesarean deliveries. Radiol Clin N Am. 2014;52(5):1117–35.

33. Chang HC, Bhatt S, Dogra VS. Pearls and pitfalls in diagnosis of ovarian torsion. Radiographics. 2008;28(5):1355–68.

34. Pedrosa I, Zeikus EA, Levine D, Rofsky NM. MR imaging of acute right lower quadrant pain in pregnant and nonpregnant patients. Radiographics. 2007;27(3):721–43. discussion 43–53.

35. Duigenan S, Oliva E, Lee SI. Ovarian torsion: diagnostic features on CT and MRI with pathologic correlation. AJR Am J Roentgenol. 2012;198(2):W122–31.

36. Rha SE, Byun JY, Jung SE, Jung JI, Choi BG, Kim BS, et al. CT and MR imaging features of adnexal torsion. Radiographics. 2002;22(2):283–94.

37. Lee EJ, Kwon HC, Joo HJ, Suh JH, Fleischer AC. Diagnosis of ovarian torsion with color Doppler sonography: depiction of twisted vascular pedicle. J Ultrasound Med. 1998;17(2):83–9.

38. Iraha Y, Okada M, Iraha R, Azama K, Yamashiro T, Tsubakimoto M, et al. CT and MR imaging of gynecologic emergencies. Radiographics. 2017;37(5):1569–86.

39. Czeyda-Pommersheim F, Kalb B, Costello J, Liau J, Meshksar A, Arif Tiwari H, et al. MRI in pelvic inflammatory disease: a pictorial review. Abdom Radiol. 2017;42(3):935–50.

40. Heverhagen JT, Klose KJ. MR imaging for acute lower abdominal and pelvic pain. Radiographics. 2009;29(6):1781–96.

41. Tukeva TA, Aronen HJ, Karjalainen PT, Molander P, Paavonen T, Paavonen J. MR imaging in pelvic inflammatory disease: comparison with laparoscopy and US. Radiology. 1999;210(1):209–16.

42. Roche O, Chavan N, Aquilina J, Rockall A. Radiological appearances of gynaecological emergencies. Insight Imaging. 2012;3(3):265–75.

43. Revzin MV, Mathur M, Dave HB, Macer ML, Spektor M. Pelvic inflammatory disease: multimodality imaging approach with clinical-pathologic correlation. Radiographics. 2016;36(5):1579–96.

44. Dohke M, Watanabe Y, Okumura A, Amoh Y, Hayashi T, Yoshizako T, et al. Comprehensive MR imaging of acute gynecologic diseases. Radiographics. 2000;20(6):1551–66.

45. Samson P, Hartman C, Palmerola R, Rahman Z, Siev M, Palmer LS, et al. Ultrasonographic assessment of testicular viability using heterogeneity levels in torsed testicles. J Urol. 2017;197(3 Pt 2):925–30.

46. Kaye JD, Shapiro EY, Levitt SB, Friedman SC, Gitlin J, Freyle J, et al. Parenchymal echo texture predicts testicular salvage after torsion: potential impact on the need for emergent exploration. J Urol. 2008;180(4 Suppl):1733–6.

47. Avery LL, Scheinfeld MH. Imaging of penile and scrotal emergencies. Radiographics. 2013;33(3):721–40.

48. Yang DM, Yoon MH, Kim HS, Jin W, Hwang HY, Kim HS, et al. Comparison of tuberculous and pyogenic epididymal abscesses: clinical, gray-scale sonographic, and color Doppler sonographic features. AJR Am J Roentgenol. 2001;177(5):1131–5.

49. Slavis SA, Kollin J, Miller JB. Pyocele of scrotum: consequence of spontaneous rupture of testicular abscess. Urology. 1989;33(4):313–6.

50. Ackerman AL, Parameshwar PS, Anger JT. Diagnosis and treatment of patients with prostatic abscess in the post-antibiotic era. Int J Urol. 2018;25(2):103–10.

51. Papanicolaou N, Pfister RC, Stafford SA, Parkhurst EC. Prostatic abscess: imaging with transrectal sonography and MR. AJR Am J Roentgenol. 1987;149(5):981–2.

52. Thornhill BA, Morehouse HT, Coleman P, Hoffman-Tretin JC. Prostatic abscess: CT and sonographic findings. AJR Am J Roentgenol. 1987;148(5):899–900.

53. Levenson RB, Singh AK, Novelline RA. Fournier gangrene: role of imaging. Radiographics. 2008;28(2):519–28.

54. Ballard DH, Mazaheri P, Raptis CA, Lubner MG, Menias CO, Pickhardt PJ, et al. Fournier gangrene in men and women: appearance on CT, ultrasound, and MRI and what the surgeon wants to know. Can Assoc Radiol J = Journal l'Association canadienne des radiologistes. 2020;71(1):30–9.

# Imaging of Nontraumatic Vascular Emergencies

# 32

Daniel R. Ludwig and Motoyo Yano

## Contents

### Abstract

Nontraumatic emergencies involving the abdominal vasculature are common and associated with significant morbidity and mortality. These conditions are almost always diagnosed or confirmed using cross-sectional imaging, and thus the radiologist plays an essential role in guiding appropriate patient management. Computed tomography (CT) angiography is the workhorse modality for evaluating patients with suspected acute vascular pathology, but magnetic resonance angiography (MRA) may be appropriate in carefully selected patients. Abdominal aortic aneurysms (AAAs) are frequently encountered in practice; however, findings of aneurysm instability or rupture may be subtle but are critically important to identify. Following open AAA repair, complications may include anastomotic pseudoaneurysm, aortoenteric and aortopancreatic fistula, graft infection, and thrombosis. After endovascular AAA repair, important complications include endoleak, rupture, stent kinking, thrombosis, and infection. Aortitis and periaortitis can occur due to a broad variety of causes. Of these, infectious aortitis is most concerning, as it can progress rapidly to infectious pseudoaneurysm and rupture. Acute aortic occlusion, while uncommon, is associated with high morbidity and mortality. Acute pathology affecting the medium-sized abdominal vessels includes vasculitis, segmental arterial mediolysis (SAM), pseudoaneurysm, and embolic or thrombotic occlusion. Complications of medium-vessel pathology present acutely and commonly include hemorrhage and visceral ischemia. The objective of this chapter is to review and illustrate the most important nontraumatic abdominal vascular emergencies and their associated complications.

### Keywords

CT angiography · Abdominal aortic aneurysm (AAA) · Aneurysm instability · Aneurysm rupture · Open aneurysm repair · Endovascular aneurysm repair (EVAR) · Infectious pseudoaneurysm · Vasculitis · Segmental arterial mediolysis (SAM) · Vascular occlusion

## Introduction

Acute nontraumatic vascular pathology involving the abdomen is common in the emergency setting and is associated with significant morbidity and mortality. Although many vascular conditions are the result of chronic processes,

D. R. Ludwig
Mallinckrodt Institute of Radiology, Washington University School of Medicine, St. Louis, MO, USA
e-mail: ludwigd@wustl.edu

M. Yano (✉)
Mayo Clinic Department of Radiology, Scottsdale, AZ, USA
e-mail: Yano.Motoyo@mayo.edu

© Springer Nature Switzerland AG 2022
M. N. Patlas et al. (eds.), *Atlas of Emergency Imaging from Head-to-Toe*,
https://doi.org/10.1007/978-3-030-92111-8_32

patients often present acutely when complications such as bleeding or thrombosis develop. In this chapter, we will review the imaging appearance and relevant clinical features of atraumatic vascular pathology affecting the abdominal aorta and major abdominal visceral arteries. Specifically, we will cover abdominal aortic aneurysm (AAA) including features of instability and rupture, acute complications of open and endovascular AAA repair, infectious and inflammatory aortitis including inflammatory AAA, acute aortic syndromes, and acute aortic occlusion. Next, we will discuss medium-vessel pathology, including vasculitis, segmental arterial mediolysis (SAM), pseudoaneurysm, and occlusion. These conditions are invariably diagnosed or confirmed using noninvasive imaging, and thus the radiologist plays an essential role in guiding patient management in the emergent setting.

## Nontraumatic Vascular Emergencies

## Imaging Approach

Computed tomography (CT) angiography is the workhorse technique for diagnosing and characterizing acute vascular pathology. CT angiography requires the injection of intravenous (IV) iodinated contrast at a rate of 3-4 mL per second into a large bore peripheral IV catheter (i.e., 20 gauge or larger) or power injectable central venous catheter, and the CT acquisition is timed for optimal arterial opacification [1]. Non-contrast CT should also be performed, as intramural or perivascular hemorrhage may be obscured by the presence of IV contrast. A delayed-phase CT acquisition (i.e., 60–90 s) is often helpful to depict active bleeding, findings of visceral malperfusion or ischemia, and identify certain complications of AAA repair such as endoleak. Magnetic resonance angiography (MRA) may be suitable in selected patients with suspected acute vascular pathology, specifically those who cannot receive iodinated contrast due to advanced renal insufficiency or severe contrast allergy [2]. Although gadolinium-based IV contrast is routinely administered during MRA, it is often not required to obtain a diagnostic evaluation. MRA, however, requires substantially more time to perform and interpret than CT angiography and cannot be used in patients who are hemodynamically unstable.

## Aorta

### Aneurysm

AAA is a relatively common condition which affects at least 5% of the population over the age of 65 [3]. AAA is typically an atherosclerotic process characterized by progressive segmental dilation of the abdominal aorta to a diameter ≥50% of normal caliber, or ≥3.0 cm. Most aneurysms are asymptomatic until they rupture which is frequently a lethal occurrence, although as many as 50% of patients who reach the hospital survive to discharge [4].

The strongest predictor of AAA rupture is aneurysm size, with an annual risk of rupture exceeding 5% when aneurysm size reaches 5.5 cm in diameter [5]. Accordingly, the Society for Vascular Surgery recommends elective repair of fusiform AAAs larger than 5.5 cm. In patients with known AAA undergoing surveillance imaging, measurements of an AAA should always be performed perpendicular to the long axis of the aorta using a double-oblique technique, as measurements made on an axial CT image often overestimate the size of the AAA [6].

Screening for AAA is performed in selected patients, although many AAAs are encountered incidentally or diagnosed in patients presenting acutely with rupture. In those whom AAA rupture is clinically apparent, CT is commonly utilized to confirm the diagnosis and guide the repair strategy. Many patients with AAA, however, present with nonspecific abdominal or back pain, and the radiologist plays in crucial role in identifying features of aneurysm instability, frank rupture, and contained rupture, some of which can appear quite subtle.

### Aneurysm Instability

Multiple CT findings have been described in the setting of aneurysm instability (i.e., impending rupture) [6, 7]. One of the most specific and worrisome features of instability is the "hyperattenuating crescent," defined as crescentic area of attenuation higher than luminal aortic blood on non-contrast CT, either within the mural thrombus or wall of the aneurysm (Fig. 1) [8]. This CT finding strongly correlates with operative findings of acute hemorrhage into the thrombus or aortic wall and is generally an indication for urgent or emergent surgical repair [9]. The high-attenuation crescent is difficult to diagnose on contrast-enhanced CT, highlighting the utility of non-contrast CT in the evaluation of the acute AAA. Importantly, the high-attenuation crescent must be distinguished from dystrophic calcification within the mural thrombus, the latter of which usually has the density of calcium, temporal stability, and a configuration that does not follow the external contour of the aortic wall, usually allowing for distinction from intimal calcifications [10].

Mural thrombus is a ubiquitous finding in AAA, and a smaller patent lumen (i.e., higher thrombus-to-lumen ratio) is considered protective against rupture [11]. Changing morphology of the mural thrombus, including an increasing size of the patient lumen or fissuring clefts within the thrombus, is associated with aneurysm instability (Fig. 2). Furthermore, various morphologic changes in the aortic wall can be seen in patients with aneurysm instability. A focal gap or discontinuity of otherwise continuous peripheral intimal

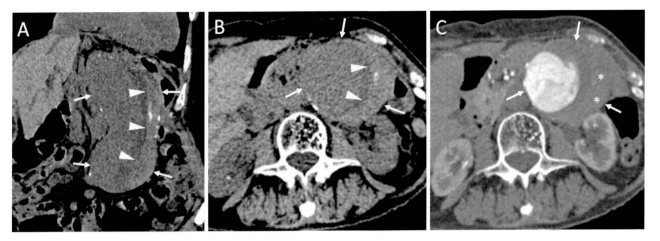

**Fig. 1** Hyperattenuating crescent in an 83-year-old woman presenting for routine evaluation of AAA. Coronal (**a**) and axial (**b**) non-contrast CT images demonstrate a large juxtarenal AAA (arrows). Along the left side of the aneurysm is a crescentic area within the mural thrombus or wall of the aneurysm (arrowheads) which has a higher attenuation than the luminal aortic blood, consistent with a hyperattenuating crescent, an indicator of aneurysm instability. The high-attenuation crescent is less conspicuous on axial contrast-enhanced CT image (**c**, asterisks), highlighting the importance of the non-contrast evaluation

**Fig. 2** Changing mural thrombus morphology in an 86-year-old woman presenting for routine follow-up of AAA. Initial non-contrast (**a**) and contrast-enhanced (**b**) axial CT images demonstrate an AAA (thin arrows), without imaging findings of instability. Non-contrast (**c**) and contrast-enhanced (**d**) axial CT image obtained 16 months later show a new high-attenuation crescent within the posterior aspect of the mural thrombus (arrowhead, C) and a new fissuring cleft within the mural thrombus (thick arrow, **d**), indicative of aneurysm instability. Additionally, the aneurysm had increased in size by 10 mm over this interval

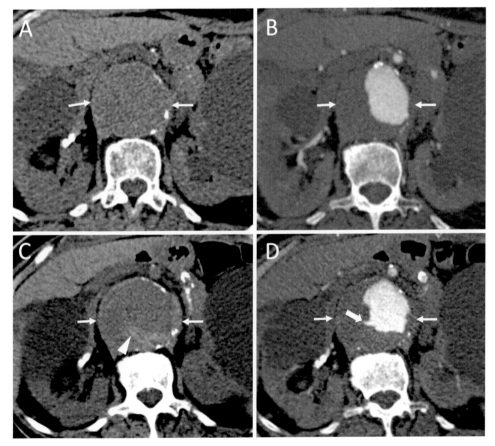

calcifications, "discontinuous calcium sign," is suggestive of weakness and/or thinning of the aortic wall at that location (Fig. 3) [8]. This feature is most specific when a prior CT is available showing complete continuity of the intimal calcifications. Progression of weakness may result in divergence of the intimal calcifications in a tangent from the expected circular contour of the aortic wall (i.e., "tangential calcium sign") (Fig. 4). A schematic of the tangential calcium sign is shown in Fig. 4d. An additional finding associated with AAA instability that may be seen in conjunction

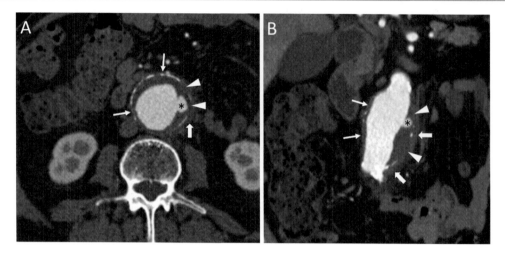

**Fig. 3** Discontinuous calcium sign in a 78-year-old man with known AAA presenting with progressively worsening back pain. Axial (**a**) and coronal (**b**) contrast-enhanced CT images show an infrarenal AAA (thin arrows), with several areas with focal discontinuity of the intimal calcifications along the left side of the aneurysm (arrowheads), indicative of aneurysm instability. Additionally, there was a small amount of periaortic stranding along the left aspect of the aneurysm (thick arrows) and a rounded area of fissuring within the mural thrombus (asterisks)

**Fig. 4** Tangential calcium sign in three different patients presenting with unstable AAAs. Axial non-contrast CT images in three different patients (**a**, **b**, and **c**, respectively) show linear areas of calcification in the aortic wall that course in a tangent to the expected contour of a circle (arrows), indicative of focal weakening of the aortic wall. Note the focal eccentric bulge of the aortic contour between the tangential calcifications (arrowheads), a relatively common finding in this setting. A schematic of the tangential calcium sign (**d**) shows wall calcifications following the tangent (dashed line) of the aortic circle, rather than continuing as an arc

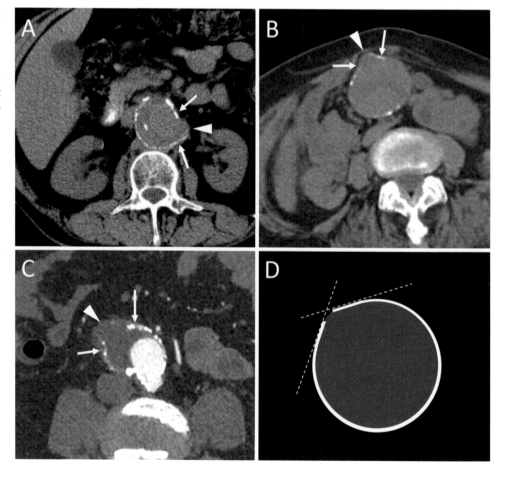

with tangential calcification is a "focal eccentric bulge" (Fig. 4a–c) [12].

Mild periaortic fat stranding is an extraluminal feature which may indicate AAA instability and may correspond to minimal retroperitoneal hemorrhage or edema (Fig. 5) [7, 13]. This finding is most helpful when seen in conjunction with additional features of aneurysm instability, as retroperitoneal edema is a nonspecific finding and may be seen in

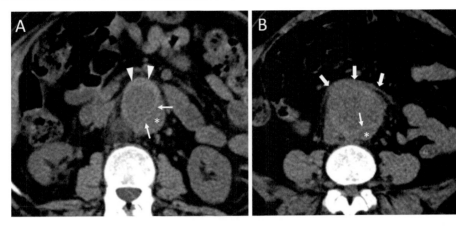

**Fig. 5** Periaortic fat stranding in a 61-year-old woman with type B aortic dissection and AAA presenting with abdominal pain. Axial non-contrast CT images at two levels through the AAA (**a** and **b**, respectively) show an intimomedial flap within the aortic lumen (thin arrows), in keeping with known aortic dissection (true lumen is denoted by asterisks). High-attenuation crescent is present along the anterior wall of the false lumen (arrowheads, **a**), and periaortic fat stranding is seen anterior to the aneurysm (thick arrows, **b**), both indicative of aneurysm instability

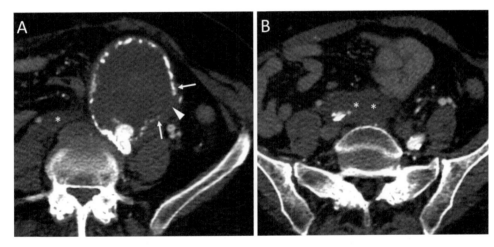

**Fig. 6** Aneurysm rupture in a 70-year-old woman presenting with abdominal pain. Sequential contrast-enhanced axial CT images (**a** and **b**) show a large AAA, with tangential calcifications along the left side of the aneurysm sac (thin arrows, **a**) and focal discontinuity of the intimal calcifications (arrowhead, **a**). Retroperitoneal hemorrhage is identified in the right retroperitoneum (asterisk, **a**), which tracks into the pelvis (asterisks, **b**), diagnostic of aneurysm rupture

volume overload. Furthermore, periaortic fat stranding is also a common feature of infectious aortitis, which will be discussed in further detail in a following section.

## Rupture

The most common imaging feature of aneurysm rupture is retroperitoneal hematoma adjacent to an AAA (Fig. 6) [8]. Hemorrhage associated with aneurysm rupture is readily identified on CT as high-density fluid (i.e., Hounsfield units of 40–80) abutting the AAA and insinuating along retroperitoneal fascial planes. Occasionally, active contrast extravasation into the hematoma is evident on contrast-enhanced CT and is indicative of active bleeding (Fig. 7). In patients with AAA rupture, the findings of aneurysm instability described above (hyperattenuating crescent, discontinuous calcium, tangential calcium) are often coexistent [7].

Although AAA rupture generally presents in the acute setting, patients may infrequently present with contained rupture in the subacute or chronic setting. Draping of the abdominal aorta against the adjacent vertebral bodies and/or musculature (i.e., draped aorta sign) is indicative of a deficient posterior aortic wall and is an imaging feature of contained rupture (Fig. 8) [14]. Flattening or scalloping of the adjacent vertebral body can occur in the setting of contained rupture if chronic [15]. It is important to differentiate the smooth vertebral body remodeling in chronic contained rupture from irregular erosion occurring in the setting of infection or neoplasm [6].

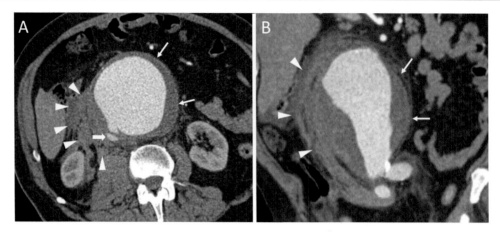

**Fig. 7** Ruptured aneurysm with active extravasation in a 74-year-old man presenting with abdominal pain and pulsatile abdominal mass. Axial (**a**) and coronal (**b**) contrast-enhanced CT images show a large AAA (thin arrows) and moderate volume right retroperitoneal hematoma (arrowheads), consistent with rupture. Active contrast extravasation is identified along the right posterolateral margin of the aneurysm sac (thick arrow, **a**). This aneurysm also demonstrates a large patent lumen and low thrombus-to-lumen ratio

**Fig. 8** Chronic contained rupture as manifested by a draped aorta in a 65-year-old man. Non-contrast axial CT image at the level of L1 (**a**) and non-contrast sagittal CT image (**b**) show a suprarenal AAA (thin arrows) which is "draped" against the L1 and L2 lumbar vertebral bodies (arrowheads), as suggested by an unidentifiable posterior aortic wall which follows the contour of the vertebral body

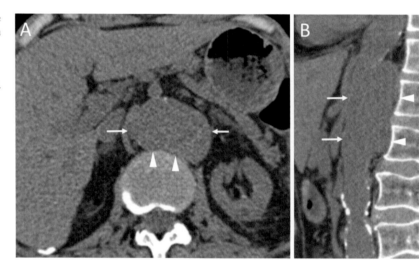

## Complications of Aneurysm Repair

Repair of an AAA can be performed with an open approach using a synthetic graft or an endovascular approach using a stent graft (i.e., endovascular aneurysm repair, EVAR) [4]. Open aortic repair carries a higher risk of perioperative mortality but is associated with lower complications, fewer re-interventions, and reduced long-term mortality [16]. Patients after EVAR require lifetime imaging surveillance due to the higher rate of complications and secondary rupture, a practice not typically performed after open repair. A broad assortment of complications can affect patients after open repair and EVAR, some of which occur in the immediate postoperative setting and others of which may present many years after the original repair. Most of these complications present acutely, and the radiologist must be knowledgeable about the normal postoperative appearance and most commonly encountered complications affecting both types of surgical repair.

## Open Repair

During open AAA repair, a bifurcated graft is anastomosed to normal aorta proximally and the common iliac arteries distally, and the aneurysm sac is closed around the graft (i.e., "aneurysmorrhaphy") [17]. The aneurysm sac should decrease in size within 6 months and is often completely collapsed around the graft within several years. The most frequently reported complication after open AAA repair is anastomotic pseudoaneurysm, which affects 1–10% of patients [18]. On CT, this manifests as a saccular outpouching of the abdominal aorta or a common iliac artery at the proximal or distal attachment sites, respectively (Fig. 9).

A feared complication after open AAA repair is aortoenteric fistula, complicating 0.3–2.5% of repairs, which carries a mortality rate of up to 50% [18]. The most common presentation of aortoenteric fistula is small volume or intermittent gastrointestinal (GI) bleeding (i.e., herald bleed) followed by massive GI hemorrhage. Fistulization

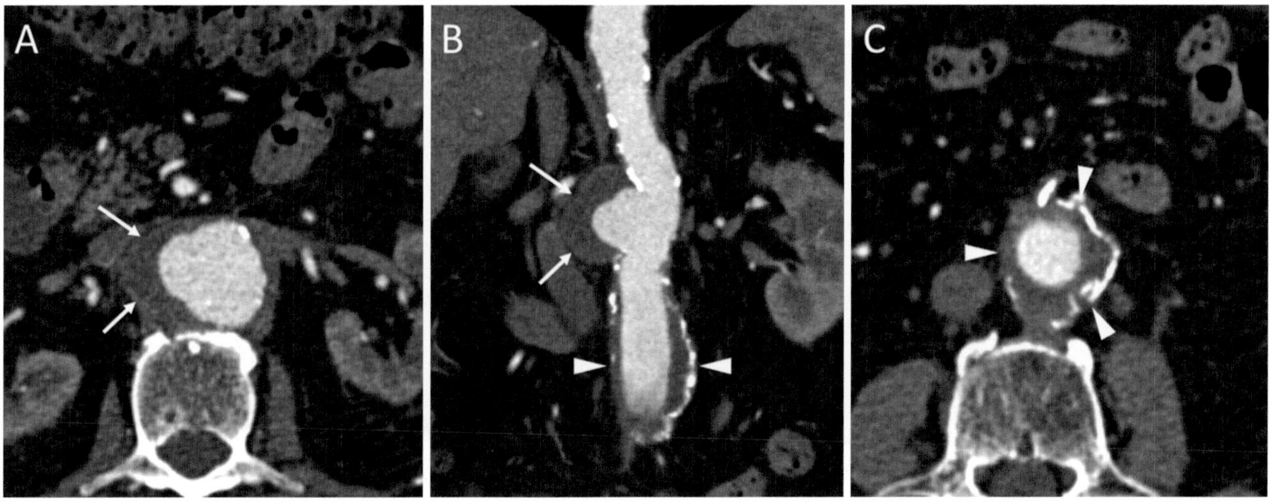

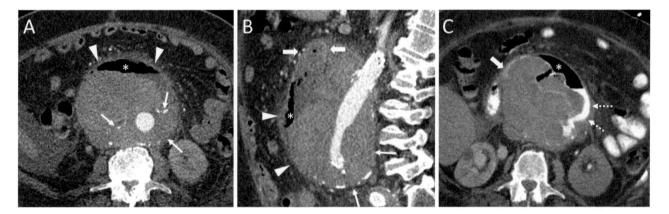

**Fig. 9** Proximal anastomotic pseudoaneurysm in an 80-year-old man with prior open repair of an AAA. Contrast-enhanced CT images at the level of the proximal anastomosis in the axial (**a**) and coronal CT planes (**b**) show a saccular outpouching arising from the right side of the abdominal aorta (arrows), diagnostic of a proximal anastomotic pseudo-aneurysm. An axial CT image more inferiorly (**c**) shows changes of prior open abdominal aortic repair consisting of a decompressed aortic sac (arrowheads) wrapped around the opacified graft

**Fig. 10** Aortoenteric fistula in a 60-year-old man with an AAA which was initially treated with endovascular repair and subsequently managed with open conversion repair, who presented with upper GI bleeding. Axial (**a**) and coronal (**b**) contrast-enhanced CT images show an AAA with changes of prior open repair (thin solid arrows). Adjacent to the aneurysm sac was a large perigraft hematoma (arrowheads) containing gas (asterisks). The transverse duodenum was tethered to the perigraft hematoma and had an indistinct inferior wall (thick arrows, **b**). Due to concern for aortoenteric fistula, subsequent axial CT image obtained with oral contrast (**c**) shows extraluminal leakage of oral contrast into the perigraft hematoma and aneurysm sac (thin dashed arrows), diag-nostic of an aortoenteric fistula. He was treated with duodenectomy, evacuation of the aortic hematoma, and omental wrapping of the aortoiliac graft

usually occurs between the aneurysm sac and transverse duodenum, and CT findings include loss of the normal fat plane and/or tethering between bowel and the aneurysm sac, disruption of the aortic wall, and gas within the aneurysm sac (Fig. 10). Infrequently, extraluminal leakage of oral contrast into the aneurysm sac may be observed (Fig. 10c). Aortoenteric fistula is treated with graft excision and extra-anatomic bypass owing to contamination of the aorta and graft with enteric bacteria, typically in an urgent fashion to prevent or treat massive GI hemorrhage. In the rare patients who develop pancreatitis in the postoperative setting, pancreatitis-related fluid collections can also fistulize to the aneurysm sac (i.e., aortopancreatic fistula) [19]. CT features

of aortopancreatic fistula include macroscopic fat within the aneurysm sac, loss of a fat plane between the aneurysm sac and the pancreas, and increase in size of the aneurysm sac (Fig. 11).

Infection of the aortic graft is another infrequently encountered complication, affecting 0.2–2% of patients after open repair [18]. Periaortic fat stranding, gas in the excluded aneurysm sac, and adjacent lymphadenopathy are highly suggestive of graft infection (Fig. 12). However, a small amount of gas in the aneurysm sac is normal within the first 4 weeks after surgical repair. Finally, graft thrombo-sis after AAA repair is an uncommon complication reported in less than 1% of patients [18]. Patients with graft

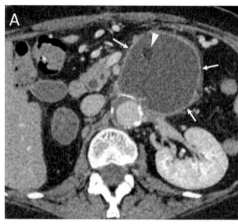
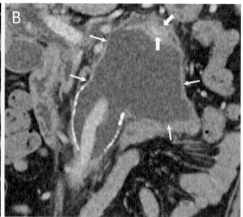

**Fig. 11** Aortopancreatic fistula in a 64-year-old woman with AAA status post open repair 1 month prior, presenting with abdominal pain. Axial (**a**) and coronal (**b**) contrast-enhanced CT images show changes of open repair, with increase in size of the excluded aneurysm sac (thin arrows). The aneurysm sac contained a locule of macroscopic fat (arrowhead, **a**) and abutted the inferior margin of the pancreas (thick arrows, **b**), highly suggestive of a fistulous connection between the aneurysm sac and a walled off necrotic collection, presumably sequela of recent necrotizing pancreatitis. This was managed conservatively, and the size of the excluded aneurysm sac decreased over multiple subsequent evaluations (not shown)

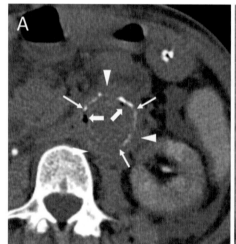
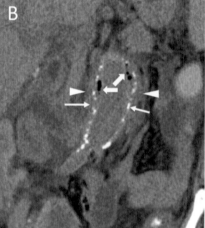
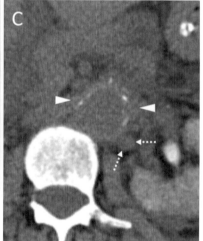

**Fig. 12** Infected abdominal aortic graft after open repair 2 years ago in a 61-year-old woman presenting with sepsis. Axial (**a**) and coronal (**b**) non-contrast CT images demonstrate changes of prior open AAA repair (thin arrows), with extensive periaortic stranding surrounding the aneurysm sac (arrowheads). Additionally, multiple foci of gas were present within the excluded aneurysm (thick arrows). Axial non-contrast CT image more superiorly (**c**) depicts a mildly enlarged retroperitoneal lymph node (dashed arrows). These findings were highly concerning for graft infection, which was confirmed at the time of surgery. Cultures from the aortic graft grew *Streptococcus anginosus*

thrombosis usually present acutely with symptoms of lower extremity malperfusion. Lack of IV contrast opacification within the graft is diagnostic (Fig. 13).

## Endovascular Repair

EVAR consists of endovascular placement of an aortobiiliac stent graft across the AAA, with the proximal attachment site in the abdominal aorta above the aneurysm and distal attachment sites typically in the common iliac arteries [20]. Similar to open repair, the AAA should slowly decrease in size after EVAR. The most common complication after EVAR is endoleak, defined as persistent blood

flow within the excluded aneurysm sac, encountered in 15–25% of patients within 1 month after EVAR [21]. Fortunately, most endoleaks are type II (i.e., retrograde blood flow from patent collateral vessel such as the inferior mesenteric artery or a lumbar artery) and are low flow, uncommonly resulting in pressurization of the aneurysm sac. These are usually managed conservatively unless the excluded AAA is increasing in size. High-flow endoleaks are more commonly associated with aortic rupture due to greater aortic sac pressurization (Fig. 14). These include type I endoleaks in which the AAA is not excluded at the proximal (type IA) or distal (type IB) attachment site and

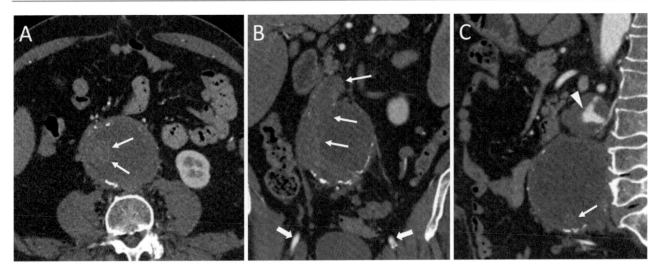

**Fig. 13** Graft thrombosis in a 65-year-old man who underwent prior open repair of an infrarenal AAA, who presented with bilateral foot numbness and pain, and who had no detectable pulses in the lower extremity on physical examination. Axial (**a**), coronal (**b**), and sagittal (**c**) contrast-enhanced CT images show no flow within the aortobiiliac graft (thin arrows), diagnostic of graft thrombosis. Contrast is seen within the aorta proximal to the graft anastomosis (arrowhead, **c**), and the common femoral arteries are reconstituted (thick arrows, **b**) via epigastric and circumflex iliac collaterals (not shown)

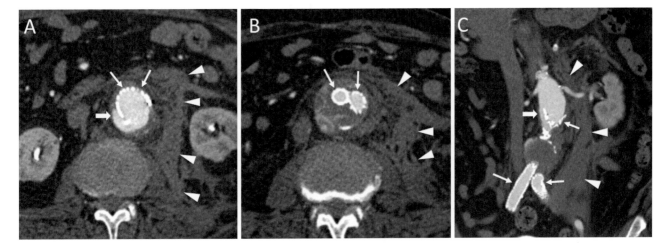

**Fig. 14** Type IA endoleak with rupture in an 80-year-old man with AAA status post endovascular repair 6 years prior. Axial contrast-enhanced CT images at the level of the proximal attachment site (**a**) and iliac limbs (**b**) show an aortobiiliac endovascular stent graft (thin arrows) with perigraft flow along the right lateral and posterior margins of the proximal attachment site (thick arrow, **a**), consistent with type IA endoleak. Coronal contrast-enhanced CT image (**c**) shows lack of apposition between the proximal endovascular graft and aorta, consistent with type IA endoleak (thick arrow, **c**). Extensive left retroperitoneal hemorrhage is present (arrowheads), diagnostic of rupture

type III endoleaks in which there is an ineffective seal between graft components.

Stent graft kinking is another relatively common complication, which occurs in up to 4% of patients after EVAR [22]. Kinking often presents with subtle angulation of one or more of the stent graft components, which can be difficult to appreciate when comparing two exams in close temporal proximity. Comparison with the initial post-stent graft CT and creation of maximum intensity projection (MIP) images are often helpful in identifying subtle changes. When occurring in the setting of component migration, stent kinking can progress to type I or III endoleak (Fig. 15). Kinking of a stent graft can also lead to thrombosis of a limb. Limb thrombosis is reported in up to 5% of patients after EVAR [23], with or without coexistent kinking.

Stent graft infection after EVAR is similar to or slightly less common than graft infection after open repair and is reported in 0.2–0.7% of patients [24]. Similar to infection after open repair, CT findings of stent graft infection include periaortic fat stranding, gas in the excluded aneurysm sac, and adjacent lymphadenopathy [25]. A small amount of gas is normal in the excluded aneurysm sac within the first 4 weeks after EVAR, provided there are no additional imaging or clinical findings supportive of infection.

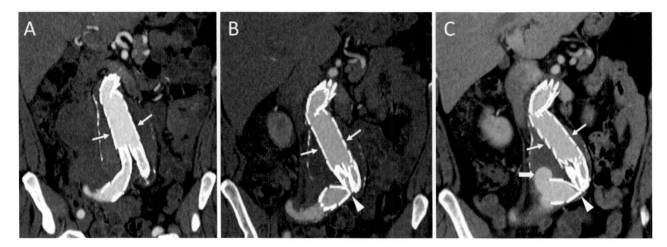

**Fig. 15** Endovascular stent graft kinking and type IB endoleak in a 53-year-old man with an AAA status post endovascular repair. Coronal contrast-enhanced CT images demonstrate the appearance of the endovascular stent (arrows) 1 month (**a**), 6 months (**b**), and 12 months (**c**) after endovascular repair. On the 6-month follow-up study, there is new kinking of the right iliac limb (arrowhead, **b**) secondary to proximal migration of the distal attachment site. At 12 months, there is progressive kinking of the right iliac limb (arrowhead, **c**) and new contrast opacification of the aneurysm sac related to incomplete opposition of the distal attachment site of the right iliac limb, consistent with type IB endoleak

## Aortitis/Periaortitis

Inflammation involving the aortic wall (i.e., aortitis) or peri-aortic soft tissues (i.e., periaortitis) can be categorized as infectious or noninfectious in etiology.

## Infectious Aortitis

Infectious aortitis is usually secondary to bacterial infection, with *Staphylococcus aureus* and *Salmonella* species representing the most common pathogens [26]. Hematogenous or direct retroperitoneal spread of a coexisting infection may occur, with the former being more common [27]. Site of preexisting aortic disease such as AAA and atherosclerotic disease is more susceptible to infection than the normal aortic wall, which is relatively resistant to infection [26]. Patients with infectious aortitis often present in the acute setting with abdominal or back pain, fever, malaise, and leukocytosis. Blood cultures are frequently positive, although up to 30% of patients will be culture negative [28].

Early findings of infectious aortitis on CT include aortic wall thickening, periaortic soft tissue stranding, adjacent reactive lymphadenopathy, and occasionally gas in the aortic wall or periaortic soft tissues [29]. As the infection progresses and destroys the aortic wall, a saccular pseudoaneurysm (i.e., infectious pseudoaneurysm) develops, often enlarging rapidly over days to weeks (Fig. 16). 18F-fluorodeoxyglucose (FDG) positron emission tomography (PET)/CT may be helpful in the diagnosis of infectious aortitis, which often shows significantly greater FDG uptake than noninfectious aortitis [30].

## Noninfectious Aortitis

Noninfectious aortitis and periaortitis is comprised of a variety of clinical entities including large-vessel vasculitis such as Takayasu and Giant cell arteritis, medium- and small-vessel vasculitis with secondary aortic involvement, radiation-induced aortitis, and idiopathic conditions such as retroperitoneal fibrosis (RPF) [26]. The most common CT manifestation of noninfectious aortitis is concentric thickening of the aortic wall (Fig. 17). Large-vessel vasculitis often involves the thoracic aorta to a greater extent than the abdominal aorta and is associated with aortic luminal narrowing and branch vascular occlusion [7]. In contrast, RPF, also known as chronic periaortitis, is characterized by more exuberant periaortic soft tissue and fibrosis and commonly involves the infrarenal abdominal aorta [31]. Although RPF may occur secondary to certain drugs or malignancy, many cases of idiopathic RPF are associated with immunoglobulin G4 (IgG4)-related disease [32]. Although noninfectious aortitis and periaortitis rarely present acutely, it is important to differentiate these entities from infectious aortitis.

## Inflammatory AAA

Inflammatory AAA is a closely related pathophysiologic entity to RPF that is depicted by an AAA and a mantle of fibrotic periaortic soft tissue, characteristically distributed along the anterolateral walls of the aneurysm with sparing of the posterior wall (Fig. 18) [33]. The periaortic soft tissue is often smooth and well defined and enhances after administration of IV contrast, in contradistinction to periaortic hematoma associated with aneurysm rupture which has irregular borders and is non-enhancing. Inflammatory AAA is treated in a similar manner to conventional AAA, although a retroperitoneal approach is often used if open surgical repair is performed [4].

**Fig. 16** Infectious aortitis with pseudoaneurysm in a 63-year-old man who underwent recent right lower lobectomy for squamous cell carcinoma. Initial contrast-enhanced coronal CT image (**a**) shows a saccular morphology to the eccentrically and irregularly dilated infrarenal aorta (thin arrows, **a**) with periaortic stranding (arrowheads, **a**), suspicious for an infectious pseudoaneurysm. Subsequent contrast-enhanced coronal CT image obtained 6 days later (**b**) shows increase in size of the irregular saccular pseudoaneurysm (thin arrows, **b**) and progression of periaortic stranding (arrowheads, **b**). Axial CT image of the chest (**c**) shows a right basilar empyema related to recent lobectomy. Axial fused PET-CT image (**d**) shows markedly increased FDG uptake associated with the infectious pseudoaneurysm (dashed arrows, **d**). Blood cultures grew *Propionibacterium (Cutibacterium) acnes*

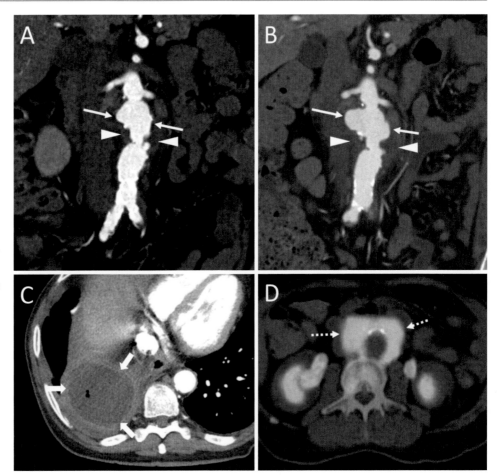

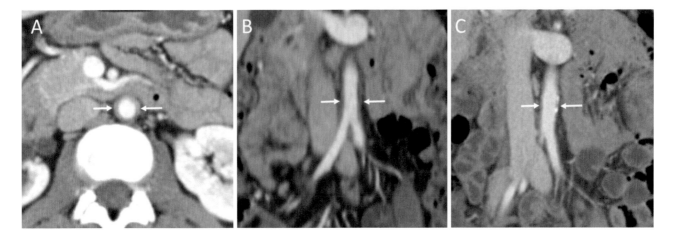

**Fig. 17** Takayasu arteritis in a 30-year-old woman with HIV presenting with abdominal pain. Axial (**a**) and coronal (**b**) contrast-enhanced CT images demonstrate long segment circumferential wall thickening of the infrarenal abdominal aorta extending into the proximal iliac arteries, highly suggestive of an inflammatory aortitis, specifically Takayasu arteritis given the patient's age. She was treated with steroids, and aortic wall thickening improved on follow-up evaluation 9 months later (coronal contrast-enhanced CT image [**c**], arrows)

## Acute Aortic Syndrome

Acute aortic syndrome includes penetrating atherosclerotic ulcer (PAU), intramural hematoma (IMH), and aortic dissection. A hallmark of these entities is disruption of the integrity of the aortic wall [34]. PAUs are focal entities which may occur within the abdominal aorta alone, while IMH and aortic dissection almost always originate in the thoracic aorta and secondarily extend into the abdominal aorta. Acute aortic

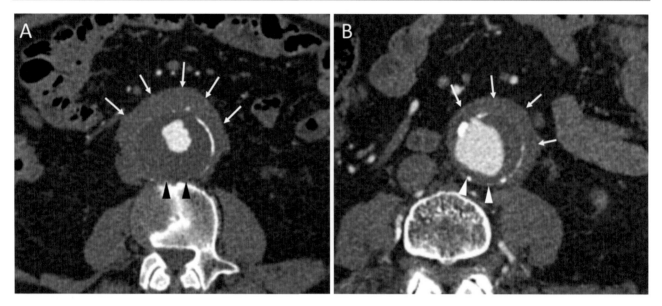

**Fig. 18** Inflammatory AAA in two different patients. Axial contrast-enhanced CT images in two different patients (**a** and **b**, respectively) show a mantle of soft tissue that surrounds the AAA (arrows) and characteristically spares the posterior wall (arrowheads). Delayed-phase images, when obtained, depict enhancement of this soft tissue (not shown), in contradistinction to periaortic hematoma which does not enhance

**Fig. 19** PAU detected incidentally in a 77-year-old man undergoing evaluation for a lung cancer. Axial (**a**) and coronal (**b**) contrast-enhanced CT images demonstrate a focal outpouching of the infrarenal abdominal aorta (arrows), which extends beyond the expected contour of the aortic wall, consistent with a PAU. Note the extensive calcified and noncalcified atherosclerosis involving the infrarenal abdominal aorta (arrowheads)

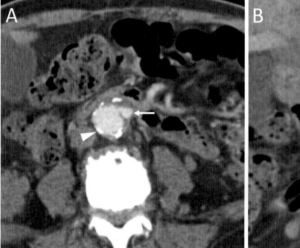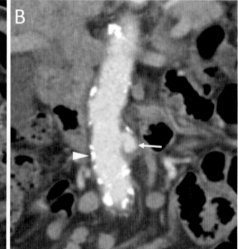

syndromes frequently present in the acute setting, and prompt diagnosis and identification of complications is important due to the high associated morbidity if not urgently treated.

## PAU

PAU is characterized by an ulceration through the intima and into the media, with a saccular outpouching beyond the expected contour of the aorta, in the setting of preexisting atherosclerotic disease (Fig. 19). Although most PAUs occur in the descending thoracic aorta, up to 30% affect the abdominal aorta [35]. PAUs may present acutely in association with chest or abdominal pain; however, an increasing number are

found incidentally during imaging for other reasons. In the chronic setting, remodeling of the aortic wall may lead to a saccular dilatation of the aorta [7]. Surgical management, consisting of EVAR or open repair, is performed for PAUs associated with refractory symptoms, a saccular configuration, and/or rupture [35].

## IMH

IMH is defined as hematoma within the aortic wall that does not communicate with the aortic lumen and is thought to be secondary to rupture of the vasa vasorum [36]. On non-contrast CT, IMH manifests as a crescentic area of high-attenuation wall thickening, almost always involving the thoracic aorta and frequently extending inferiorly to involve the abdominal aorta [37]. Intimal calcifications, when present, are displaced inward, in contradistinction to mural thrombus which forms on the luminal side of the calcified intima. The natural history of IMH is variable, and it may progress to dissection and/or rupture or may stabilize and progressively resolve. A specific feature associated with IMH progression is an ulcer-like projection (ULP), also known as a focal intimal disruption [38]. On contrast-enhanced CT, a fingerlike projection of contrast extending from the aortic lumen into the IMH with a communicating orifice > 3 mm is diagnostic of a ULP (Fig. 20). ULPs should be distinguished from intramural blood pools (i.e., tiny intimal disruptions), which are associated with intercostal or lumbar artery ostia and may have tiny (i.e., ≤3 mm) communications with the aortic lumen, and are of no prognostic significance. ULPs should also be distinguished from PAU; the former does not distort the external contour of the aorta, whereas the latter is characterized by a focal outpouching of the aortic contour.

### Aortic Dissection

Aortic dissection results from an entry tear in the intima of the aortic wall that allows pressurized blood to enter the media, with resultant anterograde and/or retrograde propagation of blood to create a false lumen [39]. Similar to IMH, isolated involvement of the abdominal aorta is rare. Accordingly, nearly all aortic dissections involving the abdominal aorta originate in the thoracic aorta and propagate antegrade. On contrast-enhanced CT, an intimomedial dissection flap separates the true and false lumen, often accompanied by one or more tears or fenestrations allowing communication between the true and false lumen [39]. The true lumen can be distinguished by its outer wall and/or eccentric flap calcifications, whereas the false lumen is typically larger and harbors an acute angle between the dissection flap and its outer wall (i.e., beak sign) [40].

A feared complication of dissection involving the abdominal aorta is visceral malperfusion, an important cause of morbidity and mortality. Ischemia may be related to static or dynamic occlusion of visceral vasculature. In static ischemia, the dissection flap extends into the origin of the branch vessels, whereas in dynamic ischemia the dissection flap transiently obstructs the ostium of a branch vessel due to oscillatory increases in pressure in the false lumen over the cardiac cycle [41].

### Acute Aortic Occlusion

Acute occlusion of the abdominal aorta may occur due to in situ thrombus in the setting of atherosclerosis or hypercoagulable state or may be the result of a saddle embolus to the aortic bifurcation (Fig. 21) [42]. Patients present acutely with symptoms and clinical findings of lower extremity ischemia. In contrast to chronic aortic occlusion, prominent collateral vessels are generally absent. Outcomes are poor despite emergent thrombectomy or aorto-bifemoral bypass, and overall survival is less than 50% [43].

### Medium Vessels

Acute pathology involving the medium-sized vessels of the abdomen, specifically the major visceral arteries and their branches, is relatively common in clinical practice. These conditions fall under the general categories of vasculitis, SAM, pseudoaneurysm, and occlusion.

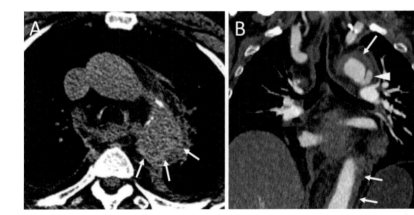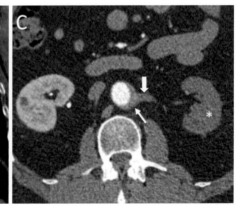

**Fig. 20** Ruptured type B IMH with a ULP and devitalization of the left kidney in a 59-year-old man presenting with chest pain. Non-contrast axial CT images at the level of the aortic arch (**a**) show a crescentic area of hyperattenuation within the wall of the proximal descending thoracic aorta (thin arrows), consistent with a type B IMH. Contrast opacification is seen within the IMH which has a clear communication with the aortic lumen (arrowhead), diagnostic of a ULP, seen to better advantage on coronal contrast-enhanced CT image (**b**). Axial contrast-enhanced CT image through the abdomen (**c**) demonstrates inferior extension of the IMH (thin arrow) into the abdominal aorta to the level of the left renal artery which is occluded (thick arrow). As a result, the left kidney no longer enhances (asterisk, **c**)

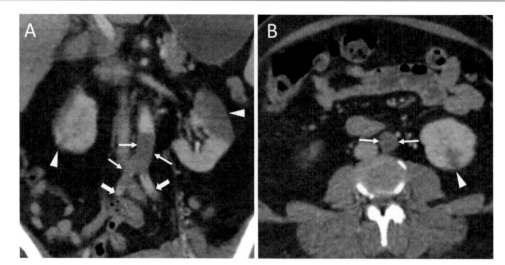

**Fig. 21** Acute aortic occlusion in a 47-year-old woman presenting with bilateral leg pain, numbness, and weakness. Coronal (**a**) and axial (**b**) contrast-enhanced CT images show acute thrombosis of the infrarenal abdominal aorta which extends into the right common iliac artery (thin arrows). There is prompt reconstitution with flow seen in both common iliac arteries (thick arrows, **a**). Notice the presence of bilateral renal infarcts (arrowheads). The patient was taken to the operating room for emergent thrombectomy, and the occlusion was presumed secondary to a hypercoagulable state

## Vasculitis

Vasculitides which primarily involve medium-sized vessels include polyarteritis nodosa (PAN) and Kawasaki disease, although the latter is uncommon after the age of 5 and most frequently involves the coronary arteries [44]. PAN is a necrotizing vasculitis affecting the visceral and renal vasculature, which is depicted on CT as vascular wall thickening, luminal irregularity or stenosis, occlusions, and multiple small aneurysms (Fig. 22). Although commonly idiopathic, PAN is associated with several viral infections including hepatitis B [45]. Small-vessel vasculitides can secondarily involve medium-sized vessels, most commonly microscopic polyangiitis (MPA). The presence of antineutrophil cytoplasmic antibody (ANCA) is a key differentiating feature of MPA, which is not present in PAN [44]. Large-vessel vasculitis can also involve medium-sized vessels but usually has concomitant aortic involvement [26]. Notably, the imaging features of vasculitis involving the main visceral arteries may overlap with those of SAM [46].

## SAM

SAM is a non-inflammatory vasculopathy characterized histologically by lysis of the smooth muscle of the arterial wall and predominantly affects the mesenteric vasculature [47]. Although the imaging features may overlap with those of vasculitis, clinical and laboratory indicators of systemic inflammation are invariably absent [48]. In the acute setting, SAM may present with spontaneous intra-abdominal hemorrhage. Additional imaging features of SAM include multifocal dissections and aneurysms or pseudoaneurysms, often much larger than those found in PAN (Fig. 23). Although vascular wall thickening, stenosis, and occlusion may occur

in SAM, these features are encountered less commonly than in vasculitis [46].

## Pseudoaneurysm

Pseudoaneurysm (i.e., false aneurysm) is defined by as a break in vascular wall with formation of a saccular outpouching continuous with the blood pool but lacking all of the layers of a normal blood vessel [49]. Imaging depicts the aneurysm morphology (i.e., saccular versus fusiform) but does not readily distinguish pseudoaneurysm from true aneurysm. CT findings that favor pseudoaneurysm include saccular morphology, lack of calcifications or mural thrombus, rapid evolution or enlargement, and surrounding hemorrhage (Fig. 24). The most common causes of atraumatic mesenteric arterial pseudoaneurysm are pancreatitis, infection (i.e., infectious pseudoaneurysms), surgical complication, and SAM. Owing to disruption in the vascular wall, mesenteric arterial pseudoaneurysms have a significant risk of rupture and are generally treated with angiography and coil embolization or stent placement.

## Arterial Thrombosis

Embolic occlusion accounts for most cases of mesenteric arterial thrombosis, which is usually from an intra-cardiac, proximal aortic source, or venous source in a patient with a patent foramen ovale. In situ thrombosis secondary to pre-existing atherosclerotic disease is another less common cause [50]. Embolic occlusion usually occurs more distally within a vessel (i.e., several centimeters from the origin), and underlying atherosclerosis is generally absent (Fig. 25), whereas in situ thrombosis is commonly found at or near the vessel origin. If an embolic etiology is suspected, the heart and aorta should be carefully evaluated to identify an embolic source (Fig. 25a).

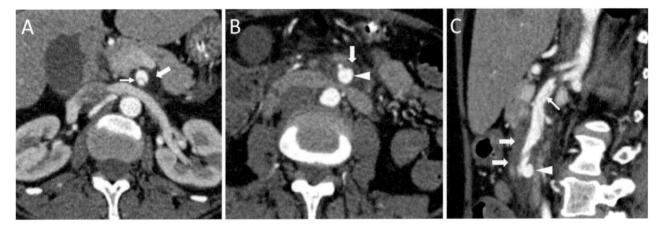

**Fig. 22** Mesenteric vasculitis in a 61-year-old man with abdominal pain and weight loss. Sequential axial (**a** and **b**) and coronal (**c**) contrast-enhanced CT images demonstrate segmental circumferential soft tissue thickening involving the celiac artery (arrows) and proximal superior mesenteric artery (arrowheads), highly suggestive of vasculitis. The patient was clinically felt to have PAN and initiated on steroid therapy

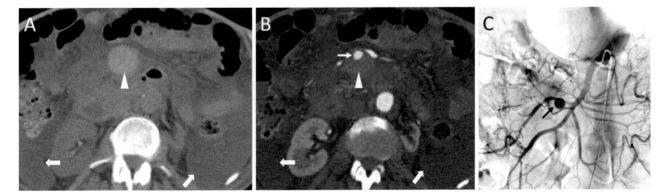

**Fig. 23** SAM presenting as superior mesenteric artery dissection and pseudoaneurysm in a 54-year-old woman presenting with tearing abdominal pain. Axial (**a** and **b**) and sagittal (**c**) contrast-enhanced CT images show a dissection involving the superior mesenteric artery (thin arrows). More distally in the superior mesenteric artery, there is a saccular outpouching of contrast consistent with a pseudoaneurysm (arrowheads). Soft tissue thickening and/or hematoma is seen tracking around the superior mesenteric artery (thick arrows). Rheumatologic evaluation was unremarkable, and findings were presumed secondary to SAM

**Fig. 24** Post-pancreatitis pseudoaneurysm in a 59-year-old man undergoing evaluation for dropping hemoglobin in the setting of acute on chronic pancreatitis. Axial non-contrast CT image (**a**) demonstrates a rounded hematoma in the mesentery (arrowheads), and axial contrast-enhanced CT image (**b**) depicts a pseudoaneurysm arising from the right colic artery (thin white arrow). Note is also made of moderate volume ascites (thick arrows). Catheter angiography (**c**) confirms the presence of a pseudoaneurysm (thin black arrow), which was treated with coil embolization (not shown)

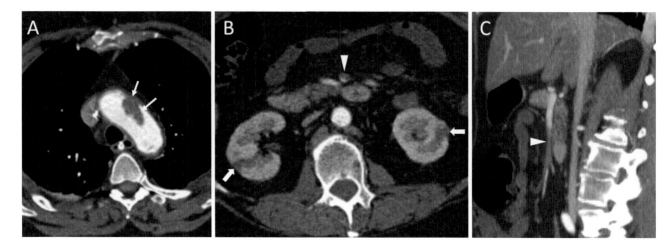

**Fig. 25** Superior mesenteric artery embolism in a 62-year-old woman with a thoracic aortic mobile thrombus. Axial contrast-enhanced CT image of the chest (**a**) demonstrates a large pedunculated intraluminal thrombus arising from the anterior aspect of the proximal aortic arch (thin arrows, **a**). Axial (**b**) and sagittal (**c**) contrast-enhanced CT images through the abdomen demonstrate an embolism in the mid- to distal superior mesenteric artery. Small bilateral renal infarcts are also present (thick arrows, **b**). The patient was taken to the operating room for urgent thrombectomy

## Conclusion/Summary

Acute nontraumatic abdominal vascular pathology is common, and effective management is based on prompt diagnosis. CT angiography is preferred for evaluating acute vascular pathology in the emergent setting, but MRA may be used in carefully selected patients. Although AAA is frequently encountered in practice, findings of aneurysm instability or rupture may be subtle but are important to identify. The most common complications after open AAA repair are anastomotic pseudoaneurysm, aortoenteric and aortopancreatic fistula, graft infection, and thrombosis. After endovascular repair, important complications include endoleak, rupture, stent kinking, thrombosis, and infection. Aortitis and periaortitis can occur due to a variety of causes, although infectious aortitis is most concerning and can progress rapidly, resulting in infectious pseudoaneurysm and rupture. Acute aortic occlusion, while uncommon, is associated with high morbidity and mortality. Acute pathology affects the medium-sized abdominal vessels including vasculitis, SAM, pseudoaneurysm, and occlusion. Complications of medium-vessel pathology present acutely and include hemorrhage and visceral ischemia. Emergent vascular conditions are readily depicted on noninvasive imaging, and accurate diagnosis is essential.

## References

1. Bae KT. Intravenous contrast medium administration and scan timing at CT: considerations and approaches. Radiology. 2010;256 (1):32–61.
2. Laissy JP, Trillaud H, Douek P. MR angiography: noninvasive vascular imaging of the abdomen. Abdom Imaging. 2002;27(5): 488–506.
3. Kent KC. Clinical practice. Abdominal aortic aneurysms. N Engl J Med. 2014;371(22):2101–8.
4. Newman JD, Motiwala A, Turin A, Chen A, Maharaj VR, Dieter RS. Abdominal aortic aneurysms. In: Diseases of the aorta. Springer; 2019. p. 199–216.
5. Parkinson F, Ferguson S, Lewis P, Williams IM, Twine CP. South East Wales Vascular Network. Rupture rates of untreated large abdominal aortic aneurysms in patients unfit for elective repair. J Vasc Surg. 2015;61(6):1606–12.
6. Wadgaonkar AD, Black JH, Weihe EK, Zimmerman SL, Fishman EK, Johnson PT. Abdominal aortic aneurysms revisited: MDCT with multiplanar reconstructions for identifying indicators of instability in the pre- and postoperative patient. Radiographics. 2015 Feb;35(1):254–68.
7. Curtis W, Yano M. Acute non-traumatic disease of the abdominal aorta. Abdom Radiol (NY). 2018;43(5):1067–83.
8. Siegel CL, Cohan RH, Korobkin M, Alpern MB, Courneya DL, Leder RA. Abdominal aortic aneurysm morphology: CT features in patients with ruptured and nonruptured aneurysms. AJR Am J Roentgenol. 1994;163(5):1123–9.
9. Arita T, Matsunaga N, Takano K, Nagaoka S, Nakamura H, Katayama S, et al. Abdominal aortic aneurysm: rupture associated with the high-attenuating crescent sign. Radiology. 1997;204(3): 765–8.
10. Torres W, Maurer D, Steinberg H, Robbins S, Bernardino M. CT of aortic aneurysms: the distinction between mural and thrombus calcification. Am J Roentgenol. 1988;150(6):1317–9.
11. Pillari G, Chang JB, Zito J, Cohen JR, Gersten K, Rizzo A, et al. Computed tomography of abdominal aortic aneurysm: an in vivo pathological report with a note on dynamic predictors. Arch Surg. 1988;123(6):727–32.
12. Hunter GC, Leong SC, Yu GS, McIntyre KE, Bernhard VM. Aortic blebs: possible site of aneurysm rupture. J Vasc Surg. 1989;10(1): 93–9.
13. Vu K-N, Kaitoukov Y, Morin-Roy F, Kauffmann C, Giroux M-F, Thérasse É, et al. Rupture signs on computed tomography, treatment, and outcome of abdominal aortic aneurysms. Insights Imaging. 2014;5(3):281–93.
14. Halliday KE, al-Kutoubi A. Draped aorta: CT sign of contained leak of aortic aneurysms. Radiology. 1996;199(1):41–3.
15. Apter S, Rimon U, Konen E, Erlich Z, Guranda L, Amitai M, et al. Sealed rupture of abdominal aortic aneurysms: CT features in

6 patients and a review of the literature. Abdom Imaging. 2010;35 (1):99–105.

16. Badger S, Forster R, Blair PH, Ellis P, Kee F, Harkin DW. Endovascular treatment for ruptured abdominal aortic aneurysm. Cochrane Database Syst Rev. 2017;26. 5:CD005261

17. Powell AR, Crowl G, Kashyap VS. Surgical treatment of the abdominal aorta. In: Diseases of the aorta. Springer; 2019. p. 293–306.

18. van Zeeland ML, van der Laan L. Late complications following aortic aneurysm repair. Diagnosis, Screening and Treatment of Abdominal, Thoracoabdominal and Thoracic Aortic Aneurysms; 2011. p. 211.

19. Tsai R, Sanchez LA, Yano M. Computed tomography identifies clinically unsuspected acute necrotizing pancreatitis complicating abdominal aortic repair. Ann Vasc Surg. 2020.

20. Buck DB, van Herwaarden JA, Schermerhorn ML, Moll FL. Endovascular treatment of abdominal aortic aneurysms. Nat Rev Cardiol. 2014;11(2):112–23.

21. Liaw JVP, Clark M, Gibbs R, Jenkins M, Cheshire N, Hamady M. Update: complications and management of infrarenal EVAR. Eur J Radiol. 2009;71(3):541–51.

22. Fransen GAJ, Desgranges P, Laheij RJF, Harris PL, Becquemin J-P, EUROSTAR Collaborators. Frequency, predictive factors, and consequences of stent-graft kink following endovascular AAA repair. J Endovasc Ther. 2003;10(5):913–8.

23. Maleux G, Koolen M, Heye S. Complications after endovascular aneurysm repair. Semin Intervent Radiol. 2009;26(1):3–9.

24. Hobbs SD, Kumar S, Gilling-Smith GL. Epidemiology and diagnosis of endograft infection. J Cardiovasc Surg. 2010;51(1):5.

25. Laser A, Baker N, Rectenwald J, Eliason JL, Criado-Pallares E, Upchurch GR. Graft infection after endovascular abdominal aortic aneurysm repair. J Vasc Surg. 2011;54(1):58–63.

26. Restrepo CS, Ocazionez D, Suri R, Vargas D. Aortitis: imaging spectrum of the infectious and inflammatory conditions of the aorta. RadioGraphics. 2011;31(2):435–51.

27. Mendelowitz DS, Ramstedt R, Yao JS, Bergan JJ. Abdominal aortic salmonellosis. Surgery. 1979;85(5):514–9.

28. Sekar N. Primary aortic infections and infected aneurysms. Ann Vasc Dis. 2010;3(1):24–7.

29. Macedo TA, Stanson AW, Oderich GS, Johnson CM, Panneton JM, Tie ML. Infected aortic aneurysms: imaging findings. Radiology. 2004;231(1):250–7.

30. Kim J, Song H-C. Role of PET/CT in the evaluation of aortic disease. Chonnam Med J. 2018;54(3):143–52.

31. Inoue D, Zen Y, Abo H, Gabata T, Demachi H, Yoshikawa J, et al. Immunoglobulin G4–related periaortitis and periarteritis: CT findings in 17 patients. Radiology. 2011;261(2):625–33.

32. Lian L, Wang C, Tian J-L. IgG4-related retroperitoneal fibrosis: a newly characterized disease. Int J Rheum Dis. 2016;19(11):1049–55.

33. Kasashima S, Zen Y. IgG4-related inflammatory abdominal aortic aneurysm, spectrum of IgG4-related chronic periaortitis. Ann Vasc Dis. 2010;3(3):182–9.

34. Corvera JS. Acute aortic syndrome. Ann Cardiothorac Surg. 2016;5 (3):188–93.

35. Nathan DP, Boonn W, Lai E, Wang GJ, Desai N, Woo EY, et al. Presentation, complications, and natural history of penetrating atherosclerotic ulcer disease. J Vasc Surg. 2012 Jan;55(1):10–5.

36. Bonaca MP. Descending aortic dissection, penetrating aortic ulcer, and intramural hematoma (acute and chronic) including Kommerell's diverticulum. In: Diseases of the aorta. Springer; 2019. p. 149–60.

37. Chao CP, Walker TG, Kalva SP. Natural history and CT appearances of aortic intramural hematoma. Radiographics. 2009 Jun;29(3):791–804.

38. Moral S, Cuéllar H, Avegliano G, Ballesteros E, Salcedo MT, Ferreira-González I, et al. Clinical implications of focal intimal disruption in patients with type b intramural hematoma. J Am Coll Cardiol. 2017;69(1):28–39.

39. McMahon MA, Squirrell CA. Multidetector CT of aortic dissection: a pictorial review. RadioGraphics. 2010;30(2):445–60.

40. LePage MA, Quint LE, Sonnad SS, Deeb GM, Williams DM. Aortic dissection: CT features that distinguish true lumen from false lumen. AJR Am J Roentgenol. 2001;177(1):207–11.

41. Meinel FG, Nikolaou K, Weidenhagen R, Hellbach K, Helck A, Bamberg F, et al. Time-resolved CT angiography in aortic dissection. Eur J Radiol. 2012;81(11):3254–61.

42. Olivia G, Anders W, Martin B. Acute aortic occlusion. Circulation. 2019;139(2):292–4.

43. Robinson WP, Patel RK, Columbo JA, Flahive J, Aiello FA, Baril DT, et al. Contemporary management of acute aortic occlusion has evolved but outcomes have not significantly improved. Ann Vasc Surg. 2016;34:178–86.

44. Hur JH, Chun EJ, Kwag HJ, Yoo JY, Kim HY, Kim JJ, et al. CT features of vasculitides based on the 2012 international Chapel Hill consensus conference revised classification. Korean J Radiol. 2017;18(5):786–98.

45. Forbess L, Bannykh S. Polyarteritis nodosa. Rheum Dis Clin N Am. 2015;41(1):33–46. vii

46. Naidu SG, Menias CO, Oklu R, Hines RS, Alhalabi K, Makar G, et al. Segmental arterial mediolysis: abdominal imaging of and disease course in 111 patients. Am J Roentgenol. 2018;210(4):899–905.

47. Slavin RE. Segmental arterial mediolysis: course, sequelae, prognosis, and pathologic-radiologic correlation. Cardiovasc Pathol. 2009;18(6):352–60.

48. Baker-LePain JC, Stone DH, Mattis A, Nakamura MC, Fye KH. Clinical diagnosis of segmental arterial mediolysis: differentiation from vasculitis and other mimics. Arthritis Care Res (Hoboken). 2010;62(11):1655–60.

49. Lee W-K, Mossop PJ, Little AF, Fitt GJ, Vrazas JI, Hoang JK, et al. Infected (mycotic) aneurysms: spectrum of imaging appearances and management. Radiographics. 2008;28(7):1853–68.

50. Shih M-CP, Hagspiel KD. CTA and MRA in mesenteric ischemia: Part 1, Role in diagnosis and differential diagnosis. Am J Roentgenol. 2007;188(2):452–61.

# Imaging of Nontraumatic Abdominal Wall and Peritoneal Emergencies

# 33

Mohamed Z. Rajput and David H. Ballard

## Contents

## Abstract

Nontraumatic abdominal wall and peritoneal emergencies comprise a spectrum of conditions ranging from those that are self-limiting and managed conservatively, to others which are potentially life-threatening and require immediate, multi-specialty levels of care and intervention. Imaging, particularly computed tomography (CT), plays an essential role in the care of patients with a suspected nontraumatic abdominal wall or peritoneal emergency. Nontraumatic emergencies of the abdominal wall include complications associated with hernias, abdominal wall fluid collections, and soft-tissue necrotizing infections (fasciitis), fistulas from the gut to the abdominal wall, rectus sheath hematomas, and complications associated with indwelling medical devices or catheters. Nontraumatic peritoneal emergencies include peritonitis, hemoperitoneum, pneumoperitoneum, peritoneal carcinomatosis, epiploic appendagitis, omental infarction, mesenteric adenitis, and mesenteric panniculitis. The emergency radiologist must be familiar with the imaging appearance of the abdominal wall and peritoneal emergencies, to help guide clinical management of these patients by establishing a diagnosis and identifying any potential complications.

## Keywords

Pneumoperitoneum · Hemoperitoneum · Peritonitis · Carcinomatosis · Hernia · Necrotizing fasciitis · Rectus sheath hematoma · Abdominal wall · Peritoneum

## Introduction

Emergencies of the abdominal wall and peritoneum comprise a wide range of severity, from those that are managed conservatively to others requiring immediate, life-saving interventions. The emergency radiologist often plays a key role in establishing the diagnosis and in determining the underlying cause, as well as guiding the clinical management of these patients. Computed tomography (CT), given its speed and wide availability, is currently the imaging modality of choice in the evaluation of patients presenting to the emergency department with a suspected abdominal wall or peritoneal emergency. Examples of specific, nontraumatic emergencies of the abdominal wall include complications associated with hernias, abdominal wall fluid collections, and soft-tissue necrotizing infections (fasciitis), fistulas from the gut to the abdominal wall, rectus sheath hematomas, and complications associated with indwelling medical devices or catheters. Examples of specific, nontraumatic peritoneal emergencies include peritonitis, hemoperitoneum, pneumoperitoneum, peritoneal carcinomatosis, epiploic appendagitis, omental infarction, mesenteric adenitis, and mesenteric panniculitis.

M. Z. Rajput (✉) · D. H. Ballard
Mallinckrodt Institute of Radiology, Washington University School of Medicine, St. Louis, MO, USA
e-mail: mrajput@wustl.edu; davidballard@wustl.edu

© Springer Nature Switzerland AG 2022
M. N. Patlas et al. (eds.), *Atlas of Emergency Imaging from Head-to-Toe*,
https://doi.org/10.1007/978-3-030-92111-8_33

This chapter reviews the common imaging findings of patients presenting with nontraumatic emergencies of the abdominal wall and peritoneal emergencies.

## Nontraumatic Emergencies of the Abdominal Wall and Peritoneum

### Abdominal Wall

The anterior abdominal wall consists of skin, subcutaneous fat, and intervening layers of superficial and deep fascia surrounding muscle groups, which include the rectus abdominis muscles along the midline and the external oblique, internal oblique, and transversus abdominis muscles laterally. The rectus abdominis muscles are enclosed within the rectus sheath formed by the aponeuroses of the lateral muscle groups. The left and right rectus sheaths fuse in the midline to form the linea alba. Cranial to the arcuate line, which is located just inferior to the umbilicus, the rectus muscles are enclosed anteriorly and posteriorly by the rectus sheath; however, caudally, the posterior layer of the rectus sheath is absent. The superior and inferior epigastric vessels run along the posterior aspect of the rectus abdominis muscles [1, 2].

Defects in the abdominal wall related to congenital deformations or prior operations lead to the development of hernias. Inguinal hernias are the most common type of abdominal wall hernia and can be classified as indirect or direct, depending on whether they are found at the internal ring located lateral to the inferior epigastric vessels (indirect inguinal hernias) or are areas of acquired weakness in the transversalis fascia medial to the inferior epigastric vessels (direct inguinal hernias). Femoral hernias occur medial to the femoral vein as it passes out of the abdomen; they are more common in older women and are associated with a greater risk of complications. Other types of hernias include umbilical hernias; Spigelian hernias, which typically occur at the lateral border of the rectus muscle; obturator hernias that occur through the obturator foramen posterior to the inguinal and femoral canals; incisional hernias; and parastomal hernias around ileostomies, colostomies, and urostomies. CT is the preferred imaging modality in the acute setting to help characterize a hernia and to assess potential complications. It is thus important for the radiologist when assessing a hernia to describe the type/location, size, and internal contents within the hernia sac, which may include fat, vessels, small or large bowel, and, less commonly, other abdominal viscera [3].

Complications of abdominal wall hernias are common causes of abdominal pain in patients presenting to the emergency department. Complications related to hernias of the abdominal wall include bowel obstruction, incarceration, and intestinal strangulation (Fig. 1) [3, 4]. Bowel obstructions caused by hernias can be readily identified by a transition point from the dilated proximal bowel to the decompressed distal bowel at the hernia defect and possibly the so-called "fecalization" of bowel contents (i.e., liquid and solid matter with interspersed gas) just proximal to the obstruction point [3–5]. Incarceration refers to a hernia that cannot be physically reduced. Although incarceration can be suggested on imaging, it remains a clinical diagnosis [3, 4]. Intestinal strangulation, the most severe complication, occurs when the vascular supply to the bowel incarcerated in the hernia defect is compromised. Strangulation can be reversible or irreversible depending on the severity and duration of the vascular compromise. Bowel contained within a strangulated hernia is obstructed in a closed-loop-type physiology, unable to be decompressed, and therefore is at high risk for ischemia and infarction [3, 4]. On CT, fluid within the hernia sac, bowel wall thickening, hypoenhancing bowel wall, and, more critically, pneumatosis and mesenteric/portal venous gas, are important signs that highly suggest a strangulated hernia with irreversible ischemia and warrant emergent surgical consultation and usually operative intervention [3, 4].

Abdominal wall cellulitis and fluid collections, including seromas and abscesses, are often seen in the postoperative setting underneath the site of a surgical incision or may result from other forms of abdominal wall inflammation (Fig. 2). Cellulitis is typically a clinical diagnosis but may manifest on imaging with skin thickening and stranding of the subcutaneous fat [6]. Seromas form when plasma/serous fluid accumulates within the abdominal wall tissues after an operation that involves dissection of the planes of the abdominal wall. Typically, seromas resolve spontaneously, although aspiration or drainage may be required in situations when they persist, grow larger in size, or become symptomatic [3, 7]. Abscesses often appear thick-walled and demonstrate rim enhancement with internal locules of air and surrounding inflammatory fat stranding [3, 8]. It may be difficult, however, to distinguish between sterile and infected collections using imaging alone; hence, percutaneous sampling of the fluid within the collection may be necessary for differentiation [3].

The small or large bowel may fistulize to the abdominal wall, most often as a complication of abdominal surgery or in the setting of penetrating Crohn's disease, diverticular disease, or malignancy (Fig. 3) [9]. Patients typically report abdominal symptoms including pain and nausea/vomiting, and enteric or fecal content often visibly drains from an abdominal wound or fistula track. The most specific CT sign of a fistula is a sinus tract of gas or enteric contrast extending directly from the bowel or an intra-abdominal collection into the tissues of the abdominal wall and may involve just the subcutaneous tissue initially or progress to penetrate the skin surface, but this may not always be visible

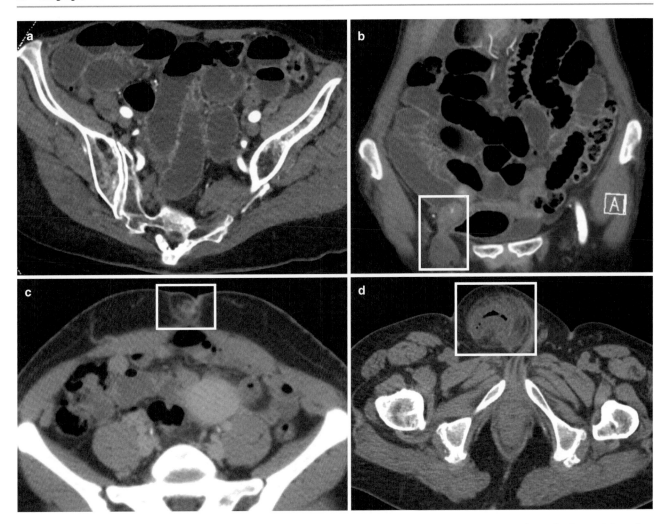

**Fig. 1** Complications of abdominal wall hernias. (**a**) and (**b**): Bowel obstruction. 55 year old woman with diffuse abdominal pain, nausea, and vomiting. Transaxial (**a**) and coronal (**b**) CT images of the abdomen and pelvis demonstrate multiple dilated, fluid-filled loops of small bowel compatible with a small bowel obstruction secondary to a right femoral hernia (box), which serves as the transition point between dilated and decompressed bowel. (**c**) Incarcerated ventral hernia. 51 year old man with epigastric abdominal pain. Transaxial CT image of the abdomen and pelvis demonstrates a small periumbilical hernia containing fat, a small amount of fluid, and accompanying fat stranding (box). The hernia could not be physically reduced on manual examination, and the patient subsequently underwent hernia repair with mesh placement. (**d**) Strangulated ventral hernia. 74 year old man with right lower quadrant abdominal pain. Transaxial CT image of the abdomen and pelvis demonstrates a right indirect inguinal hernia containing a thickened, poorly enhancing loop of small bowel with surrounding fluid and stranding (box). The hernia could not be manually reduced. The patient underwent urgent hernia repair, which revealed strangulated, ischemic small bowel requiring resection

on imaging. Indirect signs of a fistula include thickened bowel loops closely approximating an area of the abdominal wall with surrounding inflammatory stranding [8, 9]. Intramural abdominal wall or intraperitoneal abscesses may also be present (Fig. 4).

Prosthetic mesh that is often used in the repair of abdominal wall hernias can have a variable appearance on cross-sectional imaging, depending on its components and any associated infection [10]. Complications of prosthetic mesh repair include seromas, abscesses, hematomas, and mesh-associated fistulizing disease (Fig. 5) [3, 8, 11]. Mesh infection is a potentially serious complication that can ultimately lead to wound dehiscence, mesh erosion into intra-abdominal structures, or exposure of the mesh through the wound [11]. Such infections may occur ranging from days to years after the placement of the mesh. Patients with an exposed prosthetic mesh, especially those who are septic and hemodynamically unstable, require urgent surgical consultation for explantation of the mesh.

Among the causes of abdominal wall infection, necrotizing fasciitis is by far the most serious and most important for the emergency radiologist to consider (Fig. 6). As a life-threatening, rapidly progressive, polymicrobial, soft-tissue infection along the fascial planes, necrotizing fasciitis is often seen in the immunocompromised population due to poorly controlled diabetes or human immunodeficiency

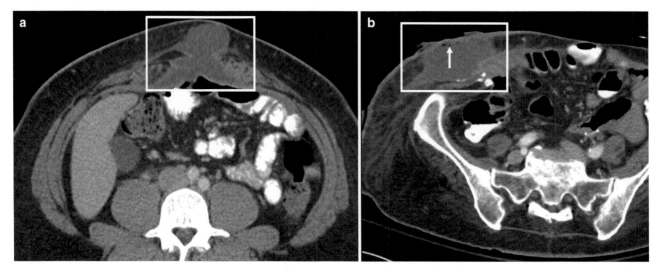

**Fig. 2** Abdominal wall fluid collections: (**a**) Seroma. 39 year old woman with a ventral hernia mesh repair 2 years prior presenting with chronic midline abdominal pain. Transaxial CT image of the abdomen and pelvis demonstrates a bilobed midline abdominal wall fluid collection extending into the subcutaneous tissues and abdominal wall musculature (box). The mesh repair itself was not distinctly visible on imaging. The patient underwent percutaneous aspiration of the collection, which contained clear, sterile fluid, compatible with a seroma. (**b**) Abscess. 62 year old woman with prior Spigelian hernia repair presenting with right lower quadrant abdominal pain, fever, and purulent discharge at the repair site. Transaxial CT image of the abdomen and pelvis demonstrates right lower anterior abdominal wall fluid collection (box) with anti-dependent gas (arrow). Aspiration revealed thick, yellow fluid which grew a mixture of aerobic and anerobic bacteria, compatible with an abscess

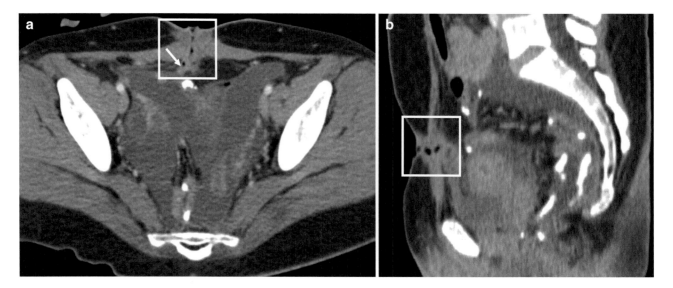

**Fig. 3** Abdominal wall enterocutaneous fistula. 27 year old woman with Crohn's disease status post total colectomy and J-pouch formation presenting with chronic abdominal pain and fluid leaking from her skin. Transaxial (**a**) and sagittal (**b**) CT images of the abdomen and pelvis demonstrate a gas-filled sinus tract (boxes) extending from a loop of small bowel (arrow) through the anterior abdominal wall to the thickened skin surface. There is no surrounding fluid collection

virus (HIV) infection [12]. When necrotizing fasciitis spreads or involves the perineum and genitalia, it is referred to as Fournier's gangrene [13]. Other CT manifestations that are associated with necrotizing fasciitis include edema along fascial planes, intramuscular edema, confluent fluid tracking along fascial planes, regional lymphadenopathy, and subcutaneous edema [13]. Necrotizing fasciitis should also not be mistaken for the expected postoperative soft-tissue gas following abdominal surgery or gas introduced via subcutaneous injections (Fig. 7). Treatment of necrotizing fasciitis includes broad-spectrum, antimicrobial therapy combined with early, aggressive, and wide operative debridement, which is necessary to improve survival in this highly morbid condition.

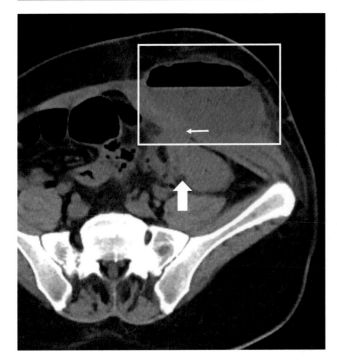

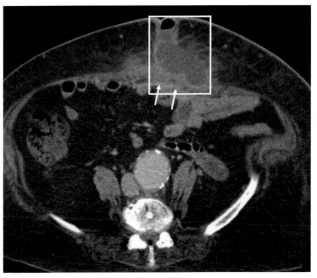

**Fig. 5** Abdominal wall abscess associated with mesh from ventral hernia repair. 72 year old woman with ventral hernia mesh repair 3 years prior presenting with left periumbilical erythema. A rim-enhancing gas and fluid collection in the left anterior abdominal wall is visualized with associated subcutaneous fat stranding, consistent with abdominal wall abscess (box). This is in close proximity to mesh from prior ventral hernia repair (arrows). Infrarenal abdominal aortic aneurysm is incidentally noted

**Fig. 4** Abdominal wall colocutaneous fistula and abscess. 45 year-old man presenting with a left abdominal wall mass and erythema. Transaxial non-contrast CT image of the abdomen and pelvis demonstrates a gas and fluid collection in the left anterior abdominal wall (box). There is loss of the fat plane in the adjacent abdominal wall musculature, suggesting possible intra-abdominal fistulization (thin arrow). There is mild thickening and pericolonic stranding surrounding the sigmoid colon (thick arrow), suggestive of possible diverticulitis versus a perforated colon cancer. Subsequent management include percutaneous drainage, where follow-up sonogram confirmed intra-abdominal fistulization. After stabilization of the abdominal abscess, and imaging resolution of the sigmoid colon thickening and pericolonic stranding, diverticulitis as the underlying etiology was confirmed on subsequent colonoscopy

Patients with bleeding diathesis, usually due to systemic anticoagulation therapy or a hematologic disorder resulting in coagulopathy, are at risk of spontaneous abdominal wall hemorrhage, often manifested by a rectus sheath hematoma. Patients with a rectus sheath hematoma present with a palpable, painful abdominal mass just lateral to the midline abdomen corresponding to the site of the hematoma [14]. IV contrast-enhanced CT can depict the extent of the hematoma and, if extravasated intravenous contrast is seen, identify sites of active bleeding (Fig. 8). It is important to note that because the posterior layer of the rectus sheath is absent below the arcuate line, a rectus sheath hematoma can extend into the extraperitoneal spaces and on occasion rupture into the peritoneum leading to pain mimicking peritonitis [1]. Typically, rectus sheath hematomas are managed conservatively, but if rapidly expanding, they may require vascular embolization of the supplying superior or inferior epigastric arteries or operative evacuation if the hemorrhage cannot be controlled with less invasive techniques [15].

Many types of medical devices are implanted in or through the abdominal wall. These include percutaneous feeding tubes (e.g., gastrostomy and jejunostomy tubes), peritoneal drainage and peritoneal dialysis catheters, intrathecal catheters and neurostimulators, or the drivelines of a ventricular-assist device. Subcutaneous stranding or fluid collections surrounding these devices in patients with fever or pain are suggestive of an underlying infection (Fig. 9) [16, 17]. Malposition and fracture of the components of the device are also important findings to communicate, because these complications are often associated with malfunction and require replacement.

## Peritoneum

The peritoneum is a serous membrane comprised of two layers: the outer, parietal peritoneum lines the abdominal wall, whereas the inner, visceral peritoneum folds to cover the greater omentum, lesser omentum, and mesentery, as well as lining the outer surface of the abdominal organs [18]. The potential space between these two layers, known as the peritoneal cavity, is typically not seen on imaging but can become visible when filled with fluid or blood, referred to as ascites. The most common cause of ascites is hepatic cirrhosis; other causes include congestive heart failure, nephrotic syndrome, peritoneal dialysis, malignancy, and bowel obstruction/ischemia [19]. Imaging assessment of ascites

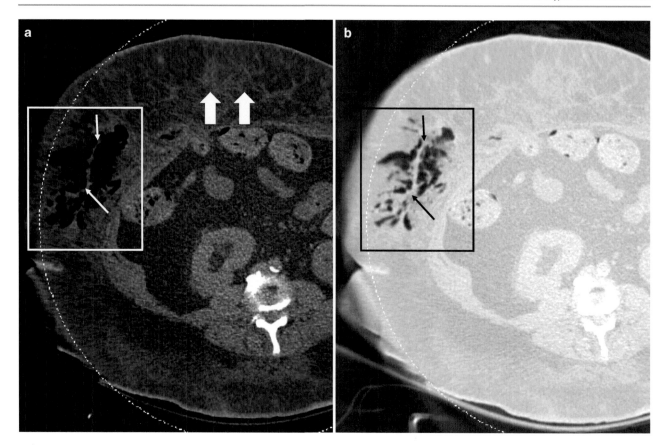

**Fig. 6** Abdominal wall necrotizing fasciitis. 65-year-old morbidly obese woman presents with leukocytosis and fever. Transaxial non-contrast CT images of the abdomen and pelvis demonstrate a large area of fascial gas to the right of midline in the anterior abdominal wall fat delineated on both soft tissue (**a**) and lung (**b**) windows (boxes).

Fascial air interdigitating demarcation of Scarpa's fascia is also noted (thin arrows). There is also diffuse stranding in the subcutaneous fat separate from the soft tissue air (thick arrows). There is no associated open wound. These findings were concerning for necrotizing fasciitis, which was confirmed at debridement

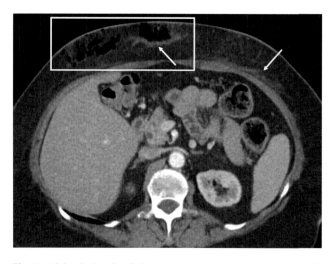

**Fig. 7** Abdominal wall soft tissue gas secondary to subcutaneous medication injection. 63 year old female with common variable immunodeficiency, presenting with elevated liver enzymes. Transaxial CT image of the abdomen demonstrates a large amount of gas (box) in the anterior abdominal wall with adjacent stranding in the subcutaneous fat (arrows). The gas was felt to be secondary to subcutaneous injections of immunoglobulin that the patient had self-administered prior to the scan. The patient was asymptomatic, afebrile, and nontoxic appearing at the time of the study. Subsequent imaging demonstrated resolution of these findings

consists primarily of abdominal sonography and CT, although the presence of ascites can be suggested on abdominal radiographs with findings including centralization of bowel loops and bulging of the flank soft tissues. Ultrasonography can be helpful in the initial evaluation of ascites by detecting septations or debris within the fluid to suggest the presence of a complex fluid collection [20]. CT may be particularly useful in helping to identify the underlying cause of ascites.

Peritonitis is a broad term referring to inflammation of the peritoneum. Peritonitis is often secondary to acute abdominal pathologies, such as hollow viscus perforation, appendicitis, diverticulitis, and pancreatitis, but peritonitis can also result from a primary bacterial infection in the setting of cirrhosis (spontaneous bacterial peritonitis), as well as from chemical irritation by extravasation of bile or barium (Fig. 10) [21]. Imaging findings of peritonitis include smooth peritoneal thickening and enhancement, which may be diffuse throughout the abdomen and pelvis, or localized near the site of primary inflammation [22]. Peritonitis and other sources of inflammation can lead to the accumulation of intraperitoneal fluid, which over time may become loculated, septated, and/or encapsulated. If large or concern exists for

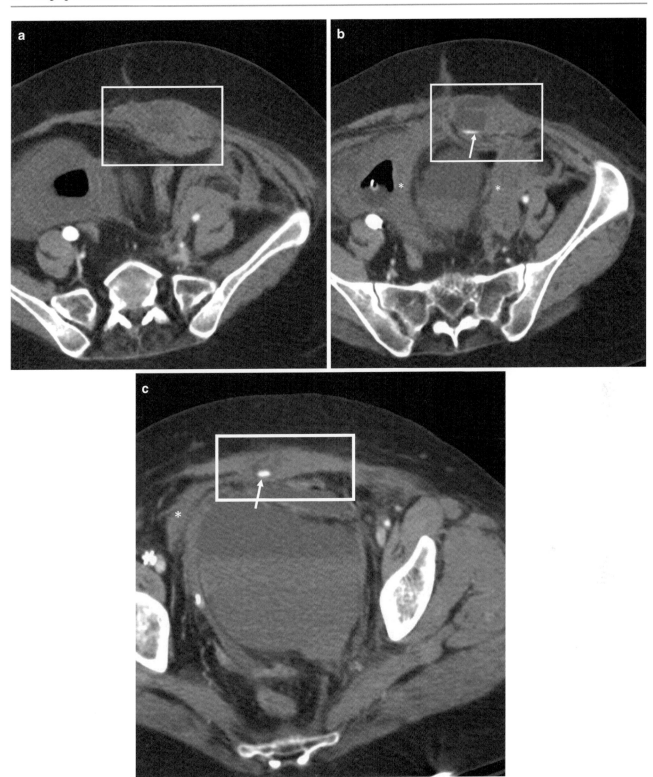

**Fig. 8** Nontraumatic rectus sheath hematoma with active extravasation above (**a** and **b**) and below (**c**) the arcuate line. 40 year old woman with an arrhythmia requiring anticoagulation presenting with dropping hemoglobin and abdominal pain. There was no preceding trauma. Serial transaxial CT images demonstrate a rectus sheath hematoma (boxes **a**–**c**) with active extravasation (arrows; **b** and **c**) and intra-abdominal extraperitoneal extension of hemorrhage (asterisks; **b** and **c**). The anatomy of the rectus sheath is demonstrated with unilateral left-sided localization of the rectus sheath hematoma above the arcuate line (**a** and **b**). As the course of the hematoma (site of active extravasation) extends below the arcuate line (**c**), the distribution crosses midline and is bilateral. This also allows access into the extraperitoneal space, allowing for intra-abdominal extension of hemorrhage. At catheter angiography, the left inferior epigastric artery was embolized

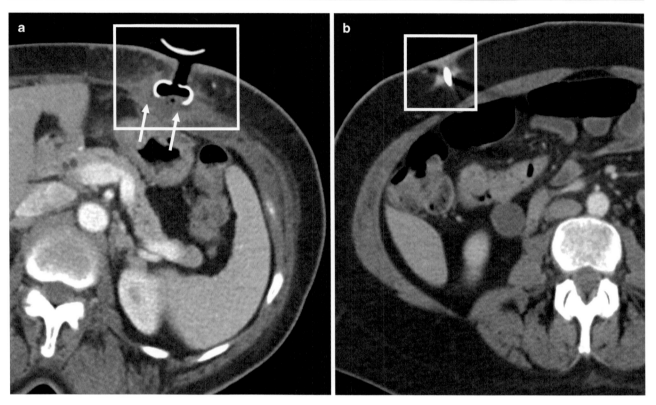

**Fig. 9** Abdominal wall medical device infections. (**a**) Gastrostomy tube infection. 66 year old woman with failure to thrive, fever, and tenderness at gastrostomy site. Transaxial non-contrast CT image of the abdomen and pelvis demonstrates retraction of a percutaneous gastrostomy catheter into the abdominal wall musculature (box) with surrounding gas and fluid (arrows), concerning for phlegmon/early abscess formation. The indwelling catheter was subsequently removed and a new gastrostomy catheter placed via the existing sinus tract into the stomach. (**b**) Driveline infection. 58 year old woman with cardiomyopathy requiring a left ventricular assist device with abdominal wall erythema and warmth. Transaxial CT image of the abdomen and pelvis demonstrates subcutaneous stranding surrounding the left ventricular assist device driveline in the right anterior abdominal wall with overlying skin thickening (box). No fluid collection surrounding the driveline was identified. The patient was treated with antibiotics, with subsequent resolution of the findings on follow-up imaging

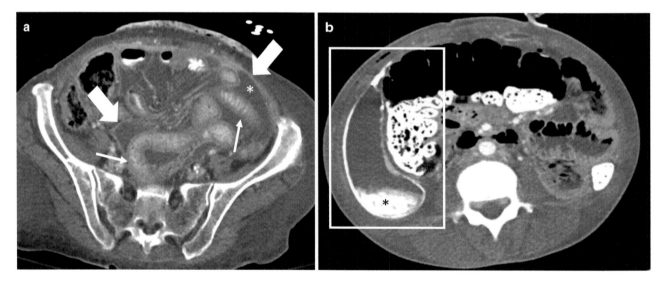

**Fig. 10** Peritonitis. (**a**) 69 year old woman with perforated gastric ulcer status post repair. Transaxial CT image of the abdomen and pelvis demonstrates diffuse smooth peritoneal thickening and enhancement (thick arrows) with simple attenuating ascites (asterisk). Thickened small bowel loops (thin arrows) represent reactive enteritis in the setting of peritoneal inflammation. (**b**) 42 year old man with achalasia status post aborted peroral endoscopic myotomy. He underwent a water-soluble and barium contrast esophagram prior to CT, which did not demonstrate any evidence of perforation. CT was ordered for worsening abdominal pain following the esophagram. Transaxial CT of the abdomen and pelvis demonstrates barium coating the peritoneal surface (box) and collecting dependently within the peritoneal cavity (asterisk), compatible with extravasated barium from an esophageal perforation following myotomy resulting in barium peritonitis

superimposed infection, these localized peritoneal fluid collections can be percutaneously aspirated or drained. A unique example of a peritoneal fluid collection is the cerebrospinal fluid (CSF) pseudocyst, which can form around the distal tip of an indwelling ventriculoperitoneal shunt catheter that has stimulated adhesions that wall off this cavity (Fig. 11) [23].

Hemoperitoneum, the accumulation of blood within the peritoneal cavity, can become life-threatening and rapidly fatal depending on the etiology and severity of the blood

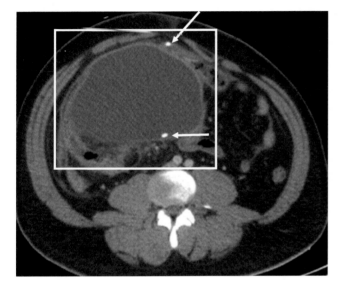

**Fig. 11** Infected peritoneal CSF pseudocyst. 44 year old man with chronic hydrocephalus requiring shunting presenting with abdominal pain, fever, and leukocytosis. Transaxial CT image of the abdomen and pelvis demonstrates a large rim-enhancing peritoneal fluid collection (box) displacing the adjacent bowel with surrounding inflammatory fat stranding. Portions of a ventriculoperitoneal shunt catheter are visualized outside and within the collection (arrows). Percutaneous drainage of the fluid collection was performed, and the ventriculoperitoneal shunt was subsequently removed

loss (Fig. 12). Unlike simple ascites, which measures near water density of -10 to 10 Hounsfield units (HU) on CT, hemoperitoneum is higher in attenuation. Clotted blood is more dense (35–70 HU) compared to unclotted blood (30–45 HU), although one should be aware that in anemic patients, these attenuation values may be artificially decreased [24, 25]. Usually, the area of the greatest density is closest to the source of bleeding and is referred to as the "sentinel clot" [26]. Additionally, a so-called hematocrit effect may be seen when dense, cellular blood products accumulate dependently; this effect can be appreciated most frequently within the pelvic cul-de-sac [27]. Identification of intravenous contrast extravasation indicative of active and brisk on-going bleeding in the setting of hemoperitoneum is crucial, because its presence often warrants endovascular and/or surgical intervention [28].

When encountering hemoperitoneum outside the setting of trauma, the emergency radiologist must also attempt to identify the underlying cause and most likely site [29] (Fig. 13). Ruptured ovarian cysts are among the most common causes in premenopausal women [30]. A ruptured ectopic pregnancy, though less common, is a much more serious, even potentially life-threatening cause of hemoperitoneum in this same age group of pre-menopausal women [30]. Correlation with results of human chorionic gonadotropin (hCG) testing for early pregnancy combined with pelvic ultrasonography is imperative in helping to differentiate a ruptured ovarian cyst, which is usually treated by nonoperative, supportive care, versus a ruptured ectopic pregnancy that requires operative intervention.

Other nontraumatic causes of hemoperitoneum include rupture of hepatic masses, particularly hepatic adenoma and hepatocellular carcinoma. The underlying mass may be obscured on initial CT by the surrounding blood and only

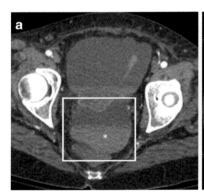
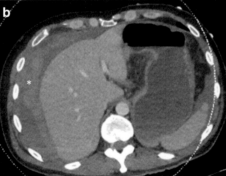
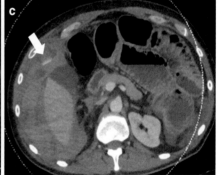

**Fig. 12** Hemoperitoneum. (**a**) 72 year old woman with dropping hemoglobin following total abdominal hysterectomy and bilateral salpingo-oophorectomy. Transaxial CT image of the abdomen and pelvis demonstrates heterogeneous fluid in the pelvic cul-de-sac compatible with hemorrhage. A hematocrit effect is observed, with dependent hyperattenuating contents representing the cellular contents of blood (asterisk). (**b** and **c**) 67 year old woman following bowel resection with dropping hemoglobin and abdominal pain. Transaxial CT images of the abdomen and pelvis demonstrates upper abdominal hemoperitoneum. A "sentinel clot" sign is present intermixed with areas of lower attenuation (asterisk), with a contrast blush (thick arrow) seen just anterior to the liver, concerning for active extravasation. The patient underwent emergent laparotomy for hematoma evacuation, which demonstrated active bleeding from an omental feeding artery

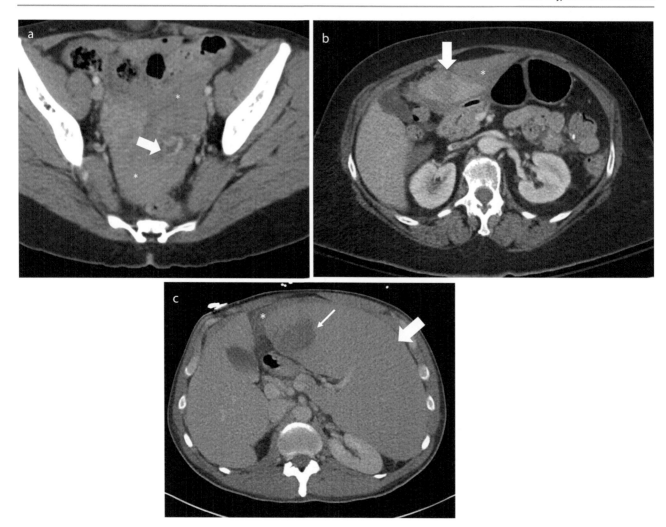

**Fig. 13** Causes of atraumatic hemoperitoneum. (**a**) Ruptured corpus luteal cyst. 31 year old woman with acute onset left lower quadrant pain. Transaxial CT of the abdomen and pelvis demonstrates moderate volume pelvic hemoperitoneum (asterisk) near an irregular, thick walled small left adnexal cystic lesion (thick arrow), compatible with a ruptured corpus luteal cyst. (**b**) Ruptured hepatocellular carcinoma. 64 year old woman with sudden onset abdominal pain and lightheadedness. Transaxial CT of the abdomen and pelvis demonstrates an ill-defined hypoattenuating mass in hepatic segment 3 (arrow) which ruptured, resulting in adjacent hemoperitoneum (asterisk). The differential at the time of CT included hepatic adenoma and hepatocellular carcinoma. The liver did not have a cirrhotic morphology. The patient underwent ultrasound-guided core biopsy of the hepatic mass, which demonstrated hepatocellular carcinoma. (**C**): Splenic rupture. 47 year old man with newly diagnosed acute myeloid leukemia presenting with abdominal pain. Transaxial CT image of the abdomen and pelvis demonstrates marked splenomegaly (thick arrow). Findings of spontaneous splenic rupture are evident with perisplenic hemorrhage (asterisk) along with an intraparenchymal hematoma (thin arrow). Given hemodynamic stability of the patient as well as the absence of active bleeding on CT, embolization and/or splenectomy was deferred, and the patient was managed conservatively

revealed on follow-up imaging after the hemorrhage has resolved [28, 31] . In such cases, the radiologist may consider recommending follow-up imaging to characterize the primary mass. Hemoperitoneum can also be seen following spontaneous, atraumatic rupture of a markedly enlarged spleen caused by infections such as mononucleosis or malaria, or a lymphoproliferative process [24, 28]. If a gynecologic, hepatic, or splenic cause is not identified, careful attention should be directed to mesenteric vessels in search for potential vascular abnormalities, such as visceral aneurysms or pseudoaneurysms, potentially in the setting of an underlying vasculitis [28]. Splenic artery aneurysms are well known to rupture during pregnancy and should be considered in any pregnant woman with a spontaneous hemoperitoneum. Spontaneous hemoperitoneum can also occur in patients with a bleeding diathesis due to anticoagulation therapy or underlying hematologic disorders [24, 28].

In addition to free fluid and hemorrhage, emergency radiologists must observe extraluminal gas in the abdomen and pelvis. Although the most serious cases of pneumoperitoneum stem from hollow viscus perforation, such as a perforated gastroduodenal ulcer or perforated

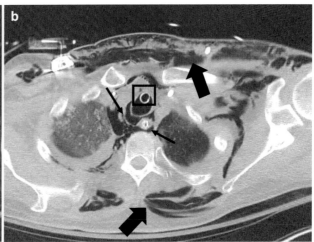

**Fig. 14** Pneumoperitoneum secondary to barotrauma from invasive mechanical ventilation. 49 year-old with diffuse large B-cell lymphoma status post stem cell transplant, admitted with graft versus host disease and subsequently diagnosed with pneumonia. Transaxial CT images of the chest and upper abdomen on lung windows demonstrate upper abdominal pneumoperitoneum (thick arrows in **a**) and pneumoretroperitoneum (thin arrows in **a**). Large volume body wall subcutaneous gas (thick arrows in **b**) as well as pneumomediastinum is also noted in the chest (thin arrows in **b**). The patient had been mechanically ventilated for several days (endotracheal tube: box in **b**). Given the patient's reported history of high positive end-expiratory pressure, barotrauma was favored to be the etiology that had resulted in subcutaneous emphysema, pneumomediastinum, and dissection of gas from the mediastinum into the peritoneal cavity resulting in pneumoperitoneum/pneumoretroperitoneum

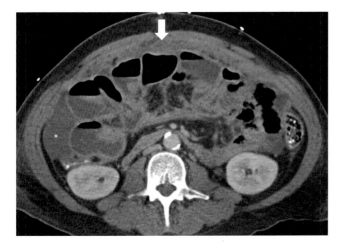

**Fig. 15** Peritoneal carcinomatosis. 53 year old man with newly diagnosed sigmoid adenocarcinoma with abdominal pain and distention. Transaxial CT image of the abdomen and pelvis demonstrates small volume ascites (asterisk) and mesenteric and omental nodular soft tissue thickening, forming an "omental cake" (arrow). Omental biopsy was performed, confirming malignancy compatible with the patient's primary colorectal cancer

diverticulitis, many other noncritical conditions can also result in intraperitoneal free air. These include the expected presence of free air in the early period after abdominal surgery, gas introduced via a recent paracentesis or access of a peritoneal dialysis catheter, or extension of a pneumothorax or pneumomediastinum, such as the setting of barotrauma from positive pressure ventilation (Fig. 14) [32]. As a result, it is important to correlate this finding with a patient's clinical status and any recent interventions. While abdominal radiographs are often obtained initially in patients with suspected pneumoperitoneum and may demonstrate the classic signs of free air under the diaphragm on an upright radiograph or anterior free air on a lateral decubitus radiograph, CT is a more sensitive modality that can also assist in identifying the underlying cause or source, which is not usually possible on abdominal radiographs alone [32, 33].

Another important peritoneal cause of abdominal pain in patients with cancer is peritoneal carcinomatosis [21]. Peritoneal carcinomatosis is often first diagnosed in the emergency department in patients with no known history of malignancy. Gastrointestinal, gynecologic, pancreatic, and lung cancers are among the most common causes of peritoneal carcinomatosis [18]. In contrast to the smooth peritoneal contour seen in peritonitis, carcinomatosis is manifested by nodular thickening and enhancement of the peritoneum accompanied by peritoneal and mesenteric soft-tissue implants. Peritoneal metastases may coalesce within the greater omentum to form a so-called "omental cake" (Fig. 15) [34]. Concomitant ascites is often present and may be loculated [34]. Metastatic peritoneal implants along the serosa, or outer surface of the small and large bowel, are important to identify, because they may be the cause of a malignant bowel obstruction (Fig. 16) [35]. Much less common processes with similar imaging findings to be mindful of that mimic carcinomatosis include infections such as actinomycosis and tuberculosis (Fig. 17) [36], primary peritoneal mesothelioma, and inflammatory conditions, such as sarcoidosis or amyloidosis.

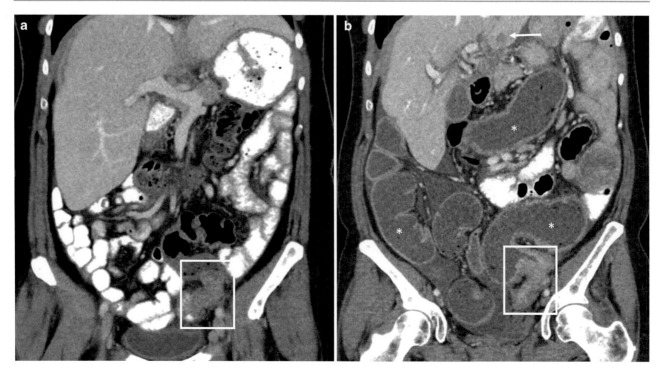

**Fig. 16** Serosal deposit resulting in bowel obstruction. 68 year old woman with metastatic ovarian cancer. (**a**) Coronal CT image of the abdomen and pelvis demonstrates a left lower quadrant soft tissue mass abutting the sigmoid colon (box), compatible with a metastatic serosal deposit. (**b**) CT performed 5 months later when the patient presented to the emergency department with acute abdominal pain, nausea, and vomiting demonstrates a malignant large bowel obstruction (asterisks) secondary to colonic invasion of the serosal mass (box), which had enlarged in the interval. Note the metastatic left hepatic lobe lesion (arrow). The patient underwent partial colectomy and end colostomy formation

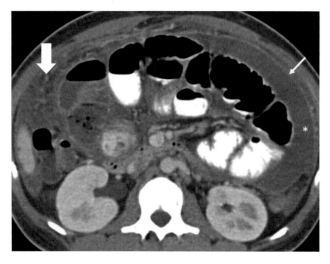

**Fig. 17** Tuberculosis peritonitis mimicking peritoneal carcinomatosis. 57 year old man, recently immigrated from China, presenting to the emergency department with several months of abdominal pain, weight loss, and intermittent fevers. Transaxial CT of the abdomen and pelvis demonstrates omental soft tissue nodularity (thick arrow) along with nodular peritoneal thickening (thin arrow) and ascites (asterisk). Omental core biopsy was performed, demonstrating necrotizing granulomatous inflammation highly suspicious for *Mycobacterium tuberculosis* infection, without evidence of malignancy

Common but generally less serious acute conditions of the peritonealized surfaces include epiploic appendagitis, omental infarction, mesenteric adenitis, and mesenteric panniculitis. Epiploic appendagitis is a self-limiting condition caused by inflammation or torsion of small, fat-filled, peritoneal outpouchings along the serosa of the colon, particularly near the sigmoid colon where a denser distribution is found [37, 38]. The clinical symptoms can simulate acute appendicitis or diverticulitis but typically in the absence of fever or leukocytosis [38].

Epiploic appendagitis can be confused with a related but distinct process known as an omental infarction, which develops following vascular compromise to a portion of the omentum. This condition often develops in the setting of a recent trauma or abdominal operation, although primary omental infarction without identifiable cause may also occur [37, 38]. Omental infarction can be distinguished from epiploic appendagitis based on its size (typically >5 cm), predominantly right-sided distribution adjacent to the proximal colon, and an overall heterogeneous, less well-demarcated appearance [37, 39] (Fig. 18). Imaging plays an essential role in diagnosing both conditions and avoiding unnecessary antibiotic therapy or operative intervention [38].

Mesenteric adenitis is a self-limiting, inflammatory condition that may be also seen in the emergency setting and

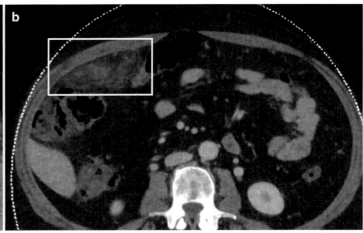

**Fig. 18** Epiploic appendagitis and omental infarction. (**a**) Epiploic appendagitis. 66 year old woman with left lower quadrant abdominal pain. Transaxial CT image of the abdomen and pelvis demonstrates an well-circumscribed, ovoid, fat-containing lesion adjacent to the junction of the sigmoid and descending colon with surrounding stranding (box). (**b**) Omental infarction. 41 year old man with right upper abdominal pain. Transaxial CT image of the abdomen and pelvis demonstrates a heterogeneous area of increased attenuation centered within the omentum adjacent to the hepatic flexure with surrounding inflammatory stranding (box). Symptoms resolved in both patients after a course of outpatient analgesic therapy

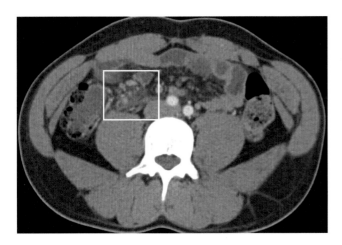

**Fig. 19** Mesenteric adenitis. 30 year old man with right lower quadrant abdominal pain. Transaxial CT of the abdomen and pelvis demonstrates several prominent subcentimeter right lower quadrant mesenteric lymph nodes with accompanying mesenteric fat stranding (box). The appendix was normal. Follow up imaging performed 1 month later demonstrated resolution of these findings

present with pain closely mimicking acute appendicitis (Fig. 19). Imaging findings include the presence of three (or more) right-lower quadrant mesenteric lymph nodes measuring ≥5 mm in patients with localized pain and/or systemic illness (e.g., fever, fatigue) [40]. Mesenteric adenitis can be associated with viral and bacterial infections, such as *Yersinia enterocolitica* and *Campylobacter jejuni*, especially when there is accompanying inflammation of the terminal ileum [41].

Lastly, mesenteric panniculitis is a benign, idiopathic, inflammatory process of the fatty tissue of the mesentery (Fig. 20). Although patients with mesenteric panniculitis are typically asymptomatic, they may present to the emergency department with abdominal symptoms, including pain and nausea/vomiting, and on occasion with increased serum levels of inflammatory markers. Imaging findings include an ill-defined, hazy fat stranding centered predominantly within the jejunal mesentery with associated, sub-centimeter mesenteric lymph nodes. A "fat halo" sign may be seen around the mesenteric vessels [42]. Historically, mesenteric panniculitis was thought to be a paraneoplastic syndrome, although more recent studies indicate it is not associated with the development of malignancy or other diseases; its precise cause remains unknown [43].

## Conclusion

Emergency radiologists must be familiar with a range of nontraumatic abdominal wall and peritoneal emergencies that can be identified on imaging. Most patients with abdominal wall hernias are asymptomatic, but complications, including incarceration and bowel strangulation, often require urgent surgical consultation and operative intervention. Fluid collections, such as seromas and abscesses, as well as bowel fistulas to the abdominal wall, are often seen in the setting of prior abdominal operations. Necrotizing fasciitis is a potentially life-threatening soft-tissue infection requiring urgent operative intervention and must be suspected in the setting of unexplainable soft-tissue gas in the abdominal wall. Rectus sheath hematomas may be a cause of abdominal wall pain, particularly in patients at an increased risk of bleeding. Additional types of abdominal wall infection are often seen in

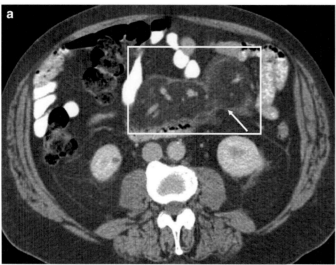 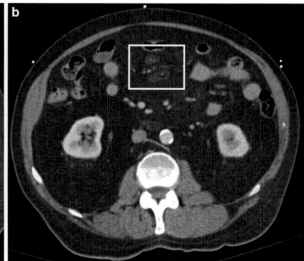

**Fig. 20** Mesenteric panniculitis in two different patients presenting with vague abdominal pain and diarrhea. (**a**) Transaxial CT of the abdomen and pelvis demonstrates ill-defined mesenteric fat stranding and mesenteric lymph nodes (box) surrounded by a thin pseudocapsule (arrow). (**b**) A "fat halo" sign (box) is demonstrated with preservation of a normal fat plane surrounding the mesenteric vessels

the setting of catheters or medical devices implanted or traversing the abdominal wall.

It is important to distinguish between simple intraperitoneal fluid and hemoperitoneum. Determining the cause of hemoperitoneum and identifying the sites of active bleeding are critical in the management of these patients. Both serious and benign etiologies may result in pneumoperitoneum; therefore, careful consideration of the clinical context and any recent abdominal intervention is necessary to determine the source of free air and guide further management of these patients. Although overall less serious and usually self-limiting, conditions such as epiploic appendagitis, omental infarction, mesenteric adenitis, and mesenteric panniculitis may also be a source of pain in patients presenting to the emergency department.

## References

1. Matalon SA, Askari R, Gates JD, Patel K, Sodickson AD, Khurana B. Don't forget the abdominal wall: imaging spectrum of abdominal wall injuries after nonpenetrating trauma. Radiographics. 2017;
2. Ballard DH, Mazaheri P, Oppenheimer DC, Lubner MG, Menias CO, Pickhardt PJ, et al. Imaging of abdominal wall masses, masslike lesions, and diffuse processes. Radiographics. 2020;
3. Aguirre DA, Santosa AC, Casola G, Sirlin CB. Abdominal wall hernias: imaging features, complications, and diagnostic pitfalls at multi-detector row CT. In: Radiographics; 2005.
4. Mirvis SE, Soto JA, Shanmuganathan K, Yu JKW. Problem solving in emergency radiology. Philadelphia: Elsevier; 2014. p. 428–31.
5. Macari M, Megibow A. Imaging of suspected acute small bowel obstruction. Semin Roentgenol. 2001;
6. Hayeri MR, Ziai P, Shehata ML, Teytelboym OM, Huang BK. Soft-tissue infections and their imaging mimics: from cellulitis to necrotizing fasciitis. Radiographics. 2016;
7. Gossios K, Zikou A, Vazakas P, Passas G, Glantzouni A, Glantzounis G, et al. Value of CT after laparoscopic repair of postsurgical ventral hernia. Abdom Imaging. 2003;

8. Lacour M, Ridereau Zins C, Casa C, Venara A, Cartier V, Yahya S, et al. CT findings of complications after abdominal wall repair with prosthetic mesh. Diagn Interv Imaging. 2017;
9. Tonolini M, Magistrelli P. Enterocutaneous fistulas: a primer for radiologists with emphasis on CT and MRI. Insight Imaging. 2017;
10. Rakic S, Leblanc KA. The radiologic appearance of prosthetic materials used in hernia repair and a recommended classification. Am J Roentgenol. 2013;
11. Gavlin A, Kierans AS, Chen J, Song C, Guniganti P, Mazzariol FS. Imaging and treatment of complications of abdominal and pelvic mesh repair. Radiographics. 2020;
12. Childers BJ, Potyondy LD, Nachreiner R, Rogers FR, Childers ER, Oberg KC, et al. Necrotizing fasciitis: a fourteen-year retrospective study of 163 consecutive patients. Am Surg. 2002;
13. Ballard DH, Mazaheri P, Raptis CA, Lubner MG, Menias CO, Pickhardt PJ, et al. Fournier gangrene in men and women: appearance on CT, ultrasound, and MRI and what the surgeon wants to know. Can Assoc Radiol J. 2020;
14. Fukuda T, Sakamoto I, Kohzaki S, Uetani M, Mori M, Fujimoto T, et al. Spontaneous rectus sheath hematomas: clinical and radiological features. Abdom Imaging. 1996;
15. Rimola J, Perendreu J, Falcó J, Fortuño JR, Massuet A, Branera J. Percutaneous arterial embolization in the management of rectus sheath hematoma. AJR Am J Roentgenol. 2007;
16. Brittenden J, Tolan DM. Radiology of the post surgical abdomen. Radiol Post Surg Abdom. 2013;
17. Carr CM, Jacob J, Park SJ, Karon BL, Williamson EE, Araoz PA. CT of left ventricular assist devices. Radiographics. 2010;
18. Levy AD, Shaw JC, Sobin LH. From the archives of the AFIP: secondary tumors and tumorlike lesions of the peritoneal cavity: Imaging features with pathologic correlation. Radiographics. 2009;
19. Jolles HCC. CT of ascites: differential diagnosis. Am J Roentgenol. 1980;135(2):315–22.
20. Rudralingam V, Footitt C, Layton B. Ascites matters. Ultrasound. 2017;
21. Patlas MN, Alabousi A, Scaglione M, Romano L, Soto JA. Cross-sectional imaging of nontraumatic peritoneal and mesenteric emergencies. Can Assoc Radiol J. 2013;
22. Elsayes KM, Staveteig PT, Narra VR, Leyendecker JR, Lewis JS, Brown JJ. MRI of the peritoneum: spectrum of abnormalities. Am J Roentgenol. 2006;

23. Wallace AN, McConathy J, Menias CO, Bhalla S, Wippold FJ. Imaging evaluation of CSF shunts. Am J Roentgenol. 2014;

24. Furlan A, Fakhran S, Federle MP. Spontaneous abdominal hemorrhage: causes, CT findings, and clinical implications. Am J Roentgenol. 2009;

25. Gayer G, Hertz M, Manor H, Strauss S, Klinowski E, Zissin R. Dense ascites: CT manifestations and clinical implications. Emerg Radiol. 2004;

26. Orwig D, Federle MP. Localized clotted blood as evidence of visceral trauma on CT: the sentinel clot sign. Am J Roentgenol. 1989;

27. Federle MP, Pan KT, Pealer KM. CT criteria for differentiating abdominal hemorrhage: anticoagulation or aortic aneurysm rupture? Am J Roentgenol. 2007;

28. Lucey BC, Varghese JC, Anderson SW, Soto JA. Spontaneous hemoperitoneum: a bloody mess. Emerg Radiol. 2007;

29. Lubner M, Menias C, Rucker C, Bhalla S, Peterson CM, Wang L, et al. Blood in the belly: CT findings of hemoperitoneum. Radiographics. 2007;

30. Hertzberg BS, Kliewer MA, Paulson EK. Ovarian cyst rupture causing hemoperitoneum: Imaging features and the potential for misdiagnosis. Abdom Imaging. 1999;

31. Casillas VJ, Amendola MA, Gascue A, Pinnar N, Levi JU, Perez JM. Imaging of nontraumatic hemorrhagic hepatic lesions. Radiographics. 2000;

32. Gayer G, Jonas T, Apter S, Amitai M, Shabtai M, Hertz M. Postoperative pneumoperitoneum as detected by CT: prevalence, duration, and relevant factors affecting its possible significance. Abdom Imaging. 2000;

33. Borofsky S, Taffel M, Khati N, Zeman R, Hill M. The emergency room diagnosis of gastrointestinal tract perforation: the role of CT. Emerg Radiol. 2015;

34. Le O. Patterns of peritoneal spread of tumor in the abdomen and pelvis. World J Radiol. 2013;

35. Gore RM, Silvers RI, Thakrar KH, Wenzke DR, Mehta UK, Newmark GM, et al. Bowel obstruction. Radiol Clin N Am. 2015;

36. Neyman EG, Georgiades CS, Fishman EK. Abdominal involvement in tuberculosis. Emerg Radiol. 2002;

37. Singh AK, Gervais DA, Hahn PF, Sagar P, Mueller PR, Novelline RA. Acute epiploic appendagitis and its mimics. Radiographics. 2005;

38. Van Breda Vriesman AC, Mol D, van Otterloo AJC, Puylaert JBCM. Epiploic appendagitis and omental infarction. Eur J Surg. 2001;

39. Kamaya A, Federle MP, Desser TS. Imaging manifestations of abdominal Fat necrosis and its mimics. Radiographics. 2011;

40. Macari M, Hines J, Balthazar E, Megibow A. Mesenteric adenitis: CT diagnosis of primary versus secondary causes, incidence, and clinical significance in pediatric and adult patients. Am J Roentgenol. 2002;

41. Lucey BC, Stuhlfaut JW, Soto JA. Mesenteric lymph nodes seen at imaging: causes and significance. Radiographics. 2005;

42. McLaughlin PD, Filippone A, Maher MM. The "misty mesentery": mesenteric panniculitis and its mimics. Am J Roentgenol. 2013;

43. Gögebakan Ö, Albrecht T, Osterhoff MA, Reimann A. Is mesenteric panniculitis truely a paraneoplastic phenomenon? A matched pair analysis. Eur J Radiol. 2013;

# Emergency Imaging of the Bariatric Surgery Patient

Daniel R. Ludwig and Christine O. Menias

## Contents

## Abstract

Bariatric surgery remains the only treatment for obesity with established outcomes and durable weight loss. Roux-en-Y gastric bypass (RYGB), sleeve gastrectomy (SG), and laparoscopic adjustable gastric band (LAGB) are the most commonly performed surgeries and constitute over 90% of the procedures currently performed. Unfortunately, complications after these surgeries are relatively common, and many patients with surgical complications present acutely in the emergent setting. Imaging, computed tomography (CT) in particular, plays an important role in the care of the bariatric surgery patient by readily depicting postoperative complications and guiding further management. The most common complications of RYGB include gastrointestinal leak, postoperative hemorrhage, anastomotic stricture or ulceration, small bowel obstruction, hernia, and intussusception. Complications after SG include leak, hemorrhage, and gastric stricture. Finally, complications after LAGB include stomal stenosis, band slippage, band erosion, and port/tubing complications. The goal of this chapter is to review the normal postoperative appearance of these bariatric surgical procedures and discuss and illustrate the most commonly encountered surgical complications of each.

## Keywords

Roux-en-Y gastric bypass · Sleeve gastrectomy · Laparoscopic adjustable gastric band · Gastrointestinal leak · Anastomotic stricture · Marginal ulcer · Small bowel obstruction · Internal hernia · Stomal stenosis · Band erosion

## Introduction

Obesity is a worldwide public health crisis, with those affected at an increased risk for developing a host of chronic diseases including type II diabetes, cardiovascular disease, and cerebrovascular disease. Bariatric surgery is the only

D. R. Ludwig (✉)
Mallinckrodt Institute of Radiology, Washington University School of Medicine, St. Louis, MO, USA
e-mail: ludwigd@wustl.edu

C. O. Menias
Mayo Clinic Department of Radiology, Scottsdale, AZ, USA
e-mail: Menias.Christine@mayo.edu

© Springer Nature Switzerland AG 2022
M. N. Patlas et al. (eds.), *Atlas of Emergency Imaging from Head-to-Toe*,
https://doi.org/10.1007/978-3-030-92111-8_34

treatment for obesity with established and durable long-term success in both weight loss and reduction of metabolic and cardiovascular complications [1]. There are multiple different types of bariatric surgery that are currently in use, which can generally be categorized as restrictive (i.e., restrict the amount a patient can eat), malabsorptive (i.e., reduce the amount of food that is digested and absorbed), or a combination of the two. Roux-en-Y gastric bypass (RYGB), sleeve gastrectomy (SG), and laparoscopic adjustable gastric band (LAGB) are the most commonly performed surgeries and together constitute over 90% of the procedures performed in the past 10 years in the United States [2].

Imaging plays an important role in the care of the bariatric surgery patient, as it is heavily relied upon to depict complications after surgery. Additionally, many patients with bariatric surgical complications present acutely, often in the emergency setting. Thus, the radiologist must be knowledgeable about normal postoperative appearance of bariatric surgical procedures and be well-versed in identifying the most common complications. In this chapter, the three most commonly used bariatric surgical procedures are covered: RYGB, SG, and LAGB. First, a basic approach to imaging the bariatric surgery patient will be presented. Next, the nature of each surgery will be discussed, and the postoperative anatomy and normal imaging appearance on various modalities will be reviewed. Finally, the most common complications of each surgical procedure will be presented and illustrated.

## Bariatric Surgery Emergencies

### Imaging Approach

Radiographs have limited utility in the evaluation of the bariatric surgery patient. The sensitivity of radiographs for the diagnosis of small bowel obstruction (SBO) is relatively poor (i.e., <50%), as fluid-filled loops of obstructed small bowel may not be visualized radiographically [3]. Furthermore, when SBO is evident, the cause is unlikely to be identified, and radiographs furthermore do not readily depict complications such as bowel ischemia. In patients after LAGB, radiographs are helpful in assessing gastric band position and ensuring continuity of the port and tubing, which will be discussed in further detail in a later section.

Upper gastrointestinal (UGI) series is commonly performed in the early postoperative setting after bariatric surgery when there is clinical suspicion for gastrointestinal leak. If leak is suspected, water-soluble contrast should be used, followed by dilute barium if no leak is identified with water-soluble contrast [4]. The sensitivity of UGI for the diagnosis of a gastrointestinal leak is somewhat limited, especially when a small contained leak is present, which may quickly fill with contrast and empty [5]. UGI may be

of higher utility in patients with subacute or chronic symptoms, as it is well suited for depicting certain complications including stomal stenosis, stricturing, and fistula, as well as for assessing the positioning and stoma size of the LAGB [6].

Computed tomography (CT) is the mainstay of emergency abdominal imaging and is the preferred imaging approach in a patient after bariatric surgery presenting acutely. Intravenous (IV) contrast should be utilized unless there is a specific contraindication, as IV contrast increases the range of pathology visible on CT and improves the confidence of the interpretation. Specifically in the bariatric surgery patient, IV contrast is necessary to assess bowel wall enhancement patterns in suspected bowel ischemia, rim enhancement of a fluid collection when abscess is suspected, and active extravasation in a patient with bleeding. Many authors additionally advocate for the routine use of oral contrast in the bariatric surgery patient [6]. Oral contrast introduces a 1–2-hour delay, which is necessary for the administered contrast to traverse the small bowel. Additionally, the positive oral contrast in the small bowel may obscure enhancement of the bowel mucosa and may not be well tolerated, especially in the setting of high-grade SBO. Thus, oral contrast should be administered on a case-by-case basis depending on the clinical context and/or acuity and may be most helpful if low-grade bowel obstruction, leak, or abscesses are suspected.

## Roux-en-Y Gastric Bypass

RYGB is the reference standard for bariatric surgery, despite the advent of several more recent techniques, and combines both restrictive and malabsorptive components. In RYGB, the stomach is first partitioned into a 15–30 mL gastric fundal pouch (in continuity with the esophagus) and a larger excluded stomach (in continuity of the duodenum). Next, a Roux or efferent limb is created by dividing the jejunum distal to the ligament of Treitz and bringing up the distal aspect of the divided jejunum to the gastric pouch either anterior to the transverse colon (i.e., antecolic) or posterior to the transverse colon via creation of a hole in the mesocolon (i.e., retrocolic). Finally, the proximal aspect of the divided jejunum is anastomosed to the more distal jejunum in a side-to-side fashion (i.e., jejunojejunal anastomosis), creating a Roux limb that is approximately 75–100 cm in length [7]. The excluded stomach, duodenum, and proximal jejunum constitute the biliopancreatic limb, as it drains biliary and pancreatic secretions, and the jejunojejunal anastomosis and adjacent small bowel is referred to as the common channel.

The expected appearance of RYGB on UGI evaluation is shown in Fig. 1, including a schematic illustrating the postsurgical anatomy (Fig. 1d). Contrast passes from the esophagus to the small gastric pouch and freely flows into the Roux limb. Contrast travels through jejunojejunal anastomosis,

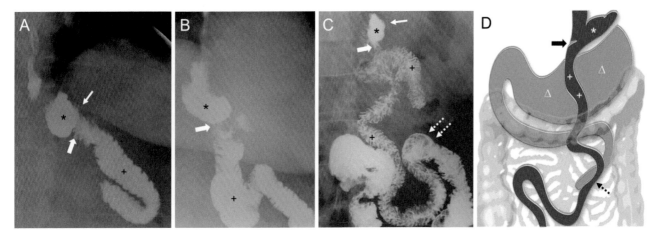

**Fig. 1** Expected appearance of Roux-en-Y gastric bypass (RYGB) on upper gastrointestinal (UGI) evaluation. Anteroposterior (**a**) and left posterior oblique views (**b**) show contrast filling the gastric pouch (asterisks) and a staple line along the left margin of the pouch (thin arrows), which divides the pouch from the excluded stomach. Contrast passes freely into the Roux limb (plus signs) through the gastrojejunal anastomosis (thick arrows). Overhead radiograph (**c**) shows contrast opacifying the Roux limb (+ signs) to the level of the jejunojejunal anastomosis in the left mid-abdomen, which is identified by its staple line (dashed arrows). A schematic (**d**) depicts the postsurgical anatomy of the RYGB, in which the excluded stomach (Δ), duodenum, and proximal jejunum are bypassed by the Roux limb (plus signs)

identified by its staple line in the left mid-abdomen, and subsequently into the common channel. The biliopancreatic limb usually does not fill with contrast on a normal UGI evaluation. Figure 2 shows the expected appearance of RYGB on CT. In contradistinction to UGI, the excluded stomach and biliopancreatic limb are readily identifiable on CT and under normal circumstances should be collapsed.

A rare complication of RYGB is the Roux-en-O misconstruction, in which the proximal aspect of the divided jejunum (i.e., the distal biliopancreatic limb) is anastomosed to the gastric pouch and the distal aspect of the divided jejunum is anastomosed to the biliopancreatic limb [18]. Patients present with bilious emesis and functional symptoms of SBO in the early postoperative setting. Although the appearance may look normal on CT, UGI shows retrograde rather than anterograde peristalsis in the Roux limb.

## Leak

Postoperative gastrointestinal leak is a serious complication of RYGB, occurring in 2–5% of patients, most commonly within 7 days after surgery [8, 9]. Leaks manifest clinically with fever, leukocytosis, tachycardia, and abdominal pain, although minor leaks may be asymptomatic [8]. If undetected, gastrointestinal leak can progress to abscess, peritonitis, and sepsis. Treatment approaches for leak include conservative management, percutaneous drainage, and surgical revision for persistent leaks [8].

The diagnosis of a leak is confirmed by the presence of extraluminal leakage of oral contrast on UGI or CT (Fig. 3). Contained leaks appear as contained collections or blind-ending tracks abutting the anastomosis [9]. Most leaks originate from the gastrojejunal anastomosis and extend into the

left upper quadrant or subphrenic space [6, 9]. Of note, UGI cannot readily demonstrate leaks associated with the excluded stomach.

## Hemorrhage

Hemorrhage following RYGB affects 1–4% of patients in the early postoperative period and is associated with significant morbidity [10]. Patients may present with hematemesis, bright red blood per rectum, melanotic stools, dropping hematocrit, and in severe cases hypotension, with the clinical picture varying depending on the rate of bleeding and whether it occurs intraluminally or extraluminally. CT angiography can be performed rapidly in the acute setting and is frequently helpful identifying the source of bleeding and directing further management. On CT, hematoma after RYGB manifests as an extraluminal high-attenuation collection adjacent to a staple line or high-attenuation fluid filling the lumen of the small bowel or the excluded stomach (Fig. 4). Treatment options for hemorrhage include conservative management, catheter angiography with embolization, upper endoscopy, and in some cases surgical exploration [10].

## Anastomotic Stricture/Ulcer

Stricturing, or stenosis, of the gastrojejunal anastomosis is a relatively common complication of RYGB, occurring in 3–16% of patients, almost always presenting >4 weeks after surgery [11]. Patients typically present with upper abdominal pain, food intolerance, excessive weight loss, and postprandial nausea and vomiting. Anastomotic strictures are readily depicted on UGI and appear as a focal area of smooth narrowing at the gastrojejunal anastomosis, with resultant dilation of the gastric pouch, and delayed passage of contrast

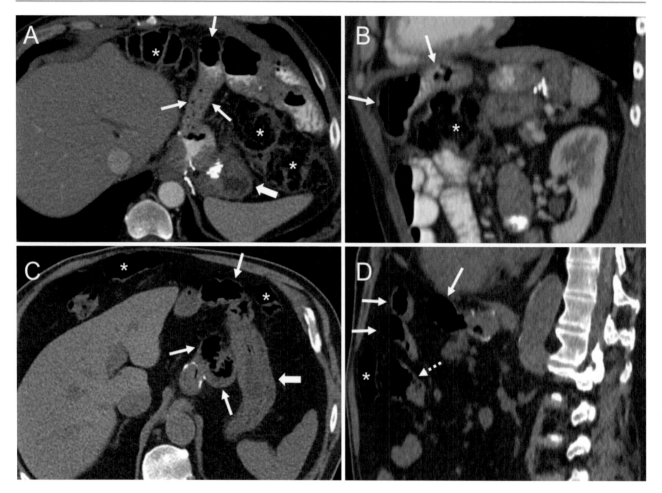

**Fig. 2** Expected appearance of antecolic and retrocolic RYGB on computed tomography (CT). Axial (**a**) and oblique sagittal (**b**) CT images with intravenous (IV) and oral contrast depict a normal antecolic RYGB, with the Roux limb (thin arrows) coursing anterior to the colon (asterisks). Axial (**c**) and oblique sagittal (**d**) non-contrast CT images in a different patient show a normal retrocolic RYGB, with the Roux limb (thin arrows) coursing posterior to the colon to the jejunojejunal anastomosis (dashed arrow, **d**). Note the presence of a relatively decompressed excluded stomach (thick arrow, **a** and **c**)

into the Roux limb [6]. In a patient presenting acutely or with symptoms of obstruction, an anastomotic stricture may instead be first encountered on CT (Fig. 5). Endoscopic balloon dilation is a highly safe and effective treatment for gastrojejunal anastomotic strictures, although some patients require more than one dilation procedure.

Ulceration at the margin of the gastrojejunal anastomosis (i.e., marginal ulcers) affects 1–7% of patients after RYGB [12]. Patients with marginal ulcers may present with dyspepsia, abdominal pain, gastrointestinal bleeding, and in rare cases perforation [12]. On UGI, marginal ulcers appear as a focal outpouching or crater, usually solitary, adjacent to the gastrojejunal anastomosis [6]. Fat stranding surrounding the ulcer crater is often evident on CT (Fig. 6). Small ulcers are not evident radiographically, and endoscopy is the standard tool for diagnosis [13]. Medical treatment with antisecretory agents and/or antibiotics in the setting of *H. pylori* is often curative [12].

## Small Bowel Obstruction

SBO after RYGB is a complication affecting 2–7% of patients and carries high attendant morbidity [14, 15]. Adhesions, jejunojejunal anastomotic strictures, internal hernias, and abdominal wall hernias account for the majority of SBOs [15], although anastomotic edema may account for many in the early postoperative setting [13]. Most patients with SBO present with a combination of nausea, vomiting, and abdominal pain. Although several classification schemes exist for SBO after RYGB, a more commonly used system is the ABC classification [16]. Type A SBO involves isolated obstruction of the Roux limb and manifests on CT and UGI as distention of the gastric pouch and Roux limb, with a decompressed biliopancreatic limb and common channel (Fig. 7). In comparison, type B SBO involves isolated obstruction of the biliopancreatic limb proximal to the jejunojejunal anastomosis, with a decompressed Roux limb and common channel (Fig. 8). Type B SBO is considered a closed-loop obstruction,

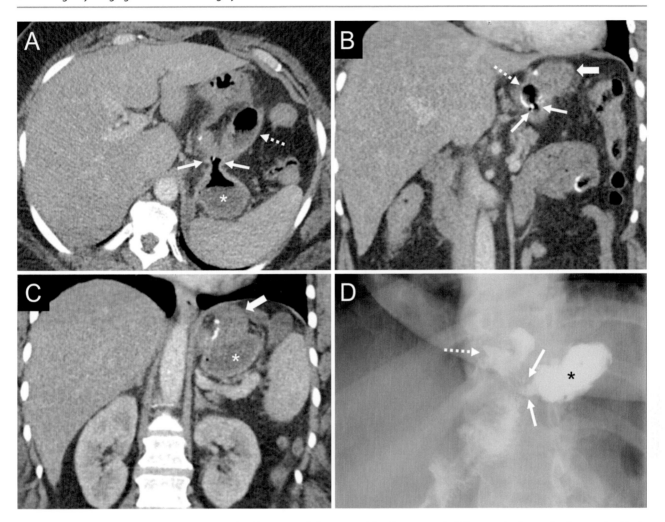

**Fig. 3** Postoperative leak arising from the gastrojejunal anastomosis in a 54-year-old woman undergoing evaluation for abdominal pain 2 weeks after RYGB. Axial (**a**) and sequential coronal (**b** and **c**) IV contrast-enhanced CT images show a small extraluminal fluid and gas collection (asterisks) which freely communicates with a dehiscent gastrojejunal anastomosis (thin arrows), diagnostic of a contained leak. The collection is inferior to the decompressed excluded stomach (thick arrows, **b** and **c**). The gastric pouch is denoted by the thin dashed arrow. A gastrointestinal leak was confirmed on subsequent single-contrast UGI evaluation (**d**)

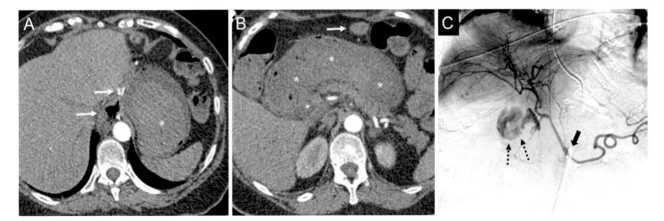

**Fig. 4** Gastrointestinal bleeding after RYGB in a 52-year-old man presenting with melena. CT angiographic images in the axial plane (**a** and **b**) show postsurgical changes of RYGB (thin arrows), with extensive blood products in the excluded stomach (asterisks). No active contrast extravasation was identified. Due to a high clinical suspicion for persistent gastrointestinal bleeding, the patient underwent catheter angiography (**c**), which showed brisk arterial contrast extravasation into the proximal duodenum (dashed arrows) via a branch of the pancreaticoduodenal artery. Note the position of the catheter tip which is positioned in the celiac artery (thick arrow). The patient was treated with transcatheter arterial embolization

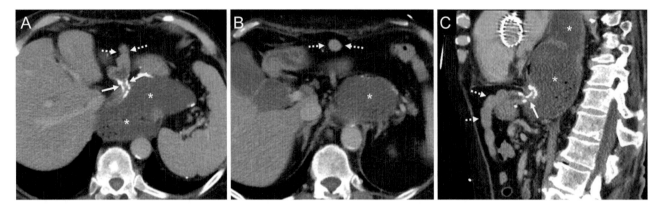

**Fig. 5** Gastrojejunal anastomotic stricture in a 72-year-old woman presenting with nausea and vomiting approximately 12 years after prior RYGB. Sequential axial (**a** and **b**) and sagittal (**c**) IV contrast-enhanced CT images show marked dilation of the distal esophagus and gastric pouch (asterisks), with narrowing at the gastrojejunal anastomosis (solid arrows) and a decompressed Roux limb (dashed arrows). Severe anastomotic narrowing was confirmed on endoscopy, and the patient was managed with balloon dilation

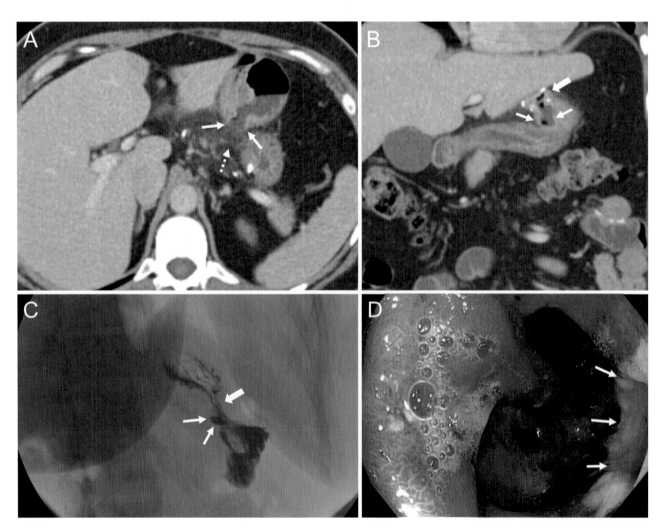

**Fig. 6** Marginal ulcer in a 43-year-old woman presenting with abdominal pain 4 years after RYGB. IV contrast-enhanced CT images in the axial (**a**) and coronal (**b**) planes show a deep ulcer crater arising posteroinferiorly from the Roux limb (thin arrows) just distal to the gastrojejunal anastomosis (thick arrow). Soft-tissue stranding involved the mesentery adjacent to the ulcer (dashed arrow, **a**). Image from UGI in the LPO orientation (**c**) also shows the presence of a marginal ulcer (thin arrows) adjacent to the gastrojejunal anastomosis (thin arrow). These findings were confirmed on upper endoscopy (**d**)

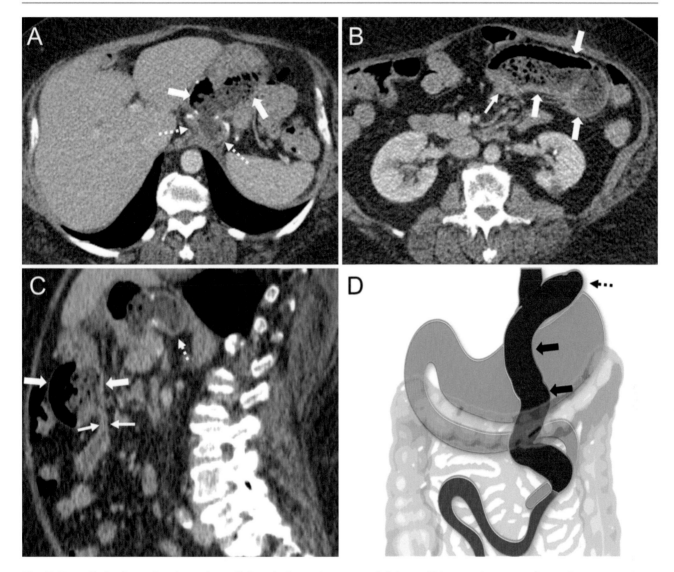

**Fig. 7** Roux limb obstruction (type A small bowel obstruction [SBO]) in a 66-year-old woman 3 weeks after RYGB. Axial IV contrast-enhanced CT images (**a** and **b**) and sagittal contrast-enhanced CT image (**c**) show moderate distention of the gastric pouch (dashed arrows) and proximal Roux limb (thick arrows). There is a transition point to the decompressed Roux limb in the central abdomen (thin arrows) corresponding to the transverse meso-colic defect of the retrocolic Roux limb. These findings were con-firmed operatively and an adhesion was identified at this location. The imaging findings are also demonstrated in a schematic (**d**), which depicts distention of the gastric pouch (dashed arrow) and Roux limb (thick arrows)

in that intraluminal pressure in the excluded stomach and duodenum cannot be relieved by emesis or nasogastric decompression, and patients with type B SBO are at substan-tially higher risk of perforation. Finally, type C SBO involves obstruction at the level of the common channel, with disten-tion of the common channel proximal to the obstruction, as well as obstruction of both the Roux and biliopancreatic limb. SBO after RYGB generally requires operative management, although a conservative approach may be attempted in the early postoperative setting [17].

**Hernia**

Hernias after RYGB include both incisional and internal hernias. Incisional hernias after laparoscopic RYGB are reported at a much lower frequency compared with open RYGB (i.e., 0.5% vs. 9%) [14]. Patients with incisional hernias may present acutely when bowel incarceration occurs [19]. Symptoms of an incarcerated incisional hernia overlap with SBO, but additional clinical features include pain local-izing to the incision site and a focal bulge on exam. Findings of an incarcerated hernia on CT include a peritoneal defect at

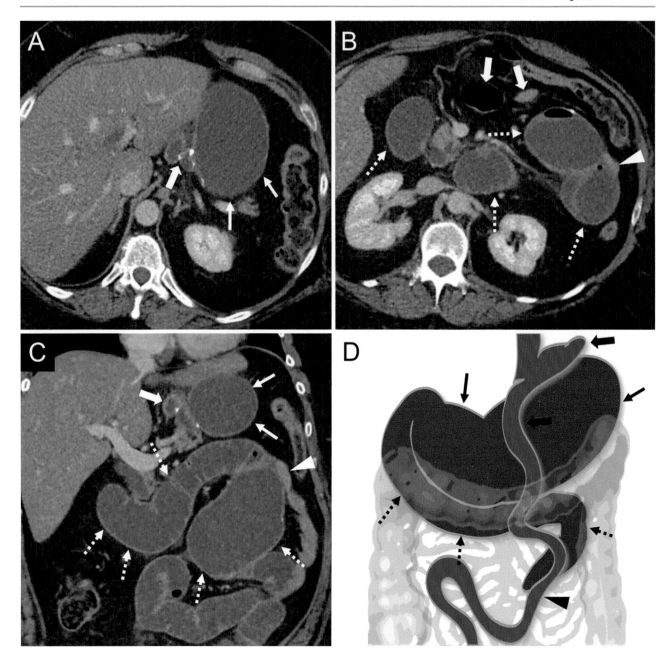

**Fig. 8** Biliopancreatic limb obstruction (type B SBO) in a 51-year-old woman with RYGB presenting with severe abdominal pain and vomiting. Sequential axial (**a** and **b**) and coronal (**c**) IV contrast-enhanced CT images show marked distention of the excluded stomach (thin arrows) and proximal small bowel (dashed arrows). There is a transition to decompressed small bowel at the location of the jejunojejunal anastomosis (arrowheads). The gastric pouch and Roux limb are largely decompressed (thick arrows). These findings are consistent with biliopancreatic limb obstruction, likely related to an adhesion. The Roux limb may also be obstructed but decompressed secondary to vomiting. The patient was managed conservatively and her symptoms improved after several days. The imaging findings are also demonstrated in a schematic (**d**), which depicts distention of the biliopancreatic limb (excluded stomach and proximal small bowel; thin solid and dashed arrows, respectively), with a decompressed Roux limb (thick arrows)

the trocar or laparotomy site, bowel within the hernia sac, and a transition point from distended to decompressed bowel at the hernia (Fig. 9). Incarcerated bowel is at risk for ischemia (i.e., strangulation), which can be suggested by the CT findings of bowel wall thickening, abnormal hyper- or hypo-enhancement, and mesenteric edema [20]. Incisional hernias present in both the early and late postoperative settings and generally require surgical management when acutely symptomatic [21].

Internal hernias, on the other hand, develop more commonly after laparoscopic RYGB and affect approximately 3% of patients [22]. It has been postulated that laparoscopic RYGB results in fewer adhesions than open RYGB, permitting increased mobility of the small bowel in the abdomen

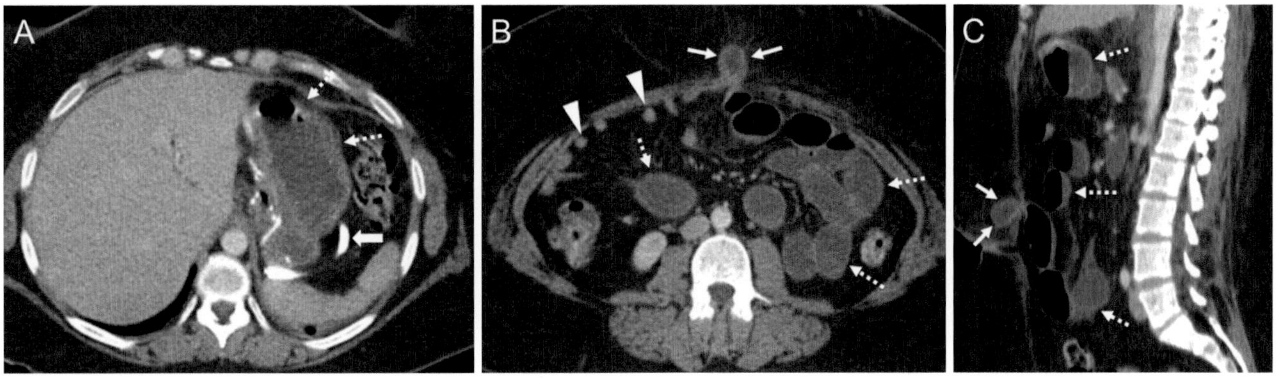

**Fig. 9** Incarcerated ventral abdominal wall hernia at prior trocar site in a 35-year-old woman 4 days after RYGB. Axial (**a** and **b**) and sagittal (**c**) IV contrast-enhanced CT images show changes of RYGB with a surgical drain in place (thick arrow, **a**). There is moderate distention of the excluded stomach (dashed arrows, **a**). More inferiorly, there are multiple dilated loops of proximal small bowel (dashed arrows) with decompressed distal small bowel in the right lower quadrant (arrowheads, **b**), consistent with a type C SBO. The transition point is an incarcerated ventral abdominal hernia containing a knuckle of the small bowel (thin arrows), just above the umbilicus at the site of prior trocar placement. The incarcerated bowel is moderately thickened (thin arrows), concerning for strangulation. The patient was taken to the operating room for reduction and repair of the abdominal wall. A portion of the incarcerated small bowel was found to be ischemic and was removed at the time of surgery

[6]. Internal hernias result from herniation of the small bowel through mesenteric defects or potential spaces, frequently resulting in vascular compromise and closed-loop obstruction. Though mesenteric defects are typically closed at the time of surgery, substantial weight loss after RYGB often leads to increase in size of these defects and potential spaces [23]. Thus, internal hernias tend to present as a late complication after RYGB [15]. Internal hernias after RYGB almost always occur at one of three locations: (1) through a defect in the transverse mesocolon (i.e., transmesocolic hernia), (2) through a potential space posterior to the Roux limb (i.e., Peterson defect), and (3) through a defect in the small bowel mesentery at the jejunojejunostomy site. Of note, transmesocolic hernias only occur in the setting of a retrocolic RYGB, whereas Peterson hernias and jejunojejunostomy site hernias may develop in either antecolic or retrocolic RYGB [15].

CT findings of internal hernia can be subtle and include swirling of the mesentery, a mushroom shape of the mesentery, displacement of the jejunojejunal anastomosis to the right of midline, and mesenteric edema [24]. Internal hernia can also be suggested when small bowel loops are seen clustered in an atypical location [25]. Although internal hernia can result in small bowel obstruction, dilated loops of the small bowel are not a requisite feature [6]. In the transmesocolic internal hernia, clustered loops of the small bowel are often seen in the left upper quadrant adjacent to the excluded stomach (Fig. 10). In a Peterson hernia, clustered loops may be found in the left or right mid-abdomen, depending on the direction of herniation (Fig. 11). Additionally, a small bowel loop other than the transverse duodenum is often located behind the superior mesenteric artery [24]. In jejunojejunostomy site hernias, displacement of the jejunojejunal anastomosis to the right of midline is a relatively common feature (Fig. 12). Although CT may show features supportive of a particular subtype, a significant overlap in findings may exist among the different internal hernias, and the role of the radiologist is primarily to suggest the presence of an internal hernia rather than identify the specific subtype. Indeed, early surgical management is vital to prevent major complications, including bowel infarction and perforation [22].

## Intussusception

Intussusception after RYGB is relatively rare, affecting less than 0.5% of patients [26, 27]. Essentially all develop at the jejunojejunal anastomosis and most are retrograde (i.e., into the Roux limb). The jejunojejunal anastomosis serves as the underlying lead point [27]. Patients with intussusception commonly present with abdominal pain, which may be episodic or recurrent, and symptoms of obstruction [27]. On CT, intussusception after RYGB is diagnosed based on the presence of a targetoid mass in the left or central abdomen associated with the jejunojejunal anastomosis which has a bowel-in-bowel configuration, often with mesenteric fat and vessels seen traveling within the intussusception (Fig. 13) [28]. Although some intussusception in RYGB reduce spontaneously, bowel ischemia, infarction, and perforation may ensue. Surgical treatment entails reduction and revision of the jejunojejunal anastomosis [29].

## Sleeve Gastrectomy

The SG is a purely restrictive procedure, in which a portion of the stomach is resected and the gastric volume is reduced by approximately 75% to roughly 100 mL [30]. In the SG, the stomach is divided in a vertical fashion, and the greater

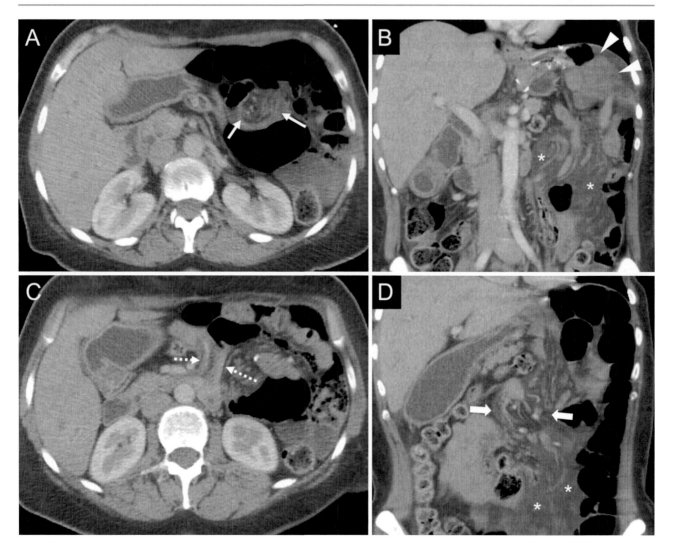

**Fig. 10** Transmesocolic hernia in a 44-year-old woman presenting with abdominal pain after retrocolic RYGB. Axial (**a**) and coronal (**b**) IV contrast-enhanced CT images depict swirling of the mesentery in the left upper quadrant (thin arrows, (**a**) and clustering of several loops of the small bowel in the left upper quadrant adjacent to the excluded stomach (arrowheads, **b**). Also note the presence of extensive mesenteric edema within the left mid- and upper quadrant (asterisks, **b**). More inferiorly, an axial IV contrast-enhanced CT image (**c**) demonstrates a stalk-like appearance of two adjacent loops of the small bowel (dashed arrows). Coronal IV contrast-enhanced CT image (**d**) shows a defect in the transverse mesocolon and upward herniation of the mesenteric fat and vessels (thick arrows). These findings are consistent with a transmesocolic internal hernia, which was confirmed at the time of surgery

curvature is removed, including nearly all of the fundus and the majority of the gastric body and antrum. The expected appearance of SG on UGI and CT is shown in Fig. 14. The gastric sleeve has a tubular or banana-shaped configuration, with a staple line present along the greater curvature. Oftentimes, a small residual fundal remnant is present and is best appreciated on UGI evaluation when the stomach is distended [31].

## Gastric Leak

Following SG, gastrointestinal leak is the most problematic early postoperative complication, presenting in 1–4% of patients [32, 33]. Similar to following RYGB, leaks manifest clinically with abdominal pain, fever, tachycardia, and leukocytosis. Leak can confidently be diagnosed on UGI or CT when there is extraluminal leakage of oral contrast (Fig. 15). A larger fundal remnant has the potential to mimic a leak on UGI, and CT may serve as a useful problem-solving tool in this setting [32]. On CT, contained leaks appear as a fluid collection abutting the staple line along the greater curvature. UGI has a limited sensitivity for the detection of leak after SG, as contrast may transit rapidly past the upper portion of the gastric remnant, where the majority of leaks occur. Although conservative management may be appropriate in selected patients, endoscopic gastroesophageal stent placement is highly effective in treating leaks and is the preferred

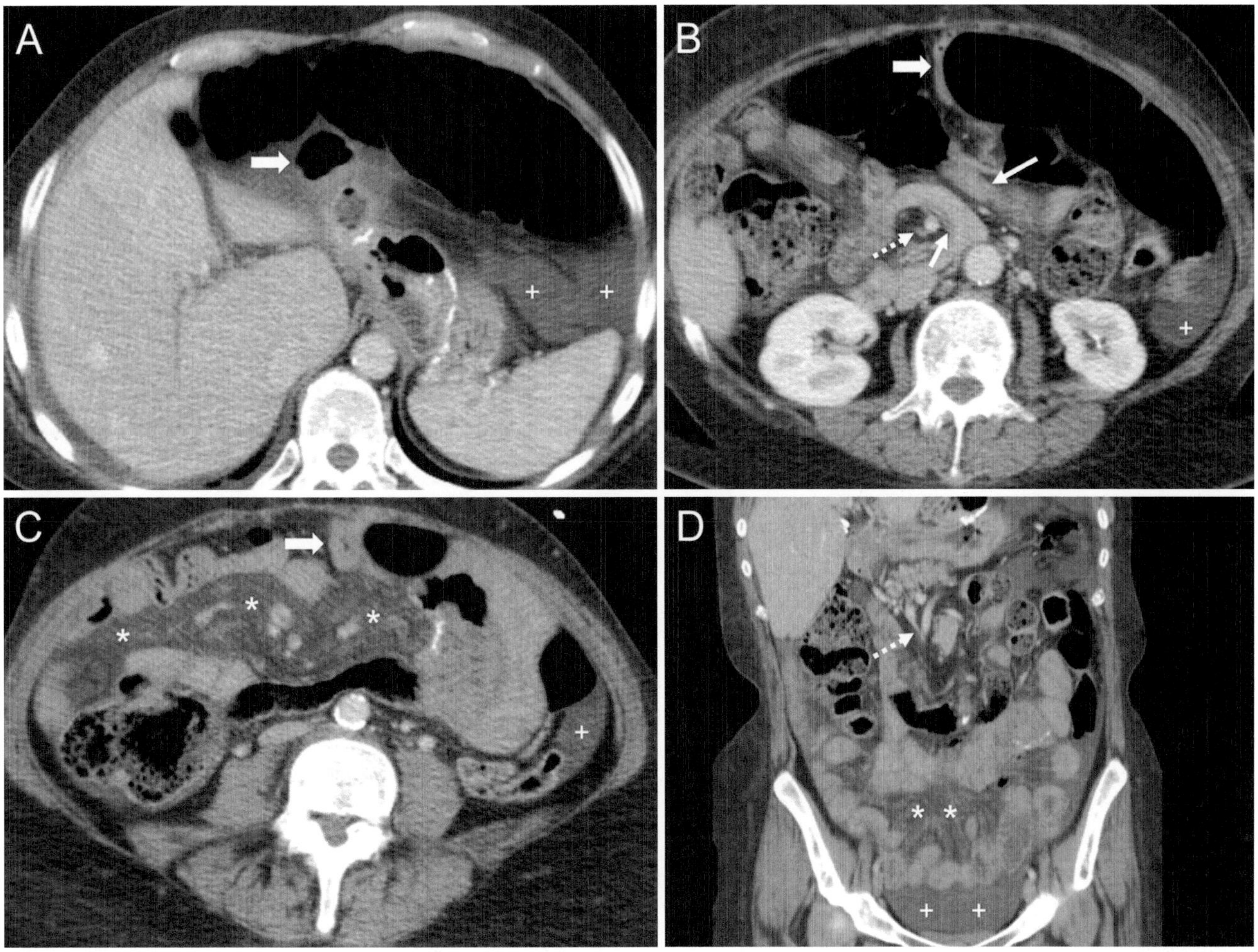

**Fig. 11** Peterson-type internal hernia in a 50-year-old woman with RYGB presenting with abdominal pain. Axial (**a–c**) and coronal (**d**) IV contrast-enhanced CT images show changes of RYGB with a retrocolic Roux limb (thick arrows). There is a mushroom-like config-uration of the mesentery with straightening of two loops of the small bowel which protrude into the right abdomen (thin arrows, **b**). Extensive mesenteric edema is present within the right mid- and lower abdomen (asterisks) along with small-volume ascites (plus sign). Additionally, there is abrupt cutoff of the superior mesenteric vein (dashed arrow, **b** and **d**) related to mass effect and/or twisting of the mesentery. These findings are diagnostic of a Peterson-type internal hernia, which was confirmed operatively

management approach in the symptomatic patient (Fig. 15d) [34].

## Hemorrhage

Postoperative hemorrhage complicates 1–4% of SG proce-dures [14]. Similar to RYGB, bleeding can occur intraluminally or extraluminally but most commonly occurs extraluminally along the greater curvature staple line [35]. Hemorrhage after SG manifests with tachycardia, hypo-tension, and dropping hematocrit, and symptoms of intraluminal bleeding additionally include hematemesis and/or melanotic stools [35]. CT is performed in patients with suspected hemorrhage, which is depicted by a high-attenuation collection adjacent to or within the gastric rem-nant (Fig. 16) [30]. Most hemorrhage after SG is self-limited,

and patients can be managed conservatively, but persistent bleeding is managed with endoscopy or catheter angiogra-phy, with laparoscopy reserved for refractory cases [32, 35].

## Gastric Stricture

Gastric stricturing or stenosis can present as a late complica-tion after SG and affects 2–4% of patients [32, 36]. However, milder forms of gastric stenosis may be asymptomatic, and radiographic evidence of stenosis may be present in up to 60% of patients [37]. Stricturing typically occurs along the greater curvature staple line, as a sequela of fibrosis and scarring [35]. Patients typically present with obstructive symptoms such as nausea, vomiting, and food intolerance [37]. UGI is the preferred approach for evaluation of a suspected gastric stricture, which shows focal or less

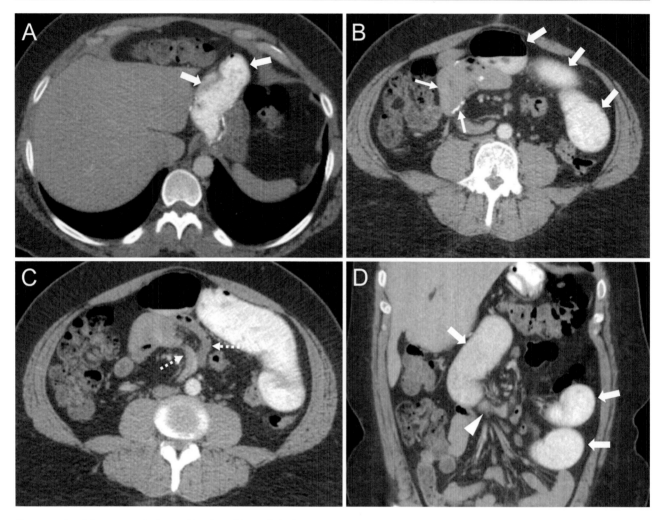

**Fig. 12** Jejunojejunostomy site internal hernia and Roux limb obstruction in a 36-year-old woman presenting with nausea, vomiting, and abdominal pain following RYGB. Axial (**a**–**c**) and coronal (**d**) IV and oral contrast-enhanced CT images show changes of RYGB, with a moderately distended antecolic Roux limb (thick arrows). The jejunojejunal anastomosis is located in the right hemiabdomen (thin arrows, **b**), displaced from its normal left-sided location. There is a stalk-like configuration of two adjacent loops of the small bowel (dashed arrows, **c**). A transition point from distended to decompressed Roux limb is seen in the central abdomen (arrowhead, **d**). Surgery confirmed the presence of a jejunojejunostomy site internal hernia

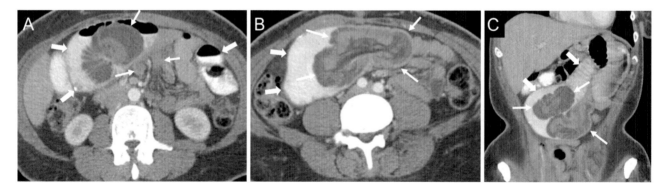

**Fig. 13** Retrograde jejunojejunal intussusception with Roux limb obstruction in a 40-year-old woman who underwent RYGB 2 years ago, presenting with abdominal pain. Axial (**a** and **b**) and coronal (**c**) IV and oral contrast-enhanced CT images show a long-segment retrograde jejunojejunal intussusception (thin arrows) with moderate distention of the Roux limb which is opacified with oral contrast (thick arrows), consistent with Roux limb obstruction. She was managed with operative revision of her jejunojejunal anastomosis

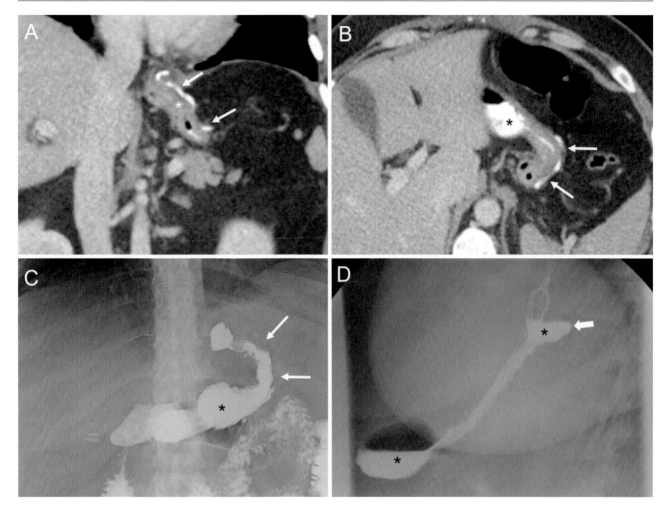

**Fig. 14** Expected appearance of sleeve gastrectomy (SG) on CT and UGI evaluation. Coronal (**a**) and axial (**b**) IV and oral contrast-enhanced CT images show changes of SG with a staple line present along the greater curvature of the stomach (thin arrows) and a thin, tubular, "banana-shaped" appearance of the remnant stomach (asterisks). Images from UGI in the anteroposterior (**c**) and lateral projections (**d**) also show similar findings, with a staple line along the greater curvature (thin arrows). Note the presence of a small fundal remnant, best appreciated on the lateral view (**d**, thick arrow)

commonly long-segment narrowing of the gastric sleeve (Fig. 17). Dilation upstream of the narrowed segment and delayed transit of contrast past the area of narrowing are also common features [37]. Endoscopic balloon dilation is frequently effective in treating gastric strictures, although multiple dilation sessions, covered stent placement, or even surgical revision may be necessary for refractory cases [36].

## Laparoscopic Adjustable Gastric Band

The LAGB is another purely restrictive bariatric surgical procedure, in which an adjustable silicone band is placed around and sutured to the gastric cardia, approximately 2 cm below the gastroesophageal junction [38]. Functionally, a small gastric pouch is created above the band, serving to promote early satiety. The gastric band is connected via tubing to a subcutaneous port in the anterior abdominal wall, in which saline can be injected to fill, or removed to collapse the inflatable sleeve situated within the gastric band [39]. Periodic adjustments are typically made to optimize the size of the band stoma, which is made progressively smaller to induce weight loss.

The normal appearance of LAGB on radiography, UGI, and CT evaluation is shown in Fig. 18. On radiographic evaluation, the gastric band is inclined at an angle (i.e., phi angle, φ) of 4–58° relative to the spinal column [40]. The gastric band appears in profile, with the anterior and posterior aspects of the band overlapping on an anteroposterior radiograph, and the band located approximately 5 cm below the left hemidiaphragm [41]. The subcutaneous reservoir and tubing are visible radiographically and should be contiguous

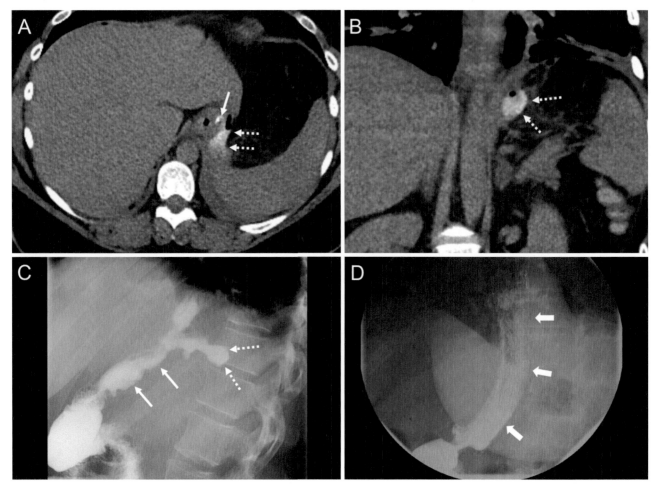

**Fig. 15** Postoperative leak in a 39-year-old woman presenting 9 days after SG, managed with gastroesophageal stenting. Axial (**a**) and coronal (**b**) CT images obtained after oral contrast administration show changes of recent SG, with a staple line along the greater curvature of the stomach (thin arrow, **a**). Arising near the proximal margin of the staple line and extending along the left lateral margin of the fundus, there is a small extraluminal fluid and gas collection containing oral contrast (dashed arrows), consistent with postoperative leak. The presence of a leak was confirmed on subsequent UGI evaluation (**c**), which shows a small contained leak (dashed arrows) coursing posteriorly from the proximal gastric remnant, which was endoscopically treated with placement of a wall stent (**d**, thick arrows)

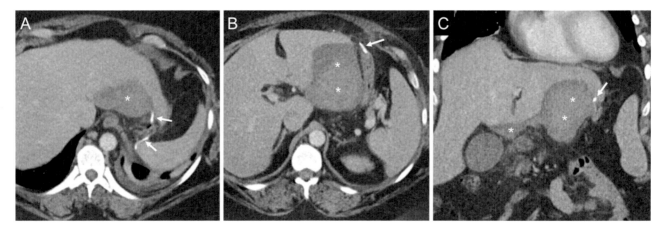

**Fig. 16** Hemorrhage after SG in a 40-year-old man presenting with hematemesis 1 week after surgery. Axial (**a** and **b**) and coronal (**c**) IV contrast-enhanced CT images show postsurgical changes of SG, with a staple line along the greater curvature (arrows). There is a large mixed attenuation hematoma in the lesser sac which tracks along the undersurface of the liver (asterisks). The patient was managed conservatively, and the hematoma decreased on follow-up evaluation (not shown)

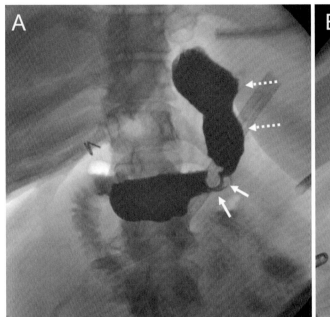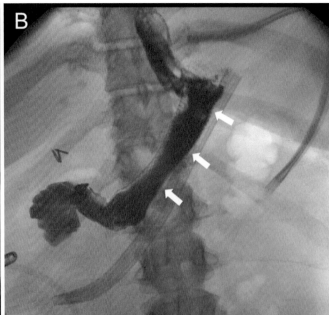

**Fig. 17** High-grade stricture of the gastric sleeve with stenting in a 45-year-old woman with feeding intolerance 1 year after SG. Fluoroscopic images obtained during UGI in the anteroposterior projection (**a**) show a high-grade stricture in the midportion of the

gastric sleeve (thin arrows, **a**). A "banana-shaped" stomach, with staple line, is seen along the greater curvature (dashed arrows, **a**), in keeping with prior SG. Subsequent fluoroscopic image (**b**) shows placement of a gastric stent (thick arrows) with resolution of the stricture

with the gastric band [41]. On UGI, contrast passes freely through the stoma which measures 3–5 mm in diameter. On CT, the gastric band encircles the proximal stomach, with the subcutaneous port visualized superficial to the rectus sheath.

## Stomal Stenosis

Stomal stenosis is a common complication after LAGB, which is thought to be due to band overinflation [41]. Patients with stomal stenosis present with nausea, vomiting, and food intolerance, although there may be more acute or severe symptoms if food impaction develops. On UGI, stomal stenosis manifests as distention of the gastric pouch and esophagus, delayed transit through the gastric band, and a narrow stomal width, generally <3 mm (Fig. 19). Stomal stenosis is managed with band deflation, which generally results in prompt symptomatic resolution [6]. Infrequently, stomal stenosis may not resolve after band deflation owing to concurrent fibrosis or scarring, and balloon dilation and/or removal of the LAGB may be required [41].

## Band Slippage

Slippage of the gastric band can be seen in up to 5% of patients after LAGB [42]. Bands can slip anteriorly, involving downward displacement of the band over the anterior stomach, or posteriorly, resulting in pouch dilatation. Patients present with nausea, vomiting, and food intolerance owing to luminal narrowing and gastric obstruction. Advanced cases may be complicated by gastric volvulus

and ischemia, which manifest with severe abdominal pain and peritonitis [43].

Band slippage can be suggested on radiographic evaluation based on an increase in φ > 58°, lack of superimposition of the anterior and posterior sides of the band (i.e., "O" sign), inferior displacement of the band, and an air-fluid level in the stomach (Fig. 20) [40]. UGI and CT depict the gastric band surrounding the gastric body or even antrum, and eccentric dilation of the gastric pouch is often evident (Fig. 20). Band slippage is managed by prompt deflation of the LAGB to relieve symptoms of gastric outlet obstruction, when present [6]. Ultimately, surgical repositioning or replacement is typically required [44].

## Band Erosion/Perforation

Intragastric band erosion is a relatively uncommon complication, affecting approximately 2% of patients with LAGB [45]. Erosion is typically a chronic process resulting from pressure necrosis of the gastric wall and subsequent erosion of the band into the lumen [41]. Clinical findings include vague abdominal pain, cessation of weight loss, recurrent infection of the port, and discoloration of the fluid in the reservoir [46]. Radiography may show abnormal positioning or an increase in the φ angle [47]. UGI and CT commonly depict the lateral margin of the band positioned within gastric lumen (Fig. 21). Oral contrast surrounding the intraluminal portion of the gastric band is diagnostic of intragastric erosion [47]. Eroded gastric bands are removed to prevent

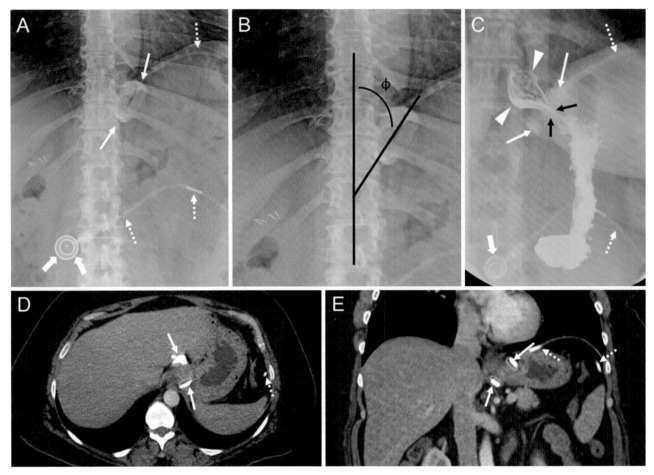

**Fig. 18** Expected appearance of a laparoscopic adjustable gastric band (LAGB) on radiography, UGI evaluation, and CT. Abdominal radiographs in the AP projection (**a** and **b**) show a gastric band just below the expected location of the gastroesophageal junction (thin white arrows, **a**), with a normal φ angle relative to the spinal column (**b**). The band is connected to a subcutaneous port (thick arrows) via catheter tubing (dashed arrows). On the UGI (**c**), the stomach is narrowed as it courses through the opening of the gastric band, creating a small stoma which should measure 3–5 mm (thin black arrows). Proximal to the gastric band is the small gastric pouch (arrowheads). Axial (**d**) and coronal (**e**) IV contrast-enhanced CT images show the LAGB in expected position (thin white arrows)

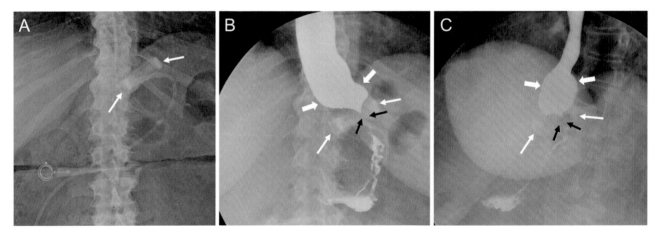

**Fig. 19** Stomal stenosis after LAGB in a 44-year-old woman undergoing evaluation or early satiety. Scout radiograph (**a**) demonstrates normal positioning of the LAGB (thin white arrows), which had a φ angle of 52°. Images from UGI in the anteroposterior (**b**) and lateral (**c**) projections show severe stomal narrowing (black arrows), with delayed transit of contrast past the gastric band (thin white arrows), and dilation of the proximal gastric pouch (thick white arrows). The gastric band was partially deflated, and the patient's symptoms resolved

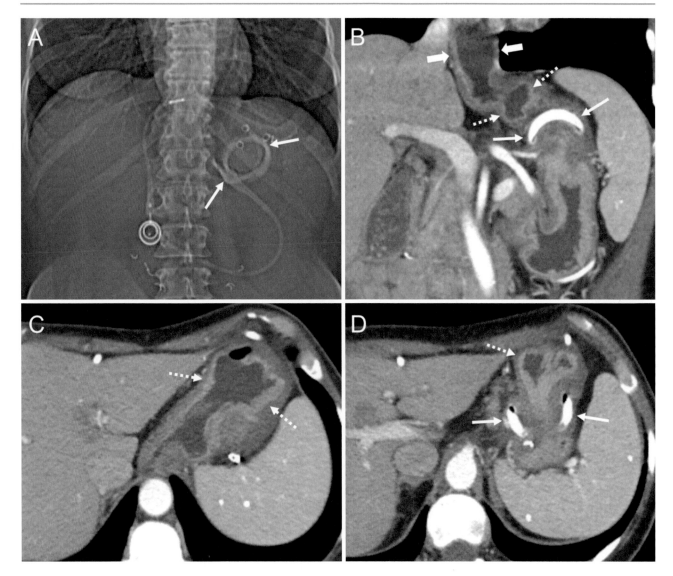

**Fig. 20** Slipped LAGB in a 51-year-old woman presenting with nausea, vomiting, and abdominal pain 4 years after initial placement. Tomogram obtained at the time of CT (**a**) shows an "O" configuration of the gastric band (thin arrows), indicative of posterior slippage. IV contrast-enhanced CT images in the coronal (**b**) and axial (**c** and **d**) planes confirm slippage of the gastric band (thin arrows), with enlargement of the gastric pouch (dashed arrows) and distention of the distal esophagus (thick arrows), suggestive of gastric outlet obstruction. The laparoscopic gastric band was removed surgically, and posterior slippage was confirmed at the time of surgery

further complication such as obstruction and gastrointestinal bleeding, and extraction via an endoscopic approach is often successful [48].

In contradistinction to intragastric band erosion, gastric perforation is rare and almost always presents acutely in the early postoperative setting [41]. Presenting signs and symptoms of gastric perforation include abdominal pain, fever, leukocytosis, and tachycardia [49]. On UGI and CT, gastric perforation can be confidently diagnosed by the presence of contained or free extraluminal leakage of oral contrast. Extraluminal fluid and gas adjacent to the stomach is highly suggestive of perforation, and abscesses may result if the diagnosis is delayed (Fig. 22).

**Port/Tubing Complications**

A more common complication involving the port and tubing is port-site infection, seen in 2–6% of patients after LAGB, and presents clinically with fever, redness, pain, and swelling at the port site [50]. Port-site infection manifests on CT as a focal fluid collection and/or soft- tissue stranding surrounding the port reservoir (Fig. 23). Localized infections may be treated with oral antibiotics, but more advanced or refractory

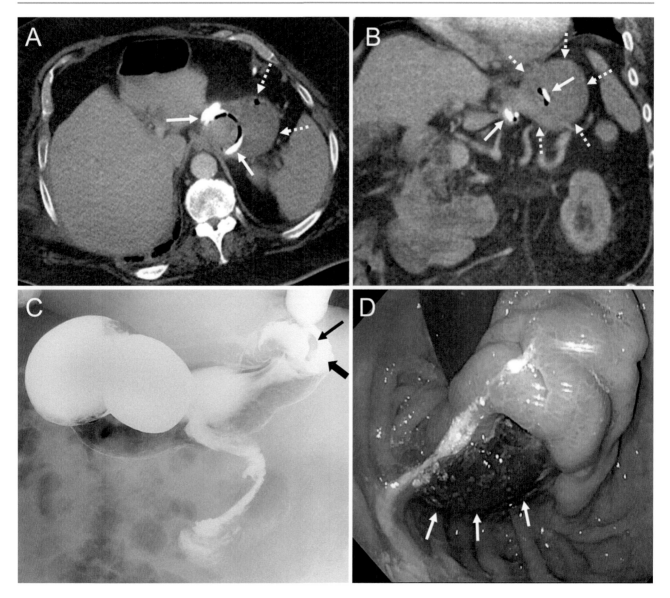

**Fig. 21** Intragastric band erosion in a 75-year-old man with a LAGB presenting with abdominal pain. Axial (**a**) and coronal (**b**) IV contrast-enhanced CT images demonstrate the left lateral aspect of the gastric band, which contains air (solid arrows), situated within the gastric fundus (dashed arrows), diagnostic of intragastric band erosion. Recent prior UGI image in the right posterior oblique projection (**c**) shows contrast filling the band (thin arrow), which confirms that it is within the gastric lumen (thick arrow). Band erosion was confirmed at upper endoscopy (**d**), and the band was subsequently removed endoscopically

infection requires port removal, antibiotic therapy, and replacement of the port once the infection subsides [41]. Infection can also involve the catheter tubing, from extension of an untreated port-site infection or occasionally as a result of intragastric band erosion (Fig. 24) [6]. Other port and tubing complications include port malfunction and catheter disconnection, the latter of which is readily depicted radiographically and on CT (Fig. 25).

## Conclusion/Summary

Bariatric surgery remains the only established treatment for durable weight loss in patients with obesity. Roux-en-Y gastric bypass (RYGB), sleeve gastrectomy (SG), and laparoscopic adjustable gastric band (LAGB) are the most commonly performed bariatric surgeries, each of which has its own set of postoperative complications. Imaging in the emergency setting, especially CT, plays an important role in the care of the post-bariatric surgery patient by readily depicting such complications and guiding further management. The most common complications of RYGB include gastrointestinal leak, postoperative hemorrhage, anastomotic stricture or ulceration, small bowel obstruction, hernia, and intussusception. Complications after SG include leak, hemorrhage, and gastric stricture. Lastly, complications after LAGB include stomal stenosis, band slippage, band erosion, and port/tubing complications. The radiologist must be well-versed in the normal postoperative appearance of these bariatric surgical procedures as well as the most commonly encountered surgical complications.

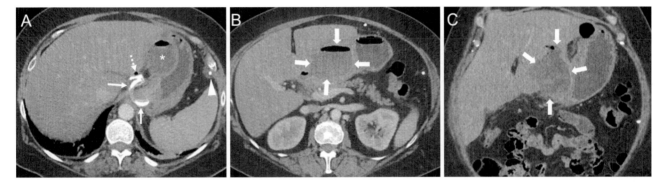

**Fig. 22** Gastric perforation with multiple intra-abdominal abscesses in a 61-year-old woman presenting with abdominal pain, nausea, and vomiting approximately 2 weeks after LAGB. Axial IV contrast-enhanced CT image (**a**) shows a gastric band surrounding the gastric cardia (solid arrows) with an adjacent focus of free gas (dashed arrow), inflammation around the proximal portion of the LAGB tubing (arrowhead), and a rim-enhancing fluid and gas collection along the lesser curvature of the stomach (asterisk). Axial (**b**) and coronal (**c**) IV contrast-enhanced CT images depict a second larger fluid and gas collection within the lesser sac, a portion of which was intrahepatic (thick arrows)

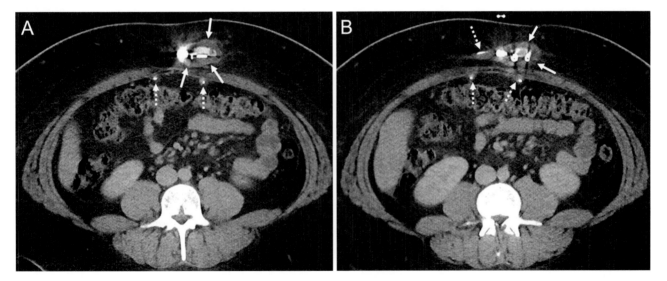

**Fig. 23** Infected LAGB port in a 23-year-old woman presenting with pain at the port site and fever. Axial IV contrast-enhanced CT images (**a** and **b**) show a small amount of fluid surrounding the gastric band port (thin arrows), with fluid tracking along the distal portion of the catheter tubing (dashed arrows). Infection of the port and catheter tubing was confirmed surgically when the gastric band and tubing was removed

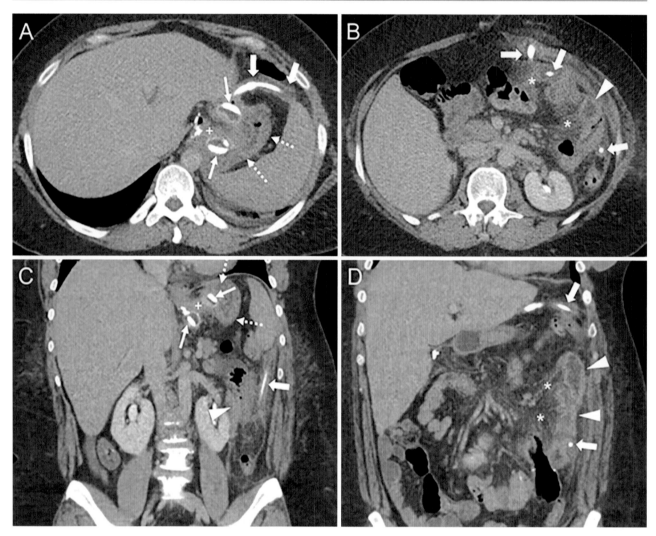

**Fig. 24** Infected laparoscopic gastric band in a 44-year-old woman with RYGB and subsequent LAGB for insufficient weight loss who presented with abdominal pain. Axial (**a** and **b**) and coronal (**c** and **d**) IV contrast-enhanced CT images demonstrate changes of prior RYGB with a gastric band (thin arrows) placed around the gastric pouch (plus signs); excluded stomach denoted by dashed arrows. There is extensive fluid tracking along the entire course of the gastric band catheter tubing (thick arrows), and resultant inflammatory changes involving the Roux limb (arrowheads), with moderate inflammatory stranding surrounding the catheter and small bowel mesentery (asterisks). Erosion of the gastric band into the gastric pouch and purulent material tracking along the catheter were found at the time of laparoscopy

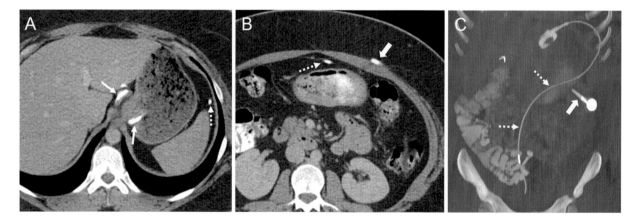

**Fig. 25** Disconnected LAGB detected incidentally in a 40-year-old woman undergoing evaluation for right lower quadrant pain. Axial IV and oral contrast-enhanced CT images (**a** and **b**) demonstrate a gastric band (thin arrows) surrounding the proximal stomach. The catheter tubing (dashed arrows) courses into the left upper quadrant and subsequently into the pelvis and is disconnected from the subcutaneous reservoir (thick arrows). Coronal maximum intensity projection image (**c**) shows the disconnected catheter to better advantage

# References

1. O'Brien PE, Hindle A, Brennan L, et al. Long-term outcomes after bariatric surgery: a systematic review and meta-analysis of weight loss at 10 or more years for all bariatric procedures and a single-centre review of 20-year outcomes after adjustable gastric banding. Obes Surg. 2019;29(1):3–14.
2. Estimate of Bariatric Surgery Numbers, 2011–2018 [Internet]. American Society for Metabolic and Bariatric Surgery. 2018. Available from: https://asmbs.org/resources/estimate-of-bariatric-surgery-numbers
3. Frager D, Medwid SW, Baer JW, et al. CT of small-bowel obstruction: value in establishing the diagnosis and determining the degree and cause. AJR Am J Roentgenol. 1994;162(1):37–41.
4. Swanson JO, Levine MS, Redfern RO, et al. Usefulness of high-density barium for detection of leaks after esophagogastrectomy, total gastrectomy, and total laryngectomy. AJR Am J Roentgenol. 2003;181(2):415–20.
5. Mbadiwe T, Prevatt E, Duerinckx A, et al. Assessing the value of routine upper gastrointestinal contrast studies following bariatric surgery: a systematic review and meta-analysis. Am J Surg. 2015;209(4):616–22.
6. Levine MS, Carucci LR. Imaging of bariatric surgery: normal anatomy and postoperative complications. Radiology. 2014;270(2):327–41.
7. Fobi MAL, Lee H, Holness R, et al. Gastric bypass operation for obesity. World J Surg. 1998;22(9):925–35.
8. Gonzalez R, Sarr MG, Smith CD, et al. Diagnosis and contemporary management of anastomotic leaks after gastric bypass for obesity. J Am Coll Surg. 2007;204(1):47–55.
9. Carucci LR, Turner MA, Conklin RC, et al. Roux-en-Y gastric bypass surgery for morbid obesity: evaluation of postoperative extraluminal leaks with upper gastrointestinal series. Radiology. 2006;238(1):119–27.
10. Nguyen NT, Longoria M, Chalifoux S, et al. Gastrointestinal hemorrhage after laparoscopic gastric bypass. Obes Surg. 2004;14(10):1308–12.
11. Pratt JSA. Roux-en-Y gastric bypass: stomal stenosis. In: Nguyen NT, De Maria EJ, Ikramuddin S, Hutter MM, editors. The sages manual: a practical guide to bariatric surgery. New York: Springer; 2008. p. 211–2.
12. Dallal RM, Bailey LA. Ulcer disease after gastric bypass surgery. Surg Obes Relat Dis. 2006;2(4):455–9.
13. Scheirey CD, Scholz FJ, Shah PC, et al. Radiology of the laparoscopic Roux-en-Y gastric bypass procedure: conceptualization and precise interpretation of results. Radiographics. 2006;26(5):1355–71.
14. Podnos YD, Jimenez JC, Wilson SE, et al. Complications after laparoscopic gastric bypass: a review of 3464 cases. Arch Surg. 2003;138(9):957–61.
15. Champion JK, Williams M. Small bowel obstruction and internal hernias after laparoscopic Roux-en-Y gastric bypass. Obes Surg. 2003;13(4):596–600.
16. Tucker ON, Escalante-Tattersfield T, Szomstein S, et al. The ABC system: a simplified classification system for small bowel obstruction after laparoscopic Roux-en-Y gastric bypass. Obes Surg. 2007;17(12):1549–54.
17. Clapp B. Small bowel obstruction after laparoscopic gastric bypass with nonclosure of mesenteric defects. JSLS. 2015;19(1).
18. Mitchell MT, Gasparaitis AE, Alverdy JC. Imaging findings in Roux-en-O and other misconstructions: rare but serious complications of Roux-en-Y gastric bypass surgery. AJR Am J Roentgenol. 2008;190(2):367–73.
19. Sunnapwar A, Sandrasegaran K, Menias CO, et al. Taxonomy and imaging spectrum of small bowel obstruction after Roux-en-Y gastric bypass surgery. AJR Am J Roentgenol. 2010;194(1):120–8.
20. Aguirre DA, Santosa AC, Casola G, et al. Abdominal Wall Hernias: imaging features, complications, and diagnostic pitfalls at multidetector row CT. RadioGraphics. 2005;25(6):1501–20.
21. Luján JA, Frutos MD, Hernández Q, et al. Laparoscopic versus open gastric bypass in the treatment of morbid obesity. Ann Surg. 2004;239(4):433–7.
22. Higa KD, Ho T, Boone KB. Internal hernias after laparoscopic Roux-en-Y gastric bypass: incidence, treatment and prevention. Obes Surg. 2003;13(3):350–4.
23. Ahmed AR, Rickards G, Husain S, et al. Trends in internal hernia incidence after laparoscopic Roux-en-Y gastric bypass. Obes Surg. 2007;17(12):1563–6.
24. Lockhart ME, Tessler FN, Canon CL, et al. Internal hernia after gastric bypass: sensitivity and specificity of seven CT signs with surgical correlation and controls. AJR Am J Roentgenol. 2007;188(3):745–50.
25. Carucci LR, Turner MA, Shaylor SD. Internal hernia following Roux-en-Y gastric bypass surgery for morbid obesity: evaluation of radiographic findings at small-bowel examination. Radiology. 2009;251(3):762–70.
26. Simper SC, Erzinger JM, McKinlay RD, et al. Retrograde (reverse) jejunal intussusception might not be such a rare problem: a single group's experience of 23 cases. Surg Obes Relat Dis. 2008;4(2):77–83.
27. Daellenbach L, Suter M. Jejunojejunal intussusception after Roux-en-Y gastric bypass: a review. Obes Surg. 2011;21(2):253–63.
28. Kim YH, Blake MA, Harisinghani MG, et al. Adult intestinal intussusception: CT appearances and identification of a causative lead point. RadioGraphics. 2006;26(3):733–44.
29. Stephenson D, Moon RC, Teixeira AF, et al. Intussusception after Roux-en-Y gastric bypass. Surg Obes Relat Dis. 2014;10(4):666–70.
30. Riaz RM, Myers DT, Williams TR. Multidetector CT imaging of bariatric surgical complications: a pictorial review. Abdom Radiol (NY). 2016;41(1):174–88.
31. Gagner M, Deitel M, Kalberer TL, et al. The second international consensus summit for sleeve gastrectomy, March 19–21. Surg Obes Relat Dis. 2009;5(4):476–85.
32. Triantafyllidis G, Lazoura O, Sioka E, et al. Anatomy and complications following laparoscopic sleeve gastrectomy: radiological evaluation and imaging pitfalls. Obes Surg. 2011;21(4):473–8.
33. Aurora AR, Khaitan L, Saber AA. Sleeve gastrectomy and the risk of leak: a systematic analysis of 4,888 patients. Surg Endosc. 2012;26(6):1509–15.
34. Puli SR, Spofford IS, Thompson CC. Use of self-expandable stents in the treatment of bariatric surgery leaks: a systematic review and meta-analysis. Gastrointest Endosc. 2012;75(2):287–93.
35. Sarkhosh K, Birch DW, Sharma A, et al. Complications associated with laparoscopic sleeve gastrectomy for morbid obesity: a surgeon's guide. Can J Surg. 56(5):347–52.
36. Deslauriers V, Beauchamp A, Garofalo F, et al. Endoscopic management of post-laparoscopic sleeve gastrectomy stenosis. Surg Endosc. 2018;32(2):601–9.
37. Levy JL, Levine MS, Rubesin SE, et al. Stenosis of gastric sleeve after laparoscopic sleeve gastrectomy: clinical, radiographic and endoscopic findings. Br J Radiol. 2018;91(1089):20170702.
38. Spivak H, Anwar F, Burton S, et al. The Lap-Band system in the United States: one surgeon's experience with 271 patients. Surg Endosc. 2004;18(2):198–202.
39. Mehanna MJ, Birjawi G, Moukaddam HA, et al. Complications of adjustable gastric banding, a radiological pictorial review. AJR Am J Roentgenol. 2006;186(2):522–34.
40. Swenson DW, Pietryga JA, Grand DJ, et al. Gastric band slippage: a case-controlled study comparing new and old radiographic signs of this important surgical complication. AJR Am J Roentgenol. 2014;203(1):10–6.
41. Sonavane SK, Menias CO, Kantawala KP, et al. Laparoscopic adjustable gastric banding: what radiologists need to know. RadioGraphics. 2012;32(4):1161–78.
42. Egan RJ, Monkhouse SJW, Meredith HE, et al. The reporting of gastric band slip and related complications; a review of the literature. Obes Surg. 2011;21(8):1280–8.

43. Kicska G, Levine MS, Raper SE, et al. Gastric volvulus after laparoscopic adjustable gastric banding for morbid obesity. AJR Am J Roentgenol. 2007;189(6):1469–72.

44. Manganiello M, Sarker S, Tempel M, et al. Management of slipped adjustable gastric bands. Surg Obes Relat Dis. 2008;4(4):534–8.

45. Cherian PT, Goussous G, Ashori F, et al. Band erosion after laparoscopic gastric banding: a retrospective analysis of 865 patients over 5 years. Surg Endosc. 2010;24(8):2031–8.

46. Chisholm J, Kitan N, Toouli J, et al. Gastric band erosion in 63 cases: endoscopic removal and rebanding evaluated. Obes Surg. 2011;21(11):1676–81.

47. Hainaux B, Agneessens E, Rubesova E, et al. Intragastric band erosion after laparoscopic adjustable gastric banding for morbid obesity: imaging characteristics of an underreported complication. AJR Am J Roentgenol. 2005;184(1):109–12.

48. Collado-Pacheco D, Rábago-Torre LR, Arias-Rivera M, et al. Endoscopic extraction of adjustable gastric bands after intragastric migration as a complication of bariatric surgery: technique and advice. Endosc Int Open. 2016;4(6):E673–7.

49. Blachar A, Blank A, Gavert N, et al. Laparoscopic adjustable gastric banding surgery for morbid obesity: imaging of normal anatomic features and postoperative gastrointestinal complications. AJR Am J Roentgenol. 2007;188(2):472–9.

50. Wiesner W, Schöb O, Hauser RS, et al. Adjustable laparoscopic gastric banding in patients with morbid obesity: radiographic management, results, and postoperative complications. Radiology. 2000;216(2):389–94.

# Emergency Imaging of Pregnant Patient

# 35

Donghoon Shin, John Lee, and Christina A. LeBedis

## Contents

### Abstract

Pregnant patients may present in the emergency setting for various reasons, and they can be broadly divided into those with trauma, pregnancy-related problems, and nonpregnancy-related problems. The spectrum of pathologies or injuries in traumas and nonpregnancy-related problems are similar in the pregnant population compared to that of the general population, but the pattern of injury, presentation, and management may differ. Radiologic examinations of pregnant patients in an emergency setting remain an important diagnostic series of tests, and present a unique set of challenges. On one hand, timely identification of the presence or absence of pathology or injury may play a critical role in management decision-making, and can affect clinical outcome for both the mother and fetus. On the other hand, it is also important to consider potential fetal and maternal risks related to the exposure to radiologic examinations, contrast agents, and contrast reaction premedication regimens (Tables 1 and 2). The aim of this chapter is to review the appropriateness of different imaging modalities, pathologies that occur in pregnant women, and important related imaging findings.

### Keywords

Emergency imaging · Pregnancy · Prengnant women · Trauma · Obstetrical emergency · Acute abdomen

## Trauma

Trauma is the leading cause of nonobstetric maternal mortality, with approximately 5–7% of pregnant women sustaining traumatic injuries at some point during their pregnancy [14]. Motor vehicle collisions are the most common cause of trauma, accounting for 50–66% of the cases [14]. Minor injuries are much more common, and are associated with lower fetal loss rates of 1–5%. For severe injuries, the fetal loss rate can be as high as 50% [14]. Initial clinical workup

D. Shin (✉) · J. Lee · C. A. LeBedis (✉)
Boston University Medical Center, Boston, MA, USA
e-mail: Donghoon.shin@bmc.org; christina.lebedis@bmc.org

**Table 1** Safety – Imaging Modality

| Modality | Recommendation | Comments |
|---|---|---|
| Ultrasound | ACR and ACOG both agree that US is generally safe, but should only be used for medical reasons [1] | Usually first line in most abdominal and pelvic conditions |
| | | Keep mechanical and thermal indexes less than 1 when examining the fetus [2] |
| CT | ACR and ACOG both agree that CT may be performed if deemed necessary after clinical workup to answer clinical question that would potentially change management [3, 4] | General consensus is that fetal doses less than 50 mGy pose negligible risks [5–9] |
| | | Fetal doses greater than 100–150 mGy have greater likelihood of adverse effects. Fetal doses from most diagnostic imaging examinations are well below 50 mGy fetal dose [3–9] |
| | | Fetal shielding is not recommended, as it may increase fetal dose due to internal scatter and automatic exposure control [10, 11] |
| MRI | ACR states MR can be used in pregnant patients regardless of gestational age when the information gained is likely to alter management and cannot be obtained through ultrasound [12] | Theoretical risk exists from energy deposition to the fetus from radiofrequency pulses and potential acoustic injury [5, 12] |
| | | Prudent strategy to limit risk is to use lower field strength ≤3 Tesla, and limiting the number of sequences obtained |

*ACR* American College of Radiology, *ACOG* American College of Obstetricians and Gynecologists

**Table 2** Safety – Contrast Agents and Common Medications [13]

| | FDA category | Comments |
|---|---|---|
| Iodine based | B | In clinical scenarios where contrast agents would be warranted in a nonpregnant patient, it may be prudent to perform an IV contrast-enhanced examination in pregnant patients to avoid nondiagnostic imaging that need to be repeated |
| Gadolinium based | C | May be used when necessary to answer clinical questions that may potentially change management. In practice, however, MR contrast is rarely needed in emergency imaging |
| Diphenhydramine | B | Premedication therapy should be administered if risks of allergic reaction is high |
| Corticosteroid | C | Premedication therapy should be administered if risks of allergic reaction are high. Prednisone and dexamethasone are preferred agents, since most of it is metabolized within the placenta before reaching the fetus |

FDA category B: No adverse effects in animal studies, but no controlled studies in pregnant women
FDA category C: Adverse effects seen in animal studies, but no controlled studies in pregnant women

and management is prioritized for maternal survival, since fetal survival is directly linked to maternal well-being [14, 15].

After the initial stabilization of the patient, imaging examinations play a pivotal role in medical decision-making. In addition to allowing for early diagnosis of severe injuries, which need to be managed aggressively, imaging studies can exclude acute injuries or identify minor injuries that can be managed medically and obviate the need for non-obstetrical laparotomy [16, 17]. This is clinically significant since laparotomy in a pregnant patient is associated with preterm labor in approximately 26% of second- trimester and 82% of third -trimester patients [16, 17].

Initial imaging workup usually involves radiographs and ultrasound (US). Radiographs can be useful in quick triage for osseous injuries and chest injuries, while US is often employed as a focused assessment with sonography in

trauma (FAST) examination and to evaluate the fetus [17–19]. Ultrasound has high specificity (95–98%) for the presence of hemoperitoneum and solid organ injury, but it has variable sensitivity (61–83%) in pregnant patients due to body habitus and the gravid uterus [20, 21]. Thus, a negative examination should not be accepted as evidence of no injury. In addition, US is less useful in the evaluation for osseous, visceral organ, and retroperitoneal injuries. Therefore, for abdominopelvic injuries in the trauma setting, IV contrast-enhanced CT remains the primary imaging modality [16–19].

## Patterns of Traumatic Injuries

Most traumatic uterine injuries occur in the third trimester when the uterus is no longer protected by the bony pelvis [14, 15, 18]. Placental abruption is the most common uterine injury, and is seen in 20–50% of the cases after severe blunt abdominal trauma, and in 1–5% of cases after minor blunt injury [22, 23]. Uterine rupture is rare, found in about ~1%, but is associated with nearly 100% fetal mortality and 10% maternal mortality [24]. Direct fetal injuries are even rarer, with a prevalence of less than 1% [24].

The range of nonuterine injuries remains the same for pregnant patients, but the likelihood of different types of injuries can vary due to the changes in anatomy that occur with pregnancy. For example, increased rates of bladder and renal injuries are seen in the third trimester as the gravid uterus displaces the bladder out of the pelvis into the abdomen [25]. Pregnancy-related hydronephrosis also predisposes for injuries to the enlarged kidneys and ureters [17, 25]. The spleen may enlarge with pregnancy and along with the liver, they are displaced toward the chest against the ribs, which predisposes them to injury [17, 22, 24]. Bowel is also displaced superiorly and is in a more compact space, which may increase the risk of multiple injuries in the setting of penetrating trauma [22, 24]. Increased pelvic vascularity related to pregnancy is also associated with increased risk of hemorrhage [17].

## Pregnancy-Related Emergencies

### Placental Abruption

Placental abruption refers to premature separation of the placenta from the uterus, and is the most common cause of vaginal bleeding in the third trimester [18]. It is seen in about 1% of all pregnancies, but is associated with relatively high mortality for the fetus, accounting for up to 25% of perinatal fetal deaths [18]. It is theorized that the placenta is more rigid than the underlying uterine wall, which predisposes it to separation in acute acceleration/deceleration injuries such as in motor vehicle collisions [23]. Patients may present with vaginal spotting to massive hemorrhage, abdominal or pelvic pain, and uterine hypertonia [18]. The magnitude of hemorrhage does not necessarily correlate with severity [17, 18]. The higher degree of placental separation is, however, associated with worse prognosis [26]. Urgent cesarean delivery may be necessary for a viable fetus in distress [26]. In stable patients with reassuring fetal assessment, expectant management may be pursued [26]. Examples of risk factors for placental abruption include preeclampsia, previous abruption, advanced maternal age, trauma, and cigarette use [17, 18]. Marginal placental abruption is the most common subtype, but retroplacental abruption has a worse prognosis [26].

Placental abruption remains largely a clinical diagnosis, with imaging done to confirm and to further characterize it, since the location and the degree of placental separation are prognostic factors. However, the initial diagnosis can be made on imaging in some cases, such as in traumas. Ultrasound remains the primary imaging modality for placental abruption despite its poor sensitivity, less than 50%, since it does not use ionizing radiation and can also be used to evaluate the fetus [17, 18, 27]. The use of magnetic resonance imaging (MRI) have been described in stable patients if the US is negative, with reported sensitivity and specificity of nearly 100%, but is not widely used in practice at present [17, 28]. In the setting of trauma, CT may be the first imaging

examination available to evaluate the placenta, and should be carefully examined. Therefore, it is important for radiologists to be familiar with imaging findings of placental abruption with different modalities.

On US, the appearance of the hematoma depends on the chronicity, size, and location of the hematoma. Acute hematomas may be iso- to hyperechoic to the placenta, and become progressively hypoechoic over time [18] (Fig. 1). However, hematoma is only detected in 20–30% of cases, and only a thickened placenta may be appreciated [17, 18, 28]. Echogenic material in the amniotic fluid is a secondary sign of placental abruption [18]. Color Doppler can be used to differentiate hematoma from normal placenta and to demonstrate areas of devascularization [18]. Uterine leiomyomas, if subjacent to the placenta, may mimic hypoechoic retroplacental clot, and focal myometrial contractions may appear as an iso- to hyperechoic mass and mimic abruption [17, 18, 28]. These, however, can be differentiated using Doppler since both of these will show blood flow.

On CT, the appearance of normal placental findings may confound the diagnosis. The placenta becomes more heterogenous and hyperattenuating to the subjacent myometrium on IV contrast-enhanced CT [29]. Cotyledons also begin to form, which can be seen as foci of rounded low attenuation surrounded by enhancing placenta, and it is important to not mistake it for area of infarction [29]. In the third trimester, venous lakes can be seen on the maternal side, which may be confused as retroplacental hematoma [28, 29]. As the pregnancy progresses, wedge-shaped age-related placental infarcts may be seen that often have no clinical significance, but may be confused with abruption [18, 28, 29]. Placental abruption on CT demonstrates contiguous retroplacental or full-thickness areas of decreased enhancement that form acute angles with myometrium [29] (Fig. 2). This is helpful in differentiating from focal myometrial contraction, which can be seen as bulging areas of hypoattenuation that form obtuse angles [29]. If there is placental infarct due to devascularization, areas of contrast extravasation may be seen as hyperattenuating foci [29]. Retroplacental hematomas may not always be identified since it may be isodense to the myometrium [18, 29]. Hyperdense material in the amniotic fluid can be seen as a secondary finding [29]. Studies have shown that the sensitivity of CT for placental infarction on the original dictated reports is low (43%), but is relatively high on retrospective review (86–100%) [29, 30]. Therefore, having a high index of suspicion and including the placenta in the search pattern, especially in trauma, may lead to improvement in the detection of placental abruption.

MRI can accurately depict placental abruption, and may be pursued if the US is negative and diagnosis could impact management. The appearance of placental hemorrhage on MR depends on the chronicity, demonstrating iso- to

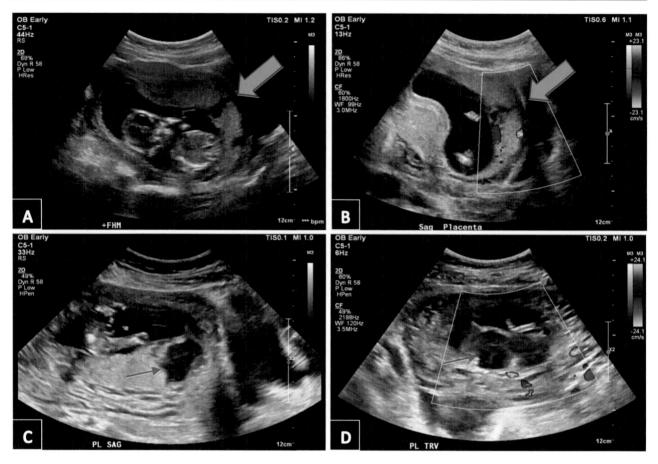

**Fig. 1 Placental Abruption on US** Ultrasound images of the uterus in two different patients show intraplacental aneochoic areas (thick arrows) and heterogeneous collection (thin arrows), consistent with placental abruption with hematoma. (A 20-year-old woman G2P0 at 15w1d pregnant presented with one-day history of vaginal spotting (Images **a** and **b**). A 31-year-old woman G1P0 at 14 weeks pregnant presented with one-day history of vaginal spotting (Images **c** and **d**))

hypointense T1 signal in the acute phase and hyperintense T1 signal in the subacute phase [28]. Hyperacute blood is hyperintense on T2-weighted images, while acute and early subacute blood tend to be T2 hypointense. Chronic hematomas are T1 and T2 hypointense [28].

## Ectopic Pregnancy

Ectopic pregnancy represents approximately 2% of all pregnancies, with the fallopian tube being the most common site accounting for 95–97% of cases [31–33]. It is one of the leading causes of maternal morbidity and mortality, accounting for up to 13% of maternal deaths in Western countries [31, 33]. Risk factors include prior ectopic pregnancy, prior tubal or uterine surgery, pelvic inflammatory disease, current intrauterine device use, and *in vitro* fertilization [31, 33]. Patients classically present with abdominal pain, usually ipsilateral to the site of ectopic, amenorrhea, and irregular vaginal bleeding [31, 33]. When intrauterine pregnancy (IUP) is not identified in

a patient with a positive pregnancy test, ectopic should remain on the differential diagnosis, and serial hCG levels and US should be pursued until an IUP can be confirmed. Serial hCG levels are helpful, since the average doubling time in a normal, viable pregnancy is about 48 h, whereas an ectopic pregnancy generally has a longer doubling time [31–33].

Early diagnosis of ectopic pregnancy is important to reduce maternal mortality and fertility complications [31, 33]. Ultrasound is the first-line imaging modality. It can be helpful to know the hCG levels, since early pregnancy may not be visualized at levels <2000 mIU/ml [31, 33]. However, not visualizing an IUP on US with a hCG >2000 mIU/ml does not definitively suggest an ectopic pregnancy; for example, twin gestation has higher hCG level and is expected to reach 2000 mIU/ml at an earlier stage [31, 33]. Therefore, the most reliable finding is visualizing an extrauterine gestation, which unfortunately is only seen 15–35% of the time [32, 33].

On US, tubal ectopic pregnancy can be seen as an adnexal mass that is separate from the ovary or an interstitial

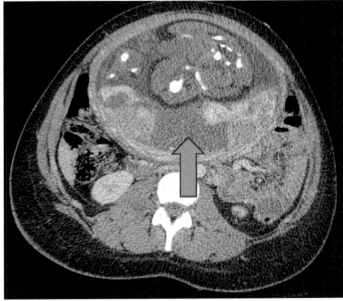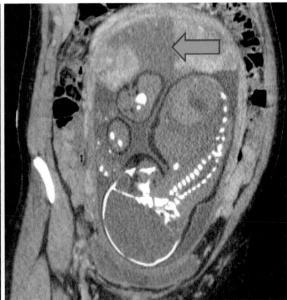

**Fig. 2** **Placental Abruption on CT** Axial and coronal CT images of the abdomen show hypoattenuating area in the placenta (arrows), highly concerning for placental abruption and infarction. Patient was taken to the operating room for emergent cesarean section after bedside ultrasound confirmed the findings, and fetal heart rate decelerations were noted. (A 23-year-old woman G1P0 at 34 weeks pregnant presented after a motor vehicle collision, complaining of abdominal and right hip pain)

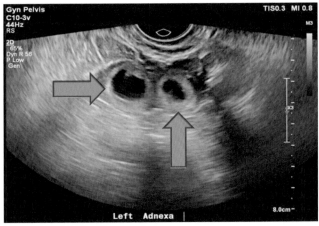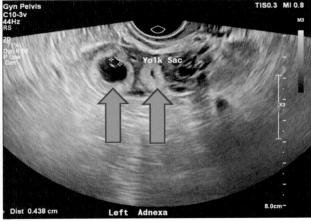

**Fig. 3** **Ectopic Pregnancy on US** Transvaginal ultrasound of the left adnexa shows two cystic structures with yolk sacs (thick arrows), diagnostic of left tubal ectopic twin pregnancy. Patient was taken to the operating room for left salpingectomy and was confirmed to have left tubal ectopic twin pregnancy. (A 38-year-old woman G6P0014 presented with no intrauterine pregnancy visualized on routine first-trimester ultrasound)

mass [32, 33] (Figs. 3 and 4). Similar to a tubal ectopic, a corpus luteum, which is often ipsilateral to the ectopic if present, can also be seen as a thick-walled cystic structure in the adnexa with peripheral hypervascularity on US [32, 33]. Therefore, separating the adnexal mass from the ovary can be helpful to confirm the diagnosis of ectopic pregnancy, by adding gentle compression using the US probe and by varying patient positioning during the examination. Additional US findings include free pelvic fluid and hematosalpinx [32, 33]. When the pelvic fluid is complex, suggesting hemorrhage, it is a more specific finding, which is associated with an 86–93% positive predictive value [32, 33]. Ovarian, cervical, caesarean scar, and abdominal ectopic pregnancies are also possible, but are rare. The presence of hemoperitoneum raises concern for a ruptured ectopic pregnancy, which is the main complication. This occurs in 15–20% of the cases, and may lead to hypovolemic shock, necessitating emergent surgical intervention [31–33]. Traumatic injuries have shown to increase the risk of rupture [31–33].

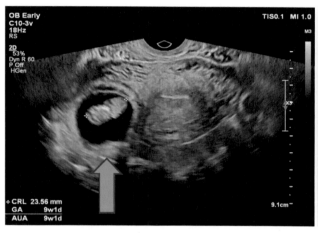
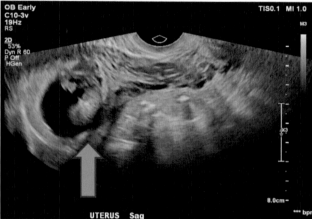

**Fig. 4** **Interstitial Ectopic Pregnancy on US** Transverse and sagittal ultrasound images of the uterus show a single live pregnancy within the right uterine cornua (arrow), highly consistent with right interstitial ectopic pregnancy. (A 36-year-old woman G5P3013 with history of ectopic pregnancy and right salpingectomy presented with one-day history of vaginal spotting and abdominal cramping)

## Preeclampsia/Eclampsia

Preeclampsia and eclampsia are hypertensive disorders of pregnancy thought to be mediated by the placenta [34]. Preeclampsia is seen in up to 8% of all pregnancies, and is associated with advanced maternal age [35, 36]. Eclampsia occurs in about 10% of those with preeclampsia, and is a dangerous condition accounting for 10–14% of pregnancy-related deaths. The only treatment is to deliver the fetus [34–36]. Hemolysis, elevated liver enzymes, and low platelets (HELLP) syndrome is a severe variant of preeclampsia characterized by laboratory abnormalities [37]. The diagnosis of preeclampisa and eclampsia is largely based on clinical findings, and patients may present to the ED for a multitude of problems including epigastric pain that may be related to hepatic dysfunction, headache, visual symptoms, stroke, seizure, pulmonary edema, and placental abruption, amongst others [34–36].

The role of imaging in the emergency setting is to identify evidence of end-organ dysfunction. Ultrasound may show evidence of intrauterine growth restriction related to placental insufficiency [34]. In severe cases, hepatic infarction or hemorrhage may be seen on ultrasound [38, 39]. In as many as 41% of the cases, US features may be present even before laboratory abnormalities in HELLP syndrome [38]. Chest radiography may demonstrate pulmonary edema [38]. Neurological complications, including seizures, strokes, and acute hypertensive encephalopathies, are best evaluated by MRI [40]. In the emergency setting, however, a CT may be done initially to assess for hemorrhage and stroke, since presentations may be similar [40]. MR findings of eclamptic encephalopathy are seen predominantly in the posterior cortex and in the subcortical white matter as T1 hypointense and T2 and FLAIR hyperintensities [40] (Fig. 5). These are related to

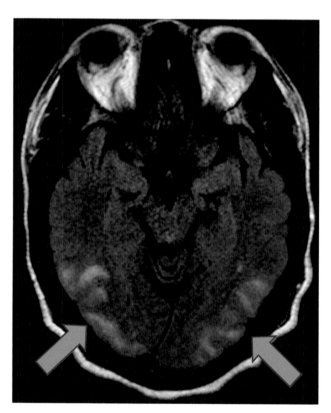

**Fig. 5** **Preeclampsia/Eclampsia** Axial MRI image of the brain shows T2/FLAIR hyperintensities in the bilateral temporal and parietal lobes (arrows), highly consistent with PRES (posterior reversible encephalopathy syndrome) secondary to eclampsia. Patient was taken to the operating room for emergent cesarean section. (A 34-year-old woman G2P0010 at 39 weeks pregnant presented with hypertension (systolic blood pressure in the 200s) and multiple episodes of seizure)

vasogenic edema, and tend to be reversible [40]. In severe cases, cortical or subarachnoid hemorrhages may also be identified as susceptibility artifacts on susceptibility-weighted or gradient-echo sequences [40].

## Molar Pregnancy

Hydatidiform mole or molar pregnancy is part of the gestational trophoblastic disease spectrum, and is considered to be premalignant for gestational trophoblastic neoplasm, particularly choriocarcinomas [41, 42]. These are rare,

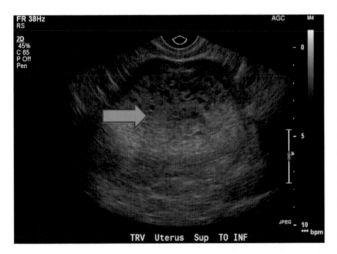

**Fig. 6 Molar Pregnancy** Ultrasound of the uterus in transverse view shows no intrauterine pregnancy and an intrauterine mass with cystic spaces and a "snowstorm" or "bunch of grapes" appearance (thick arrow). Findings were diagnostic of partial molar pregnancy on pathology. (A 26-year-old woman G3P1011 at 10 weeks pregnant presented with vaginal bleeding and elevated serum hCG level)

with a reported prevalence of 66 to 121 per 100,000 pregnancies in North America and European countries [41, 43, 44]. There are two distinct types, complete and partial moles. Patients may present to the ED often with nonspecific symptoms, including abdominal pain and cramping, hyperemesis gravidarum, and vaginal bleeding in the setting of a positive pregnancy test [42, 43]. Molar pregnancies are also associated with early onset of preeclampsia (fewer than 20 weeks of gestation) [45]. In rare cases, molar pregnancies may be complicated by ovarian hyperstimulation syndrome with increased risk of ovarian torsion, stroke, and thromboembolic disease [46] (Fig. 6). Because the hCG level is often elevated with no clear evidence of intrauterine pregnancy, patients are often presumed to have had missed abortions, and the correct diagnosis is made at a later time [41–44]. Treatment usually involves uterine evacuation or hysterectomy [41].

Complete moles are more common, characterized by the absence of embryonic tissues [43]. Ultrasound may show enlarged uterus with an intrauterine mass with cystic spaces and no associated fetal parts, classically described as a "snowstorm" or "bunch of grapes" in appearance [43, 47, 48] (Figs. 7, 8, and 9). Bilateral theca lutein cysts may be present related to ovarian hyperstimulation, seen as enlarged, multicystic ovaries with a "spoke-wheel" appearance [46]. Partial moles may demonstrate enlarged placenta, cystic spaces within the placenta associated with empty gestational sac or with an inappropriately small fetus [49]. Diagnosis based on imaging is often difficult as many partial moles can have similar appearance to complete moles, missed abortion, or even twin pregnancies [43, 49]. CT and MRI are typically not performed for initial evaluation.

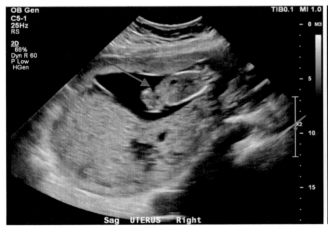

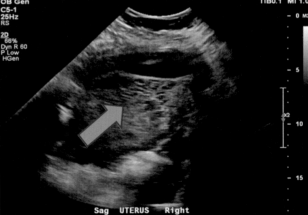

**Fig. 7 Coexistent Molar Pregnancy** Sagittal ultrasound images of the uterus show a live fetus (thin arrow) and adjacent intrauterine mass with cystic spaces and "snowstorm" or "bunch of grapes" appearance (thick arrow). Findings were diagnostic of coexistent molar pregnancy on pathology. (A 36-year-old woman G5P3013 at 16 weeks pregnant presented with vaginal bleeding, nausea, vomiting, and preeclampsia)

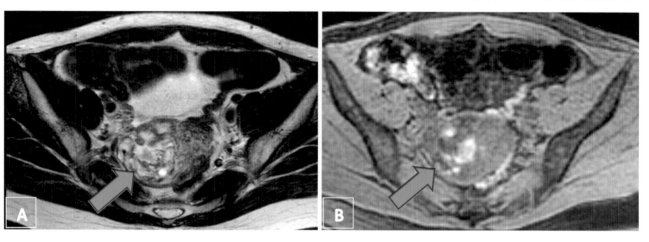

**Fig. 8 Interstitial Molar Pregnancy** Axial T2-weighted (Image **a**) and T1-weighted (Image **b**) noncontrast MR images of the pelvis show a heterogenous mass in the region of the right uterine cornua (arrows) without visualization of an intrauterine pregnancy. Findings are most consistent with interstitial pregnancy. Pathology of the surgical specimen revealed complete molar pregnancy. (A 29-year-old woman G1P0 presented with pregnancy of unknown location and elevated serum HCG)

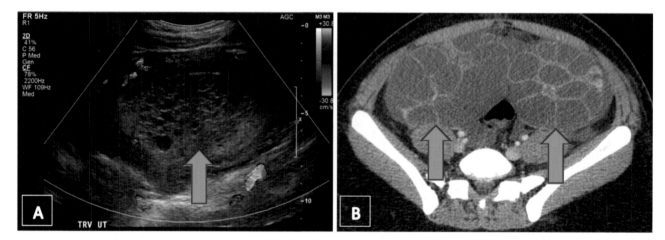

**Fig. 9 Ovarian Hyperstimulation Syndrome and Molar Pregnancy** Transverse ultrasound image of the uterus (Image **a**) shows no intrauterine pregnancy and an intrauterine mass with innumerable cystic spaces and a "snowstorm" or "bunch of grapes" appearance (thick arrow), highly consistent with molar pregnancy. Axial CT image of the pelvis with IV contrast (Image **b**) shows enlarged ovaries with multiple cysts of varying sizes, and ascites (thick arrows). These findings are due to molar pregnancy resulting in ovarian hyperstimulation syndrome, with theca lutein cysts in the enlarged ovaries. (A 19-year-old woman, G2P0010, 12 weeks pregnant, presented for elective termination, and was found to have molar pregnancy)

## Nonpregnancy-Related Emergencies

### Pulmonary Embolism (PE)

Pregnancy is associated with increased risk for deep venous thrombosis (DVT) [50]. Pulmonary embolism is associated with relatively high mortality, up to 15% [19, 50]. Unfortunately, anticoagulation therapy itself is also associated with increased maternal and fetal morbidity, and either accurately diagnosing or excluding PE remains important in management [19].

In order to reduce the radiation exposure in pregnant patients, strategies have been adopted to initially screen for DVT using US Doppler examination in patients with signs and symptoms of PE [19] (Fig. 10). Since the treatment for DVT and PE are the same, the diagnosis of DVT generally obviates the need for further imaging evaluation for PE. Unfortunately, studies in the general population have shown that up to 10% of patients with a normal US Doppler examination for DVT are found to have PE and additional imaging examinations are needed [19]. Chest radiographs, although not sensitive for PE, may be helpful in identifying alternate causes for symptoms, including pneumothorax or pulmonary edema [50]. Chest radiographs can also be used to screen patients for V/Q scintigraphy since abnormal chest radiographs tend to

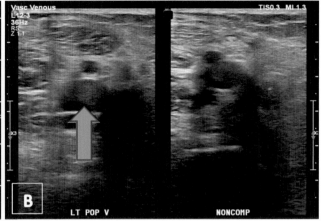

**Fig. 10 Deep Venous Thrombosis** Deep venous thrombosis extending from the left common femoral vein (Image **a**) to the left popliteal vein (Image **b**). Duplex Doppler ultrasound images demonstrate non-compressible left common femoral and popliteal veins with heterogenous material within the veins (arrows), which are areas of deep venous thrombosis. (A 30-year-old woman, G1P0, 12w2d pregnant, with left leg deep venous thrombosis and pulmonary embolism. The patient presented with nausea/vomiting and heaviness in the left leg and swelling)

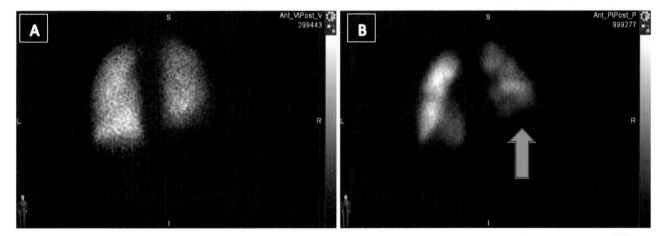

**Fig. 11 Pulmonary Embolism** Positive V/Q scan consistent with pulmonary embolus. Posterior ventilation (Image **a**) and posterior perfusion (Image **b**) images show perfusion defect at the right lung base (arrow), which was most consistent with pulmonary infarct

increase the rate of nondiagnostic V/Q scintigraphy [51]. Many studies have shown that the estimated fetal radiation exposure from CTPA and a V/Q scintigraphy are comparable; reported fetal dose from a V/Q scintigraphy is 0.1–0.8 mGy, and from a CTPA is 0.01–0.66 mGy [19]. V/Q scintigraphy has lower sensitivity and specificity for PE when compared to CTPA with sensitivity of 77% and 98% and specificity of 86% and 98%, respectively [52] (Fig. 11). Although CTPA has the added benefit of being able to evaluate for alternate causes of PE symptoms, VQ scintigraphy is favored in pregnant patients due to lower radiation to the mother's breast tissue, which is more sensitive to radiation during pregnancy [50].

## Acute Abdomen

Approximately 1 in 500 pregnancies is complicated by a nonobstetric surgical condition [53, 54]. Much of the negative outcomes are associated with delayed diagnosis of specific pathologies, which is in part due to under evaluation of pregnant patients and the high prevalence of nonspecific symptoms such as abdominal pain, nausea, vomiting, and constipation that can confound the diagnosis [53, 54]. The increased adrenocortical state seen in pregnancy can also lead to elevation of the white blood cell count, which can make the evaluation for inflammatory response difficult [54].

Acute appendicitis is the most common nontraumatic and nonobstetric surgical condition, with a prevalence of 1 in

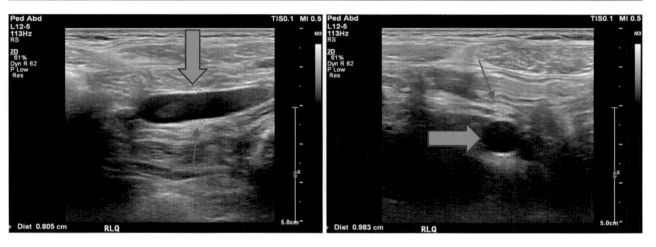

**Fig. 12 Acute Appendicitis on US** Abdominal ultrasound images show dilated appendix measuring 1 cm in diameter (thick arrow), with adjacent hyperechoic fat (thin arrow), suggestive of inflammatory changes. (A 22-year-old woman, G1P0, at 17 weeks pregnant, presented with a one-day history of generalized abdominal pain)

**Table 3** Common cross-sectional imaging findings in acute appendicitis [9, 55–58]

| Imaging findings | Modality |
| --- | --- |
| Noncompressible, dilated appendix (>6 mm) | US |
| Dilated appendix (>7 mm) | MR |
| Wall thickening (>3 mm) | US, MR |
| Periappendiceal fat infiltration | US, MR |
| Appendicolith | US, MR |
| Abscess (complicated) | US, MR |
| Free fluid (complicated) | US, MR |
| Free air (complicated) | MR |

1500 pregnancies, and accounts for 25% of operative indications [53]. There does not seem to be association with pregnancy, but presentation may be different in pregnant patients due to progressive upward displacement of the cecum and appendix (cecal tilt) due to the gravid uterus moving closer to the gallbladder, which makes the pattern of abdominal pain difficult to differentiate [53]. Prompt diagnosis is important, since fetal loss rate is significantly higher in perforated appendicitis (20–35%), while it is 1.5% in noncomplicated appendicitis [53]. Graded-compression US is the first-line imaging examination in pregnant patients, in an attempt to reduce radiation exposure [55] (Fig. 12). Aperistaltic, noncompressible, and dilated appendix (>6 mm outer diameter) with or without hyperechoic appendicolith are features of acute appendicitis on US [9]. Increased echogenicity may also be seen in the surrounding fat as well as periappendiceal fluid collections [9]. Diagnostic accuracy of US is the greatest in the first and second trimester, and decreases in the third trimester due to increasing abdominal girth and changes in anatomy related to the displacement of the appendix [55]. Unfortunately, as many as 88–92% of the examinations are nondiagnostic, and many patients end up requiring further imaging [56, 57]. Recently, MRI has become more widely used in evaluation for appendicitis with high sensitivity and specificity, 90–97% for both [56, 57] (Table 3 and Figs. 13 and 14). MR findings include a dilated appendix (>7 mm) and wall thickening (>3 mm), with fluid-sensitive sequences showing increased signal in the surrounding fat with or without discrete fluid collection [56, 57]. Blooming artifact may be helpful in identifying appendicoliths, if present [56, 57]. Commonly obtained sequences include orthogonal planes of T2-weighted single-shot fast spin-echo with and without fat saturation, 3D T1-weighted, gradient echo, and diffusion-weighted sequences. IV contrast-enhanced CT is indicated if MR is unavailable or if there is lack of expertise [56, 57] (Fig. 15).

Acute cholecystitis is the second most common cause of acute abdomen with a prevalence 1 in 1600 to 1 in 10,000 pregnancies [53, 54]. Cholelithiasis is the most common cause responsible for 90% of the cases [53, 54]. Increased incidence of acute cholecystitis in the pregnant population is theorized to be related to increased levels of progesterone, which leads to smooth muscle relaxation promoting bile stasis and lithogenesis [54]. Presentation in the pregnant patient is usually the same, and first-line evaluation remains US, followed by MRCP in select cases [19, 53, 54] (Table 4 and Fig. 16). Ultrasound classically shows cholelithiasis with a sonographic Murphy's sign with or without gallbladder wall thickening (>3 mm) and pericholecystic fluid [50, 59]. MRCP may show a calculus in the gallbladder neck or cystic duct as a filling defect in the setting of distended gallbladder, wall thickening (>3 mm), and pericholecystic fluid [50, 59]. Nonoperative management is associated with a high rate of recurrence (44–92%) and increased risk of pancreatitis (13%), which is associated with 10–20% fetal loss rate [53]. Therefore,

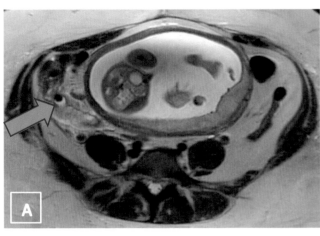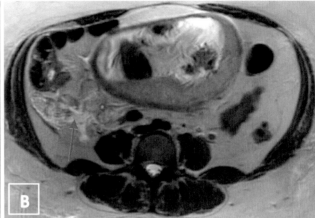

**Fig. 13 Acute Appendicitis on MR** Axial T2-weighted MR images of the abdomen show a dilated appendix with an appendicolith at the tip (thick arrow, image **a**) and periappendicial fat stranding (thin arrow, image **b**). (A 26-year-old woman, G1P0, at 22 weeks pregnant, presented with a one-day history of right upper quadrant pain)

**Fig. 14 Acute Appendicitis on MR** Sagittal T2-weighted MR images of the abdomen show a dilated appendix and a tilted cecum (arrows). The cecum routinely elevates during the course of pregnancy and may be tilted and/or positioned in the right upper quadrant. (A 27-year-old woman, G1P0, 27 weeks pregnant, presented with a two-day history of diarrhea, right lower quadrant pain, and nausea)

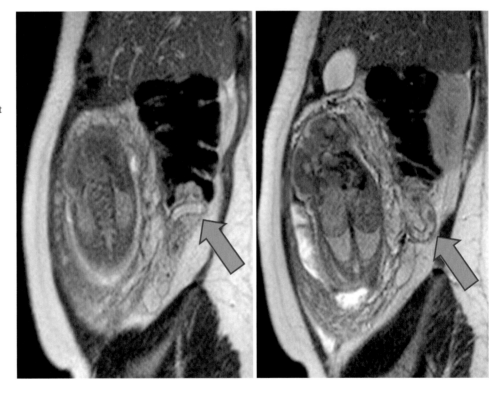

surgical management is preferred especially in the first and second trimesters [53].

Bowel obstruction complicates 1 in 1500 to 1 in 16,000 pregnancies, with increasing risk further along in pregnancy, especially from volvulus [53, 54]. The most common cause of obstruction is due to adhesions related to prior surgery or inflammatory conditions accounting for 60–70% of the cases, and intussusception is seen in 5% of the cases [53, 54]. Mortality is higher in the pregnant patients, reaching 6%, and fetal mortality is also high at 26% [54]. Serial upright radiographs, usually at 4–6 h intervals, have relatively high sensitivity (82%) for the detection of air-fluid levels and bowel dilation [53, 54]. Since oral contrast agents are not absorbed by the patient, they can be used in pregnancy, and some institutions may opt for water-soluble contrast challenge with gastrografin or its equivalent in select patients to help predict the success of conservative measures. IV contrast-enhanced CT or MR is secondarily pursued if radiographs are not typical for obstruction in the setting of a high clinical suspicion [53, 54].

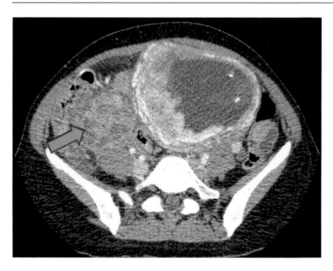

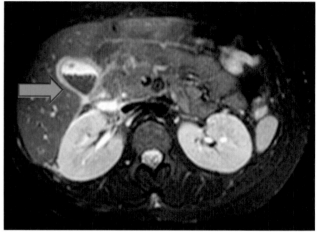

**Fig. 15** **Acute Appendicitis on CT** Axial CT image of the abdomen shows a heterogeneous collection (thick arrow) in the right lower quadrant without visualization of the appendix, indicative of a complicated appendicitis. Patient was managed with antibiotics and had uncomplicated course of hospital stay and vaginal delivery. (A 16-year-old female, G2P1, 16 weeks pregnant, presented with a two-week history of right lower quadrant pain that quickly worsened in one day. Initial workup including ultrasound and MRI failed to visualize an appendix)

**Fig. 16** **Acute Cholecystitis** Axial T2-weighted MR image of the abdomen shows gallstones and pericholecystic fluid (arrow) in a patient with right upper quadrant pain, which is highly consistent with acute cholecystitis, which was confirmed at surgery. (An 18-year-old female, G1P0, at 21 weeks pregnant, presented with a one-day history of right upper quadrant pain, anorexia, nausea, and vomiting)

**Table 4** Common cross-sectional imaging findings in acute cholecystitis [59]

| Imaging findings | Modality |
|---|---|
| Gallbladder distension | US, MR |
| Gallstone | US, MR |
| Wall thickening (>3 mm) | US, MR |
| Pericholecystic fluid | US, MR |
| Sonographic Murphy's sign | US |

## Genitourinary

Urolithiasis is seen in approximately 1 in 200 to 1 in 2000 pregnancies, with many cases being asymptomatic [19]. Approximately 75% of the calculi pass spontaneously. Ultrasound is not reliably sensitive for detecting calculi (34–95% sensitivity), particularly in the distal ureter. Ultrasound can reliably show hydronephrosis, however, which may be concerning for obstructive processes [19] (Fig. 17). This, however, is confounded by physiologic hydronephrosis in the third trimester [19]. If it would potentially affect clinical management, then noncontrast MR urography can be pursued. Otherwise, a low-dose CT protocol can be done [19].

Acute pyelonephritis is seen in 1–2% of pregnancies, and tends to be more common later in the pregnancy due to increasing degree of urinary tract obstruction from the

gravid uterus [60]. It is a clinical diagnosis, although imaging may be indicated in cases when patients fail to clinically improve after appropriate therapy [60]. Imaging may show an obstructed kidney, renal abscess, or infarction that may need to be intervened upon [61]. Although US has low sensitivity for the detection of pyelonephritis, it may play a role in the detection of renal abscess and obstruction (Table 5 and Fig. 18). Ultrasound may show renal enlargement, loss of corticomedullary differentiation, focal decrease in vascularity or abnormal echogenicity of parenchyma, and low-level echoes in the collecting system, with or without renal or perirenal abscess [61]. MRI has high sensitivity and specificity for acute pyelonephritis, 89.5 and 87.5%, respectively [61]. MRI may also demonstrate renal enlargement, perinephric fat infiltration, and focal abnormal signal in the parenchyma (decreased T1, increased T2, and increased DWI) [61]. MRI may also show fluid/fluid level in the collecting system on T2-weighted sequences [61]. MRI of the abdomen with T1-weighted, T2-weighted single-shot fast spin-echo with and without fat saturation, gradient echo, and diffusion-weighted sequences are helpful in evaluation [61].

## Conclusion

Radiologic evaluation of pregnant women in the emergency setting is an important step in clinical decision-making, and may assist in early diagnosis with improved outcomes, or

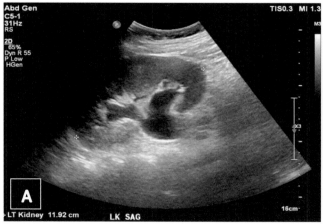

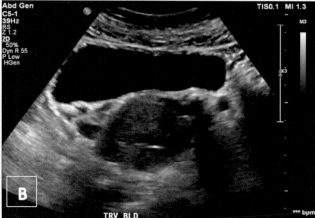

**Fig. 17  Obstructing Renal Calculus** Sagittal ultrasound image of the left kidney (Image **a**) shows moderate left hydronephrosis (thick arrow). Transverse ultrasound image of the bladder (Image **b**) shows an obstructing calculus at the left ureterovesical junction with posterior shadowing (thick arrow). (A 30-year-old woman, G2P1, at 23 weeks pregnant, presented with an eight-day history of abdominal pain, nausea, and vomiting)

**Table 5** Common cross-sectional imaging findings in acute pyelonephritis [61]

| Imaging findings | Modality |
|---|---|
| Renal enlargement | US, MR |
| Thickening of pelvicalyceal urothelium | US, MR |
| Loss of corticomedullary differentiation | US |
| Focal decrease in vascularity in the parenchyma | US |
| Perinephric fat infiltration | US, MR |
| Focal abnormal echogenicity of parenchyma | US |
| Focal decrease in T1 signal and increase in T2 and DWI signals in affected area | MR |
| Low-level echogenic debris in the collecting system | US |
| Presence of fluid-fluid level in the collecting system on T2-weighted sequences | MR |
| Renal abscesses | US, MR |

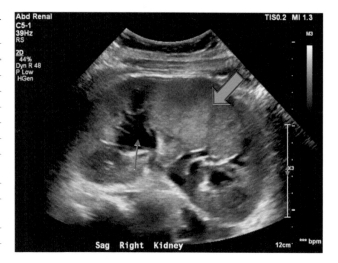

**Fig. 18  Pyelonephritis** Ultrasound of the right kidney in sagittal view shows mild hydronephrosis (thin arrow) and areas of increased echogenicity (thick arrow), a nonspecific finding which could represent a number of underlying conditions such as infection, renal amyloidosis, chronic kidney disease, and sickle cell disease. Correlation with urinalysis represented pyelonephritis. (A 19-year-old female, G1P0, at 27w2d pregnant, presented with a one-day history of headache, fever, dizziness, dysuria, and increased frequency of urination)

obviate the need for surgical interventions by excluding severe pathologies. Ultrasound generally is the first-line imaging modality followed by MRI, except in abdominal trauma, where CT is the primary imaging modality. While it is important to adopt strategies to limit ionizing radiation exposure, no imaging examination that is indicated to answer an important clinical question without a clear alternative should be withheld. It is helpful for radiologists to keep a high index of suspicion for pregnancy-specific problems, such as placental abruptions, and understand the epidemiology of nonpregnancy-related problems in the pregnant population, in order to arrive at the correct diagnosis.

## References

1. AIUM-ACR-ACOG-SMFM-SRU practice parameter for the performance of standard diagnostic obstetric ultrasound examinations. J Ultrasound Med. 2018;37(11):E13–24.

2. Torloni MR, Vedmedovska N, Merialdi M, Betrán AP, Allen T, González R, et al. Safety of ultrasonography in pregnancy: WHO systematic review of the literature and meta-analysis. Ultrasound Obstet Gynecol. 2009;33(5):599–608. Available from: http://www.ncbi.nlm.nih.gov/pubmed/19291813

3. ACR-SPR. ACR– Society of Pediatric Radiology (SPR) practice guideline for imaging pregnant or potentially pregnant adolescents and women with ionizing radiation. Am Coll Radiol. 2018;1076:1–23. Available from: https://www.acr.org/-/media/ACR/Files/Practice-Parameters/Pregnant-Pts.pdf

4. ACOG Committee on Obstetric Practice. Committee Opinion No. 723 summary: guidelines for diagnostic imaging during pregnancy and lactation. Obstet Gynecol. 2017;130(4):933–4. Available from: http://www.ncbi.nlm.nih.gov/pubmed/15339791

5. Tirada N, Dreizin D, Khati NJ, Akin EA, Zeman RK. Imaging pregnant and lactating patients. RadioGraphics. 2015;35(6):1751–65. Available from: http://pubs.rsna.org/doi/10.1148/rg.2015150031

6. McCollough CH, Schueler BA, Atwell TD, Braun NN, Regner DM, Brown DL, et al. Radiation exposure and pregnancy: when should we be concerned? RadioGraphics. 2007;27(4):909–17. Available from: https://linkinghub.elsevier.com/retrieve/pii/S0098167208791598

7. Tremblay E, Thérasse E, Thomassin-Naggara I, Trop I. Quality initiatives: guidelines for use of medical imaging during pregnancy and lactation. Radiographics. 32(3):897–911. Available from: http://www.ncbi.nlm.nih.gov/pubmed/22403117

8. Wang PI, Chong ST, Kielar AZ, Kelly AM, Knoepp UD, Mazza MB, et al. Imaging of pregnant and lactating patients: Part 1, Evidence-based review and recommendations. AJR Am J Roentgenol. 2012;198(4):778–84. Available from: http://www.ncbi.nlm.nih.gov/pubmed/22451541

9. Wang PI, Chong ST, Kielar AZ, Kelly AM, Knoepp UD, Mazza MB, et al. Imaging of pregnant and lactating patients: Part 2, Evidence-based review and recommendations. AJR Am J Roentgenol. 2012;198(4):785–92. Available from: http://www.ncbi.nlm.nih.gov/pubmed/22451542

10. Marsh RM, Silosky M. Patient shielding in diagnostic imaging: discontinuing a legacy practice. AJR Am J Roentgenol. 2019;212(4):755–7. Available from: http://www.ncbi.nlm.nih.gov/pubmed/30673332

11. American Association of Physicists in Medicine. PP32-A – AAPM Position Statement on the Use of Patient Gonadal and Fetal Shielding. 2019. Available from: https://www.aapm.org/org/policies/details.asp?id=468&type=PP&current=true

12. Expert Panel on MR Safety, Kanal E, Barkovich AJ, Bell C, Borgstede JP, Bradley WG, et al. ACR guidance document on MR safe practices: 2013. J Magn Reson Imaging. 2013;37(3):501–30. Available from: http://www.ncbi.nlm.nih.gov/pubmed/23345200

13. American College of Radiology. ACR manual on contrast media: version 10.3. Reston: American College of Radiology; 2020.

14. Mattox KL, Goetzl L. Trauma in pregnancy. Crit Care Med. 2005;33(10 Suppl):S385–9. Available from: http://www.ncbi.nlm.nih.gov/pubmed/16215362

15. Chibber R, Al-Harmi J, Fouda M, El-Saleh E. Motor-vehicle injury in pregnancy and subsequent feto-maternal outcomes: of grave concern. J Matern Fetal Neonatal Med. 2015;28(4):399–402. Available from: http://www.ncbi.nlm.nih.gov/pubmed/24866347

16. Visser BC, Glasgow RE, Mulvihill KK, Mulvihill SJ. Safety and timing of nonobstetric abdominal surgery in pregnancy. Dig Surg. 2001;18(5):409–17. Available from: http://www.ncbi.nlm.nih.gov/pubmed/11721118

17. Raptis CA, Mellnick VM, Raptis DA, Kitchin D, Fowler KJ, Lubner M, et al. Imaging of trauma in the pregnant patient. RadioGraphics. 2014;34(3):748–63. Available from: http://pubs.rsna.org/doi/10.1148/rg.343135090

18. Sadro C, Bernstein MP, Kanal KM. Imaging of trauma: Part 2, Abdominal trauma and pregnancy – a radiologist's guide to doing what is best for the mother and baby. AJR Am J Roentgenol. 2012;199(6):1207–19. Available from: http://www.ncbi.nlm.nih.gov/pubmed/23169710

19. Wieseler KM, Bhargava P, Kanal KM, Vaidya S, Stewart BK, Dighe MK. Imaging in pregnant patients: examination appropriateness. RadioGraphics. 2010;30(5):1215–29. Available from: http://pubs.rsna.org/doi/10.1148/rg.305105034

20. Richards JR, Ormsby EL, Romo MV, Gillen MA, McGahan JP. Blunt abdominal injury in the pregnant patient: detection with US. Radiology. 2004;233(2):463–70. Available from: http://www.ncbi.nlm.nih.gov/pubmed/15516618

21. Goodwin H, Holmes JF, Wisner DH. Abdominal ultrasound examination in pregnant blunt trauma patients. J Trauma. 2001;50(4):689–93. Discussion 694. Available from: http://www.ncbi.nlm.nih.gov/pubmed/11303166

22. Pearlman MD, Tintinalli JE, Lorenz RP. Blunt trauma during pregnancy. N Engl J Med. 1990;323(23):1609–13. Available from: http://www.ncbi.nlm.nih.gov/pubmed/2233950

23. Shah KH, Simons RK, Holbrook T, Fortlage D, Winchell RJ, Hoyt DB. Trauma in pregnancy: maternal and fetal outcomes. J Trauma. 1998;45(1):83–6. Available from: http://www.ncbi.nlm.nih.gov/pubmed/9680017

24. Sadro C, Bittle M, O'Connell K. Imaging the pregnant trauma patient. Ultrasound Clin. 2011;6(1):97–103. Available from: https://linkinghub.elsevier.com/retrieve/pii/S1556858X10002045

25. Goldman SM, Wagner LK. Radiologic ABCs of maternal and fetal survival after trauma: when minutes may count. Radiographics. 19(5):1349–57. Available from: http://www.ncbi.nlm.nih.gov/pubmed/10489187

26. Ananth CV, Berkowitz GS, Savitz DA, Lapinski RH. Placental abruption and adverse perinatal outcomes. JAMA. 1999;282(17):1646–51. Available from: http://www.ncbi.nlm.nih.gov/pubmed/10553791

27. Glantz C, Purnell L. Clinical utility of sonography in the diagnosis and treatment of placental abruption. J Ultrasound Med. 2002;21(8):837–40. Available from: http://www.ncbi.nlm.nih.gov/pubmed/12164566

28. Masselli G, Brunelli R, Di Tola M, Anceschi M, Gualdi G. MR imaging in the evaluation of placental abruption: correlation with sonographic findings. Radiology. 2011;259(1):222–30. Available from: http://www.ncbi.nlm.nih.gov/pubmed/21330568

29. Wei SH, Helmy M, Cohen AJ. CT evaluation of placental abruption in pregnant trauma patients. Emerg Radiol. 2009;16(5):365–73. Available from: http://www.ncbi.nlm.nih.gov/pubmed/19277736

30. Manriquez M, Srinivas G, Bollepalli S, Britt L, Drachman D. Is computed tomography a reliable diagnostic modality in detecting placental injuries in the setting of acute trauma? Am J Obstet Gynecol. 2010;202(6):611.e1–5. Available from: http://www.ncbi.nlm.nih.gov/pubmed/20223441

31. McWilliams GDE, Hill MJ, Dietrich CS. Gynecologic emergencies. Surg Clin North Am. 2008;88(2):265–83. Available from: https://linkinghub.elsevier.com/retrieve/pii/S0039610907001867

32. Rodgers SK, Chang C, DeBardeleben JT, Horrow MM. Normal and abnormal US findings in early first-trimester pregnancy: review of the Society of Radiologists in Ultrasound 2012 Consensus Panel recommendations. RadioGraphics. 2015;35(7):2135–48. Available from: http://pubs.rsna.org/doi/10.1148/rg.2015150092

33. Lin EP, Bhatt S, Dogra VS. Diagnostic clues to ectopic pregnancy. RadioGraphics. 2008;28(6):1661–71. Available from: http://pubs.rsna.org/doi/10.1148/rg.286085506

34. Gestational Hypertension and Preeclampsia: ACOG Practice Bulletin, Number 222. Obstet Gynecol. 2020;135(6):e237–60. Available from: http://www.ncbi.nlm.nih.gov/pubmed/32443079

35. Edlow JA, Caplan LR, O'Brien K, Tibbles CD. Diagnosis of acute neurological emergencies in pregnant and post-partum women. Lancet Neurol. 2013;12(2):175–85. Available from: http://www.ncbi.nlm.nih.gov/pubmed/23332362

36. Duley L, Meher S, Abalos E. Management of pre-eclampsia. BMJ. 2006;332(7539):463–8. Available from: http://www.ncbi.nlm.nih.gov/pubmed/16497761

37. Sibai BM. Diagnosis, controversies, and management of the syndrome of hemolysis, elevated liver enzymes, and low platelet count. Obstet Gynecol. 2004;103(5 Pt 1):981–91. Available from: http://www.ncbi.nlm.nih.gov/pubmed/15121574

38. Nunes JO, Turner MA, Fulcher AS. Abdominal imaging features of HELLP syndrome: a 10-year retrospective review. Am J Roentgenol. 2005;185(5):1205–10. Available from: http://www.ajronline.org/doi/10.2214/AJR.04.0817

39. Heller MT, Tublin ME, Hosseinzadeh K, Fargiano A. Imaging of hepatobiliary disorders complicating pregnancy. AJR Am J Roentgenol. 2011;197(3):W528–36. Available from: http://www.ncbi.nlm.nih.gov/pubmed/21862784

40. Kanekar S, Bennett S. Imaging of neurologic conditions in pregnant patients. RadioGraphics. 2016;36(7):2102–22. Available from: http://pubs.rsna.org/doi/10.1148/rg.2016150187

41. Berkowitz RS, Goldstein DP. Current advances in the management of gestational trophoblastic disease. Gynecol Oncol. 2013;128(1):3–5. Available from: http://www.ncbi.nlm.nih.gov/pubmed/22846466

42. Vassilakos P, Riotton G, Kajii T. Hydatidiform mole: two entities. A morphologic and cytogenetic study with some clinical consideration. Am J Obstet Gynecol. 1977;127(2):167–70. Available from: http://www.ncbi.nlm.nih.gov/pubmed/188340

43. Green CL, Angtuaco TL, Shah HR, Parmley TH. Gestational trophoblastic disease: a spectrum of radiologic diagnosis. Radiographics. 1996;16(6):1371–84. Available from: http://www.ncbi.nlm.nih.gov/pubmed/8946542

44. Altieri A, Franceschi S, Ferlay J, Smith J, La Vecchia C. Epidemiology and aetiology of gestational trophoblastic diseases. Lancet Oncol. 2003;4(11):670–8. Available from: http://www.ncbi.nlm.nih.gov/pubmed/14602247

45. Mangili G, Garavaglia E, Cavoretto P, Gentile C, Scarfone G, Rabaiotti E. Clinical presentation of hydatidiform mole in northern Italy: has it changed in the last 20 years? Am J Obstet Gynecol. 2008;198(3):302.e1–4. Available from: http://www.ncbi.nlm.nih.gov/pubmed/18177836

46. Cappa F, Pasqua C, Tobia M, Ventura T. Ascites and hydrothorax due to endogenous hyperstimulation of H.C.G. in a case of hydatidiform mole destruens with secondary irreversible kidney insufficiency due to disseminated intravascular coagulation. Riv Ital Ginecol. 56(5–6):363–8. Available from: http://www.ncbi.nlm.nih.gov/pubmed/1019550

47. Reuter K, Michlewitz H, Kahn PC. Early appearance of hydatidiform mole by ultrasound. AJR Am J Roentgenol. 1980;134(3):588–9. Available from: http://www.ncbi.nlm.nih.gov/pubmed/6766632

48. Benson CB, Genest DR, Bernstein MR, Soto-Wright V, Goldstein DP, Berkowitz RS. Sonographic appearance of first trimester complete hydatidiform moles. Ultrasound Obstet Gynecol. 2000;16(2):188–91. Available from: http://www.ncbi.nlm.nih.gov/pubmed/11117091

49. Naumoff P, Szulman AE, Weinstein B, Mazer J, Surti U. Ultrasonography of partial hydatidiform mole. Radiology. 1981;140(2):467–70. Available from: http://www.ncbi.nlm.nih.gov/pubmed/7255725

50. Pahade JK, Litmanovich D, Pedrosa I, Romero J, Bankier AA, Boiselle PM. Quality initiatives: imaging pregnant patients with suspected pulmonary embolism: what the radiologist needs to know. Radiographics. 2009;29(3):639–54. Available from: http://www.ncbi.nlm.nih.gov/pubmed/19270072

51. Forbes KP, Reid JH, Murchison JT. Do preliminary chest X-ray findings define the optimum role of pulmonary scintigraphy in suspected pulmonary embolism? Clin Radiol. 2001;56(5):397–400. Available from: http://www.ncbi.nlm.nih.gov/pubmed/11384139

52. Sostman HD, Stein PD, Gottschalk A, Matta F, Hull R, Goodman L. Acute pulmonary embolism: sensitivity and specificity of ventilation-perfusion scintigraphy in PIOPED II study. Radiology. 2008;246(3):941–6. Available from: http://www.ncbi.nlm.nih.gov/pubmed/18195380

53. Augustin G, Majerovic M. Non-obstetrical acute abdomen during pregnancy. Eur J Obstet Gynecol Reprod Biol. 2007;131(1):4–12. Available from: https://linkinghub.elsevier.com/retrieve/pii/S0301211506004842

54. Coleman MT, Trianfo VA, Rund DA. Nonobstetric emergencies in pregnancy: trauma and surgical conditions. Am J Obstet Gynecol. 1997;177(3):497–502. Available from: http://www.ncbi.nlm.nih.gov/pubmed/9322613

55. Stone MB, Chao J. Emergency ultrasound diagnosis of acute appendicitis. Acad Emerg Med. 2010;17(1):E5. Available from: http://www.ncbi.nlm.nih.gov/pubmed/19891673

56. Pedrosa I, Zeikus EA, Levine D, Rofsky NM. MR imaging of acute right lower quadrant pain in pregnant and nonpregnant patients. Radiographics. 2007;27(3):721–43. Discussion 743–53. Available from: http://www.ncbi.nlm.nih.gov/pubmed/17495289

57. Spalluto LB, Woodfield CA, DeBenedectis CM, Lazarus E. MR imaging evaluation of abdominal pain during pregnancy: appendicitis and other nonobstetric causes. RadioGraphics. 2012;32(2):317–34. Available from: http://pubs.rsna.org/doi/10.1148/rg.322115057

58. Puylaert JB. Acute appendicitis: US evaluation using graded compression. Radiology. 1986;158(2):355–60. Available from: http://www.ncbi.nlm.nih.gov/pubmed/2934762

59. Worthen NJ, Uszler JM, Funamura JL. Cholecystitis: prospective evaluation of sonography and 99mTc-HIDA cholescintigraphy. AJR Am J Roentgenol. 1981;137(5):973–8. Available from: http://www.ncbi.nlm.nih.gov/pubmed/6975025

60. Hill JB, Sheffield JS, McIntire DD, Wendel GD. Acute pyelonephritis in pregnancy. Obstet Gynecol. 2005;105(1):18–23. Available from: http://content.wkhealth.com/linkback/openurl?sid=WKPTLP:landingpage&an=00006250-200501000-00005

61. Craig WD, Wagner BJ, Travis MD. Pyelonephritis: radiologic-pathologic review. RadioGraphics. 2008;28(1):255–76. Available from: http://pubs.rsna.org/doi/10.1148/rg.281075171

Jeffrey Levine, Pamela I. Causa Andrieu, HeiShun Yu, and David D. B. Bates

## Contents

### Abstract

In the field of emergency radiology, several conditions and complications can occur specific to cancer and its therapies, which can affect the abdomen and pelvis. Familiarity with these conditions is essential for practicing emergency radiologists, as they navigate the complexities of making acute diagnoses in patients being treated for medically and surgically complex conditions. In this chapter, we present a review of several conditions related to oncologic imaging which a practicing emergency radiologist may encounter.

### Keywords

Emergency oncoradiology · Cancer imaging · Abdominal imaging · Complications

## Hepatobiliopancreatic System

### Veno-Occlusive Disease (VOD) of the Liver

The etiology of hepatic VOD is the damage to the sinusoidal endothelium of small hepatic vessels and can be due to several different etiologies. The most frequent and potentially devastating scenario occurs after hematopoietic cell transplantation

J. Levine · P. I. Causa Andrieu · D. D. B. Bates (✉)
Department of Radiology, Memorial Sloan Kettering Cancer Center, New York, NY, USA
e-mail: batesd@mskcc.org

H. Yu
Department of Radiology, Division of Emergency Radiology, Brigham and Women's Hospital/Harvard Medical School, Boston, MA, USA

© Springer Nature Switzerland AG 2022
M. N. Patlas et al. (eds.), *Atlas of Emergency Imaging from Head-to-Toe*,
https://doi.org/10.1007/978-3-030-92111-8_36

(HCT) and can result in the development of multi-organ dysfunction [1–3]. Other possible risk factors are exposure to plant pyrrolizidine alkaloids, chemotherapeutic agents, and thiopurine derivatives [1, 4].

Ultrasound (US) is the preferred modality for the initial evaluation of patients with suspected VOD, to narrow the differential diagnosis. On US, findings may include hepatomegaly, splenomegaly, gallbladder wall thickening, and/or ascites, although these findings in isolation, and even in combination, are not particularly specific vascular findings, which are more suggestive of the diagnosis, particularly if combined with other gray-scale findings, including flattening of the hepatic veins (i.e., less than 0.3 cm in diameter measured at 2 cm from the inferior vena cava), distention of the portal vein (i.e., more than 1.2 cm in adults and 0.8 cm in children), and visualization of the paraumbilical vein. Doppler imaging may show an increased resistance index of the hepatic artery (i.e., more than 0.75), monophasic flow in the hepatic veins, reversed flow at the paraumbilical vein, and decreased or reversed flow in the portal vein [2, 4] (Fig. 1). CT and MR will show similar findings to US; however, on MR, there may be reticular hypointensity of the hepatic parenchyma on delayed hepatobiliary-phase imaging, which some authors have reported as a specific finding for VOD,

although the exact pathophysiology leading to this imaging appearance is not entirely established, to our knowledge [4].

## Bacterial Acute Cholangitis

Acute bacterial cholangitis can be secondary to biliary obstruction and should be considered a life-threatening condition. Most commonly, in approximately 80% of cases, choledocholithiasis is the cause. However, other causes that can be seen are instrumentation of the biliary tract, including endoscopic retrograde cholangiopancreatography (ERCP), malignant obstruction, sclerosing cholangitis [5], and biliary sclerosis from oncologic therapy such as hepatic arterial infusion pump chemotherapy (HAIPC). The latter condition mainly occurs when floxuridine is given, causing biliary sclerosis in 2–5.5% of patients. In this setting, it most commonly involves the main hepatic duct and biliary confluence [6]. Clinically, patients classically present with right upper quadrant pain, fever, and jaundice; sepsis can also occur [5].

While no studies are available, to our knowledge, comparing CT and MR for the assessment of cholangitis, MR is preferable due to its better contrast resolution as well as the

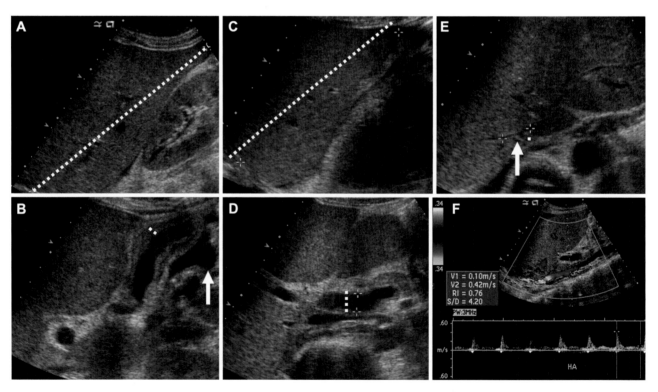

**Fig. 1 A 30-year-old man with hepatic VOD after stem cell transplant for T-cell lymphoma**. US shows (**a**) hepatomegaly, measuring 19.5 cm in the prerenal plane, with discrete heterogeneous echogenicity; (**b**) gallbladder wall thickening, 0.5 cm and trace ascites (arrow); (**c**) splenomegaly, 13 cm, with discrete heterogeneous echogenicity; (**d**) distention of the main portal vein, 1.3 cm in diameter; and (**e**) flattened

right hepatic vein, 0.17 cm (arrow). US-Doppler image shows (**f**) normal velocity and waveform with an increased resistance index of the hepatic artery, 0.76. Other images (not shown) demonstrated patent and normal flow in the portal vein, as well as normal diameters and waveforms of the main and left hepatic veins

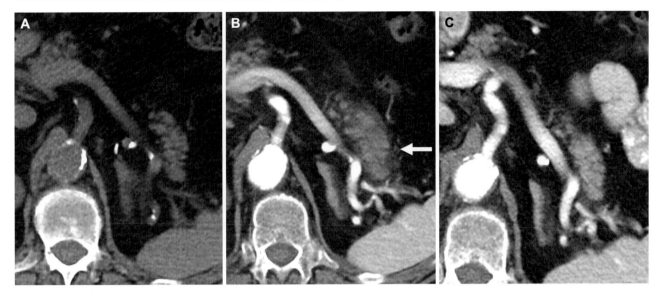

**Fig. 2** An 82-year-old man with metastatic renal cell carcinoma on pazopanib therapy, with new onset of left upper quadrant pain. Non-enhanced CT image (**a**) 1 month prior to therapy; IV contrast-enhanced CT image (**b**) with the diagnosis of pancreatitis (arrow); and IV contrast-enhanced CT image obtained 3 months later showing resolution of the findings. He had a brief pause in pazopanib therapy with an improvement of symptoms, and then he continued treatment

improved assessment of the biliary tract with magnetic resonance cholangiopancreatography (MRCP) [5].

In the acute setting, imaging findings include biliary dilatation that can be either intra- or extrahepatic, depending on the site(s) of obstruction. Concentric wall enhancement can also be seen and is better depicted on delayed post-contrast images. Furthermore, the hepatic parenchyma may demonstrate areas of T2 hyperintensity or areas of arterial hyperenhancement which are wedge-shaped, peripheral, and patchy or in a peribiliary distribution. Acute imaging complications include thrombosis of the portal or hepatic veins, development of hepatic abscesses, or infected biloma. As with many conditions, it is important to remember that acute cholangitis is primarily a clinical diagnosis, and the imaging findings are considered supportive.

## Drug-Induced Pancreatitis

Drug-induced pancreatitis is a relatively common complication and may be seen with several cytotoxic and targeted cancer therapies. Cytotoxic agents with a known propensity for drug-induced chemotherapy include L-asparaginase, which is used for acute leukemia. Targeted therapies, including sunitinib, sorafenib, and pazopanib [7] for metastatic renal cell carcinoma, are also known causes.

The imaging features of drug-induced pancreatitis are often similar to other forms of pancreatitis, with pancreatic enlargement and with diffuse or partial hypoenhancement with peri-pancreatic inflammatory changes. Increased avidity for fluorodeoxyglucose (FDG) on PET may also be seen, as

well as areas of pancreatic duct narrowing [8]. However, the affected portion of the pancreas may be focal and can mimic a metastasis on FDG-PET [9].

The time to onset from treatment, the presence of and degree of symptoms, and imaging findings are all highly variable (Fig. 2) [10]. Therefore, a high level of suspicion is needed to make the appropriate imaging findings. When diagnosed, discontinuation of the causal agent and alternative therapeutic agents may be indicated [7].

## Peritoneum and Abdominopelvic Cavity

### Peritoneal Carcinomatosis and Acute Complications

Malignancies with a propensity to metastasize to the peritoneum include primary cancers of the gastrointestinal tract, ovary, pancreas, breast, and skin [11–13]. Malignancy-related small bowel obstruction tends to occur in the setting of peritoneal metastases and is a harbinger of a poor prognosis. Closed-loop bowel obstructions may develop from serosal implants or can occur as the result of intraperitoneal adhesion following chemotherapy or debulking surgery. Malignancy-related colonic obstruction, while less common, may result from primary colorectal cancer; specifically, colorectal cancer may become obstructive due to annular growth and narrowed luminal diameter [14]. Omental metastatic disease is most commonly due to ovarian carcinoma but also can be seen with primary cancers of the colon, stomach, or breast [15].

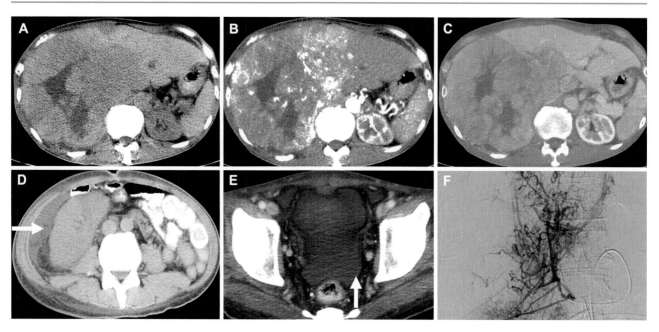

**Fig. 3** **A 50-year-old man with HCC, with a sudden onset drop in hemoglobin.** Four-phase liver CT (**a**–**c**) shows a large HCC occupying most of the right hepatic lobe. Non-contrast axial CT image (**d**) shows hemorrhage on the right flank (arrow). IV contrast-enhanced axial CT image (**e**) shows a small amount of pelvic ascites (arrow). The decision was to perform particle embolization of the tumor (**f**)

CT remains the imaging modality of choice for the evaluation of malignancy-related bowel obstruction. Small bowel obstruction is identified as dilated loops of small bowel greater than 3 cm in diameter, with either one or multiple transition points where the bowel narrows. Enhancing serosal tumor or focal asymmetric mural thickening can be seen to indicate the cause may be malignant [16, 17]. On CT, a malignant intussusception will demonstrate a "bowel-within-bowel" configuration, and at times enhancing tumor may be seen at the lead point [16]. Malignant colonic obstruction may show an enhancing polypoidal or annular tumor with abrupt focal narrowing and proximal dilated colon and small bowel. In the setting of carcinomatosis, an obstruction can be seen with nodular peritoneal thickening and the presence of bulky peritoneal tumors [12].

## Intra-abdominal Hemorrhage

Spontaneous hemoperitoneum is an emergent condition that requires prompt diagnosis and treatment. Portable US is often used as a quick screening tool in the emergency department or critically ill patients to detect free fluid. CT angiography (CTA) is highly useful to characterize the extent of hemoperitoneum and to help localize its source, namely, whether there is active bleeding from a specific vessel or organ. This is particularly useful to help guide therapy, including vascular intervention [18]. The appearance of hemorrhage on CT depends on the age of the blood products, ranging from high-attenuation ascites (i.e., 30–45 HU) to simple fluid with a hematocrit layer. The localization of a

sentinel clot or high-attenuation hematoma may be very useful to help localize the source of bleeding, if there is no active hemorrhage on CT [19].

Regarding the potential oncologic causes of spontaneous hemoperitoneum, the most common origins are the liver and spleen. In the liver, hepatic adenomas may spontaneously rupture and can be seen in the setting of adenomatosis. Hepatocellular carcinoma (HCC) (Fig. 3) or hypervascular liver metastases may also rupture into the peritoneum. Spontaneous splenic rupture can occur in the setting of lymphoproliferative disorders as well [18].

## Small and Large Bowel

### Graft-Versus-Host Disease (GVHD)

Allogeneic stem cell transplantation (allo-HCT) is a commonly used treatment for both malignant and nonmalignant hematological diseases. A potentially life-threatening complication following allo-HCT is acute GVHD [20], which can occur in up to 30–50% of patients. Early detection and treatment with immunosuppression may limit disease severity and improve prognosis. The bowel is frequently involved, and the disease can occur at any point along the length of the gastrointestinal tract.

The imaging features of GVHD enteritis are considered nonspecific and are typically a diagnosis of exclusion (Fig. 4). Although there is some overlap between GVHD and causes of small bowel inflammation, the most common imaging findings on CT are focal or diffuse wall thickening of

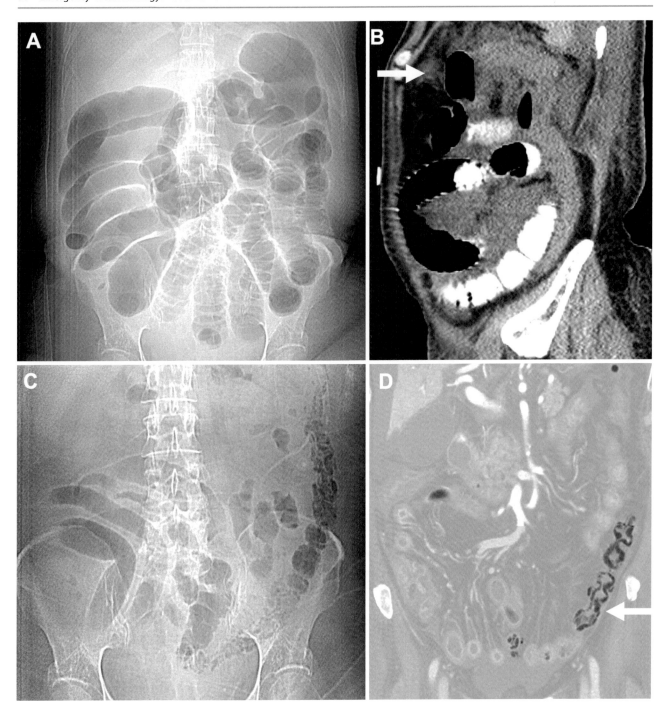

**Fig. 4** **A 45-year-old man with relapsed Hodgkin's lymphoma, following cell transplant and biopsy-proven GVHD of the colon, presenting with fever and hematochezia**. Abdominal radiograph (**a**) and sagittal non-enhanced CT image (**b**) revealed new small and large bowel obstruction, with a transition at splenic flexure from colonic wall thickening. Follow-up radiograph (**c**) and coronal IV contrast-enhanced CT image (**d**) showed new pneumatosis of the descending colon. Subsequently, the patient was diagnosed with *Enterobacter* bacteremia from gut translocation

the small bowel with or without mucosal enhancement [21, 22]. The involvement of small bowel is present in ~75% of cases. It can be useful to help exclude other pathologies that predominantly involve the colon, such as neutropenic colitis, pseudomembranous colitis, and CMV colitis, in particular [20, 22]. In some circumstances, pneumatosis intestinalis may be seen, which suggests mucosal compromise with the associated risks of ischemia and infection [23, 24]. Confirming the diagnosis of intestinal GVHD requires a biopsy; however, radiologic assessment can help to identify it and distinguish it from other posttransplant complications [20].

## Neutropenic Colitis

Neutropenic colitis occurs in immunocompromised patients, often those who are undergoing chemotherapy or receiving hematopoietic stem cell transplantation [25]. These patients are particularly susceptible to the condition due to a combination of factors, including mucosal injury by cytotoxic drugs and severe immunosuppression. The causes are multifactorial, but it is thought that the infection occurs when bacteria breach the bowel mucosa. There can be associated with bowel necrosis in life-threatening cases [26, 27].

On CT, there is often bowel distension and most commonly mural thickening of the cecum, ascending colon, and occasionally the terminal ileum (Fig. 5). Submucosal edema, mucosal hyperenhancement, and inflammatory pericolic fat infiltration [25, 28] may be seen. Although there is overlap in the imaging features with other forms of colitis, the clinical presentation and history are distinctive and critical to making the correct diagnosis [21]. CT is also useful for depicting complications that require surgical intervention in severe cases, when the inflammation progresses to ulceration, transmural necrosis, and colonic perforation [29].

## Bowel Toxicity from Chemotherapy

Oncology patients are at increased risk of bowel perforation at the site of an infiltrating or ulcerated neoplasm but also as a direct complication of the therapies which they may receive. Various molecular targeted therapies have known associations with bowel perforation [10]. For example, bowel perforation (Fig. 6) occurs in 0.9–1.7% of patients on bevacizumab. The 60-day mortality of this complication is 25% [30]. Imaging features of perforation include pneumoperitoneum and extraluminal enteric contrast, as well as fistula or abscess formation.

Pneumatosis related to cytotoxic drugs and immunotherapy can present a diagnostic challenge [31–33]. If the patient is asymptomatic, it may resolve on its own after withholding the drug. However, other imaging signs of bowel ischemia, such as bowel wall hypoenhancement or portal venous gas on CT, may be useful in determining the clinical urgency of the situation [34]. Ultimately, the clinical presentation should determine management [35].

Immune-checkpoint inhibitors used to treat advanced solid and hematologic malignancies activate the immune system and tend to have a unique toxicity profile known as immune-related adverse events (irAEs). irAEs are inherently protean and can result in several presentations, ranging from asymptomatic imaging findings to potentially life-threatening events. Patients may also develop chronic toxicities with long-term consequences [35, 36]. Colitis is the most common irAE (Fig. 7) and is characterized by bowel wall thickening, engorged mesenteric vessels, and pericolonic inflammatory changes on cross-sectional imaging. Early recognition is crucial as it may prompt cessation or modification of therapy [32]. A common causal medication for irAE colitis is ipilimumab [37].

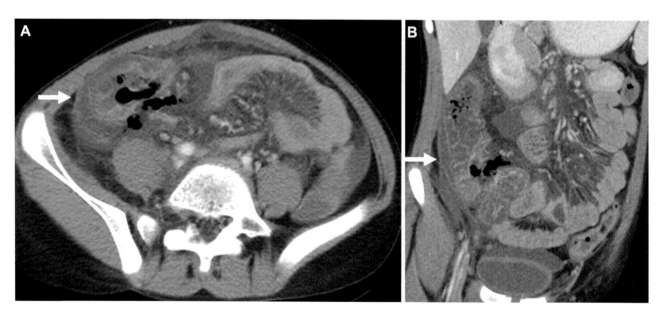

**Fig. 5 A 14-year-old boy with Ewing sarcoma, presenting with neutropenia and severe right lower quadrant pain.** Axial (**a**) and coronal (**b**) CT images reveal a diffusely edematous and thickened cecum, with focal pneumatosis and adjacent extraluminal air, highly consistent with typhlitis with pneumatosis (arrows). Due to the worsening clinical examination and acute abdomen, the patient was taken to the O.R. for diverting ileostomy. The cecum and ascending colon appeared inflamed upon direct examination, without leakage of stool or evident perforation or necrosis

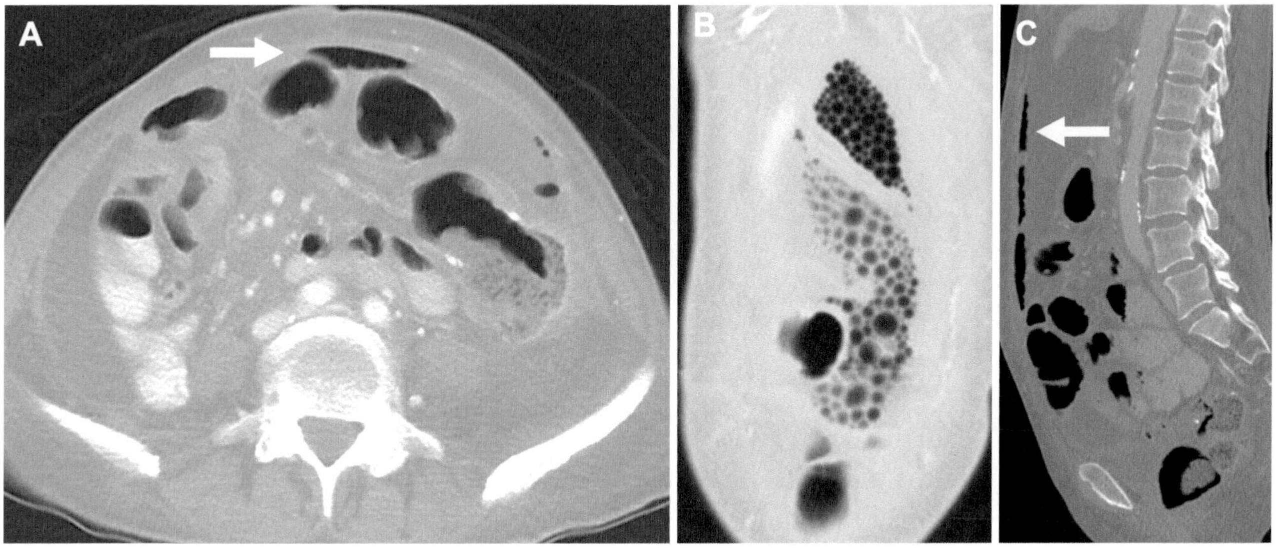

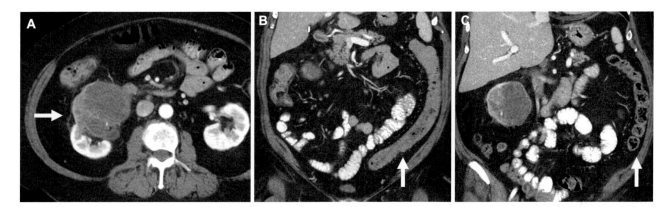

**Fig. 6** A 55-year-old woman with recurrent platinum-refractory high-grade serous ovarian cancer on chemotherapy, including bevacizumab, which was recently added to her treatment regimen, presenting with acute abdominal pain and sepsis. CT with axial (**a**), coronal (**b**), and sagittal (**c**) images revealed free air consistent with bowel perforation. The patient was not a good surgical candidate and was treated with decompression, antibiotics, fluids, and percutaneous drainage of the abscesses

**Fig. 7** A 60-year-old man with metastatic renal cell carcinoma, presenting with diarrhea and abdominal cramping. (**a**) CT reveals diffuse colitis (arrow). The patient's treating clinician suspected the colitis was a side effect of immunotherapy and subsequently reduced the dose of pembrolizumab for 2 weeks, and the patient was started on prednisone. (**b**) Subsequently, the CT findings of colitis resolved (arrow), and the patient's diarrhea correspondingly resolved

## Iatrogenic Causes of Enteritis: Radiation Induced

Radiation therapy is widely used for treatment for a variety of gastrointestinal, urological, and gynecological malignancies. Although modern radiotherapy protocols are more targeted, small bowel within a radiation port is still susceptible to injury. When this occurs, mucosal changes in the small bowel will be seen in 90% of patients, and clinically they may present with diarrhea developing within 2 to 4 weeks [38, 39]. Acute radiation enteritis is challenging to diagnose and is typically based on the CT appearance of small bowel in the setting of recent radiation exposure [40]. CT may show circumferential wall thickening and mucosal hyperenhancement, with progression to ulcers and hemorrhage [40, 41]. Whereas chemotherapy-induced enteritis tends to be more diffuse, radiation therapy-induced enteritis (Fig. 8) tends to be more focal, involving small bowel that is in or near the field of radiation. Radiation damage to the terminal ileum and rectum is common, since the terminal ileum is more fixed compared to the rest of the small bowel [41], and proctitis frequently results after radiation therapy for rectal, genitourinary, and gynecologic neoplasms [42]. Radiation-induced damage can predispose patients to bowel stricturing, fistula formation, and impaired peristalsis. Treatment is typically supportive, as the episodes are usually self-limiting. As the role of radiation therapy in the

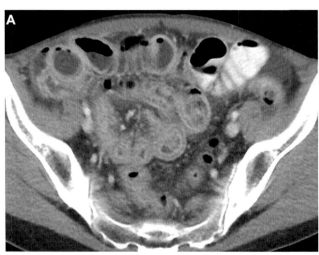

**Fig. 8** A 40-year-old woman with cervical cancer following debulking and radiotherapy a few months, before presenting with acute abdominal pain. CT (**a** and **b**) reveals diffuse wall thickening of distal small bowel segments in the mid-pelvis, consistent with radiation enteritis. One month later, dilatation of small bowel segments with air-fluid levels and a mid-pelvic transition point consistent with small bowel obstruction. Cervical brachytherapy seeds remain in situ (arrows, **b**)

management of cancer expands, recognition is helpful as these changes may be reversible [42].

## Tumor Superinfection and Postsurgical Complications

Secondary infection of a tumor can occur as a result of rapid tumor growth and spontaneous tumor necrosis. This has the potential for severe consequences, as secondary infection and systemic sepsis may result [43, 44]. Contained perforation of bowel malignancies and complex fistulas, especially rectovaginal fistulas, may present with local abscess formation [45, 46]. Intra-abdominal abscesses may also form following tumor resection and are a common cause of morbidity [47]. Uterine and cervical cancers may also become superinfected due to the proximity to vaginal flora [48].

CT with oral and intravenous contrast helps in prompt detection of the infected neoplasm and the potential communication with the gastrointestinal tract [49]. CT is both highly accurate for the identification of abscesses [44]. Perforated colonic neoplasms and ruptured pyometra from colouterine fistulas require prompt surgical attention [43]. Although it can be difficult to distinguish necrotic tumor from one that has become superinfected, clinical correlation with signs of infection can be useful. In the case of necrotic hepatic masses, some authors have found diffusion-weighted imaging to show promise in helping to make this distinction [50, 51]. Although both cystic necrotic tumors and abscesses tend to show peripheral rim enhancement, Chan et al. found that abscesses showed hyperintensity on diffusion-weighted imaging, with corresponding hypointensity on apparent diffusion coefficient (ADC) sequences [50].

## Genitourinary System

### Acute Urinary Obstruction

Urinary obstruction may be seen in up to 25% of patients with retroperitoneal or pelvic cancers due to the course of the ureters. Obstruction most commonly occurs in the distal third of the ureter and either by external compression or intraluminal obstruction. It can also occur as a complication of radiation therapy or surgery. Cross-sectional imaging modalities, either CT or MR, help to establish the diagnosis and to determine the extent of obstruction, as well as for establishing the etiology [19]. It is critical to assess for hydronephrosis/hydroureter and compromised renal function visualized as hypoenhancement of the kidney on post-contrast images, also known as a "delayed nephrogram," which can be unilateral or bilateral [52] (Fig. 9).

### Hemorrhagic Cystitis (HC)

HC may be a complication of ifosfamide and high-dose cyclophosphamide on early onset after HCT bone and soft tissue sarcoma treatment, but it may also be secondary to reactivation of latent viral infections, such as occurs with BK virus. BK virus may lay dormant in the genitourinary tract but can undergo reactivation after HCT, often around 2 weeks following therapy [53, 54]. The third cause of HC may be delayed toxicity from radiation therapy. Imaging contributes to the diagnosis, treatment planning, and follow-up, helping to exclude other etiologies [55].

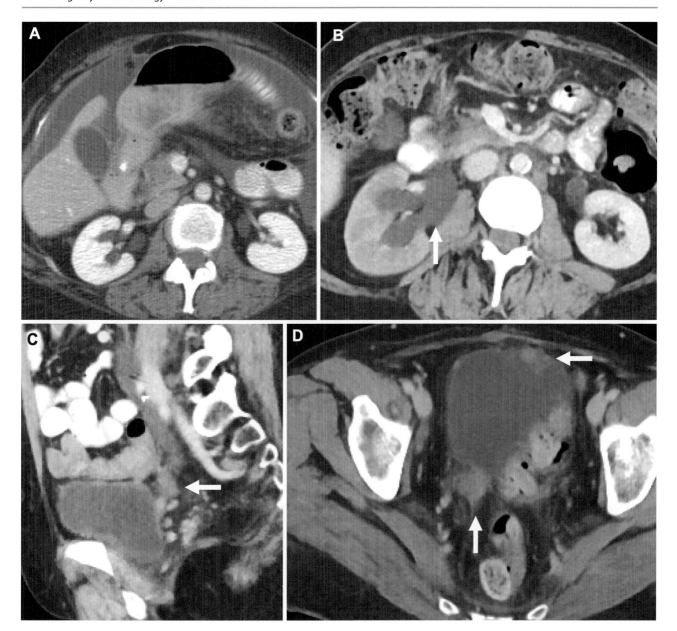

**Fig. 9** A 62-year-old woman with a history of recurrent endometrioid and serous adenocarcinoma of the endometrium, with new onset of abdominal pain. Axial IV contrast-enhanced CT image (**a**) of the first recurrence 6 months ago shows normal kidneys without hydronephrosis (arrows). Axial IV contrast-enhanced CT image of the abdomen (**b**) shows new severe right hydronephrosis with a delayed nephrogram (arrows) to the level of the bladder (arrow), better delineated on sagittal CT (**c**). Axial IV contrast-enhanced CT image of the pelvis (**b**) shows an implant on the ureterovesical junction (long arrow), as well as another implant on the bladder wall (short arrow)

In the acute phase, the urothelium is denudated and covered with fibrinous exudates which appear on imaging as thickening of the bladder wall with hyperemia, either focal or diffuse, clot formation, and decreased distensibility. On Doppler sonography, such findings appear as increased vascularity on the thickened wall and lack of Doppler signal in the clot (Fig. 10). CT shows bladder wall thickening with mucosal enhancement. Sometimes there may be perivesicular fat stranding (Fig. 11). Finally, on MRI, the wall may appear edematous with a high signal on T2. The clot may appear as non-enhancing soft tissue after contrast enhancement. In the chronic phase, there is obliterative endarteritis on the lamina propria that leads to ischemia and interstitial fibrosis, which appears as a reduced bladder volume with irregular wall thickening, and may be associated with hydronephrosis and hydroureter. Severe cases may present with bladder necrosis and fistula formation [53, 55, 56].

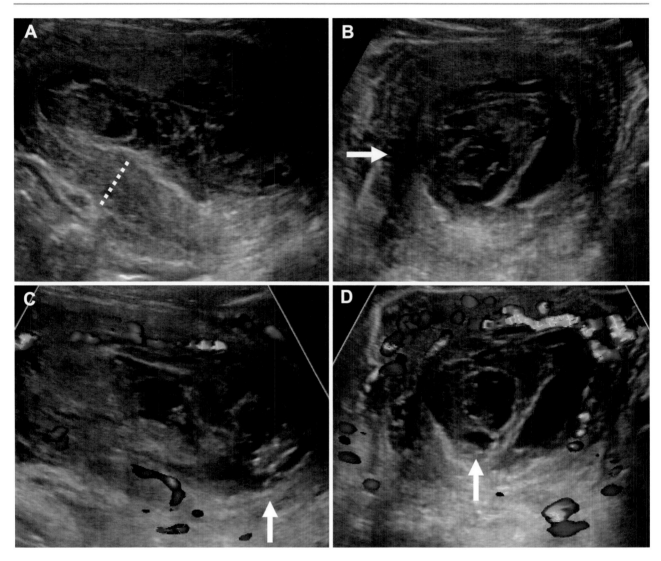

**Fig. 10** A 9-year-old boy with HC after initiating high-dose cyclo-phosphamide for medulloblastoma. US image shows diffuse and lobular thickening, up to 0.7 cm, of the bladder wall (**a** – dashes), with a retracting clot (**b** – arrow). US-Doppler image shows diffuse hyper-emia of the bladder wall (**a** – arrow) and no Doppler flow within the clot (**b** – arrow)

**Fig. 11** A 49-year-old woman with dysuria on day 59 after stem cell transplant for T-cell lymphoma. CT images with IV contrast show diffuse bladder wall thickening (**a** – dashes), with mucosal enhancement (**b** – arrow) and stranding of the surrounding fat. BK virus quantitative PCR testing of urine demonstrated markedly elevated DNA copies of BK virus, confirming the diagnosis of BK cystitis

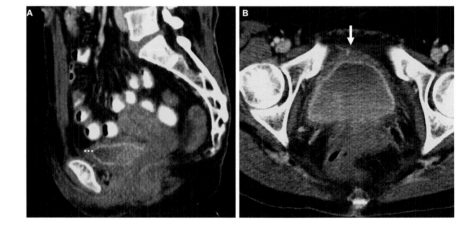

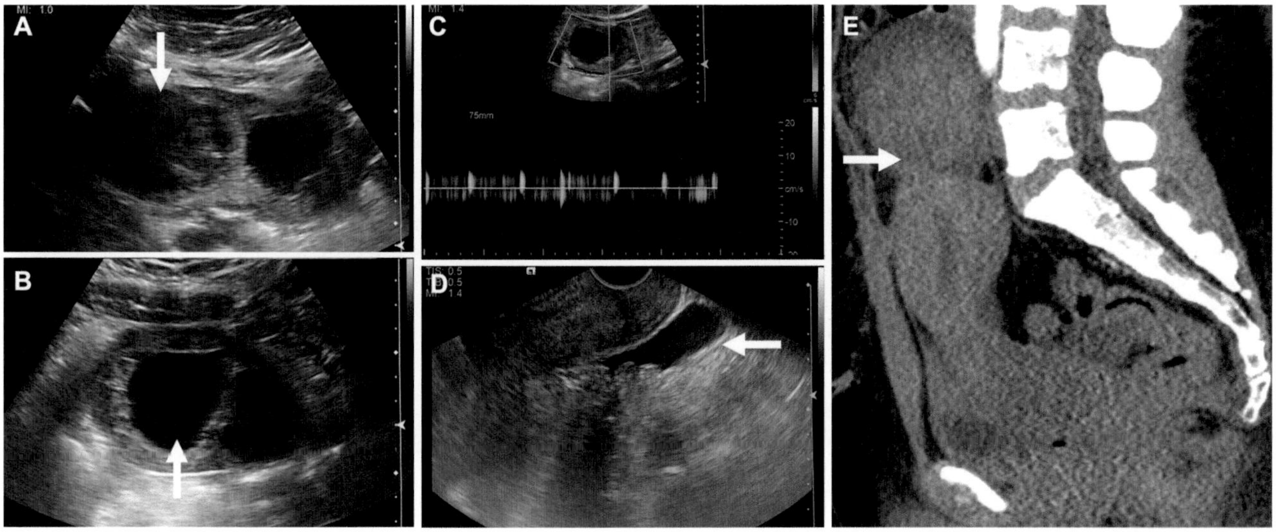

**Fig. 12** A 45-year-old woman with acute onset of abdominal pain. On tamoxifen for breast cancer. US images (**a** and **b**) show an enlarged edematous left ovary, measuring 5.8 × 13.4 cm. It has multiple cystic areas, including a probably hemorrhagic functional cyst, 2.5 × 3.8 cm (**a** – arrow), and a simple, functional cyst, 3.9 × 4.3 cm (**b** – arrow). US-Doppler image (**c**) demonstrates compromised venous (arrow) and arterial flow within the left ovary. There is trace-free ascites in the cul-de-sac (**d** – arrow). CT sagittal image (**e**) displays the displaced left ovary to the midline and above the uterus (arrow)

## Ovarian Torsion

Ovarian torsion constitutes one of the most frequent surgical emergencies in gynecology and may affect women of all ages [57]. The most substantial risk factor in adults is an underlying ovarian mass [58], usually larger than five centimeters. Almost all are benign in etiology and may include functional cyst, mature ovarian teratoma, or ovarian serous cystadenoma [57, 59]. Additional potential risk factors in female cancer patients are adhesions secondary to prior pelvic surgery, transposed ovaries [60], and ovarian hyperstimulation [58].

US is the preferred modality for the initial evaluation of any female patient with suspected ovarian torsion. US may demonstrate an asymmetrically enlarged and displaced ovary. The affected ovarian stroma may appear echogenic and heterogeneous, due to edema and hemorrhage, with displacement of small follicles to the periphery. US-Doppler findings are variable, depending on the timing and degree of torsion, as well as the integrity of the dual vascular supply. Specifically, a torsed ovary may retain arterial flow, as venous outflow may be solely obstructed at first. Alternatively, torsion may be intermittent, and normal Doppler flow is detected. Therefore, normal Doppler flow should not exclude the diagnosis. The most convincing finding is the identification of the twisted vascular pedicle [59] (Fig. 12). Finally, MRI is particularly helpful in subacute or inconclusive cases. Although not specific, the edematous stroma diffuse hyperintense on T2-weighted images is the remarkable feature, and post-contrast images can be used to assess the viability of the ovary [58, 61].

## Conclusion

There are a wide range of conditions which can result in acute abdominal presentations for oncologic patients. Some of these relate to the cancer itself, while others are due to side effects of therapy, complications of treatment, susceptibility to infection due to immunosuppression, or reactivation of latent infection. A familiarity with the range of conditions and their potential causes will help the emergency radiologist make timely diagnoses and contribute to patient care in these complex cases.

## References

1. Dhanasekaran R, Kwo PY. The liver in oncology. Clin Liver Dis. 2017;21(4):697–707.
2. Mohty M, Malard F, Abecassis M, Aerts E, Alaskar AS, Aljurf M, et al. Revised diagnosis and severity criteria for sinusoidal obstruction syndrome/veno-occlusive disease in adult patients: a new classification from the European Society for Blood and Marrow Transplantation. Bone Marrow Transplant. 2016;51(7):906–12.
3. Valla DC, Cazals-Hatem D. Vascular liver diseases on the clinical side: definitions and diagnosis, new concepts. Virchows Arch. 2018;473(1):3–13.
4. Elsayes KMSA, Rothan SM, Javadi S, Madrazo BL, Castillo RP, Casillas VJ, Menias CO. A comprehensive approach to hepatic vascular disease. Radiographics. 2017;37:813–36.
5. Catalano OASD, Forcione DG, Czermak B, Liu CH, Soricelli A, Arellano RS, Muller PR, Hahn PF. Biliary infections: spectrum of imaging findings and management. Radiographics. 2009;29:2059–80.
6. Ito K, Ito H, Kemeny NE, Gonen M, Allen PJ, Paty PB, et al. Biliary sclerosis after hepatic arterial infusion pump chemotherapy for

patients with colorectal cancer liver metastasis: incidence, clinical features, and risk factors. Ann Surg Oncol. 2012;19(5):1609–17.

7. Murtaza G, Faqah A, Konowitz N, Lu H, Kuruvilla A, Adhikari S. Acute pancreatitis related to a chemotherapy drug. World J Oncol. 2017;8(1):18–9.

8. Widmann G, Nguyen VA, Plaickner J, Jaschke W. Imaging features of toxicities by immune checkpoint inhibitors in cancer therapy. Curr Radiol Rep. 2016;5(11):59.

9. Das JP, Halpenny D, Do RK, Ulaner GA. Focal immunotherapy-induced pancreatitis mimicking metastasis on FDG PET/CT. Clin Nucl Med. 2019;44(10):836–7.

10. Torrisi JMSL, Gollub MJ, Ginsberg MS, Bosl GJ, Hricak H. CT findings of chemotherapy- induced toxicity: what radiologists need to know about the clinical and radiologic manifestations of chemotherapy toxicity. Radiology. 2011;258:41–56.

11. Manola JAM, Ibrahim J, Kirkwood J. Prognostic factors in metastatic melanoma: a pooled analysis of Eastern Cooperative Oncology Group trials. J Clin Oncol. 2000;18:3782–93.

12. Levy AD, Shaw JC, Sobin LH. From the archives of the AFIP. secondary tumors and tumorlike lesions of the peritoneal cavity: imaging features with pathologic correlation. Radiographics. 2009;29:347–73.

13. Coccolini F, Gheza F, Lotti M, Virzi S, Iusco D, Ghermandi C, et al. Peritoneal carcinomatosis. World J Gastroenterol. 2013;19(41):6979–94.

14. Ripamonti CI, Easson AM, Gerdes H. Management of malignant bowel obstruction. Eur J Cancer. 2008;44(8):1105–15.

15. Walkey MMFA, Sohotra P, Radecki PD. CT manifestations of peritoneal carcinomatosis. AJR Am J Roentgenol. 1988;150:1035–41.

16. Kim SY, Ha HK, Park SW, Kang J, Kim KW, Lee SS, et al. Gastrointestinal metastasis from primary lung cancer: CT findings and clinicopathologic features. AJR Am J Roentgenol. 2009;193(3):W197–201.

17. Silva ACPM, Guimarães LS. Small bowel obstruction: what to look for. Radiographics. 2009;2009(2):423–39.

18. Lucey BC, Varghese JC, Soto JA. Spontaneous hemoperitoneum: causes and significance. Curr Probl Diagn Radiol. 2005;34(5):182–95.

19. Katabathina VRC, Betancourt CS, Riascos R, Menias C. Imaging of oncologic emergencies: what every radiologist should know. Radiographics. 2013;33:1533–53.

20. Lubner MG, Menias CO, Agrons M, Alhalabi K, Katabathina VS, Elsayes KM, et al. Imaging of abdominal and pelvic manifestations of graft-versus-host disease after hematopoietic stem cell transplant. AJR Am J Roentgenol. 2017;209(1):33–45.

21. Kirkpatrick ID, Greenberg H. Gastrointestinal complications in the neutropenic patient: characterization and differentiation with abdominal CT. Radiology. 2003;226:668–74.

22. Mahgerefteh SYSJ, Bogot N, Shapira MY, Pappo O, Bloom AI. Radiologic imaging and intervention for gastrointestinal and hepatic complications of hematopoietic stem cell transplantation. Radiology. 2011;258:660–71.

23. Hepgur M, Ahluwalia MS, Anne N, Thomas J, Liu H, Schiff MD, et al. Medical management of pneumatosis intestinalis in patients undergoing allogeneic blood and marrow transplantation. Bone Marrow Transplant. 2011;46(6):876–9.

24. Schmit M, Bethge W, Beck R, Faul C, Claussen CD, Horger M. CT of gastrointestinal complications associated with hematopoietic stem cell transplantation. AJR Am J Roentgenol. 2008;190(3):712–9.

25. Horton KMCF, Fishman EK. CT evaluation of the colon: inflammatory disease. Radiographics. 2000;20:399–418.

26. Rodrigues FG, Dasilva G, Wexner SD. Neutropenic enterocolitis. World J Gastroenterol. 2017;23(1):42–7.

27. Wade DSNH, Douglass HO Jr. Neutropenic enterocolitis. Clinical diagnosis and treatment. Cancer. 1992;69:17–23.

28. Frick MPMC, Crass JR, Goldberg ME, Delaney JP. Computed tomography of neutropenic colitis. AJR Am J Roentgenol. 1984;143:763–5.

29. Wall SDJB. Gastrointestinal tract in the immunocompromised host: opportunistic infections and other complications. Radiology. 1992;185:327–35.

30. Thornton E, Howard SA, Jagannathan J, Krajewski KM, Shinagare AB, O'Regan K, et al. Imaging features of bowel toxicities in the setting of molecular targeted therapies in cancer patients. Br J Radiol. 2012;85(1018):1420–6.

31. Coriat R, Ropert S, Mir O, Billemont B, Chaussade S, Massault PP, et al. Pneumatosis intestinalis associated with treatment of cancer patients with the vascular growth factor receptor tyrosine kinase inhibitors sorafenib and sunitinib. Investig New Drugs. 2011;29(5):1090–3.

32. Knechtle SJ, Davidoff AM, Rice RP. Pneumatosis intestinalis. Surgical management and clinical outcome. Ann Surg. 1990;212:160–5.

33. Shinagare AB, Howard SA, Krajewski KM, Zukotynski KA, Jagannathan JP, Ramaiya NH. Pneumatosis intestinalis and bowel perforation associated with molecular targeted therapy: an emerging problem and the role of radiologists in its management. AJR Am J Roentgenol. 2012;199(6):1259–65.

34. Kernagis LY, Levine M, Jacobs JE. Pneumatosis intestinalis in patients with ischemia: correlation of CT findings with viability of the bowel. AJR Am J Roentgenol. 2003;180:733–6.

35. Wiesner W, Mortelé KJ, Glickman JN, Ji H, Ros PR. Pneumatosis intestinalis and portomesenteric venous gas in intestinal ischemia correlation of CT findings with severity of ischemia and clinical outcome. AJR Am J Roentgenol. 2001;177:1319–23.

36. Kumar V, Chaudhary N, Garg M, Floudas CS, Soni P, Chandra AB. Current diagnosis and management of immune related adverse events (irAEs) induced by immune checkpoint inhibitor therapy. Front Pharmacol. 2017;8:49.

37. O'Connor A, Marples M, Mulatero C, Hamlin J, Ford AC. Ipilimumab-induced colitis: experience from a tertiary referral center. Ther Adv Gastroenterol. 2016;9(4):457–62.

38. Potish RA. Prediction of radiation-related small-bowel damage. Radiology. 1980;135:219–21.

39. Andreyev J. Gastrointestinal symptoms after pelvic radiotherapy: a new understanding to improve management of symptomatic patients. Lancet Oncol. 2007;8(11):1007–17.

40. Sugi MD, Menias CO, Lubner MG, Bhalla S, Mellnick VM, Kwon MH, et al. CT findings of acute small-bowel entities. Radiographics. 2018;38(5):1352–69.

41. Capps GWFA, Szucs RA, Turner MA. Imaging features of radiation-induced changes in the abdomen. Radiographics. 1997;17:1455–73.

42. Do NL, Nagle D, Poylin VY. Radiation proctitis: current strategies in management. Gastroenterol Res Pract. 2011;2011:917941.

43. Viswanathan C, Truong M, Sagebiel TL, Bronstein Y, Vikram R, Patnana M, Silverman PM, Bhosale PR. Abdominal and pelvic complications of nonoperative oncologic therapy. Gastrointestinal Imaging. 2014;34(4):941–61.

44. Gore RM, Berlin JW, Yaghmai V, Mehta U, Newmark GM, Ghahremani GG. CT diagnosis of postoperative abdominal complications. Semin Ultrasound CT MR. 2004;25(3):207–21.

45. Narayanan PNM, Reynolds KM, Sahdev A, Reznek RH, Rockall AG. Fistulas in malignant gynecologic disease: etiology, imaging, and management. Radiographics. 2009;29:1073–83.

46. Tirumani SH, Fraser-Hill M, Auer R, Shabana W, Walsh C, Lee F, et al. Mucinous neoplasms of the appendix: a current comprehensive clinicopathologic and imaging review. Cancer Imaging. 2013;13:14–25.

47. Zissin R, Gayer G. Postoperative anatomic and pathologic findings at CT following colonic resection. Semin Ultrasound CT MR. 2004;25(3):222–38.

48. Ou YC, Lan KC, Lin H, Tsai CC, ChangChien CC. Clinical characteristics of perforated pyometra and impending perforation: specific issues in gynecological emergency. J Obstet Gynaecol Res. 2010;36(3):661–6.

49. Weinstein SO-BS, Aslam R, Yee J. Multidetector CT of the postoperative colon: review of normal appearances and common complications. Radiographics. 2013;33:515–32.
50. Chan JH, Tsui EY, Luk SH, Fung AS, Yuen MK, Szeto ML, et al. Diffusion-weighted MR imaging of the liver: distinguishing hepatic abscess from cystic or necrotic tumor. Abdom Imaging. 2001;26(2):161–5.
51. Holzapfel K, Rummeny E, Gaa J. Diffusion-weighted MR imaging of hepatic abscesses: possibility of different apparent diffusion coefficient (ADC)-values in early and mature abscess formation. Abdom Imaging. 2007;32(4):538–9.
52. Wolin EA, Hartman DS, Olson JR. Nephrographic and pyelographic analysis of CT urography: differential diagnosis. AJR Am J Roentgenol. 2013;200(6):1197–203.
53. Traxer ODF, Sebe P, Haab F, Le Duc A, Gattegno B, Thibault P. Hemorrhagic cystitis: etiology and treatment Prog Urol. 2001;11:591–601.
54. Schulze M, Beck R, Igney A, Vogel M, Maksimovic O, Claussen CD, et al. Computed tomography findings of human polyomavirus BK (BKV)-associated cystitis in allogeneic hematopoietic stem cell transplant recipients. Acta Radiol. 2008;49(10):1187–94.
55. McCarville M, Hoffer F, Gingrich J, Jenkins J III. Imaging findings of hemorrhagic cystitis in pediatric oncology patients. Pediatr Radiol. 2000;30(30):131–8.
56. Wong-You-Cheong JJWP, Manning MA, Davis CJ. From the archives of the AFIP: inflammatory and nonneoplastic bladder masses: radiologic-pathologic correlation. Radiographics. 2006;26:1847.
57. Houry D, Abbott JT. Ovarian torsion: a fifteen-year review. Ann Emerg Med. 2001;38(2):156–9.
58. Asch E, Wei J, Mortele KJ, Humm K, Thornton K, Levine D. Magnetic resonance imaging performance for diagnosis of ovarian torsion in pregnant women with stimulated ovaries. Fertil Res Pract. 2017;3:13.
59. Chang HCBS, Dogra VS. Pearls and pitfalls in diagnosis of ovarian torsion. Radiographics. 2008;28:1355–68.
60. Gomez-Hidalgo NR, Darin MC, Dalton H, Jhingran A, Fleming N, Brown J, et al. Ovarian torsion after laparoscopic ovarian transposition in patients with gynecologic cancer: a report of two cases. J Minim Invasive Gynecol. 2015;22(4):687–90.
61. Gao Y, Lee K, Camacho M. Utility of pelvic ultrasound following negative abdominal and pelvic CT in the emergency room. Clin Radiol. 2013;68(11):e586–92.

# Imaging of Shoulder Trauma

**37**

Yunib H. Munir and Nicholas M. Beckmann

## Contents

### Abstract

The shoulder girdle is comprised of the clavicle, scapula, and soft tissue support structures. Traumatic injuries to the shoulder girdle are common, and include injuries to the clavicle and scapula, as well as injuries to the sternoclavicular, acromioclavicular, and glenohumeral joints. These injuries can be easily missed or underdiagnosed due to the complex anatomy of the shoulder. Radiographs should be performed for initial evaluation, preferably in upright positioning to accentuate bone displacement in unstable injuries. A low threshold should be maintained for performing CT of the shoulder to further evaluate for fracture, particularly when injuries to the sternoclavicular joint or scapula are suspected. CT angiography can help assess for arterial injury, but is rarely necessary as vascular injury is very uncommon in the setting of shoulder trauma. MRI is helpful for evaluating ligament integrity in joint dislocations as well as for assessing injuries to muscles, tendons, and nerves. However, MRI is rarely performed in the emergency setting. Ultrasound is also helpful for assessing soft tissue injury, but has limited use in the acute setting due to challenges in positioning the acute injured patient as well as the high level of expertise required to accurately perform musculoskeletal ultrasound.

Y. H. Munir · N. M. Beckmann (✉)
UTHealth – McGovern School of Medicine, Houston, TX, USA
e-mail: Yunib.H.Munir@uth.tmc.edu;
Nicholas.M.Beckmann@uth.tmc.edu

© Springer Nature Switzerland AG 2022
M. N. Patlas et al. (eds.), *Atlas of Emergency Imaging from Head-to-Toe*,
https://doi.org/10.1007/978-3-030-92111-8_37

**Keywords**

Shoulder · Trauma · Fracture · Clavicle · Scapula · Acromioclavicular · Sternoclavicular · Glenohumeral

## Introduction

Shoulder trauma can occur either due to blunt or penetrating injuries. Most shoulder injuries encountered in the emergency setting are the result of blunt trauma from motor vehicle/motorcycle collisions, sports injuries, or falls [1]. Blunt trauma can be caused by either direct or indirect impaction to the shoulder, and can result in a wide variety of injuries depending on the vector of the forces applied across the shoulder. Penetrating trauma typically occurs as either gunshot or stab injuries and, although these types of injuries are less common, they have the propensity of cause devastating neurovascular injury. Evaluation of the shoulder in the emergency setting is focused on assessment of the bony and neurovascular structures. Numerous soft tissue structures contribute to the stability and function of the shoulder. However, evaluation of many of these structures requires advanced imaging with MRI, which is not routinely performed in the emergency setting. This chapter will focus primarily on the imaging evaluation of shoulder trauma routinely performed in emergency departments.

## Osseous Anatomy

The shoulder is composed of the shoulder girdle, which is the musculature and soft tissues that connect the upper extremity to the axial skeleton. The bony component of the shoulder girdle includes the clavicle, scapula, and proximal humerus.

## Clavicle

The clavicle is a long, flat bone bridging the sternum and scapula, articulating medially with the manubrium at the sternoclavicular joint, and laterally with the scapula at the acromioclavicular joint (Fig. 1). The medial two-thirds of the clavicle is tubular and along its undersurface is the attachment for the costoclavicular ligament, which attaches to a raised region called the costal tubercle or a depressed region called the rhomboid fossa. Anteriorly, the pectoralis major inserts along the medial clavicle, while the sternocleidomastoid and sternohyoid muscles insert posterosuperiorly.

The lateral third of the clavicle is more bladelike in shape, and along its inferior surface is the conoid tubercle, which serves as the attachment of the conoid band of the coracoclavicular ligament (Fig. 1). The other band of the coracoclavicular ligament is called the trapezoid band, which attaches lateral to the conoid tubercle. The coracoclavicular ligament, in conjunction with the superior and inferior acromioclavicular capsular ligaments, provides support to the acromioclavicular joint. Along the lateral clavicle, a portion of the deltoid inserts on the anterior aspect, a portion of the trapezius inserts on the posterior aspect, and the subclavius muscle inserts along the inferior aspect.

## Scapula

The scapula is a triangle-shaped bone which is composed of a body, glenoid, and two processes: the coracoid and acromion (Fig. 2). The body of the scapula has three borders (superior, medial, and lateral), and tapers laterally to form the glenoid, which articulates with the humerus via the glenohumeral joint. The glenoid neck bridges the glenoid articular surface to the scapula body. The coracoid process arises from the anterior aspect of the glenoid neck, and is the attachment site for the coracoclavicular ligament and conjoined tendon of the coracobrachialis and short head of the biceps.

Along the posterior body of the scapula is the scapular spine, which continues laterally to form the acromion process. The acromion articulates with the clavicle, and serves as an attachment site for portions of the deltoid and trapezius. The acromion contains a separate ossification center, which

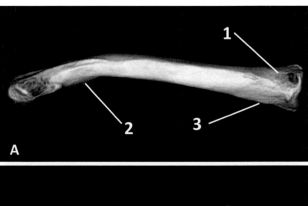

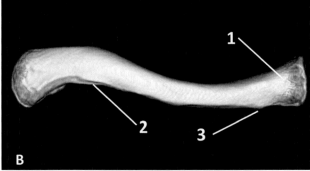

**Fig. 1** (a) Frontal and (b) Superior 3D volume render CT images of the clavicle. 1) Clavicle head. 2) Coronoid tubercle. 3) Costal tubercle

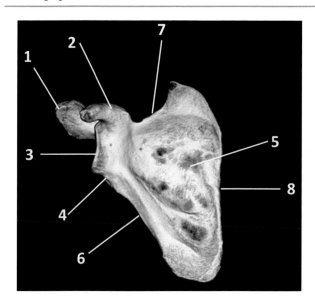

**Fig. 2** Anterior 3D volume render CT image of the scapula. 1) Acromion process. 2) Coracoid process. 3) Glenoid surface. 4) Glenoid neck. 5) Scapula body. 6) Lateral border. 7) Superior border. 8) Medial border

does not fuse in up to 15% of patients, resulting in an accessory ossicle called the os acromiale [2].

## Proximal Humerus

The proximal humerus is composed of the humeral head articular surface, neck, greater and lesser tuberosities, and shaft (Fig. 3). The greater and lesser tuberosities are the insertion sites of the rotator cuff tendons, with the subscapularis inserting on the lesser tuberosity, and the supraspinatus, infraspinatus, and teres minor inserting on the greater tuberosity. Between the two tuberosities lies the bicipital groove, through which runs the long head of the biceps tendon. The humeral head is commonly referred to having two necks: an anatomic neck, representing the division between the humeral head epiphysis and metaphysis, and a surgical neck, representing the junction between the proximal metaphysis and diaphysis.

## Imaging Protocols and Methodology

### Radiography

A shoulder series is the most common initial imaging performed in the setting of shoulder trauma. A standard shoulder series for trauma will typically include AP views in internal and external rotation, along with either a scapula-Y or axillary view (Table 1). AP views are performed in both internal and external rotation to provide orthogonal imaging

of the proximal humerus, while a scapula-Y and axillary view are added to provide orthogonal imaging of the glenohumeral joint and scapula. A standard axillary view requires 70–90 degrees of abduction, and is often not tolerated by patients with severe shoulder injury. The scapula-Y view provides orthogonal imaging of the shoulder while being better tolerated than the standard axillary view, which is why the scapula-Y view has been adopted at many emergency departments. However, some injuries (e.g., posterior shoulder dislocation) are best visualized on the axillary view. Therefore, a modified axillary view, which requires minimal abduction and is typically well tolerated, should be considered in patients unable to tolerate standard axillary imaging (Table 1) [3]. Although not commonly employed, the Stryker notch and West Point are additional shoulder views that can be useful for identifying Hill-Sachs lesions and Bankart lesions, respectively (Table 1).

A clavicle series comprised of AP and AP oblique views is commonly employed to evaluate clavicle, acromioclavicular, and sternoclavicular trauma (Table 1). Clavicle series should be performed upright, as displacement of clavicle fractures and acromioclavicular joint separations can be underestimated on supine imaging. An additional "serendipity" view can be performed on patients with suspected sternoclavicular injury to better visualize the medial clavicle (Table 1). In patients with suspected or confirmed AC joint injury, an upright AP view of the bilateral clavicles, while the patient holds 5 pound weights in each hand, can be performed to help accentuate the AC joint injury for better detection and characterization. A scapular series, comprised of AP and lateral views (Table 1), can be used for diagnosis of scapular fractures, as well as for baseline evaluation and follow-up of known scapular fractures.

## Computerized Tomography

CT has roles in the evaluation of both bony and vascular injuries in shoulder trauma. Noncontrast CT is commonly used to diagnose radiographically occult fractures and to characterize fractures identified on radiographs for preoperative planning. CT should be considered in any patient with high clinical index of suspicion for fracture and negative radiographs. In addition, a lower threshold for performing CT should be held for assessing certain regions of the shoulder which are usually difficult to evaluate with radiographs, particularly the scapula and the sternoclavicular joint. CT is also often performed for preoperative planning in patients with fractures of the humeral head or scapula, and in patients with fracture after shoulder dislocation. CT angiography (CTA) is rarely needed to evaluate for acute vascular injury in the setting of shoulder trauma, but CTA is appropriate when a patient has clinical findings (e.g., expanding hematoma), mechanism of injury (e.g., penetrating trauma), or

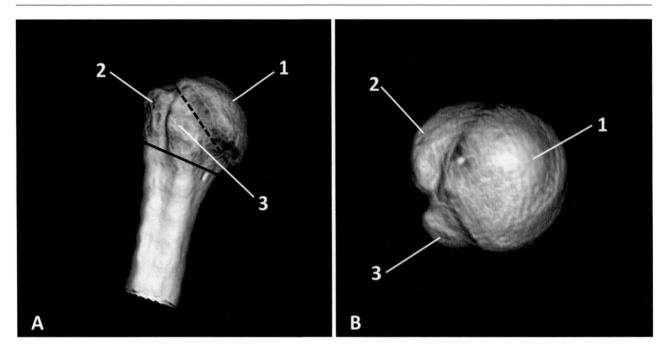

**Fig. 3** (**a**) Frontal and (**b**) Superior 3D volume render CT images of the proximal humerus. Figure A depicts the anatomic (dashed line) and surgical (solid line) necks. 1) Humeral head articular surface. 2) Greater tuberosity. 3) Lesser tuberosity

**Table 1** Positioning and indications for common shoulder projections

| Shoulder view | Patient positioning | Indications |
|---|---|---|
| AP view | Patient standing with back against the image receptor, arm is neutral | Gives overview of the entire shoulder, displaying the clavicle, AC joint, scapula, SC joint, and proximal humerus |
| Scapula-Y view | Patient sits/stands, facing the detector, and is rotating anterior oblique | This is an orthogonal view to the AP, and assesses suspected dislocations or fractures; additionally, this gives a view of the acromion and coracoid in profile |
| Modified axillary view | Patient is supine or seated, with the effected arm externally rotated and the detector placed under/behind the patient | Replaces the scapula-Y view and is preferred in the trauma setting; assesses dislocations and fractures (particularly those involving the glenoid or humeral head) |
| Stryker notch view | Patient is supine, with back against the image receptor; the patient is rotated 30–45 degrees to the affected side, with the affected arm abducted anteriorly | Specialized view which evaluates the glenohumeral articulation, and is effective in assessing for Hill-Sachs lesions |
| West Point view | Patient is prone with arm abducted 90 degrees and the beam directed 25 degrees anteriorly and 25 degrees medially | Specialized view to assess for Bankart lesions of the anterior glenoid rim |

injury pattern (e.g., scapulothoracic dissociation) indicating increased risk for vascular injury [4].

## Ultrasonography

Ultrasound has a limited role in assessment of shoulder trauma in the acute setting. However, in select patients, ultrasound offers a quicker and more cost-effective alternative to CT and MRI in the assessment of soft tissues. The clearest role for ultrasound is in the identification and quantification of hematomas. Ultrasound can also be useful in the identification and quantification of muscle tears, rotator cuff tears, or injuries to the long head of the biceps tendon. Utilization of ultrasound in these roles, however, depends

heavily on operator expertise and the patient's ability to tolerate positioning required for imaging. Due to these limitations, ultrasound evaluation of shoulder trauma is rarely performed in the emergency setting.

## Magnetic Resonance Imaging

MRI is very useful evaluating traumatic soft tissue injuries due to its high level of soft tissue contrast compared to CT, and its lower operator dependency compared to ultrasound. Limited availability of MRI, though, currently restricts the use of MRI in evaluation of shoulder trauma in the emergency setting. MRI can be helpful in identifying soft tissues that may entrap bones or inhibit complete bony reduction.

MRI is also helpful in preoperative assessment of soft tissue structures in patients with glenohumeral joint instability. Finally, MRI can be useful in identifying injuries to neurologic structures, particularly the brachial plexus. Delaying imaging for nerve injury for 4–6 weeks after trauma is preferred to allow surrounding soft tissue edema to subside. In general, contrast is not needed in MR evaluation of acute soft tissue injuries.

## Injury Patterns of the Shoulder

### Sternoclavicular Joint Injuries

Sternoclavicular (SC) joint injuries represent 1–3% of all shoulder injuries, with an incidence of 3 per 100,000 [5, 6]. These injuries usually result from high-energy trauma, either as an anterior impact to the lateral shoulder or as direct impact to the joint itself. As such, these injuries primarily occur in the younger male population [6, 7].

SC joint injuries typically occur as either an anterior or posterior dislocation of the joint (Fig. 4). Anterior dislocations occur 1.5–9 times more than posterior dislocations [5–7]. Anterior dislocations commonly occur due to an impact to the lateral shoulder, and patients usually present with a palpable lump over the sternoclavicular joint. Posterior dislocations occur either due to a direct impact to the sternoclavicular joint or by indirect blow to the posterolateral shoulder. A depression of the skin can occur in this injury, although the deformity can be masked by soft tissue swelling. Posterior sternoclavicular dislocations are at greater risk of complications due to compression of mediastinal structures. Approximately one-third of posterior sternoclavicular dislocations will report dyspnea or dysphagia, and 15% will have findings of vascular compression [8].

Sternoclavicular joint dislocations can be difficult to diagnose on radiographs, and a low threshold for CT or MR should be maintained. The cephalad angulated view of a clavicle series best demonstrates sternoclavicular malalignment, with anterior dislocation appearing as superior

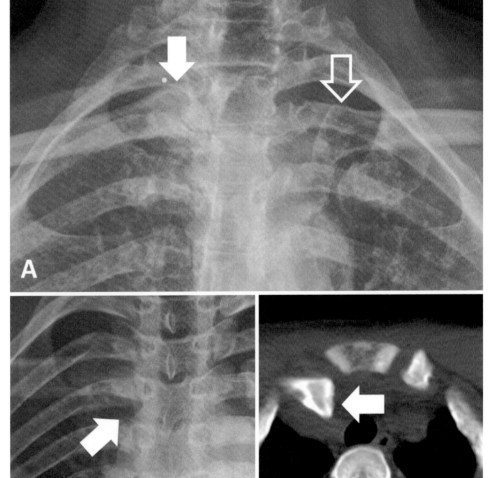

**Fig. 4** Sternoclavicular dislocations. (**a**) AP radiograph shows anterior dislocation with a dislocated right clavicular head (solid arrow) displaced superior to the uninjured left clavicle head (silhouette arrow). (**b**) Posterior dislocation. Posterior displacement of the right clavicular head (arrow) is difficult to identify on AP radiograph. C) Axial CT image clearly demonstrates posterior dislocation of the clavicular head (arrow)

displacement of the clavicular head relative to the joint, and posterior dislocation appearing as inferior displacement. IV contrast-enhanced CT is recommended for all patients will posterior dislocation to evaluate the underlying airway and vascular structures.

Another injury of the sternoclavicular joint is fracture dislocation of the medial clavicle physis. This physis typically does not fuse until 22–25 years of age, and approximately half of adolescents and young adults with sternoclavicular injuries will have fracture through the physis [9, 10]. On radiographs and CT, physeal fractures can be impossible to differentiate from true sternoclavicular joint dislocations (Fig. 5a). MRI can effectively demonstrate the displaced epiphyseal fragment, which can be useful for preoperative planning (Fig. 5b) [11].

## Acromioclavicular Joint Separations

Acromioclavicular (AC) joint separations are one of the most common injuries in the emergent setting, usually resulting from a direct impact such as a fall. The incidence of AC joint injury is 45 per 100,000 persons/year [12, 13]. AC injuries are by far most common in young men, in which the incidence is nearly ten times higher than similar-aged women. The incidence in men gradually declines until the seventh decade of life, when men have only a slightly higher incidence of injury compared with women [13].

The most commonly used system to classify AC injuries is the Rockwood classification. Rockwood types 1–3 represent injuries isolated to the acromioclavicular and coracoclavicular (CC) ligaments. Types 4–6 represent AC and CC ligament rupture, with additional soft tissue injuries (Fig. 6). Radiographs are generally adequate for diagnosing and characterizing AC separations. The normal AC joint distance varies, ranging from 3–6 mm. The coracoclavicular distance is less variable, with a normal distance of approximately 13 mm. As such, these measurements can be used when assessing for acromioclavicular joint separations. In type 1 injuries, there is minimal to no widening of the AC joint. In type 2 injuries, there is definite increase in acromioclavicular distance, seen as either widening of the joint space or vertical offset of the joint (Fig. 7a). In type 3 injuries, widening of both the AC and CC distances will be evident (Fig. 7b). In type 4 injuries, the distal clavicle is displaced posteriorly, and is entrapped in the trapezius muscle. This is best seen on an axillary view (Fig. 7c). In type 5 injuries, the coracoclavicular distance will be markedly increased due to stripping of muscle attachments to the clavicle, with the CC distance at least two times normal (>25 mm)(Fig. 7d). In type 6 injuries, the clavicle is displaced inferiorly and entrapped beneath the coracoid.

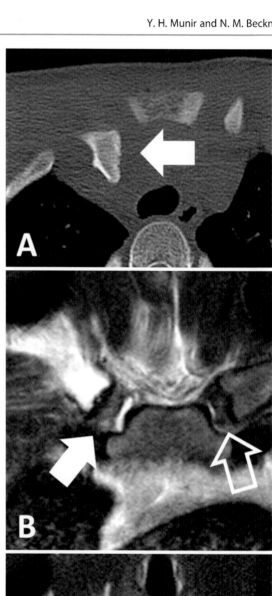

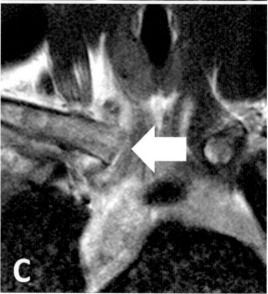

**Fig. 5** Sternoclavicular fracture dislocation. (**a**) Axial CT image shows posterior displacement of the right clavicular head without visible fracture (arrow). (**b**) Coronal fat-saturated proton density MR image shows fracture through right medial clavicular physis (solid arrow) with the intact contralateral physis (arrow silhouette) for comparison. (**c**) Additional coronal fat-saturated proton density MR image shows posteriorly displaced metaphysis without attached epiphysis (arrow)

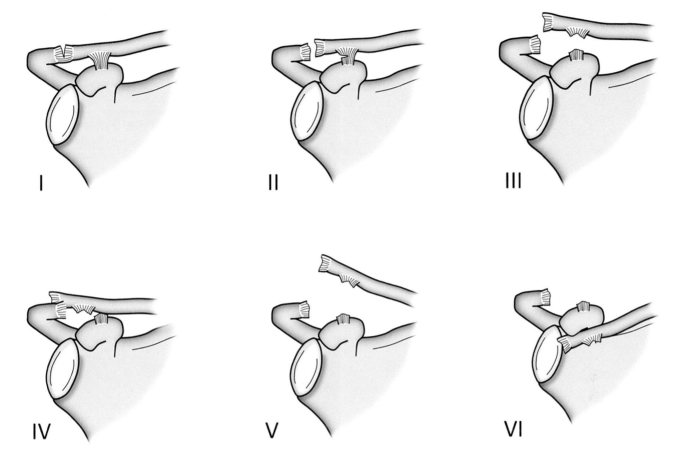

**Fig. 6** Rockwood-Altman classification of AC separations

## Clavicle Fractures

Clavicle fractures are a common shoulder injury, representing 5% of all fractures [14]. These fractures typically result from a high-energy direct blow. Clavicular fractures are described based upon which third of the clavicle is injured. Middle third clavicle fractures represent 65–76% of all clavicle fractures [15, 16]. In men, these fractures have a bimodal distribution, peaking in young adults and in the elderly. In women, these fractures follow a unimodal distribution, peaking in the elderly [14]. Lateral third fractures represent 22–30% of all clavicular fractures (Fig. 8a), and have a unimodal distribution in both men and women, with peaks in younger men and older women [14–16]. Medial third fractures represent only 2–5% of all clavicle fractures (Fig. 8b) [15, 16]. These fractures also follow a unimodal distribution in both genders, with peaks in younger men and older women [14].

Treatment of clavicle fractures depends on which third of the clavicle the fracture occurs. For the middle third, fractures displaced by greater than 1 shaft width, more than 2 cm of shortening, or those with a "z-shaped" pattern (Fig. 9) are examples of those that usually require surgical fixation. For lateral third fractures, it is important to describe displacement, comminution, involvement of the AC joint, and location relative to the insertion of the CC ligament. Medial third fractures are described similar to SC joint dislocations, with anteriorly displaced fractures being more common and likely treated conservatively, while posteriorly displaced fractures pose risk to the underlying mediastinal structures.

## Scapula Fractures

Scapular fractures represent fewer than 1% of all fractures [14]. Approximately one-third are intra-articular involving the glenoid, with the remaining being extra-articular [17]. These fractures result from direct impaction, usually secondary to high-energy trauma in young adults, or low-energy trauma in elderly patients. Both genders demonstrate a unimodal distribution, with peaks in younger men and older women [14].

The decision for surgical fixation of a scapular fracture is complex and generally revolves around which portion of the scapula is involved, the degree of displacement, the

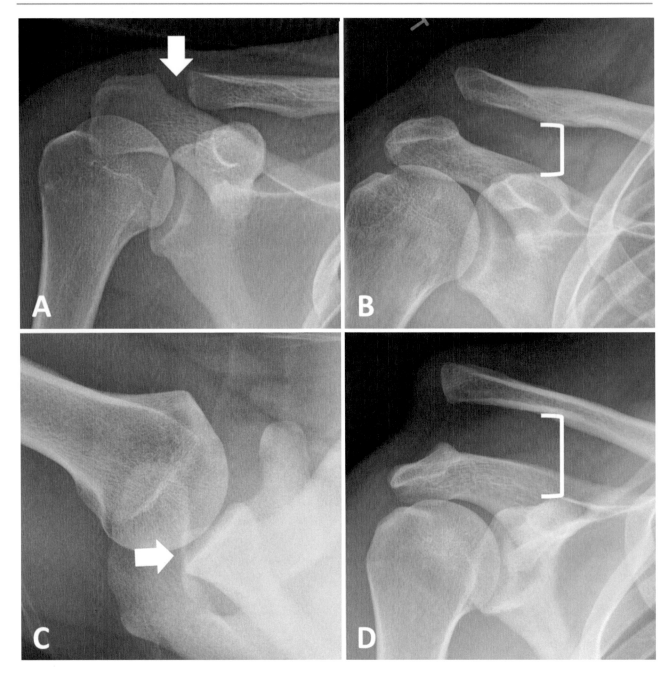

**Fig. 7** AC separations. (**a**) Type II with widened AC joint and normal CC distance on AP radiograph. (**b**) Type III with superiorly displaced clavicle and mild widening of CC distance (bracket) on AP radiograph. (**c**) Type IV with posteriorly displaced clavicle (arrow) on axillary radiograph. (**d**) Type V with superiorly displaced clavicle and widening of CC distance by more than 200% of normal distance (bracket) on AP radiograph

functional status of the patient, and other associated injuries [18–20]. Multiple classification systems have been devised to help guide management of fractures based on which portion of the scapula is involved.

The Ideberg classification is for scapula fractures involving the glenoid articular surface [17]. This system groups glenoid fractures into six types, with types 1 and 5 having additional subtypes (Fig. 10). Type 1 fractures involve the glenoid rim, and are associated with shoulder dislocations (Fig. 11a). Types 2–4 are fractures extending from the glenoid surface to one of the scapular borders (Fig. 11b). Type 5 fractures extend from the glenoid to

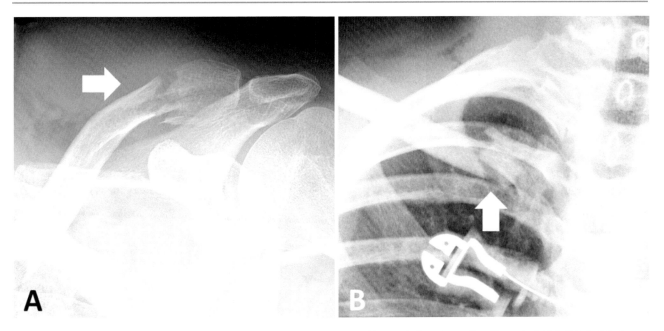

**Fig. 8** Clavicle fractures. (**a**) Lateral clavicle fracture extending lateral to coronoid tubercle (arrow) on AP radiograph. (**b**) Medial clavicle fracture extending medial to costal tubercle (arrow) on AP radiograph

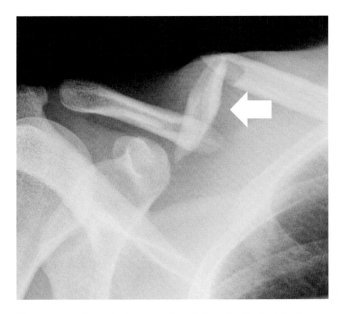

**Fig. 9** AP radiograph demonstrating Z-shaped mid clavicle fracture (arrow)

involve more than one scapula border (Fig. 11c). Type 6 fractures are comminution of the glenoid articular surface.

The Kuhn classification system is for acromion fractures (Fig. 12) [21]. Type 1 fractures are either nondisplaced complete fractures through the acromion, or an incomplete fracture that does not result in acromion instability (Fig. 13a). Type 2 fractures are displaced complete fractures that do not narrow the subacromial space (Fig. 13b). Type 3 fractures are displaced complete fractures that do cause subacromial space narrowing (Fig. 13c). As type 1 and type 2 fractures do not narrow the subacromial space, these are generally managed conservatively. Type 3 fractures may result in rotator cuff impingement; therefore, they are often treated surgically.

The Ogawa classification system is utilized for coracoid process fractures, dividing fractures based on location relative to the coracoclavicular ligament insertion (Fig. 14) [22]. Type 1 fractures occur through the base of the coracoid process, proximal to the coracoclavicular ligament insertion (Fig. 15a). These fractures can result in scapuloclavicular instability, and are usually treated surgically. Type 2 fractures are avulsion fractures distal to the coracoclavicular ligament insertion (Fig. 15b). These fractures do not result in scapuloclavicular instability, and are usually treated conservatively.

Fractures through the scapula neck are another important subtype of scapula fracture which often requires surgical treatment. There is no consensus on which glenoid neck fractures require surgical treatment, but, in general, displacement of greater than 1 cm or excessive glenopolar angle is treated with surgery [23, 24]. The glenopolar angle (GPA) is the angle between a line parallel to the glenoid articular surface and a line connecting the upper pole of the glenoid with the inferior scapular angle

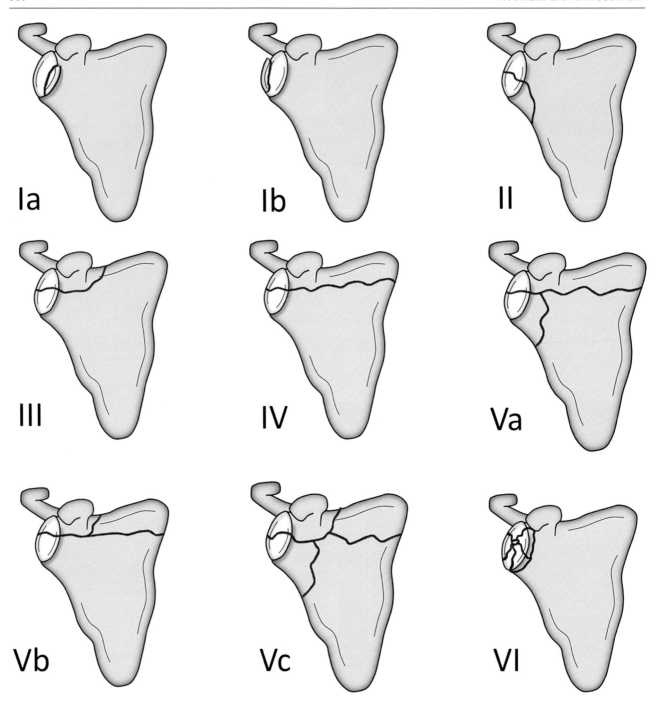

**Fig. 10** Ideberg classification of glenoid fractures

(Fig. 16a) [23]. Surgical fixation has been advocated for a GPA less than 26 or greater than 55 degrees (Fig. 16b) [24]. Entrapment of the suprascapular nerve can occur with glenoid neck fractures, and may be an additional indication for surgery [25].

## Glenohumeral Joint Dislocations

Glenohumeral (GH) joint dislocation is a common shoulder injury after trauma, with similar incidence to that of AC joint separations (17–55 per 100,000) [26, 27]. This injury has a

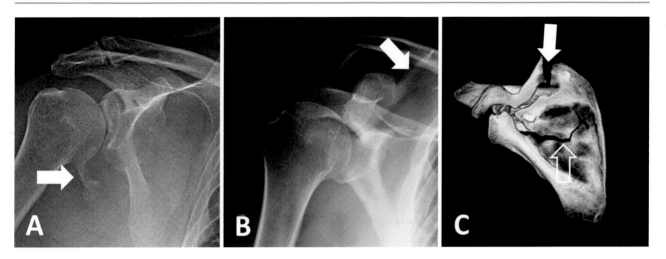

**Fig. 11** Ideberg glenoid fractures. (**a**) AP radiograph shows Ideberg 1b with a displaced fragment of the posteroinferior glenoid rim (arrow). (**b**) AP radiograph shows Ideberg 3 with displaced fracture line extending from glenoid though superior scapular border (arrow). (**c**) Three-dimensional volume-rendered CT images show Ideberg 5b with glenoid fracture lines extending though the superior (solid arrow) and medial (arrow silhouette) scapular borders

**Fig. 12** Kuhn classification of acromion fractures

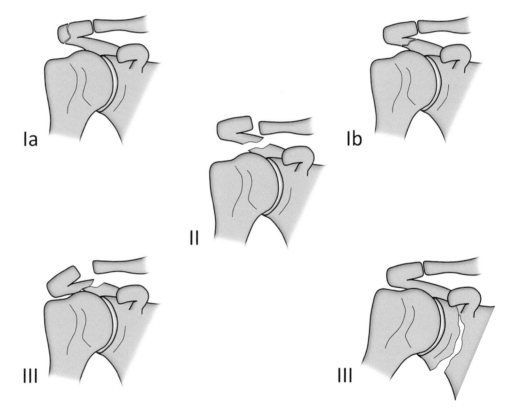

unimodal distribution in both men and women, peaking in younger men and in elderly women [12]. The direction of the displacement of the humeral head classifies the type of dislocation. Anterior dislocations comprise approximately 95% of dislocations, posterior dislocations approximately 5%, and inferior dislocations fewer than 1% [26, 27]. Rotator

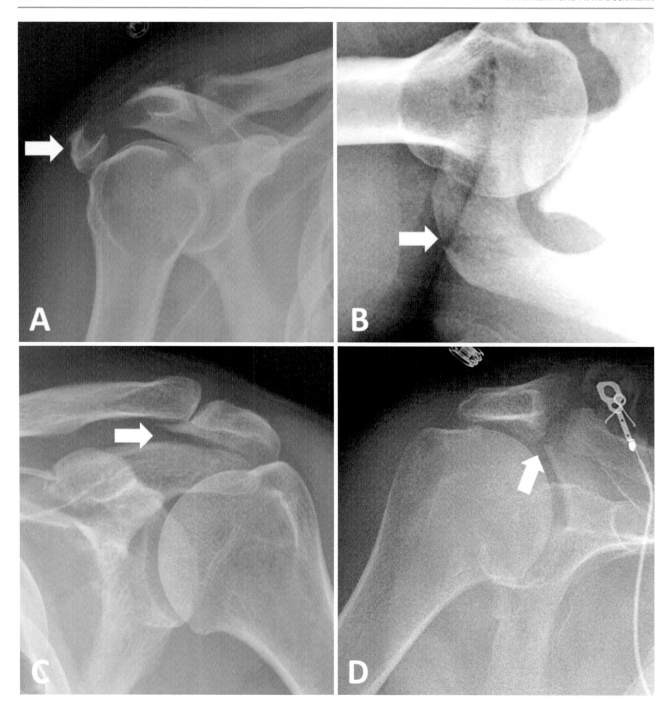

**Fig. 13** Radiograph examples of Kuhn acromion fracture patterns. (**a**) Kuhn 1a with a large avulsion fragment of the acromion (arrow). (**b**) Kuhn 1b with a nondisplaced fracture through the entire acromion (arrow). (**c**) Kuhn 2 with a mildly displaced fracture through the acromion (arrow) that does not narrow the subacromial space. (**d**) Kuhn 3 with a displaced fracture through the acromion (arrow) that does narrow subacromial space

cuff tears are frequently associated with shoulder dislocation in older patients, with a reported incidence of up to 80% in patients 60 years and older [28].

Anterior dislocations are readily visualized on an AP shoulder radiograph, demonstrating inferomedial displacement of the humeral head (Fig. 17a). Inferior dislocations

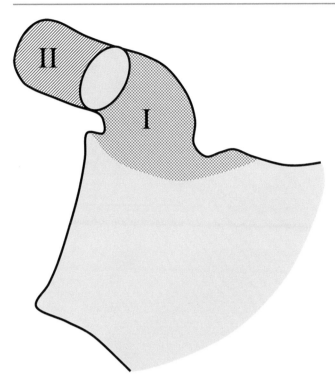

**Fig. 14** Ogawa classification of coracoid fractures

are also easily visualized, as the inferiorly displaced humeral head forces the shoulder into hyperabduction, which locks the arm in a raised position, known as "luxation erecta" (Fig. 17b). Posterior dislocations are more challenging to identify on AP radiographs as the superolateral displacement of humeral head can be subtle (Fig. 17c). A scapula-Y or axillary view can be helpful for diagnosis (Fig. 17d).

A typical injury pattern involving the humeral head and glenoid is usually present in transient shoulder dislocations. In anterior dislocations, impaction occurs along the posterolateral margin of the superior humeral head, commonly called a "Hill-Sachs lesion" (Fig. 18a). Impaction also occurs along the anterior glenoid rim, which can cause a labral tear or glenoid fracture, called a "Bankart lesion" (Fig. 18a). In posterior dislocations, the opposite pattern of injury occurs, with impaction along the anterior humeral head (reverse Hill-Sachs lesion, Fig. 18b) and along the posterior glenoid rim (reverse Bankart lesion, Fig 18b). In dislocations, it is vital to obtain postreduction radiographs in the emergency department, to ensure adequate reduction of the glenohumeral joint.

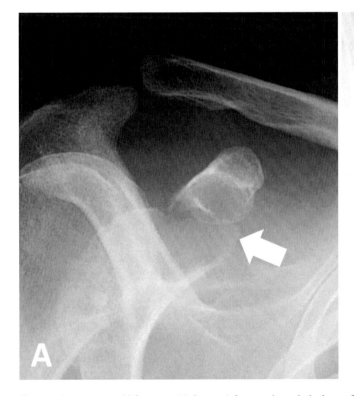
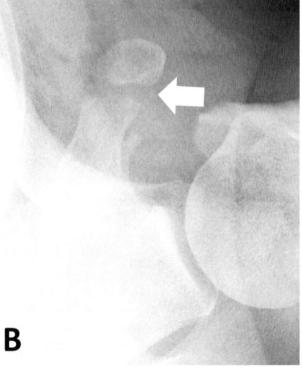

**Fig. 15** Ogawa coracoid fractures. (**a**) Ogawa 1 fracture through the base of the coracoid (arrow) on AP radiograph. (**b**) Ogawa 2 fracture distal to the coracoclavicular ligament insertion (arrow) on axillary radiograph

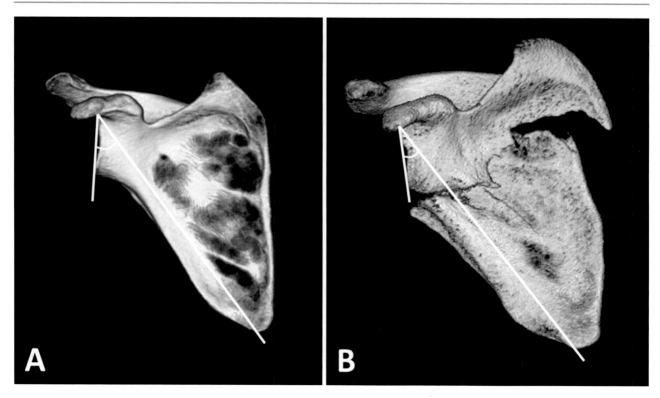

**Fig. 16** Three-dimensional volume render CT images demonstrating glenopolar angle. (**a**) Normal glenopolar angle. (**b**) Scapula fracture with medial displacement and angulation of the glenoid causing abnormally decreased glenopolar angle

## Proximal Humerus Fractures

The proximal humerus is a common site of fracture, representing approximately 6% of all fractures [14]. This type of fracture demonstrates a bimodal distribution, with a dominant peak in the elderly population usually from a fall, and a smaller peak in the younger population, usually due to high-energy trauma [29, 30].

The majority of proximal humerus fractures are treated nonoperatively [31]. Complexity of the fracture, displacement, and patient functional status all influence operative management. The Neer classification system is one of the most commonly utilized systems for describing proximal humerus fractures and can help guide management by conveying complexity and displacement of humeral head fractures. Neer's classification divides the humeral head into four major fragments (greater tuberosity, lesser tuberosity, articular surface, and shaft), with the classification based on the number of displaced fragments (Fig. 19) [32]. In the Neer classification, displacement is defined as greater than 5 mm for the greater tuberosity or 1 cm for any other major segment or more than 45 degrees of angulation of the humeral shaft.

## Scapulothoracic Dissociation/Floating Shoulder

Although rare, high-energy trauma can result in instability of the entire shoulder girdle. This instability can result in complete bony instability, called a floating shoulder, or a more severe form where there is complete bony and soft tissue instability of the girdle, termed scapulothoracic dissociation. These injuries are associated both with injuries in other regions of the body, as well as neurovascular injuries of the affected upper extremity, with up to 10% of patients having limb-threatening injury [33–35]. Further evaluation for vascular injury with CT angiography and neurologic injury with brachial plexus MRI or CT myelogram should be performed if there are clinical findings suggestive of neurovascular injury.

A floating shoulder is defined as any combination of clavicle and scapula fracture that result in complete dissociation of the glenohumeral joint from the axial skeleton (Fig. 20). In scapulothoracic disassociation, there is disruption of the clavicular bridge between the thorax and shoulder in addition to extensive soft tissue injury leading to lateral migration of the scapula (Fig. 21). This injury can be very difficult to diagnosis on initial imaging, due to most of the injury occurring in the soft tissues. Radiographically,

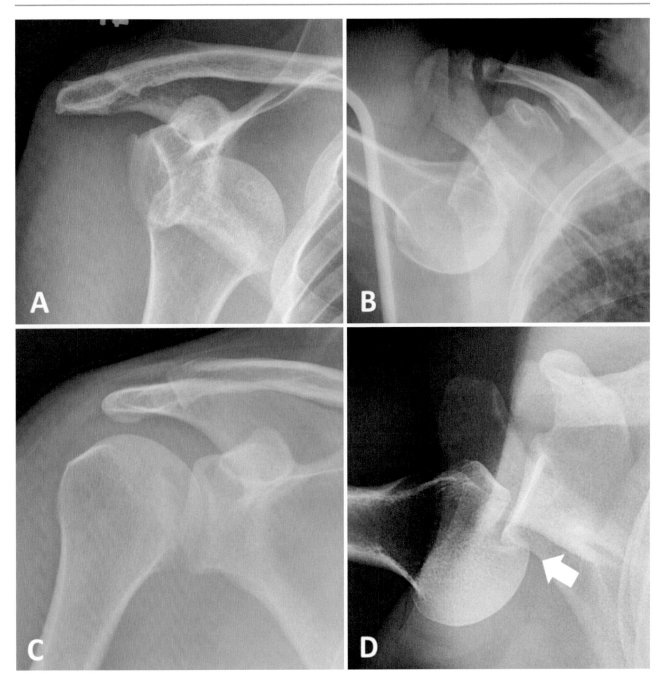

**Fig. 17** Glenohumeral dislocation types. (**a**) AP radiograph shows anterior dislocation inferior to the coracoid. (**b**) AP radiograph shows inferior dislocation with luxatio erecta. (**c**) Posterior dislocation difficult to appreciate on this standard AP radiograph. (**d**) Axillary view clearly demonstrates posterior dislocation with humeral head impacted on posterior glenoid (arrow)

scapulothoracic disassociation can be assessed by comparing the length of a line which is measured from the midline to the medial border of each scapula. An absolute difference greater than 1 cm or a ratio greater than 1.29 between the injured and uninjured side is consistent with scapulothoracic disassociation [34–36].

## Shoulder Soft Tissue Injuries

There are a variety of soft tissues at risk for injury in association with traumatic osseous injury. These include injuries to the surrounding musculotendinous structures, supporting ligaments, as well as the adjacent neurovascular structures. In

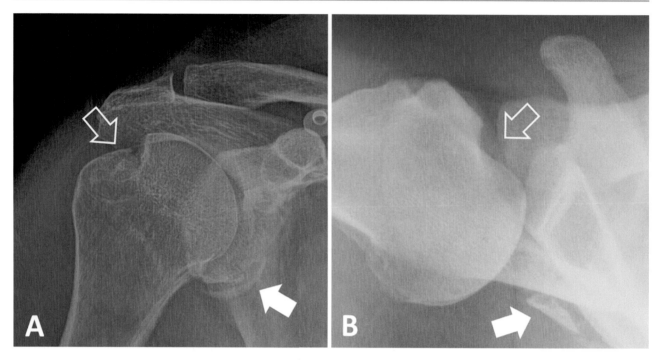

**Fig. 18** Shoulder dislocation injury patterns. (**a**) AP radiograph in patient with prior anterior shoulder dislocation after reduction shows typical Bankart fracture (solid arrow) and Hill-Sachs lesion (arrow silhouette). (**b**) Axillary radiograph in patient with prior posterior dislocation after reduction shows typical reverse Bankart fracture (solid arrow) and reverse Hill-Sachs lesion (arrow silhouette)

the emergency setting, injury to neurovascular structures is of primary concern.

Neurologic injury is relatively rare in the setting of shoulder trauma, most commonly occurring in the setting of shoulder dislocation. The most common nerve injury in the setting of shoulder dislocation is to the axillary nerve (Fig. 22a, b), with a reported incidence of 5–55% [37]. Suprascapular nerve injury has also been reported in the setting of shoulder dislocations or scapula fractures [37]. Less common nerve injuries are the spinal accessory nerve, usually due to penetrating trauma, and the musculocutaneous nerve, which can result from either penetrating trauma or blunt trauma to the coracoid [14].

Brachial plexus injuries are relatively common, particularly in the setting of high-energy trauma (Fig. 22c). Brachial plexus injuries have been reported in 1–2% of multitrauma cases [37]. Neurologic injuries can range from stretching injuries without tearing of the nerve axons (called neuropraxia) to complete rupture of the neurologic structure. In the acute setting, it can be difficult to clinically differentiate neuropraxia, which has a good prognosis for recovery with conservative management, from nerve rupture, which has a poor prognosis and may require surgical treatment. MRI of the shoulder and/or brachial plexus can be helpful for both assessing the severity of the nerve injury as well as the location of the nerve injury for surgical planning [38].

Injury to the axillary or subclavian artery is relatively rare, most commonly occurring as the result of either penetrating trauma or high-energy distraction injury to the upper extremity. Vascular injury occurs in approximately 25% of patients with osseous injuries resulting in fracture fragments displaced into the infraclavicular soft tissues [39]. Injury to the circumflex scapular artery can also occur in the setting of fracture involving the glenoid neck. Vascular injuries can range from subtle intimal injuries to complete vascular occlusion (Fig. 23a), or arterial rupture resulting in contrast

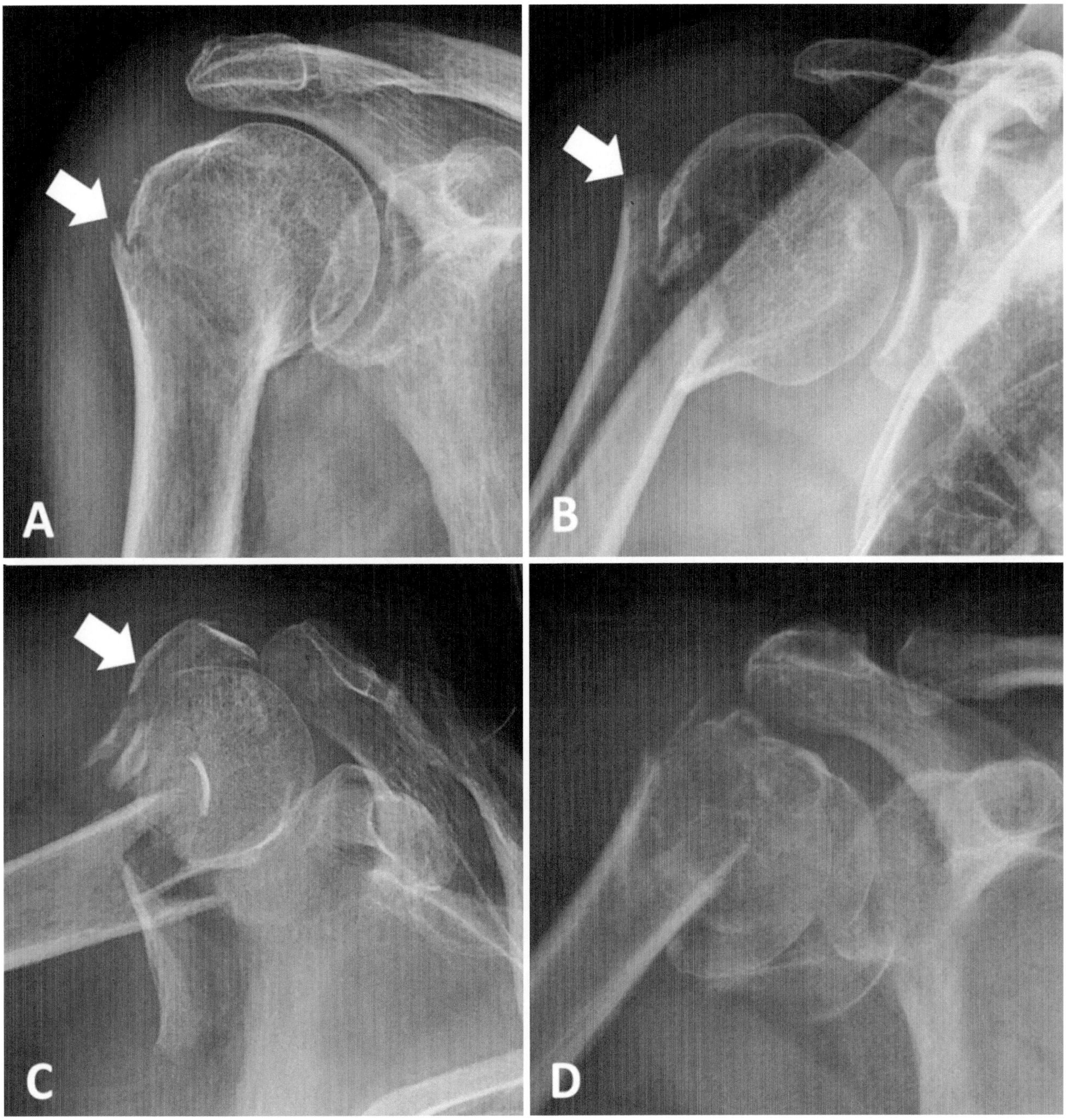

**Fig. 19** Radiographs depicting Neer classification of proximal humerus fractures. (**a**) One-part fracture through surgical neck without significant displacement (arrow). (**b**) Two-part fracture through surgical neck with significant displacement (arrow). (**c**) Three-part fracture with displaced greater tuberosity fracture (arrow), in addition to displaced articular surface and shaft fragments. (**d**) Four-part fracture with extensive displaced comminution of the humeral head

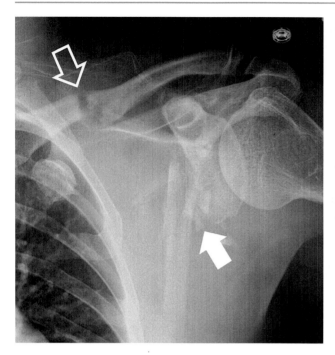

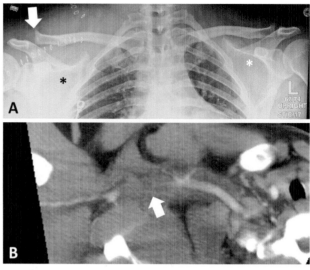

**Fig. 21** Scapulothoracic dissociation. (**a**) AP view of the clavicles demonstrating right-side AC separation (arrow), with the right scapula (black asterisks) displaced inferior to the left scapula (white asterisks). (**b**) Axial CT angiography showing focal occlusion of the axillary artery (arrow) with reconstitution distally

**Fig. 20** Floating shoulder. AP radiograph of the scapula shows fractures through the glenoid neck (sold arrow) and mid clavicle (arrow silhouette) resulting in complete bony instability of the shoulder girdle

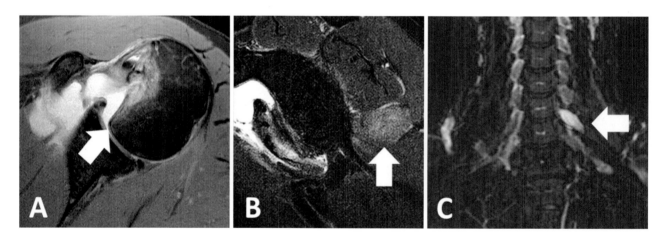

**Fig. 22** Traumatic shoulder nerve injuries. (**a**) Axial fat-saturated proton density MR image of patient with prior posterior shoulder dislocation demonstrates large reverse Hill-Sachs lesion (arrow). (**b**) Sagittal fat-saturated T2 MR image shows diffuse edema in the teres minor (arrow) consistent with denervation edema related to axillary nerve injury. (**c**) Coronal STIR MR image of the brachial plexus shows left C7 nerve root injury with pseudomeningocele formation (arrow)

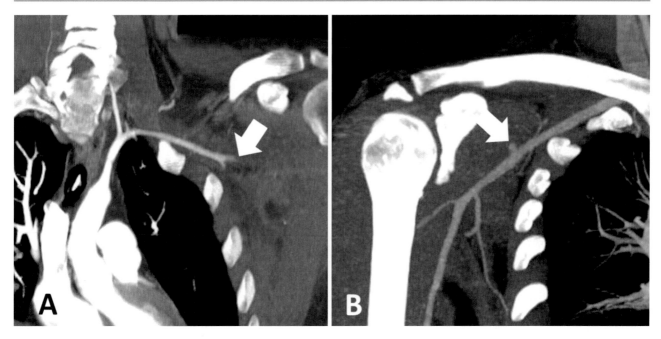

**Fig. 23** Traumatic shoulder vascular injuries. (**a**) Coronal CT angiogram image shows complete occlusion of the axillary artery (arrow). (**b**) Coronal CT angiogram maximal intensity projection image shows small pseudoaneurysm of the axillary artery (arrow)

extravasation or pseudoaneurysm formation (Fig. 23b). The axillary artery and brachial plexus are encompassed by a common connective tissue sheath. Therefore, axillary artery injury resulting in hematoma or pseudoaneurysm can lead to joint nerve injury [40].

## Summary

The shoulder girdle is a common location for trauma. Most injuries to the shoulder can be identified on radiography, but a low threshold should be maintained for performing CT, particularly in patients with suspicion for sternoclavicular or scapular injuries. CT angiography is typically not required for evaluation unless physical examination findings suggest vascular injury. MRI can be helpful for assessment of evaluating soft tissue injuries, but is rarely performed in the acute setting.

### Key Points
I. Radiographs are first-line imaging modalities for assessing shoulder trauma in the ER. However, a low threshold for CT should be maintained when fracture of the scapula or medial clavicle is suspected.
II. Modified axillary view radiographs are the preferred orthogonal shoulder radiograph in the trauma setting over a "scapula-Y" view due to patient tolerance and increased sensitivity.
III. Always maintain suspicion for possible underlying neurovascular injury, as these are generally underdiagnosed, and can pose great risk to the patient.

## References

1. Zamani A, Sharifi MD, Farzaneh R, Disfani HF, Kakhki BR, Hashemian AM. The relationship between clinical findings of shoulder joint with bone damage of shoulder joint in patients with isolated shoulder blunt trauma. Open Access Maced J Med Sci. 2018;6(11): 2101–6.
2. Sammarco VJ. Os acromiale: frequency, anatomy, and clinical implications. J Bone Joint Surg Am. 2000;82(3):394–400.
3. Senna LF, Pires E, Albuquerque R. Modified axillary radiograph of the shoulder: a new position. Rev Bras Ortop. 2016;52(1):115–8.
4. Miller-Thomas MM, West OC, Cohen AM. Diagnosing traumatic arterial injury in the extremities with CT angiography: pearls and pitfalls. Radiographics. 2005;25(Suppl 1):S133–42.

5. Gun B, Dean R, Go B, Richardson C, Waterman BR. Non-modifiable risk factors associated with sternoclavicular joint dislocations in the U.S. military. Mil Med. 2018;183(5–6): e188–93.

6. Boesmueller S, Wech M, Tiefenboeck TM, Popp D, Bukaty A, Huf W, Fialka C, Greitbauer M, Platzer P. Incidence, characteristics, and long-term follow-up of sternoclavicular injuries: an epidemiologic analysis of 92 cases. J Trauma Acute Care Surg. 2016;80(2): 289–95.

7. Glass ER, Thompson JD, Cole PA, Gause TM 2nd, Altman GT. Treatment of sternoclavicular joint dislocations: a systematic review of 251 dislocations in 24 case series. J Trauma. 2011;70(5): 1294–8.

8. Tepolt F, Carry PM, Heyn PC, Miller NH. Posterior sternoclavicular joint injuries in the adolescent population: a meta-analysis. Am J Sports Med. 2014;42(10):2517–24.

9. Wirth MA, Rockwood CA. Acute and chronic traumatic injuries of the sternoclavicular joint. J Am Acad Orthop Surg. 1996;4:268–78.

10. Lee JT, Nasreddine AY, Black EM, Bae DS, Kocher MS. Posterior sternoclavicular joint injuries in skeletally immature patients. J Pediatr Orthop. 2014;34(4):369–75.

11. Beckmann N, Crawford L. Posterior sternoclavicular Salter-Harris fracture-dislocation in a patient with unossified medial clavicle epiphysis. Skelet Radiol. 2016;45(8):1123–7.

12. Enger M, Skjaker SA, Melhuus K, Nordsletten L, Pripp AH, Moosmayer S, Brox JI. Shoulder injuries from birth to old age: a 1-year prospective study of 3031 shoulder injuries in an urban population. Injury. 2018;49(7):1324–9.

13. Clayton RA, Court-Brown CM. The epidemiology of musculoskeletal tendinous and ligamentous injuries. Injury. 2008;39(12):1338–44.

14. Court-Brown CM, Caesar B. Epidemiology of adult fractures: a review. Injury. 2006;37(8):691–7.

15. Herteleer M, Winckelmans T, Hoekstra H, Nijs S. Epidemiology of clavicle fractures in a level 1 trauma center in Belgium. Eur J Trauma Emerg Surg. 2018;44(5):717–26.

16. Kihlström C, Möller M, Lönn K, Wolf O. Clavicle fractures: epidemiology, classification and treatment of 2,422 fractures in the Swedish Fracture Register; an observational study. BMC Musculoskelet Disord. 2017;18(1):82.

17. Ideberg R, Grevsten S, Larsson S. Epidemiology of scapular fractures. Incidence and classification of 338 fractures. Acta Orthop Scand. 1995;66(5):395–7.

18. Lantry JM, Roberts CS, Giannoudis PV. Operative treatment of scapular fractures: a systematic review. Injury. 2008;39(3):271–83.

19. Anavian J, Gauger EM, Schroder LK, Wijdicks CA, Cole PA. Surgical and functional outcomes after operative management of complex and displaced intra-articular glenoid fractures. J Bone Joint Surg Am. 2012;94(7):645–53.

20. Königshausen M, Coulibaly MO, Nicolas V, Schildhauer TA, Seybold D. Results of non-operative treatment of fractures of the glenoid fossa. Bone Joint J. 2016;98-B(8):1074–9.

21. Kuhn JE, Blasier RB, Carpenter JE. Fractures of the acromion process: a proposed classification system. J Orthop Trauma. 1994;8(1):6–13.

22. Ogawa K, Yoshida A, Takahashi M, Ui M. Fractures of the coracoid process. J Bone Joint Surg (Br). 1997;79(1):17–9.

23. Bestard EA, Schvene HR, Bestard EH. Glenoplasty in management of recurrent shoulder dislocation. Contemp Orthop. 1986;12(1):47–55.

24. Bartoníček J, Tuček M, Frič V, Obruba P. Fractures of the scapular neck: diagnosis, classifications and treatment. Int Orthop. 2014;38(10):2163–73.

25. Boerger TO, Limb D. Suprascapular nerve injury at the spinoglenoid notch after glenoid neck fracture. J Shoulder Elb Surg. 2000;9(3): 236–7.

26. Krøner K, Lind T, Jensen J. The epidemiology of shoulder dislocations. Arch Orthop Trauma Surg. 1989;108(5):288–90.

27. Shields DW, Jefferies JG, Brooksbank AJ, Millar N, Jenkins PJ. Epidemiology of glenohumeral dislocation and subsequent instability in an urban population. J Shoulder Elb Surg. 2018;27(2):189–95.

28. Zanetti M, Weishaupt D, Jost B, Gerber C, Hodler J. MR imaging for traumatic tears of the rotator cuff: high prevalence of greater tuberosity fractures and subscapularis tendon tears. AJR Am J Roentgenol. 1999;172(2):463–7.

29. Chu SP, Kelsey JL, Keegan TH, Sternfeld B, Prill M, Quesenberry CP, Sidney S. Risk factors for proximal humerus fracture. Am J Epidemiol. 2004;160(4):360–7.

30. Court-Brown CM, McQueen MM. The relationship between fractures and increasing age with reference to the proximal humerus. Curr Orthop. 2002;16:213–22.

31. Schumaier A, Grawe B. Proximal humerus fractures: evaluation and management in the elderly patient. Geriatr Orthop Surg Rehabil. 2018;9:2151458517750516.

32. Carofino BC, Leopold SS. Classifications in brief: the Neer classification for proximal humerus fractures. Clin Orthop Relat Res. 2013;471(1):39–43.

33. Lee L, Miller TT, Schultz E, Toledano B. Scapulothoracic dissociation. Am J Orthop. 1998;27(10):699–702.

34. Zelle BA, Pape HC, Gerich TG, Garapati R, Ceylan B, Krettek C. Functional outcome following scapulothoracic dissociation. J Bone Joint Surg Am. 2004;86(1):2–8.

35. Sampson LN, Britton JC, Eldrup-Jorgensen J, Clark DE, Rosenberg JM, Bredenberg CE. The neurovascular outcome of scapulothoracic dissociation. J Vasc Surg. 1993;17(6):1083–8. discussion 1088-9

36. Lange RH, Noel SH. Traumatic lateral scapular displacement: an expanded spectrum of associated neurovascular injury. J Orthop Trauma. 1993;7(4):361–6.

37. Gutkowska O, Martynkiewicz J, Urban M, Gosk J. Brachial plexus injury after shoulder dislocation: a literature review. Neurosurg Rev. 2020;43(2):407–23.

38. Limthongthang R, Bachoura A, Songcharoen P, Osterman AL. Adult brachial plexus injury: evaluation and management. Orthop Clin North Am. 2013;44(4):591–603.

39. Battiston B, Vasario G, Marccocio I, Titolo P. Traumatic brachial plexus injuries. In: Peretti G, editor. Neurologic shoulder. 1st ed. Bologna: Timeo Editore; 2015. p. 57–65.

40. Stenning M, Drew S, Birch R. Low-energy arterial injury at the shoulder with progressive or delayed nerve palsy. J Bone Joint Surg (Br). 2005;87(8):1102–6.

# Imaging of Elbow Trauma

**38**

Nicholas M. Beckmann and Kimberley N. Brown

## Contents

### Abstract

The elbow is comprised of three articulations: radio-capitellar, ulnotrochlear, and proximal radioulnar joints. Soft- tissue injuries to the elbow are common, but most injuries to the elbow requiring emergency treatment involve either fracture or gross elbow instability. Radiographs are performed for initial evaluation and are typically adequate for excluding injuries requiring urgent intervention. CT of the elbow should be performed in periarticular fractures to assess for intra-articular extension and intra-articular fractures for preoperative assessment. CT angiography can help evaluate for arterial injury, but is rarely necessary as vascular injury is uncommon in the setting of elbow trauma. MRI is the preferred imaging modality for assessing most soft-tissue injuries, but is rarely performed in the emergency setting. Ultrasound can be used as an alternative to MRI for soft-tissue injury assessment, but has limited use in the acute setting due to challenges in positioning acutely injured patients, as well as the high level of expertise required to perform appropriate imaging assessment.

N. M. Beckmann (✉) · K. N. Brown
UTHealth – McGovern School of Medicine, Houston, TX, USA
e-mail: Nicholas.M.Beckmann@uth.tmc.edu;
Kimberley.Brown@uth.tmc.edu

© Springer Nature Switzerland AG 2022
M. N. Patlas et al. (eds.), *Atlas of Emergency Imaging from Head-to-Toe*,
https://doi.org/10.1007/978-3-030-92111-8_38

**Keywords**

Elbow · Trauma · Fracture · Humerus · Olecranon · Radial head · Coronoid · Dislocation

## Introduction

Elbow injuries constitute approximately 10–20% of all upper extremity injuries presenting for treatment [1, 2]. Fractures and dislocations compromise more than one-third of cases with soft-tissue injuries, including contusions and lacerations accounting for about half of cases [3]. Most elbow injuries are the result of low-energy trauma, either from axial loading during a fall on an outstretched hand (FOOSH) or a direct impaction to the elbow. Comminuted fractures or complex injury patterns are more frequently seen in high-energy trauma. Like other regions in the musculoskeletal system, the mechanism of injury greatly informs the patterns of injury seen on imaging. Therefore, knowing the mechanism of injury can aid in the detection and characterization of elbow trauma. In the emergency setting, diagnostic imaging is focused on identifying fractures or malalignment of the elbow. However, ligament injuries without malalignment or tendon injuries are common in elbow trauma and may require additional imaging assessment with MRI or ultrasound.

## Normal Anatomy

### Anatomy

The elbow is comprised of the articulation of the distal humerus with the radius and ulna, and it has three articulations: radiocapitellar, ulnotrochlear, and proximal radioulnar joints. All three of these articulations are confined in one synovial cavity. The elbow relies on osseous structures for stability more than the other major joints of the upper extremity. Increased osseous stability results in the elbow having relatively limited mobility compared to the shoulder and wrist, with the elbow only allowing motion for flexion-extension and pronation-supination.

### Distal Humerus

The distal humerus is comprised of the metaphysis, as well as medial and lateral condyles (Fig. 1). A supracondylar process or avian spur is an uncommon anatomic variant of the distal humerus metadiaphysis, occurring in up to 3% of the population (Fig. 2) [4]. This process can be mistaken for

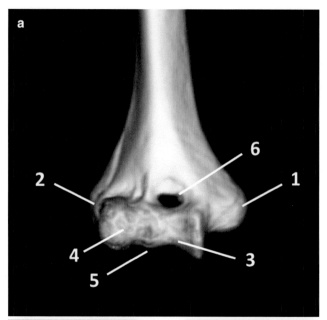

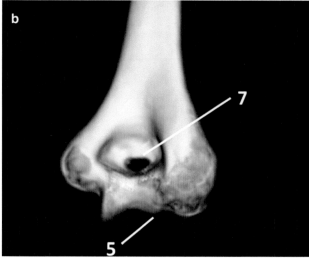

**Fig. 1** (**a**) Anterior and (**b**) posterior 3D volume-rendered CT images of the distal humerus. (*1*) Medial epicondyle. (*2*) Lateral epicondyle. (*3*) Trochlea. (*4*) Capitellum. (*5*) Trochleocapitellar groove. (*6*) Coronoid fossa. (*7*) Olecranon fossa

pathology, but can be recognized by its typical appearance as a pedunculated bony excrescence along the anteromedial distal humerus metadiaphysis directed toward the elbow joint. Supracondylar processes are usually asymptomatic, but can be symptomatic if they fracture [4].

Recesses are present at the junction of the metaphysis and condyles both anteriorly and posteriorly. These recesses accommodate the ulna coronoid and olecranon processes during elbow flexion and extension, respectively, and are termed the coronoid and olecranon fossae.

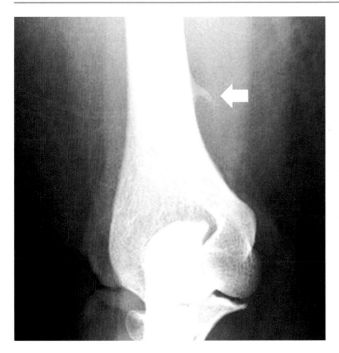

**Fig. 2** AP oblique radiograph of the elbow demonstrating a supracondylar process (arrow)

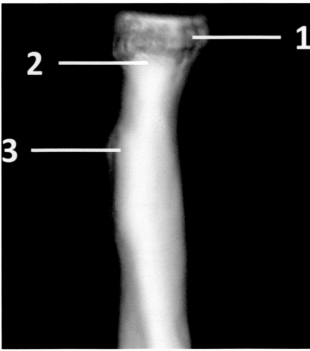

**Fig. 3** Anterior 3D volume-rendered CT image of the proximal radius. (*1*) Head. (*2*) Neck. (*3*) Radial tuberosity

The medial condyle has a large bony protuberance called the medial epicondyle, which serves as insertion sites for the ulnar collateral ligament and common flexor tendon of the forearm. The trochlea is the articular surface of the medial condyle which articulates with the trochlea. The lateral condyle contains the lateral epicondyle, which is less prominent than its medial counterpart. The lateral epicondyle is the attachment site for the common extensor tendon of the forearm, as well as the radial collateral and lateral ulnar collateral ligaments. The articular surface of the lateral condyle is the capitellum. The trochleocapitellar groove separates the trochlea and capitellar articular surface and is an important landmark when describing intra-articular fractures.

## Proximal Radius

The proximal radius is comprised of the metaphysis and radial head (Fig. 3), which articulates with the capitellum at the radiocapitellar joint and with the ulna at the proximal radioulnar joint. The radial neck forms the junction between the radial head and metaphysis. The radial head has a circular transverse morphology that allows for smooth gliding of the radial head at the proximal radioulnar joint during pronation-supination. The radial tuberosity lies along the anterolateral aspect of the proximal ulna metadiaphysis and is the insertion site for the distal biceps tendon.

## Proximal Ulna

The proximal ulna is comprised of two main processes: the olecranon proximally and coronoid anteriorly (Fig. 4). These two processes coalesce to form the greater sigmoid notch, which is the articulation between the humerus and ulna. The triceps myotendinous unit inserts along almost the entire proximal surface of the olecranon. However, the tendinous component of the triceps is confined to the posterior third of this insertion. The medial ridge of the coronoid process is called the sublime tubercle and is the distal insertion site of the ulnar collateral ligament. Along the lateral margin of the coronoid process is the radial notch, which articulates with the radial head. Slightly distal to the coronoid process along the lateral proximal metaphysis is the supinator crest, the distal insertion site of the lateral collateral ligament. The ulnar tuberosity lies along the anterior proximal metaphysis and is the insertion site for the brachialis muscle.

## Soft Tissues

The primary ligament stabilizers of the elbow are the ulnar collateral ligament medially and the radial collateral and lateral ulnar collateral ligaments laterally, which are jointly referred to as the lateral collateral ligament complex (Fig. 5).

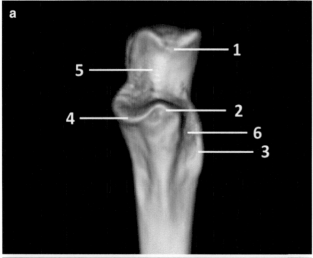

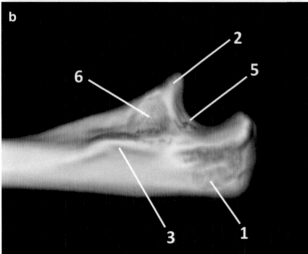

**Fig. 4** (**a**) Frontal and (**b**) lateral 3D volume-rendered CT images of the proximal ulna. (*1*) Olecranon process. (*2*) Coronoid process. (*3*) Supinator crest. (*4*) Sublime tubercle. (*5*) Greater sigmoid notch. (*6*) Radial notch

The ulnar collateral ligament stabilizes against valgus stress, while the lateral collateral ligament complex primarily resists posterolateral rotatory stress [5]. The annular ligament is an important stabilizer of the proximal radioulnar joint and can be injured in radial head dislocations. The major muscles to be considered in trauma are the triceps posteriorly, the biceps and brachialis anteriorly, the common flexor muscle mass medially, and the common extensor muscle mass laterally (Fig. 6).

The elbow has two major fat pads, the anterior fat pad lying within the coronoid fossa and the posterior fat pad within the olecranon fossa [6]. A single dominant brachial artery is typically present medial to the biceps tendon at the level of the elbow joint, which then bifurcates into radial and ulnar branches in the proximal forearm. However, a high origin of the radial artery can be seen in up to 10% of patients,

in which case separate radial and ulnar arteries will be present at the level of the elbow joint [7]. Three major nerves (radial, median, and ulnar) are present at the level of the elbow joint. The median nerve runs with the brachial artery anteriorly. The ulna nerve runs along the posteromedial elbow through a fibro-osseous tunnel posterior to the medial epicondyle, which is called the cubital tunnel. The radial nerve runs in the deep soft tissues of the anterolateral elbow just anterolateral to the brachialis muscle.

## Imaging Protocols and Methodology

### Radiography

After clinical survey, AP, lateral, and oblique radiographs are commonly used to evaluate for fractures. A radial head view can be added if there is high index of suspicion for a radial head fracture [8]. The radial head view is a modified lateral radiograph of the elbow where the x-ray beam is angled cephalad by 45°, projecting the radial head anterior to the ulna, thereby eliminating the osseous overlap between the radial head and ulna. Stress views can also be performed to evaluate for ligament instability; however, stress imaging requires a clinician proficient in stress maneuvers to be present at time of imaging. In a normally aligned elbow, a line drawn down the long axis of the radius should pass through the middle third of the capitellum on all radiograph projections (Fig. 7a). The joint space between the humerus and ulna should also be uniform, with a distance of less than 4 mm. Widening of the ulnohumeral joint to greater than 4 mm on a lateral radiograph after reduction of elbow dislocation is associated with persistent elbow instability and has been termed the "drop sign" (Fig. 7b) [9].

### Computerized Tomography

Non-contrast CT is primarily used to characterize intra-articular and periarticular fractures or to evaluate for occult fractures when there is clinical suspicion for fracture and no fracture is identified on initial radiographs. Any intra-articular fracture should undergo CT if surgical fixation is being considered in order to characterize the full extent of the fracture. Similarly, CT should be performed for any metaphyseal fractures undergoing surgical treatment, to evaluate for occult articular extension of the fracture. Elbow CT is also indicated in preoperative assessment of spiral fractures of the distal humerus diaphysis, as these fractures have a tendency to demonstrate intra-articular extension [10]. Non-contrast CT imaging of the elbow should be performed in axial, coronal, and sagittal planes with bone and soft-tissue kernels

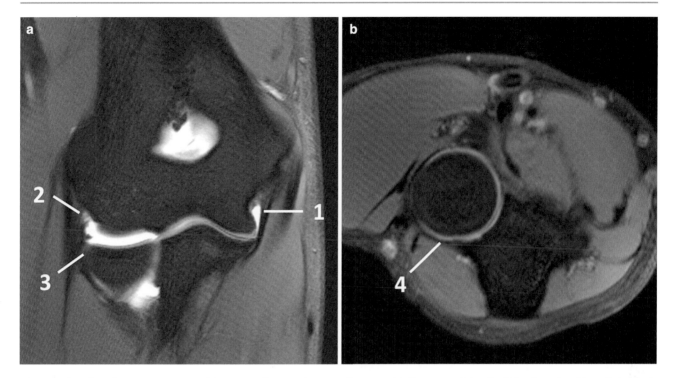

**Fig. 5** Major elbow ligaments. (**a**) Coronal fat-saturated proton density MR image through the mid-elbow and (**b**) axial fat-saturated proton density MR image at the level of the radial head. (*1*) Ulnar collateral ligament. (*2*) Common origin of radial collateral and lateral ulnar collateral ligaments. (*3*) Annual ligament. (*4*) Common insertion of the annular and lateral ulnar collateral ligaments

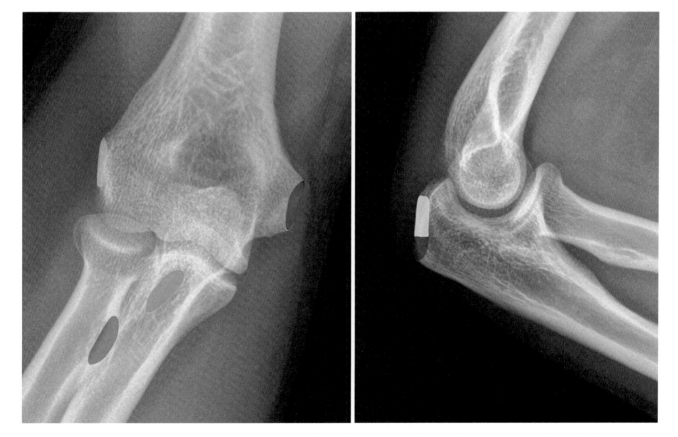

**Fig. 6** AP and lateral elbow radiographs demonstrating major muscle insertions. Common flexor (red), common extensor (orange). Biceps (purple), brachialis (green), muscle portion of triceps (yellow), tendinous portion of triceps (blue)

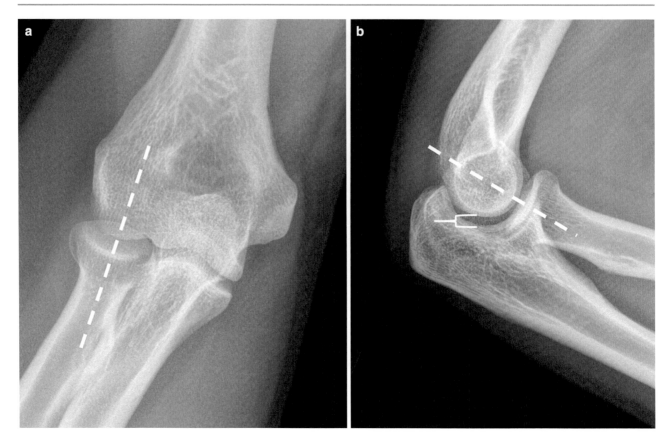

**Fig. 7** Normal elbow joint alignment. (**a**) AP and (**b**) lateral elbow radiographs. A dashed line drawn perpendicular to the center of the radial head passes through the middle third of the capitellum on both projections. On the lateral image, the ulnohumeral space is less than 4 mm (bracket)

and 2-mm or thinner slices. Three-dimensional volume-rendered images of the bones can aid in classifying fractures and for preoperative planning. CT angiography (CTA) is rarely needed to evaluate for acute vascular injury in elbow trauma, but CTA is appropriate when a patient has clinical findings, mechanism of injury, or injury pattern indicating increased risk for vascular injury [11].

## Ultrasound

Ultrasound has a limited role in assessment of elbow trauma in the acute setting, but can be a quick and cost- effective alternative to MRI in the assessment of soft-tissue injuries. Ultrasound can effectively be used to identify elbow joint effusion and soft-tissue hematomas about the joint. Ultrasound is also effective at identifying tears of the major elbow ligaments and tendons [12]. However, the accurate identification of ligament and tendon injuries relies heavily on the experience of the sonographer and the patient's ability to tolerate appropriate examination position, making

performance of diagnostic ultrasound of the elbow challenging in the emergency department setting. Dynamic ultrasound during varus and valgus stress can be performed to identify ligament instability by detecting joint widening during stress imaging [12, 13]. Again, the performance of stress imaging relies heavily on sonography expertise and patient compliance. Also, there are currently no widely accepted values to determining abnormal joint width; therefore, identifying abnormal widening typically relies on comparison to the contralateral, uninjured joint.

## Magnetic Resonance Imaging

Non-contrast MRI is very useful in evaluating soft-tissue injuries due to its high level of soft-tissue contrast compared to CT and its lower operator dependency compared to ultrasound. Limited availability of MRI, though, currently restricts the use of MRI in evaluation of elbow trauma in the emergency setting. MRI is primary used in the emergency setting to identify and quantify tears of ligaments and tendons. MRI can also be used to identify osteochondral injuries for preoperative planning in patients with elbow instability or with mechanical symptoms (e.g., popping, catching) after trauma. Although rare, MRI can be useful in identifying traumatic nerve rupture. However, delaying imaging for nerve injury for 4–6 weeks after trauma is preferred to allow surrounding soft-tissue edema to subside.

## Injury Patterns of the Elbow

### Distal Humerus Fractures

Distal humerus fractures are typically the result of high-energy trauma and are characterized based on intra-articular involvement and degree of comminution [14, 15]. Intra-articular fractures are further described based on whether they involve one of both columns of the humerus. The columns of the humerus are defined by the medial and lateral cortices of the metaphysis; the medial cortex represents the medial column, and the lateral cortex represents the lateral column. Many classification systems exist for distal humerus fractures, but the most widely used classification in adults is the Arbeitsgemeinschaft Osteosynthesefragen/Orthopedic Trauma Association (AO/OTA) classification system (Table 1) [16].

The AO/OTA classification for elbow fractures is part of a larger classification system devised to classify all bones in the human skeleton. In this system, distal humerus fractures are characterized as type "A" if they are extra-articular, "B" if they are intra-articular with single column involvement, and "C" if

**Table 1** AO/OTA classification distal humerus fractures

| Classification designation | Description |
|---|---|
| **Extra-articular (A)** | |
| **A1** | Epicondyle avulsion |
| **A2** | Simple (two-part) metaphyseal fracture |
| **A3** | Comminuted metaphyseal fracture |
| **Partial articular (B)** | |
| **B1** | Sagittal fracture through lateral column |
| **B2** | Sagittal fracture through medial column |
| **B3** | Coronal fracture through condyle articular surface |
| **Complete articular (C)** | |
| **C1** | Simple fracture (two articular fragments) involving the entire articular surface |
| **C2** | Simple articular fracture, comminuted metaphysis |
| **C3** | Comminuted (more than two articular fragments) involving the entire articular surface |

they are intra-articular, bi-columnar fractures. Each fracture type can then be subcategorized based on additional specific characteristics of the fracture (Table 1 and Figs. 8 and 9). The AO/OTA classification allows for further subclassification of fractures. For example, simple metaphyseal (A2) fractures can be further subclassified as A2.1, A2.2, or A2.3 depending on whether the fracture line is spiral, oblique, or transverse.

The AO/OTA classification system does have some general implications in surgical treatment. For example, type A fractures are more likely to be treated conservatively, and type C fractures are more likely to require olecranon osteotomy during surgical treatment [16, 17]. However, the AO/OTA classification does not consider important characteristics for fracture fixation, including degree of displacement, severity of comminution, and associated soft-tissue injuries. The greatest utility in this classification is for succinctly summarizing fracture patterns and for grouping fractures for research purposes.

## Proximal Radius Fractures

Radial head and neck fractures are the most common fracture of the elbow in adults, usually occurring as the result of a FOOSH injury [18]. The Mason-Johnston classification is most widely used to categorize radial head and neck fractures (Figs. 10 and 11) [18, 19]. Type I fractures are displaced less than 2 mm, type II fractures have more than 2 mm of displacement, type III fractures are comminuted and displaced, and type IV fractures are any radial head/neck fracture associated with elbow dislocation. Type I fractures are managed conservatively, whereas type II–IV fractures are usually treated surgically.

The radius and ulna are tightly bound together at the proximal and distal radioulnar joints. This tight binding results in the radius and ulna functioning as a single osseous ring, with injuries commonly simultaneously occurring at two points along this ring. This ring relationship results in two well-known injury patterns of the forearm that involve the radial head: Essex-Lopresti and Monteggia fracture-dislocations [20, 21]. Essex-Lopresti fracture-dislocation is a radial head fracture with dislocation of the distal radioulnar joint (Fig. 12a). A 5-mm offset of the distal radioulnar joint on a true lateral radiograph is indicative of distal radioulnar joint disruption [20]. Monteggia fracture-dislocation is dislocation of the radial head occurring with a proximal ulna diaphyseal fracture (Fig. 12b). Close inspection of both the wrist and elbow for subtle fracture or malalignment should be performed whenever an isolated fracture of the radius or ulna is identified.

**Fig. 8** AO/OTA classification distal humerus fractures

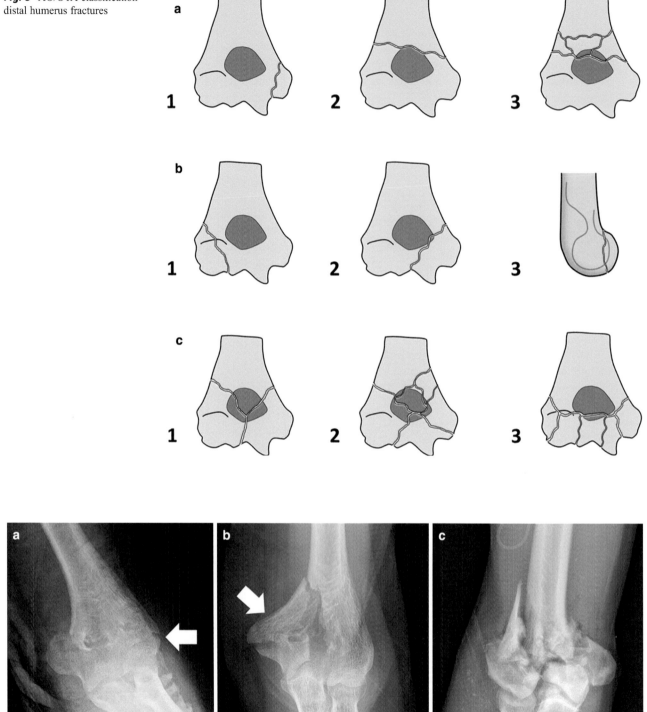

**Fig. 9** Radiographs of distal humerus fracture patterns. (**a**) Oblique extra-articular fracture through distal humerus metaphysis (AO/OTA A2). (**b**) Comminuted partial articular fracture involving the medial column (AO/OTA B2). (**c**) Complete articular fracture with comminution of the metaphysis (AO/OTA C2)

**Fig. 10** Mason-Johnston classification

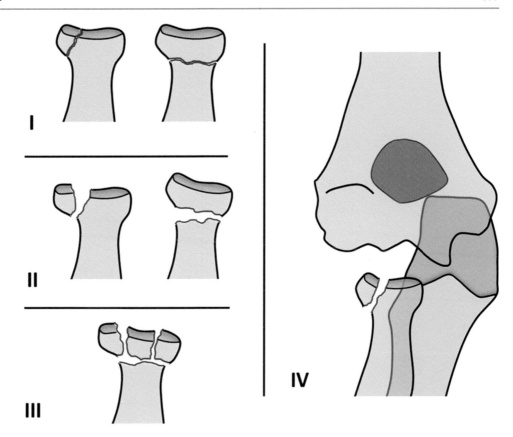

## Proximal Ulna Fractures

After radial head fractures, proximal ulna fractures are the next most common fractures occurring in adults, usually as a result of falls from standing [22]. Approximately 80% of these fractures will be olecranon fractures resulting from direct impaction by landing on the olecranon [22]. Coronoid process fractures occurring from impaction of the coronoid upon the trochlea during FOOSH injury comprise the majority of the remaining 20% of fractures.

While there is no widely used classification for olecranon fractures, to our knowledge, the Schatzker classification is one of the most commonly used classifications because it has fair inter-observer agreement on receiver-operating characteristic analysis while informing type of surgical fixation and offering some prognostic information [23, 24]. The Schatzker classification categorizes fractures based on fracture location, orientation, comminution, and associated elbow dislocation (Figs. 13 and 15) [25]. In general, the degree of olecranon comminution, fracture displacement, and fracture orientation

are important characteristics to help guide surgical treatment [26].

Coronoid process fractures can occur in insolation, but are often seen in conjunction with posterior elbow dislocations. Coronoid process fractures can be treated conservatively if small. Surgery is indicated if the fracture involves the sublime tubercle or a large portion of the coronoid process [27, 28]. The Regan-Morrey classification is a widely used classification for describing coronoid process fractures and is based on the amount of coronoid involved by the fracture (Figs. 14 and 15) [29]. Type I fractures are tiny avulsion fractures at the tip of the coronoid process, type II fractures are impaction fractures involving less than 50% of process, and type III fractures involve greater than 50% of the process. The advantage of the Regan-Morrey classification is its simplicity, which lends itself to higher inter-observer agreement. The simplicity of the Regan-Morrey classification is also a weakness of the classification, as important characteristics of coronoid process fractures

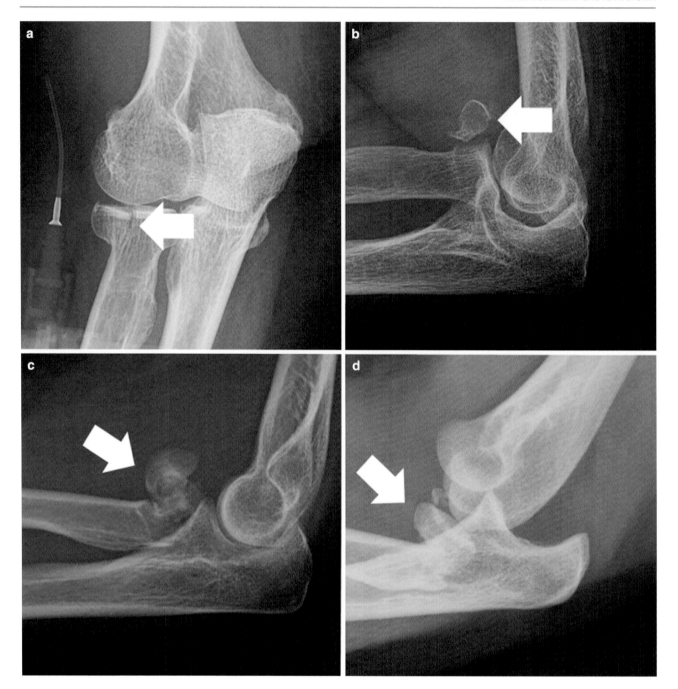

**Fig. 11** Radiographs of radial head/neck fractures. (**a**) Minimally displaced fracture (type I). (**b**) Displaced fracture (type II). (**c**) Displaced comminuted fracture (type III). (**d**) Radial head fracture with elbow joint dislocation (type IV)

which influence elbow stability, including involvement of the sublime tubercle and associated soft-tissue injuries, are not included in the classification. Furthermore, obliquity of the fracture can make quantifying the percent of coronoid involved challenging, particularly on radiographs.

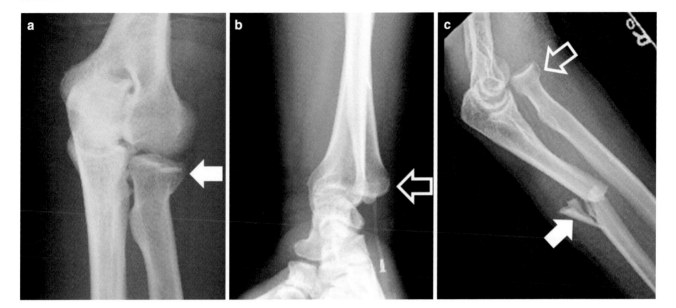

**Fig. 12** (**a** and **b**) Essex-Lopresti fracture-dislocation. AP oblique radiograph of the elbow shows fracture of the radial head (solid arrow) with dorsal dislocation of the distal radioulnar joint on lateral wrist radiograph (silhouette arrow). (**c**) Monteggia fracture-dislocation. Lateral view of the proximal forearm shows fracture of the proximal ulna diaphysis (solid arrow) with anterior dislocation of the radial head (silhouette arrow)

## Avulsion Fractures

Avulsion fractures of the elbow are a relatively rare phenomenon in adults. The most common avulsion fracture is an avulsion of the olecranon at the insertion of the tendinous portion of the triceps. These avulsions often present as a displaced fractured olecranon enthesophyte that can be easily mistaken for dystrophic soft-tissue calcification (Fig. 16a). Avulsions of the sublime tubercle (Fig. 16b) and supinator crest are rare, but can be indicators of elbow instability. Small ligament or tendinous avulsions at the epicondyles (Fig. 16c) are also rare and usually occur in the setting of larger soft-tissue injuries. More commonly, small chronic ossicles are present adjacent to the epicondyles, which can be mistaken for acute avulsion injuries (Fig. 16d).

## Instability Patterns

Elbow dislocation is the second most common joint dislocation after the shoulder and is usually classified according to the direction of movement and type of disarticulation [30, 31]. Simple dislocations are dislocations without fracture, whereas complex dislocations are accompanied by fractures. Radial head fractures and coronoid process fractures are common, warranting further cross-sectional imaging at the onset of the injury. Posterior dislocations are by far the most common dislocation type (Fig. 17). Anterior dislocations are uncommon, mostly seen in pediatric patients, and may be the result of rebound after posterior dislocation [31, 32]. A divergent dislocation is a very rare type of dislocation occurring when high-energy trauma causes interposition of the humerus between the radius and the ulna [33].

During FOOSH injuries, axial loading forces tend to drive the radial head posteriorly. The lateral ligament complex usually restrains the radial head from displacing posteriorly. However, the lateral ligament complex will sometimes rupture resulting in instability of the radiocapitellar joint and displacement of the radial head posteriorly. As the radial head moves posteriorly, a rotational force occurs across the elbow, which can lead to tearing of the joint capsule from lateral to medial. If the rotational force propagates across the entire joint, the ulnar collateral ligament can rupture as well resulting in posterior elbow dislocation. This spectrum of soft-tissue injury progression has been termed posterolateral rotatory instability and has been classified into four stages based on imaging presentation (Fig. 18) [34]. Stage 0 injuries are isolated injury to the lateral ligament complex and present with normal alignment. Stage I injuries are tears of the lateral

**Fig. 13** Schatzker classification

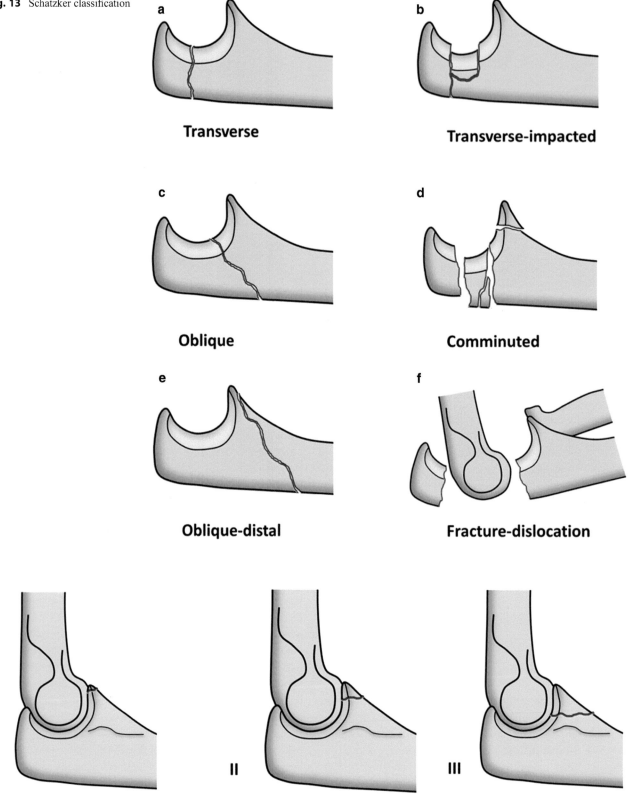

Transverse

Transverse-impacted

Oblique

Comminuted

Oblique-distal

Fracture-dislocation

I

II

III

**Fig. 14** Regan-Morrey classification

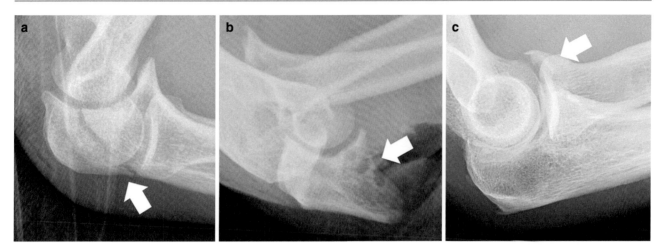

**Fig. 15**   Radiographs of proximal ulna fractures. (**a**) Oblique intra-articular olecranon fracture (Schatzker C). (**b**) Oblique extra-articular fracture (Schatzker E). (**c**) Coronoid process fracture involving less the 50% of coronoid area (Regan-Morrey II)

ligament complex and a portion of the lateral joint capsule and present with posterior radial head subluxation. Stage II injuries have near-complete tearing of the joint capsule and demonstrate subluxation of the ulnotrochlear joint in conjunction with radial head dislocation (Fig. 19). Stage III injuries have complete tearing of the medial and lateral ligament complex and present as a complete posterior dislocation.

The combination of posterior dislocation with radial head fracture and coronoid process fracture is referred to the "terrible triad" (Fig. 20). Extensive ligamentous injury complicates the surgical repair, and if restoration/reconstruction is not performed early, chronic instability and arthritis can develop [35, 36].

## Soft-Tissue Injuries

The ligament and tendon injuries are the most common surgically relevant soft-tissue injuries seen in elbow trauma. Biceps tendon injuries are one of the most common elbow tendon injuries presenting to emergency departments, typically seen in middle age to elderly patients (Fig. 21a) [37]. Biceps tendon tears are usually clinically evident and occur at the radial attachment. However, in the setting of partial tearing, imaging becomes necessary to delineate the extent of tears. Complete tearing of the biceps can also be underestimated in the setting of intact bicipital aponeurosis. Triceps tendon tearing is rare, accounting for fewer than 1% of all tendon ruptures [38]. A full-thickness tear of the entire triceps myotendinous insertion is very rare. More commonly, the superficial tendinous component comprised long and lateral heads tears, while the deep muscular insertion of the medial head remains intact (Fig. 21b). Acute isolated tears of the common flexor and common extensor tendons rarely present to emergency departments. Common flexor and common extensor tendon injuries are more often seen in the emergency department as part of a combined ligament and tendon injury occurring in unstable elbow injuries (Fig. 21c).

The most commonly injured elbow ligament is the ulnar collateral ligament (Fig. 22a) [38]. Ulnar collateral ligament injuries can occur in isolation due to hyper-valgus injuries or as a combined ligament and tendon injury in elbow dislocations. Similarly, injuries to the lateral collateral ligament complex can occur in isolation during FOOSH injuries as part of the posterolateral rotatory instability injury pattern or can occur as a complex soft- tissue injury pattern (Fig. 22b). Imaging evaluation of the ligaments is rarely performed in the emergency setting, but imaging can be useful to confirm ligament injury or assess the severity of injury in patients with clinical suspicion of elbow instability and who do not have clear evidence on instability on initial radiographic assessment.

Upper extremity nerve injuries in general are rare, comprising less than 1% of emergency visits for upper extremity trauma [39], and elbow nerve injuries comprise just a fraction of all nerve injuries of the upper limb. The ulnar nerve is the most commonly injured nerve at the elbow due to both its superficial location and intimate association with the bone in the cubital tunnel. Median nerve injuries have also been described in the setting of elbow fractures [40]. MRI can be

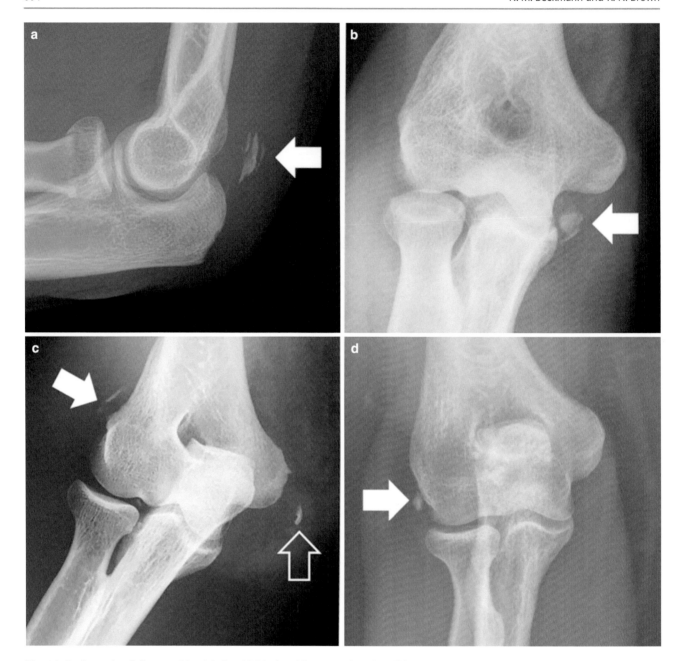

**Fig. 16** Radiographs of elbow avulsion injuries. (**a**) Displaced fracture olecranon enthesophyte at triceps insertion. (**b**) Mildly comminuted avulsion of the sublime tubercle. (**c**) Small avulsion fractures of the lateral (solid arrow) and medial (silhouette arrow) epicondyles. (**d**) Chronic ossicle adjacent to lateral epicondyle mimicking avulsion injury

useful for both defining the severity of nerve injury and determining the site of damage and degree of nerve displacement to assist in planning for surgical repair [41].

Vascular injury is a rare but well-known complication of elbow fracture and elbow dislocation [40, 42, 43]. Vascular injuries can also occur as the result of penetrating injury to the antecubital fossa. Injuries usually involve the brachial artery and can range from subtle intimal injuries to complete occlusion, pseudoaneurysm formation, or arterial transection (Fig. 23).

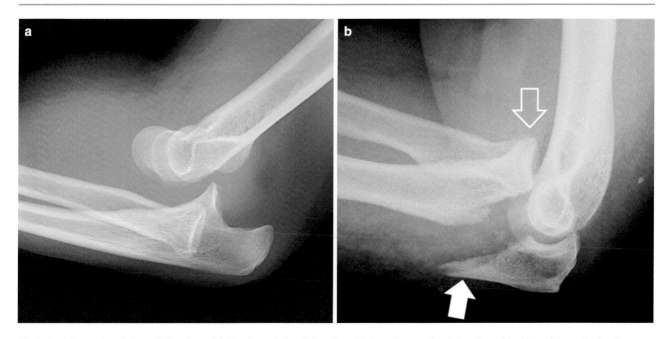

**Fig. 17**   Radiographs of elbow dislocations. (**a**) Simple posterior dislocation. (**b**) Complex anterior dislocation with oblique intra-articular olecranon fracture (solid arrow) and anterior radial head dislocation (silhouette arrow)

**Fig. 18**   Posterolateral rotatory instability stages

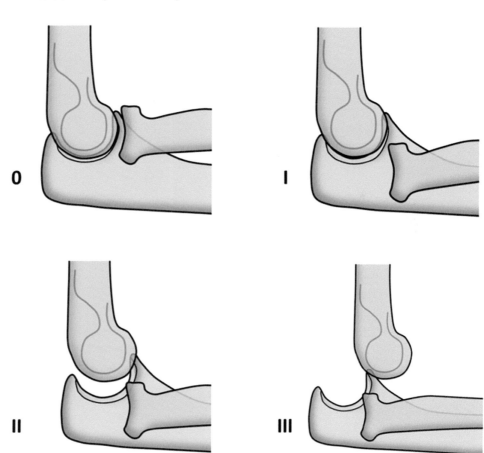

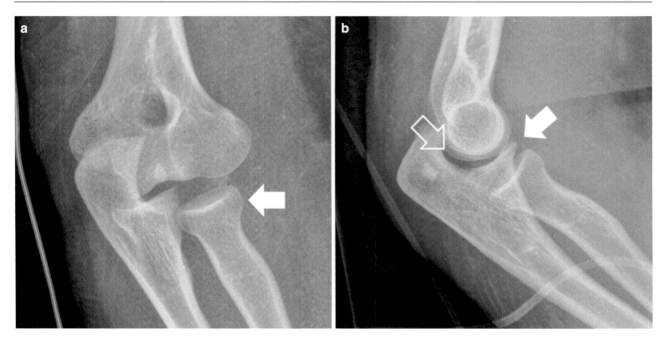

**Fig. 19** Posterolateral rotatory instability stage II. (**a**) Oblique radiograph shows posterior dislocation of the radial head (arrow) and a malaligned ulnotrochlear joint. (**b**) Lateral radiograph shows widening and posterior subluxation of radiocapitellar joint (solid arrow), with mild widening of the ulnohumeral joint (silhouette arrow)

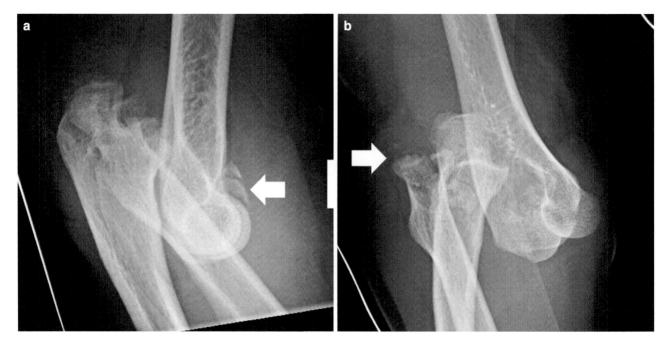

**Fig. 20** Terrible triad of elbow dislocation. (**a**) Lateral radiograph shows posterior elbow dislocation with fractures of the coronoid process (arrow. **b**) Oblique radiograph shows fracture of the radial head (arrow)

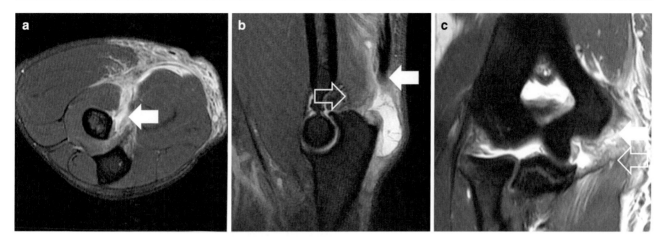

**Fig. 21** Elbow tendon injuries. (**a**) Axial fat-saturated proton density MR image shows full-thickness tear of the biceps tendon with fluidlike signal and absent tendon adjacent to the radial tubercle (arrow). (**b**) Sagittal fat-saturated proton density MR imaging shows complete tear with retraction of the tendinous component of the triceps tendon (solid arrow). The deep muscular insertion remains intact (silhouette arrow). (**c**) Coronal fat-saturated proton density MR image shows full-thickness tear of the common flexor tendon at its medial epicondyle insertion (solid arrow). Full-thickness tear of the proximal ulnar collateral ligament is present as well (silhouette arrow)

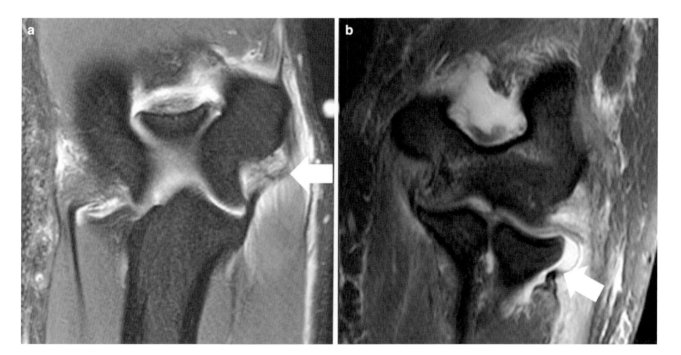

**Fig. 22** Elbow ligament injuries. (**a**) Coronal fat-saturated proton density MR image shows full-thickness tear of the proximal ulnar collateral ligament (arrow). (**b**) Coronal fat-saturated proton density MR image shows full-thickness tear of the proximal lateral collateral ligament complex with retraction to the lateral of the radial neck (arrow)

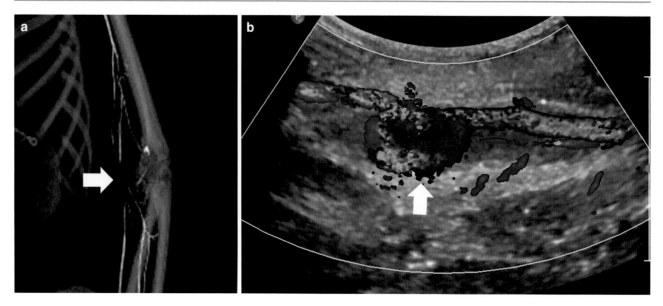

**Fig. 23** Elbow vascular injuries. (**a**) CT angiographic image demonstrating complete occlusion of a short segment of the brachial artery at the level of the antecubital fossa (arrow). (**b**) Color Doppler ultrasound image of the brachial artery showing focal outpouching with turbulent flow representing pseudoaneurysm formation (arrow)

## Summary

Elbow trauma is commonly encountered in emergency departments and is frequently due to a FOOSH mechanism of injury. Isolated soft-tissue injuries are common. However, fractures and gross elbow instability comprise a large majority of injuries requiring urgent treatment, and these injuries can usually be readily diagnosed on radiography. Purely soft-tissue instability patterns can be difficult to diagnose on radiographs and may only be apparent on MRI or stress imaging. However, this advanced imaging is typically not performed in the emergency setting. CT angiography is typically not required for evaluation unless physical examination findings suggest vascular injury.

## Key Points

I. Radiography is the first-line imaging modality for assessing elbow trauma. CT is indicated in periarticular fractures to evaluate for intra-articular extension and in intra-articular fractures for surgical planning.

II. MRI is the optimal imaging modality for assessing ligament, tendon, and nerve injuries, but is rarely performed in the emergency setting.

III. Ultrasound is an inexpensive alternative to MRI for assessing soft tissues, but is heavily reliant on operator experience for performance of imaging.

IV. Neurovascular injuries are a rare complication of elbow trauma. CT angiography should be performed in patients presenting with clinical findings, mechanism of injury, or patterns of injury suspicious for vascular injury.

## References

1. Ootes D, Lambers KT, Ring DC. The epidemiology of upper extremity injuries presenting to the emergency department in the United States. Hand. 2012;7(1):18–22.
2. Polinder S, Iordens GI, Panneman MJ, Eygendaal D, Patka P, Den Hartog D, Van Lieshout EM. Trends in incidence and costs of injuries to the shoulder, arm and wrist in The Netherlands between 1986 and 2008. BMC Public Health. 2013;13:531.
3. Pitts SR, Niska RW, Xu J, Burt CW. National hospital ambulatory medical care survey: 2006 emergency department summary. Natl Health Stat Rep. 2008;7:1–38.
4. Tomsick D, Petersen B. Normal anatomy and anatomical variant of the elbow. Semin Musculoskelet Radiol. 2010;14(4):379–93D.
5. Karbach LE, Elfar J. Elbow instability: anatomy, biomechanics, diagnostic maneuvers, and testing. J Hand Surg Am. 2017;42(2):118–26.
6. Goswami G. The fat pad sign. Radiology. 2002;222:419–20.
7. Haładaj R, Wysiadecki G, Dudkiewicz Z, Polguj M, Topol M. The high origin of the radial artery (brachioradial artery): its anatomical variations, clinical significance, and contribution to the blood supply of the hand. Biomed Res Int. 2018;2018:1520929.
8. Greenspan A, Norman A, Rosen H. Radial head-capitellum view in elbow trauma: clinical application and radiographic-anatomic correlation. AJR Am J Roentgenol. 1984;143(2):355–9.
9. Coonrad RW, Roush TF, Major NM, Basamania CJ. The drop sign, a radiographic warning sign of elbow instability. J Should Elbow Surg. 2005;14(3):312–7.
10. Updegrove GF, Mourad W, Abboud JA. Humeral shaft fractures. J Should Elbow Surg. 2018;27(4):e87–97.
11. Miller-Thomas MM, West OC, Cohen AM. Diagnosing traumatic arterial injury in the extremities with CT angiography: pearls and pitfalls. Radiographics. 2005;25(Suppl 1):S133–42.
12. Konin GP, Nazarian LN, Walz DM. US of the elbow: indications, technique, normal anatomy, and pathologic conditions. Radiographics. 2013;33(4):E125–47.

13. De Maeseneer M, Brigido MK, Antic M, et al. Ultrasound of the elbow with emphasis on detailed assessment of ligaments, tendons, and nerves. Eur J Radiol. 2015;84(4):671–81.

14. Jupiter JB, Mehne DK. Fractures of the distal humerus. Orthopedics. 1992;15(7):825–33.

15. Robinson CM. Fractures of the distal humerus. In: Rockwood CA, Green DP, Bucholz RW, editors. Rockwood and Green's fractures in adults. 6th ed. Philadelphia: Lippincott Williams & Wilkins; 2006. p. 1051–116.

16. Müller ME, Perren SM, Allgöwer M. for the Arbeitsgemeinschaft für Osteosynthesefragen. Manual of internal fixation: techniques recommended by the AO-ASIF Group. 3rd ed. Berlin: Springer; 1991.

17. Ul Islam S, Glover AW, Waseem M. Challenges and solutions in management of distal humerus fractures. Open Orthop J. 2017;11: 1292–307.

18. Mason ML. Some observations on fractures of the head of the radius with a review of one hundred cases. Br J Surg. 1954;42:123–32.

19. Johnston GW. A follow-up of one hundred cases of fracture of the head of the radius with a review of the literature. Ulster Med J. 1962;31:51–6.

20. Edwards GS Jr, Jupiter JB. Radial head fractures with acute distal radioulnar dislocation: Essex- Lopresti revisited. Clin Orthop Relat Res. 1988;234:61–9.

21. Rehim SA, Maynard MA, Sebastin SJ, Chung KC. Monteggia fracture dislocations: a historical review. J Hand Surg Am. 2014;39(7): 1384–94.

22. Duckworth AD, Clement ND, Aitken SA, Court-Brown CM, McQueen MM. The epidemiology of fractures of the proximal ulna. Injury. 2012;43(3):343–6.

23. Newman SD, Mauffrey C, Krikler S. Olecranon fractures. Injury. 2009;40(6):575–81.

24. Benetton CA, Cesa G, Junior GE, Ferreira AP, Vissoci JR, Pietrobon R. Agreement of olecranon fractures before and after the exposure to four classification systems. J Should Elbow Surg. 2015;24(3):358–63.

25. Schatzker J. Olecranon fractures. In: Schatzker J, Tile M, editors. The rationale of operative fracture care. 3rd ed. New York: Springer; 2005. p. 123–9.

26. Adams JE, Steinmann SP. Fractures of the olecranon. In: Morrey BF, Sanchez-Sotelo J, editors. The elbow and its disorders. 4th ed. Philadelphia: Saunders/Elsevier; 2009. p. 389–400.

27. Wells J, Ablove RH. Coronoid fractures of the elbow. Clin Med Res. 2008;6(1):40–4.

28. Ring D. Fractures of the coronoid process of the ulna. J Hand Surg Am. 2006;31(10):1679–89.

29. Regan W, Morrey B. Fractures of the coronoid process of the ulna. J Bone Joint Surg Am. 1989;71:1348–54.

30. O'Driscoll SW, Morrey BF, Korinek S, An KN. Elbow subluxation and dislocation: a spectrum of instability. Clin Orthop Relat Res. 1992;280:186–97.

31. Venkatram N, Wurm V, Houshian S. Anterior dislocation of the ulnar-humeral joint in a so-called 'pulled elbow'. Emerg Med J. 2006;23(6):e37.

32. O'Driscoll SW. Elbow dislocations. In: Morrey BF, Sanchez-Sotelo J, editors. The elbow and its disorders. 4th ed. Philadelphia: Saunders/Elsevier; 2009. p. 436–49.

33. Altuntas AO, Balakumar J, Howells RJ, Graham HK. Posterior divergent dislocation of the elbow in children and adolescents: a report of three cases and review of the literature. J Pediatr Orthop. 2005;25(3):317–21.

34. Camp CL, Smith J, O'Driscoll SW. Posterolateral rotatory instability of the elbow: Part I. Mechanism of injury and the posterolateral rotatory drawer test. Arthrosc Tech. 2017;6(2):e401–5.

35. O'Driscoll SW, Jupiter JB, King GJ, Hotchkiss RN, Morrey BF. The unstable elbow. Instr Course Lect. 2001;50:89–102.

36. Rodriguez-Martin J, Pretell-Mazzini J, Andres- Esteban EM, Larrainzar-Garijo R. Outcomes after terrible triads of the elbow treated with the current surgical protocols: a review. Int Orthop. 2011;35(6):851–60.

37. Clayton RA, Court-Brown CM. The epidemiology of musculoskeletal tendinous and ligamentous injuries. Injury. 2008;39(12): 1338–44.

38. Hayter CL, Adler RS. Injuries of the elbow and the current treatment of tendon disease. AJR Am J Roentgenol. 2012;199 (3):546–57.

39. Tapp M, Wenzinger E, Tarabishy S, Ricci J, Herrera FA. The epidemiology of upper extremity nerve injuries and associated cost in the us emergency departments. Ann Plast Surg. 2019;83(6):676–80.

40. Saeed W, Waseem M. Elbow fractures overview. In: StatPearls. Treasure Island: StatPearls Publishing; 2020.

41. Chhabra A, Andreisek G, Soldatos T, Wang KC, Flammang AJ, Belzberg AJ, Carrino JA. MR neurography: past, present, and future. AJR Am J Roentgenol. 2011;197(3):583–91.

42. Ayel JE, Bonnevialle N, Lafosse JM, Pidhorz L, Al Homsy M, Mansat P, Chaufour X, Rongieres M, Bonnevialle P. Acute elbow dislocation with arterial rupture. Analysis of nine cases. Orthop Traumatol Surg Res. 2009;95(5):343–51.

43. Lim SM, Chua GG, Asrul F, Yazid M. Posterior elbow dislocation with brachial artery thrombosis treated non-surgically: a case report. Malays Orthop J. 2017;11(3):63–5.

# Imaging of Hand and Wrist Trauma

**39**

Jordan R. Pollock, Thomas Wong, Jeremiah Long, and Jonathan Flug

## Contents

### Abstract

Imaging of the hand and wrist has been a staple of radiology, beginning with the first performed radiograph of Dr. Wilhelm Roentgen's wife in 1895. The first clinical radiograph was performed 1 year later for wrist trauma and depicted a Colles' fracture [1]. Injuries to the hand and wrist reportedly account for approximately 20% of visits to the emergency department [2], totaling approximately 3.5 million hand and wrist injuries in 2009 with an incidence of 1130 injuries per 100,000 persons per year in the United States [3].

Evaluation of the hand and wrist can involve assessment of as many as 29 bones and 29 joints. The ability of the hand to perform delicate maneuvers requires coordination of these bones, along with numerous ligaments, tendons, and nerves. Hand and wrist injuries can be associated with substantial disability and morbidity. They may carry

J. R. Pollock
Mayo Clinic Alix School of Medicine, Scottsdale, AZ, USA
e-mail: Pollock.jordan@mayo.edu

T. Wong
Vanderbilt University Medical Center, Department of Radiology, Nashville, TN, USA

J. Long · J. Flug (✉)
Mayo Clinic Arizona, Department of Radiology, Phoenix, AZ, USA
e-mail: Long.Jeremiah@mayo.edu; Flug.Jonathan@mayo.edu

© Springer Nature Switzerland AG 2022
M. N. Patlas et al. (eds.), *Atlas of Emergency Imaging from Head-to-Toe*,
https://doi.org/10.1007/978-3-030-92111-8_39

long-term socialand economic consequences, particularly if the diagnosis isinitially missed or if treatment is delayed.

**Keywords**

Hand · Wrist · Fracture · Imaging

## Teaching Points

1. A minimum of three radiographic views is recommended for evaluation of acute trauma of the hand and wrist, with a fourth view recommended when there is concern for scaphoid fracture, hook of hamate fracture, and scapholunate ligament injuries.
2. In the case of suspected acute hand or wrist trauma with negative or equivocal initial radiographs, MRI without contrast, repeat radiography in 10–14 days, or CT without contrast are all appropriate next best imaging options.
3. The three carpal arcs of Gilula should be continuous and will be disrupted in cases of carpal dislocation or carpal fracture-dislocation.
4. Evaluation of distal radial fractures should include a description including the location of the fracture, any articular involvement, comminution, displacement, and dorsal or volar tilt of the radial articular surface.

## Typical Clinical Scenarios

Hand and wrist trauma is a common presenting complaint and injury to the emergency department, spanning patients of all ages. A common mechanism of injury for hand and wrist trauma involves a fall on an outstretched hand, or "FOOSH." Fractures and dislocations may present after high-energy trauma, such as motor vehicle collisions, or low-energy trauma, especially in osteoporotic patients. Occupational injuries are common, including digit amputation, crush injuries, and foreign bodies, and often present with specific clinical treatment challenges. The physical examination, and, in particular, the exact location of pain and symptoms, will often guide the clinical assessment toward the presumed diagnosis.

## Imaging Protocols/Methodology

For most patients with hand and wrist trauma, standard trauma series radiographs provide adequate evaluation and information for the referring provider to derive their treatment plan. The American College of Radiology (ACR) Appropriateness Criteria for acute hand and wrist trauma recommend radiographs initially as usually appropriate and grade all other imaging modalities as usually not appropriate [4]. In the case of suspected acute hand or wrist trauma with negative or equivocal initial radiographs, MRI without contrast, repeat radiography in 10–14 days, and CT without contrast are the usually appropriate imaging options. For suspected penetrating trauma with a foreign body in the soft tissues in hand or wrist with negative radiographs, ultrasound and CT without contrast are usually the appropriate imaging options.

## Radiographs

Standard radiographs of the hand and wrist in the setting of trauma will generally include a total of three views, including posteroanterior (PA), oblique, and lateral projections. The field of view of a wrist radiographic examination should cover the distal radius to the metacarpal bases, while the hand radiographic examination will include the distal radius to the distal fingertips. When added to the PA and lateral views, the oblique view has been shown to alter diagnosis in 5% of cases [5]. In general, the wrist should be imaged in a neutral position with no flexion, extension, or deviation. The hand is placed palm down on the cassette with the fingers extended. The lateral view is obtained with the elbow flexed to 90°, with the wrist in a neutral position so that the axes of the radius, lunate, capitate, and third metacarpal are all in alignment (Fig. 1a, b). The oblique view is obtained by pronating the wrist 45° from the lateral position.

Additional views of the hand or wrist may help address specific clinical concerns. PA views of the wrist in radial and ulnar deviation help reduce osseous overlap to visualize the carpal bones on the ulnar and radial sides, respectively, and can be helpful in subtle fracture identification and in elucidating carpal mobility and potential instability. Specifically, the ulnar-deviated view causes dorsal and ulnar rotation of the distal pole of the scaphoid, thereby elongating the scaphoid to allow for easier detection of scaphoid fractures (Fig. 2) [6]. The radial-deviated view improves visualization of the ulnar-sided carpal interspaces. A clenched fist view can be obtained to aid in the detection of scapholunate widening, by driving the capitate toward the scapholunate interval (Fig. 3). A comparison view of the contralateral wrist can also be helpful in evaluating scapholunate interval asymmetry. When thumb injuries are suspected clinically, dedicated PA, lateral, and oblique radiographs of the thumb should be obtained to provide coned-down views of the thumb's bones and articulations. Likewise, additional coned-down views of the other individual fingers can be obtained to

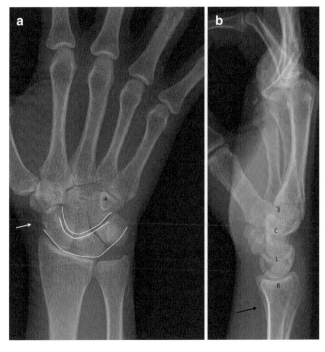

Fig. 1 (a) Standard PA view of the wrist. The carpal arcs of Gilula outline the margins of the proximal and distal carpal rows and can be disrupted in cases of dislocation (white lines). The ring of the hook of the hamate will be disrupted in hook of hamate fractures (black asterisk). The navicular fat pad can be obliterated as a secondary sign of scaphoid fracture or other fracture (white arrow). (b) Standard lateral view of the wrist. The base of the third metacarpal [3], the capitate (C), lunate (L), and distal radius (R), should be aligned. The pronator fat pad can be obliterated as a secondary sign of distal radius fracture (black arrow)

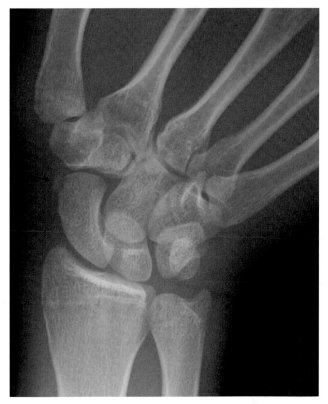

Fig. 2 Ulnar-deviated scaphoid view of the wrist showing a minimally displaced fracture of the scaphoid tubercle (black arrow)

improve visualization of subtle fractures and aid in assessment of the soft tissues. A carpal tunnel view can be obtained with the wrist dorsiflexed and the beam angled to profile the carpal tunnel, to primarily assess for fractures of the pisiform, hook of the hamate, and trapezial ridge (Fig. 4).

## Computed Tomography (CT)

General indications for CT of the hand and wrist include suspected fractures despite normal radiographs, suspected penetrating foreign bodies, or CT examinations obtained for surgical planning for known fractures. In this setting, CT is generally performed without intravenous contrast. A CT angiogram with intravenous contrast would be required if there is concern for a vascular injury in the setting of acute trauma and can be used to accurately diagnose arterial spasm, dissection, occlusion, pseudoaneurysm, and external vascular compression [7].

Ideal positioning of patients for CT of the wrist and hand involves the "superman" position, with the patient prone on the CT table and the affected arm extended over the head in the center of the gantry. In the setting of trauma, this patient positioning may not be possible, and, in these cases, the hand and wrist can be scanned resting on the abdomen or at the side of the body. The scan is generally performed in the axial plane to the body, with coronal and sagittal reformatted images subsequently created at the scanner parallel to the long axis of the radius. Additionally, oblique-sagittal reformats can also be made along the axis of the scaphoid, to evaluate scaphoid fractures and fragment alignment (Fig. 5) [8]. Bone algorithm reformatted images, which enhance the sharpness of the osseous structures, should be created by the scanner in three planes, and soft tissue algorithm images which soften the edges of images should be reformatted in at least one plane (typically axial) to assist in the diagnosis of associated soft tissue injuries. CT coverage depends on the area of clinical concern and may include only the wrist or the entire hand. Dual-energy CT scanning technique can be used to improve detection of bone marrow edema by subtracting the calcium from bone. This can result in improved detection of occult fractures, with a reported sensitivity of 100% and a specificity of 99.5% [9]. This technique can also be used for assessment of gout and uric acid deposition, utilizing a different set of post-processing tools.

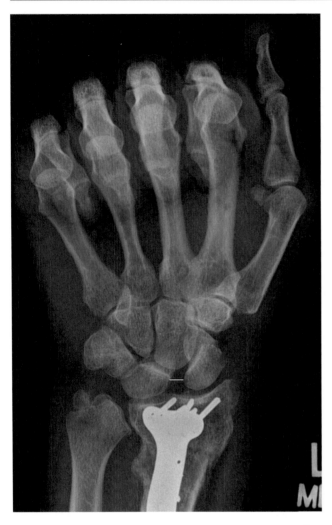

**Fig. 3** Clenched fist view of the wrist stresses the scapholunate ligament and can display scapholunate widening due to ligament insufficiency (yellow line)

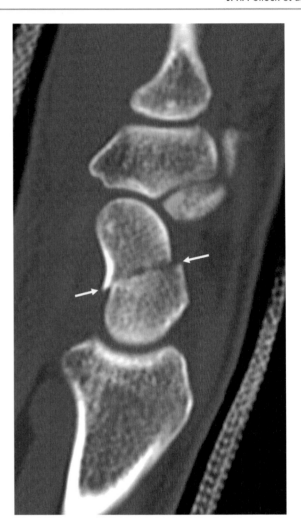

**Fig. 5** Sagittal oblique scaphoid reformatted CT image without contrast, showing a minimally displaced fracture through the waist of the scaphoid (white arrows). These images are oriented to the long axis of the scaphoid and may assist in fracture evaluation. The fracture was not seen on initial radiographs

## Magnetic Resonance Imaging (MRI)

MRI of the hand and wrist without contrast plays a limited role in evaluating acute trauma. This examination may be a helpful addition if a gamekeeper's thumb (injury to the ulnar collateral ligament of the thumb metacarpophalangeal [MCP] joint) is suspected clinically or if a radiographically occult distal radius or scaphoid fracture is suspected. Often in the emergency department setting, thumb radiographs, as well as repeat radiographs in 10–14 days, are also appropriate in those respective settings [4]. MRI without contrast would be an appropriate test in the setting of ligamentous injury in the fingers and wrist, pulley injuries involving the flexor tendon sheaths, or triangular fibrocartilage complex injuries.

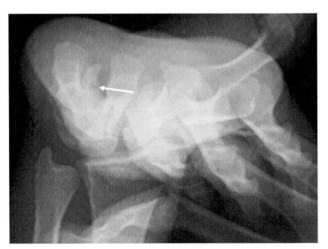

**Fig. 4** Carpal tunnel view of the wrist shows a non-displaced fracture through the hook of the hamate (white arrow)

The ideal positioning of the patient during MRI is similar to CT. A surface coil is utilized, and multi-planar imaging with T1-weighted and fat-suppressed fluid-sensitive

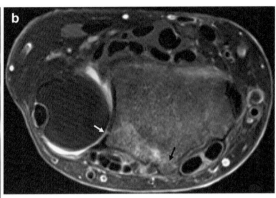

**Fig. 6** (**a**) Coronal T1-weighted MR image, showing a low signal transverse metaphyseal distal radial fracture (asterisks), which was occult on radiographs (not shown). The low signal fracture line replaces the normal fatty marrow, which is hyperintense on T1. (**b**) Axial proton-density fat-saturated MR image shows the hyperintense bone marrow edema within the entire radius, with extension of the fracture into Lister's tubercle (white arrow) and the sigmoid notch (black arrow)

sequences are best to evaluate for fracture and other associated tendinous and ligamentous injuries (Figs. 6a, b and 7).

## Anatomy

### Phalanges

The distal phalanx has a base, shaft, and distal tuft. The base has a similar width as the adjacent head of the middle phalanx. The distal tuft has a wide ridge of bone with a crescent shape which supports the fingernail complex, including the germinal matrix along the dorsal surface of the tuft [10].

The middle and proximal phalanges are similarly shaped with several slight differences. These phalanges consist of a base, shaft, and a head. The shaft has an hourglass shape when seen in the AP plane. The articular surfaces extend more prominently along the palmar surface, allowing for greater flexion than extension at the DIP and PIP joints.

The thumb has only two phalanges. The proximal phalanx of the thumb resembles the proximal phalanx in the remaining digits but is generally shorter.

### Metacarpals

The metacarpal axis is parallel on a lateral view of the hand but forms an arch when viewed axially, with an individualized shape to each metacarpal base (Panchal). The thumb metacarpal is pronated relative to the other metacarpals, requiring dedicated obliquity to image the thumb. The base of the thumb metacarpal is saddle-shaped, allowing for flexion, extension, adduction, and abduction. The first, fourth,

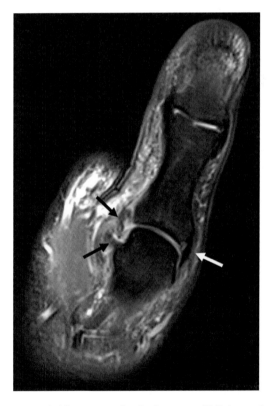

**Fig. 7** Coronal oblique proton-density fat-saturated MR image shows a torn thumb MCP joint ulnar collateral ligament with discontinuous fibers (black arrows). Proximally, these are oriented perpendicular to the axis of metacarpal that are displaced by the adductor aponeurosis. The radial collateral ligament is intact (white arrow)

and fifth metacarpals form mobile borders with the second and third forming a stiffer central pillar, with minimal motion at these respective CMC joints. The small finger metacarpal articulates with the hamate and has a somewhat saddle-shaped articulation, allowing for grasping objects of varying sizes. The head of the thumb metacarpal is rounded and less spherical than the other metacarpals, resulting in hinged motion. The articular surface extends further palmarly than dorsally, resulting in greater flexion than extension.

## Carpal Bones

There are a total of eight carpal bones, organized into proximal and distal carpal rows. The carpal bones are contained within the wrist joint capsule. With the exception of the pisiform, there are no tendinous attachments to the carpal bones.

The proximal carpal row consists of the scaphoid, lunate, triquetrum, and pisiform. The scaphoid is the largest bone in the proximal carpal row and has a "boat shape." The scaphoid sits on a plane 45° to the long axis of the wrist. The bone consists of a tuberosity, body, and proximal pole. The majority of the bone is covered with cartilage, with the dominant blood supply through a dorsal branch of the radial artery which enters at the waist of the scaphoid, providing retrograde blood flow to the proximal pole [10].

The lunate is a "hemi-moon"-shaped bone which articulates proximally with the lunate fossa of the distal radius and distally with the capitate. The triquetrum has a pyramid shape and is located on the ulnar side of the proximal carpal row, abutting the triangular fibrocartilage complex. The pisiform is a sesamoid bone within the flexor carpi ulnaris tendon sheath, articulating with the triquetrum.

The distal carpal row consists of the trapezium, trapezoid, capitate, and hamate. The trapezium is the most radial of the carpal bones and sits at the base of the thumb metacarpal. There is a ridge along the palmar margin of the bone which serves as the attachment site for the transverse carpal ligament. There is general instability of the thumb CMC joint allowing for the multi-planar range of motion, requiring 16 ligaments to provide additional support of the joint.

The trapezoid is the smallest bone of the distal row and is rarely fractured as it is well surrounded by a deep notch formed from the base of the index metacarpal. The capitate is the largest and most central of the carpal bones, articulating proximally with the lunate and scaphoid. The hamate consists of a body, proximal pole, and hook, located on the palmar surface of the bone, serving as an attachment for the transverse carpal ligament.

## Distal Radius and Ulna

The distal aspect of the radius articulates with the scaphoid and lunate. There is concave ulnar notch along the medial side of the distal radius, allowing for articulation with the ulna. The distal end of the ulna contains a small round head and a styloid process. Distally the ulna articulates with the triangular fibrocartilage complex.

## Radiographic Evaluation of the Hand and Wrist

Radiographic evaluation of the hand and wrist in the setting of trauma should begin with a thorough evaluation of the osseous structures for overt fracture lines, more subtle cortical discontinuity, avulsion fracture fragments, and associated soft tissue swelling. It is important to evaluate each view closely as small or subtle fractures may be visible on a single view alone. In particular, the decrease in cortical bone and the relative increase in weaker cancellous bone predispose the metaphyseal widening of the distal radius to fracture [11]. This area begins approximately 2 cm proximal to the radiocarpal joint and should be closely evaluated in all three plains. However, an epiphyseal scar can persist in the distal radius until at least 50 years of age and should not be mistaken for a non-displaced fracture (Fig. 8) [12]. Evaluation of the distal radius should also include precise assessment of the radiocarpal articulation and distal radioulnar joint (DRUJ), as these may impact clinical referral and treatment.

The three carpal "arcs of Gilula" should be assessed for continuity. Arc disruptions suggest carpal dislocation or fracture-dislocation. The proximal arc outlines the proximal convex surfaces of the scaphoid, lunate, and triquetrum, while the second arc outlines the distal concave surfaces of those carpal bones. The third arc outlines the proximal convexity along the surface of the capitate and hamate [13]. Interosseous intervals should be approximately equal in spacing, and each arc should appear in parallel [14]. The scapholunate interval should measure less than 3 mm and will be increased in the setting of scapholunate ligamentous injury [15].

The lateral radiograph of the wrist should be examined for the normal collinearity of the distal radial articular surface, lunate, capitate, and third metacarpal. A pronator fat pad can be seen as a thin radiolucent triangle along the volar margin of the distal radius. It is normally seen approximately 90% of the time and may be displaced, anteriorly bowed, or obliterated in the setting of a distal radius or ulna fracture. The sensitivity of this finding ranges from 26% to 98% [16].

In the setting of a distal radius fracture, measurements which have a substantial role in clinical treatment include radial height, radial inclination, radial tilt, and the degree of cortical step-off in intra-articular fractures [11]. Radial height is measured on a PA radiograph as the distance between a line perpendicular to the long axis of the radius passing through the distal tip of the radial styloid and a second parallel line intersecting the distal articular surface of the ulnar head

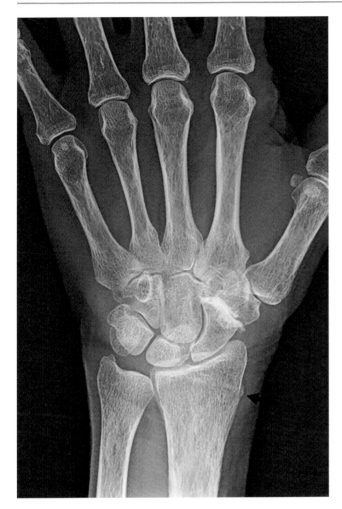

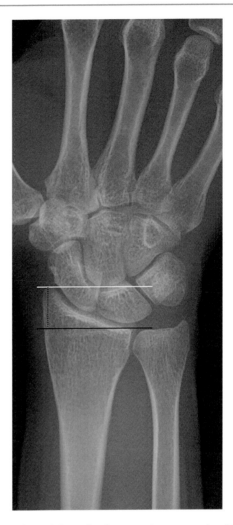

**Fig. 8** PA view of the wrist in an 89-year-old-female with diffuse atraumatic wrist pain shows a physeal scar (black arrow), a normal anatomic variant which can be confused for a distal radial fracture

**Fig. 9** PA view of the wrist demonstrating a normal radial height measured as the distance (dashed line) between a line perpendicular to the long axis of the radius passing through the distal tip of the radial styloid (white line) and a second parallel line intersecting the distal articular surface of the ulnar head (black line)

(Fig. 9). This should normally measure 10–13 mm. The radial inclination is measured on a PA radiograph as the angle between a line connecting the radial styloid tip and the ulnar aspect of the distal radius, with a second line perpendicular to the longitudinal axis of the radius. This should normally measure between 21° and 25°. A decrease in this value increases contact pressures across the lunate. The radial tilt is measured on a lateral projection and reflects the angle between a line across the distal radial articular surface and a line perpendicular to the longitudinal axis of the radius (Fig. 10a, b). Normal radial tilt should range from 2° to 20° of volar tilt. Lastly, incongruity at the articular surface of the distal radius, demonstrating greater than 2 mm of step-off, is a general indication for surgical fixation.

Radiographic evaluation of the fingers should include PA, oblique, and lateral views of the fingers and soft tissues. If trauma is suspected in a specific finger, coned- down lateral views may help evaluation by decreasing osseous overlap. If

thumb trauma is suspected, radiographs should be performed relative to the axes of the thumb.

## Fractures

### Wrist Trauma

Distal radial fractures represent approximately one-sixth of all fractures seen acutely in the emergency department [17]. The mechanism of injury usually involves a fall on an outstretched hand; however, high-energy trauma, such as in the case of a motor vehicle collision, contributes as well. This area is particularly at risk for fracture due to the decreased amount of cortical bone in the metaphyseal widening of the distal radius. Evaluation of the distal radius in the setting of trauma requires close attention to the radial cortex on all

**Fig. 10** (**a**) Lateral view of the wrist demonstrating a normal radial tilt measured as the angle between a line across the distal radial articular surface (white line) and a line perpendicular to the longitudinal axis of the radius (black line). (**b**) Lateral view of the wrist in a patient with an acute Colles' fracture. There is abnormal radial tilt measuring approximately 45° in the dorsal direction

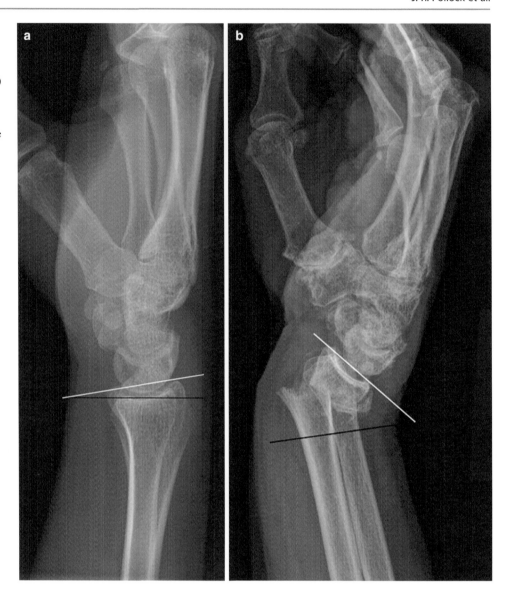

views, as many fractures may only be apparent on a single view. It is critical to note the location of the fracture, any articular involvement, comminution, displacement, and dorsal or volar tilt of the radial articular surface. Multiple eponyms exist for distal radial fractures, which are outlined in Table 1 (Fig. 11). Indications for surgical fixation in distal radius fractures include dorsal tilt >10°, articular step-off >2 mm, radial shortening >5 mm, and radial inclination <15° [18].

Fractures of the distal radius are often accompanied by fractures of the distal ulna and/or ulnar styloid process. Avulsion fractures involving the tip of the ulnar styloid process are generally considered stable fractures and are not associated with significant instability of the DRUJ. Unstable fractures generally involve the base of the distal ulna and are associated with disruption of the major stabilizing ligaments of the distal ulna and triangular fibrocartilage complex. Subluxation of the ulnar head should be noted and requires reduction to avoid chronic instability.

The scaphoid is the most frequent site of carpal fracture, accounting for an estimated 70% of all carpal fractures [19]. The most common mechanism is a fall on an outstretched hand, and patients generally present with pain in the anatomical snuffbox. The Herbert classification is the most commonly used classification system and is based on fracture stability (Fig. 12) [20]. Scaphoid tubercle fractures and incomplete waist fractures are type A, acute stable fractures. Comminuted fractures, fracture-dislocations, oblique distal pole fractures, proximal pole fractures, and complete/displaced waist fractures are all considered acute unstable,

**Table 1** Common eponyms for distal radius fractures as described by fracture location and displacement

| Eponym | Location | Displacement | Specific considerations |
|---|---|---|---|
| Colles' | Extra-articular, distal metaphysis | Dorsal | Evaluate for displacement affecting the articular space: radial shortening, inclination, tilt, distal radial ulnar joint involvement |
| Smith's | Extra-articular, distal metaphysis | Volar | Often derived from the impact on volarly flexed wrist, increasing risk for comminution and intra-articular extension |
| Dorsal Barton's | Intra-articular, dorsal rim of distal radius | Dorsal, radiocarpal dislocation | Sheared radial fragment, which may be comminuted, may maintain carpal articulation causing radiocarpal dislocation |
| Volar Barton's | Intra-articular, volar rim of distal radius | Volar, radiocarpal dislocation | Similar to dorsal-type Barton fractures but are usually more common |
| Hutchinson's/ Chauffeur's | Radial styloid process | Uncommon | May present alongside intra-articular communitive fractures, involving injury to the scapholunate ligament |
| Die-punch | Intra-articular, radiolunate fossa | Depression of radiolunate fossa | Associated with proximal displacement of the lunate fossa, often disrupting the first carpal arc of Gilula |

type B fractures [21]. Type C fractures are those with delayed union after at least 6 weeks of treatment, and type D are those that have progressed to nonunion. All bi-cortical fractures under this system are considered unstable and may be candidates for surgical treatment. Pediatric patients are more likely to fracture the distal scaphoid tuberosity, while adult patients are more likely to fracture the scaphoid waist [22].

At least four views are recommended for radiographic evaluation when scaphoid fractures are suspected [23]. Despite these multiple views, fractures can be occult on initial radiographs in 5–20% of cases in the acute setting [24]. If one suspects an acute scaphoid fracture and initial radiographs are interpreted as normal, the ACR Appropriateness Criteria deems that it is usually appropriate to follow with either an MRI without contrast, CT without contrast, or repeat radiographs within 10–14 days, depending on local preference [4]. Additional pertinent findings include the location of the fracture, the involvement of articular surfaces, fragment displacement, scaphoid humpback deformity, scapholunate interval alignment, and other associated fractures. The humpback deformity results from apex dorsal angulation of the proximal and distal poles of the scaphoid resulting in a palpable abnormality in the anatomic snuffbox. In the setting of a subacute or chronic fracture, the presence of avascular necrosis appears as sclerosis, fragmentation, and collapse involving the proximal pole fragment (Fig. 13). Avascular necrosis is a late complication of a scaphoid fracture nonunion. The proximal pole receives its blood supply in a retrograde fashion from the dorsal carpal branch of the radial artery, which enters the bone distally.

The navicular fat stripe is a lucency located between the distal pole of the scaphoid and the radial collateral ligament related to radiolucent fat between the ligament and the common tendon sheath of the extensor pollicis brevis and abductor pollicis longus muscles [25]. The presence of a navicular fat stripe has been shown to have a 95% negative predictive

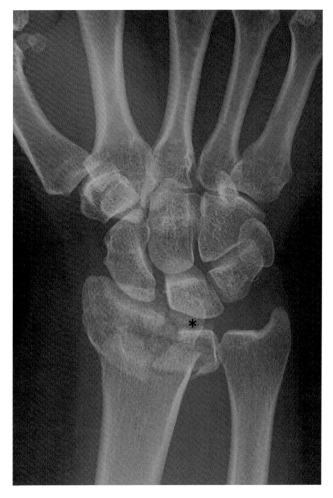

**Fig. 11** PA view of the wrist shows a comminuted distal radial fracture extending to the articular surface. There is depression of the lunate fossa consistent with a die-punch distal radial fracture (asterisk)

value for fracture, with only a positive predictive value of 15%, and therefore may be a useful indicator to exclude a scaphoid fracture [26].

**Fig. 12** Herbert classification of scaphoid fractures based on fracture stability. Type A fractures are stable and can generally be treated nonoperatively. Types B, C, and D fractures are unstable and generally require surgical treatment

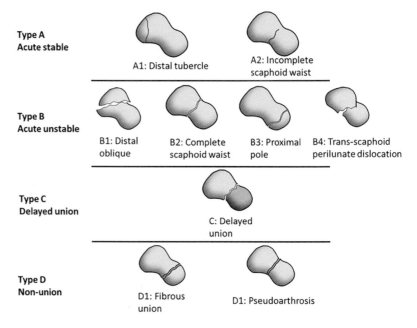

Type A
Acute stable

A1: Distal tubercle          A2: Incomplete
                             scaphoid waist

Type B
Acute unstable

B1: Distal      B2: Complete      B3: Proximal      B4: Trans-scaphoid
oblique         scaphoid waist    pole              perilunate dislocation

Type C
Delayed union

C: Delayed
union

Type D
Non-union

D1: Fibrous          D1: Pseudoarthrosis
union

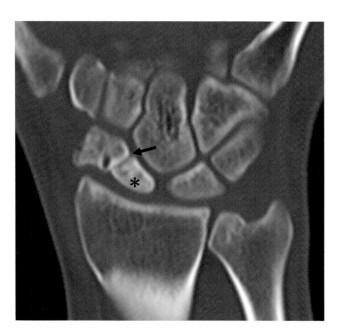

**Fig. 13** Coronal reformatted CT image of the wrist shows a chronic ununited fracture through the waist of the scaphoid (arrow). There is sclerosis in the proximal pole fragment caused by avascular necrosis (asterisk)

Triquetral fractures represent the second most common carpal fracture (Fig. 14) [14]. Most fractures demonstrate an avulsion of the dorsal cortex, which is suspected to be caused by injury at the ligamentous insertion of the dorsal intercarpal and radiotriquetral ligaments. Lateral projections of the wrist best depict these dorsal avulsions. Fractures of the body of the triquetrum and cortical palmar fractures have been described but are rare [27].

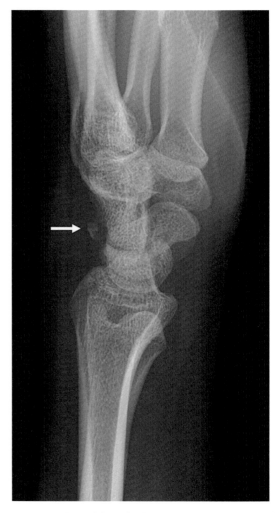

**Fig. 14** Lateral view of the wrist shows a minimally displaced dorsal fragment (arrow) with soft tissue swelling, consistent with an acute triquetral fracture

The most common fracture of the hamate involves the hook of the hamate along the palmer margin of the bone. These occur from blunt trauma, falls, and trauma in sports which require swinging, including golf, baseball, and tennis. The absence of the hook cortical ring on the PA view of the wrist suggests injury to the hamate; however, these are best seen radiographically on a carpal tunnel view of the wrist. Wrist radiographs, including a carpal tunnel view in a cadaver study, showed a sensitivity of 72.2% and a specificity of 88.8% for the depiction of hamate fractures [28]. CT and MRI would be the next best tests in the setting of normal radiographs and a suspected hamate fracture [4].

Carpal dislocations involve a spectrum of injuries to the carpal ligaments. The injury generally involves falling on an outstretched hand with a fixed, pronated forearm, causing hyperextension and supination of the carpus. Evaluation for these types of injuries focuses on evaluating the carpal arcs of Gilula on the PA view of the wrist and assessing the radius-lunate-capitate relationship on the lateral view. These injuries may range from purely ligamentous injuries to injuries encompassing fracture of one or more carpal bones with or without ligamentous injuries (Table 2, Fig. 15). These injuries are classified by the Mayfield classification and progress in severity from stage I to IV. Stage I injuries involve disruption of the scapholunate joint and manifest as scapholunate joint space widening on the frontal view only. Stage II injuries disrupt the capitolunate joint and result in a perilunate dislocation. These manifest with a dorsally dislocated

**Table 2** General categories of carpus dislocations according to carpus involvement and displacement or disruption of the radius-lunate-capitate axis

| Carpal dislocation | Carpus involvement | Displacement | Specific considerations |
|---|---|---|---|
| Perilunate | Carpus dislocation around stationary lunate | Dorsal displacement of carpus, coaxial disruption of capitate from radius-lunate axis | Often involves ligamentous injury, manifesting as disruption to the second carpal arc of Gilula |
| Midcarpal | Dislocation of all carpi | Volar displacement of lunate with dorsal displacement of surrounding carpi, no linearity among radius-lunate-capitate on lateral radiograph | May appear similar to perilunate dislocations that mobilize the carpus surrounding the lunate |
| Lunate | Lunate dislocation around stationary carpus | Volar displacement of lunate, coaxial disruption of lunate from radius-capitate axis | Stems from injury to dorsal ligamentous attachments to the lunate |

**Fig. 15** Mayfield classification of perilunate injuries. Expected findings on frontal and lateral radiographs in each progressive stage. The dashed line represents the axis of the radius, highlighting the changes in alignment in each stage

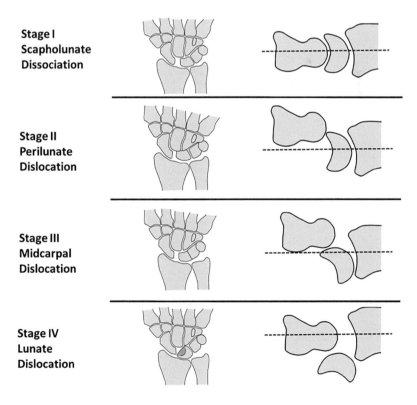

Stage I
Scapholunate
Dissociation

Stage II
Perilunate
Dislocation

Stage III
Midcarpal
Dislocation

Stage IV
Lunate
Dislocation

**Fig. 16** (**a**) PA view of the wrist shows disruption of the carpal arcs of Gilula outlining the proximal (white lines) and distal (black lines) surfaces of the proximal carpal row. (**b**) Lateral view of the wrist shows malalignment of the base of the third metacarpal [3], capitate (C), lunate (L), and distal radius (R). The carpus is dorsally dislocated relative to the lunate, which indicates a perilunate dislocation

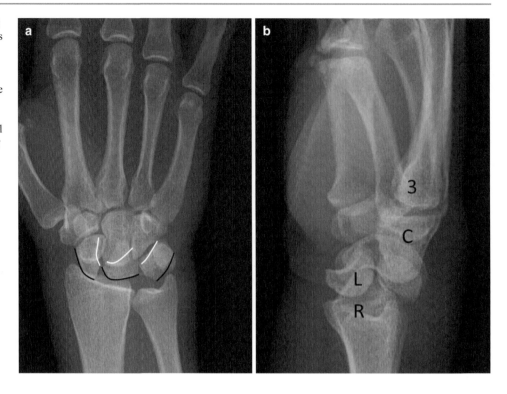

capitate with preserved collinearity of the lunate and radius. Stage III injuries disrupt the lunotriquetral joint and result in a midcarpal dislocation. These manifest with volar tilt and volar subluxation of the lunate with dorsal subluxation of the capitate. Stage IV injuries completely mobilize the lunate and result in a lunate dislocation, which manifests with volar dislocation and tilt of the lunate while maintaining collinearity of the capitate and radius. This results in a "pie-shaped" or triangular lunate. These injuries may be missed clinically and radiographically in up to 25% of cases [29] (Fig. 16a, b).

## Finger Trauma

Metacarpal fractures account for 40% of all hand injuries, and, in particular, 80% of thumb fractures involve the metacarpal base (Fig. 17) [30]. The most common fracture of the thumb is the Bennett fracture-dislocation, which consists of an intra-articular two-part fracture of the base of the first metacarpal. There is dorsolateral dislocation of the fragment with lateral retraction of the first metacarpal shaft by the abductor pollicis longus. These injuries will generally require surgical treatment when there is greater than 2 mm of displacement between the fracture fragments. A Rolando fracture is a comminuted intra-articular fracture of the base of the thumb metacarpal involving more than two parts, which has a worse long-term prognosis and usually requires surgical fixation. Extra-articular factures at the base of the first metacarpal can occur and will generally require surgical fixation if

post-reduction angulation is greater than 30°. Extra-articular metacarpal fractures have the best long-term outcome.

A gamekeeper's thumb or skier's thumb refers to an injury to the ulnar collateral ligament of the thumb MCP joint. Imaging when this injury is suspected begins with radiographs, which may show an avulsion fragment at the ulnar base of the thumb proximal phalanx. If there is a ligament tear without an osseous avulsion, the ulnar side of the MCP joint may be slightly widened. An MRI can be obtained to evaluate the ligaments and tendons at this articulation, but this generally occurs outside of the emergency department setting.

A fracture-dislocation of the base of the fifth metacarpal is known as the reverse Bennett fracture-dislocation. A lateral view with supination can allow for improved visualization of the ring and small finger metacarpal bases. This fracture is generally unstable due to unopposed extensor carpi ulnaris force on the fragment, which causes migration and subluxation of the fragment, which can be seen as offset between the base of the metacarpal and hamate bone on the lateral view. Treatment generally requires surgical fixation. Fourth and fifth metacarpal neck fractures are also known as Boxer's fractures and generally occur due to the direct impact of the clenched fist on a solid object. Apex dorsal angulation of up to 40° is considered an acceptable reduction for the fifth metacarpal [31]. Open fractures and closed irreducible fractures will need open reduction and internal fixation for treatment.

Phalangeal fractures account for 10% of all fractures, and the distal phalanx is the most common fractured bone in the hand [32]. Fractures extending to the articular surface may

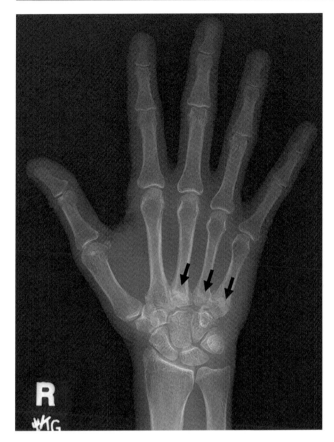

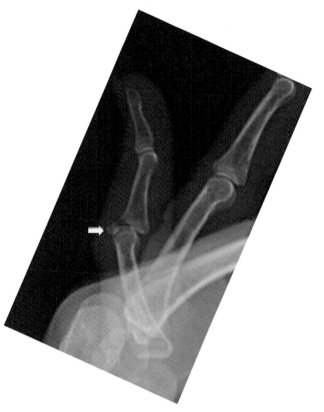

**Fig. 17** PA view of the wrist in a 64-year-old female with a fall while hiking 5 weeks prior to the examination. There is transverse sclerosis spanning the bases of the third, fourth, and fifth metacarpals (black arrows), which is consistent with non-displaced fractures. These were not seen on initial radiographs but were more evident on follow-up 4 weeks later

**Fig. 18** Acute displaced fracture of the base of the small finger middle phalanx in a 62-year-old female who fell and tripped, landing on her hand and jamming her small finger (arrow). The central slip of the extensor tendon inserts on the fragment causing displacement. The middle phalanx is subluxed with a boutonnière deformity consisting of flexion at the PIP joint and extension at the DIP joint

result in fracture-dislocations. Proximal phalanx deformities are generally apex volar. Middle phalanx fractures usually have a deformity apex dorsal if the fracture is proximal to the flexor digitorum superficialis tendon insertion or apex volar if distal to the tendon insertion. Crush injuries to the distal phalanx can result in multiple comminuted fragments which frequently fail to completely unite. Extensive soft tissue abnormality in the setting of a comminuted distal phalanx fracture may suggest an associated nail bed injury. Distal phalangeal fractures with nail bed disruption may be treated as open fractures and should, therefore, be reported if identified.

A mallet finger is a deformity caused by disruption of the terminal extensor tendon at its insertion on the dorsal base of the distal phalanx and presents with an inability to actively extend the DIP joint. These may be associated with an osseous fracture or purely tendinous injury, often secondary to blunt force trauma, causing forced DIP flexion. The percentage of articular surface involvement, the amount of widening along the articular surface, and the presence of

palmar displacement of the distal phalanx should be reported and may determine the need for fixation [22]. In contrast, a jersey finger deformity results from the avulsion of the flexor digitorum profundus tendon at its insertion on the distal phalanx and occurs from forced hyperextension of the DIP joint while it is actively flexed. This most commonly involves the ring finger. The injury may occur as a solely tendinous injury or along with an avulsion fracture or fracture of a larger piece of bone. Radiographs can help detect bone fragments which may require open reduction and internal fixation [33].

Disruption of the central slip of the extensor digitorum tendon at its insertion on the base of the middle phalanx causes a boutonnière deformity (Fig. 18). These patients will present with a flexed PIP joint and a hyperextended DIP joint. A small dorsal chip fracture may occur and be seen radiographically, but the majority of cases will not have an osseous fracture fragment [34].

A coach's finger injury involves a dorsal dislocation of the PIP joint. These may occur in conjunction with a volar plate injury of the joint, which would require subsequent MR or ultrasound imaging for diagnosis. These injuries generally occur as a result of hyperextension at the PIP joint.

Amputation of the distal margins of the fingers is a common injury. Radiographs obtained in the setting of an amputation should be examined for potential associated fracture or bony avulsion. Up to 30% of these injuries may involve more than one finger, and most involve a complete amputation of the fingertip [35] (Fig. 19).

Fractures associated with human or animal bites need to be treated aggressively with antibiotics to prevent infection. Bite injuries distal to the wrist are at a higher risk for infection due to the proximity of superficial spaces, tendons, and joints. The MCP joint and the adjacent tissues are the most commonly involved as the teeth of the opponent are often struck with the knuckle of the clenched fist.

## Soft Tissue Injuries

Soft tissue injuries in the hand and wrist are common, and many do not require imaging. Compartment syndrome remains one of the most critical surgical emergencies in the hand where imaging plays a limited role.

Finger amputation injuries, including those involving only soft tissue defects, are frequently evaluated with radiographs and should be assessed for bony involvement along with the soft tissue amputation, as this will determine whether a soft tissue closure will suffice or if a bony amputation is required prior to closure. Nail plate and nail bed injuries may present with a subungual hematoma and may be imaged to evaluate for an underlying distal phalanx fracture.

Foreign bodies, including wood, glass, metal, bullets, or plant thorns, are a common problem in the emergency setting. Some foreign bodies may be unnoticed for days or years before presentation with symptoms. These most commonly present with symptoms of infection, but neurovascular or tendinous injury may also occur. These are often initially evaluated with radiographs. Metallic foreign bodies are relatively radiopaque, while glass, wood, acrylics, and plastic foreign bodies are less dense in comparison. Ultrasound has become a critical modality for the detection of these foreign bodies when a targeted evaluation with a high-frequency linear array probe is used to target the area of concern [36] (Fig. 20).

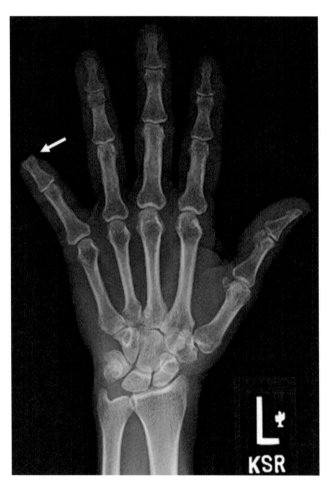

**Fig. 19** PA view of the hand showing an amputation of the fifth finger distal phalanx caused by a roping injury. The distal margin of the middle phalanx is exposed beyond the soft tissues (arrow). This will require further amputation of the middle phalanx before soft tissue closure due to the exposed bone

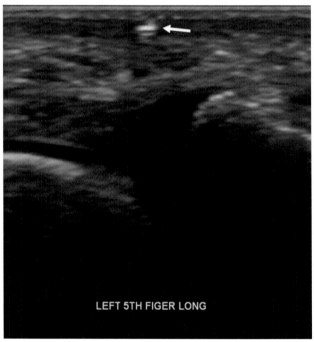

LEFT 5TH FIGER LONG

**Fig. 20** Longitudinal ultrasound image with a high-frequency linear transducer in the palmar region of the fifth MCP joint shows a linear hyperechoic foreign body (arrow) in the superficial subcutaneous tissues corresponding to the area of pain which turned out to be a glass fragment

## Summary

Traumatic injuries of the hand and wrist are common reasons for presentation to the emergency department. Many of these injuries can be accurately diagnosed by radiographs tailored to the area of concern, based on presenting symptoms and clinical diagnosis. However, many of these injuries may remain radiographically occult and may require appropriate follow-up imaging to obtain a diagnosis. Delayed or missed diagnoses in this setting can potentially lead to significant long-term morbidity and disability. By being aware of common injury patterns and common occult injuries, radiologists can provide optimal care and guidance to the treating team in the emergency setting.

## References

1. Spiegel PK. The first clinical X-ray made in America – 100 years. Am J Roentgenol. 1995;164(1):241–3.
2. de Putter CE, Selles RW, Polinder S, et al. Epidemiology and healthcare utilisation of wrist fractures in older adults in The Netherlands, 1997-2009. Injury. 2013;44(4):421–6.
3. Ootes D, Lambers KT, Ring DC. The epidemiology of upper extremity injuries presenting to the emergency department in the United States. Hand (N Y). 2012;7(1):18–22.
4. Expert Panel on Musculoskeletal Imaging, Torabi M, Lenchik L, et al. ACR appropriateness criteria® acute hand and wrist trauma. J Am Coll Radiol. 2019;16(5S):S7–S17.
5. De Smet AA, Doherty MP, Norris MA, Hollister MC, Smith DL. Are oblique views needed for trauma radiography of the distal extremities? Am J Roentgenol. 1999;172(6):1561–5.
6. Bhat AK, Kumar B, Acharya A. Radiographic imaging of the wrist. Indian J Plast Surg. 2011;44(2):186.
7. Bozlar U, Ogur T, Norton PT, et al. CT angiography of the upper extremity arterial system: part 1 – anatomy, technique, and use in trauma patients. Am J Roentgenol. 2013;201:745–52.
8. Mallee WH, Doornberg JN, Ring D, et al. Computed tomography for suspected scaphoid fractures: comparison of reformations in the plane of the wrist versus the long axis of the scaphoid. Hand (N Y). 2014;9(1):117–21.
9. Ali IT, Wong WD, Liang T, et al. Clinical utility of dual-energy CT analysis of bone marrow edema in acute wrist fractures. Am J Roentgenol. 2018;210(4):842–7.
10. Panchal-Kildare S, Malone K. Skeletal anatomy of the hand. Hand Clin. 2013;29:459–71.
11. Goldfarb CA, Yin Y, Gilula LA, Fisher AJ, Boyer MI. Wrist fractures: what the clinician wants to know. Radiology. 2001;219(1):11–28.
12. Davies C, Hackman L, Black S. The persistence of epiphyseal scars in the distal radius in adult individuals. Int J Legal Med. 2016;130(1):199–206.
13. Gilula L. Carpal injuries: analytic approach and case exercises. Am J Roentgenol. 1979;133(3):503–17.
14. Loredo RA, Sorge DG, Garcia G. Radiographic evaluation of the wrist: a vanishing art. Semin Roentgenol. 2005;40(3):248–89.
15. Griffith JF, Nin Chan DP, Ho PC, Zhao L, Hung LK, Metreweli C. Sonography of the normal scapholunate ligament and scapholunate joint space. J Clin Ultrasound. 2001;29(4):223–9.
16. Moosikasuwan JB. The pronator quadratus sign. Radiology. 2007;244(3):927–8.
17. Owen RA, Melton LJ, Johnson KA, Ilstrup DM, Riggs BL. Incidence of Colles' fracture in a North American community. Am J Public Health. 1982;72(6):605–7.
18. Arora R, Gabl M, Gschwentner M, Deml C, Krappinger D, Lutz M. A comparative study of clinical and radiologic outcomes of unstable Colles type distal radius fractures in patients older than 70 years: nonoperative treatment versus volar locking plating. J Orthop Trauma. 2009;23(4):237–42.
19. Rettig AC. Athletic injuries of the wrist and hand. Am J Sports Med. 2003;31(6):1038–48.
20. Ten Berg PW, Drijkoningen T, Strackee SD, Buijze GA. Classifications of acute scaphoid fractures: a systematic literature review. J Wrist Surg. 2016;5(2):152–9.
21. Fowler JR, Hughes TB. Scaphoid fractures. Clin Sports Med. 2015;34(1):37–50.
22. Cockenpot E, Lefebvre G, Demondion X, Chantelot C, Cotten A. Imaging of sports-related hand and wrist injuries: sports imaging series. Radiology. 2016;279(3):674–92.
23. Cheung GC, Lever CJ, Morris AD. X-ray diagnosis of acute scaphoid fractures. J Hand Surg Br. 2006;31(1):104–9.
24. Pines JM, Carpenter CR, Raja AS, Schuur JD. Evidence-based emergency care: diagnostic testing and clinical decision rules. The Atrium, Southern Gate, Chichester, West Sussex, PO19 8SQ, UK, Wiley; 2012. 474 p.
25. Corfitsen M, Christensen SE, Cetti R. The anatomical fat pad and the radiological "scaphoid fat stripe". J Hand Surg Br Eur Vol. 1989;14(3):326–8.
26. Kirk M, Orlinsky M, Goldberg R, Brotman P. The validity and reliability of the navicular fat stripe as a screening test for detection of navicular fractures. Ann Emerg Med. 1990;19(12):1371–6.
27. Becce F, Theumann N, Bollmann C, et al. Dorsal fractures of the triquetrum: MRI findings with an emphasis on dorsal carpal ligament injuries. Am J Roentgenol. 2013;200(3):608–17.
28. Andresen R, Radmer S, Sparmann M, Bogusch G, Banzer D. Imaging of hamate bone fractures in conventional X-rays and high-resolution computed tomography. An in vitro study. Investig Radiol. 1999;34(1):46–50.
29. Herzberg G, Comtet JJ, Linscheid RL, Amadio PC, Cooney WP, Stalder J. Perilunate dislocations and fracture-dislocations: a multicenter study. J Hand Surg Am. 1993;18(5):768–79.
30. Kamath JB, Harshvardhan, Naik DM, Bansal A. Current concepts in managing fractures of metacarpal and phalanges. Indian J Plast Surg. 2011;44(2):203–11.
31. Wieschhoff GG, Sheehan SE, Wortman JR, et al. Traumatic finger injuries: what the orthopedic surgeon wants to know. Radiographics. 2016;36(4):1106–28.
32. Barton NJ. Fractures of the shafts of the phalanges of the hand. Hand. 1979;11(2):119–33.
33. Freilich AM. Evaluation and treatment of Jersey finger and pulley injuries in athletes. Clin Sports Med. 2015;34(1):151–66.
34. Clavero JA, Alomar X, Monill JM, et al. MR imaging of ligament and tendon injuries of the fingers. Radiographics. 2002;22(2):237–56.
35. Conn JM, Annest JL, Ryan GW, Budnitz DS. Non–work-related finger amputations in the United States, 2001–2002. Ann Emerg Med. 2005;45(6):630–5.
36. Jarraya M, Hayashi D, de Villiers RV, et al. Multimodality imaging of foreign bodies of the musculoskeletal system. Am J Roentgenol. 2014;203(1):W92–W102.

# Imaging of Pelvis and Hip Trauma

**40**

Jake M. Adkins and Nicholas M. Beckmann

## Contents

**Abstract**

Pelvis and hip trauma has a bimodal distribution, occurring most commonly due to high-energy trauma in young patients and as low-energy fragility fractures in the elderly. Radiography is usually adequate for assessing acute hip trauma, although MRI or CT should be considered to evaluate for occult femoral neck fractures in patients with a high index of suspicion for injury. CT is usually required for assessment of pelvic fractures due to the complex bony anatomy osteology of the pelvis. Intravenous contrast is not needed to assess for fractures on CT but should be used in high-energy trauma to characterize soft tissue injuries. MRI is the best modality for identifying most soft tissue injuries; however, it is rarely utilized in the acute trauma setting because musculoskeletal soft tissue injuries rarely require urgent management. Avulsion fractures are common in pelvis and hip trauma. It is important to be familiar to attachment sites of major muscle groups in order to identify these injuries. Pathologic fractures of the hip are also common. Particularly, low-energy fractures of the subtrochanteric femur or avulsion of the lesser trochanter in adults should be considered highly suspicious for an underlying osseous malignancy focus and should undergo further imaging and clinical evaluation.

J. M. Adkins · N. M. Beckmann (✉)
UTHealth – McGovern School of Medicine, Houston, TX, USA
e-mail: Jake.M.Adkins@uth.tmc.edu;
Nicholas.M.Beckmann@uth.tmc.edu

**Keywords**

Pelvis · Hip · Sacrum · Trauma · Fracture · Pelvic ring · Acetabulum · Musculoskeletal · Bone

© Springer Nature Switzerland AG 2022
M. N. Patlas et al. (eds.), *Atlas of Emergency Imaging from Head-to-Toe*,
https://doi.org/10.1007/978-3-030-92111-8_40

## Introduction

Pelvic and hip fractures are both rare injuries in young patients, predominately occurring as the result of high-energy blunt trauma. The incidence of pelvic and hip fractures begins to increase around 50 years of age due to an increase in fragility fractures related to osteoporosis, with a marked increase in fragility fractures in patients over 65 years of age [1, 2]. The morbidity and mortality of pelvis and hip fractures is substantial. The mortality of pelvic and hip fragility fractures has been found to be 23% at 1 year [3, 4]. Patients who survive these fractures often cannot recover to a state of prior functioning after sustaining a pelvic or hip fracture.

Over the last few decades, there has been very substantial improvement in the diagnosis and treatment of pelvic and hip injuries. Surgical decision-making is related to the presence and severity of pelvic and hip injuries diagnosed on imaging, and, thus, hospital course and duration can be substantially influenced by identifying and appropriately classifying these injuries.

## Osseous Anatomy

The bony anatomy of the pelvis is complex with many cortical reflections and superimposed bony structures, making diagnosis of pelvic fractures challenging. Fortunately, there are many consistent cortical lines which can be systematically analyzed to improve the sensitivity in identifying pelvic ring and acetabular fractures on radiographs.

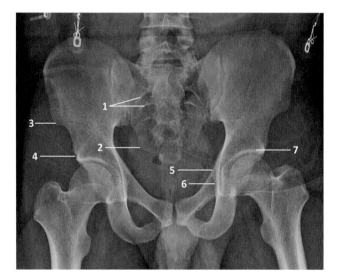

**Fig. 1** Key bony landmarks on AP pelvic radiograph. (1) Arcuate lines, (2) sacral spine, (3) anterosuperior iliac spine, (4) anterior inferior iliac spine, (5) iliopectineal line, (6) ilioischial line, and (7) sourcil

## Pelvic Ring

The pelvic ring is the osseous ring that provides architectural structure to the pelvis. The pelvic ring is comprised of the sacrum and iliac bones posteriorly, the acetabulum laterally, and the pubic bones anteriorly. The sacral body is the central portion of the sacrum medial to the neuroforamina. The cortical reflections of these neuroforamina form what are known as the "arcuate lines" on radiographs, best seen at the S1–S2 levels (Fig. 1). Disruption or buckling of arcuate lines is commonly seen with sacral fractures. Lateral to the neuroforamina are the sacral alae. The sacral alae of S1 and S2 articulate with the iliac bones and bear most of the weight-bearing force. The lower (S3–S5) sacral alae offer little structural support for the pelvis but do serve as ligament attachment sites at the sacral spine (Fig. 1).

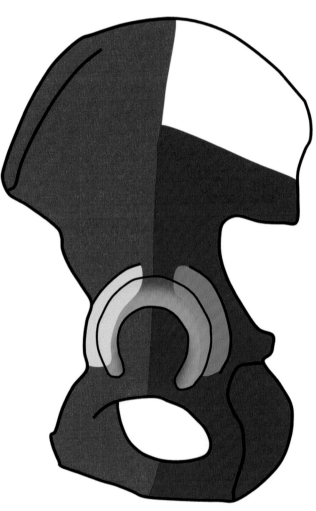

**Fig. 2** Lateral view of the acetabulum showing basic acetabular anatomy. Anterior column (red), posterior column (blue), anterior wall (yellow), posterior wall (green), and sciatic buttress (purple)

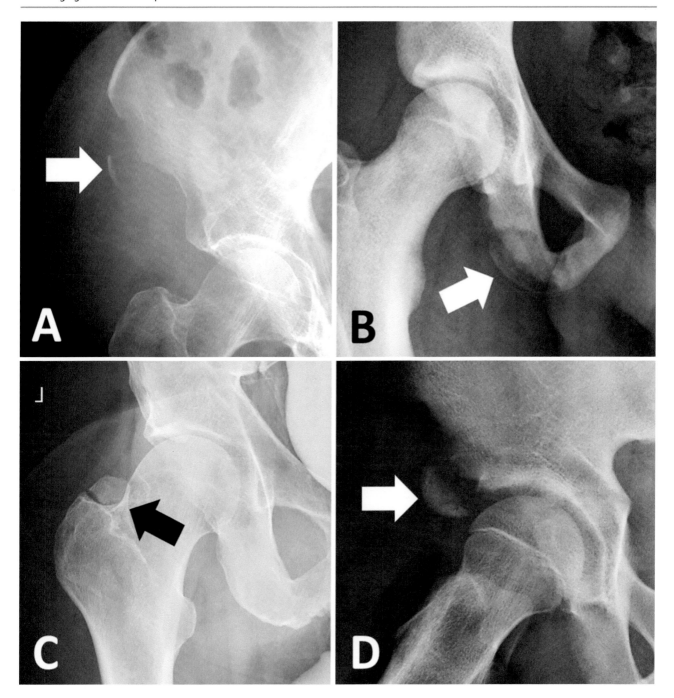

**Fig. 3** Common avulsion injuries of the pelvis on AP radiographs. (**a**) Anterosuperior iliac spine, (**b**) ischial tuberosity, (**c**) greater trochanter, and (**d**) anteroinferior iliac spine

On either side of the sacrum are the sacroiliac joints. The sacroiliac joints have thick posterior and less robust anterior capsular ligaments. The large iliac bones extend laterally from the sacroiliac joints, providing attachment sites for abdominal musculature. Anteriorly, the bony protuberances of the iliac bone called the anterosuperior and anteroinferior iliac spines serve as attachment sites for the anterior thigh musculature (Fig. 1).

Anteriorly, the obturator ring is comprised of the pubic rami superior and inferiorly, the pubic body medially, and the ischium laterally. The cortical margin of the obturator ring typically has a smooth continuous contour, and

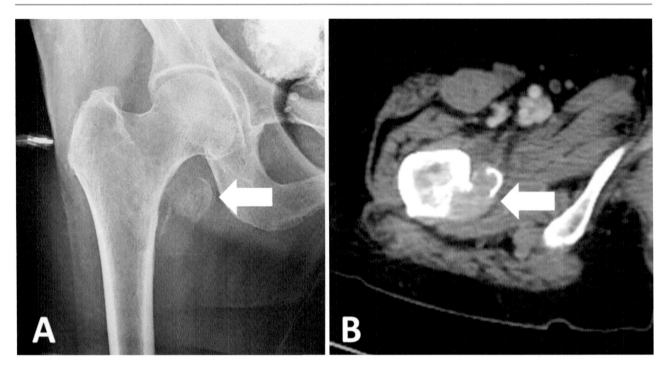

**Fig. 4** A 38-year-old female with giant cell tumor resulting in pathologic avulsion fracture of the lesser trochanter. (**a**) Avulsed lesser trochanter fracture visible on a frontal radiograph (arrow) without a visible underlying bone tumor. (**b**) Enhancing bone tumor representing a metastasis is visible on a post-contrast axial CT image (arrow)

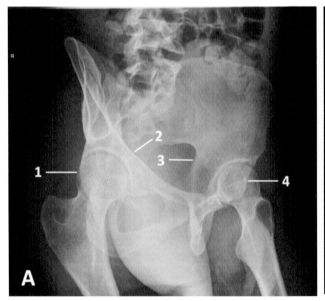
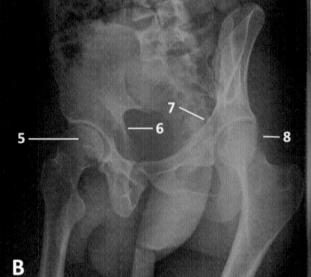

**Fig. 5** Judet radiograph anatomy. (**a**) Right obturator view: (1) right posterior acetabular wall, (2) right anterior acetabular column, (3) left posterior acetabular column, and (4) left anterior acetabular wall. (**b**) Right iliac view: (5) right anterior acetabular wall, (6) right posterior acetabular column, (7) left anterior acetabular column, (8) and left posterior acetabular wall

buckling or interruption of this cortical margin is suspicious for fracture. At midline, the pubic bones meet to form the pubic symphysis. The normal width of the pubic symphysis varies depending on patient age and gender; however, in general, a pubic symphyseal distance of more than 6 mm is considered suggestive of injury, while a distance greater than 10 mm is considered diagnostic of injury [5].

## Acetabulum

The acetabulum is formed by the confluence of the iliac, ischial, and pubic bones and provides the framework for transfer of forces from the spine to the lower extremity. The acetabulum consists of four basic components: the anterior wall, anterior column, posterior wall, and posterior column (Fig. 2). The anterior and posterior walls help keep the femoral head contained within the joint, while the anterior and posterior columns comprise the weight-bearing struts of the pelvis. The anterior and posterior columns can be identified on AP radiographs by curvilinear reflections of cortical bone called the iliopectineal and ilioischial lines, respectively (Fig. 1). The weight-bearing surface of the acetabulum is represented on radiographs by a thick, sclerotic line along the acetabular roof, known as the sourcil (Fig. 1). The acetabular columns are joined to the axial skeleton by the sciatic buttress, the piece of cortical bone that comprises the margin of the greater sciatic notch (Fig. 2).

## Femoral Head and Neck

The femoral head sits within the acetabulum and forms the hip joint. The femoral head should be spherical, with a focal notch medially at the ligamentum teres insertion, termed the fovea capitis. Most of the blood supply to the femoral head is from the medial circumflex femoral artery via the femoral neck. This blood supply is tenuous and at risk for disruption in femoral neck fractures, resulting in femoral head avascular necrosis and poor fracture healing.

## Muscle and Ligament Attachments

Soft tissue insertion sites about the pelvis are complex. However, a few sites comprise the large majority of avulsion-type injuries in the pelvis. The sartorius insertion on the anterosuperior iliac spine (Fig. 3a) and the hamstring insertion on the ischial tuberosity (Fig. 3b) are the two most common avulsion injuries. Avulsion of the gluteal tendons at the greater trochanter (Fig. 3c) is another relatively common injury, particularly in older patients. Less commonly, avulsion of the rectus femoris at the anterior inferior iliac spine (Fig. 3d) or iliopsoas at the lesser trochanter can occur, predominately in children. An avulsion of the lesser trochanter in an adult should prompt evaluation for underlying pathologic bone process, classically a metastatic focus (Fig. 4). Three common sites of ligament avulsion in the pelvis are the sacrospinous and sacrotuberous ligaments at the sacral spine, the anterior sacroiliac ligament at the sacral ala, and the iliolumbar ligament at the L5 transverse process.

## Imaging Protocols and Methodology

### Radiography

An AP pelvic radiograph is the imaging examination of choice in all patients presenting with acute pelvic trauma. However, the sensitivity of pelvic radiographs for identifying pelvic fractures is poor, ranging from 50% to 68% [6]. Additional views of the pelvis can be added to improve detection of pelvic fractures. Inlet and outlet views can help assess pelvic ring injuries. The outlet view is particularly useful for assessing vertical translation of the pelvis. Bilateral Judet views, termed obturator and iliac oblique projections, help evaluate acetabular fractures. The obturator oblique allows optimal visualization of the anterior column and posterior wall on the side of injury, while the iliac oblique allows optimal visualization of the anterior wall and posterior column (Fig. 5). With the widespread availability of CT, these additional pelvic views are primarily used today for follow-up of known pelvic fractures.

Diagnosis of sacral fractures with radiography is frequently challenging due to overlying bowel. However, for suspected isolated sacral trauma, collimated AP oblique (Ferguson view) and lateral radiographs of the sacrum are often used in place of standard pelvic radiographs. The Ferguson view optimizes evaluation of the sacroiliac joints, and the lateral radiograph is helpful in detecting transverse sacral fractures.

For acute hip injuries, a hip radiograph series can be performed comprised of an AP view of the pelvis and an abduction (i.e., "frog-leg") view of the injured hip. AP and lateral femur radiographs should be included in all acute hip fractures to evaluate for additional injuries of the femur. The sensitivity of radiographs for proximal femur fractures is at least 90% [7]. Radiographically occult femoral neck fractures are common in patients with osteoporosis or presenting with high-velocity femoral shaft fractures [8, 9]. In these patients, a low threshold should be maintained for performing CT or MRI.

### Computerized Tomography

A CT scan of the pelvis is the preferred method for assessing pelvic fractures after the initial AP pelvic radiograph is performed. CT aids in surgical planning and detection of radiographically occult fractures. CT has a nearly 100%

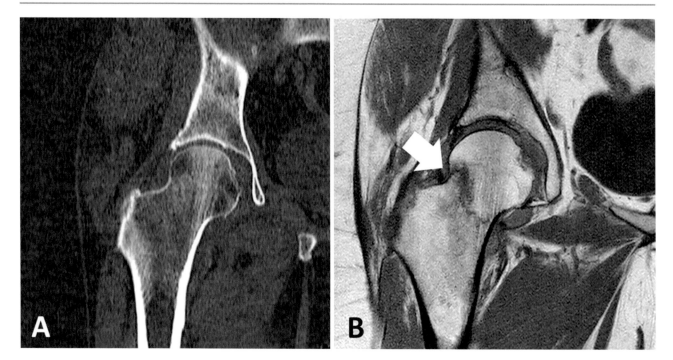

**Fig. 6** Occult CT femoral neck fracture visible on MRI. (**a**) No femoral neck fracture visible on coronal noncontrast CT image. (**b**) Coronal T1 MR image showing incomplete fracture line through lateral femoral neck (arrow)

sensitivity for identifying pelvic fractures and a nearly 90% sensitivity for identifying radiographically occult hip fractures when compared to MRI [9–11]. Despite the slightly lower sensitivity, CT is often preferred to MRI in the acute setting of pelvic trauma due to CT having shorter acquisition time and fewer contraindications [12].

Standard CT imaging of the pelvis should be performed in axial, coronal, and sagittal planes with bone and soft tissue kernels. In general, 2-mm-thick slices are adequate for identifying pelvic fractures [13]. Addition of 3D volume-rendered images can help surgeons conceptualize fracture patterns and degree of fracture displacement for preoperative planning. The use of intravenous contrast is not necessary for the diagnosis of fractures with pelvic CT. However, intravenous contrast is recommended in the setting of high-energy trauma to assess for vascular injuries, organ injuries, and hemorrhage.

### Magnetic Resonance Imaging

MRI has a limited role in the evaluation of traumatic pelvic and hip injuries in the emergency setting. MRI can be beneficial in identifying occult pelvic and hip fractures and does have higher sensitivity than CT for the identification of these injuries (Fig. 6) [9, 11]. However, MRI is constrained by length of examination time and limited

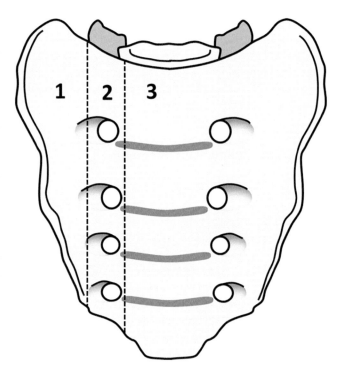

**Fig. 7** Denis classification system of sacral fractures

availability of MRI in emergency departments. An abbreviated pelvis MRI protocol comprised of coronal STIR and T1 sequences can be performed to screen for pelvic

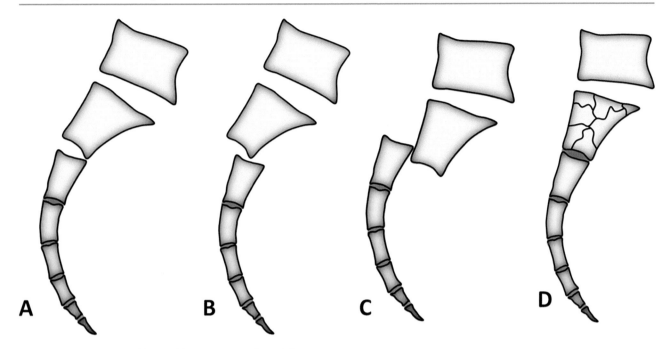

**Fig. 8** Modified Roy-Camille classification system of sacral fractures

fractures, which can significantly reduce examination time. Although not commonly employed in the emergency setting, pelvis MR neurography can also be beneficial in evaluating cauda equina compression or impingement of the lumbosacral plexus in the setting of pelvic trauma. Many other soft tissue injuries, including injuries to tendons, muscles, and cartilage, are best assessed on MRI. However, MRI is not routinely utilized in the emergent setting to assess these injuries since urgent intervention is usually not required.

## Injury Patterns of the Pelvis and Hip

### Sacrum

The sacrum is an important keystone transferring forces between the spine and the pelvic ring. Fractures of the sacrum can result in spinopelvic and/or pelvic ring instability. For instability to occur, fractures need to involve the upper two segments (S1–S2) of the sacrum which articulate with the iliac bones [14]. The probability of neurologic injury from sacral fracture is difficult to predict. However, there are several imaging findings that are associated with increased likelihood for neurologic injury: central canal or neuroforminal involvement, increased fracture displacement, increased central canal/neuroforminal stenosis, and severity of comminution [15, 16].

The sacrum typically fractures either along the long axis of the sacrum (longitudinal fractures) or perpendicular to the long axis (transverse fractures). Longitudinal fractures are a component of over 85% of sacral fracture patterns [14, 17]. Transverse fractures are present in a little more than 10% of sacral fracture patterns, although they are substantially more common in falls from height [17, 18]. Rarely, avulsion fractures of the sacral spine or the anterior sacroiliac ligaments can occur as part of a larger pelvic ring injury pattern, most commonly related to an AP compression mechanism [17].

The complexity of sacral fracture management is reflected in the multiple classification systems devised for sacral fractures. Each of these classification systems addresses one facet of sacral injury but fails to comprehensively describe clinically substantial components of sacral fractures. In 2016, the AO society put forth a classification system designed to capture the most clinically relevant features of sacral fractures [19].

**Denis Classification** The Denis classification is based on fracture location relative to the neuroforamen [16]. This classification divides the sacrum into three zones (Fig. 7). Zone 1 fractures are lateral to the neuroformina, zone 2 fractures through the neuroforamina, and zone 3 fractures medial to the neuroforamina. Zone 1 fractures are the least likely to result in nerve injury and typically result in L5 nerve root injuries. Zone 2 fractures have an intermediate risk for nerve injury and typically result in injury of whichever nerve root passes through the fractured neuroforamen. Zone 3 fractures have the highest association with neurologic injury, with cauda equina syndrome being the most common neurologic deficit.

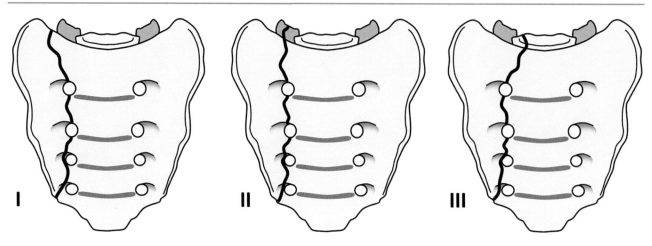

**Fig. 9** Isler classification system of sacral fractures involving the lumbosacral junction

While both longitudinal and transverse sacral fractures involving the central canal are classified as zone 3 injuries, the risk of neurologic deficit with longitudinal zone 3 fractures is considerably less compared to transverse fractures [20].

**Modified Roy-Camille classification** The modified Roy-Camille classification system specifically describes transverse sacral fractures of the upper sacrum (Fig. 8) [21, 22]. Type 1 fractures demonstrate kyphotic angulation without translation, type 2 fractures have kyphosis with retrolisthesis, type 3 fractures have complete anterior translation, and type 4 fractures are comminution of either the S1 or S2 vertebral body. Fracture types carry both management and prognosis implications [14, 22]. Type 1 fractures are generally considered stable and have a low risk for neurologic injury. Type 2 fractures are often unstable and carry a higher incidence of neurologic injury. Type 3 and 4 fractures are uniformly unstable and carry the highest risk of neurologic injury.

**Isler classification** The Isler classification predicts the risk for a sacral fracture creating instability at the lumbosacral junction and is based on the relationship of the sacral fracture to the S1 facet (Fig. 9) [23]. Type 1 fractures extend lateral to the S1 facet, type 2 fractures extend into the facet, and type 3 fractures extend medial to the facet. In Isler I fractures, lumbosacral stability is considered preserved, and only pelvic ring instability needs to be addressed. In Isler II and Isler III fractures, the lumbosacral junction is considered unstable and needs to be addressed along with pelvic ring instability.

**Spinopelvic Dissociation** Spinopelvic dissociation is the term given to any combination of upper sacral fractures resulting in complete separation of the spine from the pelvis.

These injury patterns uniformly result in pelvic instability along with significant neurologic injury in most patients [14]. Many different fracture patterns can result in spinopelvic dissociation (Fig. 10), with the H-shaped and U-shaped fracture patterns being most common.

**AOSpine Classification** The AO spine classification incorporates many of the fracture patterns and concepts described in previous classification systems [20]. The AOSpine classification considers three components of sacral fractures: morphology, neurologic status, and clinical modifiers. Injury morphology is divided into three types, with each type having three to four subtypes (Table 1) (Fig. 11). Type A fractures do not result in spinopelvic or pelvic ring instability but may result in neurologic injury if substantial displacement occurs. Type B fractures are associated with pelvic ring instability, while spinopelvic stability is preserved. Type B injuries are further subtype based on location of the fracture line relative to the neuroforamina, as this has implications for probability of nerve root injury. Type C injuries are fractures which result in spinopelvic instability.

## Pelvic Ring

Pelvic ring factures occur in a bimodal distribution occurring from high-energy trauma in young patients and as fragility fractures in older patients [24]. The mortality rate of pelvic ring injuries is approximately 15% and is substantially higher in complex or open pelvic injuries [24–26]. Restoration of pelvic ring stability is the primary goal in treatment of pelvic ring fractures. Instability can occur in both the horizontal and vertical axes. Several classification systems have been created to characterize pelvic ring injuries, but the two most

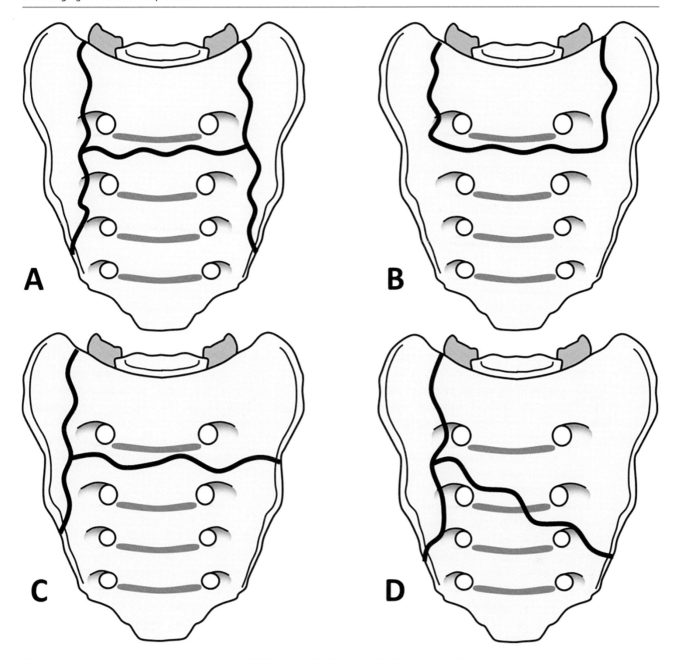

**Fig. 10** Spinopelvic dissociation fracture patterns. (**a**) H-shaped, (**b**) U-shaped, (**c**) T-shaped, and (**d**) lambda-shaped

widely used systems are the Young-Burgess classification and the Tile classification, which both have utility for predicting transfusion/fluid requirements and mortality [27].

**Young-Burgess Classification** The Young-Burgess classification is the most utilized classification system in orthopedic literature for describing pelvic ring injuries [28]. This is likely due to the system being simple and based on mechanism of injury, which has implications for associated injuries. The Young-Burgess classification separates pelvic

injuries into three mechanisms: anteroposterior compression (APC), lateral compression (LC), and vertical sheer (VS) (Fig. 12).

LC injuries are due to compression forces from the lateral direction, leading to transverse pubic rami fractures with sacral, iliac wing, and/or contralateral open-book injuries. LC injuries make up 57–77% of pelvic ring fractures [29, 30]. The LC mechanism is most commonly due to a fall on the side, followed by laterally directed motor vehicle

**Table 1** AOSpine classification system of sacral fractures

| Type A | Lower sacrum (S3–S5) and/or coccyx fractures | **A1.** Sacral compression, coccyx fractures, or ligamentous avulsion fractures (Tile A1 equivalent) | **A2.** Nondisplaced lower transverse fractures (S3–S5) (Roy-Camille type 1) | **A3.** Displaced lower transverse fractures (S3–S5) (Roy-Camille type 2 or 3) | |
|---|---|---|---|---|---|
| Type B | Posterior pelvic fractures | **B1.** Longitudinal sacral body fracture involving spinal canal (Denis III equivalent) | **B2.** Longitudinal transalar fracture lateral to the neuroforamen (Denis I equivalent) | **B3.** Transforaminal longitudinal fracture not extending to spinal canal (Denis II equivalent) | |
| Type C | Spinopelvic fractures | **C0.** Nondisplaced sacral U-type variant (nondisplaced U- or H- type spinopelvic dissociation) | **C1.** Alternative- sacral U-type variant without posterior pelvic instability (Isler I, II, or III equivalent) | **C2.** Bilateral complete type B injuries without transverse fracture | **C3.** Displaced U-type sacral fracture (displaced U- or H-type spinopelvic dissociation) |

collision force [31]. The LC mechanism is associated with sacral fractures in up to 88% of patients [30]. LC I mechanism causes horizontally directed transverse pubic rami fracture with longitudinal sacral compression fracture. LC II injuries are similar to LC I, with the addition of an ipsilateral crescent iliac wing fracture (Fig. 13a). LC III fractures produce ipsilateral transverse pubic rami and longitudinal sacral fractures with contralateral open-book injury, which is commonly referred to as a "wind-swept pelvis" (Fig. 13b).

APC injuries make up 18% of pelvic injury mechanisms [29]. They are commonly seen in single rider accidents and crush injuries. APC I injuries result in anterior ring disruption with an intact posterior ring. APC II injuries result in complete anterior and partial posterior ring injuries. Differentiating APC I and APC II injuries can be difficult on static imaging; however, widening of the pubic symphysis to >2.5 cm and/or avulsions of the sacral spine or sacral ala strongly favor APC II injury. APC III injuries result in complete disruption of the anterior and posterior pelvic ring (Fig. 13c). APC II and III injuries are referred to as "open-book" fracture patterns, due to external rotation of the pelvis anteriorly and the resultant increase in pelvic volume.

Vertical shear injuries are the result of an asymmetric axial loading mechanism and are defined by vertical displacement of the injured hemi-pelvis (Fig. 13d). The VS mechanism is the most infrequently observed injury, representing 1–2% of pelvic fracture mechanisms [29]. Unlike APC and LC injuries, VS injuries result in both horizontal and vertical instability. Rarely (~3%), a combination pelvic ring injury occurs combining multiple fracture patterns [29].

**Tile Classification** The Tile classification divides the pelvis into anterior and posterior arches and grades injuries into three categories based on pelvic stability (Table 2) (Fig. 14) [32, 33]. The Tile classification categorizes fractures as stable (A), rotationally unstable but vertically stable (B), or both rotationally and vertically unstable (C). The relative frequency of each injury type is 55% for type A, 25% for type B, and 20% for type C injuries [24]. Since they do not result in pelvic ring instability, type A fractures often do not require surgery. Type B and C fractures both require surgical stabilization of the pelvic ring, with fixation of type B fractures only needing to address rotational instability, while fixation of type C fractures needs to address vertical and rotational instability.

## Acetabulum

A large majority (81%) of acetabular fractures are the result of high-energy motor vehicle collisions [34]. Treatment of acetabular fractures must address restoring the weight-bearing columns of the acetabulum, as well as the congruency of the acetabular articular surface, to minimize post-traumatic osteoarthrosis of the hip. Severity of articular surface comminution and displacement as well as the presence of intra-articular bone fragments are important characteristics that can contribute to post-traumatic osteoarthrosis. Acetabular fractures often occur in conjunction with fracture of the ipsilateral femoral head/neck or, less commonly, as part of a pelvic ring injury pattern [35, 36]. The Judet-Letournel system is by far the most commonly used classification for acetabular fractures [34].

**Judet-Letournel Classification** The Judet-Letournel classification was devised to aid communication of acetabular fracture patterns and to guide treatment [37, 38]. Historically, this classification system helped surgeons determine anterior or posterior approach for open fixation of acetabular

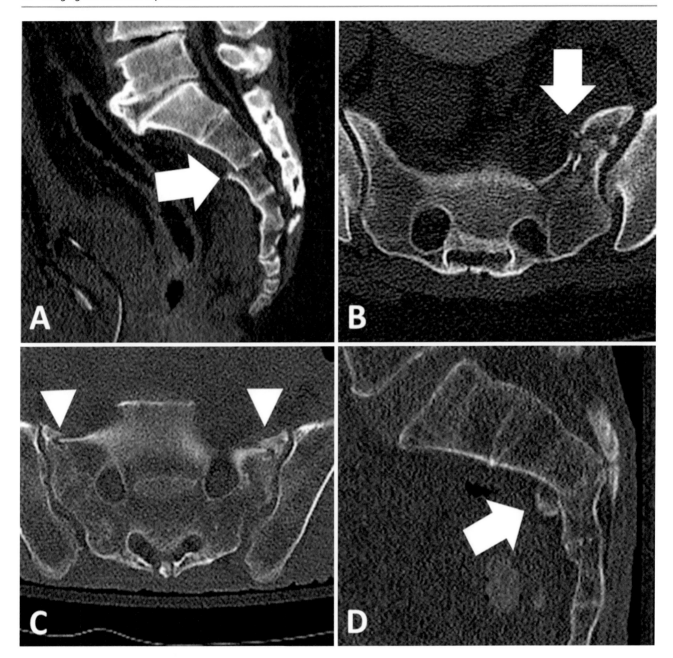

**Fig. 11** Examples of AOSpine sacral fracture morphologies. (**a**) Sagittal CT image shows displaced lower sacral fracture (AOSpine A3). (**b**) Axial CT image shows longitudinal fracture through the S2 neuroforamen (AOSpine B3). (**c**) Axial CT and (**d**) sagittal CT images show bilateral longitudinal fractures (arrowheads) and S3 transverse fracture (arrow) (AOSpine C3)

fractures. With increasing use of percutaneous techniques, this classification guiding open surgical approach has become less relevant. However, this classification is still widely used because of its relative simplicity, reliability among surgeons, and association with prognostic outcomes [39].

The Judet-Letournel classification divides acetabular fractures into ten patterns: five elementary and five associated (Fig. 15). Elementary fractures involve a single element of the acetabulum, while associated fractures are the five most common patterns involving combinations of the elementary fractures. Elementary patterns comprise 31–42% of acetabular fractures, with over half being posterior wall fractures [40, 41]. Overall, 80% of fractures observed are made up of five patterns: posterior wall, transverse fractures, transverse with posterior wall fracture (Fig. 16a), T-shaped (Fig. 16b), and both columns (Fig. 16c) [34].

## AP Compression

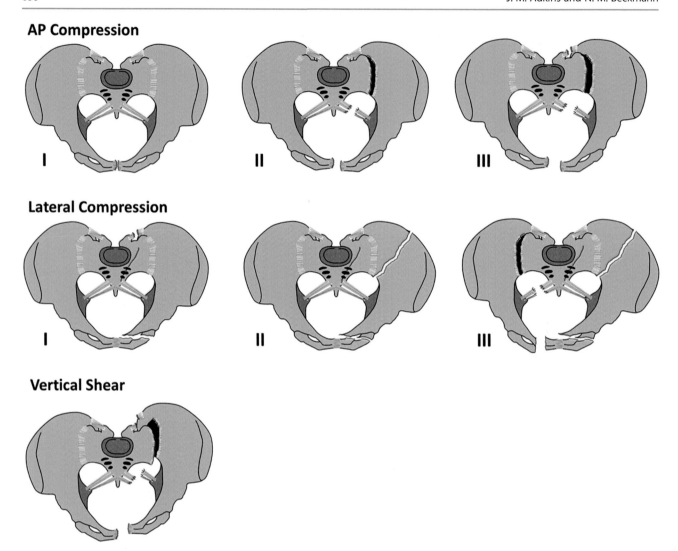

## Lateral Compression

## Vertical Shear

**Fig. 12** Young-Burgess classification system of pelvic ring injuries

## Femoral Neck

Femoral neck fractures commonly present as fragility fractures in geriatric patients and carry a high mortality rate of 22–33% at 1 year [42]. Most femoral neck fractures in younger patients are due to high-energy trauma, and neck fractures in young patients without high-energy trauma are very suspicious for a pathologic fracture. There is a strong association between high-energy femoral neck and shaft fractures, with 5–10% of high-energy femoral shaft fractures having an associated neck fracture (Fig. 17). Subtrochanteric femur fractures are rare in the absence of high-energy trauma at any age. Pathologic fracture should be considered in patients with low-energy subtrochanteric fractures. This is particularly true in patients with a history of bisphosphonate use, as the subtrochanteric region is a common location for bisphosphonate-related stress

fractures (Fig. 18a). When bisphosphonate fracture is suspected, the contralateral femur should be imaged, as bisphosphonate-related stress fractures are frequently bilateral (Fig. 18b).

The Garden classification describes femoral neck fractures based on their degree of displacement (Fig. 19) [43]. Increased displacement of femoral neck fractures is associated with increased rates of avascular necrosis and nonunion; therefore, the Garden classification is used as a general prognostic indicator for these common complications.

## Femoral Head

Femoral head fractures most commonly occur in association with other fractures. Femoral head fractures occur in approximately 20% of acetabular fractures and 70% of

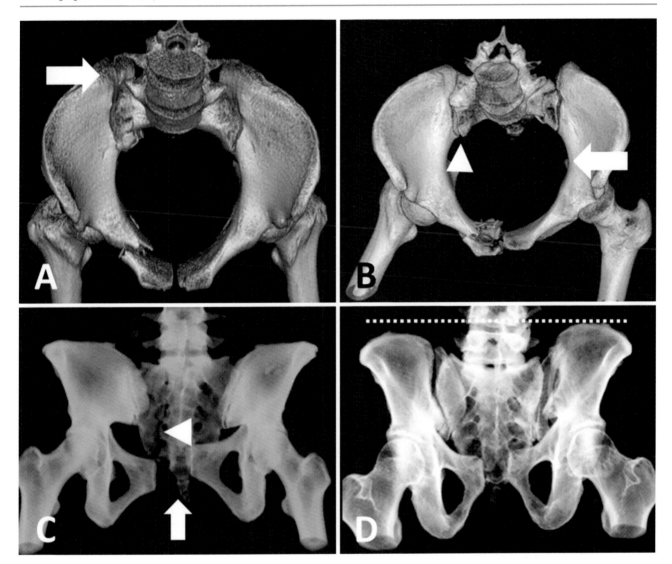

**Fig. 13** Examples of Young-Burgess fracture patterns. (**a**) 3D volume-rendered CT image shows LC II injury with crescent fracture of posterior ilium (arrow). (**b**) 3D volume-rendered CT image shows LC III injury with narrowing of the left pelvic inlet (arrow) and contralateral diastasis of the anterior sacroiliac joint (arrowhead). (**c**) Outlet view on virtual radiograph CT reformat shows AP III injury with diastasis of the pubic symphysis (arrow) and right zone 2 sacral fracture (arrowhead). (**d**) AP view on virtual radiograph CT reformat shows VS injury with mild vertical offset of the iliac crests (dashed line)

**Table 2** Tile classification system of pelvic ring injuries

|  | Tile A | Tile B | Tile C |
|---|---|---|---|
| Pelvic ring | Vertically intact and rotationally intact | Vertically intact and rotationally disrupted | Vertically disrupted and rotationally disrupted |
| Posterior arch | Intact | Partially intact posterior structures | Disrupted |
| Stability | Stable | Partially stable | Complete – unstable |
| Tile category subclassifications *each tile classification has three subtypes | Avulsions and iliac bone fractures (A1) | Open book (B1) | Unilateral (C1) |
|  | Minimally displaced pelvic ring fractures (A2) | LC, ipsilateral (B2) | Bilateral – one side rotationally and one side vertically unstable (C2) |
|  | Low transverse sacral/coccygeal fractures (A3) | LC, contralateral (B3) | Associated with acetabular fracture (C3) |

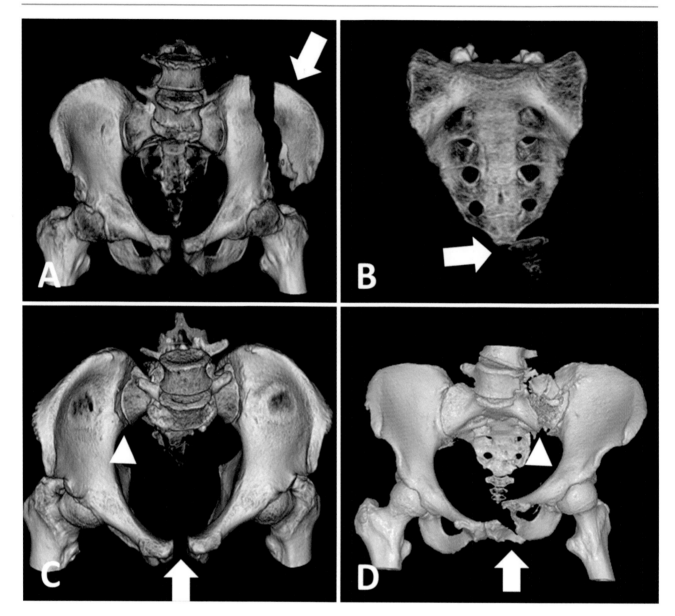

**Fig. 14** 3D volume-rendered images of the pelvis demonstrating examples of the Tile classification. (**a**) Iliac wing fracture (Tile A1). (**b**) Transverse coccyx fracture (Tile A3). (**c**) Pubic symphysis diastasis (arrow) with partial disruption of right SI joint (arrowhead) (Tile B1). (**d**) Unilateral pubic rami (arrow) and sacral ala (arrowhead) fractures with vertical instability (Tile C1)

hip dislocations. Most femoral head fractures are impaction-type fractures (Fig. 20a,b), with fewer than 10% of femoral head fractures being shear-type fractures (Fig. 20c, d).

The Pipkin classification is based on four commonly observed femoral head fracture patterns (Fig. 21) [44]. Originally, this classification system was designed to help guide surgical management. However, the utility of this classification for management has diminished over time. Studies have also found the Pipkin classification to be unreliable as a prognostic indicator for avascular necrosis or osteoarthrosis [45]. The longevity of this classification system is likely a factor of its simplicity and reproducibility rather than its actual clinical utility.

A large majority of hip dislocations occur in young males [46]. Over 90% of hip dislocations occur in the posterior direction, with anterior dislocations comprising less than 10%. Anterior hip dislocations can be further divided into inferior (90%) and superior (10%) subtypes [47]. Up to 70% of hip dislocations cause acetabular fractures [48]. Impaction fractures of the femoral head are also common. The most common associated injuries are avascular necrosis of the femoral head, post-traumatic osteoarthrosis, and sciatic nerve injuries.

## Elementary patterns

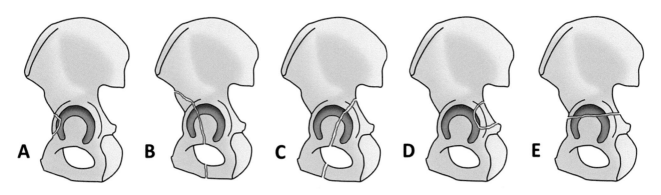

## Associated patterns

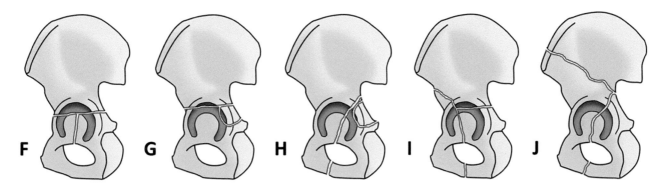

**Fig. 15**   Judet-Letournel classification system of acetabular fractures

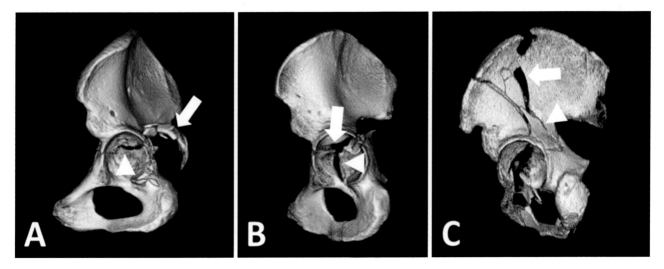

**Fig. 16**   Lateral 3D volume-rendered images of the acetabulum demonstrating common acetabular fracture patterns. (**a**) Transverse with posterior wall. Transverse fracture line (arrowhead) and displaced posterior wall fracture (arrow). (**b**) T-shaped. Transverse fracture line (arrow) with connecting vertical fracture line extending into obturator foramen (arrowhead). (**c**) Both columns. Anterior column fracture line extending into iliac wing (arrow), with posterior column fracture line (arrowhead) creating complete separation of the acetabular cup from the sciatic buttress

**Fig. 17** Occult high-velocity femoral neck fracture associated with femur diaphyseal fracture. (**a**) AP radiograph of the proximal left femur shows a comminuted proximal femur diaphyseal fracture from high-energy trauma, with no visible femoral neck fracture. (**b**) Axial CT image of the left femoral neck in the same patient shows a nondisplaced transcervical femoral neck fracture (arrow)

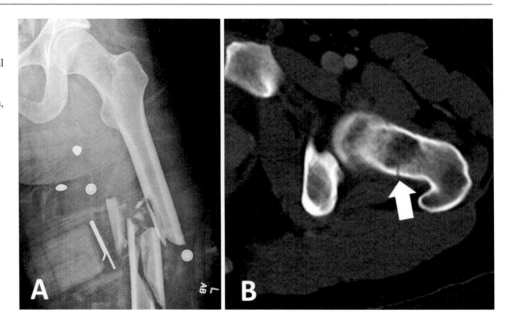

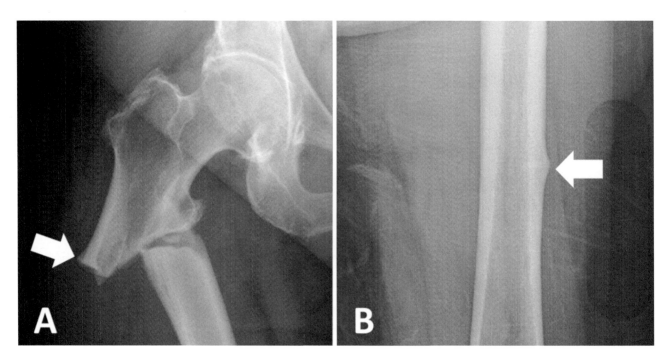

**Fig. 18** Pathologic subtrochanteric fracture related to chronic bisphosphonate use. (**a**) AP radiograph of the proximal right femur shows a subtrochanteric fracture with subtle focal periosteal reaction (a.k.a. cortical "beak") typically seen in bisphosphonate-related fractures. (**b**) AP radiograph of the mid-left femur in the same patient shows a similar cortical beak present along the lateral cortex of the femur

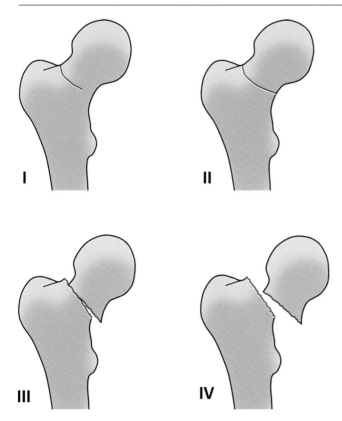

**Fig. 19** Garden classification system of femoral neck fractures

## Pelvis and Hip Soft Tissue Injuries

Soft tissue trauma of the pelvis and hips is common and represents a substantial source of morbidity and mortality. For example, up to 63% of patients with pelvic fractures can have associated injuries of the bladder and/or urethra [24]. Extraperitoneal bladder rupture (Fig. 22a) is commonly seen with urine extravasation into the prevesical space of Retzius and is typically managed nonoperatively. Intraperitoneal bladder rupture (Fig. 22b), typically diagnosed by intraperitoneal contrast after CT or fluoroscopic cystography, requires emergent surgical management. The most injured area of the urethra is the posterior urethra (Fig. 22c), which is seen in up to 25% of patients with pelvic fractures [49]. This occurs more commonly in men; however, urethral injury in women can occur in association with vaginal and rectal trauma [50]. Although uncommon, colon and rectum injuries resulting from pelvic fractures often require primary repair or diverting colostomy.

Superficial soft tissue injuries include abrasions/lacerations, degloving injuries, and hematoma formation. Internally, when the pelvic floor is torn, large amounts of hemorrhage into the pelvis are possible (Fig. 23a–c). Venous and arterial sources of bleeding are both common, occurring with a frequency of approximately 80% and 20%, respectively [24, 51]. Additionally, soft tissue degloving or shearing injuries along the layers of subcutaneous tissues can create a potential space allowing for the accumulation of fluid, which is referred to as a Morel-Lavallee lesion and commonly occurs along the proximal lateral thigh (Fig. 23d).

## Summary

Pelvic and hip fractures most commonly present as high-energy trauma in younger patients and fragility fractures in older patients. These injuries can result in substantial morbidity and mortality, particular if they are missed on initial assessment. Pelvic fractures in general are notoriously difficult to identify on radiographs; therefore, a low threshold should be maintained for performing CT in patients presenting with pelvic trauma. CT imaging is also indicated in patients with pelvic fractures diagnosed on radiographs as CT is superior to radiographs in characterizing pelvic injury patterns, which can help guide management. Intravenous contrast should be given in the setting of high-energy trauma to assess for associated soft tissue injuries. MRI is superior to CT for assessing most soft tissue injuries but is rarely required in an emergent setting.

**Key Points** I. Radiographs are typically adequate for evaluating acute hip trauma, but due to complex osteology, CT should be performed when there is clinical concern for a pelvic fracture.

II. CT should be performed in patients with pelvic ring or acetabulum fracture diagnosed on radiographs to completely characterize the injury pattern and help guide preoperative planning.

III. Avulsion fractures of the hip and pelvis are common. Being familiar with the attachment points of major muscles of the hip and pelvis can help aid in diagnosing these injuries.

IV. Pathologic fractures of the pelvis and hip are common. Particularly, low-energy fractures of the subtrochanteric femur and avulsion fracture of the lesser trochanter in adults should be considered pathologic until proven otherwise.

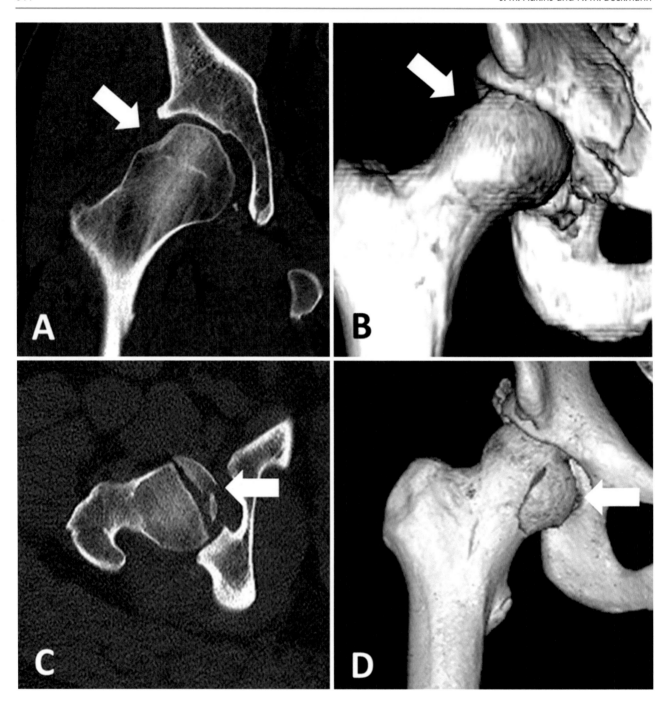

**Fig. 20** Femoral head fractures. (**a**) Coronal CT and (**b**) 3D volume-rendered CT images show an impaction fracture of the superolateral right femoral head (arrows). (**c**) Axial CT and (**d**) 3D volume-rendered CT images show a shear-type fracture of the anteroinferior femoral head (arrows)

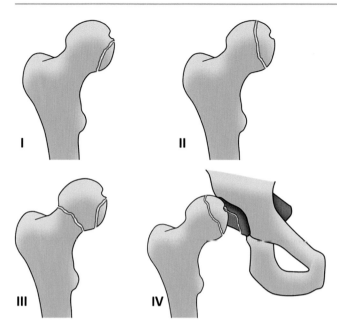

**Fig. 21** Pipkin classification system of femoral head fractures

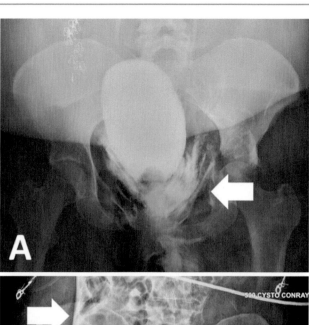

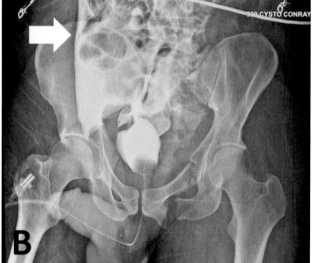

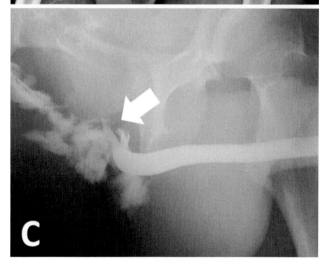

**Fig. 22** Common genitourinary injuries in pelvic trauma. (**a**) Fluoroscopic cystogram demonstrating extraperitoneal bladder rupture with contrast leak into the space of Retzius (arrow). (**b**) Fluoroscopic cystogram demonstrating intraperitoneal bladder rupture with a loop of bowel outlined by intraperitoneal contrast (arrow). (**c**) Retrograde urethrogram demonstrating posterior urethral injury with contrast extravasation at the level of the membranous urethra (arrow)

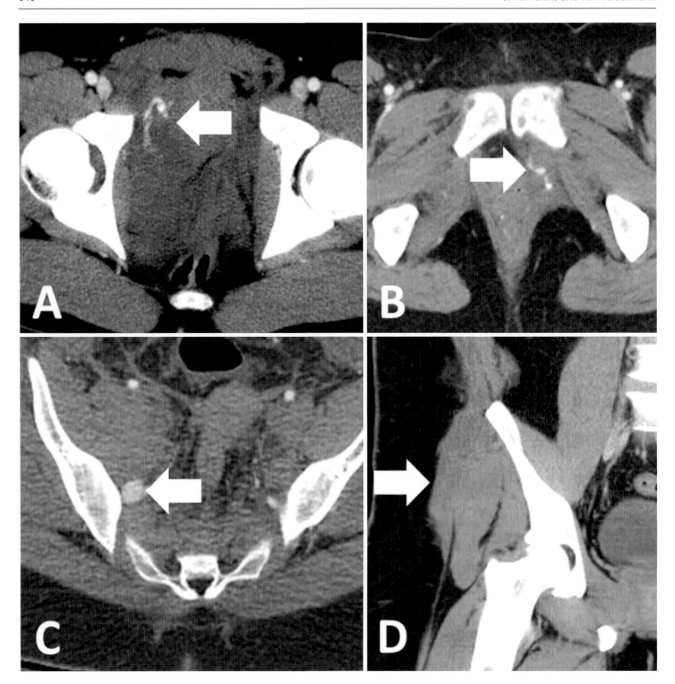

**Fig. 23** Pelvic traumatic hemorrhage. (**a**) Axial CT angiogram shows obturator artery extravasation (arrow). (**b**) Axial CT angiogram shows pudendal artery extravasation (arrow). (**c**) Axial CT angiogram shows gluteal artery pseudoaneurysm (arrow). (**d**) Coronal CT with contrast shows Morel-Lavallee lesion along lateral fascia of hip (arrow)

## References

1. Pasco JA, Lane SE, Brennan-Olsen SL, Holloway KL, Timney EN, Bucki-Smith G, Morse AG, Dobbins AG, Williams LJ, Hyde NK, Kotowicz MA. The epidemiology of incident fracture from cradle to senescence. Calcif Tissue Int. 2015;97(6):568–76.

2. Burge R, Dawson-Hughes B, Solomon DH, Wong JB, King A, Tosteson A. Incidence and economic burden of osteoporosis-related fractures in the United States, 2005-2025. J Bone Miner Res. 2007;22(3):465–75.

3. Mears SC, Berry DJ. Outcomes of displaced and nondisplaced pelvic and sacral fractures in elderly adults. J Am Geriatr Soc. 2011;59(7):1309–12.

4. Mundi S, Pindiprolu B, Simunovic N, Bhandari M. Similar mortality rates in hip fracture patients over the past 31 years. Acta Orthop. 2014;85(1):54–9.
5. Vix VA, Ryu CY. The adult symphysis pubis: normal and abnormal. Am J Roentgenol Radium Therapy, Nucl Med. 1971;112(3):517–25.
6. Paydar S, Ghaffarpasand F, Foroughi M, Saberi A, Dehghankhalili M, Abbasi H, Malekpoor B, Bananzadeh AM, Vahid Hosseini M, Bolandparvaz S. Role of routine pelvic radiography in initial evaluation of stable, high-energy, blunt trauma patients. Emerg Med J. 2013;30(9):724–7.
7. Dominguez S, Liu P, Roberts C, Mandell M, Richman PB. Prevalence of traumatic hip and pelvic fractures in patients with suspected hip fracture and negative initial standard radiographs-a study of emergency department patients. Acad Emerg Med. 2005;12:366–9.
8. Rodriguez-Merchan EC, Moraleda L, Gomez-Cardero P. Injuries associated with femoral shaft fractures with special emphasis on occult injuries. Arch Bone Jt Surg. 2013;1(2):59–63.
9. Sadozai Z, Davies R, Warner J. The sensitivity of CT scans in diagnosing occult femoral neck fractures. Injury. 2016;47(12):2769–71.
10. Haubro M, Stougaard C, Torfing T, Overgaard S. Sensitivity and specificity of CT- and MRI-scanning in evaluation of occult fracture of the proximal femur. Injury. 2015;46(8):1557–61.
11. Mandell JC, Weaver MJ, Khurana B. Computed tomography for occult fractures of the proximal femur, pelvis, and sacrum in clinical practice: single institution, dual-site experience. Emerg Radiol. 2018;25(3):265–73.
12. Eggenberger E, Hildebrand G, Vang S, Ly A, Ward C. Use of CT Vs. MRI for diagnosis of hip or pelvic fractures in elderly patients after low energy trauma. Iowa Orthop J. 2019;39(1):179–83.
13. Beckmann NM, Chinapuvvula NR. Sacral fractures: classification and management. Emerg Radiol. 2017;24(6):605–17.
14. Robles LA. Transverse sacral fractures. Spine J. 2009;9(1):60–9.
15. Khan JM, Marquez-Lara A, Miller AN. Relationship of sacral fractures to nerve injury: Is the Denis classification still accurate? J Orthop Trauma. 2017;31(4):181–4.
16. Denis F, Davis S, Comfort T. Sacral fractures: an important problem. Retrospective analysis of 236 cases. Clin Orthop Relat Res. 1988;227:67–81.
17. Beckmann N, Cai C. CT characteristics of traumatic sacral fractures in association with pelvic ring injuries: correlation using the Young-Burgess classification system. Emerg Radiol. 2017;24(3):255–62.
18. Kim MY, Reidy DP, Nolan PC, Finkelstein JA. Transverse sacral fractures: case series and literature review. Can J Surg. 2001;44(5):359–63.
19. Bellabarba C, Schroeder GD, Kepler CK, Kurd MF, Kleweno CP, Firoozabadi R, Chapman JR, Kandziora F, Schnake KJ, Rajasekaran S, Holstein JH, Sagi HC, Marcel FD, Vialle LR, Oner FC, Vaccaro AR, Krieg JC. The AOSpine sacral fracture classification. Global Spine J. 2016;6(1suppl):s-0036-1582696-6.
20. Bellabarba C, Stewart JD, Ricci WM, DiPasquale TG, Bolhofner BR. Midline sagittal sacral fractures in anterior-posterior compression pelvic ring injuries. J Orthop Trauma. 2003;17(1):32–7.
21. Roy-Camille R, Saillant G, Gagna G, Mazel C. Transverse fracture of the upper sacrum. Suicidal jumper's fracture. Spine. 1985;10:838–45.
22. Strange-Vognsen HH, Lebech A. An unusual type of fracture in the upper sacrum. J Orthop Trauma. 1991;5:200–3.
23. Isler B. Lumbosacral lesions associated with pelvic ring injuries. J Orthop Trauma. 1990;4:1–6.
24. Gansslen A, Hildebrand F, Pohlemann T. Management of hemodynamically unstable patients "in extremis" with pelvic ring fractures. Acta Chir Orthop Traumatol Cechoslov. 2012;79:193–202.
25. Wong JM, Bucknill A. Fractures of the pelvic ring. Injury. 2017;48(4):795–802.
26. Perry K, Chauvin BJ. Pelvic ring injuries. 2020 Aug 15. In: StatPearls [Internet]. Treasure Island (FL): StatPearls Publishing; 2020 Jan.
27. Osterhoff G, Scheyerer MJ, Fritz Y, Bouaicha S, Wanner GA, Simmen HP, Werner CM. Comparing the predictive value of the pelvic ring injury classification systems by Tile and by Young and Burgess. Injury. 2014;45(4):742–7.
28. McCormack R, Strauss EJ, Alwattar BJ, Tejwani NC. Diagnosis and management of pelvic fractures. Bull NYU Hosp Jt Dis. 2010;68(4):281–91.
29. Manson T, O'Toole RV, Whitney A, Duggan B, Sciadini M, Nascone J. Young-Burgess classification of pelvic ring fractures: does it predict mortality, transfusion requirements, and non-orthopaedic injuries? J Orthop Trauma. 2010;24(10):603–9.
30. Young JW, Burgess AR, Brumback RJ, Poka A. Pelvic fractures: value of plain radiography in early assessment and management. Radiology. 1986;160:445–51.
31. Weaver MJ, Bruinsma W, Toney E, Dafford E, Vrahas MS. What are the patterns of injury and displacement seen in lateral compression pelvic fractures? Clin Orthop Relat Res. 2012;470(8):2104–10.
32. Tile M, Pennal GF. Pelvic disruption: principles of management. Clin Orthop Rel Res. 1980;151:56–64.4.
33. Tile M. Pelvic fractures: operative versus nonoperative treatment. Orthop Clin North Am. 1980;11:423–64.
34. Scheinfeld MH, Dym AA, Spektor M, Avery LL, Dym RJ, Amanatullah DF. Acetabular fractures: what radiologists should know and how 3D CT can aid classification. Radiographics. 2015;35(2):555–77.
35. Beckmann NM, Chinapuvvula NR, Cai C. Association of femoral head and acetabular fractures on computerized tomography: correlation with the Judet-Letournel classification. Emerg Radiol. 2017;24(5):531–9.
36. Osgood GM, Manson TT, O'Toole RV, Turen CH. Combined pelvic ring disruption and acetabular fracture: associated injury patterns in 40 patients. J Orthop Trauma. 2013;27(5):243–7.
37. Letournel E, Judet R. Fractures of the acetabulum. Second ed. Berlin: Springer-Verlag; 1993.
38. Letournel E. Acetabulum fractures: classification and management. Clin Orthop Relat Res. 1980;151:81–106.
39. Butler BA, Lawton CD, Hashmi SZ, Stover MD. The relevance of the Judet and Letournel acetabular fracture classification system in the modern era: a review. J Orthop Trauma. 2019;33(Suppl 2):S3–7.
40. Giannoudis PV, Grotz MR, Papakostidis C, Dinopoulos H. Operative treatment of displaced fractures of the acetabulum: a meta-analysis. J Bone Joint Surg (Br). 2005;87(1):2–9.
41. Geijer M, El-Khoury GY. Imaging of the acetabulum in the era of multidetector computed tomography. Emerg Radiol. 2007;14(5):271–87.
42. Brauer CA, Coca-Perraillon M, Cutler DM, Rosen AB. Incidence and mortality of hip fractures in the United States. JAMA. 2009;302:1573–9.
43. Garden RS. Low-angle fixation in fractures of the femoral neck. J Bone Joint Surg (Br). 1961;43:647–63.
44. Pipkin G. Treatment of grade IV fracture-dislocation of the hip. J Bone Joint Surg Am. 1957;39-A(5):1027–42. passim
45. Romeo NM, Firoozabadi R. Classifications in brief: the Pipkin classification of femoral head fractures. Clin Orthop Relat Res. 2018;476(5):1114–9.

46. Graber M, Marino DV, Johnson DE. Anterior hip dislocation. 2020 Aug 25. In: StatPearls [Internet]. Treasure Island (FL): StatPearls Publishing; 2020 Jan–.

47. Clegg TE, Roberts CS, Greene JW, Prather BA. Hip dislocations: epidemiology, treatment, and outcomes. Injury. 2010;41:329–34.

48. Hak DJ, Goulet JA. Severity of injuries associated with traumatic hip dislocation as a result of motor vehicle collisions. J Trauma. 1999;47(1):60–3.

49. Patel U. Lower urinary tract trauma. In: Patel U, Rickards D, editors. Imaging and urodynamics of the lower urinary tract. London: Taylor & Francis; 2005. p. 115–21.

50. Kommu SS, Illahi I, Mumtaz F. Patterns of urethral injury and immediate management. Curr Opin Urol. 2007;17:383–9.

51. Goslings JC, Ponsen KJ, van Delden OM. Injuries to the pelvis and extremities. In: Ashley SW, editor. ACS surgery: principles and practice. Toronto: Decker Intellectual Properties; 2013.

# Imaging of Knee Injuries

**41**

Pritish Bawa and Vaeman Chintamaneni

## Contents

P. Bawa (✉) · V. Chintamaneni
Department of Diagnostic and Interventional Imaging, McGovern
Medical School at UT Health, Houston, TX, USA
e-mail: pritish.bawa@uth.tmc.edu; vaeman.chintamaneni@uth.tmc.edu

© Springer Nature Switzerland AG 2022
M. N. Patlas et al. (eds.), *Atlas of Emergency Imaging from Head-to-Toe*,
https://doi.org/10.1007/978-3-030-92111-8_41

## Abstract

The knee is one of the most injured joints in the human body, accounting for an estimated 1.3 million visits to the emergency department annually in the United States and approximately 6% of all acute injuries in a prospective European study. Radiographs have low yield for the diagnosis of clinically relevant fractures and are often negative despite significant internal derangement of the knee. Computed tomography (CT) allows for a fast and accurate examination of patients for whom there is a high clinical suspicion of a radiographically occult fracture and to determine the intra-articular extent of the injury for presurgical planning. CT angiography is indicated in cases of supracondylar fracture or knee dislocation, even if spontaneously reduced, as there is a higher incidence of popliteal artery injury. Soft tissue injuries and internal derangements of the knee are best evaluated on MRI given its high soft tissue spatial resolution.

## Keywords

Acute knee trauma · Knee injury · Knee dislocation · Patellofemoral · Tibiofemoral · Tibia · Fibula · Femur · Patella

## Introduction

The knee is one of the largest joints in the human body. It has complex anatomy, comprised of two hinge-type joints at the tibiofemoral compartment between the medial and lateral tibial plateaus and the femoral condyles, and a gliding-type joint between the patella and the trochlear groove of the distal femur [1]. The proximal tibiofibular joint is a plane-type synovial joint. The knee joint serves to provide balance while standing and mobility during physical activities. Stabilization of the knee is provided by multiple soft tissue structures. Primary stabilization arises from ligaments about the knee including the cruciate ligaments and the medial and lateral ligament complexes. The menisci, which primarily serve as shock absorbers, also improve the stability of the knee joint. Secondary stabilization of the knee is from the muscles around the knee.

The knee is also one of the most injured joints in the body. It comprises the second most common musculoskeletal complaint, and the most common sport-related injury seen in emergency departments for children and adolescents [2]. An estimated 1.3 million visits to the emergency department occur annually in the United States for acute knee trauma accounting for approximately 6% of all acute injuries in a prospective European study [3, 4]. Most of such injuries are caused by athletic activities, motor vehicle collisions (MVCs), or falls commonly involving both the bones and the soft tissues, including the ligaments, cartilage, and menisci, with over 50,000 of these injuries requiring surgical intervention [5]. Radiographic evaluation, supplemented by CT, thus plays a major role in the diagnosis and evaluation of knee injuries, as there is relatively limited availability of MRI in the emergency setting.

## Anatomy

### Osseous Structures

The knee is formed by the articulation between the femoral condyles and the tibial plateaus, with interposed C-shaped fibrocartilaginous medial and lateral menisci [6]. The patella articulates with the femur and is part of the extensor mechanism where the quadriceps and patellar tendon attach. The fibular head and proximal tibia articulate at the proximal tibiofibular joint [7].

### Ligaments

Ligaments and musculotendinous structures provide stability to the knee joint. The anterior cruciate ligament (ACL) resists anterior displacement and internal rotation of the tibia on the femur. The posterior cruciate ligaments (PCL) resist posterior displacement of the tibia on the femur and help resist external rotation and varus movement of the knee. The medial and lateral collateral ligaments stabilize against valgus and varus stress, respectively [7].

### Neurovascular

The popliteal neurovascular bundle includes the popliteal artery and nerve, sural veins, and tibial nerve.

## Epidemiology

In a Swiss epidemiologic study reporting the incidence of knee injuries in the general population of a European setting, roughly 6% of all injuries treated at an emergency department were found to involve the knee joint. This corresponds with an incidence of 2.3 knee injuries per 1000 persons per year. Approximately one-third of these injuries occurred during sports. In terms of demographics, 30% were between the ages of 15 and 24, and men were more likely to be injured during sports, while women were more likely injured during transportation [8].

## Mechanisms of Injury

Knee injuries can be caused by a single force acting on the knee or by a complex mechanism involving a combination of multiple forces. In the direct contact mechanism, there can be injury caused by an external object, such as an opponent's helmet or boot in case of a sports injury, or a dashboard in case of a motor vehicle injury. If there is a "non-contact" mechanism, there can be an injury caused by twisting or buckling of the knee especially as a pivot shift in soccer. The location and severity of the injury depend on the location and direction of the force, as well as the position of the knee at the time of injury.

## Imaging

When indicated, radiographs are the mainstay of the initial imaging for suspected knee injury. Knee injury patients with a high clinical suspicion of fracture or soft tissue injury based on initial clinical review, which is not apparent on the radiographs, can be further assessed with either computed tomography (CT) or with magnetic resonance imaging (MRI). The mainstay of imaging in the emergency setting is radiographs and CT, so this will be discussed in more detail.

## Radiography

Although radiography is commonly used to evaluate patients following acute knee trauma, it has a low yield for the diagnosis of clinically relevant fractures. In a retrospective review of 1967 patients with acute knee injuries, 74% of patients underwent knee radiography, but only approximately 5% demonstrated a fracture [9]. As a result, several clinical prediction rules have been developed to reduce the number of radiographs ordered without missing a clinically relevant

fracture. Two of the rules most utilized include the Ottawa knee rules and the Pittsburgh decision rules. The Ottawa rules have a 100% sensitivity for identifying knee fractures while allowing for a 28% relative reduction in the number of knee radiographs ordered [2].

The standard initial radiographic examination includes anteroposterior and lateral projections. Either the cross-table or standing lateral view may allow identification of a fat-fluid level, which is indicative of an intra-articular fracture. The articular surface involvement of a fracture might not be apparent on radiographs and should be further evaluated with CT [2]. A knee joint effusion is demonstrated on a lateral radiograph as an oval density obscuring the suprapatellar fat pad. Additional views including a sunrise view of the patella should also be obtained if a patellar injury is suspected. A tunnel view of the knee, for instance, is indicated for suspected fracture of the posterior aspect of the distal femur. Stress radiographs with valgus and varus stress can help in the assessment of an unstable injury of the medial or lateral supporting structures. PCL stress views are sometimes required to assess for partial or complete PCL tear. The PCL stress views are performed with weight applied to the proximal tibia while imaging with the lateral view. Both knees are compared to assess the posterior translation of the tibia [3].

Despite these varying views and techniques, many injuries remain radiographically occult including tibial plateau and tibial spine fractures, transient dislocation of the patella, and bone contusions. Part of the low sensitivity of radiographs can be explained with difficulty in the optimal positioning of the patients with severely injured knees; however, the majority is due to the inherent limitations of the modality [2].

Of note, anatomical variants which can be mistaken for fractures include the fabella, bipartite patella, and patella alta. Common radiological signs to recognize on radiographs are as follows:

## Lipohemarthrosis

The presence of both fat and the blood in the joint is referred to as lipohemarthrosis. It is indirect but very strong evidence of the intra-articular presence of a fracture, as the fat and blood escapes through the fracture into the joint. It occurs in approximately 40% of intra-articular fractures of the knee and appears within 3 hours of the injury [10]. The fracture may be sometimes occult on radiographs. A fat-fluid level with layering appearance in the horizontal lateral knee radiographs (cross-table lateral view) is characteristic (Fig. 15b). In the case of a radiographically occult fracture with a fat-fluid level, a CT should be obtained as the next step for diagnosis.

## Deep Lateral Femoral Sulcus

The lateral femoral condyle has a normal small indentation which divides it into anterior and posterior halves. This indentation, called the lateral femoral sulcus, normally measures 0.45 mm in depth. A sulcus measuring 1.5 mm or deeper (deep lateral femoral sulcus) corresponds to the fracture of the lateral femoral condyle (Fig. 1a and b) and has a high correlation with acute ACL tear [11] (Fig. 1c).

## Segond Fracture

A Segond fracture is a vertical avulsion fracture along the anterolateral aspect of the proximal tibial capsular attachment, which is also referred to as the anterolateral ligament in the literature. It is associated with an ACL injury in 75–100% of cases and meniscus tears in 42–67% of cases [12]. It is seen as an elliptic bone fragment 3–6 mm distal to the tibial plateau along the lateral aspect of the tibia on an AP radiograph (Fig. 2).

## Reverse Segond Fracture

The reverse Segond fracture is an avulsion of the capsular ligament along the medial side of the tibia, opposite to the avulsion seen in the Segond fracture (Fig. 3). It is associated with PCL injury, as well as medial meniscus tear.

## Pellegrini-Stieda Disease

Pellegrini-Stieda "lesions" are calcified post-traumatic foci along the medial femoral collateral ligament. They are often curvilinear and are seen about the border of the femoral cortex. They are a sequela of avulsion injury to the medial collateral ligament from its insertion at the medial femoral condyle. Typically, they form several weeks after the inciting trauma (Fig. 4).

## Patella Alta/Baja

The term patella alta describes the superior displacement of the patella with respect to the femur and can be an indicator of patellar tendon tear (Fig. 5) or a morphological variant. Patella baja, on the other hand, is an inferior displacement of the patella with respect to the femur and can indicate quadriceps tendon tear in the setting of trauma (Fig. 6).

## CT

CT allows for a fast and accurate examination of patients with a history of trauma for whom there is a high clinical suspicion of a fracture involving the knee joint which is not apparent on radiographs [13]. CT with three-dimensional reformations is particularly useful to demonstrate the position of fracture fragments and the intra-articular extension of complex fractures, particularly of the tibial plateau,

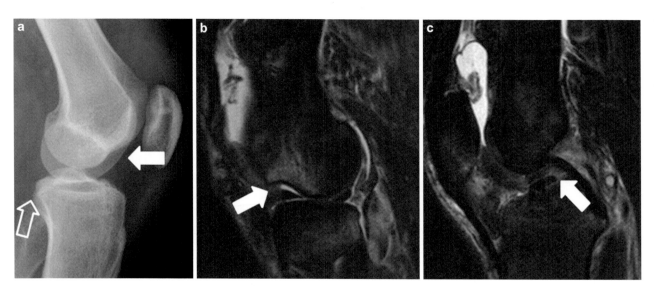

**Fig. 1** A 23 years old man who presented after fall with knee pain and swelling. Lateral radiograph of the knee (**a**) shows the deep lateral femoral sulcus (white arrows on **a** & **b**). A subtle fracture of the posterior aspect of lateral tibial plateau is also seen (hollow arrow). Fat suppressed T2 weighted sagittal MR images (**b** & **c**) confirms deep sulcus with pivot shift contusion pattern and tear of the anterior cruciate ligament (arrow in **c**)

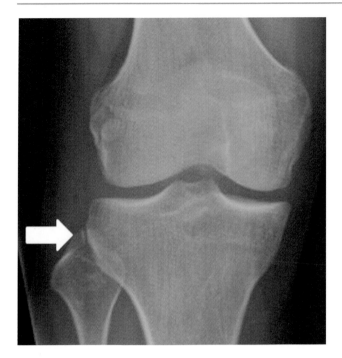

Fig. 2 35 years old man with knee injury. AP radiograph of the right knee demonstrating avulsion fracture along lateral aspect of tibia consistent with Segond fracture (arrow)

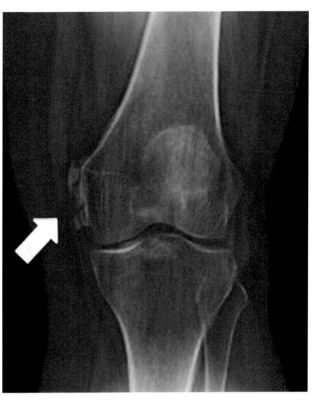

Fig. 4 A 63 years old woman with knee pain. AP radiograph of the left knee demonstrating Pellegrini-Stieda lesion along the medial aspect of the medial femoral condyle (arrow) from remote avulsion injury of the medial collateral ligament

which is helpful for surgical planning of internal fixation. In one study, CT was more accurate for the evaluation of the severity of tibial plateau fractures in 43% of cases compared to radiographs and led to modification of the surgical plan in 59% of cases [8]. The use of dual-energy CT scans further allows for the evaluation of bone marrow edema/contusions [14]. CT and especially CT arthrography can also be used to detect osteochondral injuries by identifying a loose intra-articular body and defect(s) of the articular cartilage.

## MRI

Apart from clinically relevant fractures, soft tissue injuries must also be considered in the evaluation of patients with acute knee pain. In fact, up to 93.5% of patients who present to the emergency department with acute knee pain have soft tissue rather than osseous injuries [2]. MRI is the modality of choice given its high soft tissue spatial resolution for evaluating the cartilage, menisci, ligaments, and tendons. MRI is also more sensitive than CT in depicting non-displaced trabecular fractures and bone

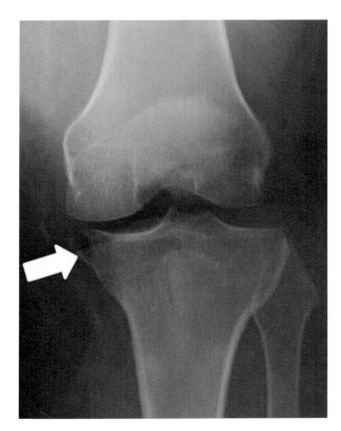

Fig. 3 39 years old woman with unknown trauma. AP radiograph of the knee showing avulsion fracture along the medial aspect of the tibia consistent with reverse segond fracture

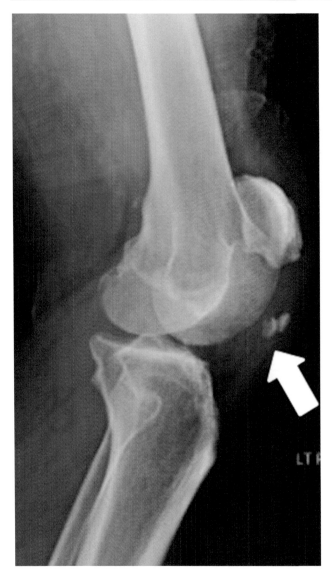

**Fig. 5** 59 years old man presented with left knee pain post fall. Lateral radiograph of the knee demonstrating avulsion of the inferior patellar pole (arrow) at the patellar tendon attachment resulting in patella alta

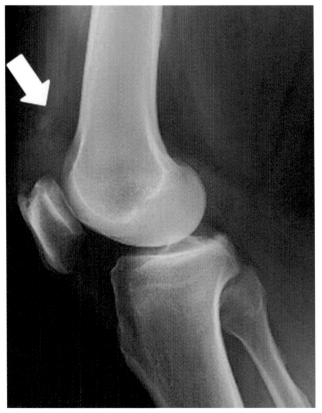

**Fig. 6** 58 years old man presented with left knee pain after fall. On physical examination, there was downward displacement of the patella and decreased extension movement. Lateral radiograph of the knee demonstrating avulsion of the superior patellar pole (arrow) at the quadriceps tendon attachment resulting in patella baja. Small joint effusion and overlying soft tissue swelling is present

bruises [15]. In cases of radiographically occult hip fractures with high clinical suspicion, routine limited MRI is performed for detection. In addition, MRI is valuable in diagnosing transient dislocation of the patella, as it shows the typical pattern of bone contusion and associated soft tissue injury.

## Angiography

In supracondylar fracture or knee dislocation, even if spontaneously reduced, there is a potential threat to the popliteal artery. Studies have suggested that the isolated presence of abnormal pedal pulses on initial examination after knee dislocation is not sensitive enough to detect a vascular injury that necessitates surgery and that the workup should, therefore, include angiography with conventional or cross-sectional imaging like CT angiography [3].

## Ultrasonography

Although not routinely used, sonographic detection of effusion in an acutely injured knee has a 91% positive predictive value for internal derangement [2]. It has also been highly accurate for the detection of ACL tears within 10 weeks of an acute hemarthrosis in the absence of bony abnormalities. A study evaluating 30 consecutive patients with traumatic knee injuries who received same-day sonography and MRI had a reported sensitivity of 91% and specificity of 100% [8].

## Fractures

### Distal Femur

Distal femur fractures represent less than 1% of all fractures and 3–6% of all femoral fractures [16]. The mechanism of injury commonly involves high-energy trauma to the flexed knee as seen in dashboard injuries during MVCs. The AO classification system by Muller and associates (Fig. 7) is the most accepted way to describe such fractures [17]. Type A fractures are extra-articular involving varying degrees of comminution of the distal femoral shaft. Type B fractures are partially articular and unicondylar, involving a sagittal split of the lateral (B1) or medial (B2) condyles, or a coronal fracture (B3). Fractures of the femoral condyles in the coronal plane are also referred to as a Hoffa fracture (Fig. 11) and are usually seen with high-energy trauma. The type B fractures are typically treated with open reduction and internal fixation with a lag screw. Type C fractures are the most severe and are complete articular fractures with the articular fragment fully separated from the femoral shaft with varying degrees of comminution. These fractures typically require open reduction followed by articular surface reconstruction and locking plate stabilization [18]. Some of the examples of distal femoral fractures are shown in Figs. 8, 9, 10, 11 and 12.

### Proximal Tibia

The proximal tibia consists of the articular surfaces of the medial and lateral tibial plateau and is separated by the non-articular intercondylar eminence which contains the tibial spines and footprint for the cruciate ligaments. The lateral tibial plateau normally has a small posterior slope. It is also smaller and more cranial compared to the medial tibial plateau. It has a relatively more convex articular surface and has a slight valgus mechanical axis. The medial tibial plateau is larger and more concave and transmits about 60% of the body weight. It has a stronger and denser subchondral plate.

Fractures of the tibial plateau comprise about 1% of all fractures. Men aged less than 50 years sustain tibial plateau fractures from high-energy trauma, and women over the age of 70 years have fractures from a fall [18] which are then related to osteoporosis. The fractures involve cortical disruption, depression, or displacement of the articular surfaces of the proximal tibia. There are multiple fracture classification systems for the proximal tibia, with the more commonly used classification systems including the Schatzker classification, AO/OTA (AO foundation and orthopedic trauma association) classification system, and three-column classification system. In the AO/OTA

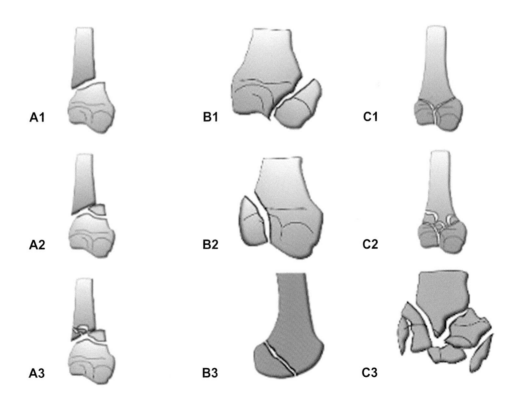

**Fig. 7** Schematic showing classification of distal femoral fracture

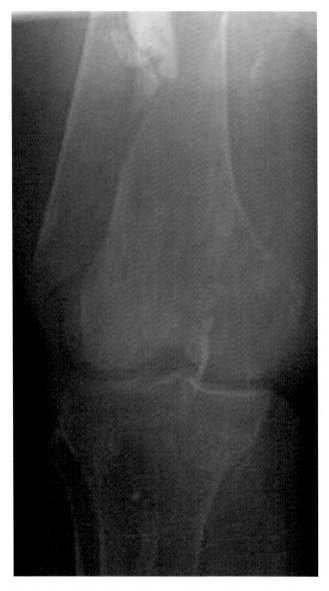

**Fig. 8** Type A2 distal femoral fracture. 59 years old man with unknown trauma. AP radiograph of the right knee shows a displaced fracture of the distal femoral metadiaphysis with small wedge

management and clinical prognosis. Types I–III typically occur due to low-energy trauma, while types III–VI commonly occur due to high-energy trauma. Type III is the most common type occurring in 36% of all tibial plateau fractures [20].

Both the AO and Schatzker classification systems are based on the AP radiographs, which are limited in their evaluation. The coronal plane and posterior fracture fragments are not well defined on radiographs. Improper treatment of the coronal fractures and posterior tibial plateau fractures results in malunion and nonunion. The three-column classification system is based on the axial CT scan of the proximal tibia, which divides the tibia into three pillars (Fig. 20). It bisects the tibia in the coronal plane in anterior and posterior parts at the level anterior to the fibular head. A central line through the anterior intercondylar eminence is drawn joining the coronal plane dividing the anterior tibia into the lateral and medial columns. There are resultant three columns: medial, lateral, and posterior.

Based on this classification, there are four types of fractures, from zero columns to three columns. Schatzker type III fractures are considered zero-column fractures as there is only articular surface depression without a break of the column wall. Schatzker types I and II are considered one-column fractures involving the lateral wall. Additional one-column fractures not described on the Schatzker classification include articular depression and break of the posterior column. Two-column fractures typically involve either an anterolateral fracture and separate posterolateral articular depression and break of the posterior wall (Fig. 19) or an anteromedial fracture with a separate posteromedial fragment (i.e., Schatzker type IV medial condylar fracture). Three-column fractures most commonly present as a bicondylar fracture (Schatzker type V or VI) and a separate posterolateral articular fragment (Fig. 18) [21]. Utilizing this classification system stresses posterior column fixation when the fractures involve the posterior aspect of the tibial plateau, compared to the traditional medial and lateral aspects via the Schatzker classification.

Dedicated trauma series radiographs are usually recommended for the initial evaluation of proximal tibial fractures. CT is required for preoperative planning and provides more detailed information regarding the fracture pattern, degree of depression, and comminution. Complex injuries of the proximal tibia which can have fractures in the coronal plane, median eminence fractures, and posterior tibial plateau fractures, which are better defined on CT. Some ligament tears can also be evaluated on the soft tissue window settings of the CT and especially if it is associated with bony avulsion.

classification system, there are three types of proximal tibial fractures, which are labeled as 41A, 41B, and 41C. The type 41A fractures are extra-articular and 41B fractures are partially articular, involving one condyle. Type 41C fractures involve the articular surface, and the articular surface is completely separated from the diaphysis [19]. The Schatzker classification system (Figs. 14, 15, 16, 17, 18 and 19) is more commonly used in the radiology literature and ranks common injury patterns of the tibial plateau into six types in order of increasing severity (Fig. 13), therefore helpful for assessment of surgical

**Fig. 9** Type A3 distal femoral fracture. 63 years old woman pedestrian involved in motor vehicle accident. AP (**a**) and lateral (**b**) radiographs of the right knee show a displaced comminuted fracture of the distal femoral metadiaphysis without intraarticular extension

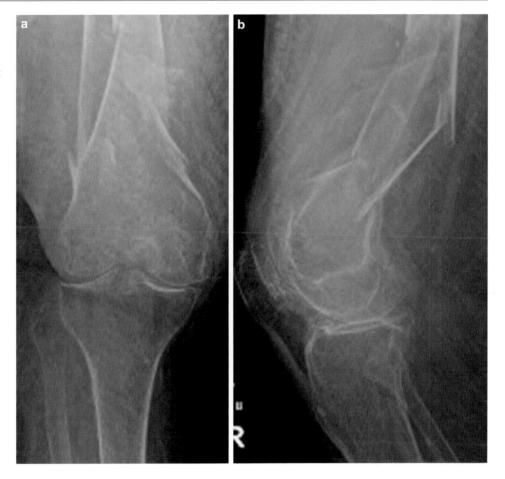

## Proximal Fibula

Avulsion fractures of the fibular head typically involve the styloid process and are an important indicator of posterolateral instability of the knee. The styloid process is the site of attachment of several ligaments, including the fabellofibular, popliteofibular, and arcuate ligaments, which collectively are called the "arcuate complex." The "arcuate" sign describes the characteristic radiographic appearance of the triangular-shaped avulsed bone fragment in relation to the insertion site of the arcuate complex (Fig. 21). Given its strong correlation with tears of the PCL, MR imaging should be recommended in cases where the arcuate sign is detected radiographically [22].

## Patella

Patellar fractures are a common injury caused by either direct blow to the anterior knee, from a fall or dashboard injury, or excessive tension through the extensor mechanism. They can be classified as either non-displaced or displaced (>2–3-mm step-off and >1–4 mm of displacement) [23]. Non-displaced

fractures may be managed conservatively, whereas surgical fixation is recommended for displaced fractures. Additional descriptors are used to describe patellar fractures but do not direct treatment and can be subdivided as transverse, vertical, upper or lower pole, multi-fragmented (Fig. 22), or osteochondral. The Sinding-Larsen-Johansson disease demonstrates one or multiple bone fragments along the inferior aspect of the patella. It is differentiated from the patellar sleeve avulsion fracture by the lack of cartilaginous injury to the lower pole of the patella on MRI. This differentiation is important for management, as the former is treated non-operatively, while the latter requires open reduction.

## Joint Instability

### Patellofemoral Dislocation

Acute dislocation of the patella typically occurs in young athletes. Approximately 60% of first-time dislocations occur during sporting events [23]. Dislocations commonly occur in

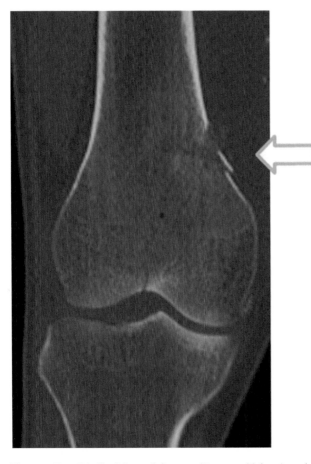

**Fig. 10** Type B1 distal femoral fracture. 32 years old female patient with history of fall from height. Coronal CT reconstruction of the right knee demonstrates obliquely oriented fracture with comminution at the medial cortex (arrow) of the distal femoral metaphysis extending to the femoral notch

the lateral direction and are usually transient. Typically, they occur as a result of a twisting motion of the knee while the knee is in a state of flexion [25]. A flexed knee with an internally rotated femur on a fixed tibia results in lateral dislocation of the patella out of the trochlear groove when the quadriceps are flexed [22]. The patella thus dislocates laterally, with a resultant injury of the medial soft tissue patellofemoral restraints.

Radiographs acquired after patellar dislocation may only demonstrate a large effusion, as the knee has been reduced by the time the radiographs are acquired. The sunrise view may show patellar tilt or subluxation or sometimes an intra-articular bone fragment. A tiny intra-articular bone fragment is seen in approximately 15% of affected patients and is described as a "sliver sign" in the literature [26]. This results from the shearing of the articular surface of the patella or lateral femoral condyle during dislocation or relocation injury, resulting in linear or curvilinear osteochondral fracture fragment.

If clinically suspected, MRI is utilized to identify kissing osseous contusions or fractures involving the inferomedial pole of the patella and anterolateral aspect of the lateral femoral condyle (Fig. 23). The most common findings on MRI are joint effusion and medial retinacular tears, which occur in 95% of patients [24]. Rarely the adductor tubercle can get avulsed at the attachment of the medial patellofemoral ligament (MPFL). Patellofemoral dislocation is commonly associated with osteochondral injury of the knee. It is critical to identify the osteochondral defect or free fragment, as it may be an indication for surgery [27].

Rare forms of patellar dislocations are horizontal and vertical axis dislocation and medial and superior patellofemoral dislocation [24]. A horizontal axis dislocation results from a direct impact on the flexed knee, usually seen

**Fig. 11** Type B3 distal femoral fracture. 30 years old man with history of gunshot injury. (**a**) Lateral radiograph of the left knee demonstrating non-displaced coronally oriented Hoffa's fracture of the lateral femoral condyle (arrows). Lipohemarthrosis is seen as fat fluid level (hollow arrow). (**b**) Sagittal reconstruction CT scan of the knee confirmed the intra-articular fracture of lateral femoral condyle in coronal plane

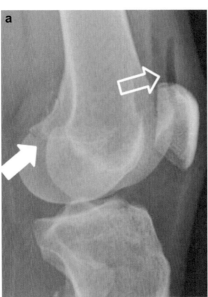
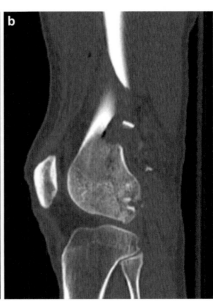

**Fig. 12** Type C2 distal femoral fracture. 46 years old man involved in motor vehicle accident. AP radiograph of the right knee (**a**) demonstrates comminution of the distal femoral metadiaphysis with obliquely oriented fracture from the lateral cortex extending to the femoral notch. Axial CT image (**b**) better defines the intraarticular extension of the fracture (white arrow)

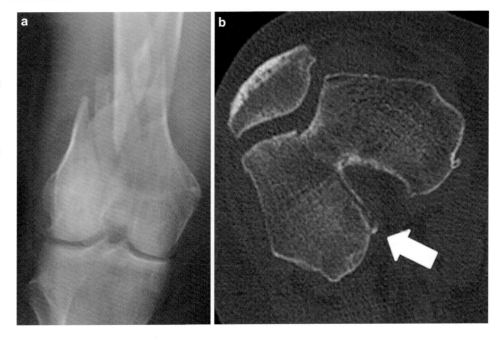

**Fig. 13** Schematic showing Schatzker classification of proximal tibial fracture

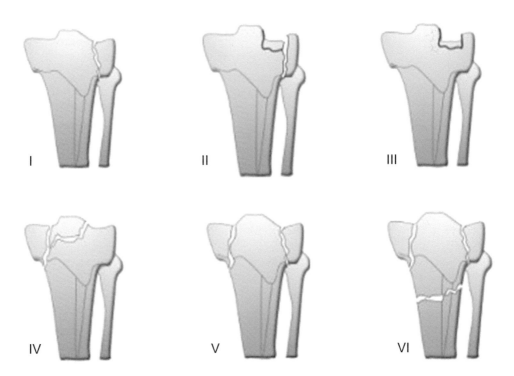

in adolescent patients. A vertical axis dislocation results from a blow to the lateral or medial aspect of the knee. The patella rotates 90 degrees about the vertical axis, and it can become lodged into the intercondylar femoral notch. Extremely rare superior patellofemoral dislocations can result from hyperextension or a direct blow to the lower pole of the patella. Osteoarthritis may be a predisposing factor [28].

**Tibiofemoral Dislocation**

Tibiofemoral dislocations are uncommon but often devastating injuries, with an estimated incidence between .001 and .013% of all orthopedic injuries [29]. The knee dislocations are thought to be underreported, as many of these dislocations are spontaneously reduced and do not present as a frankly dislocated knee when clinically examined. They occur most commonly due to high-energy trauma, as in automobile and motorcycle collisions, but can also occur in lower-energy traumas such as sports injuries, or even as a simple fall in obese or morbidly obese patients. High-energy injuries are commonly associated with poly-trauma and multiple other injuries, including open fractures and life-threatening head injury.

Several classification systems have been defined in the literature for knee dislocations. The French Society of Orthopedic Surgery and Traumatology combined direction of dislocation and pattern of ligament injury, to describe a

pathophysiological classification of knee dislocation. The most common pattern of injury is anterior dislocation, accounting for approximately 40% of all tibiofemoral dislocations [23] resulting from hyperextension injury. Posterior dislocations accounting for about 33% of cases are caused by posteriorly applied forces to the tibia, as with dashboard injuries, in particular.

As in patellofemoral injuries, the tibiofemoral dislocations may be transient, with radiographs often only demonstrating a large joint effusion. The radiographs may demonstrate the direction of dislocation and associated fractures including a Segond fracture, PCL avulsion fragment, tibial tubercle or plateau fracture (Fig. 24a), or osteochondral injury. Even the joint effusion may not be seen sometimes due to capsular tears. Associated vascular injuries can be evaluated with CT angiography as discussed. Nerve injuries are better evaluated with MRI.

## Proximal Tibiofibular Dislocation

Proximal tibiofibular joint injury is a rare, often isolated injury and can be classified into four main types: subluxation, anterolateral dislocation, posteromedial dislocation, and superior dislocation [30]. Anterolateral dislocation is the most common, usually resulting from an indirect injury such as fall onto flexed knee while the foot is inverted and plantar-flexed [30, 31]. The injuries are seen in various sports activities and parachute descents, with most being able to be treated with closed reduction. Posteromedial dislocations occur from direct injuries, such as from a car bumper [30]. These are frequently associated with peroneal nerve palsy. Superior dislocations are the least common of the proximal tibiofibular joint dislocations and are associated with high-energy ankle injuries and associated tibial shaft

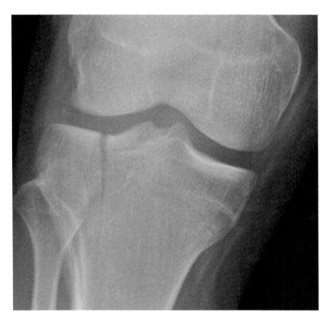

**Fig. 14** 28 years old man who jumped a fence and sustained right knee injury. AP radiograph of the knee demonstrating minimally displaced split fracture of the lateral tibial plateau (Schatzker type I)

**Fig. 15** 24 years old woman with a history of polytrauma due to motor vehicle collision. (**a**) AP and (**b**) lateral radiographs of the knee demonstrating Schatzker type II fracture of the lateral tibial plateau. A large depressed fragment is present along the posterior tibial plateau (solid arrows in a and b). Large lipohemarthrosis is present in the lateral radiograph (hollow arrow)

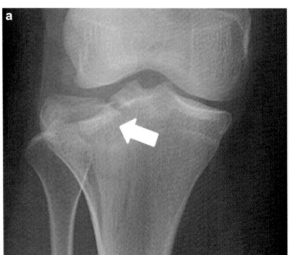
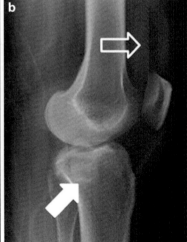

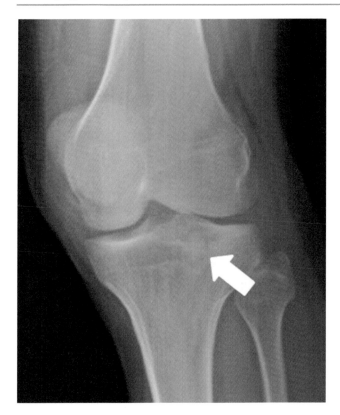

**Fig. 16** A 38 years old man presented with knee pain after motor vehicle collision. Oblique radiograph of the knee demonstrating Schatzker type III fracture of the lateral tibial plateau (arrow). The fracture was not seen on the AP view (not shown)

fractures [29]. Radiographs are usually enough for diagnosis of the proximal tibiofibular joint dislocation. A CT may show subtle fractures. MRI may be required for the evaluation of potential nerve injuries and the evaluation of ligamentous structures.

## Soft Tissue Injuries

The most common soft tissue injuries of the knee include the supporting ligaments and menisci, which can be best imaged with MRI. These are usually not imaged in the emergency settings and are thus beyond the scope of this chapter. There are, however, radiographic findings which can indicate the presence of associated ligamentous injuries. These include a deep lateral femoral sulcus (Fig. 1) and a Segond fracture (Fig. 2) along the anterolateral tibial rim. An avulsion fracture at the tibial footprint may also be evident on radiographs (Fig. 25), especially in the adolescent age group. The sensitivity of radiographs for the evaluation of such fractures is limited, however, but when present these fractures are highly specific for ACL injury. The PCL injuries may be occult on initial radiographs. Posterior translation of the tibia with respect to the femoral condyles may be seen on the lateral views with or without stress radiography. In comparison with the unaffected knee, a side-to-side difference of 5 to 12 mm on stress radiographs is indicative of isolated PCL tear, while

**Fig. 17** 33 years old woman presented after fall. (**a**) AP radiograph of the knee demonstrating poorly delineated vertical fracture of the medial tibial plateau (arrow). (**b**) Coronal 3D volume rendered CT image of the knee confirmed mildly displaced vertical fracture of medial tibial plateau

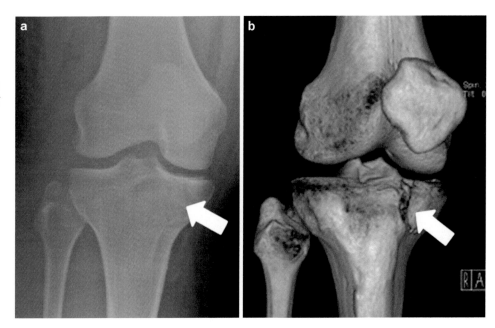

**Fig. 18** A 23 years old man involved in severe high speed accident with multiple bilateral lower extremity injuries. (**a**) AP radiograph of the right knee demonstrating highly comminuted bicondylar proximal tibial fracture, Schatzker type V. (**b**) Axial CT image in bone window better defines the intra-articular fracture planes and involvement of all the three columns

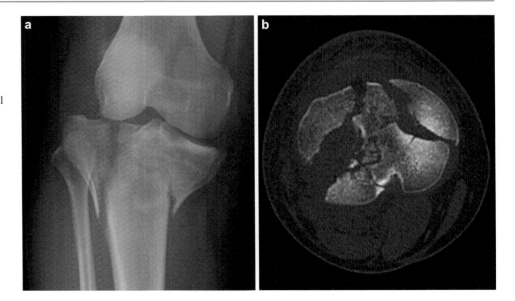

**Fig. 19** Same patient as in fig. 18 (**a**) Axial CT image of the left knee showing the intra-articular sagittal and coronal fracture planes and involvement of the lateral and posterior columns. (**b**) Coronal reconstruction of the knee shows separation of the tibial metaphysis and diaphysis consistent with Schatzker VI fracture

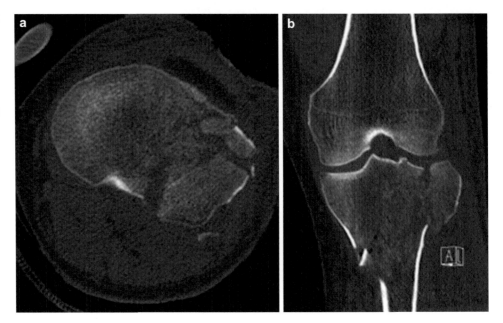

a difference of more than 20 mm is indicative of injury to multiple ligaments [32]. Avulsion fractures of the PCL attachment on tibia can be seen on radiographs (Fig. 26) but are more accurately assessed on CT.

## Neurovascular Injuries

Post-traumatic neurovascular compromise of the tibial nerve and popliteal artery may result in irreversible nerve damage or ischemia if not quickly addressed. The popliteal

artery, for instance, may be injured in approximately 40% of dislocations, with amputation rates up to 85% for injuries not corrected within 8 hours. The popliteal artery has a fixed position proximally at the adductor canal and distally at the soleal arch, thus making it vulnerable to a high risk of injury [33]. Posterior knee dislocation results in popliteal artery dissection or transection (Fig. 24b), and anterior dislocations more commonly result in traction or stretching injury of the popliteal artery with intimal trauma [34]. Although catheter angiography is the reference standard to assess the popliteal artery injury, Doppler ultrasound and CT

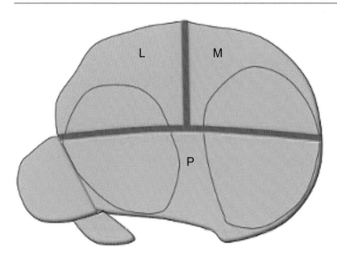

**Fig. 20** Schematic demonstrating division of proximal tibia into medial (M), lateral (L) and posterior (P) columns

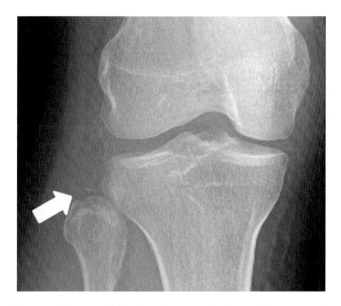

**Fig. 21** 32 years old female with auto-pedestrian accident presented with right lower extremity pain. Oblique radiograph of the knee demonstrating arcuate fracture of the fibular head (arrow)

angiography are less invasive and are also highly sensitive and specific for vascular injury. MR angiography is an alternative to define vascular anatomy and asymptomatic vascular abnormalities.

The common peroneal nerve is injured in one-third of patients and is more common with injury to the posterolateral structures [24]. Peroneal nerve injury presents with paresis, diminished motor or sensory function, or both. The fixed position of the peroneal nerve around the fibular neck is responsible for its vulnerability in a knee injury.

## Other Soft Tissue Injuries of the Knee

### Morel-Lavallée Lesions (MLLs)

The MLL is a closed soft tissue degloving injury in which the skin and subcutaneous fat are separated off the underlying deep fascia after sustaining an abrupt shearing force, most commonly in the setting of high-speed MVCs, and contact sports including football and wrestling. The radiographs may just show soft tissue swelling of the knee. Classically, the MLL appears as an oval or fusiform cystic structure, with varying degrees of internal complexity on cross-sectional images [35].

## Injuries of the Muscles and Tendons

The musculotendinous injuries around the knee can be categorized as muscle contusions, myotendinous strain, or tendon avulsion. The contusions are in the deep muscle belly and tend to be less symptomatic compared to the strains which are more superficial. A tear or avulsion of the distal quadriceps tendon can result in patella baja (Fig. 6), while a tear or avulsion of the patellar tendon can result in patella alta (Fig. 5). There can be blurring of the tendon margins and increased soft tissue density around the femoral condyles or Hoffa fat pad. Small avulsion fractures can be better depicted on CT. MRI is the modality of choice for evaluation of these traumatic contusions, strains, and tendon avulsions [36].

## Conclusion

The knee has complex anatomy comprising bony articulations and surrounding ligaments and musculotendinous structures which provide stability to the joint. It is one of the most injured joints in the body. An initial evaluation is performed via radiographs, despite their low yield for depicting clinically relevant fractures. Important radiological signs of more severe injury or internal derangement of the knee include lipohemarthrosis, Segond and reverse Segond fractures, Pellegrini-Stieda disease, and patella alta. CT is often the next step in the examination of patients with high clinical suspicion of a fracture which is radiographically occult. Distal femur fractures represent fewer than 1% of all fractures classified using the Muller system. Proximal tibia fractures, on the other hand, are commonly classified using the Schatzker or AO/OTA system. Joint instability including tibiofemoral dislocation is associated

**Fig. 22** 21 years old man presented after fall from a skateboard. (**a**) AP radiograph and (**b**) volume rendered CT image of the knee shows stellate patellar fracture

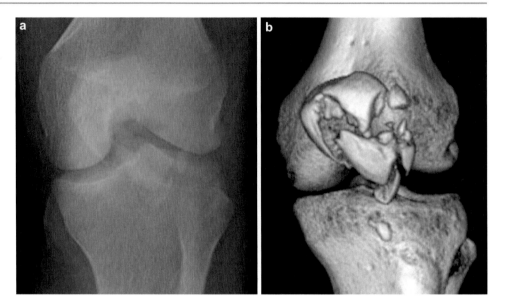

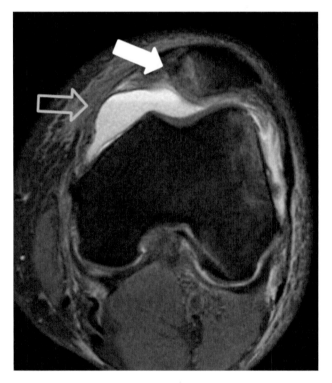

**Fig. 23** 29 years old man presented with knee pain after basketball injury. Axial fat-saturated proton density MR image of the knee demonstrating minimally displaced fracture of the medial patella along the inferior pole (solid white arrow) with contusion of the peripheral anterior aspect of lateral femoral condyle, pattern consistent with lateral patellar dislocation relocation injury. MPFL is otherwise intact in this patient. There is large hemarthrosis with fluid level as shown by the hollow arrow

with a higher incidence of neurovascular compromise and may be irreversible if not quickly diagnosed with angiography and appropriately treated. Ultrasonography, although not routinely used, can be used to detect knee effusions in an acutely injured knee, with a 91% positive predictive value for internal derangement [9]. MRI plays an important role in the evaluation of internal derangements of the knee and soft tissue injuries.

**Key Learning Points**
- Knee injuries are a common and increasing cause of presentation to the emergency department.
- Radiographs have low yield for the diagnosis of clinically relevant fractures and are often negative despite significant internal derangement of the knee.
- Important radiological signs signifying further injury include lipohemarthrosis, Segond and reverse Segond fractures, Pellegrini-Stieda disease, and patella alta.
- CT is indicated when there is a high clinical suspicion for fracture and to determine the intra-articular extent of the injury for presurgical planning.
- Supracondylar fractures or knee dislocation, even if transient, has a higher incidence of popliteal artery injury, requiring angiography, cross-sectional or catheter, for diagnosis.

**Fig. 24** 25 years old man involved in motor vehicle collision. (**a**) Lateral radiograph of the right knee shows highly comminuted fracture of the proximal tibia with posterior dislocation of the tibia with respect to the femur. (**b**) Maximum intensity projection (MIP) CT image of the knee shows occlusion of the right popliteal artery (arrow) in the region of displaced fracture with reconstitution of the tibioperoneal trunk

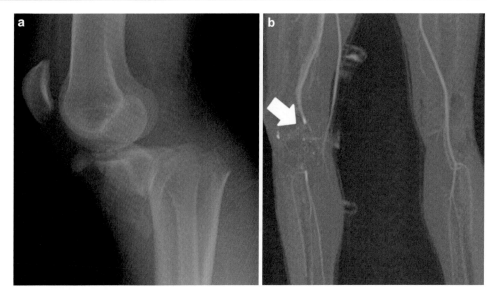

**Fig. 25** 33 years old man presents with pain and instability of the knee after a heavy object fell on the left lower extremity. AP (**a**) and lateral (**b**) radiographs of the knee demonstrating ACL avulsion fracture at the tibial footprint (arrows)

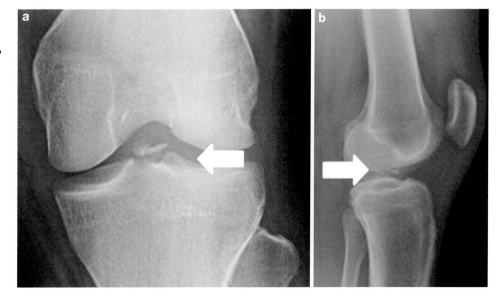

**Fig. 26** 49 years old man involved in a motor vehicle collision. (**a**) Lateral radiograph of the left knee demonstrating PCL avulsion fracture at the tibia (arrow). It was not visualized on the AP view (not shown). Also note displaced fracture of the distal femoral condyle and soft tissue defect in the prepatellar region. (**b**) Sagittal T1 MR image shows the displaced PCL avulsion. There is metal artifact from intramedullary nail fixation of the femur

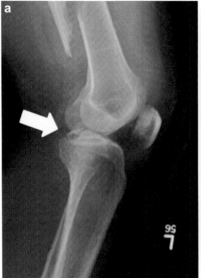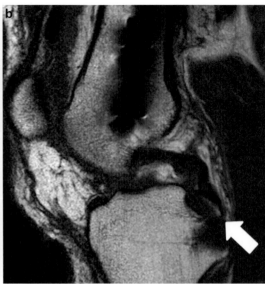

# References

1. Frick MA, Wenger DE, Adkins M. MR imaging of synovial disorders of the knee: an update. Magn Reson Imaging Clin N Am. 2007 Feb 1;15(1):87–101. https://doi.org/10.1016/j.mric.2007.02.008.
2. Tuite MJ, Kransdorf MJ, Beaman FD, et al. ACR appropriateness criteria acute trauma to the knee. J Am Coll Radiol. 2015;12(11): 1164–72. https://doi.org/10.1016/j.jacr.2015.08.014.
3. Tandeter HB, Shvartzman P, Stevens MA. Acute knee injuries: use of decision rules for selective radiograph ordering. Am Fam Physician. 1999;60(9):2599–608.
4. Nielsen AB, Yde J. Epidemiology of acute knee injuries: a prospective hospital investigation. J Trauma. 1991 Dec;31(12):1644–8. https://doi.org/10.1097/00005373-199112000-00014.
5. Roberts DM, Stallard TC. Emergency department evaluation and treatment of knee and leg injuries. Emerg Med Clin North Am. 2000;18(1):67–vi. https://doi.org/10.1016/s0733-8627(05)70108-5.
6. Gimber LH, Hardy JC, Melville DM, Scalcione LR, Rowan A, Taljanovic MS. Normal magnetic resonance imaging anatomy of the capsular ligamentous supporting structures of the knee. Can Assoc Radiol J. 2016;67(4):356–67. https://doi.org/10.1016/j.carj.2015.11.004.
7. Knutson T, Bothwell J, Durbin R. Evaluation and management of traumatic knee injuries in the emergency department. Emerg Med Clin North Am. 2015;33(2):345–62. https://doi.org/10.1016/j.emc.2014.12.007.
8. Ferry T, Bergström U, Hedström EM, et al. Epidemiology of acute knee injuries seen at the emergency department at Umeå University Hospital, Sweden, during 15 years. Knee Surg Sports Traumatol Arthrosc. 2014;22:1149–55. https://doi.org/10.1007/s00167-013-2555-3.
9. Teh J, Kambouroglou G, Newton J. Investigation of acute knee injury. BMJ. 2012;344:e3167. Published 2012 May 25. https://doi.org/10.1136/bmj.e3167.
10. Schick C, Mack MG, Marzi I, Vogl TG. Lipohemarthrosis of the knee: MRI as an alternative to the puncture of the knee joint. Eur Radiol. 2003;13(5):1185–7. https://doi.org/10.1007/s00330-002-1375-5.
11. Garth WP, et al. The Lateral Notch Sign Associated with Acute Anterior Cruciate Ligament Disruption. Am J Sports Med. 2000;28(1):68–73. https://doi.org/10.1177/03635465000280012301.
12. Goldman AB, Pavlov H, Rubenstein D. The Segond fracture of the proximal tibia: a small avulsion that reflects major ligamentous damage. AJR Am J Roentgenol. 1988;151(6):1163–7. https://doi.org/10.2214/ajr.151.6.1163.
13. Mustonen AO, Koskinen SK, Kiuru MJ. Acute knee trauma: analysis of multidetector computed tomography findings and comparison with conventional radiography. Acta Radiol. 2005;46(8): 866–74. https://doi.org/10.1080/02841850500335135.
14. Pache G, Krauss B, Strohm P, et al. Dual-energy CT virtual noncalcium technique: detecting posttraumatic bone marrow lesions–feasibility study. Radiology. 2010;256(2):617–24. https://doi.org/10.1148/radiol.10091230.
15. Ciuffreda P, Lelario M, Milillo P, et al. Mechanism of traumatic knee injuries and MRI findings. Musculoskelet Surg. 2013;97(Suppl 2): S127–35. https://doi.org/10.1007/s12306-013-0279-7.
16. Coon MS, Best BJ. Distal Femur Fractures. In: StatPearls. Treasure Island (FL): StatPearls Publishing; 2020.
17. Kanakeshwar RB, Kamal CA, Dheenadayalan J. Classification of distal femur fractures and their clinical relevance. Trauma Int. 2016;2:3–6.
18. Elsoe R, Larsen P, Nielsen NP, Swenne J, Rasmussen S, Ostgaard SE. Population-based epidemiology of tibial plateau fractures. Orthopedics. 2015;38(9):e780–6.
19. Meinberg EG, Agel J, Roberts CS, Karam MD, Kellam JF. Fracture and dislocation classification compendium-2018. J Orthop Trauma. 2018;32(Suppl 1):S1–S170. https://doi.org/10.1097/BOT.0000000000001063.
20. Markhardt BK, Gross JM, Monu JU. Schatzker classification of tibial plateau fractures: use of CT and MR imaging improves assessment. Radiographics. 2009;29(2):585–97. https://doi.org/10.1148/rg.292085078.
21. Luo CF, Sun H, Zhang B, Zeng BF. Three-column fixation for complex tibial plateau fractures. J Orthop Trauma. 2010 Nov;24(11):683–92. https://doi.org/10.1097/bot.0b013e3181d436f3.
22. Huang GS, Yu JS, Munshi M, et al. Avulsion fracture of the head of the fibula (the "arcuate" sign): MR imaging findings predictive of injuries to the posterolateral ligaments and posterior cruciate

ligament. AJR Am J Roentgenol. 2003;180(2):381–7. https://doi.org/10.2214/ajr.180.2.1800381.

23. Melvin JS, Mehta S. Patellar fractures in adults. J Am Acad Orthop Surg. 2011;19(4):198–207.

24. Kapur S, Wissman RD, Robertson M, Verma S, Kreeger MC, Oostveen RJ. Acute knee dislocation: review of an elusive entity. Curr Probl Diagn Radiol. 2009;38(6):237–50. https://doi.org/10.1067/j.cpradiol.2008.06.001.

25. Kirsch MD, Fitzgerald SW, Friedman H, Rogers LF. Transient lateral patellar dislocation: diagnosis with MR imaging. AJR Am J Roentgenol. 1993;161(1):109–13. https://doi.org/10.2214/ajr.161.1.8517287.

26. Haas JP, Collins MS, Stuart MJ. The "sliver sign": a specific radiographic sign of acute lateral patellar dislocation. Skelet Radiol. 2012;41(5):595–601. https://doi.org/10.1007/s00256-011-1262-8.

27. Rorabeck CH, Bobechko WP. Acute dislocation of the patella with osteochondral fracture: a review of eighteen cases. J Bone Joint Surg (Br). 1976;58(2):237–40.

28. Gruber H, Peer S, Meirer R, Bodner G. Peroneal nerve palsy associated with knee luxation: evaluation by sonography–initial experiences. AJR Am J Roentgenol. 2005;185(5):1119–25. https://doi.org/10.2214/AJR.04.1050.

29. Johnson ME, Foster L, DeLee JC. Neurologic and vascular injuries associated with knee ligament injuries. Am J Sports Med. 2008;36(12):2448–62. https://doi.org/10.1177/0363546508325669.

30. Ogden JA. Subluxation and dislocation of the proximal tibiofibular joint. J Bone Joint Surg Am. 1974;56(1):145–54.

31. Iosifidis MI, Giannoulis I, Tsarouhas A, Traios S. Isolated acute dislocation of the proximal tibiofibular joint. Orthopedics. 2008;31(6):605.

32. Schulz MS, Russe K, Weiler A, Eichhorn HJ, Strobel MJ. Epidemiology of posterior cruciate ligament injuries. Arch Orthop Trauma Surg. 2003;123(4):186–91. https://doi.org/10.1007/s00402-002-0471-y.

33. Becker EH, Watson JD, Dreese JC. Investigation of multiligamentous knee injury patterns with associated injuries presenting at a level I trauma center. J Orthop Trauma. 2013;27(4):226–31. https://doi.org/10.1097/BOT.0b013e318270def4.

34. Medina O, Arom GA, Yeranosian MG, Petrigliano FA, McAllister DR. Vascular and nerve injury after knee dislocation: a systematic review. Clin Orthop Relat Res. 2014;472(9):2621–9. https://doi.org/10.1007/s11999-014-3511-3.

35. Diviti S, Gupta N, Hooda K, Sharma K, Lo L. Morel-Lavallee lesions-review of pathophysiology, clinical findings, imaging findings and management. J Clin Diagn Res. 2017;11(4):TE01–4. https://doi.org/10.7860/JCDR/2017/25479.9689.

36. Diederichs G, Issever AS, Scheffler S. MR imaging of patellar instability: injury patterns and assessment of risk factors [published correction appears in Radiographics. 2011 Mar-Apr;31(2):624]. Radiographics. 2010;30(4):961–81. https://doi.org/10.1148/rg.304095755.

# Imaging of Ankle and Foot Injuries

42

Joshua Gu, Saagar Patel, and Manickam Kumaravel

## Contents

### Abstract

The ankle and foot is one of the most frequently injured regions in the body. Injuries in this region may lead to significant long-term morbidity, even despite accurate diagnosis and treatment. Imaging plays a crucial role in the diagnosis and management of ankle and foot injuries. Non-weight-bearing radiography is usually the first step in evaluation of ankle and foot injuries, but weight-bearing or stress imaging of the ankle or foot can help identify subtle injuries. CT is typically reserved for characterizing known fractures of the tibial plafond or posterior foot. However, CT can also be useful for diagnosing radiographically occult fractures. MRI is excellent for identifying injuries to soft tissue structure, but it has a limited role in the acute imaging of foot and ankle injuries due to availability. Ultrasound can also be an excellent modality for identifying soft tissue injuries of the ankle and foot.

### Keywords

Imaging · Ankle · Foot · Trauma · Talus · Calcaneus · Lisfranc · Fracture · Musculoskeletal · Bone

## Introduction

The ankle and foot contain some of the least stable joints in the body due to most of the joints relying more on extrinsic support from soft tissues than intrinsic support from bony anatomy. This natural instability coupled with the critical role the foot and ankle play in ambulation places this region of the musculoskeletal system at particular risk for sustaining injuries. In 2017, foot and ankle trauma accounted for over

J. Gu · S. Patel · M. Kumaravel (✉)
UTHealth – McGovern School of Medicine, Houston, TX, USA
e-mail: Joshua.L.Gu@uth.tmc.edu; Saagar.Patel@uth.tmc.edu;
Manickam.Kumaravel@uth.tmc.edu

© Springer Nature Switzerland AG 2022
M. N. Patlas et al. (eds.), *Atlas of Emergency Imaging from Head-to-Toe*,
https://doi.org/10.1007/978-3-030-92111-8_42

**Fig. 1** Ligament and retinaculum attachment sites of the ankle. AITFL (yellow), PITFL (dark blue), deltoid ligament (red), lateral ankle complex (green), superior peroneal retinaculum (light blue), flexor retinaculum (orange)

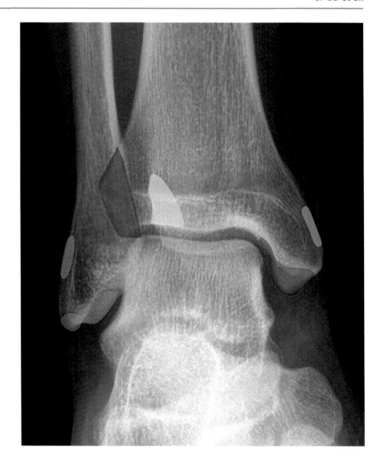

2.3 million emergency department visits in the USA and was almost 9% of all emergency department visits [1]. The estimated incidence of fracture or sprain is 78 cases per 100,000 person/years for the foot and 255 cases per 100,000 person/years for the ankle [2].

The foot and ankle can be injured in a myriad of patterns, and these injuries are often purely soft tissue injuries. While isolated soft tissue injuries often heal without surgical treatment, failure to identify these injuries can lead to long-term morbidity and potential recurrent injury. Imaging plays a critical role in evaluating injuries and elucidating the likely mechanism. Determination of the injury mechanism allows for the diagnosis of occult injuries and surgical planning which can lead to better clinical outcomes.

## Anatomy

### Osseous Anatomy

#### Ankle

The ankle is comprised of two major joints, the tibiotalar joint and distal tibiofibular syndesmosis. The syndesmosis is stabilized by three main ligaments, the anteroinferior

tibiofibular ligament (AITFL), interosseous ligament, and posteroinferior tibiofibular ligament (PITFL) (Fig. 1) [3]. The AITFL inserts on the anterolateral tubercle of the talus, while the PITFL inserts on the posterior malleolus. The tibiotalar joint is comprised of the weight-bearing surface of distal tibia (termed the tibial plafond) and medial, lateral, and posterior malleoli. The tibiotalar joint is stabilized by medial (as called "deltoid") and lateral ligament complexes (Fig. 1). The deltoid ligament inserts along the medial and inferior aspect of the medial malleolus, while the lateral ligament complex inserts at the tip of the lateral malleolus. The flexor retinaculum and the superior peroneal retinaculum insert along the outer cortex of the medial and lateral malleolus, respectively (Fig. 1). The flexor retinaculum holds the flexor tendons in place behind the medial malleolus, while the superior peroneal retinaculum holds the peroneal tendons in place.

### Hind Foot

The hind foot is comprised of the talus and calcaneal. The talus consists of the head and body, which are joined by the neck (Fig. 2). The superior articular surface of the body is commonly referred to as the talar dome. The lateral process serves as the attachment site of the lateral ligament complex. The talus also has a posterior process that is divided into

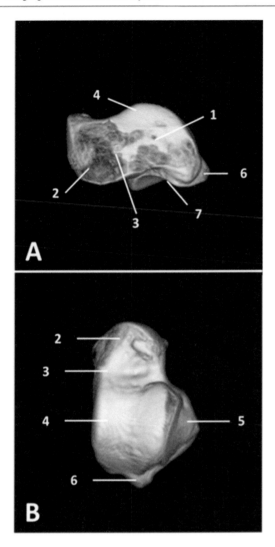

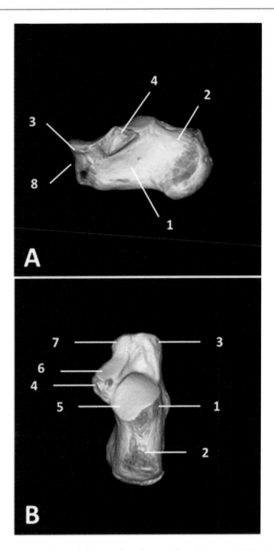

**Fig. 2** (**a**) Medial and (**b**) superior views of the talus. (*1*) Body. (*2*) Head. (*3*) Neck. (*4*) Dome. (*5*) Lateral process. (*6*) Posterior process. (*7*) Posterior facet

**Fig. 3** (**a**) Medial and (**b**) superior views of the calcaneus. (*1*) Body. (*2*) Posterior process. (*3*) Anterior process. (*4*) Sustentaculum tali. (*5*) Posterior facet. (*6*) Middle facet. (*7*) Anterior facet. (*8*) Cuboid facet

medial and lateral tubercles [4, 17], which form a groove for the flexor hallucis longus tendon.

The main components of the calcaneal are the body and three major processes: anterior, posterior, and Stieda processes (Fig. 3). The central body contains the posterior subtalar facet, which bears a large portion of the weight-bearing force. The middle subtalar facet is contained within the Stieda process, and the anterior subtalar facet lies along the dorsal aspect of the anterior process. Anterior lies the articular facet for the cuboid.

## Midfoot

The midfoot is comprised of the navicular, cuboid, and three cuneiform bones (Fig. 4). Medially, the navicular has an elongated tubercle serving as the insertion site of the posterior tibial tendon. The cuboid contains the peroneal groove inferiorly which contains the peroneus longus tendon as it

passes inferior to the cuboid. The medial, intermediate, and lateral cuneiforms articulate with the first, second, and third metatarsal bases, respectively. Each of the cuneiforms lies flush with their respective metatarsal base along the dorsal and medial aspect of the first–third tarsometatarsal joints. Between the medial cuneiform and second metatarsal base is the Lisfranc interval which houses the Lisfranc ligament complex.

## Imaging Protocols and Methodology

### Radiography

Standard ankle radiographs include AP, lateral, and mortise views with the foot internally rotated 20°. On the mortise view, the tibiotalar joint space (medial clear space)

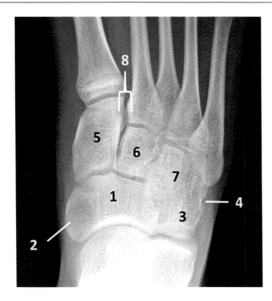

**Fig. 4** Normal midfoot bony anatomy. (*1*) Navicular. (*2*) Navicular tubercle. (*3*) Cuboid. (*4*) Peroneal groove. (*5*) Medial cuneiform. (*6*) Intermediate cuneiform. (*7*) Lateral cuneiform. (*8*) Lisfranc interval

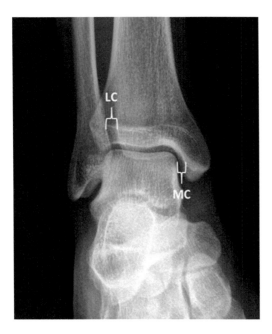

**Fig. 5** Normal medial (MC) and lateral (LC) clear spaces of the ankle

and distal tibiofibular joint space (lateral clear space) are visible (Fig. 5), representing the medial tibiotalar joint space and distal syndesmosis, respectively. Normally, the tibiotalar joint space is less than 4–5 mm and distal tibiofibular joint space is less than 6 mm [5, 6]. Widening of these distances suggests injury to the deltoid or syndesmotic ligaments. Mortise views during adduction or external rotation of the ankle can be performed to identify ligament injuries of the tibiotalar and syndesmotic joints.

An additional axial (or "Harris") view of the hind foot can be performed to help identify and characterize calcaneal fractures, although, with the widespread use of CT, axial views are primarily used for follow-up of known calcaneal fractures. Weight-bearing or stress views of the foot are rarely performed in the acute trauma setting, but they can be very helpful in identifying injuries to the Lisfranc ligament. In general, a Lisfranc interval greater than 2 mm is suggestive of Lisfranc ligament injury, although significant variability exists between patients, and comparison with the contralateral foot is often helpful to confirm widening [7].

## Computerized Tomography

CT imaging is not indicated in the initial evaluation of ankle and foot fractures. CT should be considered whenever there is high clinical suspicion for fracture without fracture visible on radiographs. This is particularly true in patients with hind foot and midfoot trauma since fractures in this region are easily obscured by the complex bone anatomy. CT should also be used to characterize all high-energy trauma fractures of the midfoot and hind foot, including the Lisfranc joint, as well as all fractures resulting in comminution of the tibial plafond articular surface. Intravenous contrast is not indicated for evaluating fractures, but CT angiography should be performed in patients with clinical findings of vascular injury. For calcaneal fractures, oblique reformats oriented parallel and perpendicular to the posterior facet of the subtalar joint can allow optimal visualization of intra-articular fracture lines [8]. Similarly, sagittal and long axis oblique reformats aligned to the Lisfranc joint can help identify subtle malalignments in Lisfranc joint injuries. Three-dimensional volume-rendered images of the bones can aid in categorizing fracture patterns and in preoperative planning.

## Ultrasonography

In select patients, ultrasound offers a quicker and more cost-effective alternative to CT and MRI in the assessment of soft tissues. Ultrasound is excellent for assessing ankle tendon and ligament injuries [9, 10]. Ultrasound can also identify hematomas and foreign bodies and should be considered in patients presenting with laceration and sensation of retained foreign body as wood and plastic foreign bodies may not be visible on radiographs [11].

## Magnetic Resonance Imaging

MRI is the best modality for assessing ankle and foot soft tissues including tendons, ligaments, and cartilage. Cost and availability are factors that commonly limit the use of MRI in the emergent trauma setting. In addition, most soft tissue injuries do not require urgent surgical treatment, allowing patients with suspected soft tissue injury to have MRI performed in a routine outpatient setting. However, MRI may be performed in the emergent setting as an alternative to stress imaging in patients unable to tolerate a stress exam or for preoperative planning in patients undergoing urgent surgical treatment of unstable foot and ankle injuries. Intravenous contrast is not required to diagnose acute traumatic injuries on MRI.

## Injuries

## Ankle

### Twisting Injuries

Twisting is by far the most common mechanism of ankle injury. There are two commonly used classifications for twisting injuries: Danis-Weber and Lauge-Hansen. The Danis-Weber system describes lateral malleolus fractures and is based on the level of the fracture relative to the syndesmosis (Figs. 6 and 7). The Danis-Weber classification is useful in its simplicity and ability to predict syndesmosis disruption: Weber A injuries have low probability, Weber B intermediate

probability, and Weber C high probability of syndesmosis disruption. While the Danis-Weber system is simple, it is limited due to its inability to classify fractures not involving the fibula and is often erroneously applied to fibula fractures that did not occur as part of a twisting mechanism.

The Lauge-Hansen system more comprehensively describes ankle twisting injuries than the Danis-Weber system, although this comes at the cost of the Lauge-Hansen system being much more complex. In the Lauge-Hansen system, injuries are classified by four injury mechanisms based on the position of the foot at the time of injury and the direction of the deforming force (Table 1 and Figs. 8 and 9) [12]. The Lauge-Hansen system is based on the notion that certain ligamentous injuries must precede certain fractures, and therefore fracture patterns may be used to predict ligamentous injuries [12].

Occasionally, the force from a pronation-exorotation mechanism of injury will travel up the shaft of the fibula and create a proximal fibula shaft fracture, which is a variant of a Weber C lateral malleolus fracture. This proximal fibula fracture is referred to as a Maisonneuve fracture and is associated with syndesmosis disruption and an unstable ankle joint (Fig. 9e) [13]. Radiographs of the entire tibia/fibula are recommended in addition to ankle radiographs in patients presenting with twisting ankle injuries in order to identify this potentially occult injury.

**Fig. 6** Danis-Weber classification of lateral malleolus fractures. Type **a**) Transverse fractures below the syndesmosis. Type **b**) Oblique fractures at the level of the syndesmosis. Type **c**) Oblique fractures above the syndesmosis

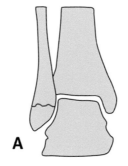
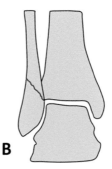
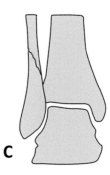

**Fig. 7** Danis-Weber Fractures. (**a**) Weber A fracture (arrow). (**b**) Weber B fracture (arrow). (**c**) Weber C fracture (solid arrow). A small avulsion of the medial malleolus is also present (silhouette arrow)

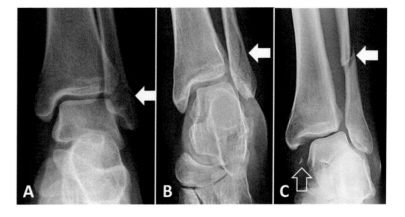

**Table 1** Lauge-Hansen classification system

| Supination with adduction | |
|---|---|
| Stage 1 | Transverse lateral malleolar fracture or lateral collateral ligament rupture |
| Stage 2 | Vertical medial malleolar fracture |
| **Supination with external rotation** | |
| Stage 1 | AITFL rupture |
| Stage 2 | Lateral malleolus spiral fracture at the level of the joint |
| Stage 3 | PITFL rupture or posterior malleolar fracture |
| Stage 4 | Medial malleolar fracture or deltoid ligament rupture |
| **Pronation with external rotation** | |
| Stage 1 | Medial malleolus avulsion fracture or deltoid ligament rupture |
| Stage 2 | Anterior syndesmosis injury (AITFL) |
| Stage 3 | Spiral or oblique fibular fracture above the talotibial joint |
| Stage 4 | Posterior syndesmosis injury – PITFL or posterior malleolar fracture |
| **Pronation with abduction** | |
| Stage 1 | Medial malleolus avulsion fracture or deltoid ligament rupture |
| Stage 2 | Rupture of syndesmosis or posterior malleolar fracture |
| Stage 3 | Oblique fibular fracture above the talotibial joint |

**Fig. 8** Lauge-Hansen classification of ankle injuries

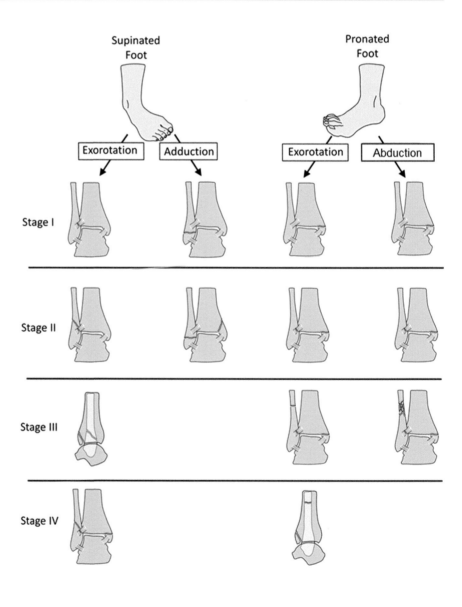

**Fig. 9** Lauge-Hansen fracture patterns. (**a**) Supination-adduction stage II with vertical medial malleolus (solid arrow) and transverse lateral malleolus (silhouette arrow) fractures. (**b**) Supination-exorotation stage IV with oblique lateral malleolus fracture at the level of the syndesmosis (solid arrow) and avulsion of the medial malleolus (silhouette arrow). Posterior malleolus fracture is not shown. (**c–e**) Pronation-exorotation stage IV with posterior malleolus fracture (solid arrow), widened tibiotalar joint space representing deltoid ligament rupture (silhouette arrow), and a proximal fibula diaphyseal (i.e., Maisonneuve) fracture

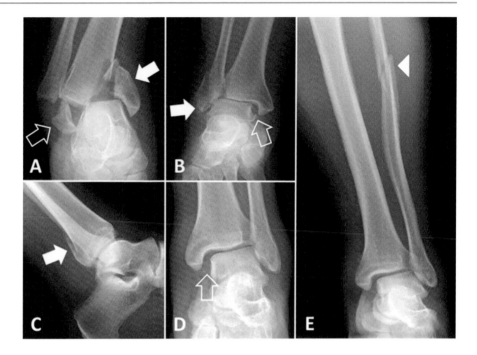

## Pilon Fractures

A pilon fracture is a comminuted intra-articular fracture involving the tibial plafond (Fig. 10) caused by high-energy axial compression, most commonly due to motor vehicle accidents or falls from height. These injuries comprise approximately 5% of all lower leg fractures and are frequently associated with fibular/talar fractures and ankle dislocations [13]. Posttraumatic complications such as arthritis and malunion are common. In addition, frequent soft tissue compromise leaves patients vulnerable to infection. Even with prompt surgical intervention, function may not be fully restored, and complications are common. The most commonly used classification for pilon fractures is the Ruedi-Allgower classification, which classifies pilon fractures based on displacement and comminution [14] (Fig. 11). Pilon fractures should not be confused with trimalleolar fractures. Features of pilon fractures that differentiate pilon from trimalleolar fractures include significant comminution, involvement of the tibial plafond, talar fracture, and preservation of the syndesmosis [15].

## Tillaux Fracture

A Tillaux fracture is defined as a fracture of the anterolateral distal tibia through the epiphysis (Fig. 12). These are most commonly seen in adolescents, often as a consequence of an external rotation injury (10). Growth plate fusion occurs gradually from medial to lateral, leading to a predisposition for lateral Salter-Harris III injury. An important imaging consideration is displacement of lateral fragments by more than 2 mm (3). The AITFL may cause an avulsion of the anterior lateral tubercle of the tibia.

## Avulsion Fractures

Avulsion fractures of the ankle are a frequent injury, most commonly involving the insertions of the syndesmosis, lateral ankle ligament complex, or deltoid ligament (Fig. 13a, b).

Avulsion fractures can be very small or subtle, or the injury can be purely soft tissue without associated fracture. Widening of the tibiotalar or distal tibiofibular joint spaces of the ankle can be indirect evidence of injury to the deltoid or syndesmotic ligaments, respectively. Accessory ossicles are occasionally present at the tip of the medial (os subtibiale, Fig. 12c) and lateral (os subfibulare, Fig. 12d) malleoli and should not be confused for avulsion injuries.

The retinacula of the ankle are deep fascial condensations which bind tendons, thus facilitating gliding and preventing bowstringing. These include the superior/inferior extensor, flexor, and superior/inferior peroneal retinacula. By far the most common retinaculum to be injured is the superior peroneal retinaculum with the flexor retinaculum the next most commonly injured. The superior peroneal retinaculum can be injured in isolation or in association with calcaneal fractures [16]. Soft tissue injury of the peroneal retinaculum is best visualized on MRI or ultrasound. Bony avulsions of the retinaculum can be appreciated as small vertical bone fragments along the lateral cortex of the lateral malleolus, called the "fleck" sign (Fig. 13e) [17]. Although much less common, flexor retinaculum avulsions present with similar imaging findings as superior peroneal retinaculum avulsions, a small vertical piece of bone adjacent to the medial cortex of the medial malleolus (Fig. 13f). Avulsions of the tendon retinacula are crucial to identify as retinacular disruption can lead to tendon entrapment (Fig. 14).

**Fig. 10** Pilon fracture. (**a**) Radiograph showing comminuted fracture of the tibial plafond (arrow), indicative of a pilon fracture. (**b**) Coronal and (**c**) sagittal CT image of the same patient demonstrates an area of impaction at the anterior tibial plafond (arrows), which is usually present in pilon fractures

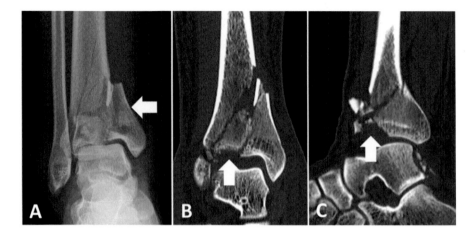

**Fig. 11** Ruedi-Allgower classification of pilon fractures. Type I) Nondisplaced fractures of the tibial plafond. Type II) Simple (i.e., two-part) displaced fractures of the tibial plafond. Type III) Comminuted, displaced fractures of the tibial plafond

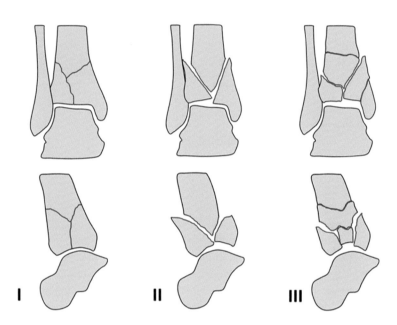

## Hind Foot

### Talus

Talar fractures account for only 3–6% of foot fractures. Of these, talar neck fractures are the most common [18]. The mechanism of injury of talar neck fracture is a combination of high-energy axial force and dorsiflexion of the talus, which causes rupture of the posterior subtalar ligaments followed by impact against the anterior aspect of the tibia. If this force is continued, subtalar and tibiotalar dislocations may result. These fractures are most commonly encountered in motor vehicle collisions and falls from height. The talus serves as a critical link between the leg and foot and has a tenuous vascular supply that is primarily extra-osseous. Therefore, talar neck fractures often lead to significant long-term morbidity, such as osteoarthritis and avascular necrosis [19]. The

Hawkins-Canale classification system is employed to categorize talar neck fractures based on the presence and location of vertical fracture components (Figs. 15 and 16a) [20]. Fracture type is strongly correlated with progression to avascular necrosis [20]. The risk of avascular necrosis for type I, II, III, and IV fractures is 0–20%, 20–50%, 30–100%, and 50–100%, respectively [21].

Lateral (Fig. 16b) and posterior (Fig. 16c) talar process fractures are also relatively common fractures. Both are caused by high-energy forced dorsiflexion/inversion of a pronated foot with some posterior process fractures also caused by forced plantarflexion of the foot [19]. Lateral and posterior talar process fractures can be difficult to visualize on radiographs, and they often present with localized pain and swelling that can be easily mistaken for an ankle sprain. An accessory ossicle is often present at the posterior aspect of

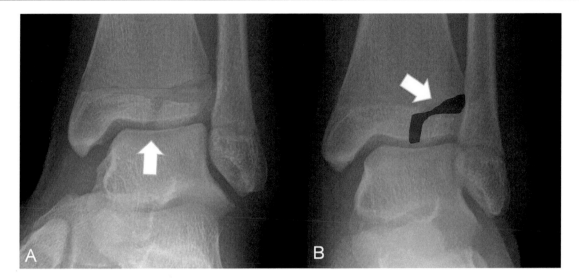

**Fig. 12** AP radiograph with internal rotation (**a**) and external rotation (**b**) views. Solid white arrow shows a juvenile Tillaux fracture through the lateral tibial growth plate. Green shaded area shows progressive widening of the epiphysis for increased predisposition for lateral-sided injury. Red shaded area shows the extension of the fracture through the growth plate down to the articular surface

| Types of Tillaux fracture | |
|---|---|
| Lateral malleolar fracture | Low severity |
| Lateral malleolus with syndesmosis involvement | Medium severity |
| Lateral and medial malleolar fracture | Medium severity |
| Lateral malleolar fracture with fibular fracture above the syndesmosis | High severity |

the talus (os trigonum, Fig. 16d), which should not be mistaken for a posterior process fracture.

Another potential talus injury is the osteochondral fracture (Fig. 17), which occurs via impaction. They present with deep ankle pain with weight bearing and ambulation, often impairing sports participation and daily activities in young patients [19]. These fractures affect the articular hyaline cartilage and subchondral bone of the talus, manifesting as detached bone surrounded by radiolucency on routine radiographs. However, radiographs may miss small or posteriorly located injuries, so more sensitive modalities such as CT and MRI may provide more information, especially regarding the cartilage [13].

## Calcaneus

Calcaneal fractures account for 60% of all tarsal fractures and occur bilaterally in about 10% of cases [22]. Calcaneal fractures can be classified as intra-articular or extra-articular based on the involvement of the subtalar joint posterior facet. Calcaneal fractures are commonly caused by falls from height and are frequently associated with other fractures, particularly of the thoracolumbar spine.

Extra-articular calcaneal fractures are comprised of impaction- and avulsion-type injuries. Achilles avulsion fractures are rare and typically result in complete avulsion of the Achilles tendon requiring surgical fixation. The avulsion fracture may just involve the Achilles attachment, but often the fracture line propagates horizontally along the entire length of the posterior calcaneal tuberosity in what is commonly referred to as a "tongue-type" fracture (Fig. 18a). Small avulsion fractures of the anterior process (Fig. 18b) are common and can be easily mistaken for an accessory ossicle (os calcaneal secundaris, Fig. 18c) that often occurs in this region. The two most common locations for extra-articular impaction fractures are the cuboid facet (Fig. 18d) and posterior calcaneal tuberosity.

Intra-articular fractures are characterized as having a primary fracture line that extends vertically from the posterior subtalar facet through the inferior calcaneal body and a secondary fracture line extending from the calcaneal body either through the superior cortex of the posterior tuberosity ("joint-depression type," Fig. 19a) or through the posterior cortex below the Achilles insertion ("tongue type," Fig. 19b). Tongue-type fractures need special surgical consideration to address the unstable tongue of calcaneal bone containing the Achilles insertion. Intra-articular calcaneal fractures can be easily missed on radiographs due to the complex osteology of the calcaneal. If CT is utilized to evaluate for intra-articular calcaneal fractures, oblique reformats parallel and perpendicular to the posterior facet of the subtalar joint should be obtained so as to optimally evaluate the intra-articular fracture lines.

Bohler's angle and angle of Gissane can both be used to help identify intra-articular calcaneal fractures [23, 24]

**Fig. 13** Avulsion fractures of the
ankle. (**a**) Deltoid ligament
avulsion. (**b**) Lateral ligament
complex avulsion. (**c**) Os
subtibiale. (**d**) Os subfibulare. (**e**)
Superior peroneal retinaculum
avulsion. (**f**) Flexor retinaculum
avulsion

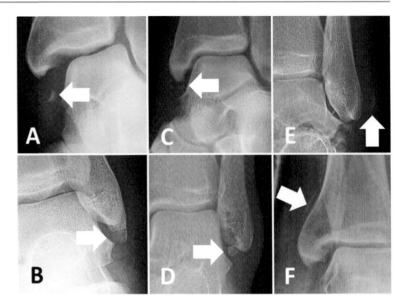

**Fig. 14** Superior peroneal
retinacular avulsion fracture with
common peroneal tendon
entrapment. (**a**) Bone window. (**b**)
Soft tissue window

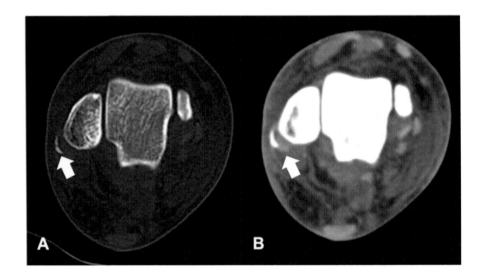

(Fig. 19a, c). A Bohler's angle <20° indicates collapse of the posterior facet from an impacted intra-articular fracture. An angle of Gissane greater than 130° also indicates an impacted intra-articular fracture. These measurements are of limited utility as the measurements will not be abnormal in all intra-articular calcaneal fractures, and most fractures can be identified without the use of these measurements [25].

The Sanders classification system is the most commonly used classification for intra-articular calcaneal fractures (Figs. 19d and 20) [26]. In this classification, the posterior facet is divided by three lines (A, B, C). The classification is based on the number and location of displaced fracture lines at the posterior facet which is used for both prognosis and to guide surgical treatment. Type I fractures have no displaced posterior facet fracture lines, type II fractures have one displaced fracture line, type III have two displaced fracture

lines, and type IV have more than two displaced fracture lines. Type II and III fractures can be further subcategorized based on which fracture lines are displaced.

Another complication of intra-articular calcaneal fracture is the involvement of the sustentaculum tali. This medial process of the calcaneal is an integral support to the subtalar joint with close proximity to the flexor hallucis longus. Nearly one-half of patients with an intra-articular calcaneal fracture demonstrate a sustentacular fracture. Twelve percent of these fractures showed a displacement of >2 mm. Although misalignment of the sustentaculum tali is rare, special consideration should be given to displaced fractures as they can cause misalignment and entrapment of the flexor bundle. This injury is more prevalent in high-grade Sanders calcaneal fractures. This is often best visualized on an axial view of the calcaneal on CT.

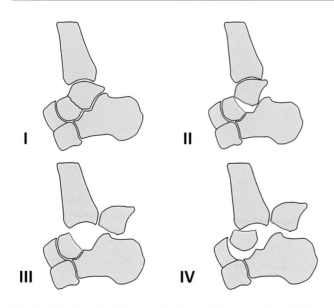

**Fig. 15** Hawkins classification of talar neck fractures. Type I) Non-displaced fracture through the talar neck. Type II) Displaced neck fracture with subluxation of the subtalar joint. Type III) Displaced neck fracture with subluxation of the subtalar and tibiotalar joints. Type IV) Displaced neck fracture with subluxation of the subtalar, tibiotalar, and talonavicular joints

# Midfoot

## Cuboid

Cuboid fractures are relatively rare, comprising less than 3% of foot and ankle fractures [27]. Most cuboid fractures are caused by direct compression of the cuboid between the calcaneal and the fourth and fifth metatarsal bases. This has been likened to the crushing of a walnut between the leavers of a nutcracker, and these types of cuboid compression fractures have been called "nutcracker" fractures [19]. Almost all cuboid fractures occur in the setting of high-energy trauma; therefore, cuboid fractures are often associated with other foot injuries [28]. Like many mid- and hind foot fractures, cuboid fractures are often difficult to recognize on radiographs, leading to frequent misdiagnosis.

Cuboid fractures can generally be categorized as avulsion- (Fig. 21a) or compression-type fractures with compression-type fractures further subdivided based on whether they involve the entire length of the cuboid (Fig. 21b) or just a portion of the length (Fig. 21c). Other important characteristics of cuboid fractures to assess are degree of fracture displacement and comminution of the fracture. Cuboid fractures also tend to result in shortening of the lateral column of the

**Fig. 16** Talus fractures. (**a**) Hawkins III fracture with dislocated tibiotalar and subtalar joints with displaced talus body. (**b**) Lateral talar process fracture. (**c**) Posterior talar process fracture. (**d**) Os trigonum

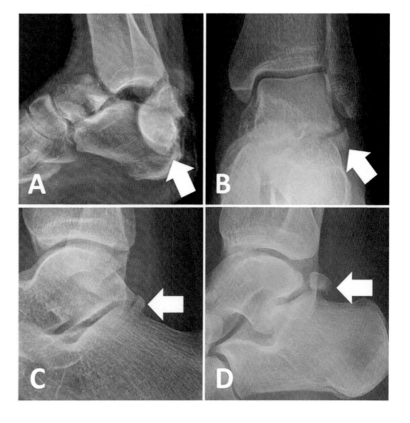

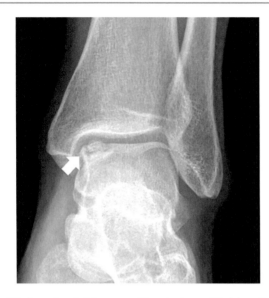

**Fig. 17** Osteochondral fractures of the talar dome: AP plain radiograph of the ankle showing displaced fragment of the medial talar dome. Special consideration should be given to any small fleck of bones

foot, particularly cuboid fractures involving the entire cuboid length, so degree of cuboid length loss is also important. Particular note should also be made of displaced fragments involving the peroneal groove as the peroneus longus tendon can become entrapped as it courses beneath the cuboid.

## Navicular

Navicular fractures are slightly less common than cuboid fractures, comprising approximately 2% of all foot and ankle fractures [27]. Multiple classification systems for navicular fractures exist, but there is no single widely used classification system. Navicular fractures can be generally categorized as capsular avulsion fractures (Fig. 22a), fractures of the navicular tubercle (Fig. 22b), and fractures of the navicular body. Fractures of the navicular body can occur as simple sagittal (Fig. 22c) or coronal fractures through the mid-body or present as comminution of the body (Fig. 22d). Most navicular fractures are the result of high-energy trauma; however, navicular fractures can occur in

**Fig. 18** Extra-articular calcaneal fractures. (**a**) Tongue-type Achilles tendon avulsion. (**b**) Anterior process avulsion. (**c**) Os calcaneus secundaris. (**d**) Impaction of the cuboid facet

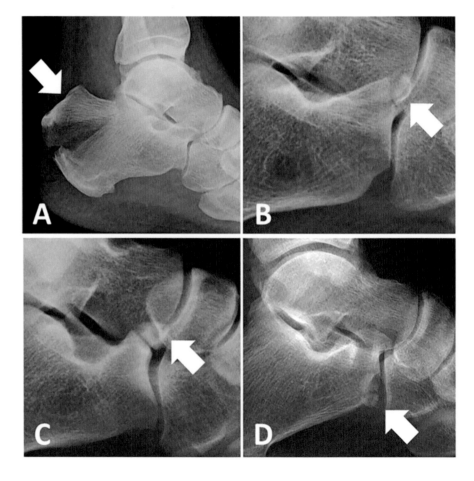

**Fig. 19** Intra-articular calcaneal fractures. (**a**) Joint-depression fracture with secondary fracture line extending through superior calcaneus cortex (arrow). Bohler's angle is decreased to less than 20°. (**b**) Tongue-type fracture with secondary fracture line extending through the posterior cortex inferior to the Achilles tendon insertion. (**c**) Joint-depression fracture with increase in angle to Gissane to greater than 130°. (**d**) Sanders 2B calcaneal fracture with single displaced intra-articular fracture line at the junction of the medial and middle thirds of the articular surface

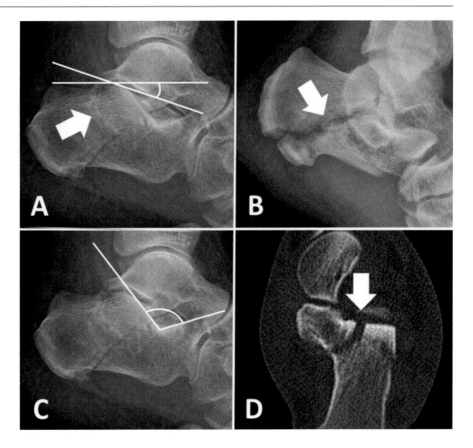

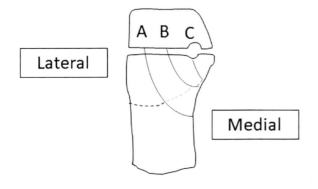

Two Fragments:
    Type IIA: -- and A
    Type IIB: --, -- and B
    Type IIC: --, --, --, and C
Three Fragments:
    Type IIIAB: --, A and B
    Type IIIAC: --, A and C
    Type III BC: --, --, B and C
Four Fragments:
    Type IV: --, A, B, and C

**Fig. 20** Sanders classification of intra-articular calcaneal fractures

low-energy twisting injuries [37], usually in conjunction with forced plantar flexion or dorsiflexion of the midfoot [29]. Similar to shortening of the lateral foot column seen in cuboid fractures, fractures of the navicular are at risk for shortening of the medial foot column. Important characteristics of navicular fractures to describe are orientation of the fracture line (coronal vs. sagittal), comminution, degree of displacement, involvement of the navicular tubercle, and presence of midfoot subluxation. Note should be made of the portion of the navicular body involved, as the middle one-third of the bone is relatively avascular, and fracture here carries the largest potential for long-term complications.

### Lisfranc Joint

The Lisfranc joint consists of the articulation between the tarsal bones and metatarsals. Lisfranc joint dislocation is the most common dislocation of the foot. The major ligament stabilizer of the Lisfranc joint is the Lisfranc ligament complex, which spans the Lisfranc interval, the space between the medial cuneiform and base of the second metatarsal. In addition to the Lisfranc ligament complex, strong intermetatarsal ligaments span the bases between the second and fifth metatarsal. These intermetatarsal ligaments rarely

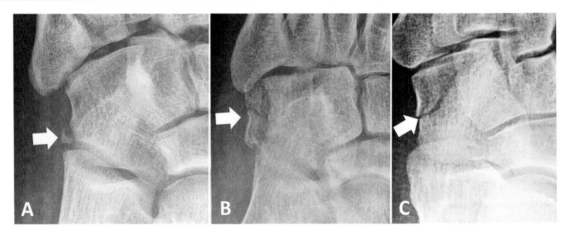

**Fig. 21** Cuboid fractures. (**a**) Avulsion fracture of the calcaneocuboidal joint capsule. (**b**) Comminuted fracture spanning the entire length of the lateral cuboid. (**c**) Oblique fracture isolated to the distal half of the cuboid

**Fig. 22** Navicular fractures. (**a**) Avulsion fracture of the navicular. (**b**) Fracture of the navicular tubercle. (**c**) Nondisplaced sagittal fracture of the navicular body. (**d**) Comminuted fracture of the body with dorsal dislocation

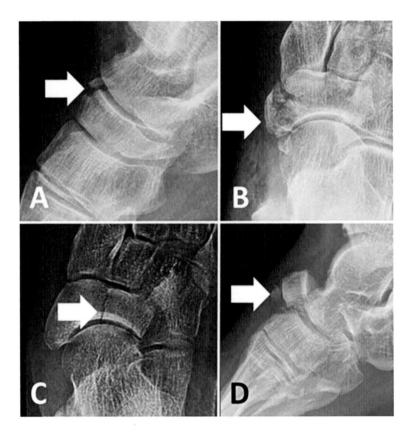

tear; as a result, the second through fifth metatarsal bases typically displace in the same direction during Lisfranc injuries.

Lisfranc joint injuries can be divided between high-impact fracture-displacements and low-impact midfoot sprains. High-impact injuries are usually due to direct force, such as in motor vehicle accidents or crush injuries. Low-impact injuries are usually due to indirect forces and are more commonly encountered in sports [28].

The most consistent indicator of a Lisfranc injury is lateral displacement of the second metatarsal base relative to the middle cuneiform, resulting in a step-off along the medial borders of these bones and a diastasis between the bones measuring >2 mm on AP radiographs [28]. Often, a small avulsion fracture of the Lisfranc ligament can be seen in the Lisfranc interval (Fig. 23a); however, it should be noted an accessory ossicle (os intermetatarseum) is often in this region and can be mistaken for an acute avulsion injury. Slight step-

**Fig. 23** Lisfranc joint injuries. (**a**) Small avulsion fracture of the Lisfranc ligament with widening of the Lisfranc interval. (**b**) Subtle dorsal step-off at the second tarsometatarsal joint. (**c**) Total incongruent Lisfranc joint (Hardcastle-Myerson type A) with lateral displacement. (**d**) Complete, divergent Lisfranc joint injury (Hardcastle-Myerson type C)

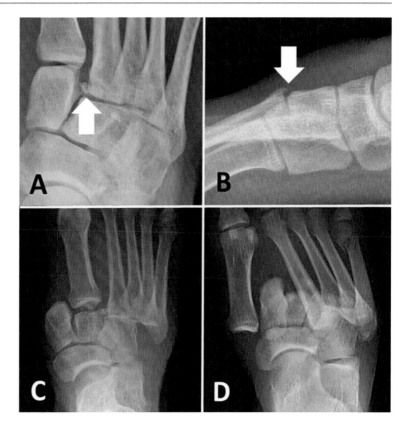

off along the dorsal (Fig. 23b) and medial aspect of the tarsometatarsal joints can also be a subtle finding of Lisfranc injury, which can be accentuated with weight-bearing imaging. It is important to remember that small avulsion fractures or malalignments of the Lisfranc joint can be a "tip-of-the-iceberg" finding indicating a much more severe soft tissue injury to the joint.

The most widely used classification system for Lisfranc injuries is the Hardcastle-Myerson system [30]. This system divides Lisfranc injuries into three types based on whether there is complete or partial Lisfranc joint disruption and the direction of displacement (Figs. 23c, d and 24). The Hardcastle-Myerson system is useful to provide a simple, unified set of terminology for describing Lisfranc fracture-dislocations. However, the system has little utility in gauging prognosis or guiding surgical management.

## Forefoot

### Metatarsals

The most common fractures of metatarsals involve the head or shaft of the bone. Approximately 80% of metatarsal fractures will be minimally displaced and can be treated conservatively [31]. General indications for surgery include displacement of more than 3–4 mm, more than 10° of dorsoplantar angulation, and fracture or multiple metatarsals [32]. The first metatarsal bears a disproportionate amount of load-bearing force during ambulation compared to the other four "lesser" metatarsals, and because of this, surgical treatment is more aggressive for first metatarsal fractures.

Fractures at the base of the fifth metatarsal are another common forefoot fracture. Fifth metatarsal base fractures are typically described based on whether the fracture involves the tarsometatarsal joints (Fig. 25a) or is extra-articular (Fig. 25b). Extra-articular fractures, also called "Jones" fractures, are most commonly located 2 cm distal to the proximal tuberosity and are at increased risk for nonunion compared to their intra-articular, "pseudo-Jones," counterpart. As such, Jones fractures are often treated surgically, while pseudo-Jones fractures typically heal with only conservative management [33]. Fractures of the other metatarsal bases are typically managed conservatively unless there is excessive displacement or the fracture occurs as part of a larger Lisfranc joint injury pattern.

### Soft Tissue Injuries

There are many soft tissue injuries that can occur in the foot and ankle. However, in the emergency setting, the most important injuries to consider are injuries to the ligaments, tendons, and neurovascular structures. As previously discussed, the most important joints to evaluate for ligament

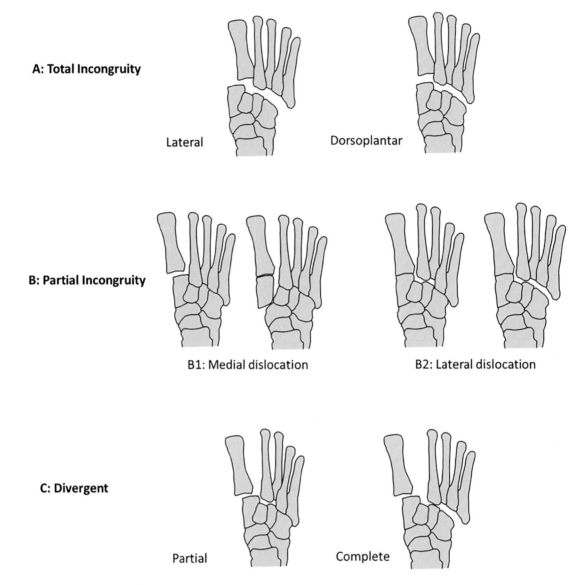

**A: Total Incongruity**

Lateral          Dorsoplantar

**B: Partial Incongruity**

B1: Medial dislocation          B2: Lateral dislocation

**C: Divergent**

Partial          Complete

**Fig. 24** Hardcastle-Myerson classification of Lisfranc fracture-dislocations

**Fig. 25** Fifth metatarsal base fractures. (**a**) Intra-articular fracture of the metatarsal base (pseudo-Jones fracture). (**b**) Extra-articular fracture of the metatarsal base (Jones fracture)

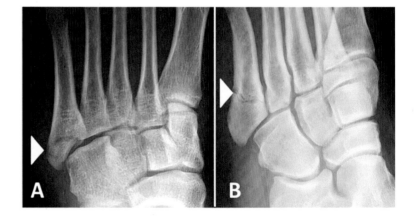

instability are the tibiotalar, ankle syndesmosis, and Lisfranc joints, and stability of these joints can usually be adequately assessed on routine and stress radiography. MRI is excellent at depicting acute rupture of the major ligaments of the ankle and foot (Fig. 26) [34], and MRI can be helpful for diagnosing ligament injuries in patients with equivocal stress

**Fig. 26** MRI of ankle and foot ligaments. (**a**) Normal band-like appearance of ATFL extending from lateral malleolus to lateral process of the talus (arrow). (**b**) Thickened and increased signal of ATFL (arrowhead) representing a high-grade partial tear. (**c**) Normal striated appearance of Lisfranc ligament extending between the medial cuneiform and base of the second metatarsal (arrow). (**d**) Slight widening of the Lisfranc interval with high signal and irregular appearance of the Lisfranc ligament (arrowhead) representing ligament rupture

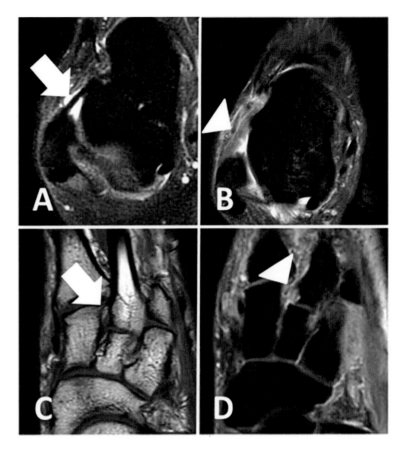

**Fig. 27** Achilles tendon rupture. (**a**) Sagittal MRI and (**b**) sagittal ultrasound in the same patient demonstrating full-thickness tear of Achilles tendon (arrows) with 5 cm of intact distal tendon (asterisks)

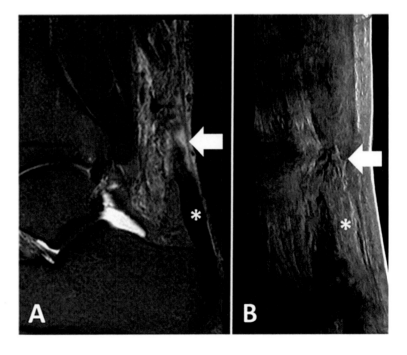

imaging or who are unable to tolerate stress exams. Ultrasound is another alternative for assessing ligaments.

MRI and ultrasound are also excellent at identifying acute injuries to the tendons of the ankle and foot. The Achilles tendon is the most commonly injured ankle tendon and it is a frequent cause of emergency center visits [35]. Achilles tendon rupture most commonly (75%) occurs at the vascular watershed area located 2–6 cm proximal to the calcaneal insertion [36]. MRI (Fig. 27a) and ultrasound (Fig. 27b) are optimal for evaluation of the Achilles tendon. Approximation of the level of retraction of the two ruptured ends of the tendon and degree of cross-sectional involvement are two key factors in management [36].

## Summary

Ankle and foot injuries are commonly encountered and carry the potential for significant long-term morbidity and complications. Numerous structures in the ankle and foot can undergo a variety of mechanisms of injury, slight variations of which may have significant implications in management and prognosis. Imaging evaluation is crucial in the diagnosis and treatment of ankle and foot injuries. Radiography is the most common and typically first tool used in imaging assessment of ankle injuries. However, other modalities such as CT and MRI have roles in assessing radiographically occult injuries, and imaging evaluation beyond routine radiographs is usually indicated in patients presenting with a functionally limiting injury to the ankle or foot.

## Key Points

I. Radiographs are usually adequate for evaluating fractures of the ankle and foot. However, CT is often beneficial for characterizing known pilon and midfoot/hind foot fractures and for identifying occult fractures when a high clinical suspicion for fracture is present.

II. Stressed or weight-bearing images of the ankle and foot can help identify unstable injuries of the ankle and midfoot that may not be visible on initial non-weight-bearing imaging.

III. Avulsion fractures of the ankle and foot are very common. A basic knowledge of soft tissue anatomy of the ankle and foot can help identify these injuries.

## References

1. Rui P, Kang K. National Hospital Ambulatory Medical Care Survey: 2017 emergency department summary tables. National Center for Health Statistics. Available from: https://www.cdc.gov/nchs/data/nhamcs/web_tables/2017_ed_web_tables-508.pdf

2. Lambers K, Ootes D, Ring D. Incidence of patients with lower extremity injuries presenting to US emergency departments by anatomic region, disease category, and age. Clin Orthop Relat Res. 2012;470(1):284–90.

3. Hermans JJ, Beumer A, De Jong TA, Kleinrensink G. Anatomy of the distal tibiofibular syndesmosis in adults: a pictorial essay with a multimodality approach. J Anat. 2010;217(6):633–45.

4. Peace K, Hillier J, Hulme A, Healy J. MRI features of posterior ankle impingement syndrome in ballet dancers: a review of 25 cases. Clin Radiol. 2004;59(11):1025–33.

5. Park SS, Kubiak EN, Egol KA, Kummer F, Koval KJ. Stress radiographs after ankle fracture: the effect of ankle position and deltoid ligament status on medial clear space measurements. J Orthop Trauma. 2006;20(1):11–8.

6. Harper MC. An anatomic and radiographic investigation of the tibiofibular clear space. Foot Ankle. 1993;14(8):455–8.

7. Sivakumar BS, An VVG, Oitment C, Myerson M. Subtle lisfranc injuries: a topical review and modification of the classification system. Orthopedics. 2018;41(2):e168–75.

8. Egol KA, Koval KJ, Zuckerman JD. Handbook of fractures. Lippincott Williams & Wilkins; 2010.

9. Hetta WM, Niazi G. Concordance of US and MRI for diagnosis of ligamentous and tendinous injuries around the ankle. Egypt J Radiol Nucl Med. 2018;49(1):131–7.

10. Morvan G, Busson J, Wybier M, Mathieu P. Ultrasound of the ankle. Eur J Ultrasound. 2001;14(1):73–82.

11. Horton LK, Jacobson JA, Powell A, Fessell DP, Hayes CW. Sonography and radiography of soft-tissue foreign bodies. AJR Am J Roentgenol. 2001;176(5):1155–9.

12. Okanobo H, Khurana B, Sheehan S, Duran-Mendicuti A, Arianjam A, Ledbetter S. Simplified diagnostic algorithm for Lauge-Hansen classification of ankle injuries. Radiographics. 2012;32(2):E71–84.

13. Greenspan A. Orthopedic imaging: a practical approach. Lippincott Williams & Wilkins; 2014.

14. Rüedi TP, Allgöwer M. The operative treatment of intra-articular fractures of the lower end of the tibia. Clin Orthop Relat Res. 1979;138:105–10.

15. Mainwaring BL, Daffner RH, Riemer BL. Pylon fractures of the ankle: a distinct clinical and radiologic entity. Radiology. 1988;168(1):215–8.

16. Golshani A, Zhu L, Cai C, Beckmann NM. Incidence and association of CT findings of ankle tendon injuries in patients presenting with ankle and hindfoot fractures. AJR Am J Roentgenol. 2017;208(2):373–9.

17. Davda K, Malhotra K, O'Donnell P, Singh D, Cullen N. Peroneal tendon disorders. EFORT Open Rev. 2017;2(6):281–92.

18. Hak DJ, Lin S. Management of talar neck fractures. Orthopedics. 2011;32(9):715–21.

19. Melenevsky Y, Mackey RA, Abrahams RB, Thomson NB. Talar fractures and dislocations: a radiologist's guide to timely diagnosis and classification. Radiographics. 2015;35(3):765–79.

20. Alton T, Patton DJ, Gee AO. Classifications in brief: the hawkins classification for talus fractures. Clin Orthop Relat Res. 2015;473(9):3046–9.

21. Metzger MJ, Levin JS, Clancy JT. Talar neck fractures and rates of avascular necrosis. J Foot Ankle Surg. 1999;38(2):154–62.

22. Badillo K, Pacheco JA, Padua SO, Gomez AA, Colon E, Vidal JA. Multidetector CT evaluation of calcaneal fractures. Radiographics. 2011;31(1):81–92.

23. Boehler L. Diagnosis, pathology and treatment of fractures of the os calcis. J Bone Joint Surg. 1931;13:75–89.

24. Gissane W. Discussion on fractures of the os calcis. Proceedings of the British Orthopedic Association. J Bone Joint Surg. 1947;29:254–5.

25. Knight JR, Gross EA, Bradley GH, Bay C, LoVecchio F. Boehler's angle and the critical angle of Gissane are of limited use in diagnosing calcaneal fractures in the ED. Am J Emerg Med. 2006;24(4):423–7.

26. Sanders R, Fortin P, DiPasquale T, Walling A. Operative treatment in 120 displaced intraarticular calcaneal fractures. Results using a prognostic computed tomography scan classification. Clin Orthop Relat Res. 1993;290:87–95.

27. Shibuya N, Davis ML, Jupiter DC. Epidemiology of foot and ankle fractures in the United States: an analysis of the National Trauma Data Bank (2007 to 2011). J Foot Ankle Surg. 2014;53(5):606–8.

28. Siddiqui NA, Galizia MS, Almusa E, Omar IM. Evaluation of the tarsometatarsal joint using conventional radiography, CT, and MR imaging. Radiographics. 2014;34(2):514–31.

29. Ramadorai MU, Beuchel MW, Sangeorzan BJ. Fractures and dislocations of the tarsal navicular. J Am Acad Orthop Surg. 2016;24(6): 379–89.

30. Mahmoud S, Hamad F, Riaz M, Ahmed G, Al Ateeq M, Ibrahim T. Reliability of the Lisfranc injury radiological classification (Myerson-modified Hardcastle classification system). Int Orthop. 2015;39(11):2215–8.

31. Cakir H, Van Vliet-Koppert ST, Van Lieshout EM, De Vries MR, Van Der Elst M, Schepers T. Demographics and outcome of metatarsal fractures. Arch Orthop Trauma Surg. 2011;131:241–24.

32. Bica D, Sprouse RA, Armen J. Diagnosis and management of common foot fractures. Am Fam Physician. 2016;93(3):183–91.

33. Richli WR, Rosenthal DI. Avulsion fracture of the fifth metatarsal: experimental study of pathomechanics. AJR Am J Roentgenol. 1984;143(4):889–91.

34. Gaebler C, Kukla C, Breitenseher MJ, et al. Diagnosis of lateral ankle ligament injuries. Comparison between talar tilt, MRI and operative findings in 112 athletes. Acta Orthop Scand. 1997;68(3): 286–90.

35. Miller TT. Common tendon and muscle injuries: lower extremity. Ultrasound Clin. 2007;2(4):595–615.

36. Pedowitz D, Kirwan G. Achilles tendon ruptures. Curr Rev Musculoskelet Med. 2013;6(4):285–93.

37. Harris G, Harris C. Imaging of tarsal navicular stress injury with a focus on MRI: a pictorial essay. J Med Imaging Radiat Oncol. 2016;60(3):359–64.

# Imaging of Nontraumatic Musculoskeletal Conditions

**43**

Gregg W. Bean and Michael A. Davis

## Contents

G. W. Bean (✉) · M. A. Davis
University of Texas Health San Antoni, San Antonio, TX, USA
e-mail: beang@uthscsa.edu; davism8@uthscsa.edu

© Springer Nature Switzerland AG 2022
M. N. Patlas et al. (eds.), *Atlas of Emergency Imaging from Head-to-Toe*,
https://doi.org/10.1007/978-3-030-92111-8_43

### Abstract

A wide variety of musculoskeletal conditions can present to the emergency department. In addition to trauma and internal derangement, infectious diseases of the musculoskeletal system are a common occurrence, especially in centers with a large diabetic population. These infections can involve the superficial soft tissues, as in cellulitis, or can extend to the deep soft tissues, bones, and joints. Of these, necrotizing fasciitis is the most feared and a true surgical emergency. If left untreated, some of these relatively nonaggressive soft-tissue infections can progress and result in abscess, osteomyelitis, and septic arthritis.

Bursitis, presenting with pain or as a palpable abnormality, is another condition which can present emergently. This is usually caused by an underlying inflammatory process or repetitive microtrauma, although this could also have an infectious etiology. An imbedded foreign body from recent minor trauma is an infrequent complaint of patients. Imaging examinations can determine if a retained foreign body is present and allows for preoperative planning.

### Keywords

Abscess · Bursitis · Diabetic myonecrosis · Necrotizing fasciitis · Septic arthritis · Osteomyelitis · Bisphosphonate · Pathologic fracture

## Introduction

Patients present to the emergency department with a wide variety of acute musculoskeletal complaints, other than trauma. Chief among these conditions are the infectious processes of the extremities, many of which are more common in the diabetic population. Some of these entities can be potentially life and limb-threatening. Infectious and noninfectious bursitis and retained foreign bodies are other conditions which are sometimes encountered in the emergency department. When presented with an imaging examination, the radiologist must be mindful of these diagnoses, and not limit their search pattern to trauma only. In addition, there are a couple unique fractures which deserve discussion, namely, pathologic fractures associated with bisphosphonate use or underlying bone tumor.

## Cellulitis

Knowledge of the anatomy of the soft tissues is essential to understand the spread of infection and imaging findings. Infections of the epidermis and dermis include erysipelas and cellulitis. The hypodermis is composed of the deeper soft tissues, including the subcutaneous fat. The term superficial fascia is applied to the fascia within this subcutaneous fat. The deep fascia is composed of the peripheral deep fascia, which is contiguous with the epimysium, and is at the interface between the subcutaneous fat and the underlying muscle, and the deep intermuscular fascia which separates muscles into compartments (Fig. 1, Illustration 1).

## Epidemiology and Clinical Features

Cellulitis, a superficial soft tissue infection confined to the dermis and subcutaneous fat, is the most common musculoskeletal infection encountered in clinical practice [1–3]. Cellulitis manifests clinically as pain, swelling, erythema, and warmth. Systemic manifestations may also be present. Infection most commonly occurs following disruption of the skin, and *Staphylococcus aureus* is the most common causative organism. Susceptibility is increased by peripheral vascular disease, diabetes, and immunodeficiency. Uncomplicated cellulitis is most commonly diagnosed clinically and is treated with systemic antibiotics.

## Diagnostic Investigations

Radiographs typically show nonspecific subcutaneous soft-tissue thickening and increased density. Ultrasound demonstrates skin thickening with variable subcutaneous edema and

**Fig. 1** Extremity soft-tissue fascial compartmental anatomy

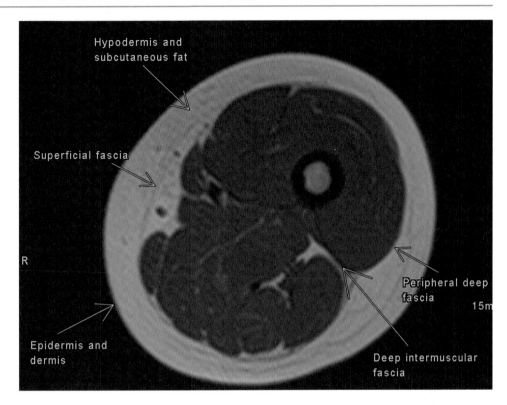

**Illustration 1** Layers of soft tissue. Anatomic structures relevant to soft-tissue infection, including skin, subcutaneous tissue, deep fascia, and muscle

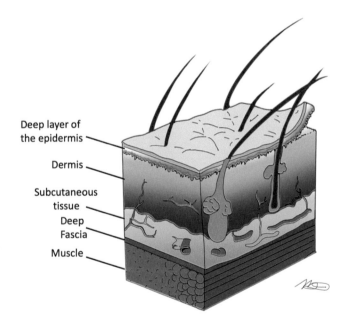

fluid. In some cases, small linear fluid collections tracking along interlobular septa and between echogenic fat lobules give a characteristic "cobblestone" appearance [4]. Non-infectious conditions such as heart failure, venous insufficiency, or lymphedema can have a similar appearance, but color or power Doppler ultrasound can be used to demonstrate hyperemia, increasing the specificity for cellulitis (Fig. 2) [5]. Ultrasound is helpful for differentiating cellulitis from venous thrombosis, although the two entities may coexist [3].

CT and MRI are useful when there is rapid progression or concern for abscess formation or deeper infection. CT demonstrates skin thickening, reticular abnormal soft-tissue attenuation, and variable soft-tissue enhancement (Fig. 3) [6]. MR demonstrates subcutaneous high-signal intensity on fluid-sensitive sequences and low signal intensity on T1-weighted images. Enhancement after IV gadolinium administration is helpful to differentiate cellulitis from non-infectious causes of edema

## Conclusions/Summary

- Cellulitis is confined to the dermis and subcutaneous fat.
- Noninfectious conditions such as heart failure, venous insufficiency, and lymphedema can have a similar appearance.
- CT and MRI are useful when there is rapid progression or concern for abscess formation or deep infection.

## Bursitis

### Epidemiology and Clinical Features

Bursitis, or inflammation of a bursal cavity, is usually non-infectious and results from trauma, repetitive stress, crystal-line arthropathy, or inflammatory arthropathy. When infectious, *Staphylococcus aureus* is the most common

agent. The olecranon and prepatellar bursae are most commonly infected, due to their superficial location and suscep-tibility to minor trauma [6]. Infection of deeper bursae including the iliopsoas bursa and subacromial-subdeltoid bursa often result from extension of inflammation from an adjacent joint. Treatment of an infectious bursitis is typically with antibiotic therapy, although complicated cases may require surgery [4].

### Diagnostic Investigations

Radiographs typically show nonspecific soft-tissue fullness [3]. MRI is sensitive for fluid distension of the bursa and surrounding edema (Fig. 4). The bursal wall is typically thick-ened and enhances. Similarly, CT demonstrates distension of the bursa and wall enhancement. CT and MRI are also useful for detecting adjacent bone and joint involvement. Ultrasound demonstrates bursal wall thickening and fluid distension of the bursa with mixed echogenicity material and sometimes debris. Color Doppler will show bursal wall hyperemia.

There is substantial imaging overlap between reactive or inflammatory bursitis and infectious bursitis. The sole reli-able distinguishing finding is emphysema, which can result from a gas-forming organism. If infection is suspected based on clinical and laboratory findings, fluid sampling should be performed [3, 4].

**Fig. 2** Cellulitis on ultrasound. A 32-year-old man with cellulitis. Ultrasound longitudinal image demonstrates diffuse edema in the subcutaneous soft tissues, with small linear fluid collections tracking along the interlobular septa and between fat lobules. Color Doppler demonstrates hyperemia

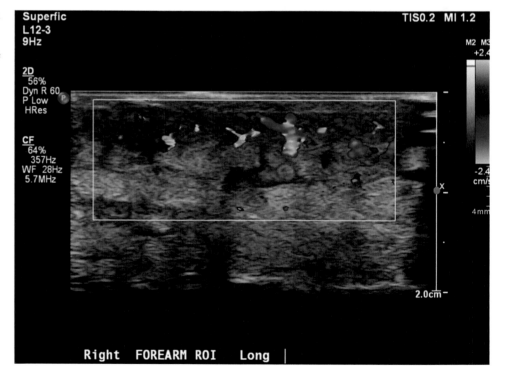

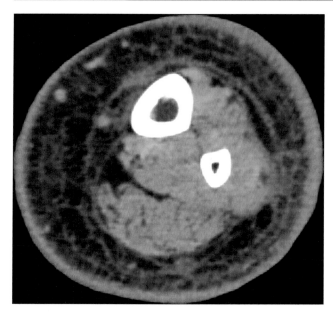

**Fig. 3** Cellulitis on CT. A 31-year-old man with cellulitis. Axial CT image of the left calf demonstrates skin thickening and extensive subcutaneous soft-tissue edema in a reticular pattern

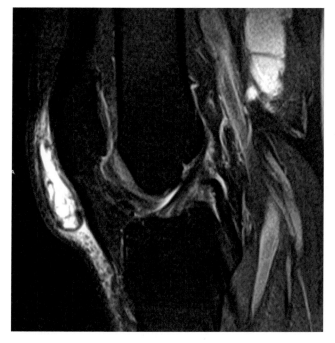

**Fig. 4** Prepatellar bursitis. A 39-year-old man with prepatellar bursitis. Sagittal T2-wighted fat-suppressed MR image reveals hyperintense signal within a complex, well-defined collection. Regional soft-tissue edema is present

## Conclusions/Summary

- Bursitis is most commonly noninfectious.
- The olecranon and prepatellar bursae are most commonly involved due to their superficial location.

- If infection is clinically suspected, fluid sampling should be performed.

## Foreign Bodies

### Epidemiology and Clinical Features

Retained foreign bodies are a common presenting problem in the emergency department and may present in an acute or delayed fashion. The most common materials are wood, glass, and metal. Complications include infection, nerve or vascular injury, and granulomatous reaction [7].

### Diagnostic Investigations

Radiographs are a good initial screening examination for suspected foreign bodies. High-density objects such as those made of metal are easily detected (Fig. 5). Other materials such as plastic, wood, and other organic matter are often radiolucent [5]. It is a misconception that glass is not detectable with radiography, or that only lead-containing glass can be detected [8].

Ultrasound is ideal for detecting superficial foreign bodies, particularly of radiolucent material. A high-frequency (7.5 mHz or higher) linear array transducer should be used. A foreign body produces "clean" posterior shadowing if the object has an irregular or curved surface and "dirty shadowing" (posterior reverberation) if the object has a flat, smooth surface (Fig. 6) [11]. A hypoechoic rim surrounding the object represents inflammatory reaction and granulation tissue and may be present as soon as 24 h after the object is embedded. Ultrasound also allows the evaluation of tendons and vascular structures and can be used to guide object removal.

CT has excellent spatial resolution and can be used to precisely localize radiopaque foreign bodies. Non-radiopaque foreign bodies such as wood can be detected with wide window settings [7]. MRI is less commonly used; however, the soft-tissue resolution of MRI is ideal for evaluating soft-tissue complications including abscess, sinus tract, and vascular compromise. Foreign bodies typically demonstrate hypointense signal, signal void, or susceptibility artifact. Granulomatous reaction may have variable appearance and enhancement.

## Conclusions/Summary

- Radiographs are good for initial screening for foreign bodies.
- It is a misconception that glass is not detectable with radiography.

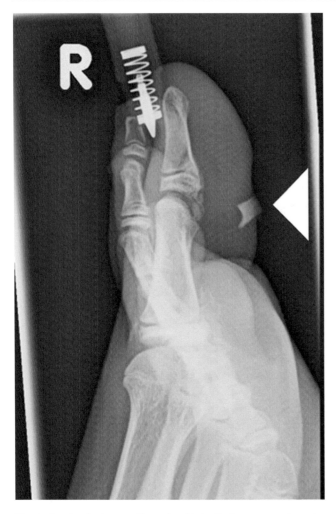

**Fig. 5** Foreign body on radiography. Skeletally immature patient who stepped on glass. Computed radiography lateral image of the patient's right foot demonstrates glass within the superficial soft tissues at the plantar aspect of the great toe (arrowhead)

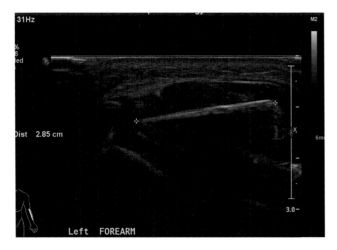

**Fig. 6** Foreign body on ultrasound. A 27-year-old man presenting with retained foreign body. Ultrasound longitudinal image demonstrates a linear echogenic wood splinter within the soft tissues of the left forearm

- Ultrasound is ideal for superficial foreign bodies, particularly of radiolucent material.

## Abscess

### Epidemiology and Clinical Features

An abscess is a localized collection of necrotic tissue, bacteria, and inflammatory exudate within subcutaneous tissue or muscle [5]. The infectious agent is frequently *Staphylococcus aureus* and more than 50% may be methicillin-resistant. Abscesses require drainage in addition to antibiotic treatment.

### Diagnostic Investigations

Radiographic findings of abscess are nonspecific; however, soft-tissue emphysema may be identified. IV contrast-enhanced CT demonstrates a rim-enhancing, thick-walled, fluid collection with variable internal density (Fig. 7a) [4]. On MRI, an abscess demonstrates uniform or heterogeneous high-signal intensity on fluid-sensitive sequences and intermediate to low signal intensity on T1-weighted sequences, as well as peripheral enhancement on post-contrast images. Internal necrotic contents do not enhance. Foci of signal void within the collection representing emphysema may be present. The surrounding tissues are typically edematous [4]. The ultrasound appearance of abscess is a complex fluid collection with mixed echogenicity and a thick, hyperechoic, and hyperemic wall (Fig. 7b). Increased through transmission is typical, and internal air bubbles may be seen [4].

Abscess formation within skeletal muscle, or pyomyositis, is usually the result of hematogenous spread. Healthy muscle is resistant to infection, so pyomyositis generally occurs in the setting of a predisposing factor, particularly diabetes, IV drug use, trauma, or immunodeficiency [3]. The muscles of the lower extremity are most commonly involved. Early muscle infection is characterized by muscle enlargement, edema, and effacement of fat planes on MR and CT. Mature intramuscular abscesses demonstrate extensive surrounding inflammatory changes, which help differentiate them from differential considerations including neoplasm, intramuscular hematoma, and diabetic myonecrosis.

## Conclusions/Summary

- IV contrast-enhanced CT and MRI demonstrate a rim-enhancing, thick-walled fluid collection with non-enhancing contents.

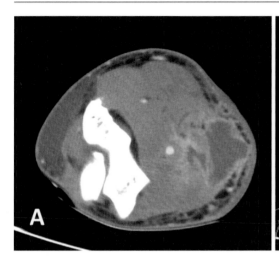 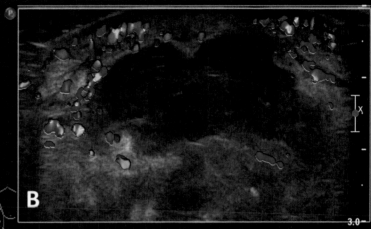

**Fig. 7** Abscess. A 57-year-old man with history of IV drug abuse and swelling about the elbow. (**a**) IV contrast-enhanced axial CT image through the right elbow demonstrates an intramuscular fluid collection with peripheral enhancement consistent with pyomyositis. (**b**) Concurrent transverse ultrasound image with color Doppler demonstrates the abscess cavity with complex fluid and surrounding hyperemia

- Intramuscular abscess often occurs in the setting of diabetes, IV drug abuse, trauma, or immunodeficiency.
- Extensive surrounding inflammatory changes help differentiate pyomyositis from neoplasm, hematoma, and diabetic myonecrosis.

## Diabetic Myonecrosis

### Epidemiology

On the list of differential diagnoses for pyomyositis is diabetic myonecrosis, which is due to thrombosis and embolism of the small intramuscular vessels [1]. The mortality rate is 10%, not due to myonecrosis, but due to the complications of long-term diabetes including cardiovascular disease [10].

### Clinical Features

Long-standing type 1 and 2 diabetics present with acute pain, swelling, and induration of the involved muscles. A palpable mass may be present. The anterior muscle compartment of the thigh, especially the vastus muscles, and the calf are the most commonly involved [10]. Often multiple, noncontiguous and bilateral muscles are affected.

Laboratory values are mostly normal except for glucose, hemoglobin A1c, and ESR. Creatinine kinase is sometimes mildly elevated [10]. Although the patient may be mildly febrile, the white blood cell count is normal, differentiating between diabetic myonecrosis and pyomyositis.

### Diagnostic Investigations

CT demonstrates nonspecific subcutaneous and muscular edema (Fig. 8a). MRI can be helpful to distinguish between diabetic myonecrosis, pyomyositis, and other causes of myositis. T1-weighted images demonstrate enlargement of the involved muscles with loss of the normal intramuscular fatty streaks [11]. Hyperintensity can be seen on T1-weighted images when there is hemorrhagic necrosis. Intramuscular, fascial, and subcutaneous edema is demonstrated as hyperintensity on T2-weighted/STIR sequences (Fig. 8b). Although the patient's nephropathy may preclude administering contrast, the classic enhancement pattern is either diffuse or peripheral rim-like, with some areas of linear enhancement traversing the central areas of non-enhancement (Fig. 8c). These linear areas of enhancement are strands of inflamed tissue in between the areas of necrosis [11].

The diagnosis is confirmed using the patient presentation, history of diabetes, and laboratory values. Treatment is conservative, with aggressive control of blood glucose, analgesics, anti-inflammatories, and antiplatelet therapy. Biopsy should not be performed given the potential for complications and can actually increase the chance of recurrence [10].

### Conclusions/Summary

- Diabetic myonecrosis involves the anterior muscular compartment of the thigh and calf.
- MRI findings include enlargement and edema of the involved muscles with either heterogeneous diffuse or peripheral rim-like enhancement.

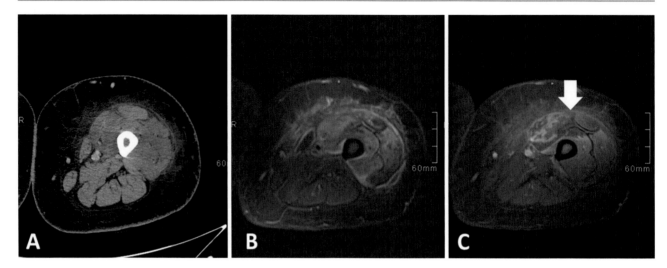

**Fig. 8** Diabetic myonecrosis. A 42-year-old afebrile woman with uncontrolled diabetes presenting to the ER with left lower extremity pain for 3 weeks. Blood glucose was 548 mg/dL. (**a**) CT axial image through the mid-thigh demonstrating enlargement and hypodensity (edema) of the vastus musculature. (**b**) MR T2-weighted with fast suppression axial image, showing hyperintensity in the vastus muscles and rectus femoris with surrounding subcutaneous and superficial fascial edema. (**c**) Post-contrast T1-weighted axial MR image with fat suppression demonstrating heterogenous but predominantly peripheral enhancement (arrow)

- Diagnosis is based on history of present illness, long-term diabetes, and laboratory values.
- Treatment is conservative.

## Necrotizing Fasciitis

### Epidemiology

In the USA each year, there are approximately 700–1200 cases of necrotizing fasciitis [12]. In Western Europe, there is approximately 1 case in 100,000 individuals compared to 0.4 cases in 100,000 individuals in the USA [13]. The most commonly affected regions are the extremities, trunk, and perineum [3]. The reported mortality rate varies from 22% to as high as 80% [14, 15] and correlates with a delay in diagnosis and surgical debridement [16]. The most common organisms to infect the soft tissues are *Staphylococcus aureus* and *Streptococcus pyogenes* [3].

### Clinical Features

Initially, symptoms are similar to cellulitis, with erythema and tenderness to palpation. The proliferation of bacteria results in microvascular invasion and thrombosis, resulting in necrosis [16]. Necrosis manifests as bullae and blisters, and later as hemorrhagic bullae, skin anesthesia and discoloration, and crepitus [16].

Patients present with fever, hypotension, and septic shock. However, in immunocompromised patients, these symptoms may be absent [16]. Pain is out-of-proportion to the findings on physical examination and are elicited beyond the region of erythema.

Necrotizing fasciitis is a clinical diagnosis. However, distinguishing between cellulitis and a deep soft-tissue infection can be difficult. Wong et al. developed the Laboratory Risk Indicator for Necrotizing Fasciitis (LRINEC) score in 2004 (Table 1) [17]. A score of 5 or less confers a low risk, 6–7 is intermediate, and 8 or greater confers a high risk. A LRINEC score cutoff of 6 or greater suggests the presence of necrotizing fasciitis with a PPV of 92% and NPV of 96% [17].

### Diagnostic Investigations

Imaging can provide useful information in determining the extent of infection and expedite patient management.

Radiographs are relatively insensitive, often demonstrating only soft-tissue edema. The percentage of patients that exhibit soft-tissue emphysema on radiographs varies from 13% to 55% (Fig. 9a) [14, 15]. However, radiographs often demonstrate soft-tissue emphysema before crepitus is discovered on physical examination [15].

Given the availability in emergency departments and fast acquisition time, CT is often performed, and has a sensitivity of 80% for diagnosing necrotizing fasciitis [15]. The diagnosis is suggested by identifying deep, thick intermuscular fascial edema (Fig. 9c). Soft-tissue emphysema tracking along the fascial planes is better appreciated on CT than radiography (Fig. 9b, c) [4].

**Table 1** The Laboratory Risk Indicator for Necrotizing Fasciitis (LRINEC) score; score of $\leq 5$ = low risk, 6–7 = intermediate risk, $\geq 8$ = high risk

| Parameter | Score |
|---|---|
| C-reactive protein (mg/L) | |
| <150 | 0 |
| $\geq 150$ | 4 |
| WBC count (mm$^3$) | |
| <15 | 0 |
| 15–25 | 1 |
| >25 | 2 |
| Hemoglobin (g/dL) | |
| >13.5 | 0 |
| 11–13.5 | 1 |
| <11 | 2 |
| Sodium (mmol/L) | |
| $\geq 135$ | 0 |
| <135 | 2 |
| Creatinine (mg/dL) | |
| $\leq 1.6$ | 0 |
| >1.6 | 2 |
| Glucose (mg/dL) | |
| $\leq 180$ | 0 |
| >180 | 1 |

Adapted from Wong CH et al. [18]

Although MR imaging is considered the imaging reference standard for the diagnosis, with a sensitivity of 93% [15], it is often not performed due to the long acquisition time. An MR should not delay treatment. If an MR is performed, the key finding is thick, 3 mm or more, T2-/STIR-hyperintensity in the deep intermuscular fascia involving multiple compartments. A lack of deep intermuscular edema virtually excludes necrotizing fasciitis [16]. If contrast is administered, enhancement of the deep intermuscular fascia is variable [3, 14].

Urgent surgical debridement is the cornerstone of treatment. The diagnosis of necrotizing fasciitis can be confirmed by the presence of foul-smelling "dishwater" fluid, grayish fascia, loss of resistance to blunt dissection, and absence of bleeding [16, 18].

## Conclusions/Summary

- Although necrotizing fasciitis is a clinical diagnosis, imaging can help confirm the diagnosis and assess the degree of extent.
- Tracking soft-tissue emphysema along the fascia and deep intermuscular fascial edema are the hallmarks of the imaging diagnosis.
- MRI should not delay surgical treatment.

- Prognosis worsens with a delay in diagnosis and surgical debridement. Necrotizing fasciitis is a surgical emergency.

## Septic Arthritis

## Epidemiology

Although a joint can become infected through direct inoculation or contiguous spread from an overlying soft-tissue infection, a septic joint is most often due to hematogenous dissemination. There were approximately 16,000 emergency department visits in the USA for septic arthritis in 2012 [19] with an incidence of 4–10/100,000 patient-years/year in Western Europe [20]. The mortality rate is approximately 3–25% [21]. The risk factors include prior joint surgery, recent joint injection, rheumatoid arthritis, immunocompromise (including diabetes), IV drug use, and adjacent soft tissue or osseous infection. Of note, a therapeutic joint injection carries as much as a 0.04% chance of developing septic arthritis [22]. *Staphylococcus aureus* is the most common etiologic bacteria, followed by streptococci [22].

## Clinical Features

About 80% of patients present classically with erythema, edema, and limited range of motion of the involved joint [19]. Although patients usually have elevated WBC, ESR, and CRP, others are afebrile and have relatively normal laboratory values. Given the variability in presentation, imaging can aid in narrowing the differential diagnosis.

## Diagnostic Investigations

Imaging evaluation should begin with a radiograph [23]. Initially, the radiograph may be normal or show soft-tissue swelling and joint effusion. Hyperemia presenting as diffuse demineralization is sometimes present. As the infection progresses, cartilage loss with resultant joint space narrowing and osseous erosions representing osteomyelitis can be identified (Fig. 10a). On MRI, a joint effusion is common but is absent in almost a third of cases, more commonly present in larger joints (Fig. 10b) [24]. The joint effusion is often complex with surrounding synovial thickening and enhancement (Fig. 10b). Diffuse or focal T2-weighted hyperintensity in the adjacent bone is often present (Fig. 10c) [24]. Obtaining an MRI prior to aspiration can yield unsuspected findings such as an overlying abscess which can alter management. However, the diagnosis of septic arthritis is confirmed by joint aspiration.

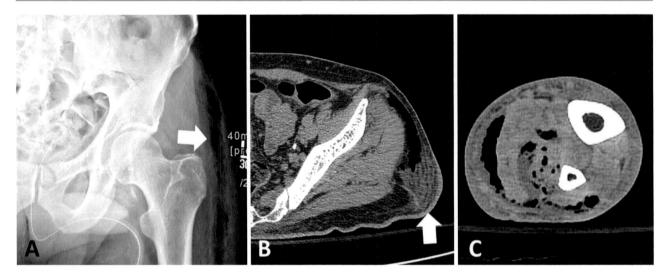

**Fig. 9** Necrotizing fasciitis. A 63-year-old man found down with altered mental status. On physical examination, he was found to have gangrenous toes with cellulitis and crepitus extending proximally to the level of the hip. The patient was taken to the OR, where upon incision, there was pus and dishwater-appearing fluid. LRINEC = 10. (**a**) AP pelvic radiograph demonstrating soft-tissue emphysema along the left lateral hip (arrow). (**b**) CT axial image at the same level with emphysema tracking along the peripheral deep muscular fascia (arrow). (**c**) CT axial image at the level of the mid-tibial diaphysis demonstrating fluid and emphysema in the deep intermuscular fascia

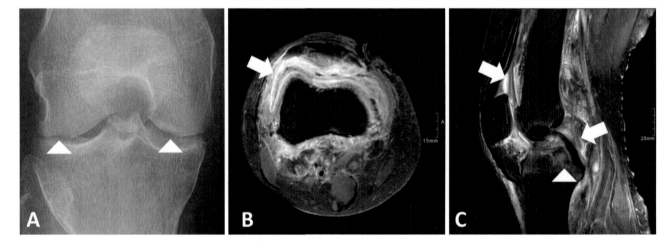

**Fig. 10** Gonococcal septic arthritis of the right knee in a 38-year-old woman. (**a**) AP knee radiograph demonstrating erosions along the weight-bearing surfaces of the medial and lateral femoral condyle (arrowheads). There was no joint effusion on the lateral radiograph (not shown). (**b**) Post-contrast T1-weighted-fat suppressed axial MR image at the level of the distal quadriceps tendon demonstrating synovial thickening and enhancement (arrow), peri-synovial soft-tissue enhancement, and a lack of joint effusion. (**c**) T2-weighted with fat suppression sagittal MR image demonstrating tibial plateau bone marrow edema (arrowhead), lack of joint effusion, and edema in the synovium and peri-synovial soft tissues (arrows)

## Conclusions/Summary

- In almost a third of patients with septic arthritis, a joint effusion is absent.
- An MRI can demonstrate overlying abscesses which can change management.
- MRI findings include an effusion with synovial thickening and enhancement. Bone marrow edema is common.
- The diagnosis is confirmed with aspiration.

## Pedal Osteomyelitis

### Epidemiology

An estimated 435 million people have diabetes throughout the world with the prevalence quadrupling since 1980 [25]. Approximately 75 million of these will develop a foot infection sometime during their life [25].

## Clinical Features

The most common sites of pedal osteomyelitis are the small toe metatarsal, hallux metatarsal head, hallux distal phalanx, and calcaneus [26]. Although most ulcerations are along the plantar surface, clawtoe deformities or ill-fitting shoes can result in dorsal ulcerations due to friction and pressure of the toes along the top of the footwear. Osteomyelitis in the foot is due to contiguous spread from an adjacent ulcer. Therefore, knowledge of the location of the ulcer is key.

## Diagnostic Investigations

Radiographs are low in sensitivity. Findings may not be present in adults for 10–14 days, and only after approximately 30–50% of bone mineral content has been eroded [27]. Changes on radiographs include erosion, loss of the normal cortical white stripe, and aggressive periosteal reaction (Fig. 11a).

On MRI, a geographic, intramedullary region of confluent T1-iso to hypointense (equal to or less than muscle) represents osteomyelitis (Fig. 11b). Subcortical or hazy, reticular signal abnormality should not be diagnosed as osteomyelitis [28]. Although there should be corresponding T2-hyperintense signal equal to joint fluid, this hyperintensity extends beyond the region of infected bone. Therefore, T1-weighted images should be used to make the diagnosis. IV-contrast administration is used to characterize findings in the adjacent soft tissues, including abscess, sinus tracks, and necrosis, but not to diagnose osteomyelitis.

The field of view of the MR examination should only include the area adjacent to the ulcer. Therefore, protocols should be developed to image the hindfoot, midfoot, or forefoot, not the entire foot.

## Conclusions/Summary

- Pedal osteomyelitis occurs due to contiguous spread of infection from an ulcer. Knowing the location of the ulcer is essential.
- Although radiographs are relatively insensitive, they may demonstrate erosion, loss of the normal cortical white strip, or aggressive periosteal reaction.
- Osteomyelitis can be diagnosed on MRI using T1-weighted images. Intramedullary, geographic, confluent T1 iso- to hypointense signal represents infection.
- The MRI should only include the region adjacent to the ulcer. The field of view should not include the entire foot.

## Bisphosphonate-Associated Fractures

### Epidemiology and Clinical Features

Osteoporosis is a major public health issue worldwide with an estimated 10–21 million women affected and approximately 9 million osteoporotic fractures annually [29]. Bisphosphonates are the preferred form of treatment and have been shown in randomized trials to improve bone mineral density and lower fracture risk. The mechanism of bisphosphonates involves osteoclast apoptosis resulting in inhibition of bone resorption.

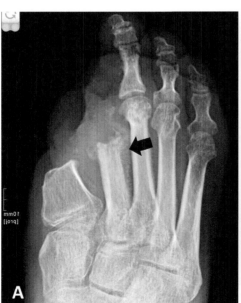
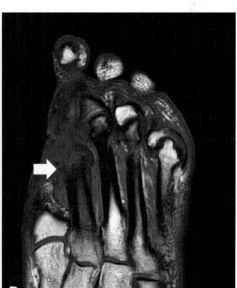

**Fig. 11** Pedal osteomyelitis. A 44-year-old man with a history of amputations, now wound dehiscence with drainage. (**a**) AP radiograph of the left foot shows spiculated, aggressive periosteal reaction about the second toe metatarsal diaphysis (arrow). (**b**) Axial (long axis) T1-weighted MR image of the forefoot demonstrating geographic, intramedullary T1-iso to hypointense signal consistent with osteomyelitis (arrow)

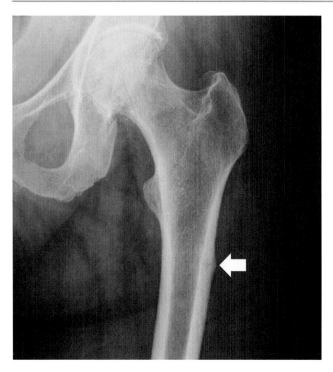

**Fig. 12** Bisphosphonate-associated fracture of the femur. Anteroposterior radiograph of a 63-year-old woman with a characteristic bisphosphonate-related fracture demonstrating focal lateral cortical thickening and a subtle transverse fracture orientation in the subtrochanteric femur (arrow)

Osteoclast inhibition results in decreased bone turnover as normal osteoclast resorption is followed by repair and remodeling of bone by osteoblasts [29]. Over-suppression of bone turnover leads to microdamage accumulation and atypical skeletal fragility [30]. A strong association has been found between bisphosphonate usage and what are called "atypical femur fractures (AFFs)" involving the lateral cortex of the femoral shaft, an area of high tensile stress.

The absolute risk of AFFs is low and increases with long-term bisphosphonate use. The ASBMR reported an incidence of 2/100,000 cases/year after 2 years of bisphosphonate use, increasing to 78/100,000 cases/year after 8 years of use [31].

## Diagnostic Investigations

Atypical femur fractures have characteristic features which have been described by the American Society for Bone and Mineral Research (ASBMR) Task Force. They include location along the lateral cortex of the femur distal to the lesser trochanter, a transverse fracture line at the lateral cortex associated with focal lateral cortical thickening, no comminution, and minimal or no trauma mechanism (Fig. 12). Atypical femur fractures are often bilateral and may be associated with prodromal symptoms of dull or aching pain in the groin or thigh (Fig. 13) [32].

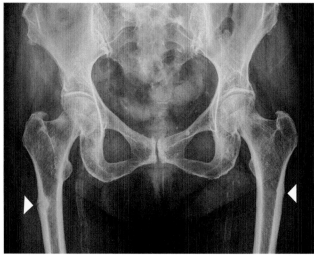

**Fig. 13** Bisphosphonate-associated fractures of the bilateral femurs. Anteroposterior radiograph of the pelvis in a 67-year-old woman with bilateral atypical femoral fractures in the subtrochanteric region (arrowheads)

Recognizing atypical femoral fractures and distinguishing them from typical traumatic fractures is critical to management. Bisphosphonates typically must be stopped, and imaging of the contralateral femur is indicated. Completed fractures are treated with intramedullary rod fixation, and when present, incomplete contralateral fractures are often treated with surgical stabilization as well to avoid the trauma and morbidity of a completed fracture.

## Conclusions/Summary

- A strong association exists between bisphosphonate usage and "atypical femoral fractures."
- Characteristic findings include location distal to the lesser trochanter, a transverse fracture line at the lateral cortex associated with focal lateral cortical thickening, no comminution, and minimal or no trauma mechanism.
- Bilateral fractures are common, and imaging of the contralateral femur is indicated.
- Incomplete fractures are often prophylactically treated with intramedullary fixation.

## Pathologic Fractures

### Epidemiology

An infrequent, but not-to-be-missed diagnosis in the emergency department is a possible pathologic fracture. Pathologic fractures occur in approximately 9–29% of patients with bone metastases [33]. Although a pathologic fracture

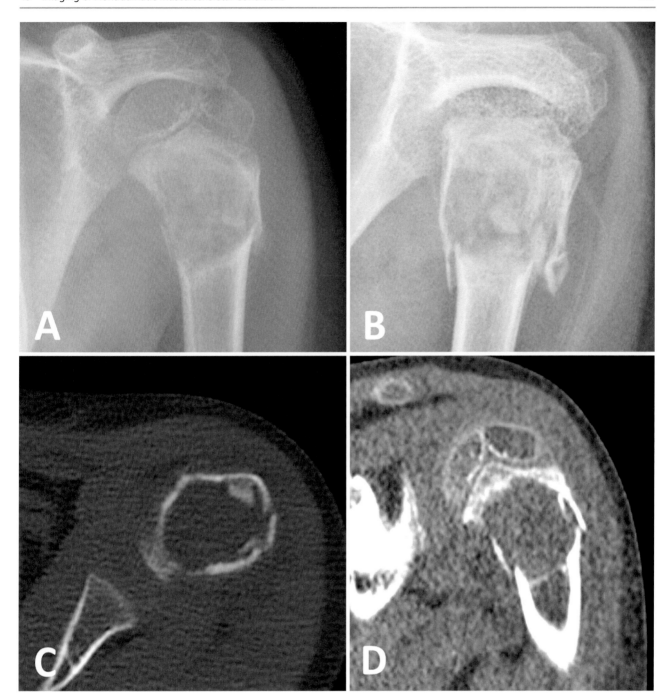

**Fig. 14** Pathologic fracture of the proximal humeral diaphysis. A 6-year-old boy tripped over his dog and fell onto his left upper extremity with immediate pain. Imaging demonstrated a lucent focus in the proximal humerus, with a differential diagnosis favoring a simple or aneurysmal bone cyst. The patient has been treated conservatively. (**a**) AP radiograph in external rotation of the left humerus demonstrating a circumscribed, lucent focus in the proximal humeral diaphysis, with a non-displaced fracture along the medial aspect. (**b**) AP radiograph in internal rotation redemonstrating the pathologic fracture along the anterior and posterior margins. (**c**) CT axial image of the left humerus using bone algorithm demonstrating the fracture with internal displacement of cortical fragments. (**d**) CT coronal image of the left humerus using soft tissue algorithm demonstrating soft-tissue attenuation of the benign tumor, compared to the intramedullary yellow fatty marrow of the proximal humeral diaphysis

can be due to any underlying abnormality, a recent review of hospitalized patients with known malignancy found that metastatic foci from hepatobiliary and renal carcinoma and multiple myeloma are strongly associated with pathologic fractures [33]. In that same review, the most common sites of fractures in decreasing frequency are the vertebrae, hip or

**Table 2** Mirels scoring system. Each abnormality is assigned values (1–3) based on the site, associated pain, tumor characteristic, and size. The sum of these values is used to identify impending pathologic fractures, which necessitates prophylactic nailing. A score of ≤7 = conservative therapy; 8 = equivocal; ≥ 9 = prophylactic nailing

| Score | 1 | 2 | 3 |
|---|---|---|---|
| Site | Upper extremity | Lower extremity | Femoral peritrochanteric region |
| Pain | Mild | Moderate | With use |
| Lesion | Sclerotic | Mixed lucent and sclerotic | Lucent |
| Size (diameter of shaft) | <1/3 | 1/3–2/3 | >2/3 |

femur, humerus, tibia or fibula, and radius. As patient management and prognosis may differ from that of a typical traumatic fracture, correctly diagnosing a pathologic fracture is essential for optimal patient care.

## Clinical Features

A pathologic fracture is a fracture through an existing bone tumor, benign, or malignant. The underlying tumor causes destruction and weakening of the trabecular and/or cortical bone, which can result in a fracture (Fig. 14a, b). The fracture may occur spontaneously due to the weakened bone or as a result of trauma, however trivial.

## Diagnostic Investigations

Often a multimodality approach is used to diagnose pathologic fractures. Initially, radiographs of the fracture site can demonstrate a bone tumor (lucent, mixed lucent and sclerotic, or sclerotic), endosteal scalloping, aggressive periosteal reaction, and a soft-tissue mass, in addition to the fracture. CT (Fig. 14c, d) can aid in confirming the diagnosis, by demonstrating an increased attenuating intramedullary tumoral focus compared to the normal yellow fatty marrow, cortical and endosteal erosion, and improved identification of a soft-tissue mass. In addition, CT allows the radiologist to accurately measure the size of the tumor with respect to the diameter of the shaft of bone.

Compared to CT, MRI can improve diagnostic confidence by identifying a circumscribed T1-hypointense signal abnormality representing the bone tumor. In the absence of a T1- or T2-signal abnormality, a stress fracture is more likely [34]. In addition, MRI can better demonstrate an associated soft-tissue mass and additional metastatic bone foci.

In the case of a patient presenting with pain and known bone metastases, an impending pathologic fracture is a possible diagnosis. Although there are several imaging features which suggest an impending pathologic fracture, the Mirels scoring system is often employed (Table 2). The tumoral focus in question is given a score based on the location (upper or lower extremity, peritrochanteric region), tumor

characteristics (sclerotic, mixed lucent, and sclerotic, or lucent), tumor size (<1/3, 1/3–2/3, or >2/3 the diameter of the bone), and whether or not the tumoral focus is causing pain [35]. A score of 9 or greater is diagnostic of an impending fracture and should be prophylactically nailed, whereas a score of 7 or less is usually treated conservatively. A score of 8 has a 15% chance of going on to fracture and is equivocal [35].

## Conclusions/Summary

- Pathologic fractures are infrequent in the Emergency Department, but their diagnosis is essential for proper patient management.
- Radiographs, CT, and MR all have role in evaluating potential pathologic fractures, with MR best demonstrating the underlying bone involvement.
- The Mirels scoring system is often used to direct patient management, with a score of ≥9 indicating prophylactic fixation.

## References

1. Yu JS, Habib P. MR imaging of urgent inflammatory and infectious conditions affecting the soft tissues of the musculoskeletal system. Emerg Radiol. 2009;16(4):267–76.
2. Fayad LM, Carrino JA, Fishman EK. Musculoskeletal infection: role of CT in the emergency department. Radiographics. 2007;27(6):1723–36.
3. Hayeri MR, Ziai P, Shehata ML, Teytelboym OM, Huang BK. Soft-tissue infections and their imaging mimics: from cellulitis to necrotizing fasciitis. Radiographics. 2016;36(6):1888–910.
4. Turecki MB, Taljanovic MS, Stubbs AY, Graham AR, Holden DA, Hunter TB, Rogers LF. Imaging of musculoskeletal soft tissue infections. Skelet Radiol. 2010;39(10):957–71.
5. Chau CL, Griffith JF. Musculoskeletal infections: ultrasound appearances. Clin Radiol. 2005;60(2):149–59.
6. Yadavalli S. Radiologic evaluation of musculoskeletal soft tissue infections: a pictorial review. Curr Radiol Rep. 2015;3:40.
7. Jarraya M, Hayashi D, de Villiers RV, Roemer FW, Murakami AM, Cossi A, Guermazi A. Multimodality imaging of foreign bodies of the musculoskeletal system. AJR Am J Roentgenol. 2014;203(1): W92–102.
8. Horton LK, Jacobson JA, Powell A, Fessell DP, Hayes CW. Sonography and radiography of soft-tissue foreign bodies. AJR Am J Roentgenol. 2001;176(5):1155–9.

9. Boyse TD, Fessell DP, Jacobson JA, Lin J, van Holsbeeck MT, Hayes CW. US of soft-tissue foreign bodies and associated complications with surgical correlation. Radiographics. 2001;21(5):1251–6.

10. Huang BK, Monu JUV, Doumanian J. Diabetic myopathy: MRI patterns and current trends. Am J Roentgenol. 2010;195:198–204.

11. Glauser SR, Glauser J, Hatem SF. Diabetic muscle infarction: a rare complication of advanced diabetes mellitus. Emerg Radiol. 2008;15:61–5.

12. Centers for Disease Control: Necrotizing fasciitis: all you need to know. 2019. https://www.cdc.gov/groupastrep/diseases-public/necrotizing-fasciitis.html. Accessed 3 May 2020.

13. Maya SP, Beltran DD, Lemercier P, Leiva-Salinas C. Necrotizing fasciitis: an urgent diagnosis. Skelet Radiol. 2014;43:577–89.

14. Yu J. Emergent soft tissue conditions. In: Mirvis S, editor. Problem solving in emergency radiology. Philadelphia: Elsevier; 2015. p. 551–7.

15. Tso DK, Singh AK. Necrotizing fasciitis of the lower extremity: imaging pearls and pitfalls. Br J Radiol. 2018;91:2–6.

16. Wong CH, Wang YS. The diagnosis of necrotizing fasciitis. Curr Opin Infect Dis. 2005;18:101–6.

17. Wong CH, Khin LW, Heng KS, Tan KC, Low CO. The LRINEC (Laboratory Risk Indicator for Necrotizing Fasciitis) score: a tool for distinguishing necrotizing fasciitis from other soft tissue infections. Crit Care Med. 2004;32(7):1535–41.

18. Yoon MA, Chung HW, Yeo Y, Yoo HJ, Kang Y, Chee CG, Lee MH, Lee SH, Shin MJ. Distinguishing necrotizing from non-necrotizing fasciitis: a new predictive scoring integrating MRI in the LRINEC score. Eur Radiol. 2019;29:3414–23.

19. Goldenberg DL, Sexton DJ. Septic arthritis in adults. In: UpToDate. 2020. Available via http://www.uptodate.com. Accessed 25 May 2020.

20. Mathews CJ, Weston VC, Jones A, Field M, Coakley G. Bacterial septic arthritis in adults. Lancet. 2010;375(9717):846–55.

21. Long B, Koyfman A, Gottlieb M. Evaluation and management of septic arthritis and its mimics in the emergency department. West J Emerg Med. 2019;20(2):331–41.

22. Mathews CJ, Weston VC, Jones A, Field M, Coakley G. Bacterial septic arthritis in adults. Lancet. 2010;375:846–55.

23. Beaman FD, von Herrmann PF, Kransdorf MJ, Adler RS, Amini B, Appel M, Arnold E, Bernard SA, Greenspan BS, Lee KS, Tuite MJ, Walker EA, Ward RJ, Wessell DE, Weissman BN: ACR Appropriateness Criteria® suspected osteomyelitis, septic arthritis, or soft tissue infection (excluding spine and diabetic foot). 2016. Available via https://acsearch.acr.org/docs/3094201/Narrative/. Accessed 25 May 2020.

24. Karchevsky M, Schweitzer ME, Morrison WB, Parellada JA. MRI findings of septic arthritis and associated osteomyelitis in adults. Am J Roentgenol. 2004;182:119–22.

25. Chastain CA, Klopfenstein N, Serezani CH, Aronoff DM. A clinical review of diabetic foot infections. Clin Podiatr Med Surg. 2019;36(3):381–95.

26. Ledermann HP, Morrison WB, Schweitzer ME. MR image analysis of pedal osteomyelitis: distribution, patterns of spread, and frequency of associated ulceration and septic arthritis. Radiology. 2002;223:747–55.

27. Pineda C, Espinosa R, Pena A. Radiographic imaging in osteomyelitis: the role of plain radiography, computed tomography, ultrasonography, magnetic resonance imaging, and scintigraphy. Semin Plast Surg. 2009;23(2):80–9.

28. Collins MS, Schaar MM, Wenger DE, Mandrekar JN. T1-weighted MRI characteristics of pedal osteomyelitis. AJR Am J Roentgenol. 2005;185:386–93.

29. Feldman F. Atypical diaphyseal femoral fractures-new aspects. Skelet Radiol. 2012;41(1):75–81.

30. Rosenberg ZS, La Rocca Vieira R, Chan SS, Babb J, Akyol Y, Rybak LD, Moore S, Bencardino JT, Peck V, Tejwani NC, Egol KA. Bisphosphonate-related complete atypical subtrochanteric femoral fractures: diagnostic utility of radiography. AJR Am J Roentgenol. 2011;197(4):954–60.

31. Unnanuntana A, Saleh A, Mensah KA, Kleimeyer JP, Lane JM. Atypical femoral fractures: what do we know about them?: AAOS Exhibit Selection. J Bone Joint Surg Am. 2013;95(2):e8. 1–13

32. Shane E, Burr D, Abrahamsen B, Adler RA, Brown TD, Cheung AM, Cosman F, Curtis JR, Dell R, Dempster DW, Ebeling PR, Einhorn TA, Genant HK, Geusens P, Klaushofer K, Lane JM, McKiernan F, McKinney R, Ng A, Nieves J, O'Keefe R, Papapoulos S, Howe TS, van der Meulen MC, Weinstein RS, Whyte MP. Atypical subtrochanteric and diaphyseal femoral fractures: second report of a task force of the American Society for Bone and Mineral Research. J Bone Miner Res. 2014;1:1–23.

33. Jairam V, Lee V, Yu JB, Park HS. Nationwide patterns of pathologic fractures among patients hospitalized with bone metastases. Am J Clin Oncol. 2020; https://doi.org/10.1097/COC.0000000000000737.

34. Fayad LM, Kawamoto S, Kamel IR, Bluemke DA, Eng J, Frassica FJ, Fishman EK. Distinction of long bone stress fractures from pathologic fractures on cross-sectional imaging: how successful are we? AJR Am J Roentgenol. 2005;185:915–24.

35. Mirels H. Metastatic disease in long bones: a proposed scoring system for diagnosing impending pathologic fractures. Clin Orthop Relat Res. 1989;249:256–64.

# Imaging of Pediatric Traumatic and Nontraumatic Brain Emergencies

Prakash Muthusami, Adam A. Dmytriw, and Manohar M. Shroff

## Contents

**Abstract**

Neuroimaging plays a central role in the initial diagnosis, follow-up, prognosis, and decision-making for various acute intracranial pathologies in children. Whereas the rarity of several of these conditions in children, poorly understood natural histories, limited representation in the literature, nonspecificity of clinical signs, and heterogeneity of treatment responses make frequent neuroimaging desirable, this has to be counterbalanced against associated risks and costs. Considerations which are usually relatively straightforward and minor in adult patients can lead to substantial morbidity and anxiety in pediatric hospitals, for instance, extravasation of even a small amount of IV contrast agent can result in limb edema and/or compartment syndrome. Imaging examinations in small children often require general anesthesia. Similarly, procedures that entail ionizing radiation, i.e., CT and digital subtraction angiography, necessitate diligent

P. Muthusami (✉) · A. A. Dmytriw · M. M. Shroff
Neuroradiology and Image Guided Therapy, Diagnostic Imaging, The Hospital for Sick Children, and University of Toronto, Toronto, ON, Canada
e-mail: prakash.muthusami@sickkids.ca; manohar.shroff@sickkids.ca

© Springer Nature Switzerland AG 2022
M. N. Patlas et al. (eds.), *Atlas of Emergency Imaging from Head-to-Toe*,
https://doi.org/10.1007/978-3-030-92111-8_44

justification with dialogue between the neuroradiologist and the clinical team, with every effort made to ensure that callback examinations are eliminated. This also implies that alternative imaging be performed when feasible for obtaining similar information, for instance, awake bedside transcranial Doppler or alternative fast sequence MR protocol under adequate clinical indications, to assess ventricular size in infants. In yet other cases, established adult pipelines for neuroimaging are not necessarily suitable in children, such as multiphasic CTA for adult stroke patients for triaging of endovascular therapy. Lastly, the availability of pediatric-trained nurses and technologists in a radiology department is fundamental to minimizing morbidity and obtaining high-quality images and for the care of pediatric patients undergoing interventional procedures.

### Keywords

Pediatric Brain Emergencies · Traumatic Brain Injury · Pediatric Stroke · Intracranial hemorrhage · Congenital Infections

## Introduction

Pediatric brain emergencies present with diverse and often nonspecific symptoms. An antecedent history can be revealing, such as headache in the presence of a ventricular shunt suggesting obstruction, or an obvious history of trauma. However, these can often be absent, unreliable, hard to characterize, or evident only after meticulous history-taking from family members. This can lead to delays in referral and diagnosis. Some characteristic presentations in adult patients can be absent in children with similar findings, including hemiplegia following large arterial occlusion, whereas some lesions are specific to the pediatric population, such as in the setting of abusive head trauma (AHT), requiring a keen understanding of neuroanatomy and physiology at different pediatric ages. Acute presentations in children can sometimes bring a longer-standing pathology such as brainstem tumor or moyamoya disease to the fore, be a manifestation of systemic disease including vasculitis or hepatic/hyperammonemic encephalopathy, or be the initial presentation of a syndrome such as intracranial hemorrhage (ICH) in hereditary hemorrhagic telangiectasia (HHT).

In this chapter, we discuss the neuroimaging of common pediatric brain emergencies under specific categories, acknowledging a not-infrequent overlap of presentations and neuroimaging features between these categories.

## Pediatric Traumatic Brain Injury

### Accidental Trauma

Traumatic brain injury (TBI) is the leading cause of death and disability in children [1]. Imaging of TBI includes the assessment of the primary injury (fractures, contusions, cortical lacerations, and hemorrhage) as well as secondary injuries (cerebral edema, ischemia, and vasospasm). Children exhibit distinct pathophysiological responses to neurotrauma depending on severity. In addition, age-specific neuroanatomy and neurophysiology dictate distinctive intra- and extracranial injuries, for instance, large head-body ratio, weak neck muscles, ligamentous laxity, large subarachnoid spaces, thin skull, and flat skull base [2].

### Birth-Related

Delivery using vacuum extraction or forceps is associated with an increased rate of intracranial hemorrhages as compared to unassisted vaginal delivery and caesarian section [3]. Predisposing feto-maternal factors include macrosomia, shoulder dystocia, maternal diabetes, and fetopelvic disproportion. Subdural hemorrhage (SDH) is common on MRI (Fig. 1a), most often infratentorial, but also in the interhemispheric fissures and over the convexities [4]. Proposed mechanisms include shearing or tearing of bridging cortical veins due to sudden pressure changes or overstretching [5]. The prevalence of SDH in asymptomatic neonates ranges between 6.9% and 46% [6] and, often, has no clinical consequences [3]. Most SDH resolve in 4–6 weeks, and SDH seen after 3 months is unlikely to be related to birth-injury [5]. Subarachnoid and intraparenchymal hemorrhages are less frequent.

Extracranial injuries can occur during delivery ranging from clinically inconsequential subperiosteal cephalhematomas to sizeable subgaleal hematomas requiring surgical evacuation, vascular injury with stroke (Fig. 1b), and skull fractures. Molding and deformation in the birth canal can distort skull base synchondroses, potentially resulting in basilar or nuchal impression, or occipital osteodiastasis [7].

### Traumatic Brain Injury in Older Children

Motor vehicle injuries, pedestrian injuries, falls, and sports are common causes of TBI in children [8]. CT is the imaging modality of choice, allowing evaluation of intra- and extracranial injuries (Fig. 2a). MRI can be used to better characterize parenchymal injury, including contusions and cortical lacerations. High brain water content in children can result in substantial edema, setting up a cycle with ischemia and hypoxia. Diffuse axonal injury, when not evident clinically, can be diagnosed on MRI (Fig. 2b) and is associated with poor clinical and cognitive outcomes. Cranial sutures being yet unfused, one must look for sutural diastasis in addition to fractures. Fractures are usually linear, but depressed/ping-pong (Fig. 2c) and compound fractures can present in up to two-thirds of patients. In cases of fractures overlying or indenting a dural sinus, contrast CT venography should be performed. Basal skull fractures can result in cerebrospinal fluid leaks, cranial nerve, or vascular injury [9].

Blunt or penetrating trauma can lead to vascular injury: dissection, occlusion, pseudoaneurysm, or arteriovenous

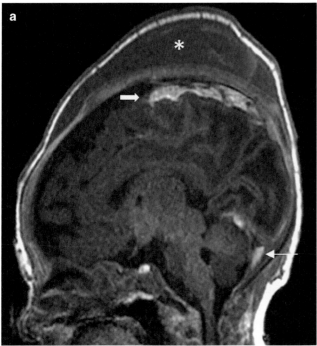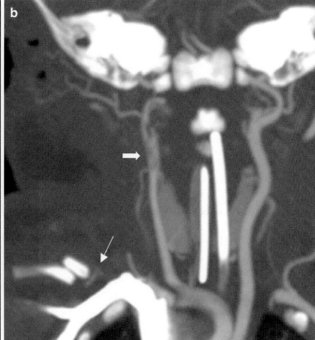

**Fig. 1 Birth-related trauma**: (**a**) neonate, first day of life, following difficult instrumental delivery. Sagittal T1WI showing a large subgaleal hematoma (asterisk), infratentorial (solid arrow), and convexity (block arrow) subdural hemorrhages; (**b**) right clavicular fracture (solid arrow) in another neonate with traumatic delivery seen on a coronal CTA image, with dissection at the carotid bulb (block arrow) that caused a large arterial territorial embolic infarction (not shown here)

fistula formation. The mobile neck in children and "fixed" portions predispose certain arterial segments to injury, e.g., the internal carotid artery at the skull base, the anterior cerebral artery against the falx (Fig. 2d), and the posterior cerebral artery against the tentorium. Secondary effects of TBI can include vasospasm, microcirculatory dysfunction secondary to edema, and raised intracranial pressure [10].

## Pediatric Abusive Head Trauma

Abusive head trauma (AHT) has an incidence of 30 per 100,000 infants and is the most common cause of death from nonaccidental trauma in children [11]. The diagnosis is often challenging with nonspecific clinical and imaging signs. The unique anatomic predispositions to intracranial injury are also relevant to AHT.

The most common intracranial finding in AHT is subdural hemorrhage (SDH), which is often multicompartmental and of differing CT densities (Fig. 3a). Inward displacement of leptomeningeal vessels and effacement of sulci can help to differentiate SDH from benign enlargement of the subarachnoid spaces. CT density alone is relatively unreliable to determine the age of SDH. Acute SDH may be characterized by rapid change in attenuation over serial imaging, redistribution of hemorrhage, and sedimentation of blood products [12], whereas enhancing membranes are considered indicative of chronic SDH [13]. SDH can be associated with bridging vein thrombosis (Fig. 3b), seen as CT density with lack of contrast enhancement, or as blooming on gradient-echo or susceptibility-weighted images: the "tadpole" or "lollipop" signs [14]. Posterior fossa SDH can also be associated with gravitational spinal SDH (Fig. 3c), and with retroclival hematoma, which could indicate craniocervical junction injury [15].

Skull fractures are usually linear and parietal, but multiple, complex, comminuted, diastatic, or depressed fractures, or occipital fractures, should increase the suspicion for AHT [16]. One particular challenge is to distinguish skull fractures from accessory sutures in the developing skull [13]. Although skull radiographs are performed as part of the skeletal series, CT is the modality of choice to definitively exclude fractures. Low-dose CT with 3D surface-shaded or volume-rendered reconstructions are useful (Fig. 3d).

Parenchymal injury can account for major morbidity in AHT. Hypoxic ischemic injury is seen in one-third of AHT patients. It is postulated to be related to shear and stretch injuries at the cervicomedullary junction, although reduced CBF from edema, and large vessel occlusion from herniation, can contribute to morbidity [17]. This is often represented as diffuse supratentorial ischemia with posterior fossa sparing (reversal sign, Fig. 3e).

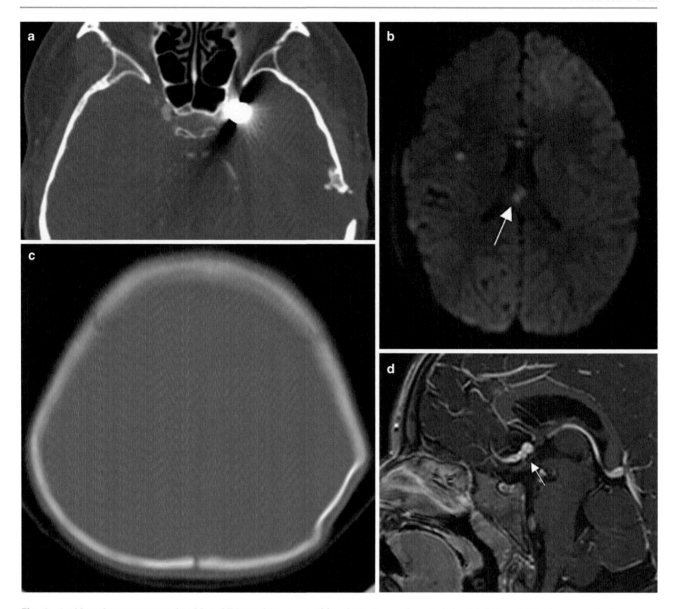

**Fig. 2** **Accidental neurotrauma in older children**: (**a**) teenage girl with shrapnel related to projectile injury. Axial CT image showing the metallic density in the left cavernous sinus. CT is useful to look for foreign bodies that might preclude MRI; (**b**) diffuse axonal injury on axial diffusion-weighted image in an 8-year-old boy following a fall from a height. Multiple punctate foci of diffusion restriction at the corticomedullary junctions and splenium of the corpus callosum (arrow) are characteristic; (**c**) left parietal ping-pong fracture in an 8-month girl with blunt trauma to the skull from an object falling from a height. Axial CT image showing the characteristic flattening associated with inward buckling of the calvarium; and (**d**) sagittal post-gadolinium T1WI in a 7-year-old boy following fall from a height, showing a fusiform aneurysm (arrow) in the A2-anterior cerebral artery, presumably caused by acute arterial dissection against the falx

Diffuse axonal injury can also be seen, with the characteristic appearance of restricted diffusion and microhemorrhages at gray-white interfaces, the corpus callosum, and the brainstem.

(AVM), coagulopathies (32%), and brain tumors (13%), are other causes of nontraumatic pediatric ICH.

## Spontaneous Intracranial Hemorrhage in Children

ICH accounts for half of pediatric stroke and is associated with high mortality and disability [18]. Vascular abnormalities (40–60%), such as an arteriovenous malformation

## Spontaneous ICH in Neonates

Neonatal hemorrhagic stroke is often idiopathic but can be secondary to sinovenous thrombosis, hypoxic/ischemic encephalopathy, or arterial ischemic stroke [19]. In preterm neonates, ICH is most often related to germinal matrix

**Fig. 3** **Abusive head trauma (AHT)**: (**a**) axial CT image in a 9-month girl with AHT showing multicompartmental subdural hemorrhages of differing densities; (**b**) axial susceptibility-weighted image in an 11-month boy with AHT showing blooming artifact related to thrombosis of bridging veins (arrow), with a characteristic "tadpole" appearance; (**c**) sagittal T2WI in a 2-year-old boy with AHT showing a large hypointense lumbar spinal subdural hemorrhage; (**d**) volume-rendered reconstruction from CT in a 2-year-old girl with suspected AHT, showing a complex parietal skull fracture; and (**e**) axial CT image showing the "white cerebellum" or "reversal" sign in severe hypoxic injury in an 18-month boy AHT

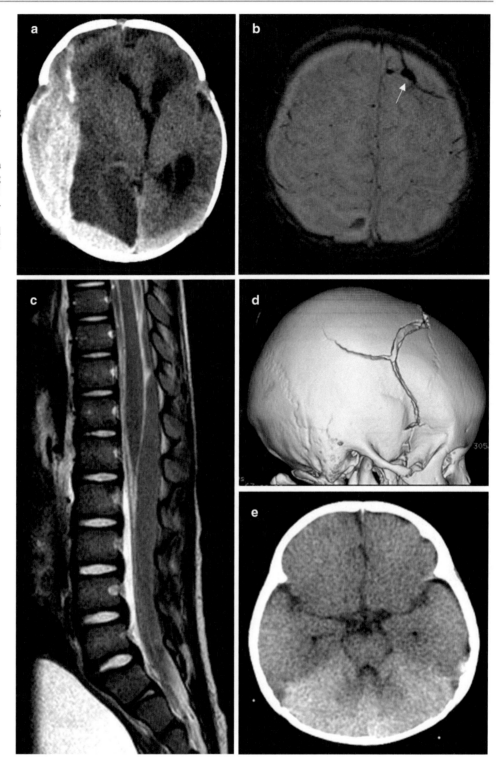

hemorrhage. These are assessed and followed with Doppler sonography and/or MRI. IV contrast-enhanced CT and digital subtraction angiography (DSA) are rarely required, and the decision to perform this entails risk-benefit discussion on an individual case basis.

## Arteriovenous Malformations in Children

The annual risk for brain AVM rupture in children is 2–10% (2–4% across all ages), with a mortality rate up to 25% per event [20]. Risk factors for rupture include previous hemorrhage, infratentorial location, deep venous drainage, nidal aneurysms, venous stenosis, and associated aneurysms. Presentation with multiple AVM, pial arteriovenous fistulae, and capillary malformations (CM) raises the possibility of hereditary hemorrhagic telangiectasia or CM-AVM syndrome (RASA-1 mutation) [21].

CT angiography and MRI allow better characterization of nidus location and brain parenchymal changes (Fig. 4a), whereas CA is the reference standard for AVM characterization and treatment planning. Although early treatment is indicated, a compressive hematoma could necessitate awaiting resorption. High spatial resolution post-gadolinium MRI, with time-of-flight MRA and cone-beam CTA, can provide valuable information and be integrated (Fig. 4b) into intraoperative neuro-navigation software [22].

## Pediatric Intracranial Aneurysms

Intracranial aneurysms in children are rare (<5% of all brain aneurysms) and have different etiologies compared with their adult counterparts, commonly being traumatic, dissecting (Fig. 4c), mycotic, AVM-related, or dysplastic [23]. The terminal internal carotid artery (ICA), cavernous ICA, and posterior circulation are common locations in children. Certain locations such as the proximal MCA and PCA have a propensity for fusiform-dissecting aneurysms. Mycotic aneurysms can be seen in immunocompromised children or in the presence of systemic infection and are often small and distally located. Giant aneurysms (>25 mm) are also more frequent in children [24], as is association with vascular syndromes such as Marfan and Ehler-Danlos, sickle cell anemia, or neurofibromatosis-1.

Although aneurysm growth in childhood years is uncommon [24], long-term follow-up is indicated to monitor for growth or new aneurysm formation [23]. This is ideally performed with TOF-MRA; however, spatial resolution can be limiting, with infundibula being mistaken for aneurysms, requiring CTA [25]. Subarachnoid hemorrhage from aneurysmal rupture in children exhibits a bimodal age distribution, between ages 2 and 5 and after age 15 years [26]. Treatments (surgical, endovascular, or a combination thereof) can be either deconstructive or reconstructive.

## Arterial Ischemic Stroke (AIS)

Pediatric AIS has a diverse etiology, without traditional adult stroke risk factors, and is often under- or misdiagnosed. Increased recent awareness, along with increased survival of children with risk factors including congenital heart disease, sickle cell disease, infections, prothrombothic disorders, and leukemia, has resulted in an increased reported incidence of pediatric AIS [27]. Approximately a third are due to cardioembolism, and approximately half are related to intracranial arteriopathy. Other causes comprise infections, dissection, prothrombotic states, and chronic systemic diseases. Neuroimaging is important for differentiation from stroke mimics, which have been reported in 20–50% of children. These include mitochondrial encephalopathy, lactic acidosis, and stroke-like episodes (MELAS, Fig. 5a), hypoglycemia, demyelinating disorders, tumors, infections, metabolic syndromes, posterior reversible leukoencephalopathy syndrome, and complex migraine (Fig. 5b) [28].

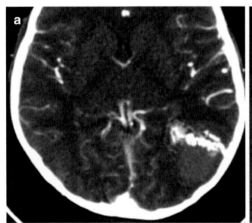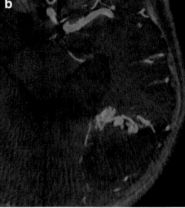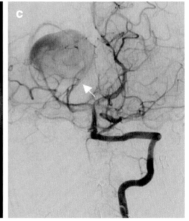

**Fig. 4 Spontaneous intracranial hemorrhage in children**: (**a**) 10-year-old boy with left posterior temporal hematoma related to a compact nidus arteriovenous malformation. The mass effect on the nidus, which is displaced anteriorly, is evident; (**b**) fusion following coregistration of 3D-T1W MRI with CTA reconstruction from 3D-rotational angiography (MRI-DSA fusion) in the same patient showing detailed angioarchitecture and neuroanatomical relations prior to resection; and (**c**) frontal DSA image in a 6-year-old boy with a dissecting aneurysm of the posterior cerebral artery (arrow), presenting with subarachnoid hemorrhage. The site of dissection, at the P1/2 junction, is characteristic and represents microtrauma against the tentorium cerebelli

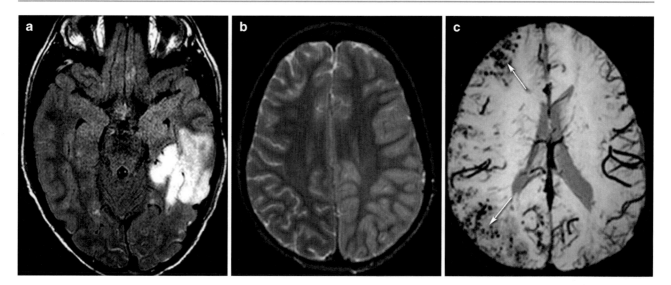

**Fig. 5** **Arterial ischemic stroke in children**: (**a**) axial FLAIR image in a 10-year-old boy with MELAS showing a large area of hyperintensity with edematous swelling in the posterior left temporal region. This showed heterogeneous diffusion restriction, in keeping with a combination of cytotoxic and vasogenic edema. Other smaller infarcts were also seen in the bilateral frontal and left occipital regions (not shown); (**b**) axial T2WI in a 7-year-old boy presenting to the emergency department

with acute hemiplegia, showing diffuse left-sided cortical swelling. This was associated with (not shown) prominent arteries, in keeping with hyperperfusion, and mild gyriform enhancement; and (**c**) axial susceptibility-weighted MR image in a 14-year-old boy with sickle cell disease who presented with stroke. Multiple punctate foci of gyral blooming (arrows) on this axial susceptibility-weighted MR image represent thrombotic microangiopathy

MRI is the modality of choice for children presenting with stroke-like symptoms. DWI can depict acute infarct, while FLAIR depicts subacute and chronic infarcts. TOF-MRA is useful to exclude large vessel occlusion (LVO) and to assess for arteriopathies including focal cerebral arteriopathy, moyamoya disease, or sickle cell arteriopathy. Targeted sequences can help narrow the differential such as vessel wall imaging (VWI) for mural hematoma and wall enhancement, SWI for thrombotic microangiopathy (Fig. 5c), postgadolinium FLAIR for leptomeningeal enhancement, and neck imaging for dissection. When MRI is contraindicated or unavailable, and in certain cases including dissection, CT angiography might provide additional information. DSA is useful in the acute or subacute phase for evaluating cryptogenic stroke, when vasculitis is suspected, and electively for planning revascularization surgery.

## Endovascular Therapy (EVT) for Hyperacute Stroke in Children

The role of endovascular revascularization pediatric hyperacute ischemic stroke is uncertain at present to our knowledge, despite current extensive evidence of benefit in adults. This is partly due to the rarity of clot-related LVO in children but also reflects the challenges in diagnosis and prognostication in pediatric AIS. An individual approach is key, ideally within a dedicated pediatric stroke service. A recent meta-analysis of EVT in pediatric stroke showed approximately

90% successful recanalization rate, and good long-term neurological outcomes, and suggested that EVT be considered for AIS from LVO in patients aged 2–18 years [29].

## Cerebral Sinovenous Thrombosis

Cerebral sinovenous thrombosis (CSVT) can occur in all childhood age groups, 30–50% occurring in neonates [30]. Diverse underlying risk factors, varied clinical presentations, and nonspecific imaging findings make diagnosis challenging. Associated risk factors should be sought, including head and neck infections such as mastoiditis or sinusitis, dehydration, chronic diseases including nephrotic syndrome, and malignancy. With acute presentation, CT (noncontrast CT if a low index of suspicion; CTV for more accuracy) is the modality of choice. MRI is usually reserved for neonates, for assessing secondary changes from ischemia, hemorrhage, cerebral edema and mass effect, and for follow-up. Phasecontrast and time-of-flight MRV provide reliable and often complementary information for diagnosis, while IV gadolinium-enhanced MRV has been shown to be superior noncontrast techniques [31]. Although head ultrasound/Doppler can demonstrate abnormal venous sinus flow in neonates, it is not sensitive enough for excluding smaller or cortical venous clots.

Classical imaging signs are well described: the "dense triangle" sign (clot in dural venous sinus) on noncontrast CT and associated "empty delta" sign on CECT or CT venography, the "cord sign" on CECT (cortical venous clot), or flow void in expected regions of venous flow on MR venography. Venous thrombosis can be detected as hyperdensity on CT (Fig. 6), T1-hyperintensity on MRI, loss of T2-flow void, or blooming on T2*-weighted sequences, indicating deoxyhemoglobin, methemoglobin, or hemosiderin. Indirect signs include white matter edema, hemorrhagic infarction, or cortical subarachnoid hemorrhage. There are several imaging pitfalls, artifacts, and normal variations, including dural sinus hyperattenuation due to high

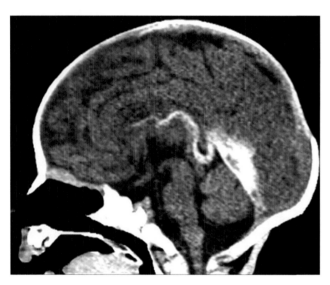

**Fig. 6** **Cerebral sinovenous thrombosis (CSVT) in children.** Sagittal midline noncontrast CT image in a toddler with extensive CSVT showing hyperdense clot in the deep veins

hematocrit, flow gaps related to intravoxel dephasing, skull molding or involuting torcular soft tissue in neonates, encoding velocity ranges for phase-contrast MRV, arachnoid granulations, and persistence of embryonic venous channels. Table 1 summarizes the imaging modalities for venography.

## Intracranial Infections

The severity of brain infections in children is determined by the stage of CNS development, virulence of the pathogen, and immune status. MRI is the modality of choice for investigating infections and their complications.

### Congenital Viral Infections (TORCH: Toxoplasmosis, Other, I.E., Syphilis and HIV, Rubella, Cytomegalovirus, Herpes Simplex Virus)

Infections acquired early in fetal development can generally lead to malformations, while those at the later stages cause destructive foci [32]. Infections can also be transmitted during labor. Fetal and postnatal MRI can help to evaluate CNS anomalies and is of prognostic value.

Common congenital CNS infections including cytomegalovirus, toxoplasmosis, and rubella typically do not present as emergencies and are out of the scope of this chapter. Neonatal herpesvirus infection (usually HSV2 transmitted during labor, or HSV1 postnatally) is typically meningoencephalitis, with or without gyral or leptomeningeal enhancement. Parenchymal herpetic

**Table 1** Comparison of imaging modalities for cerebral sinovenous thrombosis

| Technique | Sequence | Advantages | Disadvantages |
|---|---|---|---|
| MR venography | Time-of-flight | No contrast or ionizing radiation<br>Relatively short acquisition times<br>Maximum intensity projections for global assessment | Prone to motion and saturation effects from in-plane flow<br>False negatives from methemoglobin and other intrinsically T1-hyperintense structures |
| | Phase-contrast | Better background suppression<br>Flow quantification if needed | "Contamination" from arteries<br>Needs setting of optimal encoding velocity according to vessel of interest |
| | Gadolinium Enhanced | Better anatomical visualization<br>Less susceptible to slow or complex flow<br>Can be reformatted in required plane | Need intravenous access<br>Need to inject gadolinium, recent concerns with contrast deposition<br>Longer scan time than noncontrast sequences |
| CT venography | | Rapid assessment, widely available<br>Less prone to motion artifacts<br>More accessible for critical patients or in case of MRI incompatibility | Uses ionizing radiation<br>Requires iodinated contrast agent<br>Artifacts at skull base and posterior fossa<br>Less sensitive to early secondary changes (infarction, edema) |
| Doppler | | Useful for screening in neonates and infants<br>Can be performed at the bedside<br>No ionizing radiation | Low sensitivity<br>Cannot depict all dural sinuses<br>Operator dependent |
| Digital subtraction angiography | | Reference standard for vascular assessment<br>Can guide therapeutic interventions | Invasive, requires general anesthesia in children<br>Uses ionizing radiation<br>Training and expertise needed |

abnormalities are frequent in bilateral cerebral cortices, cerebellum, or deep gray structures [33], best evaluated by DWI, which can also be used to identify remote watershed ischemia. Hemorrhage can be associated with parenchymal abnormalities.

## Acute Viral Infections

MRI is the imaging modality of choice for the investigation of acute viral CNS encephalitis. Findings can include focal or diffuse edema, diffusion restriction from cytotoxic edema, hemorrhagic foci, necrosis, and enhancement.

Herpesvirus infection (HSV1) is an important cause of childhood viral encephalitis, infecting the trigeminal nerve branches through nasopharyngeal mucosa. Resultant abnormalities are T2-FLAIR hyperintense and/or diffusion restricting, involving the cortical and the subcortical regions of bilateral temporal and frontal lobes and insula asymmetrically (Fig. 7a), with basal ganglia sparing [34]. Enhancement is unusual and mild if present, and petechial hemorrhages can develop within affected regions. Extratemporal and brainstem involvement is unusual. Focal abnormalities can progress into cystic encephalomalacia.

Viral cerebellitis (commonly, varicella, Epstein-Barr virus, and enterovirus) can be identified on MRI as areas of cerebellar cortical T2-FLAIR hyperintenstity with or without swelling (Fig. 7b). Varicella and flaviviral (e.g., Japanese encephalitis virus, West Nile virus, and dengue virus)-related abnormalities can also be seen in the basal ganglia and thalami and can be associated with hemorrhages or immune-mediated (Bickerstaff) brainstem encephalitis, potentially mimicking infiltrative tumor or vascular disease [35].

## Bacterial Infections

Common causes of bacterial meningitis vary by age group: group B *Streptococcus* and *S. pneumoniae* in neonates, and *S. pneumoniae* and *Neisseria meningitidis* in infants and older children. MRI is more sensitive than CT for leptomeningeal or ependymal enhancement, seen in more than half of patients [36]. Meningeal inflammation can extend to the cerebral parenchyma, causing cerebritis reflected as T2-FLAIR hyperintensity, gyral swelling with patchy enhancement. Parenchymal abscess formation shows internal diffusion restriction, surrounding edema, rim enhancement, and MR spectroscopic lipid-lactate peak. Vascular involvement can lead to small vessel vasculitis and vasospasm leading to infarction. Subdural empyema is less common but can cause rapid clinical deterioration warranting neurosurgical evacuation. This has higher T1 and FLAIR signal than CSF, with diffusion restriction. Basal cisternal leptomeningeal enhancement should raise the suspicion of tuberculous meningoencephalitis (Fig. 7c), often with perforating artery infarcts [37].

## Acute Encephalopathies

### Hypoxic Ischemic Injury

Global hypoxic/ischemic injury (HII) is a significant cause of neonatal mortality and neurologic disability. The severity of injury and imaging findings is dependent on the stage of brain maturity, duration and severity of insult, and timing of imaging. Neuroimaging, particularly MRI, can show specific patterns of injury.

In severe HII in term neonates, the deep gray structures (putamen, ventrolateral thalamus, hippocampi, and dorsal

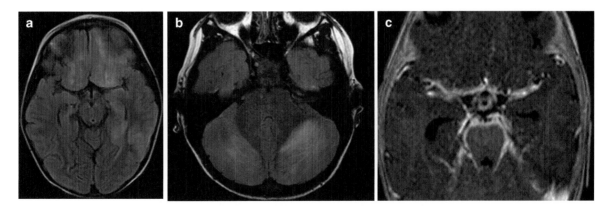

**Fig. 7 Pediatric intracranial infections**: (**a**) teenage boy with HSV1 encephalitis, axial FLAIR image showing bilateral asymmetric confluent hyperintensities with a predilection for the inferior frontal, medial temporal, and insular regions, but relatively sparing the basal ganglia; (**b**) axial FLAIR image from MRI in an 8-year-old boy with acute viral cerebellitis shows ill-defined cerebellar cortical hyperintensity associated with swelling, identified as effacement of folia and the fourth ventricle; and (**c**) axial post-gadolinium T1W MR image showing extensive and rind-like basal enhancement in a 11-month boy with tuberculous meningitis

**Fig. 8** Hypoxic ischemic injury (HII): (**a**) DWI in a term neonate with severe HII showing diffusion restriction in the bilateral posterolateral putamen, thalami, and perirolandic cortices; (**b**) T1-hyperintensity in the setting of HII in a term neonate at day 6, with characteristic locations in the basal ganglia and thalamus (arrows), and missing the normal hyperintensity in the posterior limb of the internal capsule

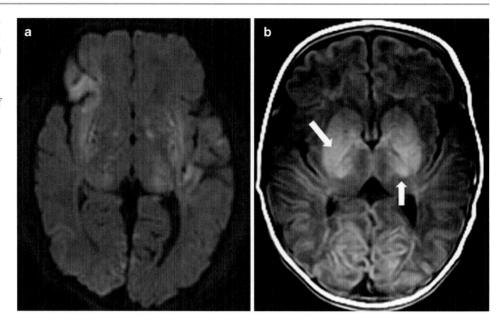

brainstem), and the perirolandic cortex are preferentially involved (Fig. 8a) as these are actively myelinating and metabolically active areas [38]. Diffuse involvement of the cerebral cortices suggests a more prolonged insult, a total anoxic pattern, whereas mild-to-moderate HII results in parasagittal watershed territory infarcts, sparing the deep gray structures [39].

MRI findings evolve over the first few days following an anoxic episode. In the first 24 h, DWI is most sensitive for the detection of HII but can under-reveal the extent, which becomes more apparent at 3–5 days, following which DWI signal "pseudonormalizes" at 7–10 days. At this stage, T1-shortening and, subsequently, T2-shortening become more reliable for assessing HII (Fig. 8b).

In postnatal infants and young children, the pattern of HII is reflective of rapid ongoing brain maturation.

Severe infantile asphyxia results in injury to basal ganglia, hippocampi, and frontal/parieto-occipital cortex with relative sparing of the perirolandic cortex and thalami. Hemorrhagic infarction of the basal ganglia can occur. Profound HII in older children affects the basal ganglia, thalami, sensorimotor, and visual cortices, hippocampi, and cerebellum. Diffuse edema with raised intracranial pressure and redistribution of blood can result in the CT "reversal" (Fig. 3f) or "white cerebellum" sign.

## Acute Inflammatory Demyelinating Disorders

Acute disseminated encephalomyelitis (ADEM), an autoimmune condition triggered by environmental stimuli (most often a viral infection) in genetically susceptible individuals, presents as a monophasic disorder with multifocal neurological symptoms and encephalopathy (mild lethargy to coma) [40]. T2-WI and FLAIR sequences are most sensitive, while DWI and IV contrast enhancement can identify acute abnormalities. The findings are typically bilateral and asymmetrically distributed, poorly defined T2/FLAIR hyperintensities, with a propensity for the thalami and basal ganglia (Fig. 9a). Multiple subcortical white matter abnormalities are common, relatively sparing the periventricular white matter. Foci of involvement can range in size from a few millimeters to over 3 cm. Spinal cord abnormalities in ADEM are typically multisegmental and confluent. Whereas the presence of encephalopathy at onset is useful to distinguish ADEM from clinically isolated syndromes such as optic neuritis and neuromyelitis optica (Devic disease), sequential MRI is also important to exclude multiphasic ADEM and multiple sclerosis (MS), characterized by new abnormalities more than 3 months after the inciting episode (dissemination in time). The presence of periventricular T2-hyperintense abnormalities, T1-hypointense abnormalities, and IV gadolinium enhancement, in a clinically silent abnormality, is unusual for ADEM and could represent the first attack of MS. In addition, dissemination in space is represented by abnormalities in at least two of juxtacortical, infratentorial, periventricular white matter, and spinal cord [41].

Acute hemorrhagic leukoencephalopathy (AHLE) is a rare, severe monophasic inflammatory disorder with rapid progression of fulminant demyelination and a 70% mortality rate. Extensive and rapidly progressive confluent T2-FLAIR hyperintensities are seen on MRI, with edema, mass effect, and areas of hemorrhage secondary to necrotizing vasculitis and perivascular demyelination [42].

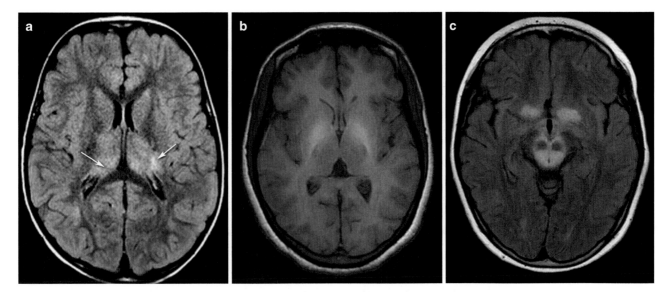

**Fig. 9 Acute inflammatory and toxic-metabolic encephalopathies in children:** (**a**) axial FLAIR image in a teenage boy with ADEM, showing poorly defined hyperintensity in bilateral thalami (arrows) and caudate nuclei, with more scattered white matter hyperintensities; (**b**) axial T1W image in a 13-year-old girl demonstrating marked basal ganglia hyperintensity in hyperammonemic encephalopathy; and (**c**) axial FLAIR image in a 5-year-old girl with Wilson disease, showing T2-hyperintensity in the deep grey nuclei, as well as in the midbrain tegmental around the red nuclei and substantia nigra, with the characteristic "face of the giant panda" sign

## Toxic-Metabolic Encephalopathies in Children

Systemic metabolic dysfunction (e.g., renal or hepatic impairment), electrolyte disturbances, deficiency syndromes, and exogenous substance toxicity can result in encephalopathy with nonspecific neurological presentations. Neuroimaging features can be specific or contributory to diagnosis, e.g., bilateral symmetrical T1-hyperintensity (Fig. 9b) in the globus pallidus, with cortical cytotoxic edema (T2-hyperintensity and diffusion restriction) in the insula and cingulate gyrus, with increased MR spectroscopic glutamate/glutamine and relative occipital/perirolandic sparing, and in acute hyperammonemic encephalopathy [43]. Alternatively, central pontine and thalamic T2-hyperintensity with/without hemispheric white matter involvement can occur in osmotic (noninflammatory) demyelination which is associated with rapidly corrected hyponatremia, organ transplant, or diuretic use [44].

Wilson disease, an inborn error of copper metabolism, can present with neurological manifestations secondary to neurotoxic cerebral levels of copper. Whereas CT can show basal ganglia atrophy, MRI abnormalities are more specific and can be used for monitoring treatment effects. T2-hyperintensity in bilateral putamina is classical, not associated with T1-hyperintensity. Abnormalities in the midbrain ("face of the giant panda" sign) and pons ("panda cub"), together called the "double panda" sign (Fig. 9c), are considered highly characteristic.

Cocaine abuse in adolescents and teenagers can result in stroke, related to vasospasm and vasculitis, or can present as multifocal metabolic leukoencephalopathy, with confluent T2-FLAIR hyperintensities in cerebral and cerebellar white matter, as well as brainstem abnormalities, with raised lactate levels on MR spectroscopy, patchy diffusion restriction, and heterogeneous IV gadolinium enhancement less commonly described. Levamisole contamination in cocaine can also cause acute and recurrent white matter abnormalities of an inflammatory demyelinating nature. Heroin leukoencephalopathy can have similar MRI findings, with an occipital-cerebellar preponderance.

## High-Flow Arteriovenous Shunts in Neonates/Infants with Congestive Cardiac Failure

### Arteriovenous Fistulae

Pial (non-Galenic) arteriovenous fistulae (AVF) are abnormal arterial connections to a vein without an intervening nidus. These vascular abnormalities more commonly present in infancy, or early childhood, and can be associated with genetic vascular syndromes including HHT [21], and less likely are traumatic/iatrogenic AVF. Presentation can be incidental, hemorrhagic, with neurological deficit or seizures. Cardiac decompensation occurs in more than half of neonates with pial AVF, and in up to 16% of infants [45]. High-flow

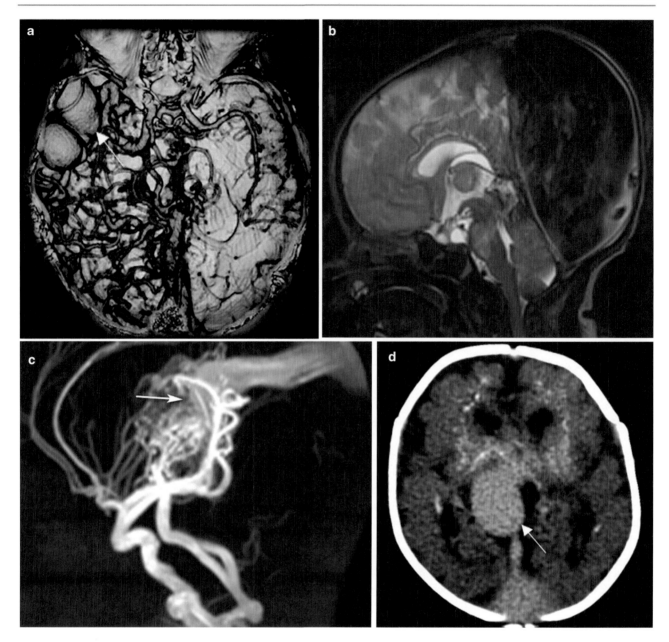

**Fig. 10 High-flow intracranial arteriovenous shunts presenting with congestive cardiac failure**: (a) volume-rendered reconstruction from CTA in an infant with hereditary hemorrhagic telangiectasia (HHT) presenting with heart failure, showing a right middle cerebral arteriovenous fistula (AVF) with large venous pouches (arrow); (b) sagittal T2-WI in a term boy with dural sinus malformation (DSM), showing a T2-hypointense torcular lake compressing the posterior fossa structures. This was treated with staged embolization starting on day 3 of life, followed by prolonged heparinization; (c) sagittal maximum intensity projection image from time-of-flight MRA showing a mixed-type VGAM. A choroidal network into the vein can be seen, as well as a direct mural shunt (arrow); and (d) neonate with VGAM (arrow), axial CT image showing generalized parenchymal volume loss, with extensive calcifications often referred to as the "melting brain" syndrome

AVF can be associated with palpable varices, bruit, skull erosion, macrocephaly, raised intracranial pressure, and hydrocephalus from hydrodynamic failure [21]. MRI (Fig. 10a) can show dilated feeding arteries, draining veins, any parenchymal changes (venous edema, steal-related ischemia, and hemorrhages), and hydrocephalus, but because of flow-related artifacts on routine sequences, IV gadolinium administration and/or CT angiography are required. CA is indicated in all cases for assessing flow dynamics, the presence of aneurysms and venous sacs, arterial steal, cortical and dural sinus reflux, and the type of fistula (single- or multi-hole). Treatment is either by surgical or, more commonly, endovascular disconnection, with good long-term outcomes in two-thirds of patients [46].

Infantile dural arteriovenous fistulae and dural sinus malformations are rare, and their etiology is incompletely understood, to our knowledge, with structural weaknesses and intrauterine dural sinus thrombosis believed to be underlying [47]. These direct communications between meningeal and pial arteries to the dural sinuses typically present as neonates with an aggressive clinical course, either from cardiac failure, hypertensive venopathy, or massively dilated dural venous sinuses with thrombosis. Fistulae are commonly multifocal and commonly involve the transverse and superior sagittal sinuses. On imaging, these can be identified as large branches of the occipital and/or middle meningeal arteries, with large flow voids representing arterialized dural venous sinuses or dural lakes (Fig. 10b). Dilated dural sinuses with T1-hyperintensity suggest thrombosis. Midline involvement of the torcular is associated with poor prognosis. Parenchymal infarcts related to chronic venous hypertension can occur. Endovascular therapy targeted to areas of shunting is the mainstay of treatment, but close follow-up is required to assess for dural sinus thrombosis with consumptive thrombocytopenia, and recruitment of arterial feeders.

## Vein of Galen Aneurysmal Malformations (VGAM)

The majority of VGAM, which represent arteriovenous shunts between the choroidal arterial system and the fetal median prosencephalic vein, are diagnosed in the intrauterine and neonatal periods, and the remainder during early childhood [48]. The typical presentation is a neonate with congestive cardiac failure, pulmonary hypertension, cyanosis, and multiorgan failure but can present later with hydrocephalus from hydrodynamic dysfunction, or developmental delay. Presentation with hemorrhage is uncommon, either due to feeding artery microaneurysms or progressive dural sinus stenosis from arterialization. In milder forms, neonates present with tachycardia, feeding difficulty, and radiographic cardiomegaly. Whereas medical management of cardiac and systemic signs is the first-line approach, emergent endovascular embolization is required in refractory or more severe cases [48].

Angiographically, VGAM are classified into mural, choroidal, and mixed types. Mural VGAM refer to high-flow shunts directly into the wall of the prosencephalic vein; in the choroidal type, an extensive network of feeders from the choroidal, pericallosal, subependymal, and perforating arteries shunt into the vein (Fig. 10c). Endovascular treatment typically consists of transarterial embolization with liquid embolic agent (n-butyl cyanoacrylate or Onyx), with a multistaged approach. Arterial access can be challenging in the neonatal period, with increased risk of access site complications and procedure-related morbidity. When feasible, endovascular embolization is deferred until 4–6 months of life. In the newborn, access through the umbilical artery is an alternative. Although there have been substantial advances in mortality rates since the use of embolization therapy, procedures are high-risk, and long-term outcomes are guarded [49]. Long-standing arterial steal and congestive venopathy can result in cerebral ischemia, with infarction multifocal encephalomalacia with calcifications, the "melting-brain" syndrome [50] (Fig. 10d).

## References

1. Exo J, Smith C, Smith R, Bell M. Emergency treatment options for pediatric traumatic brain injury. Pediatr Health. 2009;3(6):533–41.
2. Case ME, Graham MA, Handy TC, Jentzen JM, Monteleone JA. National Association of medical examiners ad hoc committee on Shaken Baby syndrome. Position paper on fatal abusive head injuries in infants and young children. Am J Forensic Med Pathol. 2001;22(2):112–22.
3. Kumpulainen V, Lehtola SJ, Tuulari JJ, Silver E, Copeland A, Korja R, et al. Prevalence and risk factors of incidental findings in brain MRIs of healthy neonates – the FinnBrain birth cohort study. Front Neurol. 2020;10:1347.
4. Poussaint TY, Moeller KK. Imaging of pediatric head trauma. Neuroimaging Clin N Am. 2002;12(2):271–94.
5. Rooks VJ, Eaton JP, Ruess L, Petermann GW, Keck-Wherley J, Pedersen RC. Prevalence and evolution of intracranial hemorrhage in asymptomatic term infants. Am J Neuroradiol. 2008;29(6):1082–9.
6. Looney CB, Smith JK, Merck LH, Wolfe HM, Chescheir NC, Hamer RM, et al. Intracranial hemorrhage in asymptomatic neonates: prevalence on MR images and relationship to obstetric and neonatal risk factors. Radiology. 2007;242(2):535–41.
7. Chaturvedi A, Chaturvedi A, Stanescu AL, Blickman JG, Meyers SP. Mechanical birth-related trauma to the neonate: an imaging perspective. Insights Imaging. 2018;9(1):103–18.
8. Popernack ML, Gray N, Reuter-Rice K. Moderate-to-severe traumatic brain injury in children: complications and rehabilitation strategies. J Pediatr Health Care. 2015;29(3):e1–7.
9. Wang H, Zhou Y, Liu J, Ou L, Han J, Xiang L. Traumatic skull fractures in children and adolescents: a retrospective observational study. Injury. 2018;49(2):219–25.
10. Armin SS, Colohan ART, Zhang JH. Vasospasm in traumatic brain injury. Acta Neurochir Suppl. 2008;104(13):421–5.
11. Paul AR, Adamo MA. Non-accidental trauma in pediatric patients: a review of epidemiology, pathophysiology, diagnosis and treatment. Transl Pediatr. 2014;3(3):195–207.
12. Vezina G. Assessment of the nature and age of subdural collections in nonaccidental head injury with CT and MRI. Pediatr Radiol. 2009;39(6):586–90.
13. Gunda D, Cornwell BO, Dahmoush HM, Jazbeh S, Alleman AM. Pediatric central nervous system imaging of nonaccidental trauma: beyond subdural hematomas. Radiographics. 2018;39(1):213–28.
14. Orman G, Kralik SF, Meoded A, Desai N, Risen S, Huisman TAGM. MRI findings in pediatric abusive head trauma: a review. J Neuroimaging. 2020;30(1):15–27.
15. Silvera VM, Danehy AR, Newton AW, Stamoulis C, Carducci C, Grant PE, et al. Retroclival collections associated with abusive head trauma in children. Pediatr Radiol. 2014;44(4):621–31.
16. Wright JN. CNS injuries in abusive head trauma. AJR Am J Roentgenol. 2017;208(5):991–1001.
17. Khan NR, Fraser BD, Nguyen V, Moore K, Boop S, Vaughn BN, et al. Pediatric abusive head trauma and stroke. J Neurosurg Pediatr. 2017;20(2):183–90.

18. Lo WD, Lee J, Rusin J, Perkins E, Roach ES. Intracranial hemorrhage in children: an evolving Spectrum. Arch Neurol. 2008;65(12): 1629–33.

19. Cole L, Dewey D, Letourneau N, Kaplan BJ, Chaput K, Gallagher C, et al. Clinical characteristics, risk factors, and outcomes associated with neonatal hemorrhagic stroke: a population-based case-control study. JAMA Pediatr. 2017;171(3):230–8.

20. El-Ghanem M, Kass-Hout T, Kass-Hout O, Alderazi YJ, Amuluru K, Al-Mufti F, et al. Arteriovenous malformations in the pediatric population: review of the existing literature. Intervent Neurol. 2016;5(3–4):218–25.

21. Walcott BP, Smith ER, Scott RM, Orbach DB. Pial arteriovenous fistulae in pediatric patients: associated syndromes and treatment outcome. J NeuroIntervent Surg. 2013;5(1):10–4.

22. Jhaveri A, Amirabadi A, Dirks P, Kulkarni AV, Shroff MM, Shkumat N, et al. Predictive value of MRI in diagnosing brain AVM recurrence after angiographically documented exclusion in children. AJNR Am J Neuroradiol. 2019;40(7):1227–35.

23. Päivi K-P, Mika N, Hanna L, Riku K, Jussi N, Aki L, et al. De novo and recurrent aneurysms in pediatric patients with cerebral aneurysms. Stroke. 2013;44(5):1436–9.

24. Bisson D-A, Dirks P, Amirabadi A, Shroff MM, Krings T, Pereira VM, et al. Unruptured intracranial aneurysms in children: 18 years' experience in a tertiary care pediatric institution. J Neurosurg Pediatr. 2019;24(2):184–9.

25. Dmytriw AA, Bisson D-A, Phan K, Amirabadi A, Branson H, Dirks PB, et al. Locations, associations and temporal evolution of intracranial arterial infundibular dilatations in children. J Neurointervent Surg. 2020;12(5):495–8.

26. Krings T, Geibprasert S, terBrugge KG. Pathomechanisms and treatment of pediatric aneurysms. Childs Nerv Syst. 2010;26(10): 1309–18.

27. Tsze DS, Valente JH. Pediatric stroke: a review. Emerg Med Int. 2011; [cited 2020 Apr 25]. Available from: https://www.ncbi.nlm.nih.gov/pmc/articles/PMC3255104/

28. Mirsky DM, Beslow LA, Amlie-Lefond C, Krishnan P, Laughlin S, Lee S, et al. Pathways for neuroimaging of childhood stroke. Pediatr Neurol. 2017;69:11–23.

29. Bhatia K, Kortman H, Blair C, Parker G, Brunacci D, Ang T, et al. Mechanical thrombectomy in pediatric stroke: systematic review, individual patient data meta-analysis, and case series. J Neurosurg Pediatr. 2019:1–14.

30. Grunt S, Wingeier K, Wehrli E, Boltshauser E, Capone A, Fluss J, et al. Cerebral sinus venous thrombosis in Swiss children. Dev Med Child Neurol. 2010;52(12):1145–50.

31. Rollins N, Ison C, Reyes T, Chia J. Cerebral MR venography in children: comparison of 2D time-of-flight and gadolinium-enhanced 3D gradient-Echo techniques. Radiology. 2005;235(3):1011–7.

32. Triulzi F, Doneda C, Parazzini C. Neuroimaging of pediatric brain infections. Expert Rev Anti-Infect Ther. 2011;9(6):737–51.

33. Okanishi T, Yamamoto H, Hosokawa T, Ando N, Nagayama Y, Hashimoto Y, et al. Diffusion-weighted MRI for early diagnosis of neonatal herpes simplex encephalitis. Brain and Development. 2015;37(4):423–31.

34. Jayaraman K, Rangasami R, Chandrasekharan A. Magnetic resonance imaging findings in viral encephalitis: a pictorial essay. J Neurosci Rural Pract. 2018;9(4):556–60.

35. Park JY, Ko KO, Lim JW, Cheon EJ, Yoon JM, Kim HJ. A pediatric case of Bickerstaff's brainstem encephalitis. Korean J Pediatr. 2014;57(12):542–5.

36. Oliveira CR, Morriss MC, Mistrot JG, Cantey JB, Doern CD, Sánchez PJ. Brain magnetic resonance imaging of infants with bacterial meningitis. J Pediatr. 2014;165(1):134–9.

37. Pienaar M, Andronikou S, van Toorn R. MRI to demonstrate diagnostic features and complications of TBM not seen with CT. Childs Nerv Syst ChNS Off J Int Soc Pediatr Neurosurg. 2009;25(8):941–7.

38. Grant PE, Yu D. Acute injury to the immature brain with hypoxia with or without hypoperfusion. Radiol Clin N Am. 2006;44(1): 63–77, viii

39. Huang BY, Castillo M. Hypoxic-ischemic brain injury: imaging findings from birth to adulthood. Radiographics. 2008;28(2): 417–39.

40. Tardieu M, Banwell B, Wolinsky JS, Pohl D, Krupp LB. Consensus definitions for pediatric MS and other demyelinating disorders in childhood: table. Neurology. 2016;87(9 Suppl 2):S8–11.

41. Banwell B, Arnold DL, Tillema J-M, Rocca MA, Filippi M, Weinstock-Guttman B, et al. MRI in the evaluation of pediatric multiple sclerosis. Neurology. 2016;87(9 Suppl 2):S88–96.

42. Gibbs WN, Kreidie MA, Kim RC, Hasso AN. Acute hemorrhagic leukoencephalitis: neuroimaging features and neuropathologic diagnosis. J Comput Assist Tomogr. 2005;29(5):689–93.

43. Reis E, Coolen T, Lolli V. MRI findings in acute hyperammonemic encephalopathy: three cases of different etiologies. J Belg Soc Radiol. 2020;104(1):9.

44. Abbott R, Silber E, Felber J, Ekpo E. Osmotic demyelination syndrome. BMJ. 2005;331(7520):829–30.

45. Pillai A, Rajeev K, Unnikrishnan M. Surgical management of a pial arteriovenous fistula with giant varix in an infant. Neurol India. 2006;54(4):434–6.

46. Madsen PJ, Lang S-S, Pisapia JM, Storm PB, Hurst RW, Heuer GG. An institutional series and literature review of pial arteriovenous fistulas in the pediatric population: clinical article. J Neurosurg Pediatr. 2013;12(4):344–50.

47. Morales H, Jones BV, Leach JL, Abruzzo TA. Documented development of a dural arteriovenous fistula in an infant subsequent to sinus thrombosis: case report and review of the literature. Neuroradiology. 2010;52(3):225–9.

48. Hoang S, Choudhri O, Edwards M, Guzman R. Vein of Galen malformation. Neurosurg Focus. 2009;27(5):E8.

49. Bhatia K, Mendes Pereira V, Krings T, Ter Brugge K, Kortman H, Dirks P et al. Factors contributing to major neurological complications from vein of Galen malformation embolization. JAMA Neurol. 2020.

50. Lasjaunias P. Vein of Galen aneurysmal malformation. In: Lasjaunias P, editor. Vascular diseases in neonates, infants and children: interventional neuroradiology management [Internet]. Berlin/Heidelberg: Springer; 1997. p. 67–202. https://doi.org/10.1007/978-3-662-10740-9_2. [cited 2020 May 27].

# Imaging of Pediatric Head and Neck Emergencies

Elka Miller ⓘ, Claudia Martinez-Rios ⓘ, Laura Acosta-Izquierdo, and Sara R. Teixeira ⓘ

## Contents

E. Miller (✉) · C. Martinez-Rios · L. Acosta-Izquierdo
Medical Imaging Department, CHEO, Department of Radiology,
University of Ottawa, Ottawa, ON, Canada
e-mail: emiller@cheo.on.ca; cmartinezrios@cheo.on.ca

S. R. Teixeira
Radiology Department, Children's Hospital of Philadelphia, University
of Pennsylvania, Philadelphia, PA, USA
e-mail: sarat@alumni.usp.br

© Crown 2022
M. N. Patlas et al. (eds.), *Atlas of Emergency Imaging from Head-to-Toe*,
https://doi.org/10.1007/978-3-030-92111-8_45

## Abstract

Acute emergencies of the head and neck in children are wide-ranging. Frequently, these conditions are challenging to diagnose, mainly because clinical history and physical examinations are limited, particularly in younger children. The spectrum of conditions seen in the emergency setting can be divided depending on the specific area of involvement, as congenital, infectious, inflammatory, neoplastic, and traumatic conditions. Diagnostic imaging plays an important role in identifying the correct diagnosis. Understanding the spectrum of the different clinical presentations, imaging findings, and potential associated complications of the commonly encountered acute head and neck conditions in children may help to tailor a specific imaging protocol, to reach a prompt diagnosis, and to help to guide management.

frequent clinical scenarios and awareness of the imaging spectrum of the most common acute congenital, infectious, inflammatory, neoplastic, and traumatic head and neck emergencies encountered in children is paramount. Integrating these findings would help to achieve an appropriate and prompt diagnosis to guide further management, avoiding potentially life-threatening complications.

## Keywords

Children · Orbit · Sinonasal · Neck · Congenital · Inflammation · Infection · Trauma · Neoplasia · Imaging

## Introduction

Imaging plays an important role in the diagnostic workup of pediatric head and neck emergencies. The clinical and imaging algorithm for children with emergencies of the head and neck will vary, depending on the clinical scenario, location, extension of the findings, and potential complications.

This chapter describes the clinical features, diagnostic investigations, and imaging findings of relevant pediatric head and neck emergencies. Familiarity with the most

## Acute Rhinosinusitis (AR)

### Epidemiology

Approximately 6–7% of children with respiratory symptoms have AR. An estimated 5–10% of viral rhinosinusitis (VRS) will develop bacterial infections in children [1–6].

### Clinical Features

In children, AR is caused by rhino-, adeno-, influenza, and parainfluenza viruses, which resolve spontaneously [4–6]. Acute bacterial rhinosinusitis (ABRS) should be considered when persistent illness, with nasal discharge lasting for >10 days, or severe purulent nasal discharge for at least 3 consecutive days, with coexisting high fever ($\geq 39\ °C$), is present. Common pathogens in ABRS are *Streptococcus pneumoniae* (38%), *Haemophilus influenzae* (36%), and *Moraxella catarrhalis* (16%) [1–8]. Although rare, fungal infections can cause AR, mostly in immunocompromised patients [4, 9].

Complications of AR are rare (1 / 1000 cases) but carry significant morbidity and mortality [3, 4, 8–12]. Sinus infections may spread to the orbit, bone, or intracranial structures causing pre- or post-septal orbital cellulitis, abscess, and osteomyelitis (Fig. 1). *Pott puffy tumor*, a frontal osteomyelitis with a subperiosteal abscess, is most commonly associated with frontal sinusitis. Intracranial extension with an intra-axial abscess, meningitis, cerebritis, or vascular involvement with venous or cavernous sinus thrombosis

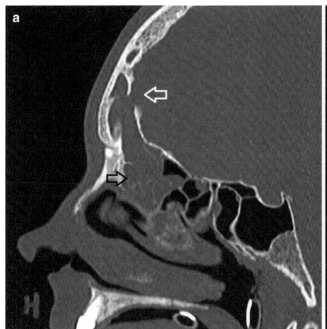
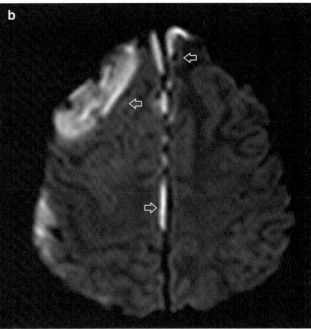

**Fig. 1  Intracranial complications of rhinosinusitis**. A 17-year-old boy admitted to PICU for intracranial abscess in the context of 1.5-month history of sinus disease with rhinosinusitis complicated with intracranial empyemas and cerebritis. NECT in sagittal plane (**a**) shows extensive opacification of the ethmoid and frontal sinuses (open black arrow) with a focal bone defect (open white arrow) in the posterior wall of the left frontal sinus. Axial DWI (**b**) shows restricted diffusion involving the extra-axial spaces of the right frontal, parietal, and anterior interhemispheric fissure (white arrows), consistent with subdural empyemas (abscesses)

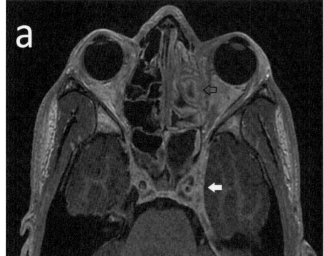
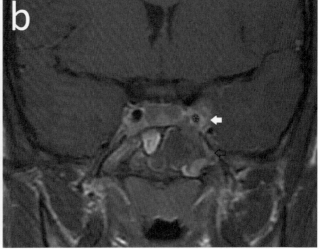

**Fig. 2  Sphenoid sinusitis and cavernous sinus thrombosis**. A 14-year-old boy with left ethmoidal and sphenoid sinusitis, with ipsilateral cavernous sinus thrombosis. Axial (**a**) and coronal (**b**) T1 CEMRI show enhancing mucosal thickening involving the left ethmoidal and sphenoidal sinuses (open black arrow), with bulging, asymmetric enhancement, and filling defect of the left cavernous sinus (white arrow), as well as narrowing of the left carotid artery

(Fig. 2) or vasculitis can occur and should be excluded as potential complications [1, 3–11].

## Diagnostic Investigations

- Imaging is not recommended for children with uncomplicated AR [4, 5]. An IV contrast-enhanced computed tomography (CECT) should be performed if complicated sinus disease is suspected. IV contrast-enhanced magnetic resonance imaging (CEMRI) is advised when there is clinical concern for intracranial complications or potential meningitis. CEMRI, when compared to CECT, has higher sensitivity (93% versus 63%) and accuracy (97% versus 82%), respectively [5, 8–10]. In the acute setting, imaging findings of fungal sinonasal disease are nonspecific.

## Summary

- Imaging should not be performed in noncomplicated AR.
- If concerned for complicated rhinosinusitis, a contrast-enhanced CT is advised for initial workup. Contrast-enhanced MRI is warranted to assess for intracranial complications.

- In the acute setting, imaging findings of fungal sinonasal disease are nonspecific.

## Orbital Infection

### Epidemiology

Infections of the orbits are frequent in children. Preseptal (periorbital) cellulitis accounts for 84–87% of orbital infections. The incidence of orbital cellulitis in children ranges from 1.6 to 6/100000 [4, 5, 11–17].

### Clinical Features

Differentiation of preseptal and post-septal orbital cellulitis is limited based on clinical information. However, this distinction is important due to their unique potential complications and management. The clinical course of preseptal cellulitis is typically self-limited, unlike post-septal cellulitis, which requires a more aggressive management and carries higher risk of complications. The most common cause of post-septal cellulitis is sinusitis (60% to 91%), but also via hematogenous, or contiguous spread of infections, dental abscesses, penetrating injuries, or a

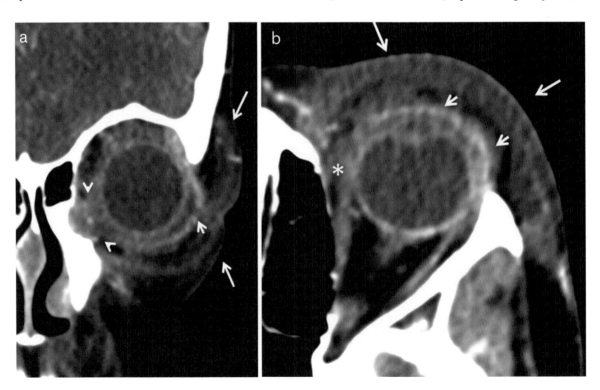

**Fig. 3 Preseptal cellulitis and dacryocystitis.** A 7-year-old girl with recurrent left preseptal cellulitis and dacryocystitis, papillary conjunctivitis, and rhinitis. Underwent left external dacryocystorhinostomy. Coronal (**a**) and axial (**b**) CECT show edema of the left preseptal soft tissue (long arrows) superficial to the orbital septum (*), with associated conjunctival chemosis (short arrows) and left dacryocystitis (arrowheads)

nasolacrimal duct mucocele [1, 4, 5, 11–18]. Complications of post-septal cellulitis include a subperiosteal or orbital abscess, extraocular myositis, intracranial infection (epidural, subdural, or intra-axial abscess, meningitis, cerebritis), cavernous sinus thrombosis (via superior ophthalmic vein thrombosis), septic thrombophlebitis, and vasculitis [11–19]. Ocular complications may include endophthalmitis, retinitis, retinal detachment, and optic neuropathy [11–16, 20–22].

## Diagnostic Investigations

CECT is the imaging of choice for the initial assessment of orbital infections [4–8]. In preseptal cellulitis, CT shows edema of the soft tissues located superficial to the orbital septum (Fig. 3) [11–22]. In post-septal cellulitis, the inflammatory changes extend posterior to the orbital septum, with proptosis and often ipsilateral (or bilateral) mucosal thickening in the sinuses (Fig. 4). If complicated orbital cellulitis is suspected, CEMRI is the modality of choice, including MR angiography to exclude vasculitis [4, 5, 9–11, 13, 14].

## Summary

- Contrast-enhanced CT scans are warranted to differentiate between preseptal and orbital cellulitis.
- Preseptal cellulitis is a self-limited condition. Post-septal cellulitis requires more aggressive management.
- Complications of orbital cellulitis may require to be assessed with contrast-enhanced MRI.

## Pharyngeal and Retropharyngeal Processes

### Epidemiology

*Tonsillitis/pharyngitis* accounts for nearly 2% of infections in adults and children and typically occurs in school-age children and adolescents. It can be caused by viral and bacterial etiologies, with group A *Streptococcus* (GAS) infection in approximately 20–30% of cases [11, 21–25].

*Peritonsillar abscess (PTA)* is a suppurative infection of the tonsils, with an incidence of 9.4/100,000 in patients, with an average age of 13 years [23].

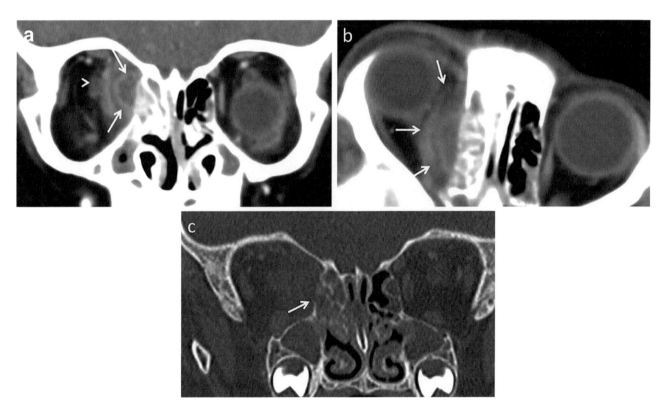

**Fig. 4  Post-septal cellulitis and subperiosteal abscess.** A 2-year-old boy with complicated right post-septal cellulitis with a subperiosteal abscess. Coronal (**a**) and axial (**b**) CECT show right proptosis associated with mucosal thickening of the right ethmoidal and maxillary sinuses and a rim-enhancing post-septal subperiosteal abscess causing lateral displacement of the medial rectus muscle (long arrows). There is surrounding edema as well as mild optic neuritis (arrowhead). Coronal (**c**) CT in bone window shows small defect in the right lamina papyracea (arrow)

Retropharyngeal abscess (RPA) is a deep neck infection, with an incidence of 4.1/100,000 in < 20 years of age. RPA can result from a *suppurative retropharyngeal adenopathy (SRA)*, trauma, or iatrogenic [11, 21–25].

## Clinical Features

*Tonsillitis/pharyngitis* may present with nonspecific findings, including fever and throat pain [11–25]. The presence of a pharyngeal and/or tonsillar exudate, vomiting, and tender cervical nodes increase the likelihood of GAS infection in more than 50% [23]. Associated cough, rhinorrhea, hoarseness, and/or evidence of oropharyngeal vesicles may suggest a viral etiology [23].

*PTA* and *SRA* show associated neck pain, dysphagia, trismus, halitosis, bulging of the tonsils or pharyngeal asymmetry, and adenopathy [11, 21–25]. In *RPA*, children have significant pain and torticollis. Due to its anatomic relations, RPA can rapidly progress to life-threatening complications, including sepsis and the spread of infection to the mediastinum [11, 21–25]. Therefore, prompt identification of RPA is critical.

## Diagnostic Investigations

Imaging is not always recommended, unless there is clinically suspected abscess, for preoperative assessment, in patients without improvement with medical treatment, and when the diagnosis is questionable [23]. Radiographs fail to reveal the type of process in the retropharyngeal space (i.e., cellulitis, PTA, SPA, or RPA) [21–25].

CECT is the first-line imaging examination for the evaluation of retropharyngeal infection [11, 21–25]. In *acute noncomplicated tonsillitis*, CECT shows tonsillar enlargement and increased enhancement, occasionally with a striated pattern. In a *PTA*, CECT shows a rim-enhancing fluid collection between the palatine tonsil capsule and the pharyngeal muscles, associated with tonsil enlargement, hyperenhancement, and edema of the surrounding tissues, with possible narrowing of the airway (Fig. 5a). In *SRA*, CECT shows a smaller rim-enhancing, hypodense fluid collection within an enlarged node. These nodes are generally lateral in the retropharyngeal space and do not cross the midline (Fig. 5b) [11, 21–25]. In an *RPA*, CECT shows a rim-enhancing fluid collection with mass effect on the surrounding structures and airway narrowing. RPA can

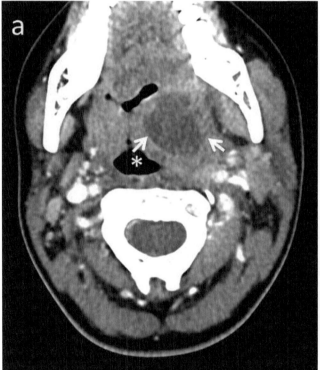
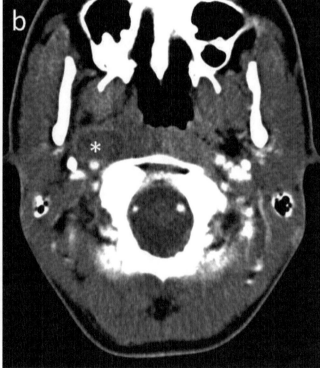
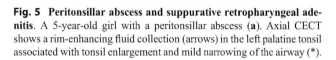

**Fig. 5 Peritonsillar abscess and suppurative retropharyngeal adenitis**. A 5-year-old girl with a peritonsillar abscess (**a**). Axial CECT shows a rim-enhancing fluid collection (arrows) in the left palatine tonsil associated with tonsil enlargement and mild narrowing of the airway (*).

A 15-year-old boy with suppurative lymphadenopathy (**b**). Axial CECT shows a small, focal, rim-enhancing hypodense fluid collection (*) in the right lateral retropharyngeal space

**Fig. 6** RPA. A 5-month-old boy with cervical lymphadenopathy and torticollis. Lateral radiograph of the neck (**a**) shows marked thickening of the prevertebral soft tissue (long arrows). CECT in sagittal (**b**), coronal (**c**), and axial (**d**) planes show a large retropharyngeal and right paravertebral rim-enhancing fluid collection (long arrows), causing mass effect on the surrounding structures, and marked narrowing of the airway (asterisk). Note how the retropharyngeal collection is crossing the midline anterior to the spine (arrowheads)

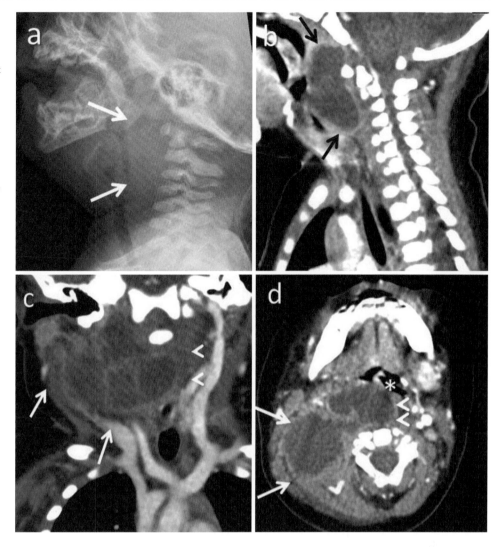

cross the midline (Fig. 6) [11]. CECT can help to delineate the extent of the abscess, identify changes on the airway, exclude the involvement of the danger space with the potential risk for mediastinitis, and assess for vascular complications (i.e., jugular vein thrombosis-Lemierre syndrome, pseudoaneurysms, or vasospasm) (Fig. 7) [11, 21–25].

## Summary

- *Peritonsillar abscess* is a rim-enhancing fluid collection between the palatine tonsil capsule and the pharyngeal muscles.
- *SRA* is a smaller and lateral rim-enhancing fluid collection, not crossing the midline.

- *RPA* is a rim-enhancing fluid retropharyngeal collection that may cross the midline. Always exclude potential complications: mediastinitis, jugular vein thrombosis, pseudoaneurysms, or vasospasm.

## Larynx and Upper Trachea

### Epidemiology

*Laryngotracheobronchitis or croup* is the most common cause of upper airway obstruction between 6 months and 3 years old, usually due to parainfluenza viruses [11, 22, 24, 25].

*Epiglottitis* is a potentially life-threatening airway condition that results in marked enlargement of the epiglottis and

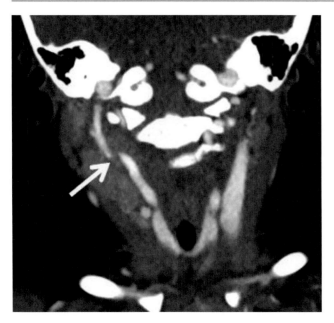

**Fig. 7 RPA and vasospasm.** A 2-year-old girl with RPA. Coronal CECT shows also abrupt tapering and occlusion of the cervical segment of the right internal carotid artery (long arrow), between the lower C2 level and the skull base, consistent with vasospasm secondary to the adjacent inflammatory process. After the drainage and resolution of the RPA, there was improvement in the caliber of the right ICA (not shown)

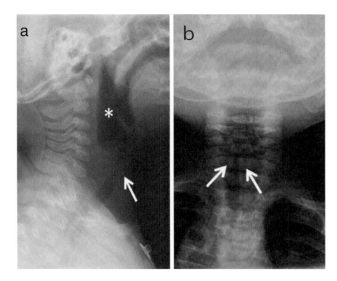

**Fig. 8 Croup.** A 5-month-old boy with a history of stridor and barky cough. Lateral (**a**) and frontal (**b**) radiographs show loss of the normal "shoulders" of the subglottic airway (long arrows) causing the steeple sign. There is prominence of the hypopharynx (*)

aryepiglottic folds. Before vaccination, it was common in children around 3 years. It is now seen in teenagers (mean 14.6 years of age) [11, 22, 24, 25].

Most non-infectious processes obstructing the upper airway are due to *foreign body aspiration (FB)*, with a rate of

20.4/100,000 in children between 1 and 3 years of age. The most common aspirated objects include food, coins, toys, and balloons. They can lodge anywhere in the airway, but the right main bronchus is the most common site [24].

## Clinical Features

*Croup* presents with gradual onset of fever, inspiratory stridor, hoarseness, and a classic "barking" cough [11, 22, 24, 25].

*Epiglottitis* presents with acute onset of high fever, sore throat, drooling, dysphagia, dysphonia and dyspnea (4Ds), and the classical "tripod position" in respiratory distress, with rapid deterioration over hours [11, 24, 25]. Prompt recognition and airway management are vital.

*Aspirated FB* may present with sudden respiratory distress, cough, wheeze, and unilaterally reduced breath sounds in nearly 60% of cases [24].

## Diagnostic Investigations

Croup and epiglottitis are clinical diagnoses. Radiographs can be performed for clinically unclear cases [11, 22, 24, 25].

*Croup* The classical radiograph findings are the "steeple sign" with loss of the normal "shoulders" of the subglottic airway and tapered narrowing up to the glottis. Lateral radiographs show a narrowing of the subglottic airway (Fig. 8). Approximately 50% of children will have a normal radiograph.

*Epiglottitis* Radiographs are performed only on airway-stable children. The classical finding is the "thumb sign" with the thickening of the epiglottis and aryepiglottic folds (Fig. 9).

*Aspirated FB* Frontal and lateral radiographs of the neck are routinely obtained. While metallic FBs are easily identified (Fig. 10), the majority are non-radiopaque which limits their visualization on the radiographs. A button-shaped battery is radiographically distinct by its beveled margins and peripheral radiolucent rim. It can cause early caustic injury, mucosal erosion, perforation, and mediastinitis.

## Summary

- "Steeple sign" and loss of normal "shouldering" are classic radiographic findings in croup.
- "Thumb sign" is the classic radiographic finding in epiglottitis.

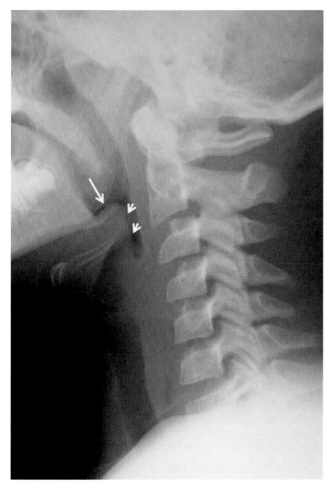

**Fig. 9 Epiglottitis.** An 11-year-old boy with acute onset of high fever, sore throat, drooling, dysphagia, dysphonia, and dyspnea. Lateral radiograph of the neck shows classical thickening (long arrow) of the epiglottis ("thumb sign") and aryepiglottic folds (shorts arrows). Courtesy of Dr. Rita Putnins, Pediatric Radiologist, CHEO

- Button-shaped batteries can cause caustic injury with mucosal erosion, perforation, and mediastinitis. On radiographs, they have a beveled margin and radiolucent rim.

# Cystic Lesions of the Neck

## Thyroglossal Duct Cyst (TGDC)

### Epidemiology
TGDC is the most common midline suprahyoid or infrahyoid cystic neck mass, accounting for 70% of congenital anomalies of the neck in children [11, 22, 26–28].

### Clinical Features
TGDC presents as a painless, round, midline, or paramedian compressible neck mass that moves with tongue protrusion or swallowing. If infected, it may become symptomatic. It can be found in any place between the foramen cecum at the base of the tongue to the thyroid. The most locations are suprahyoid (20–25%), at the hyoid bone (50%), and infrahyoid (25%) [26–28].

### Diagnostic Investigations
Ultrasonography (US) is the modality of choice to assess neck lumps (cystic or solid). CECT or CEMRI can be performed if suspected superimposed infection or the diagnosis is uncertain. On US, *TGDC* is an anechoic or hypoechoic cystic mass but can contain internal echoes/ hemorrhage. It is usually firmly embedded in the strap muscles (Fig. 11). It is important to reassure the presence of a normal thyroid. Differential diagnosis includes a dermoid cyst or a lymphatic malformation (Fig. 12) [11, 22, 24, 26–28].

## Branchial Cleft Cysts (BCC)

### Epidemiology
Branchial cleft cysts are benign congenital neck cysts due to the persistence of the branchial cleft or pouches. They are located along the anterior border of the sternocleidomastoid muscle (SCM) from the tragus to the clavicle [11, 21, 22, 24–31].

BCC Types:

- First BCC (<10%): above the level of the mandible near the external auditory canal or near the parotid.
- Second BCC (90–95%): posterolateral to the submandibular gland, lateral to the carotid space, anterior or anteromedial to the SCM (Fig. 13) [30].
- Third BCC (3%): most common upper posterior triangle, close to the carotid sheath.
- Fourth BCC (rare): from the apex of the pyriform sinus to the left thyroid lobe (Fig. 14).

### Clinical Features
BCC may become symptomatic when infected. Children show a painful, fluctuant mass, rarely with purulent drainage. The third and fourth BCC are difficult to distinguish one from another. They may involve the thyroid, with associated thyroiditis.

### Diagnostic Investigations
In **BCC** imaging shows a cyst in the corresponding anatomic location. If infected, the cyst may show a thickened wall and surrounding inflammatory changes. Associated sinus tracts are important to define in imaging [11, 22, 28–31].

## Summary

- TGDC is the most common midline/paramedian cystic mass in children. Always confirm the presence of a normal thyroid.

- Consider branchial cleft anomalies in recurrent fluctuant neck masses.

## Cervical Lymphadenopathy

### Epidemiology

Cervical lymphadenopathy is the most common solid neck mass in children. It may be due to infections, inflammation, or neoplasia [22, 26, 28, 32, 33].

### Clinical Features and Diagnostic Investigations

Normal lymph nodes (LNs) are <10 mm in the long axis. Except in level IB and level IIA, nodes may measure ≤15 mm in diameter, and the retropharyngeal nodes <8 mm in diameter [11, 33].

*Suppurative adenopathy* is pus within a node or an intranodal abscess. Imaging shows nodal enlargement with ill-defined margins, loss of the echogenic hilum, and surrounding inflammation (myositis, arterial vasospasm). If central hypoechogenicity (US) or hypodensity (CT) are present, suspect an abscess, with risk for rupture. In MRI, look for restricted diffusion on diffusion- weighted imaging (Fig. 15a).

*Nontuberculous mycobacteria (NTM) cervical lymphadenitis* is most often due to *Mycobacterium* avium complex (MAC), affecting healthy children <5 years of age. Imaging shows rim-enhancing, necrotic lymphadenopathy with skin changes and discoloration (Fig. 15b) [32].

*Neoplastic nodes* are nonmobile, painless and enlarged, or round nodal masses with variable vascularity. They can contain necrosis or calcifications. Imaging alone cannot be used

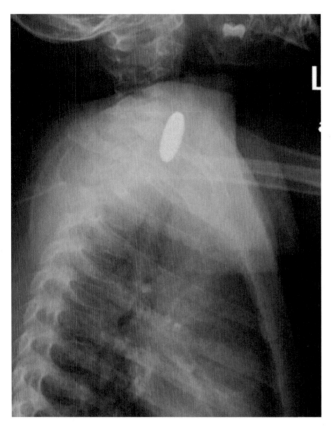

**Fig. 10  FB**. A 3-year-old boy who swallowed a coin, at presentation there was no breathing difficulty. Lateral radiograph shows a rounded radiopaque FB projected over the upper esophagus, consistent with the swallowed coin. Lateral radiograph is critical to determining the location (esophagus vs airway) of the FB

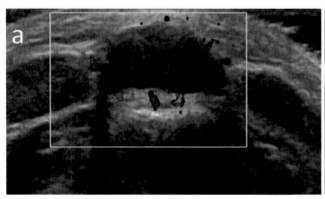
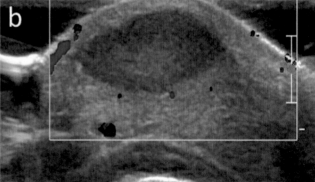

**Fig. 11  TGDC**. Color Doppler US image in a 7-year-old girl with small, barely palpable, mobile, midline round neck lump (**a**) shows a well-defined, avascular, thin-walled cystic structure with posterior acoustic enhancement. No surrounding inflammatory changes. Color Doppler US image in 6-year-old girl with neck lesion that moves with swallowing (**b**) shows a slight off-midline, predominantly hypoechoic, complex cystic lesion with internal low-level echoes, embedded in the strap muscles with thickening and increased echogenicity of the superficial subcutaneous tissues, in keeping with an infected TGDC

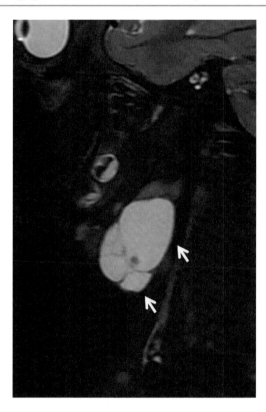

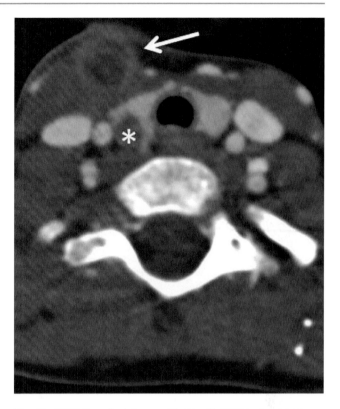

**Fig. 12  Lymphatic malformation**. A 4-year-old girl with left-sided neck mass with some fluctuation. Sagittal STIR image demonstrates a well-defined, hyperintense, multiloculated, multicompartment cystic mass, with thin hypointense septations (arrows)

**Fig. 13  BCC Type 2**. A 3-year-old girl with BCC in the right lower neck. Axial CECT shows a rim-enhancing, septated, cystic lesion with surrounding inflammatory changes (long arrow) located in the right lower neck, anteromedial to the SCM muscle and anterior the right thyroid lobe. Incidentally, there is an ectopic intrathyroid thymic tissue in the right thyroid lobe (*), which can be better characterized with ultrasound

to distinguish among the following etiologies: lymphoma/leukemia, metastases (neuroblastoma, thyroid), Langerhans cell histiocytosis (LCH) (Fig. 16), or Castleman disease (Fig. 17) [11, 22, 26, 28, 32].

## Summary

- Suppurative nodes can rupture and may require drainage.
- Consider NTM adenitis in painless nodal mass with skin involvement, not responding to standard antibiotics.

## Acute Mastoiditis

### Epidemiology

Acute mastoiditis is a suppurative inflammation of the mastoid bone, most frequently a complication of acute otitis media, with peak prevalence at the age of 2 years [34], and an incidence of 1.2 and 4.2/100,000 children/year [34–37].

## Clinical Features

The most common presentation is fever and postauricular swelling. *Streptococcus pneumonia* is the most prevalent pathogen. Complications range between 5% and 29% [34–37] and include:

- Subperiosteal abscess or periauricular fluid collection
- Bezold abscess: collection around the SCM
- Middle and/or posterior cranial fossa abscess and meningitis
- Thrombosis of the sigmoid sinus and/or jugular vein (Fig. 18)

## Diagnostic Investigations

Acute confluent mastoiditis often manifest after acute otitis media resolves [37]. CECT defines the bone changes and most of the complications. CEMRI is more sensitive for revealing intracranial complications.

## Summary

- Contrast-enhanced CT should be considered in the emergency setting for acute mastoiditis even after the use of antibiotics.
- Contrast-enhanced MRI is better for assessment of intracranial complications.

## Benign Neoplasms

### Epidemiology

**Benign tumors** Most pediatric neck masses are benign (90%). **Infantile hemangioma** (IH) is the most common benign vascular tumor of infancy, with an incidence of 4–10% [11, 22, 26, 28].

### Clinical Findings

*IH* is asymptomatic at birth and then during the first week of life undergoes a proliferating phase with rapid growth, followed by spontaneous involution. Common locations are the parotid gland (Fig. 19) or the subglottic region. Infants <6 months of age may present with inspiratory stridor. IH may be seen in PHACE syndrome (acronym describing the association of anomalies which together comprise: posterior fossa, hemangioma, arterial lesions, cardiac abnormalities, eye or endocrine abnormalities). Other common cervical benign masses are teratoma and ectopic thymus.

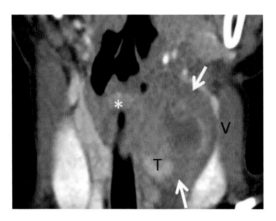

**Fig. 14 BCC type 4**. A 4-year-old boy with a fluctuant mass in the left lower neck and abnormal thyroid function. Coronal CECT shows and ill-defined, inflammatory mass-like soft tissue lesion (arrows) centered in the left thyroid lobe bed (T) causing heterogeneity and displacement of the left thyroid lobe, with a small central rim-enhancing hypodense abscess formation. There is surrounding inflammation and mass effect to the deeper soft tissue of the neck, including the ipsilateral internal jugular vein (V) and carotid artery which are displaced. There is narrowing of the left pyriform sinus, larynx (*), and proximal trachea with a shift of the central airway to the right

### Diagnostic Investigations

On US, IH shows a well-circumscribed, lobulated, hypervascular soft tissue mass, with high vessel density (proliferating phase). On CECT, IH shows soft tissue attenuation with avid enhancement. On CEMRI, IH is isointense to muscle on T1 and hyperintense on T2 and shows homogeneous hyperenhancement. Flow voids can be seen within the mass. A subglottic hemangioma can cause asymmetric subglottic narrowing on frontal radiographs.

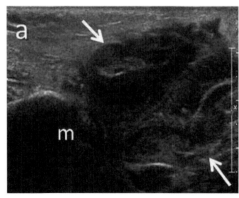
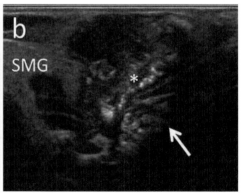
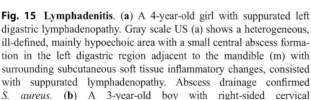

**Fig. 15 Lymphadenitis**. (**a**) A 4-year-old girl with suppurated left digastric lymphadenopathy. Gray scale US (a) shows a heterogeneous, ill-defined, mainly hypoechoic area with a small central abscess formation in the left digastric region adjacent to the mandible (m) with surrounding subcutaneous soft tissue inflammatory changes, consisted with suppurated lymphadenopathy. Abscess drainage confirmed *S. aureus*. (**b**) A 3-year-old boy with right-sided cervical lymphadenopathy without response to three courses of antibiotics. Gray scale US shows a right cervical bilobed complex lesion of heterogeneous echotexture that shows internal coarse calcifications (*) with a superficial mainly hypoechoic component adjacent to the submandibular gland (SMG), and a second deeper component (arrow) extending in the soft tissues underneath the SCM. Excisional biopsy showed necrotizing granulomatous atypical mycobacterial lymphadenitis

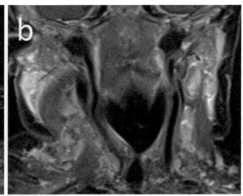

**Fig. 16 Neoplastic lymphadenopathy.** Gray scale US image in a 3-month-old boy with bilateral neck swelling (**a**) demonstrates multiple enlarged, heterogeneous neoplastic LNs, with loss of their normal configuration and fatty hilum. These nodes show a rounded configuration and diffuse hypoechogenicity. CEMR coronal T1 WI with fat saturation (**b**) demonstrates multiple enhancing enlarged bilateral cervical nodes, corresponding to the nodal mass in a patient with confirmed LCH

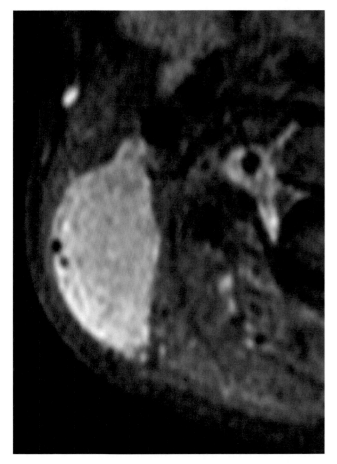

**Fig. 17 Castleman disease.** A 15-year-old girl with a palpable right posterior LN mobile and non-tender consistent with Castleman disease. Axial T1-weighted with fat saturation after contrast administration demonstrates an oval-shaped, well-defined, soft tissue mass lesion located in the right posterior cervical space, posterior to the jugular vein, posteromedial to the SCM muscle, and lateral to the right paravertebral muscles. The lesion demonstrates similar signal intensity to the surrounding cervical LNs with avid enhancement

## Malignant Neoplasms

### Epidemiology

*Lymphoma* is the third most common cancer in children. It accounts for 50% of all head and neck cancers in childhood and occurs rarely in the neck region <3 years of age [26].

*Leukemia* is the most common spectrum of stem cell hematopoietic malignancies in children <15 years of age, accounting for approximately 35–40% [26].

*Cervical neuroblastoma* (CNB): Malignant tumor of primitive neural crest cells. *NB* is the most common solid extracranial tumor in children <5 years of age. It corresponds to 8–10% of all childhood cancers [38]. Primary CNB is rare and *occurs* in 1–5% of cases [28, 38].

*Rhabdomyosarcoma* (RMS): The most common childhood soft tissue tumor, accounting for approximately 3% of pediatric cancers. Nearly 60% of RMS are seen in children <6 years of age, with nearly 40% occurring in the neck. Of cases, 20% show distant metastases at the time of diagnosis [11, 28].

*Langerhans cell histiocytosis (LCH)* encompasses a group of entities, better understood as neoplastic processes, divided into groups based on the number of foci, and systems involved. LCH typically presents in children <2 years of age, with a male predominance [11, 22, 26, 28, 39].

### Clinical Findings

*Lymphoma* should be suspected in painless, enlarged, non-necrotic nodes persisting for >6 weeks. Extranodal

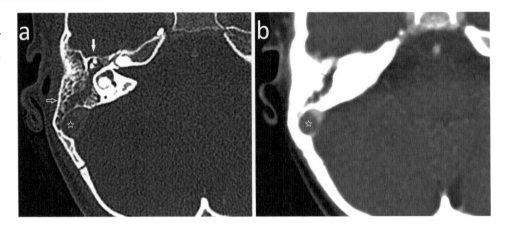

**Fig. 18** **Acute otomastoiditis and dural venous thrombosis**. A 4-year-old girl admitted for right otitis media. Axial CECT in bone (**a**) and soft tissue (**b**) windows show complete opacification of the right mastoid air cells (open arrow) and middle ear cavity (white arrow) with a non-occlusive thrombus (star) in the right sigmoid sinus

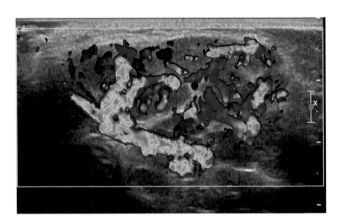

**Fig. 19** **Intraparotid hemangioma**. A 6-month-old girl with a right periauricular lump that has grown over time, consistent with intraparotid hemangioma. Color Doppler US demonstrates a complex hypoechoic solid mass with thick hyperechoic septations involving the parotid gland and high-density vascularity with venous and arterial vessels within the mass

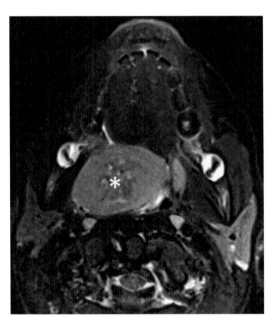

**Fig. 20** **Tonsillar lymphoma**. A 9-year-old boy with right tonsillar Burkitt's lymphoma. Axial T2 with fat saturation (FS) shows a well-defined oval mass (*) centered in the right tonsillar fossa. The mass is hyperintense on T2 with mild heterogeneous and central necrosis. It showed increased enhancement and restricted diffusion (not shown). The mass is extending to the level of hypopharynx obliterating the right vallecula and is causing marked narrowing of the pharyngeal airway

involvement (i.e., nasopharynx, oral cavity) is more common in non-Hodgkin's lymphoma (Fig. 20).

*Leukemia* may manifest as lytic, blastic, or mixed osseous tumoral foci, with an associated aggressive periosteal reaction. It may involve the skull base, face, orbit, sinonasal, nasopharynx, tonsil, mouth, lacrimal gland, or the salivary glands. Foci of leukemic cells behave like localized malignancy, with a soft tissue mass, known as a granulocytic sarcoma or chloroma (Fig. 21). Cervical adenopathy is a common initial finding in acute lymphocytic leukemia [26].

*Metastatic NB* usually involves the skull base, calvarium, and orbit and can manifest with proptosis, Horner syndrome, and periorbital soft tissue masses or hematomas ("raccoon eyes").

*RMS* can occur in parameningeal (middle ear, nasal/paranasal, nasopharynx) or non-parameningeal sites and in the orbit.

*LCH:* Lytic bone foci are the most common manifestation in 80–95% of children. The calvarium is the most common osseous site of involvement, followed by the mastoid portion of temporal bone, mandible, orbits, and facial bones [11, 22, 26, 28, 39]. Children may present with extensive adenopathy (Fig. 16).

## Diagnostic Investigations

Malignant tumors may appear heterogeneous on CT, but due to their high cellularity, CT may show a hyperdense soft

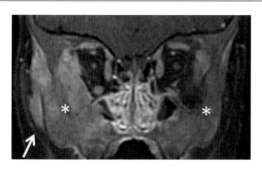

**Fig. 21 Acute lymphocytic leukemia**. A 3-year-old boy with acute lymphocytic leukemia and right proptosis. Coronal contrast-enhanced T1-WI with FS shows an enhancing soft tissue mass (arrow) centered in the right zygomatic bone, with an intraorbital extraconal extension causing mass effect over the lateral rectus muscle with secondary proptosis (not shown). There is thickening and increased enhancement in the bilateral zygomatic bones and maxilla in keeping with bone marrow infiltration (*)

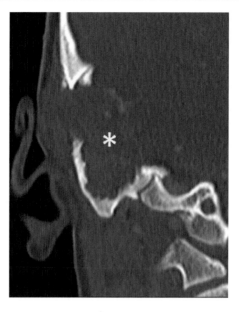

**Fig. 22 LCH**. A 5-year-old girl with a mass behind right ear consistent with LCH. Coronal CECT shows a lytic lesion involving the inner and outer tables of the right temporal bone with an associated solid soft tissue component extending into the right mastoid air cells (*)

tissue mass, associated with aggressive bone changes (permeative appearance, "hair-on-end" or spiculated periosteal reaction and new bone formation). MRI delineates and characterizes neck masses and assesses their intracranial, orbital, perineural, and bone marrow involvement.

LCH foci appear as sharply marginated, "punched-out" lytic defects, with beveled edges, associated with an enhancing soft tissue mass. LCH orbital disease is typically unifocal. Temporal bone LCH is usually bilateral but may be unilateral (Fig. 22).

## Summary

- Consider an IH in a well-defined, vascular, growing mass in the neck, sinonasal, or airway in children <1 year. This may be part of the PHACE syndrome.
- The most common aggressive mass in the pediatric neck includes *RMS*, leukemia/lymphoma, and metastatic neuroblastoma. Look for osseous erosions.
- Think about *LCH* in children with well-defined, sharply marginated, lytic defects.

## Trauma

## Epidemiology

Facial fractures are relatively uncommon in children, accounting for nearly 15% of all facial fractures (56.4% < 5 years, 50% between 6 and 11 years, and 44.6% between 12 and 18 years) [40, 41]. Facial fractures are more common in males. In serious trauma, the most common associated injury is brain trauma (47%). Blindness has only been reported in 0.5% as sequelae of orbital fracture [41]. Other significant traumatic facial injuries include

foreign bodies, animal bites, globe injury, and retrobulbar collections (air, hematoma).

## Clinical Features

Trauma in children differs from adults due to their distinct craniofacial skeleton proportion, more plasticity of facial bones, and developing paranasal sinuses. The most common fractures in younger children are isolated orbital roof "blow-in" fractures, while orbital floor/"blow-out"-type fractures are more common in >5 years of age. The latter are associated with a secondary orbital functional unit injury [40–43]. A retrobulbar collection is an emergency, since it may compress the optic nerve causing blindness.

## Diagnostic Investigations

Radiography is not indicated for facial or orbital trauma. NECT is the imaging modality of choice to assess orbital trauma in the acute setting. Imaging findings together with an ophthalmologic examination should be performed. CT shows site, extent, and type of fractures and associated soft tissue or nerve injury (Fig. 23). If concerned for vascular injury, a CECT is required.

## Summary

- Isolated orbital roof "blow-in" fractures are seen in younger children.

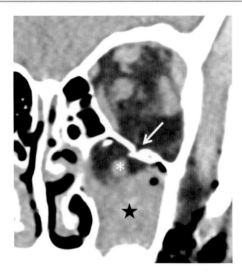

**Fig. 23 Trauma**. A 13-year-old boy with multiple facial fractures. Coronal NECT shows a comminuted, slightly depressed, left orbital floor fracture causing mild distortion of the infraorbital foramen (long arrow), with associated orbital fat and inferior rectus muscle herniation into the maxillary antrum and inferior rectus muscle entrapment (*). There is hemosinus (star) with air-fluid levels and hyperdense content of the left maxillary sinus

- Trap-door "blow-out" orbital fractures are a medical emergency due to the risk of orbital functional unit injury.
- CT is the modality of choice to assess head and neck trauma. Consider CECT if a vascular injury is suspected.

## References

1. Wald ER, Applegate KE, Bordley C, et al. Clinical practice guideline for the diagnosis and management of acute bacterial sinusitis in children aged 1 to 18 years. Pediatrics. 2013;132(1):e262–80.
2. American Academy of Pediatrics. Subcommittee on Management of Sinusitis and Committee on Quality Improvement. Clinical practice guideline: management of sinusitis. Pediatrics. 2001;108(3):798–808.
3. DeMuri GP, Wald ER. Clinical practice. Acute bacterial sinusitis in children. N Engl J Med. 2012;367(12):1128–34.
4. Romero C, Bardo D. Patient-friendly summary of the ACR appropriateness criteria: sinusitis–child. J Am Coll Radiol. 2019;16(8):e35.
5. Expert Panel on Neurologic Imaging, Kirsch CFE, Bykowski J, et al. ACR appropriateness criteria® sinonasal disease. J Am Coll Radiol. 2017;14(11S):S550–9.
6. Meltzer EO, Hamilos DL. Rhinosinusitis diagnosis and management for the clinician: a synopsis of recent consensus guidelines. Mayo Clin Proc. 2011;86(5):427–43.
7. Aring AM, Chan MM. Current concepts in adult acute rhinosinusitis. Am Fam Physician. 2016;94(2):97–105.
8. Chow AW, Benninger MS, Brook I, et al. IDSA clinical practice guideline for acute bacterial rhinosinusitis in children and adults. Clin Infect Dis. 2012;54(8):e72–e112.
9. Din-Lovinescu C, Mir G, Blanco C, et al. Intracranial complications of pediatric rhinosinusitis: identifying risk factors and interventions affecting length of hospitalization. Int J Pediatr Otorhinolaryngol. 2020;131:109841.
10. Hicks CW, Weber JG, Reid JR, et al. Identifying and managing intracranial complications of sinusitis in children: a retrospective series. Pediatr Infect Dis J. 2011;30(3):222–6.
11. Ludwig BJ, Foster BR, Saito N, et al. Diagnostic imaging in non-traumatic pediatric head and neck emergencies. Radiographics. 2010;30(3):781–99.
12. Çelik M, Kaya KH, Yegin Y, et al. Anatomical factors in children with orbital complications due to acute rhinosinusitis. Iran J Otorhinolaryngol. 2019;31(106):289–95.
13. Rudloe TF, Harper MB, Prabhu SP, et al. Acute periorbital infections: who needs emergent imaging? Pediatrics. 2010;125(4):e719–26.
14. LeBedis CA, Sakai O. Nontraumatic orbital conditions: diagnosis with CT and MR imaging in the emergent setting. Radiographics. 2008;28(6):1741–53.
15. Nguyen VD, Singh AK, Altmeyer WB, et al. Demystifying orbital emergencies: a pictorial review. Radiographics. 2017;37(3):947–62.
16. Ekhlassi T, Becker N. Preseptal and orbital cellulitis. Dis Mon. 2017;63(2):30–2.
17. Sharma A, Liu ES, Le TD, et al. Pediatric orbital cellulitis in the Haemophilus influenzae vaccine era. J AAPOS. 2015;19(3):206–10.
18. Jabarin B, Eviatar E, Israel O, et al. Indicators for imaging in periorbital cellulitis secondary to rhinosinusitis. Eur Arch Otorhinolaryngol. 2018;275(4):943–8.
19. Le TD, Liu ES, Adatia FA, et al. The effect of adding orbital computed tomography findings to the Chandler criteria for classifying pediatric orbital cellulitis in predicting which patients will require surgical intervention. J AAPOS. 2014;18(3):271–7.
20. Chandler JR, Langenbrunner DJ, Stevens ER. The pathogenesis of orbital complications in acute sinusitis. Laryngoscope. 1970;80(9):1414–28.
21. Capps EF, Kinsella JJ, Gupta M. Emergency imaging assessment of acute, nontraumatic conditions of the head and neck. Radiographics. 2010;30(5):1335–52.
22. Vaughn J. Emergency imaging of the nontraumatic pediatric head and neck. Semin Ultrasound CT MR. 2019;40(2):147–56.
23. Bochner RE, Gangar M, Belamarich PF. A clinical approach to tonsillitis, tonsillar hypertrophy, and peritonsillar and retropharyngeal abscesses. Pediatr Rev. 2017;38(2):81–92.
24. Chapman T, Sandstrom C, Parnell S. Pediatric emergencies of the upper and lower airway. Appl Radiol. 2012;41(4):10–7. Available via https://www.appliedradiology.com/communities/Pediatric-Imaging/pediatric-emergencies-of-the-upper-and-lower-airway. Accessed May 31 2020.
25. Mandal A, Kabra SK, Lodha R. Upper airway obstruction in children. Indian J Pediatr. 2015;82(8):737–44.
26. Bansal AG, Oudsema R, Masseaux JA, et al. US of pediatric superficial masses of the head and neck. Radiographics. 2018;38(4):1239–63.
27. Inarejos Clemente E, Oyewumi M, Propst EJ, et al. Thyroglossal duct cysts in children: sonographic features every radiologist should know and their histopathological correlation. Clin Imaging. 2017;46:57–64.
28. Kadom N, Lee EY. Neck masses in children: current imaging guidelines and imaging findings. Semin Roentgenol. 2012;47(1):7–20.
29. Bi J, Chen X, Zhou Z, et al. Diagnosis and treatment of deep neck abscess due to congenital pyriform sinus fistula in children. Braz J Otorhinolaryngol. 2020;S1808-8694(20)30009–4.
30. Adams A, Mankad K, Offiah C, et al. Branchial cleft anomalies: a pictorial review of embryological development and spectrum of imaging findings. Insights Imaging. 2016;7(1):69–76.
31. Thomas B, Shroff M, Forte V, et al. Revisiting imaging features and the embryologic basis of third and fourth branchial anomalies. AJNR Am J Neuroradiol. 2010;31(4):755–60.
32. Moe J, Rajan R, Caltharp S, et al. Diagnosis and management of children with Mycobacterium abscessus infections in the head and neck. J Oral Maxillofac Surg. 2018;76(9):1902–11.

33. Ahuja AT, Ying M. Sonographic evaluation of cervical lymph nodes. AJR Am J Roentgenol. 2005;184(5):1691–9.
34. Loh R, Phua M, Shaw CL. Management of paediatric acute mastoiditis: systematic review. J Laryngol Otol. 2018;132(2):96–104.
35. Van Zuijlen DA, Schilder AG, Van Balen FA, et al. National differences in incidence of acute mastoiditis: relationship to prescribing patterns of antibiotics for acute otitis media? Pediatr Infect Dis J. 2001;20(2):140–4.
36. Benito MB, Gorricho BP. Acute mastoiditis: increase in the incidence and complications. Int J Pediatr Otorhinolaryngol. 2007;71 (7):1007–11.
37. Mansour T, Yehudai N, Tobia A, et al. Acute mastoiditis: 20 years of experience with a uniform management protocol. Int J Pediatr Otorhinolaryngol. 2019;125:187–91.
38. Csanády M, Vass G, Bartyik K, et al. Multidisciplinary management of cervical neuroblastoma in infants. Int J Pediatr Otorhinolaryngol. 2014;78(12):2103–6.
39. Rodriguez DP, Orscheln ES, Koch BL. Masses of the nose, nasal cavity, and nasopharynx in children. Radiographics. 2017;37(6): 1704–30.
40. Vyas RM, Dickinson BP, Wasson KL, et al. Pediatric facial fractures: current national incidence, distribution, and health care resource use. J Craniofac Surg. 2008;19(2):339–50.
41. Grunwaldt L, Smith DM, Zuckerbraun NS, et al. Pediatric facial fractures: demographics, injury patterns, and associated injuries in 772 consecutive patients. Plast Reconstr Surg. 2011;128(6):1263–71.
42. Yoo YJ, Yang HK, Kim N, et al. Pediatric orbital wall fractures: prognostic factors of diplopia and ocular motility limitation. PLoS One. 2017;12(11):e0184945.
43. Cobb AR, Jeelani NO, Ayliffe PR. Orbital fractures in children. Br J Oral Maxillofac Surg. 2013;51(1):41–6.

# Imaging of Pediatric Traumatic and Nontraumatic Spinal Emergencies

**46**

Matthias W. Wagner and Birgit B. Ertl-Wagner

## Contents

### Abstract

Pediatric spinal emergencies differ from adult spinal emergencies. The developing spinal column is more mobile and deformable and absorbs traumatic forces differently compared to the adult spine. Moreover, each pediatric age group has its own patterns of injury. Knowledge about the normal developing spinal anatomy is essential to correctly diagnose traumatic injury. Non-traumatic spinal cord injury has many heterogeneous causes. These include spinal tumors (including astrocytoma and ependymoma) and inflammatory/autoimmune conditions (including multiple sclerosis [MS] and neuromyelitis optica). Cord infarction is rare in childhood. While CT is commonly the modality of choice to initially evaluate suspected spinal injury, MRI is better suited to assess spinal cord injury and potential disruption of ligamentous structures. MRI is usually the modality of choice to investigate nontraumatic spinal emergencies. In this chapter, a summary of the epidemiology, clinical features, and diagnostic investigations of traumatic and nontraumatic pediatric spinal emergencies is given in the context of the normal anatomical variations.

### Keywords

Spine · Trauma · Pediatric · Imaging · Infection · Spinal cord

### Abbreviations

| | |
|---|---|
| ADEM | Acute disseminated encephalomyelitis |
| AFM | Acute flaccid myelitis |
| AQP4 | Aquaporin-4 |
| ATM | Acute transverse myelitis |
| C | Cervical |

M. W. Wagner
Division of Neuroradiology, The Hospital for Sick Children, Toronto, ON, Canada
e-mail: matthias.wagner@sickkids.ca

B. B. Ertl-Wagner (✉)
Division of Neuroradiology, The Hospital for Sick Children, Toronto, ON, Canada

Department of Medical Imaging, University of Toronto, Toronto, ON, Canada
e-mail: BirgitBetina.Ertl-Wagner@sickkids.ca

© Springer Nature Switzerland AG 2022
M. N. Patlas et al. (eds.), *Atlas of Emergency Imaging from Head-to-Toe*,
https://doi.org/10.1007/978-3-030-92111-8_46

| | |
|---|---|
| CNS | Central nervous system |
| GCS | Glasgow Coma Scale |
| L | Lumbar |
| MS | Multiple sclerosis |
| NEXUS | National Emergency X-Radiography Utilization Study |
| NMOSD | Neuromyelitis optica spectrum disorder |
| PECARN | Pediatric Emergency Care Applied Research Network |
| S | Sacral |
| SCIWORA | Spinal cord injury without radiographic abnormality |
| T | Thoracic |
| WI | Weighted imaging |

## Traumatic Spinal Emergencies

Pediatric spinal trauma differs from adult spinal trauma. Key factors include the initially predominantly cartilaginous pediatric spine with relatively lax ligaments, the comparatively weak neck and paraspinal musculature, a large head-to-torso ratio, shallow occipital condyles, horizontal orientation of the facet joints (30° in infants vs. 60–70° in adults), small uncinate processes and immature uncovertebral joints, increased elasticity of the posterior joint capsules, the cartilaginous junction between the vertebral bodies and their endplates, increased transverse (extension/flexion) and rotational mobility, and less well-developed protective reflexes [1]. The pediatric spine is therefore (1) more mobile and deformable and (2) absorbs traumatic forces differently compared to the adult spine. Consequently, dislocations, ligamentous injuries, epiphyseal detachments, and focal abnormalities of the ossification centers are more frequent in children than in adults, whereas vertebral fractures are less often encountered. There is a gradually decreasing influence of these key factors with advancing age from the neonate to the adolescent. In the 0–2-year age group, most spinal injuries occur in conjunction with motor vehicle collisions (42%), followed by falls (29%) and child abuse (18%). Motor vehicle collisions and falls are also the most frequent causes in the 3–12-year and in the 13–20-year age groups (52%, 26% and 66%, 13%, respectively) [2].

## Traumatic Spinal Injury: Craniocervical Junction and Cervical Spine

### Epidemiology

In the 0–2-year age group, approximately 52% of spinal trauma admissions occur for injuries in the cervical (C) spine [2], with 38% of injuries found at the C1–4 level. The frequency of C-spine trauma admissions decreases to 34% in the 3–12-year age group and 33% in the 13–20-year age group [2].

## Clinical Features

In the 2019 Consensus Statement from the Pediatric Cervical Spine Clearance Working Group, best practice guidelines for pediatric C-spine clearance are divided into three pathways depending on the Glasgow Coma Scale (GCS) [3]. The National Emergency X-Radiography Utilization Study (NEXUS) trial identified five high-risk criteria for pediatric C-spine injury including (1) midline cervical tenderness, (2) evidence of intoxication, (3) altered level of alertness, (4) focal neurologic deficit, and (5) painful distracting injury [4]. The presence of one or more of these criteria placed a patient into the high-risk group, where about 1% of patients were found to have C-spine injury [4, 5]. The absence of all criteria defined a patient as low risk where no patient had C-spine injury [4]. The results of the NEXUS criteria may be less applicable in young children and infants, in whom clinical examinations may be challenging and methods of spine injury may be different [5].

The Pediatric Emergency Care Applied Research Network (PECARN) identified eight high-risk factors associated with C-spine injury which are partially overlapping with the NEXUS criteria: altered mental status, focal neurologic findings, neck pain, torticollis, substantial torso injury, conditions predisposing to C-spine injury, diving, and high-risk motor vehicle collision [6]. Having one or more of these risk factors was 98% sensitive and 26% specific for C-spine injury [6].

Pieretti-Vanmarcke et al. reviewed 12,537 patients younger than 3 years from 22 level I or II trauma centers [7]. Four independent predictors of C-spine injury were identified and weighted with risk points: GCS <14 (3 points), GCS (EYE) = 1 (2 points), motor vehicle collision (2 points), and age 2 years or older (1 point). A score of <2 had a negative predictive value of 99.93% in excluding C-spine injury, and a score of 2–8 points was considered high risk [7].

## Diagnostic Investigations

### Imaging Guidelines

The 2019 Consensus Statement from the Pediatric Cervical Spine Clearance Working Group recommends a radiograph with a lateral view and flexion/extension radiographs (>30 degrees of flexion/extension) for patients with GCS 14 or 15 when clinical history and physical examination cannot "clear" the C-spine. For patients with GCS 9–13, a radiograph with a lateral view was recommended when there was the potential for improvement of the level of consciousness. If not, a CT of the C-spine was recommended; if this was interpreted as normal and the patient was not anticipated to improve to GCS14/15 within 72 hours, an additional C-spine MRI should be performed. For a GCS below 8 and reasonable suspicion for C-spine injury, a CT of the C-spine was recommended as the initial imaging modality of choice. When interpreted as normal, the pathway followed the one outlined for GCS 9-13.

The 2019 update of the American College of Radiology's (ACR) Appropriateness Criteria [8] differentiated four variants, with the first three variants concerning C-spine imaging, and the fourth variant thoracic (T) and lumbar (L) spine imaging. **Variant 1:** Initial imaging was not recommended for the 3–16-year age group with acute C-spine trauma with absent high-risk criteria based on PECARN or NEXUS. **Variant 2:** Initial C-spine radiographs were appropriate for the 3–16-year age group with acute C-spine trauma with at least one risk factor and with a reliable clinical examination based on PECARN or NEXUS. CT or MRI of the C-spine without intravenous contrast may be appropriate as the initial imaging method but was considered controversial due to insufficient literature to conclude whether or not these patients benefit from these procedures. **Variant 3:** Radiographs of the C-spine were considered appropriate for initial imaging of children <3 years with acute C-spine trauma with a Pieretti-Vanmarcke weighted score of 2–8 points. CT or MRI of the C-spine without intravenous contrast may be appropriate as initial imaging method but was considered controversial due to insufficient literature to conclude whether or not these patients would benefit from these procedures [8].

## Measurements

Craniocervical junction injury is more common in young children than in adults. Several measurements can indicate craniocervical junction injury [5]. Generally accepted normal values are (1) basion-dens interval <12 mm (distance from tip of basion to superior tip of the dens); (2) atlanto-occipital joint space <5 mm (tangential distance from occipital condyle to C1 massa lateralis); (3) atlanto-axial joint space line <4 mm (tangential distance from inferior border of C1 massa lateralis to superior border of C2 vertebral body); (4) anterior atlanto-dental interval <5 mm (in children ≤8 years) and <3 mm (in children >8 years) (also known as the predental interval: from the posterior aspect of the inferior margin of the anterior arch of the C1 to the dens); (5) the Wackenheim clival line (line along the posterior aspect of the clivus toward the odontoid process), which should normally barely touch the tip of the dens; (6) C1–C2 laminar line <12 mm (distance from the posterior-inferior aspect of the C1 posterior ring to the superior aspect of the C2 posterior elements); and (7) Powers ratio <1 (ratio of the distance from the basion to the posterior aspect of the spinolaminar line of the atlas divided by the distance from the anterior tubercle of the atlas to the opisthion) (Fig. 1) [5].

## Traumatic Abnormalities at the Craniocervical Junction

Traumatic abnormalities at the craniocervical junction are encountered within a spectrum of severity. Depending on the force and mechanism, translational, flexion/extension, distraction, and compression injuries and/or fractures may occur. At the mild end of the spectrum, ligaments such as the alar, apical, interspinous, or transverse ligaments are stretched, but aside from straightening of the physiological cervical lordosis, radiographs and CT can be unremarkable [1, 9]. Retroclival and/or intraspinal hematomas may be visible on CT (Fig. 2). They can displace the tectorial membrane and extend into the epidural space of the cervical spinal canal and should be specifically looked for. At the severe end of the spectrum, traumatic injuries can involve the atlanto-occipital joint, where C1 may become axially dislocated in relation to the occiput (atlanto-occipital dislocation, Fig. 3). A dislocation can also be seen between C1 and C2 (atlanto-axial dislocation) [1, 10]. In an atlanto-occipital dislocation, a complete rupture of the ligaments between the occiput and C1/C2 separates the spinal column vertically from the skull. Usually, the spinal cord is severely injured, and the prognosis is poor.

Sagittal CT reformations help in demonstrating potential widening of the vertebral body synchondroses (particularly in children <7 years), epiphyseal detachments, and fractures and are also helpful in visualizing retroclival and intraspinal hematomas (Fig. 2a). CT also allows measuring the craniocervical distances. T2-weighted MRI with or without fat saturation may show thinning and/or increased signal of the injured ligaments and in the immediate vicinity. T2-hyperintense edematous signal may also be seen at the epiphyseal plates, at the insertion of the ligaments with the subchondral bone, and within the adjacent prevertebral and posterior nuchal soft tissues [1]. High-spatial-resolution 3D-T2-weighted sequences with or without fat saturation can directly display the disrupted ligaments and allow visualization of injured cervical nerve roots.

Depending on the severity of the injury, further investigations including CT- or MR-angiography need to be considered to exclude concomitant vascular injuries, i.e., vertebral artery dissection. In addition, coexisting spinal and intracranial soft tissue injury (i.e., transection and/or diffuse axonal injury) may be present in more severe cases and will need to be assessed with MRI if clinically indicated.

Dynamic CT can be performed to differentiate atlanto-axial rotatory subluxation from fixation. The examination requires a controlled setting, where the patient is at rest and then rotates the head to each side. This is performed independently by the patient alone in order to prevent worsening of any underlying spinal injury. If the C1/C2 levels are fixed, they will not rotate independently [5, 11].

SCIWORA (spinal cord injury without radiographic abnormality) is defined as objective clinical signs of spinal

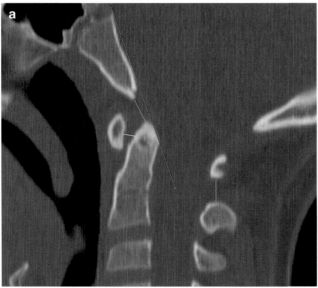

**Fig. 1** (**a**) Normal example of measurement lines. Sagittal reformation of a CT of the craniocervical junction demonstrates the basion-dens interval (green line), the predental interval (orange line), the C1-C2 laminar line (blue line), and the Wackenheim clival line (red line). (**b**) Coronal reformation of a CT of the craniocervical junction demonstrates the atlanto-axial joint space (red lines) and the atlanto-occipital joint space (blue lines)

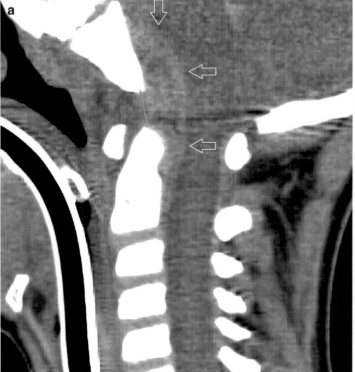
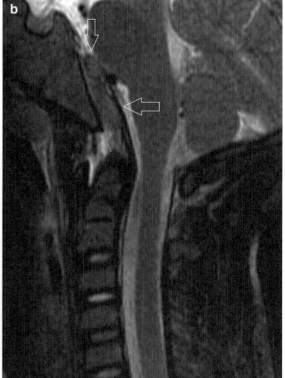

**Fig. 2** An 8-year-old boy with retroclival hematoma after a motor vehicle collision. Sagittal CT reformation (**a**) and sagittal T2-weighted MR image (**b**) demonstrate a large retroclival hematoma (arrows), a widened basion-dens interval (green line), and multiple ligamentous injuries including a rupture of the tectorial membrane

cord injury without evidence of injury on radiographs. This entity most often affects the C-spine and is most common in children under the age of 9 years [1, 5]. Fat-saturated T2-weighted sequences and heavily T2-weighted, high-spatial-resolution (e.g., FIESTA or CISS) MRI sequences are used as a problem-solving examination and usually

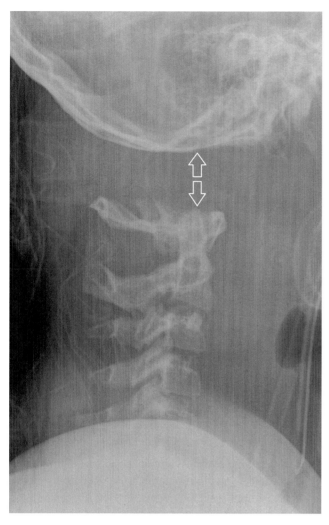

**Fig. 3** A 10-year-old boy with atlanto-occipital dissociation after a motor vehicle collision. Lateral radiograph of the cervical spine demonstrates extensive atlanto-occipital dissociation with extensive widening of the basion-dens interval (arrows)

provide the necessary soft tissue contrast to reveal spinal cord injury, nerve root injury, paraspinal plexus injury, and accompanying ligamentous injury [12].

Cervical fractures are similar in appearance compared to the spectrum encountered in the adult population. Various trauma mechanisms lead to respective types of injury [1, 5]. C3 to C7 compression fractures are typically encountered after traumatic hyperflexion. Sagittal CT reformations usually facilitate the assessment of the degree of anterior wedging and other concomitant C-spine fractures, including fractures of the spinous processes.

## Summary

Pediatric cervical spine injury is different from adult C-spine injury with regard to distribution and incidence. Radiographs and CT are used to predominantly assess the osseous injury, while MRI is the modality of choice to depict spinal cord

injury including SCIWORA as well as ligamentous injury. Depending on the severity of injury, CT- or MR-angiography should be considered to exclude or diagnose concomitant vascular injuries.

## Key Points

- The pediatric spine is more mobile and deformable and absorbs traumatic forces differently compared to the adult spine.
- Dislocations, ligamentous injuries, epiphyseal detachments, and abnormalities of the ossification centers are more frequent in children – whereas vertebral fractures are less often encountered.
- In the 0–2-year-old age group, most spinal injuries occur in conjunction with motor vehicle collisions (42%), followed by falls (29%) and child abuse (18%).

## Traumatic Spinal Injury: Thoracic and Lumbosacral Spine

### Epidemiology

At the 0–2-year age group, approximately 55% of admissions for spinal trauma occur in the T/L/sacral (S) spine [2]. This increases to 74% in the 3–12-year age group and 85% in the 13–20-year age group [2]. Fractures are typically encountered at the T/L junction and in the L spine; they occur less frequently in the thoracic spine because of the stabilizing effects of the rib cage. Compression fractures are the most frequently encountered type of T/L fractures in children [13].

### Clinical Features

Clinical assessment only has an estimated 81% sensitivity and 68% specificity for T/L spine fractures [8]. Consequently, there is a low threshold for obtaining radiographs to screen for injury independent of the clinical symptoms. When assessment of mental status, positive physical examination findings, trauma mechanism, and age are included in clinical decision-making, sensitivity improves to 99% for clinically relevant spinal injury in adults, while the specificity decreases to 29% [14]. The ACR Criteria recommend the use of MRI to evaluate patients with neurologic deficits, abnormal CT scans, and high clinical suspicion despite negative radiographic evaluation [8, 15].

Sacral fractures account for only approximately 0.2% of all fractures in pediatric trauma patients [8, 16]. In a review of 89 patients, all sacral fractures were lateral to the neural element (Denis zone 1) [16]. CT and MRI are the recommended modalities to assess sacral fractures since radiographs were shown to not demonstrate 35% of sacral fractures [17].

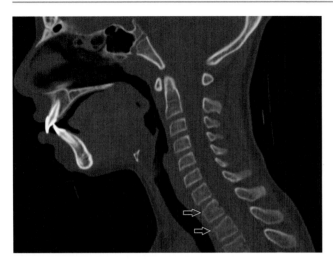

**Fig. 4** A 12-year-old boy with compression fractures after a motor vehicle collision. Sagittal CT reformation demonstrates mild anterior compression fractures of T1 and T2 (arrows), which were confirmed on MRI. Note that the mild anterior wedging of C3 to C6 vertebral bodies is physiologic for age

## Diagnostic Investigations

### Imaging Guidelines

The 2019 update of the ACR Appropriateness Criteria [8] recommends imaging for suspected spinal injuries using the four variants discussed above, with the first three variants covering on C-spine imaging and the fourth variant covering T/L spine imaging. In this **Variant 4**, radiographs of the T/L spine were considered appropriate for initial imaging of children <16 years with suspected T/L spine trauma. CT or MRI may be appropriate as initial imaging, but this was considered controversial due to insufficient literature.

### Focal Injuries of the Thoracic and Lumbosacral Spine

Compression, burst, and Chance fractures are among the typically encountered injuries. Compression fractures are characterized by a wedge-shaped deformity of the vertebral body (Fig. 4). Burst fractures are a severe type of compression fracture where the anterior and posterior vertebral body cortices are disrupted, and bony fragments may be dislocated into the spinal canal (Fig. 5). Compression or laceration of the adjacent neural structures needs to be excluded. Further dislocations may be seen with increase of the axial loading. Chance fractures [18], also known as seat belt fractures, are unstable fractures and are characterized by a transverse or oblique fracture which involves all three vertebral columns due to a flexion-distraction injury [1] (Fig. 6). The typical mechanism of injury is that of a back-seat passenger restrained by a seat belt without shoulder strap. The flexion or compression injury occurs at the vertebral body (first and second vertebral column), and the distraction force is exerted at the posterior elements (third column). Approximately 50%

of these fractures occur at the thoracolumbar junction [19], with the upper and mid-lumbar regions being affected less frequently. Whereas the anterior compression fracture may be obvious on CT, the injury to the posterior elements may only be depicted using MRI. Secondary signs, including increased interspinous distance and widened facet joints, may be visible on CT and should be specifically looked for. MRI is warranted to directly visualize ligamentous injury, including distraction or disruption of the posterior longitudinal ligament and interspinous ligament. Chance fractures have a high incidence of concomitant intra-abdominal injury, particularly pancreatic and/or duodenal laceration in both adults and children. Imaging should therefore also be used to evaluate the chest, abdomen, and pelvis, and its vasculature.

## Summary

Imaging is crucial in the detection and classification of traumatic spinal injuries in children. With descent of the fulcrum and shift of injury toward the thoracic and lumbar spine with advancing age, the ACR Appropriateness Criteria apply adult clinical decision rules to the pediatric population. Compression, burst, and Chance fractures are commonly encountered injuries of the thoracolumbar spine in children.

## Key Points

- Burst fractures are a severe type of compression fracture where the anterior and posterior vertebral body cortex is disrupted, and bony fragments may be dislocated into the spinal canal. Subsequent compression and/or laceration of the adjacent neural structures need to be excluded.
- Chance fractures are unstable fractures and are characterized by a transverse or oblique fracture which involves all three vertebral columns due to a flexion-distraction injury.
- Secondary signs, including increased interspinous distance and widened facet joints, may be visible on CT, but MRI is warranted to directly visualize ligamentous injury, including distraction or disruption of the posterior longitudinal ligament and interspinous ligament.
- Chance fractures have a high incidence of concomitant intra-abdominal injury, particularly pancreatic and/or duodenal laceration.

## Birth-Related Injury

### Epidemiology

Birth trauma is reported to occur in fewer than 3% of all live births in the United States [20]. Neonatal spinal cord injury is rare, with an estimated prevalence of 1 per 29,000 live births

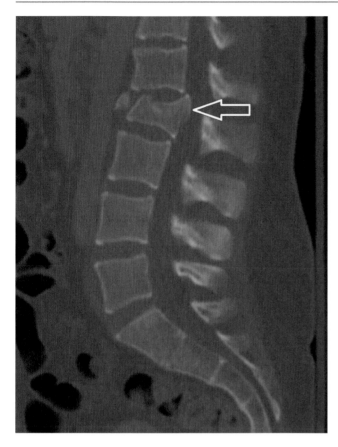

**Fig. 5** A 14-year-old girl with burst fracture after a skiing accident. Sagittal CT reformation demonstrates a burst fracture of L2, with the retropulsion of bony fragments into the narrowed spinal canal (arrow)

[21]. Birth-related brachial plexus injuries include Erb und Klumpke palsies. The most common cause is excessive lateral traction or stretching of the head and neck.

### Clinical Features

Spinal cord injury during delivery likely results from excessive traction, rotation, or hyperextension, with the most frequent sites of injury being the lower cervical and upper thoracic region for breech delivery and the upper and mid C-spine for vertex delivery [22–24]. Direct spinal cord injuries are rare but should be suspected if the neonate is hypotonic with flaccid quadriplegia or paraplegia [20].

### Diagnostic Investigations

The spectrum of birth-related spinal injuries ranges from ligamentous, cartilaginous, and osseous focal abnormalities to nerve root avulsions, brachial plexus injuries, focal cord hemorrhages, complete cord transections, and extraspinal hematomas [1]. Carotid dissections are a very rare complication of dystocic labor [25]. Doppler ultrasound, CT, and MRI can play a role in the diagnosis. Lateral radiographs of the spine can be obtained to demonstrate vertebral fracture and subluxation [26]. MRI is the modality of choice for the evaluation of newborn spinal cord injury and nerve root avulsions due to C-spine trauma [27]. Dedicated plexus imaging can be considered for birth-related plexus injuries. Depending on the severity, brachial plexus injuries present with edema and an avulsion pseudomeningocele. The "cele" is located at the site of the avulsed nerve root and does not contain neural elements. Hematomyelia may be present. In

**Fig. 6** A 14-year-old girl with Chance fracture after a motor vehicle collision. Sagittal CT reformation (**a**) and sagittal fat-saturated T2-weighted MR image (**b**) demonstrate a Chance fracture of L2 involving all three columns (arrows). MRI also demonstrated pronounced degloving injury posteriorly

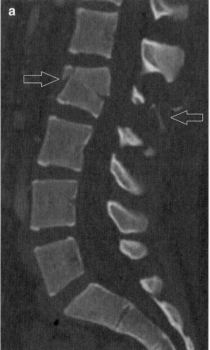
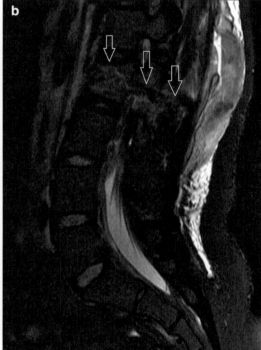

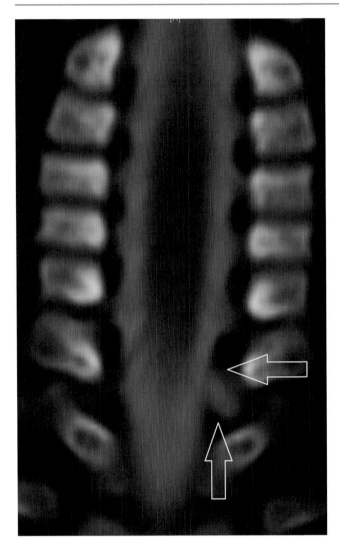

**Fig. 7** A 10-month-old girl after birth-related C8 injury. Coronal reformation of a CT myelography demonstrating left-sided C8 injury with discontinuity (arrows) of the nerve roots

rare instances, CT myelography can be considered for surgical planning (Fig. 7).

## Summary

Birth-related spinal cord injury is rare. MRI is the modality of choice for evaluation. The spectrum of birth-related spinal injuries ranges from ligamentous and cartilaginous and osseous injuries to nerve root avulsions, brachial plexus injuries, focal cord hemorrhages, complete cord transections, and extraspinal hematomas.

## Key Points

- Spinal cord injury should be suspected if a newborn presents with hypotonia, flaccid quadriplegia, or high thoracic paraplegia after a difficult delivery.
- MRI is the modality of choice to investigate birth-related spinal cord injury.

## Non-accidental Spinal Injury

### Epidemiology

It is estimated that between 2.4% and 23.8% of all pediatric blunt trauma is due to non-accidental injury (NAI) [28]. Non-accidental spinal injury is frequently overlooked, likely due to its overall low incidence and its often occult clinical presentation. However, it was found to be relatively common in children under the age of 2 years [28]. In suspected NAI, a complete diagnostic workup including physical examination, psychosocial evaluation, and a skeletal survey is recommended [27].

### Clinical Features

The presence of spinal injury in the setting of NAI is associated with a relatively high risk of long-term neurological impairment [29]. Kemp et al. described two patterns of injury with cervical spinal injuries being more commonly encountered in younger infants (median age 5 months) who presented with signs of impaired consciousness and respiratory distress [29]. Thoracolumbar injury was more common in older infants (median age 13.5 months) with a visible spinal deformity or focal neurological signs [29].

### Diagnostic Investigations

There are no pathognomonic injury patterns to confirm the non-accidental etiology of the trauma mechanism [1, 5]. Isolated fractures of the spinous processes may raise suspicion of NAI, particularly in the absence of an adequate trauma history [1]. In addition, spinal subdural hemorrhages are more common in children with NAI compared to children with accidental trauma [30]. The most common type of spinal injury in NAI is cervical spinal ligamentous disruption followed by compression fractures, spinal cord injury, nerve root injury, and subdural hematomas [5, 29–31]. Choudhary et al. showed that the presence of injury of the cervical ligaments correlated with evidence of hypoxic-ischemic brain injury [32]. Jacob et al. suggested including C-spine MRI in the battery of tests performed while working up a child with NAI [31]. While fractures, ligamentous, or soft tissue injury can be secondary to a wide range of mechanisms, detection of occult injury could be clinically and forensically valuable [33]. Also, a thorough evaluation for associated injuries remote to the spine, neurological deficits, and multilevel spine injury should be performed [28].

### Summary

Spinal trauma can occur in NAI and can be radiographically occult. There is no pathognomonic imaging feature of spinal NAI.

## Key Points

- The frequency of spinal trauma in NAI is higher in children under the age of 2 years.
- Spinal subdural hematoma is more frequent in children with NAI.
- Cervical spinal ligamentous disruption, compression fractures, spinal cord injury, nerve root injury, and subdural hematomas can all occur in non-accidental spinal injury.

## Normal Development: Mimicker of Traumatic Spinal Injury

### Epidemiology

Misinterpretation of normal development may result in misdiagnosis of traumatic spinal injury. The variable appearance of ossification centers with cartilaginous components, complex synchondroses, physiologic subluxation, and the different shape of vertebral bodies related to development may contribute. Moreover, less common diseases including metabolic disorders, segmentation/formation anomalies, connective tissue disorders, chromosomal anomalies, or genetic skeletal dysplasias can be associated with skeletal deformities suggesting traumatic injuries [1].

### Clinical Features

Vertebral bodies in children have a more oval appearance compared to the rectangular shape of adult vertebral bodies [5]. Anterior wedging of the vertebral bodies up to 3 mm should not be confused with a compression fracture [11] (Fig. 4). Whereas a ventral tilt of the odontoid is concerning for traumatic injury, a dorsal dental tilt represents an anatomic variant [5]. The unossified odontoid appears often hyperattenuating on CT and should not be misinterpreted as hematoma. Compared to adults, a straightened appearance of the cervical lordosis can often be a normal finding in children up to 16 years [5].

One of the most commonly encountered mimickers of traumatic injury is the physiologic anterolisthesis (pseudosubluxation) of the C2 relative to the C3 vertebral body (Fig. 8). In addition to that, there is variable angulation of the individual intervertebral spaces [5]. In children, widening of the prevertebral space depends more on the degree of inspiration and may show a significant physiological variability [1, 11]. Additionally, the adenoids and cervical lymphatic tissues are more prominent in children compared to adults.

A limbus vertebra can be misdiagnosed as an acute fracture (Fig. 9). The apophysis of the vertebral ring ossifies before the remainder of the vertebral body. In the event of disk herniation before the fusion of the physis, isolation and non-fusion of the ring apophysis results in a limbus vertebra either anteriorly or less commonly also posteriorly [5].

### Diagnostic Investigations

To avoid misinterpretation of the commonly encountered pseudosubluxation of C2 relative to C3, a line can be drawn from the posterior arch of C1 to the posterior arch of C3 (Fig. 8). If this line is more than 2 mm from the posterior arch of C2, traumatic listhesis should be suspected in younger children [5].

On lateral radiographs, physiologic prevertebral soft tissue thickening may be misinterpreted as acute ligamentous injury. CT or MRI may be needed to assess the presence of true prevertebral edema and to help differentiate traumatic soft tissue thickening from adenoidal hypertrophy or other etiologies [5].

CT is helpful to differentiate an acute dens fracture from an os odontoideum. Well-corticated, smooth sclerotic margins, which are separated from a hypoplastic dens, suggest an orthotopic os odontoideum. A dystopic os odontoideum is located near the foramen magnum. Imaging with flexion and extension positioning may be helpful to assess the stability of an os odontoideum [5].

### Summary

Interpretation of pediatric spine studies requires familiarity with the imaging appearance of the physiologic development of the pediatric spine. Knowledge of the most important measurements helps to differentiate normal variants from spinal injury.

### Key Points

- Physiologic anterolisthesis of the C2 relative to the C3 vertebral body is a common mimicker of traumatic injury.
- A limbus vertebra should be differentiated from a traumatic injury.
- Typical imaging features of an orthotopic os odontoideum are well-corticated, smooth sclerotic margins, which are separated from a hypoplastic dens.

## Nontraumatic Spinal Emergencies

Nontraumatic spinal cord damage has many heterogeneous causes [34]. Compared with traumatic spinal cord injury, there are fewer publications on nontraumatic spinal emergencies, and only a small number of these involve the pediatric age group [34]. The median incidence rates in various global regions are as follows: Australasia 6.5/million population/year, Western Europe 6.2/million population/year, and North America 2.1/million population/year [35]. The most common causes of spinal cord damage are tumors (30–63%) and inflammatory/autoimmune causes (28–35%) [35].

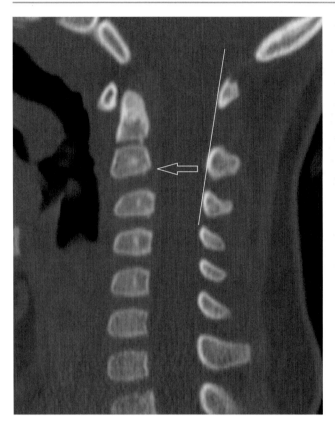

**Fig. 8** A 3-year-old boy presenting after fall. Sagittal CT reformation demonstrates a physiologic anterolisthesis (pseudo-subluxation) of the C2 relative to the C3 vertebral body (arrows). A line is drawn from the posterior arch of C1 to the posterior arch of C3 with the posterior arch of C2 reaching less than 2 mm anterior to it. Also note the physiologic more oval appearance of the vertebral bodies compared to an adult spine

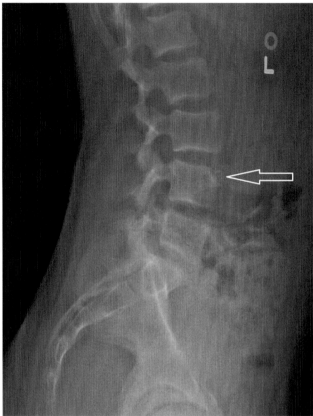

**Fig. 9** A 14-year-old girl with back pain. Lateral radiograph demonstrates a limbus vertebra of L4 (arrow)

## Neoplastic Disease

### Epidemiology

Duong et al. reported on the epidemiology of adult and pediatric malignant and nonmalignant tumors of the spinal cord, spinal meninges, and cauda equina in the United States [36]. Of the 869 pediatric patients with spinal tumors, 51% were malignant and 49% were nonmalignant primary spinal tumors. More than 90% of spinal cord tumors were of glial origin, with pilocytic and anaplastic astrocytomas being the most common (60% and 30%, respectively) [37]. Non-glial tumors are rare and include a variety of histologic subtypes such as hemangioblastoma, subependymoma, ganglioglioma, paraganglioma, lymphoma, neurocytoma, or oligodendroglioma [37].

### Clinical Features

In most children with **disease** spinal cord tumors, the diagnosis is made relatively late after the initial onset of clinical symptoms. Many such children present with a long history of exacerbation and remission of symptoms, which is believed to be related to fluctuating degrees of spinal cord edema [37]. Key neurological symptoms include progressive motor weakness, progressive scoliosis, gait disturbance, and muscle rigidity with paraspinal muscle spasm, while sensory deficits are less common. Approximately 20–30% of children with a spinal cord tumor present with back pain as the leading complaint [37]. More acute clinical presentation with loss of neurologic function can be seen with intramedullary tumors [5].

### Diagnostic Investigations

#### Intramedullary: Spinal Astrocytoma

Spinal astrocytomas are the most common spinal cord tumors in children. Of these, 50% are in the cervicothoracic region. The majority are low-grade tumors (75–80%), with anaplastic astrocytomas and glioblastoma multiforme being less frequent. Due to the infiltrative nature, their margin is often not well defined. The location is often eccentric within the spinal cord and may show an asymmetric spinal cord expansion. On MRI, spinal astrocytomas are typically hyperintense on T2WI (Fig. 10) and iso- to hypointense on T1WI and may demonstrate mild to moderate IV contrast enhancement. Polar or intratumoral cysts with or without peripheral contrast enhancement are encountered in around 20–40% of patients (Fig. 10), frequently accompanied by a rostral and/or caudal

**Fig. 10** A 14-year-old girl with spinal astrocytoma. Sagittal (**a**) and axial (**b**) T2-weighted MR images demonstrate an extensive tumor with ill-defined spinal cord signal abnormalities and intratumoral cysts (arrows)

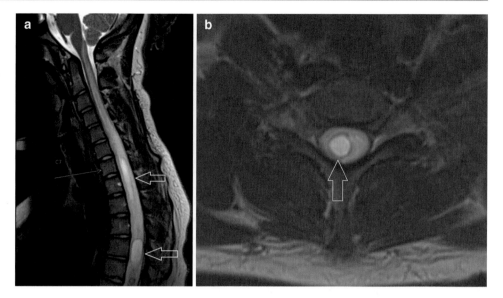

syrinx. Exophytic tumor components or internal hemorrhage are less frequent [37, 38].

### Intramedullary: Spinal Ependymoma

Spinal ependymomas are the second most frequent pediatric spinal cord tumor. Ependymomas are often more centrally located around the central canal and are most frequently encountered in the cervical spinal cord [37]. Ependymomas are less infiltrative than astrocytomas and tend to compress and displace the adjacent spinal cord tissue. Polar cysts and a clear cleavage plane may be more commonly seen (Fig. 11). Another imaging feature is a stronger contrast enhancement due to the high vascularity of the tumor with multiple small feeding vessels. The high vascularity increases the risk of intratumoral (Fig. 11) and subarachnoid hemorrhage. The "cap" sign (a rim of hypointense hemosiderin on T2WI below and/or above the tumor) has been described with ependymoma, but it is not pathognomonic [37]. Myxopapillary ependymomas are predominantly encountered in the area of the conus medullaris and filum terminale. They often fill the spinal canal and may lead to scalloping of the adjacent vertebra. Due to their location, they tend to present with lower back pain, leg weakness, and sphincter dysfunction [37, 38].

### Extramedullary

Intradural extramedullary and extradural tumors may present with symptoms due to spinal cord or cauda equina compression. MRI is the modality of choice to assess the compression and to narrow the differential diagnosis [5]. Typical extramedullary intradural tumors in children include schwannomas and neurofibromas. Extradural tumors can arise from the vertebrae and soft tissues and include neuroblastoma (Fig. 12), rhabdomyosarcoma, leukemia/lymphoma, Ewing sarcoma,

and others [5]. Several nonneoplastic masses may also mimic malignancy. These include dermoids, epidermoids, and teratomas [5, 37].

### Summary

Most children with spinal cord tumors are diagnosed relatively late after initial onset of symptoms and then may present in the emergency setting. Astrocytomas are the most common pediatric spinal cord tumors, with pilocytic and anaplastic astrocytomas being the most common. Spinal ependymomas are the second most common spinal cord tumor in children, while they are the most common in adults. Non-glial tumors are rare and include a variety of histologic subtypes. MRI is the modality of choice to assess the degree of cord compression and to help narrow the differential diagnosis.

### Key Points

- Spinal astrocytomas are the most common pediatric spinal cord tumor, followed by spinal ependymomas.
- The most common location of a spinal cord tumor in children is the cervical spine.

## Inflammatory and Infectious Diseases

### Epidemiology

Various inflammatory conditions involve the cord and may be indistinguishable from other etiologies on imaging. They can be classified as (1) demyelinating disorders, (2) infections, and (3) miscellaneous disorders including granulomatous disease, connective tissue disease, compressive myelopathy, and nutritional deficiency [39].

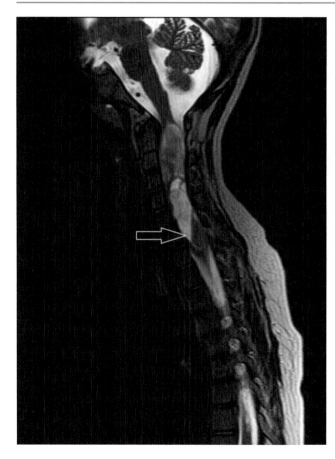

**Fig. 11** An 8-year-old boy with spinal ependymoma. Sagittal T2-weighted MR image demonstrates an expansile tumor of the cervical spinal cord with relatively well-circumscribed borders and intratumoral hemorrhage (arrow)

## Clinical Features

### Demyelinating Disorders: Multiple Sclerosis (MS)

The prevalence of MS onset in childhood and adolescence varies between 2% and 4% of all MS patients [40]. About 2.3 million people worldwide have MS, with 2.7–10% of these being younger than 18 years of age and fewer than 1% being younger than 10 years of age [40]. Involvement of the spinal cord is relatively uncommon. A clinical central nervous system (CNS) event attributable to MS must last for at least 24 hours and can include optic neuritis, transverse myelitis, and/or hemispheric/brainstem-related syndromes. Once MS is suspected during a first demyelinating episode, an MRI of the spine is suggested [40].

### Demyelinating Disorders: Neuromyelitis Optica Spectrum Disorder (NMOSD)

NMOSD is a relapsing autoimmune demyelinating disorder that affects the optic nerves and spinal cord. Initially, most pediatric patients present with optic neuritis (75%) and/or transverse myelitis (30%). Prognosis is better in children than in adults, with 77% versus 18% complete recovery. The course can be multiphasic with recurrence intervals ranging from less than 6 months to up to 5 years after initial presentation [38]. Further key features of the initial clinical presentation include area postrema syndrome with otherwise unexplained hiccups, nausea and vomiting, and narcolepsy [38]. About 60% of children with the classic clinical onset are tested positive for anti-aquaporin-4 (AQP4) antibodies (NMO-IgG) [41]. In children with AQP4 seronegative NMOSD, the presence of anti-myelin oligodendrocyte glycoprotein (MOG) can serve as a diagnostic and potentially a prognostic tool [42].

### Demyelinating Disorders: Acute Disseminated Encephalomyelitis (ADEM)

ADEM typically presents as a monophasic demyelinating disease with multi-focal neurological symptoms associated with encephalopathy [43]. Children may develop ADEM after a viral or bacterial infection (more often mycoplasma); less common precursors include immunizations or drug ingestion [38]. Clinically, children present with encephalopathy with behavioral changes, headache of rapid onset, vomiting, impaired level of consciousness, and nuchal rigidity. Focal neurological signs include long tract signs, cerebellar ataxia, cranial nerve palsy, and visual loss [38]. Multiphasic ADEM is defined as two episodes consistent with ADEM separated by an interval of at least 3 months [43]. Further recurrence of symptoms beyond two episodes is not consistent with multiphasic ADEM and can indicate MS or NMOSD [43]. MOG-IgG can be found in up to 40% of monophasic and up to 100% of multiphasic ADEM patients [40].

### Demyelinating Disorders: Idiopathic Acute Transverse Myelitis (ATM)

ATM presents with acute or subacute static or ascending bilateral motor or sensory symptoms and autonomic symptoms including bowel and bladder dysfunction. Similar to ADEM, a preceding infection or immunization may or may not be present [39]. Idiopathic ATM is a diagnosis of exclusion, and consideration must be given to differential diagnoses including ATM seen with MS, NMOSD, or ADEM, acute flaccid myelitis (AFM), and ATM associated with autoimmune rheumatologic disorder including system lupus erythematosus, Sjogren syndrome, and sarcoidosis [39, 44].

### Demyelinating Disorders: Guillain-Barré Syndrome

Guillain-Barré syndrome is an inflammatory demyelinating polyradiculopathy which presents with ascending weakness and hyporeflexia [5]. Progression of symptoms is rapid and may include facial nerve palsy, autonomic dysfunction, pain, numbness, and respiratory failure [45]. In approximately 75% of affected patients, clinical history reveals a preceding

**Fig. 12** A 4-year-old girl with spinal metastasis of a relapsed neuroblastoma. Sagittal T2-weighted MR image (**a**) and axial contrast-enhanced T1-weighted MR image with fat saturation (**b**) demonstrates a large expansile mass of the posterior elements of L4, with compression of the cauda equina fibers (arrows)

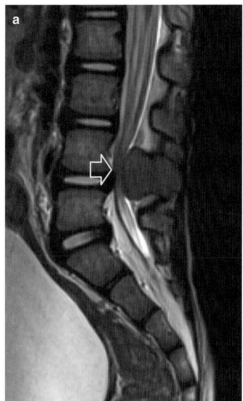
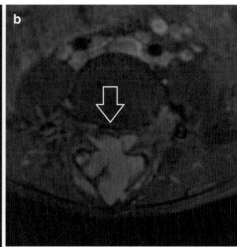

respiratory or gastrointestinal infection [45]. *Campylobacter jejuni* and cytomegalovirus infections are most frequently reported.

### Infectious Disorders: AFM

Similar to ATM, the presentation of AFM often follows a respiratory illness. Over 90% of patients had a mild viral respiratory illness or fever before the onset of symptoms [46]. Important clinical signs of AFM include asymmetric onset of flaccid limb weakness and complaints of pain or paresthesia in the affected limb without an apparent sensory deficit [47]. Autonomic symptoms are less commonly seen in AFM compared to ATM [47]. The clinical and radiological phenotype of AFM is similar to poliomyelitis. A temporal and geographical correlation with enterovirus infections detected in respiratory specimens has led to enterovirus (types D68 and A71) being the most favored causative agent [46, 47]. Experimental mouse models have confirmed the presence of active infectious virus in the spinal cord [47].

### Infectious Disorders: Various Spinal Infections

Other spinal infectious processes include spondylodiscitis, epidural abscess, meningitis, and spinal cord abscess or granuloma [5]. Spondylodiscitis is less common in the pediatric age group compared to adults.

### Diagnostic Investigations

### Demyelinating Disorders: MS

The typical pattern of spinal cord involvement in MS is usually shorter than two cord segments. Demyelinating foci are hyperintense on T2WI and can have a peripheral and ovoid appearance in a paracentral location. The simultaneous presence of multiple demyelinating foci over time and space in the brain and spinal cord is characteristic. The cervical cord and the dorsal aspect of the cord are more commonly affected. Active foci can be seen with restricted diffusion and ring-like IV contrast enhancement.

### Demyelinating Disorders: NMOSD

In contrast to MS, spinal cord focal abnormalities in NMOSD typically involve three or more cord segments (Fig. 13), although this is somewhat less specific for children [38]. Similar to MS, focal abnormalities are hyperintense on T2WI but have a more heterogeneous appearance. They commonly involve almost the entire cross-sectional area of the cord with a central predilection [38]. Often, cervical and thoracic cord segments are involved. Swelling of the affected cord is seen in the acute phase, but spinal cord necrosis ultimately may develop [38]. IV contrast-enhancing foci are observed in approximately 20% of patients [38]. Signal hypointensity on T1WI is suggestive of a chronic relapsing demyelinating

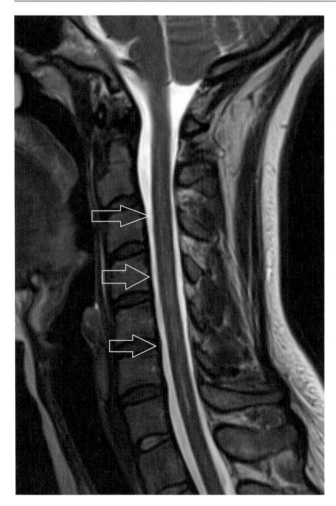

**Fig. 13** A 17-year-old girl with NMOSD. Sagittal T2-weighted MR image demonstrates the ill-defined signal hyperintensity of the cervical spinal cord spanning multiple segments (arrows)

process, which includes both MS and NMOSD. Cord cavitations are more suggestive of NMOSD [47]. Apart from the pertinent imaging findings at the optic nerves, the area of the dorsal brainstem/area postrema is commonly involved [38].

### Demyelinating Disorders: ADEM

Spinal cord involvement in ADEM is seen in 30–50% of patients. Abnormalities are commonly located in the central gray matter with long segments of the cord (>3 vertebral segments) being affected. This differentiates ADEM from MS but not from NMOSD. Petechial hemorrhage may be present in spinal foci, and this can be best seen on T2W gradient-echo or susceptibility-weighted MR images. In the acute phase, diffusion-weighted imaging shows reduced diffusivity in the area of demyelination. In the subacute phase, abnormal foci can show various patterns of IV contrast enhancement, including nodular, ring-like, or diffuse enhancement. Simultaneous large and confluent white matter abnormalities are a typical imaging feature of ADEM [38].

### Demyelinating Disorders: ATM

The affected cord is hyperintense on T2WI in patients with ATM with minimal expansion and variable IV contrast enhancement. Typically, focal abnormalities are longitudinally extensive (>2 segments) and involve more than two-thirds of the cross-sectional area of the spinal cord [47]. The signal abnormality in ATM is often centrally located with abnormal signal seen involving central gray matter and adjacent white matter [44]. The majority of abnormalities are located in the cervical and cervicothoracic spine. Asymptomatic focal abnormalities in the brain are seen in more than 40% of children. In up to 6% of patients with clinical ATM, MRI will not demonstrate any cord abnormality [44].

### Demyelinating Disorders: Guillain-Barré Syndrome

IV contrast-enhanced MRI in patients with Guillain-Barré syndrome typically shows surface thickening and contrast enhancement of the conus medullaris and anterior cauda equina nerve roots [48] (Fig. 14). Enhancement of the posterior nerve roots may also be present.

### Infectious Disorders: AFM

AFM is characterized by injury to the anterior horn cells of the spinal cord. MRI may demonstrate hyperintensity of spinal cord gray matter, particularly the anterior horns, on T2WI (Fig. 15) with variable IV contrast enhancement. Similar to Guillain-Barré syndrome, IV contrast-enhanced MRI may also show smooth enhancement of the anterior cauda equina nerve roots. Hyperintense foci on T2WI and anterior nerve root enhancement may occur throughout the spinal cord [47].

### Infectious Disorders: Various Spinal Infections

Imaging abnormalities in spondylodiscitis, discitis, osteomyelitis, and epidural abscesses are usually best appreciated on fat-saturated sequences. Characteristic imaging features include signal hyperintensity on T2WI and IV contrast enhancement of the affected area, including the disk, bone, and paraspinal soft tissues (Fig. 16). Depending on their size, abscesses can be visualized as peripherally enhancing or irregular ring-enhancing fluid collections. In the very rare instance of an intramedullary cord abscess, the spinal cord appears expanded at the affected site and demonstrates IV contrast enhancement and diffusion restriction.

### Summary

MRI is the mainstay of diagnosis of inflammatory and infectious spinal emergencies. T1W and T2W sequences with or without fat saturation and before and after the IV administration of a gadolinium-based contrast agent should be acquired to properly assess the cord for acute demyelinating or infectious conditions. Once abnormal findings are identified, care

**Fig. 14** A 14-year-old girl with Guillain-Barré syndrome presenting with progressive extremity weakness. Sagittal (**a**) and axial (**b**) contrast-enhanced T1-weighted MR images demonstrate extensive enhancement of the anterior cauda equine nerve roots (arrows)

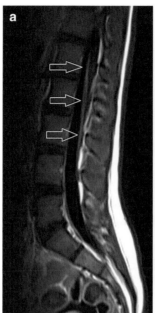
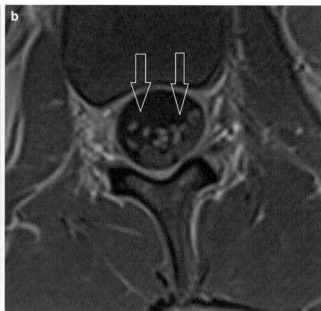

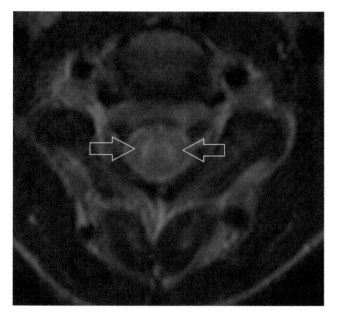

**Fig. 15** A 12-year-old girl with AFM presenting with progressive extremity weakness. Axial T2-weighted MR image demonstrates signal hyperintensity of the spinal cord grey matter (arrows)

should be taken to assess the brain for concomitant abnormalities, which narrows the differential diagnosis.

## Key Points
- In contrast to MS, spinal cord abnormalities in NMOSD typically involve three or more cord segments. In patients with suspected NMOSD, closely look at the area postrema.

- ADEM can also present with multi-segment cord involvement.
- Typical findings of Guillain-Barré syndrome are surface thickening and IV contrast enhancement of the conus medullaris and anterior cauda equina nerve roots.
- AFM is characterized by injury to the anterior horn cells of the spinal cord.

## Vascular Disease

### Epidemiology
Spinal emergencies from vascular causes are rare in children [5]. Potential etiologies include systemic hypotension, poor autoregulation of spinal blood flow in premature children, local shunting due to arteriovenous malformations with subsequent decreased perfusion, trauma and vascular compromise due to aortic dissection or congenital cardiovascular abnormalities, thromboembolic disease, infection, hyperflexion injury with reactive vasospasm, and cerebellar herniation secondary to lumbar puncture [49].

### Clinical Features
Acute infarction of the cord presents with acute (within minutes or few hours) onset of back pain, weakness and paralysis, loss of reflexes, loss of pain and temperature sensation, and incontinence.

### Diagnostic Investigations
The clinical history is important to differentiate infarction from ATM. MRI of the cord reveals hyperintense signal on

**Fig. 16** A 2-year-old girl with spondylodiscitis. Sagittal (**a**) and coronal (**b**) IV contrast-enhanced T1-weighted MR images demonstrate irregularity and avid enhancement of the vertebral bodies and disk space of T 11/12, as well as paravertebral fluid collections (arrows)

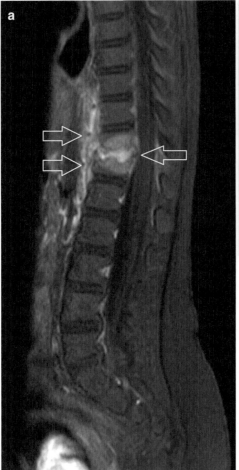
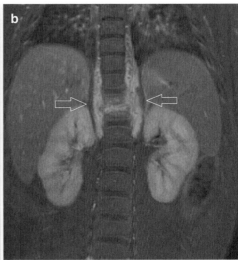

T2WI with associated diffusion restriction within hours after the event. The pattern of signal abnormality depends on the vascular territory. On axial imaging, anterior spinal artery infarctions involve the anterior and central aspects of the cord, bilaterally. If the anterior horn cells are predominantly involved, this can give rise to the "owl eye" or "snake eye" appearance [50] (Fig. 17). This is not specific for a spinal cord infarction and has been described in other entities including NMOSD. The acquisition of an axial and/or sagittal DWI sequence can be helpful to establish the infarct. However, motion artifacts and CSF flow-induced artifacts can decrease the diagnostic utility.

## Summary

Various rare etiologies may cause spinal cord infarction in children. T2W and diffusion-weighted sequences are the most important sequences to assess for spinal cord infarction. However, the underlying cause in children

presenting with acute spinal cord infarction often remains unclear [49].

## Key Points
- Spinal cord infarctions are relatively rare in children.
- Axial T2W and diffusion-weighted MR sequences facilitate the imaging-based diagnosis of spinal cord infarction.

In anterior spinal artery infarctions, the anterior and central aspects of the cord are involved bilaterally, which may lead to an "owl eye" or "snake eye" appearance.

In summary, pediatric spinal emergencies may markedly differ from adult spinal emergencies. The biomechanical properties of the spine change with age, and the patterns of traumatic injury change accordingly. Nontraumatic spinal cord injury may have various causes in children, including spinal cord tumors and inflammatory/autoimmune conditions. MRI is usually the modality of choice to assess

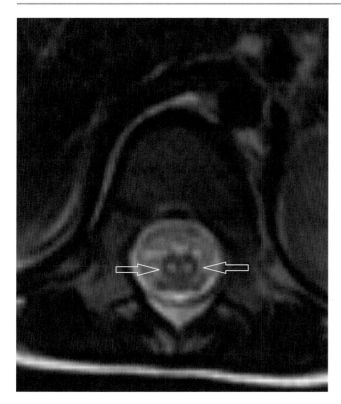

**Fig. 17** A 1-year-old girl with anterior spinal artery infarction with acute lower extremity weakness. Axial T2-weighted MR image demonstrates the characteristic "owl eye" or "snake eye" appearance of signal abnormality (arrows)

traumatic disruption of the ligaments and spinal cord injury and to investigate nontraumatic spinal emergencies.

# References

1. Huisman TA, Wagner MW, Bosemani T, Tekes A, Poretti A. Pediatric spinal trauma. J Neuroimaging. 2015;25(3):337–53.
2. Piatt JH. Pediatric spinal injury in the US: epidemiology and disparities. J Neurosurg Pediatr. 2015;16(4):463–71.
3. Herman MJ, Brown KO, Sponseller PD, Phillips JH, Petrucelli PM, Parikh DJ, et al. Pediatric cervical spine clearance: a consensus statement and algorithm from the pediatric cervical spine clearance working group. JBJS. 2019;101(1):e1.
4. Viccellio P, Simon H, Pressman BD, Shah MN, Mower WR, Hoffman JR, et al. A prospective multicenter study of cervical spine injury in children. Pediatrics. 2001;108(2):e20–e.
5. Traylor KS, Kralik SF, Radhakrishnan R, editors. Pediatric spine emergencies. Seminars in ultrasound, CT and MRI. Elsevier; 2018.
6. Leonard JC, Kuppermann N, Olsen C, Babcock-Cimpello L, Brown K, Mahajan P, et al. Factors associated with cervical spine injury in children after blunt trauma. Ann Emerg Med. 2011;58(2):145–55.
7. Pieretti-Vanmarcke R, Velmahos GC, Nance ML, Islam S, Falcone RA Jr, Wales PW, et al. Clinical clearance of the cervical spine in blunt trauma patients younger than 3 years: a multi-center study of the American Association for the Surgery of Trauma. J Trauma Acute Care Surg. 2009;67(3):543–50.
8. Kadom N, Palasis S, Pruthi S, Biffl WL, Booth TN, Desai NK, et al. ACR appropriateness criteria® suspected spine trauma-child. J Am Coll Radiol. 2019;16(5):S286–S99.
9. Roche C, Carty H. Spinal trauma in children. Pediatr Radiol. 2001;31(10):677–700.
10. Martínez-Lage JF, Alarcón F, Alfaro R, Gilabert A, Reyes SB, Almagro M-J, et al. Severe spinal cord injury in craniocervical dislocation. Case-based update. Childs Nerv Syst. 2013;29(2):187–94.
11. Lustrin ES, Karakas SP, Ortiz AO, Cinnamon J, Castillo M, Vaheesan K, et al. Pediatric cervical spine: normal anatomy, variants, and trauma. Radiographics. 2003;23(3):539–60.
12. Mahajan P, Jaffe DM, Olsen CS, Leonard JR, Nigrovic LE, Rogers AJ, et al. Spinal cord injury without radiologic abnormality in children imaged with magnetic resonance imaging. J Trauma Acute Care Surg. 2013;75(5):843–7.
13. Srinivasan V, Jea A. Pediatric thoracolumbar spine trauma. Neurosurg Clin. 2017;28(1):103–14.
14. Inaba K, Nosanov L, Menaker J, Bosarge P, Williams L, Turay D, et al. Prospective derivation of a clinical decision rule for thoracolumbar spine evaluation after blunt trauma: an American Association for the Surgery of Trauma Multi-Institutional Trials Group Study. J Trauma Acute Care Surg. 2015;78(3):459–67.
15. Diaz JJ Jr, Cullinane DC, Altman DT, Bokhari F, Cheng JS, Como J, et al. Practice management guidelines for the screening of thoracolumbar spine fracture. J Trauma Acute Care Surg. 2007;63(3):709–18.
16. Dogan S, Safavi-Abbasi S, Theodore N, Chang SW, Horn EM, Mariwalla NR, et al. Thoracolumbar and sacral spinal injuries in children and adolescents: a review of 89 cases. J Neurosurg Pediatr. 2007;106(6):426–33.
17. White J, Hague C, Nicolaou S, Gee R, Marchinkow L, Munk P. Imaging of sacral fractures. Clin Radiol. 2003;58(12):914–21.
18. Chance GQ. Note on a type of flexion fracture of the spine. Br J Radiol. 1948;21(249):452.
19. Bernstein MP, Mirvis SE, Shanmuganathan K. Chance-type fractures of the thoracolumbar spine: imaging analysis in 53 patients. AJR Am J Roentgenol. 2006;187(4):859–68.
20. Huisman TA, Phelps T, Bosemani T, Tekes A, Poretti A. Parturitional injury of the head and neck. J Neuroimaging. 2015;25(2):151–66.
21. Rehan V, Seshia M. Spinal cord birth injury–diagnostic difficulties. Arch Dis Child. 1993;69(1 Spec No):92.
22. Towbin A. Central nervous system damage in the human fetus and newborn infant. Mechanical and hypoxic injury incurred in the fetal-neonatal period. Am J Dis Child. 1970;119(6):529–42.
23. Surendrababu NR, Rao A. Clinical image. Transection of the spinal cord: a rare birth-related trauma. Pediatr Radiol. 2006;36(7):719.
24. Vialle R, Piétin-Vialle C, Vinchon M, Dauger S, Ilharreborde B, Glorion C. Birth-related spinal cord injuries: a multicentric review of nine cases. Childs Nerv Syst. 2008;24(1):79–85.
25. Hamida N, Hakim A, Fourati H, Thabet B, Walha L, Bouraoui A, et al. Neonatal cervical artery dissection secondary to birth trauma. Arch Pediatr. 2013;21(2):201–5.
26. Chaturvedi A, Chaturvedi A, Stanescu AL, Blickman JG, Meyers SP. Mechanical birth-related trauma to the neonate: an imaging perspective. Insights Imaging. 2018;9(1):103–18.
27. Kadom N, Khademian Z, Vezina G, Shalaby-Rana E, Rice A, Hinds T. Usefulness of MRI detection of cervical spine and brain injuries in the evaluation of abusive head trauma. Pediatr Radiol. 2014;44(7):839–48.
28. Knox J, Schneider J, Wimberly RL, Riccio AI. Characteristics of spinal injuries secondary to nonaccidental trauma. J Pediatr Orthop. 2014;34(4):376–81.

29. Kemp AM, Joshi AH, Mann M, Tempest V, Liu A, Holden S, et al. What are the clinical and radiological characteristics of spinal injuries from physical abuse: a systematic review. Arch Dis Child. 2010;95(5):355–60.

30. Choudhary AK, Bradford RK, Dias MS, Moore GJ, Boal DK. Spinal subdural hemorrhage in abusive head trauma: a retrospective study. Radiology. 2012;262(1):216–23.

31. Jacob R, Cox M, Koral K, Greenwell C, Xi Y, Vinson L, et al. MR imaging of the cervical spine in nonaccidental trauma: a tertiary institution experience. AJNR Am J Neuroradiol. 2016;37(10): 1944–50.

32. Choudhary AK, Ishak R, Zacharia TT, Dias MS. Imaging of spinal injury in abusive head trauma: a retrospective study. Pediatr Radiol. 2014;44(9):1130–40.

33. Rabbitt AL, Kelly TG, Yan K, Zhang J, Bretl DA, Quijano CV. Characteristics associated with spine injury on magnetic resonance imaging in children evaluated for abusive head trauma. Pediatr Radiol. 2020;50(1):83–97.

34. New PW. A narrative review of pediatric nontraumatic spinal cord dysfunction. Top Spinal Cord Inj Rehabil. 2019;25(2):112–20.

35. New PW, Lee BB, Cripps R, Vogel LC, Scheinberg A, Waugh M-C. Global mapping for the epidemiology of paediatric spinal cord damage: towards a living data repository. Spinal Cord. 2019;57(3): 183–97.

36. Duong LM, McCarthy BJ, McLendon RE, Dolecek TA, Kruchko C, Douglas LL, et al. Descriptive epidemiology of malignant and nonmalignant primary spinal cord, spinal meninges, and cauda equina tumors, United States, 2004-2007. Cancer. 2012;118(17): 4220–7.

37. Huisman TAGM. Pediatric tumors of the spine. Cancer Imaging. 2009;9 Spec No A(Special issue A):S45–S8.

38. Raybaud C, Barkovich AJ. Pediatric neuroimaging. Lippincott Williams & Wilkins; 2012.

39. Baruah D, Chandra T, Bajaj M, Sonowal P, Klein A, Maheshwari M, et al. A simplified algorithm for diagnosis of spinal cord lesions. Curr Probl Diagn Radiol. 2015;44(3):256–66.

40. Padilha IG, Fonseca AP, Pettengill AL, Fragoso DC, Pacheco FT, Nunes RH, et al. Pediatric multiple sclerosis: from clinical basis to imaging spectrum and differential diagnosis. Pediatr Radiol. 2020;50(6):776–792.

41. Absoud M, Lim MJ, Appleton R, Jacob A, Kitley J, Leite MI, et al. Paediatric neuromyelitis optica: clinical, MRI of the brain and prognostic features. J Neurol Neurosurg Psychiatry. 2015;86(4):470–2.

42. Pröbstel A-K, Rudolf G, Dornmair K, Collongues N, Chanson J-B, Sanderson NSR, et al. Anti-MOG antibodies are present in a subgroup of patients with a neuromyelitis optica phenotype. J Neuroinflammation. 2015;12(1):46.

43. Alroughani R, Boyko A. Pediatric multiple sclerosis: a review. BMC Neurol. 2018;18(1):27.

44. Absoud M, Greenberg BM, Lim M, Lotze T, Thomas T, Deiva K. Pediatric transverse myelitis. Neurology. 2016;87(9 Supplement 2):S46–52.

45. Zuccoli G, Panigrahy A, Bailey A, Fitz C. Redefining the Guillain-Barré spectrum in children: neuroimaging findings of cranial nerve involvement. Am J Neuroradiol. 2011;32(4):639–42.

46. Wang C, Greenberg B. Clinical approach to pediatric transverse myelitis, neuromyelitis optica spectrum disorder and acute flaccid myelitis. Children (Basel). 2019;6(5):70.

47. Theroux LM, Brenton JN. Acute transverse and flaccid myelitis in children. Curr Treat Options Neurol. 2019;21(12):64.

48. Alkan O, Yildirim T, Tokmak N, Tan M. Spinal MRI findings of guillain-barré syndrome. J Radiol Case Rep. 2009;3(3):25–8.

49. Sheikh A, Warren D, Childs A-M, Russell J, Liddington M, Guruswamy V, et al. Paediatric spinal cord infarction-a review of the literature and two case reports. Childs Nerv Syst. 2017;33(4): 671–6.

50. Masson C, Pruvo JP, Meder JF, Cordonnier C, Touzé E, De La Sayette V, et al. Spinal cord infarction: clinical and magnetic resonance imaging findings and short term outcome. J Neurol Neurosurg Psychiatry. 2004;75(10):1431–5.

# Imaging of Pediatric Traumatic Musculoskeletal Emergencies

# 47

Colin Brown and Rebecca Stein-Wexler

## Contents

C. Brown · R. Stein-Wexler (✉)
University of California Davis Health Department of Radiology and
Shriners Hospital for Children Northern California, Sacramento, CA,
USA
e-mail: cobrown@ucdavis.edu; rsteinwexler@ucdavis.edu

© Springer Nature Switzerland AG 2022
M. N. Patlas et al. (eds.), *Atlas of Emergency Imaging from Head-to-Toe*,
https://doi.org/10.1007/978-3-030-92111-8_47

### Abstract

Musculoskeletal injuries are a common and important reason for pediatric emergency department visits. Due to the unique properties of the developing bones of children, pediatric musculoskeletal injuries often differ from those that occur in adults. It is essential for radiologists involved in the emergency care of children to be familiar with common pediatric bony injuries. This chapter reviews a number of the most important musculoskeletal injuries which can occur in children, including pediatric fracture types, distal radius and forearm fractures, elbow fractures, slipped capital femoral epiphysis (SCFE), avulsion fractures of the pelvis and knee, toddler and trampoline fractures (TRFs), transitional ankle fractures (TAFs), and nonaccidental trauma (NAT).

### Keywords

Radiology · Pediatric · Emergency · Musculoskeletal · Fracture · Forearm · Elbow · Ankle · Avulsion · Nonaccidental trauma

### Abbreviations

| | |
|---|---|
| AP | Anteroposterior |
| CML | Classic metaphyseal lesion |
| CT | Computed tomography |
| DRUJ | Distal radioulnar joint |
| GFD | Galeazzi fracture-dislocation |
| JTF | Juvenile Tillaux fracture |
| LCHF | Lateral condylar humerus fracture |
| MEAF | Medial epicondylar avulsion fracture |
| MFD | Monteggia fracture-dislocation |
| MRI | Magnetic resonance imaging |
| NAT | Nonaccidental trauma |
| PSAF | Patellar sleeve avulsion fracture |
| SCFE | Slipped capital femoral epiphysis |
| SCHF | Supracondylar humerus fracture |
| SH | Salter-Harris |
| TAF | Transitional ankle fracture |
| TF | Toddler fracture |
| TRF | Trampoline fracture |
| TrPF | Triplane fracture |
| TSAF | Tibial spine avulsion fracture |
| TTAF | Tibial tubercle avulsion fracture |

## Pediatric Fractures - Introduction

### Epidemiology

Fractures are a leading cause of pediatric emergency department visits. While fractures can occur at any age, the incidence of childhood fractures peaks during adolescence. On average, boys sustain fractures nearly twice as often as girls. Accidents at home and school and sports injuries are leading causes of fractures in children [1].

### Clinical Features

The bones of children differ from those of adults in several respects. Pediatric bones are less mineralized and are more flexible [2]. The open physes are mechanically weak compared to ligaments and tendons and are therefore particularly vulnerable to injury [3]. As a result, some bony injury types are unique to or predominantly seen in the pediatric population. These include fractures involving the physes, buckle and greenstick fractures, and plastic bowing deformities [4, 5].

Fractures involving the physes are of special significance due to the potential for subsequent growth arrest or physeal bar formation, leading to growth disturbance including limb length asymmetry and angular deformity. Physeal fractures are most often categorized using the Salter-Harris (SH) classification (Fig. 1). SH-I fractures are characterized by transverse disruption of the physis. SH-II fractures involve both the physis and metaphysis and are the most common type of physeal fracture. SH-III fractures involve the physis and epiphysis. SH-IV fractures involve the metaphysis, physis, and epiphysis. Both SH-III and SH-IV fractures are

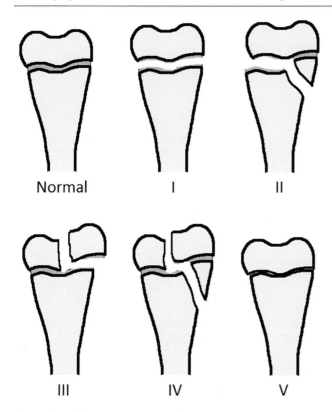

Normal        I        II

III        IV        V

**Fig. 1** Illustration of the Salter-Harris classification of physeal fractures

often intra-articular. SH-V fractures are rare axial crush injuries of the physis [6].

Buckle fractures, also known as torus fractures, are characterized by compressive deformity of the cortex on one side of the bone and typically occur at long bone metaphyses and metadiaphyses. Greenstick fractures are distinguished by bending of the bone with cortical disruption at the tension side, typically occurring at long bone diaphyses. Plastic bowing deformities are longitudinal compression injuries of long bone diaphyses, most commonly affecting the radius, ulna, and fibula. Although microscopic fractures are present with plastic bowing deformities, there is no macroscopic fracture, and the periosteum is intact [5, 7].

## Diagnostic Investigations

Radiographs are the primary imaging test for fracture [5]. Fractures involving the physes are seen as widening of the affected portion of the growth plate, with variable involvement of the adjacent bony segments depending on type (Fig. 2a). Buckle fractures appear as convex cortical deformity and lack a distinct fracture lucency (Fig. 2b). Greenstick fractures demonstrate bending of the bone with fracture lucency at the convex side (Fig. 2c). Plastic bowing deformities are seen as abnormal curvature of the affected

bone, typically with long-segment diaphyseal involvement, without fracture lucency (Fig. 2d) [5, 7].

## Summary and Key Points

- Fractures are a common reason for pediatric emergency department visits.
- Fracture types unique to or predominantly seen in children include physeal (Salter-Harris), buckle, and greenstick fractures, as well as plastic bowing deformities.
- Radiographs are the primary imaging test for pediatric fractures.

## Pediatric Wrist and Forearm Fractures

### Epidemiology

Fractures of the distal radius and forearm are among the most common fractures in children [1]. Additionally, the distal radial physis is one of the most frequent sites of fracture involving the growth plate [7]. Monteggia fracture-dislocation (MFD) injuries account for approximately 1% of pediatric forearm fractures and typically occur in children aged 4–10 years [8]. Galeazzi fracture-dislocation (GFD) injuries account for up to 3% of forearm fractures in children, with a peak age range of 9–13 years [9].

### Clinical Features

Distal radius and forearm fractures most often result from indirect trauma; a fall on an outstretched hand is the typical mechanism [10]. At the distal radius, there is a high potential for remodeling of fracture deformity, and growth disturbance is uncommon [7]. Diaphyseal forearm fractures in children can occur as complete fractures, greenstick fractures, plastic bowing deformities, or a combination of these fracture types [7].

The forearm acts as a bony ring. As a result, trauma tends to produce disruption in the form of either fracture or dislocation at two locations [11]. Fracture of a single forearm long bone is less common and is usually due to direct trauma. Detection of an apparent isolated radius or ulna fracture should prompt careful scrutiny of bony alignment to search for an associated dislocation [10]. Failure to recognize the dislocation component of a fracture-dislocation injury can lead to poor functional outcomes and may necessitate surgery for injuries which could otherwise be managed nonoperatively [12, 13].

MFDs consist of an ulnar fracture and dislocation of the radiocapitellar joint [5]. GFDs consist of fracture of the radius and malalignment at the distal radioulnar joint (DRUJ)

**Fig. 2** (**a**) A 6-year-old girl hit by car. AP right femur radiograph with Salter-Harris II fracture. (**b**) A 7-year-old girl with fall from skateboard. Lateral left wrist radiograph with distal radius buckle fracture. (**c**) A 7-year-old girl with fall onto outstretched hand. Lateral right wrist radiograph with greenstick fracture of the radius. (**d**) A 16-year-old boy after motocross crash. AP right forearm radiograph with plastic bowing deformity of the distal ulna (*arrows*) and radius fracture

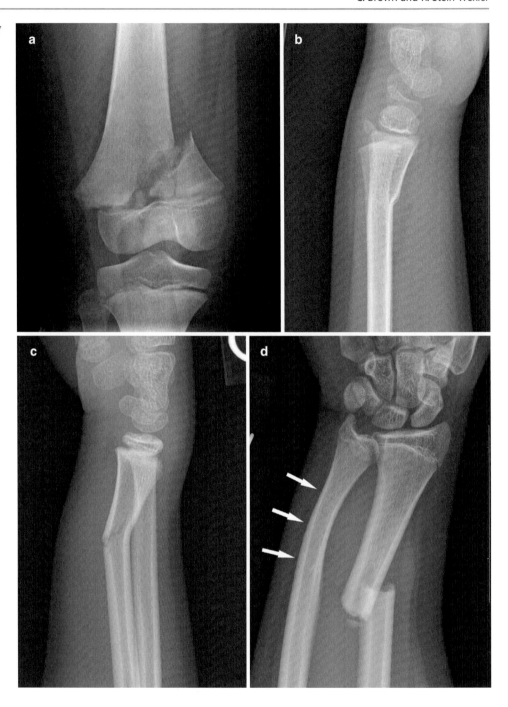

[14]. In children with open growth plates, a related injury termed a Galeazzi equivalent can occur, with fracture of the radius and accompanying displaced fracture through the distal ulnar physis [3].

## Diagnostic Investigations

Radiographs are the primary diagnostic test for distal radius and forearm fractures in children and depict the location and type of fracture as well as the presence and magnitude of angulation, displacement, and bayonet apposition (side-by-side overlap of fragments) [7].

In patients with MFD, the ulnar fracture is often the most conspicuous feature on radiographs (Fig. 3). The use of the radiocapitellar line (described in Sect. "Pediatric Elbow Fractures") is important to detect the dislocation component of a MFD. Likewise, with typical GFD, the radius fracture may be the most apparent radiographic finding. In most cases of GFD, the distal ulna is dorsally displaced relative to the radius [14]. Obtaining a true lateral view of the wrist is important for evaluating alignment at the DRUJ [13].

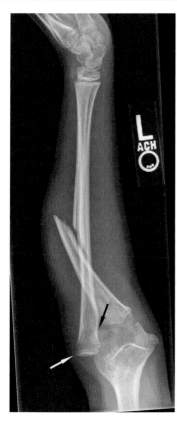

**Fig. 3** A 12-year-old boy with fall. AP left forearm radiograph with MFD with ulnar fracture and dislocation of the radial head (*white arrow*) relative to the capitellum (*black arrow*)

**Fig. 4** A 12-year-old boy with fall. (**a**) Posteroanterior and (**b**) lateral left wrist radiographs with Galeazzi equivalent injury, with a fracture of the distal radius and displaced Salter-Harris II fracture of the ulna

Galeazzi equivalent injuries are seen as radius fracture as well as a SH fracture of the distal ulna (Fig. 4) [3].

## Summary and Key Points

- Distal radius and forearm fractures are among the most common pediatric fractures.
- The forearm acts as a bony ring – carefully scrutinize for an associated malalignment injury if an apparent isolated radius or ulna fracture is seen.

## Pediatric Elbow Fractures

### Epidemiology

Pediatric elbow fractures are common and differ from those which occur in adults. Supracondylar humerus fractures (SCHFs) account for more than 50% of elbow fractures in children and are typically seen at the ages of 3–10 years [15]. Lateral condylar humerus fractures (LCHFs) are considered the second most frequent pediatric elbow fracture, with a usual age range of 6–10 years [4, 16]. Medial epicondyle avulsion fractures (MEAFs) are an additional important fracture type and typically occur at 7–15 years of age [15, 16].

### Clinical Features

Elbow fractures present with pain, swelling, deformity, decreased range of motion, and/or point tenderness [17].

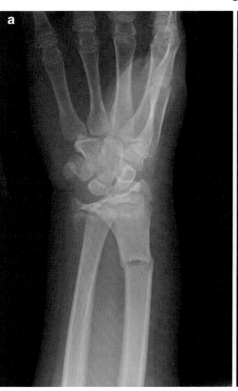
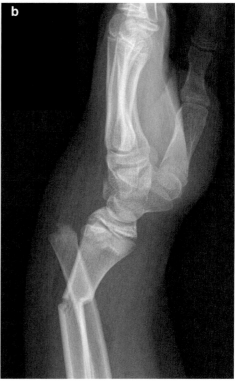

**Fig. 5** An 11-year-old boy. (**a**) AP and (**b**) lateral left elbow radiographs demonstrating the secondary ossification centers – capitellum (*C*), radial head (*R*), medial epicondyle (*M*), trochlea (*T*), olecranon (*O*), and lateral epicondyle (*L*)

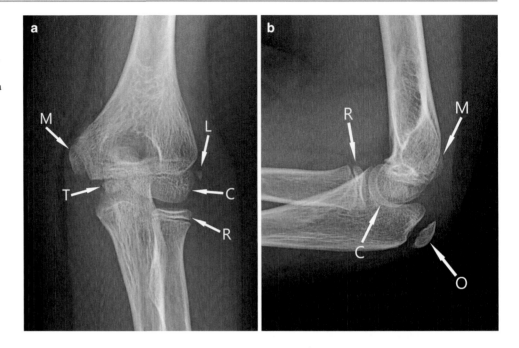

**Table 1** Ossification centers of the elbow

| Ossification center | Approximate age of appearance (years) |
|---|---|
| Capitellum | 1 |
| Radial head | 3 |
| Medial epicondyle | 5 |
| Trochlea | 7 |
| Olecranon | 9 |
| Lateral epicondyle | 11 |

**Fig. 6** (**a**) A 10-year-old girl. Lateral right elbow radiograph with normal anterior fat pad (*arrow*). (**b**) A 4-year-old girl with fall from sofa. Lateral left elbow radiograph with positive fat pad sign with elevation of the anterior (*arrow*) and posterior (*double arrows*) fat pads

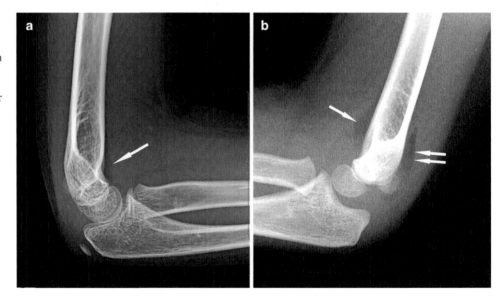

SCHFs are often caused by a fall on an outstretched hand, producing extension-type injury of the relatively weak supracondylar region of the distal humerus [4, 15]. SCHFs with displacement or substantial angulation are usually treated surgically [5].

LCHFs extend horizontally from the lateral aspect of the metaphysis and then distally through the cartilage medial to the developing capitellum or less commonly through the capitellum itself [18]. Lateral condylar fractures with >2 mm displacement typically require surgical treatment [15].

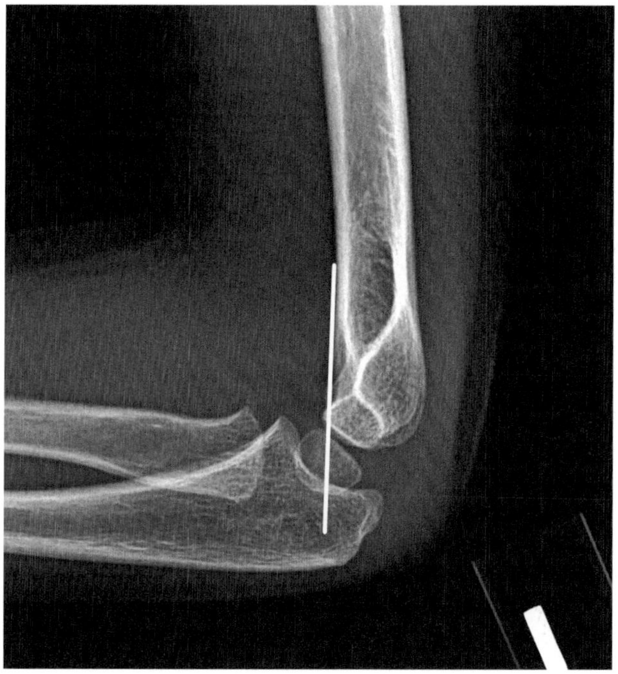

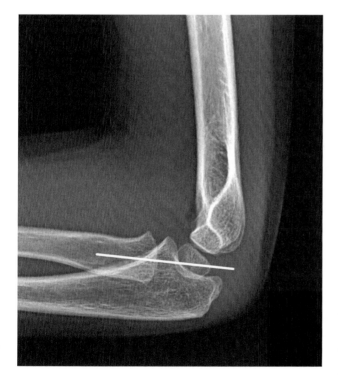

**Fig. 7** A 6-year-old boy. Lateral left elbow radiograph with normal anterior humeral line (*white line*) passing through the middle third of the capitellum

**Fig. 8** A 6-year-old boy. Lateral left elbow radiograph with normal radiocapitellar line (*white line*) passing through the capitellum

Approximately 50% of MEAFs occur in the setting of elbow dislocation, although the dislocation may reduce spontaneously prior to presentation [4, 15, 18]. There is potential for the displaced medial epicondylar apophysis to become

entrapped in the ulnohumeral articulation, particularly when the fracture is associated with a dislocation. If fragment entrapment is not recognized and addressed surgically, substantial morbidity including decreased range of motion and ulnar nerve injury can result [4, 18, 19].

## Diagnostic Investigations

Radiographs are the primary imaging test used in pediatric elbow trauma. Frontal and lateral radiographs of the elbow should be obtained routinely. Additional projections including oblique and radial head views are often helpful. Comparison views of the contralateral elbow can be used as a problem-solving technique [18].

There are six secondary ossification centers at the elbow which undergo ossification in a predictable sequence (Fig. 5). The typical order of ossification is as follows: capitellum, radial head, medial epicondyle, trochlea, olecranon, and lateral epicondyle [18]. The mnemonic "CRITOE" (**c**apitellum, **r**adial head, (**i**nternal) medial epicondyle, **t**rochlea, **o**lecranon, (**e**xternal) lateral epicondyle) is often used to aid in remembering this order of ossification [4]. The respective ages of ossification of these centers can be approximated as 1, 3, 5, 7, 9, and 11 years (Table 1) [18]. Knowledge of the normal order of ossification is important to help detect pathology, including the presence of a displaced MEAF.

On the lateral radiograph of a normal elbow, the anterior fat pad is visible as a thin, vertical band of lucency anterior to the distal humerus, and the posterior fat pad is located in the olecranon fossa and not visible (Fig. 6a). A positive "fat pad sign" is present when the fat pads are elevated on the lateral view by hemarthrosis or other joint effusion (Fig. 6b). When elevated, the anterior fat pad is displaced anteriorly and superiorly, acquiring a triangular "sail sign" appearance, and the posterior fat pad becomes visible [11]. A positive fat pad sign is present in most intra-articular fractures, although it can be absent when there is an associated tear of the joint capsule. Occult fracture is present in many, but not all, children who have trauma with fat pad elevation but no visible fracture [15].

A line drawn along the anterior cortex of the distal humerus on a lateral radiograph, referred to as the anterior humeral line, should intersect the middle third of the developing capitellum in children older than 2.5 years and can pass through the anterior third of the capitellum in children younger than 2.5 years (Fig. 7). Failure of the anterior humeral line to intersect the expected portion of the capitellum is a reliable sign of fracture, most commonly a supracondylar fracture with the line passing anterior to its expected position [15].

The radiocapitellar line, drawn along the central long axis of the radial neck, is used for evaluating radiocapitellar alignment. Although an imperfect rule, in general the radiocapitellar line should pass through the capitellum regardless

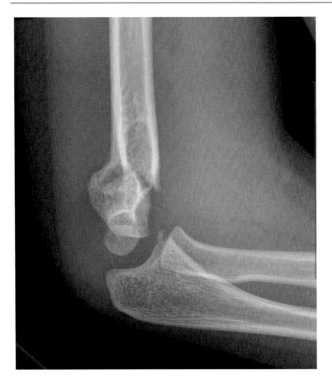

**Fig. 9** A 5-year-old girl with fall from monkey bars. Lateral right elbow radiograph with supracondylar fracture

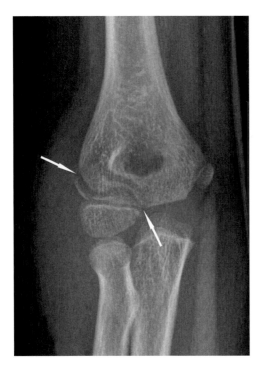

**Fig. 10** A 7-year-old boy with fall from aboveground swimming pool. AP right elbow radiograph with lateral condylar fracture (*arrows*)

of the projection (Fig. 8). If this relationship is not maintained, radiocapitellar malalignment should be suspected [11, 20].

The lateral view is the most useful projection for depicting SCHFs (Fig. 9). When there is posterior angulation of the distal portion of the bone, the anterior humeral line will be abnormal. On the anteroposterior (AP) view, SCHFs can often be seen as a transverse lucency through the distal humeral metaphysis at the level of the olecranon fossa. Fat pad elevation may be the only radiographic sign of injury with non-displaced SCHFs [4, 15].

With LCHFs, the metaphyseal bony fragment seen on radiographs is often small and fails to depict the full extent of these intra-articular fractures (Fig. 10). LCHFs can be poorly visible on AP radiographs and are often better seen when oblique images are obtained [18]. As with other intra-articular fractures, a positive fat pad sign will usually be present [15].

To identify apophyseal entrapment from MEAF, it is important to carefully evaluate for the presence of a normally positioned medial epicondyle ossification center (Fig. 11). If the ossification center is not seen after the age of 6–7 years, if there appears to be trochlear ossification without medial epicondylar ossification, or if ulnohumeral joint alignment remains incongruent following dislocation reduction, then fragment entrapment may be present [4, 15].

## Summary and Key Points

- Supracondylar, lateral condylar, and medial epicondylar avulsion fractures are among the most common pediatric elbow injuries.
- When reviewing pediatric elbow radiographs, it is important to evaluate the anterior humeral and radio-capitellar lines, the presence and location of the medial epicondylar apophysis, and the presence of fat pad elevation.

## SCFE

### Epidemiology

SCFE occurs prior to closure of the proximal femoral growth plate, which fuses on average around 15 years [21]. The age range for SCFE in boys is 10–17 years, with a peak at 13–14 years. In girls, the age range is 8–15 years, with a peak at 11–12 years. SCFE is more common in boys and is strongly associated with obesity, although not all patients are overweight [22–24]. SCFE is said to be atypical when it occurs in the presence of an underlying endocrine disorder (e.g., hypothyroidism) or metabolic disease (e.g., renal osteodystrophy) [25].

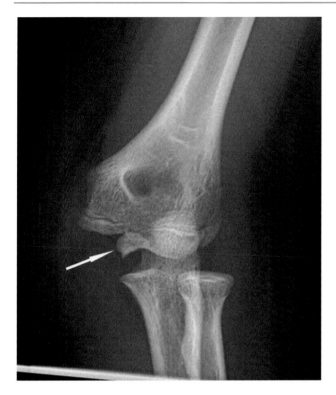

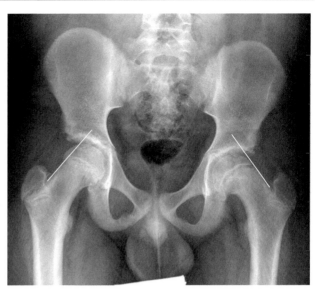

**Fig. 12** An 11-year-old boy with 4 months of left hip pain. AP pelvis radiograph with left SCFE. On the left, Klein's line (*white lines*) fails to intersect the medially displaced femoral head epiphysis, and the growth plate is widened. On the normal right side, Klein's line passes through the lateral aspect of the epiphysis

**Fig. 11** An 11-year-old girl with fall from bicycle. AP left elbow radiograph with medial epicondylar avulsion fracture, with displaced and entrapped ossification center (*arrow*), as well as malalignment

## Clinical Features

SCFE is characterized by disruption of the proximal femoral growth plate with displacement of the epiphysis and is an important cause of premature osteoarthritis at the hip. The typical presentation of SCFE is hip pain of variable severity and chronicity. However, a substantial proportion of patients present with a chief complaint of knee pain, sometimes causing diagnostic confusion and delay [23]. About one-third of patients with SCFE have bilateral disease, which can be synchronous or metachronous [25]. SCFE is most commonly treated with in situ screw fixation of the femoral head, as reduction of the slip is associated with a high rate of subsequent femoral head avascular necrosis [23].

## Diagnostic Investigations

Radiographs are the primary diagnostic test for SCFE. The initial evaluation should include AP and frog-leg lateral or true lateral radiographs of both hips [23, 25]. The main radiographic findings in SCFE are displacement of the epiphysis and widening of the proximal femoral growth plate. Epiphyseal slippage is usually posteromedial

[23]. On AP radiographs, medial slippage can be detected using Klein's line, a line drawn along the lateral aspect of the femoral neck (Fig. 12). Failure of the line to intersect a portion of the epiphysis is suggestive of slippage [25]. However, the sensitivity of Klein's line is imperfect as mild slippage can be predominantly posterior. In these cases, displacement of the epiphysis is better visualized on the lateral view [22, 23]. In some early cases, there is no displacement of the epiphysis, and the only finding is the subtle widening of the proximal femoral physis, referred to as "pre-slip" [22].

Computed tomography (CT) and magnetic resonance imaging (MRI) have a relatively minor role in the diagnosis and preoperative evaluation of SCFE and are more commonly used to evaluate complications in patients who have already undergone surgical treatment [22, 23].

## Summary and Key Points

- SCFE most commonly affects adolescent boys and is strongly associated with obesity.
- A substantial proportion of patients present with knee pain, which can delay diagnosis.
- On frontal radiographs, Klein's line is used to assess for epiphyseal slippage.
- Early slippage is often posterior and better appreciated on lateral images.

## Apophyseal Avulsion Fractures at the Pelvis and Hips

### Epidemiology

Apophyseal avulsion fractures at the pelvis and hip are usually seen in adolescents and are more common in boys [26, 27].

### Clinical Features

Pelvis/hip avulsion injuries typically occur during vigorous athletic activities involving running and kicking. Many but not all patients present with acute onset of pain following a specific inciting event. These injuries are usually treated conservatively with good outcome [26, 27].

There are five sites at the pelvis/hip region where avulsion injuries typically occur. The ischial tuberosity (hamstring tendon origin) is the most common site. The anterior superior iliac spine (sartorius muscle origin), anterior inferior iliac spine (rectus femoris straight head origin), and the lesser trochanter of the femur (iliopsoas tendon insertion) are also frequently affected [26–28]. Iliac crest (attachment site of the lateral abdominal wall muscles) avulsion is less common [27].

### Diagnostic Investigations

An AP pelvis radiograph is typically adequate to depict these avulsions, although minimally displaced fractures can be

better seen with oblique views. In the acute setting, radiographs demonstrate an avulsion fragment, often crescentic in morphology, with a variable degree of displacement from the donor site in the direction of muscular traction force (Fig. 13) [27]. During the healing phase, pelvic avulsions can exhibit exuberant bony proliferative change, in some cases producing an aggressive appearance which can mimic neoplasm; chronic avulsions can have prominent associated heterotopic ossification [28].

### Summary and Key Points

- Apophyseal avulsion fractures of the pelvis and hip usually occur in adolescents during athletic activity.
- The ischial tuberosity is the most common location. The anterior superior iliac spine, anterior inferior iliac spine, and lesser trochanter are also frequently affected. Iliac crest avulsion is less common.
- Healing avulsion fractures can have exuberant callus which should not be mistaken for a more aggressive process.

## Pediatric Avulsion Fractures at the Knee

### Epidemiology

Children can sustain avulsion fractures at several locations in the knee, including the tibial spine, patella, and tibial tubercle. Tibial spine avulsion fractures (TSAFs) can occur in

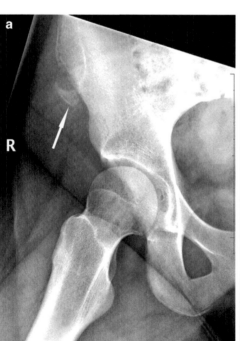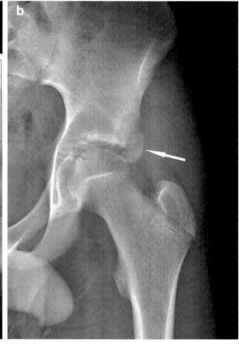

**Fig. 13** (**a**) A 14-year-old boy with athletic injury. Frog-leg lateral right hip radiograph with anterior superior iliac spine avulsion (*arrow*). (**b**) A 14-year-old boy with hip pain after playing football. AP left hip radiograph with anterior inferior iliac spine avulsion (*arrow*)

adults but are more common in children [29]. Patellar sleeve avulsion fractures (PSAFs) occur exclusively in children and are typically encountered in patients aged 8–12 years [30]. Tibial tubercle avulsion fractures (TTAFs) usually occur in adolescent males and are associated with athletic activities involving jumping [30, 31].

## Clinical Features

TSAFs are avulsion injuries of the tibial attachment of the anterior cruciate ligament (ACL). When displaced, TSAFs are treated with surgical reduction and fixation [29]. PSAFs are characterized by avulsion of a variable amount of cartilage and bone from the inferior pole of the incompletely ossified patella. TTAFs occur with varying degrees of displacement and can extend into the proximal tibial epiphysis and involve the tibial plateau articular surface. With the exception of non-displaced fractures confined to the tubercle, TTAFs are typically treated surgically [30].

## Diagnostic Investigations

In patients with TSAF, radiographs reveal a bony fragment avulsed from the tibial spine with a variable degree of displacement (Fig. 14). As this fracture is intra-articular, joint effusion is expected in the acute setting. MRI can be performed to evaluate the integrity of the ACL and to depict additional injuries, which are frequently present [29].

With PSAF, radiographs reveal bony avulsion from the patellar lower pole, often with associated patella alta, joint effusion, and soft tissue edema (Fig. 15). The extent of cartilage injury and degree of displacement can be underestimated using radiographs, and MRI can better demonstrate all components of the injury [30].

Radiographs are the initial imaging modality for the evaluation of TTAFs (Fig. 16) [30]. CT and MRI can be useful to fully evaluate fracture morphology and the extent of intra-articular involvement [31].

## Summary and Key Points

- TSAFs occur at the ACL attachment and are more common in children than in adults.
- PSAFs occur at the lower pole of the patella; radiographs demonstrate the bony fragment but often fail to fully depict the extent of the cartilaginous injury.
- TTAFs usually occur in adolescent males, can involve the tibial plateau articular surface, and often require surgical fixation.

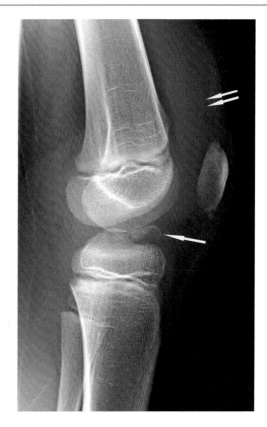

**Fig. 14** A 9-year-old boy hit in knee while playing soccer. Lateral left knee radiograph with TSAF (*arrow*) with associated hemarthrosis (*double arrows*)

## Toddler Fractures (TFs) and Trampoline Fractures (TRFs)

### Epidemiology

TFs occur in children aged approximately 1–4 years [32]. The typical age range for TRFs is 2–5 years [33, 34].

### Clinical Features

TF is one of the primary diagnostic considerations in a young child with limping or refusal to bear weight. TFs were originally described as non-displaced spiral or oblique fractures of the distal shaft of the tibia, often occurring without recognized trauma or following minor trauma [32, 35, 36]. However, other lower extremity fractures (e.g., tibial and fibular buckle fractures and tarsal/metatarsal fractures) can have a similar clinical presentation [35, 36].

TRFs are fractures of the proximal tibial metaphysis which classically occur when a small child is jumping on a trampoline at the same time as a second, larger individual.

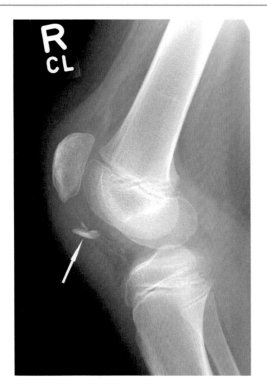

**Fig. 15** A 10-year-old boy with football injury. Lateral right knee radiograph with PSAF, with a displaced fragment (arrow) and patella alta

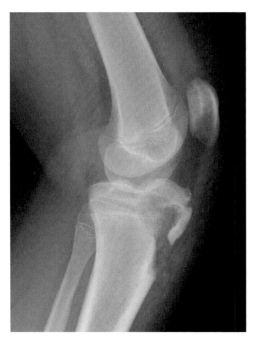

**Fig. 16** A 13-year-old boy who tripped and fell while running. Lateral left knee radiograph with displaced TTAF

Other axial loading injuries can also produce this type of fracture [33].

Both TFs and TRFs are managed with casting and immobilization and have excellent outcomes [33, 35].

## Diagnostic Investigations

As TFs are typically non-displaced, they often appear on radiographs as a subtle lucency, and up to 40% are radiographically occult initially (Fig. 17) [35, 36]. The addition of an internal oblique view increases the rate of fracture visualization, and follow-up images will demonstrate evidence of fracture healing in some patients with negative initial radiographs [32, 35]. Radionuclide bone scintigraphy is sensitive for depiction of radiographically occult TFs but is not routinely advised due to the relatively substantial radiation dose and the lack of specificity [35]. In the proper clinical setting, radiographically occult TFs can be diagnosed presumptively, and imaging confirmation is not mandatory [35].

TRFs appear on radiographs as transverse linear or buckling fractures of the proximal tibial metaphysis (Fig. 18). As with TFs, TRFs are in some cases subtle and difficult to detect [34].

## Summary and Key Points

- TFs are non-displaced oblique or spiral distal tibial fractures which occur in young children with minor trauma, although the fractures can be radiographically occult, and other lower extremity fractures can have a similar presentation.
- TRFs are axial loading injuries of the proximal tibial metaphysis, also occurring in young children.

## Transitional Ankle Fractures (TAFs)

### Epidemiology

Triplane fractures (TrPFs) and juvenile Tillaux fractures (JTFs), together referred to as TAFs, are unique to adolescents and occur during the process of closure of the distal tibial growth plate. The fusion of the growth plate in general progresses from medial to lateral over about 1.5 years, occurring last at the anterolateral portion [37, 38]. TAFs typically occur at 10–16 years of age, with most in the midportion of this range [39, 40]. On average, patients with JTFs are slightly older than those with TrPFs, as JTFs occur at a more advanced stage of physeal fusion [41].

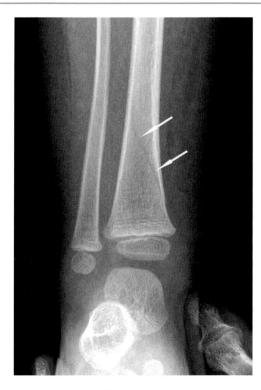

**Fig. 17** A 2-year-old girl with leg swelling and refusal to bear weight. AP right lower leg radiograph with TF (*arrows*)

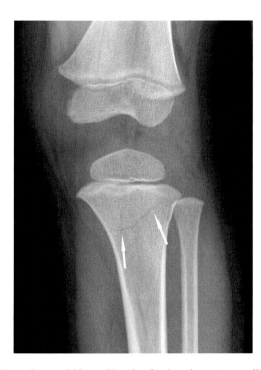

**Fig. 18** A 2-year-old boy with pain after jumping on trampoline. AP left lower leg radiograph with TRF (arrows)

## Clinical Features

TrPFs are complex Salter-Harris IV fractures, named "triplane" because the fracture classically has components in three anatomic planes: an oblique coronal fracture at the posterior metaphysis, a transverse fracture through the lateral portion of the physis, and fracture with sagittal orientation through the epiphysis extending to the articular surface (Fig. 19). However, multiple variants of this pattern have been described [42]. JTFs are intra-articular Salter-Harris III fractures, with separation of an anterolateral epiphyseal fragment (Fig. 20) [43]. About one-third of TrPFs are accompanied by a fibular fracture; concomitant fibular fractures are uncommon with JTFs [37, 39].

Substantial growth disturbance is uncommon following TAFs, as they occur when there is little potential for growth remaining. However, except for certain extra-articular TrPF variants, these fractures are intra-articular and can, therefore, lead to premature osteoarthritis [41, 43]. In general, an articular surface gap or step-off of greater than 2 mm persisting after attempted closed reduction is an indication for surgery [43].

## Diagnostic Investigations

Radiographs are the initial imaging modality for evaluating ankle fractures [40]. However, CT is often used to evaluate TAFs as it allows a better understanding of complex fracture morphology and more precise quantification of fragment displacement [38, 39].

## Summary and Key Points

- TrPFs and JTFs, together referred to as TAFs, occur in adolescents during closure of the distal tibial growth plate.
- These fractures are intra-articular and often require surgical reduction.
- CT is useful for evaluating TAFs.

## Nonaccidental Trauma (NAT)

### Epidemiology

Nonaccidental trauma (NAT), also known as abusive trauma, is a substantial cause of morbidity and mortality in young children and is commonly encountered in the emergency department setting, accounting for 10% of injury-related visits for children under the age of 5 [44].

**Fig. 19** A 12-year-old boy with fall while roller skating. (**a**) AP and (**b**) lateral right ankle radiographs with TrPF. Note epiphyseal (*arrow on a*), physeal (*double arrows on a*), and metaphyseal (*arrow on b*) fracture components

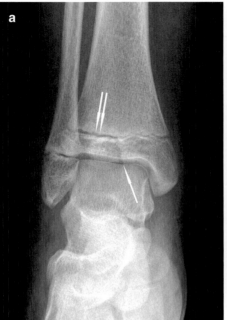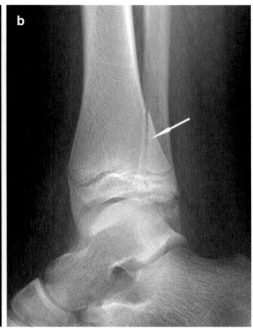

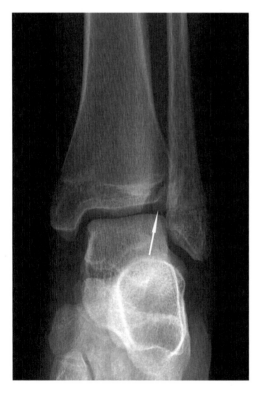

**Fig. 20** A 13-year-old girl with ice-skating injury. AP left ankle radiograph with JTF with displaced anterolateral epiphyseal fragment (*arrow*)

## Clinical Features

While any fracture can potentially be due to NAT, certain fractures and injury patterns should arouse greater suspicion.

Most significant among these are classic metaphyseal lesions (CMLs) and rib fractures [45, 46]. The presence of multiple fractures and/or fractures in different stages of healing should also raise concern [45, 46].

CMLs are transverse fractures at the zone of provisional calcification along the growth plates at the ends of developing long bones. These fractures are highly specific for NAT in the first year of life and are believed to occur as a result of forceful shaking of an infant [46, 47]. The most common locations include the distal femur, proximal and distal tibia and fibula, and proximal humerus [48].

Rib fractures are strongly associated with NAT in children under the age of 3 and are often the only skeletal manifestation of abusive injury [49]. Posterior rib fractures in infants are especially suspicious and are believed to occur when an adult grabs the child's chest with two hands and squeezes, applying AP compressive force [46].

## Diagnostic Investigations

A complete skeletal survey is the primary imaging test for fracture in the setting of suspected NAT and should be obtained in any child younger than 2 years of age for whom there is concern for physical abuse. In children who are 2 years of age or older, radiographs targeted to sites of suspected injury should be obtained although a skeletal survey is appropriate in some cases (e.g., if the child is unable to localize pain). The American College of Radiology has published guidelines specifying the components of a skeletal survey (Table 2) [45]. Notably, oblique views of the ribs should be included

**Table 2** Components of a radiographic skeletal survey for NAT

| Axial skeleton | Extremities |
|---|---|
| Skull – AP and lateral | Humerus – bilateral AP |
| Cervical spine – AP and lateral | Forearm – bilateral AP |
| Thorax including ribs, thoracic spine, and upper lumbar spine – AP and lateral | Hand – bilateral posteroanterior |
| Ribs – bilateral oblique | Femur – bilateral AP |
| Pelvis and lumbar spine – AP | Lower leg – bilateral AP |
| Lumbosacral spine – lateral | Foot – AP or posteroanterior bilateral |

Modified from Ref. [45]

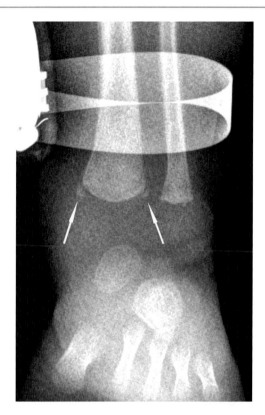

**Fig. 22** A 4-week-old boy with lower extremity swelling. AP left ankle radiograph with CML of the distal tibia (*arrows*) with "corner fracture" appearance

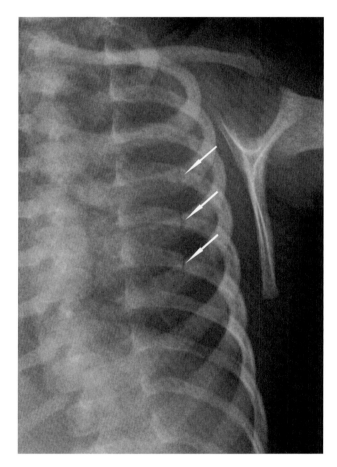

**Fig. 21** A 3-month-old girl seen in emergency department with chief complaint of vomiting; possible rib fractures noted on AP chest radiograph (not shown). Oblique left rib radiograph with acute posterior rib fractures (*arrows*)

morphology (Fig. 21) [46]. CMLs typically have a "corner fracture" appearance when imaged in a plane orthogonal to the fracture and with obliquity have a "bucket-handle" appearance (Fig. 22) [47].

## Summary and Key Points

- NAT is a substantial cause of morbidity and mortality in infants and young children.
- Rib fractures are strongly associated with NAT in children under the age of 3.
- CMLs are highly specific for NAT and can have a "corner fracture" or "bucket-handle" appearance.
- A complete skeletal survey should be performed in children younger than age 2 years when physical abuse is suspected.

to increase detection of rib fractures [45, 50]. A "babygram" which includes most or all of the infant's body is not adequate for evaluation of suspected NAT [46].

Acute rib fractures appear as linear lucencies and when healing demonstrate associated callus with fusiform

## References

1. Naranje SM, Erali RA, Warner WC Jr, Sawyer JR, Kelly DM. Epidemiology of pediatric fractures presenting to emergency departments in the United States. J Pediatr Orthop. 2016;36 (4):e45–8.

2. Forestier-Zhang L, Bishop N. Bone strength in children: understanding basic bone biomechanics. Arch Dis Child Educ Pract Ed. 2016;101(1):2–7.

3. Maloney E, Zbojniewicz AM, Nguyen J, Luo Y, Thapa MM. Anatomy and injuries of the pediatric wrist: beyond the basics. Pediatr Radiol. 2018;48(6):764–82.

4. Delgado J, Jaramillo D, Chauvin NA. Imaging the injured pediatric athlete: upper extremity. Radiographics. 2016;36(6):1672–87.

5. Arora R, Fichadia U, Hartwig E, Kannikeswaran N. Pediatric upper-extremity fractures. Pediatr Ann. 2014;43(5):196–204.

6. Cepela DJ, Tartaglione JP, Dooley TP, Patel PN. Classifications in brief: Salter-Harris classification of pediatric physeal fractures. Clin Orthop Relat Res. 2016;474(11):2531–7.

7. Bae DS. Pediatric distal radius and forearm fractures. J Hand Surg Am. 2008;33(10):1911–23.

8. Bae DS. Successful strategies for managing Monteggia injuries. J Pediatr Orthop. 2016;36(Suppl 1):S67–70.

9. Eberl R, Singer G, Schalamon J, Petnehazy T, Hoellwarth ME. Galeazzi lesions in children and adolescents: treatment and outcome. Clin Orthop Relat Res. 2008;466(7):1705–9.

10. Pace JL. Pediatric and adolescent forearm fractures: current controversies and treatment recommendations. J Am Acad Orthop Surg. 2016;24(11):780–8.

11. Grayson DE. The elbow: radiographic imaging pearls and pitfalls. Semin Roentgenol. 2005;40(3):223–47.

12. Gleeson AP, Beattie TF. Monteggia fracture-dislocation in children. J Accid Emerg Med. 1994;11(3):192–4.

13. Walsh HP, McLaren CA, Owen R. Galeazzi fractures in children. J Bone Joint Surg Br. 1987;69(5):730–3.

14. Perron AD, Hersh RE, Brady WJ, Keats TE. Orthopedic pitfalls in the ED: Galeazzi and Monteggia fracture-dislocation. Am J Emerg Med. 2001;19(3):225–8.

15. Iyer RS, Thapa MM, Khanna PC, Chew FS. Pediatric bone imaging: imaging elbow trauma in children – a review of acute and chronic injuries. AJR Am J Roentgenol. 2012;198(5):1053–68.

16. Emery KH, Zingula SN, Anton CG, Salisbury SR, Tamai J. Pediatric elbow fractures: a new angle on an old topic. Pediatr Radiol. 2016;46(1):61–6.

17. Dubrovsky AS, Mok E, Lau SY, Al Humaidan M. Point tenderness at 1 of 5 locations and limited elbow extension identify significant injury in children with acute elbow trauma: a study of diagnostic accuracy. Am J Emerg Med. 2015;33(2):229–33.

18. Townsend DJ, Bassett GS. Common elbow fractures in children. Am Fam Physician. 1996;53(6):2031–41.

19. Lima S, Correia JF, Ribeiro RP, Martins RM, Alegrete N, Coutinho J, et al. A rare case of elbow dislocation associated with unrecognized fracture of medial epicondyle and delayed ulnar neuropathy in pediatric age. J Shoulder Elbow Surg. 2013;22(3):e9–e11.

20. Kunkel S, Cornwall R, Little K, Jain V, Mehlman C, Tamai J. Limitations of the radiocapitellar line for assessment of pediatric elbow radiographs. J Pediatr Orthop. 2011;31(6):628–32.

21. Parvaresh KC, Upasani VV, Bomar JD, Pennock AT. Secondary ossification center appearance and closure in the pelvis and proximal femur. J Pediatr Orthop. 2018;38(8):418–23.

22. Umans H, Liebling MS, Moy L, Haramati N, Macy NJ, Pritzker HA. Slipped capital femoral epiphysis: a physeal lesion diagnosed by MRI, with radiographic and CT correlation. Skeletal Radiol. 1998;27(3):139–44.

23. Boles CA, el-Khoury GY. Slipped capital femoral epiphysis. Radiographics. 1997;17(4):809–23.

24. Obana KK, Siddiqui AA, Broom AM, Barrett K, Andras LM, Millis MB, et al. Slipped capital femoral epiphysis in children without obesity. J Pediatr. 2020;218:192–7 e1.

25. Loder RT, Skopelja EN. The epidemiology and demographics of slipped capital femoral epiphysis. ISRN Orthop. 2011;2011:486512.

26. Sundar M, Carty H. Avulsion fractures of the pelvis in children: a report of 32 fractures and their outcome. Skeletal Radiol. 1994;23(2):85–90.

27. Fernbach SK, Wilkinson RH. Avulsion injuries of the pelvis and proximal femur. AJR Am J Roentgenol. 1981;137(3):581–4.

28. Stevens MA, El-Khoury GY, Kathol MH, Brandser EA, Chow S. Imaging features of avulsion injuries. Radiographics. 1999;19(3):655–72.

29. Gottsegen CJ, Eyer BA, White EA, Learch TJ, Forrester D. Avulsion fractures of the knee: imaging findings and clinical significance. Radiographics. 2008;28(6):1755–70.

30. Dupuis CS, Westra SJ, Makris J, Wallace EC. Injuries and conditions of the extensor mechanism of the pediatric knee. Radiographics. 2009;29(3):877–86.

31. Pandya NK, Edmonds EW, Roocroft JH, Mubarak SJ. Tibial tubercle fractures: complications, classification, and the need for intra-articular assessment. J Pediatr Orthop. 2012;32(8):749–59.

32. Tenenbein M, Reed MH, Black GB. The toddler's fracture revisited. Am J Emerg Med. 1990;8(3):208–11.

33. Boyer RS, Jaffe RB, Nixon GW, Condon VR. Trampoline fracture of the proximal tibia in children. AJR Am J Roentgenol. 1986;146(1):83–5.

34. Stranzinger E, Leidolt L, Eich G, Klimek PM. The anterior tilt angle of the proximal tibia epiphyseal plate: a significant radiological finding in young children with trampoline fractures. Eur J Radiol. 2014;83(8):1433–6.

35. Halsey MF, Finzel KC, Carrion WV, Haralabatos SS, Gruber MA, Meinhard BP. Toddler's fracture: presumptive diagnosis and treatment. J Pediatr Orthop. 2001;21(2):152–6.

36. John SD, Moorthy CS, Swischuk LE. Expanding the concept of the toddler's fracture. Radiographics. 1997;17(2):367–76.

37. Duchesneau S, Fallat LM. The Tillaux fracture. J Foot Ankle Surg. 1996;35(2):127–33. discussion 89

38. Horn BD, Crisci K, Krug M, Pizzutillo PD, MacEwen GD. Radiologic evaluation of juvenile tillaux fractures of the distal tibia. J Pediatr Orthop. 2001;21(2):162–4.

39. Brown SD, Kasser JR, Zurakowski D, Jaramillo D. Analysis of 51 tibial triplane fractures using CT with multiplanar reconstruction. AJR Am J Roentgenol. 2004;183(5):1489–95.

40. Liporace FA, Yoon RS, Kubiak EN, Parisi DM, Koval KJ, Feldman DS, et al. Does adding computed tomography change the diagnosis and treatment of Tillaux and triplane pediatric ankle fractures? Orthopedics. 2012;35(2):e208–12.

41. Leary JT, Handling M, Talerico M, Yong L, Bowe JA. Physeal fractures of the distal tibia: predictive factors of premature physeal closure and growth arrest. J Pediatr Orthop. 2009;29(4):356–61.

42. Karrholm J. The triplane fracture: four years of follow-up of 21 cases and review of the literature. J Pediatr Orthop B. 1997;6(2):91–102.

43. Crawford AH. Triplane and Tillaux fractures: is a 2 mm residual gap acceptable? J Pediatr Orthop. 2012;32(Suppl 1):S69–73.

44. Hobbs CJ, Bilo RA. Nonaccidental trauma: clinical aspects and epidemiology of child abuse. Pediatr Radiol. 2009;39(5):457–60.

45. Expert Panel on Pediatric I, Wootton-Gorges SL, Soares BP, Alazraki AL, Anupindi SA, Blount JP, et al. ACR appropriateness criteria((R)) suspected physical abuse-child. J Am Coll Radiol. 2017;14(5S):S338–S49.
46. Dwek JR. The radiographic approach to child abuse. Clin Orthop Relat Res. 2011;469(3):776–89.
47. Kleinman PK, Marks SC Jr. Relationship of the subperiosteal bone collar to metaphyseal lesions in abused infants. J Bone Joint Surg Am. 1995;77(10):1471–6.
48. Offiah A, van Rijn RR, Perez-Rossello JM, Kleinman PK. Skeletal imaging of child abuse (non-accidental injury). Pediatr Radiol. 2009;39(5):461–70.
49. Barsness KA, Cha ES, Bensard DD, Calkins CM, Partrick DA, Karrer FM, et al. The positive predictive value of rib fractures as an indicator of nonaccidental trauma in children. J Trauma. 2003;54(6):1107–10.
50. Ingram JD, Connell J, Hay TC, Strain JD, Mackenzie T. Oblique radiographs of the chest in nonaccidental trauma. Emerg Radiol. 2000;7(1):42–6.

Kayla Cort and Rebecca Stein-Wexler

## Contents

### Abstract

This chapter explores the more common causes of pediatric, nontraumatic musculoskeletal emergencies, thus largely focusing on infectious entities. The spectrum of diseases discussed ranges from mild to severe and includes cellulitis, septic arthritis, osteomyelitis, soft tissue abscess, pyomyositis, and necrotizing fasciitis. As the pediatric population encompasses a large age range from the neonatal period to adolescence, the variability in predisposing factors and clinical presentations among this demographic is highlighted, as well as the differences when compared to the adult population. Imaging, for the majority of the discussed entities, serves as an important tool for guiding diagnosis and management, especially in this young demographic where clinicians often face the unique challenge of the patient's inability to verbally communicate and/or adequately localize pain. Thus, in addition to elaborating on the details of characteristic imaging appearances of multiple disease processes across different modalities, there is also discussion of when imaging should be considered and how imaging findings can potentially alter patient management.

K. Cort (✉)
University of California Davis health and Shriners Hospitals for Children Northern California, Sacramento, CA, USA
e-mail: kcort@ucdavis.edu

R. Stein-Wexler
University of California Davis Health Department of Radiology and Shriners Hospital for Children Northern California, Sacramento, CA, USA
e-mail: rsteinwexler@ucdavis.edu

### Keywords

Osteomyelitis · Pyomyositis · Abscess · Cellulitis · Septic arthritis · Necrotizing fasciitis

© Springer Nature Switzerland AG 2022
M. N. Patlas et al. (eds.), *Atlas of Emergency Imaging from Head-to-Toe*,
https://doi.org/10.1007/978-3-030-92111-8_48

## Introduction

As with traumatic musculoskeletal emergencies, the importance of managing the infectious entities lies in making both accurate and timely diagnoses. However, with these infectious entities, there are additional risks of rapidly progressing disease and the increasing likelihood of postinfectious complications when diagnoses are not efficiently made. Joint destruction and growth plate abnormalities are some of the postinfectious complications that can be devastating in a growing child. With invasive, community-acquired methicillin-resistant *Staphylococcus aureus* (*S. aureus*) infection becoming more prevalent, it is critical that clinicians and radiologists become familiar with its varying clinical presentations and imaging characteristics in children to optimize patient outcomes.

## Osteomyelitis

### Epidemiology

Osteomyelitis is defined as an infection of the bone or bone marrow. Its frequency has increased over the years, with an incidence of 8–10 per 100,000 children in developed countries [1, 2]. Neonates are more prone to developing osteomyelitis because of an immature immune system. However, all children from neonates to adolescents are susceptible. Pediatric osteomyelitis usually results from hematogenous spread. Less common routes include direct inoculation and direct spread from soft tissue infections. *S. aureus* is most commonly implicated in pediatric osteomyelitis, followed by respiratory pathogens *Streptococcus pyogenes* (*S. pyogenes*), *Streptococcus pneumoniae* (*S. pneumoniae*), and *Kingella kingae* (*K. kingae*). Infections with methicillin-resistant *S. aureus* (*MRSA*) have become more prevalent in the last few years, causing a more severe disease characterized by extensive soft tissue involvement, multifocality, and increased incidence of subperiosteal abscess [2].

Infectious pathogens and distribution of disease vary with age and background medical conditions. *K. kingae* commonly affects neonates and infants, with a tendency for epiphyseal involvement. In fact, this is the most common pathogen in young children with osteomyelitis and septic arthritis. Although *S. aureus* is the most common cause of osteomyelitis overall, *Salmonella* is often implicated in children with sickle cell disease [3, 4].

The rich vascularity of the metaphysis renders it the primary site of infection in pediatric patients. Sluggish flow within the metaphyseal intramedullary venous sinusoids creates an optimal environment for the deposition and growth of pathogens circulating in the blood [2, 5, 7]. In neonates and toddlers, epiphyseal spread is relatively common since, until about age 18 months, communication between metaphyseal and epiphyseal vasculature across the physis facilitates the spread of infection (Fig. 1) [8].

Metaphyseal equivalents are also predisposed to develop osteomyelitis. Metaphyseal equivalents are defined as the junction of cartilage and bone in round bones, flat bones, and epiphyseal ossification centers in skeletally immature patients. A few examples of metaphyseal equivalents include multiple sites in the pelvis, such as the bones adjacent to the triradiate cartilage and sacroiliac joints. The vascular supply to these regions is similar to that of the metaphysis, so these areas are equally susceptible to infection [2, 7].

## Clinical Features

Osteomyelitis is defined as acute if symptom duration is less than 2 weeks, subacute when the duration is between 2 weeks and 3 months, and chronic when symptom duration exceeds 3 months. Classic symptoms are focal tenderness and swelling around the affected long bone, fever, and in older children, refusal to bear weight or walk. Spinal osteomyelitis commonly presents with back pain, while tenderness upon digital rectal examination can be present with sacral osteomyelitis [9]. Young children and neonates may present with irritability, poor feeding, and pseudoparalysis of a limb, with or without fever as their developing immune systems may render them unable to mount a response [1]. Epiphyseal osteomyelitis in young children, often caused by *K. kingae*, has a subacute presentation with mild clinical symptoms and lack of white blood cell count elevation in almost two-thirds of patients [2].

Chronic nonbacterial osteomyelitis/chronic recurrent multifocal osteomyelitis (CNO/CRMO) is a noninfectious form of osteomyelitis that should also be considered in the differential diagnosis. Defined as an inflammatory condition of unclear etiology affecting children and adolescents, characterized by periodic exacerbations and remissions, its presentation is insidious, and symptoms are typically less acute than with infectious osteomyelitis. The most common symptoms are bone pain, malaise, and low-grade fever [8]. Because CNO/CRMO is inflammatory rather than infectious, the treatment differs from that of bacterial osteomyelitis, making differentiation essential. Like its infectious counterpart, CNO/CRMO more commonly affects the metaphysis and metaphyseal equivalents and causes bone destruction. The lower extremities, pelvis, and spine are commonly affected in CNO/CRMO, and involvement is frequently multifocal [2]. The prevalence of CNO/CRMO may be underreported as it is a diagnosis of exclusion [10]. Thus, it is important to consider this entity as alternate diagnosis, particularly when the clinical presentation deviates from that of bacterial osteomyelitis.

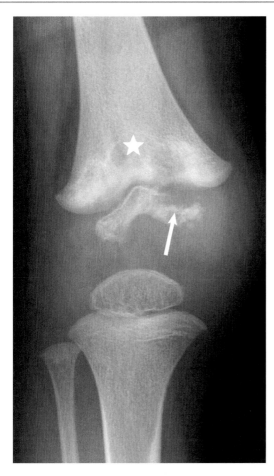

**Fig. 1** A 1-year-old boy with resolving osteomyelitis, with extension into the epiphysis. Anteroposterior radiograph of the right knee demonstrates sclerotic and lucent regions in the distal femoral metaphysis (star) and a focal lucent region at the medial aspect of the distal femoral epiphysis (arrow)

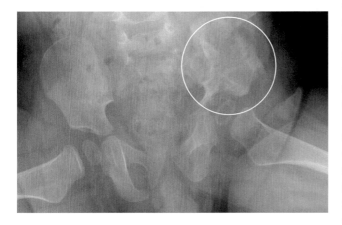

**Fig. 2** An 11-month-old boy with left hip septic arthritis complicated by osteomyelitis. Anteroposterior radiograph of the pelvis shows a permeative appearance of the left iliac wing with irregularity of the left acetabulum (circle). At presentation, the pelvis radiograph was unremarkable (not shown)

## Diagnostic Investigations

Imaging plays a very important role in the diagnosis of osteomyelitis as well as its management. It is also important for excluding osteomyelitis, since this diagnosis can present in a variety of nonspecific manners in the pediatric age group. Noninfectious or traumatic etiologies involving the bones and soft tissues may present similarly. If soft tissue infectious or inflammatory etiologies are suspected, imaging can aid in determining osseous involvement.

After establishing the diagnosis of osteomyelitis, it is critical to determine the presence and severity of complications. Subperiosteal abscess, intraosseous abscess, and soft tissue abscess all warrant surgical drainage and can shift the treatment from exclusively medical to surgical [2, 6, 11]. The various modalities for assessing and diagnosing osteomyelitis include radiography, computed tomography (CT), magnetic resonance imaging (MRI), ultrasound (US), and nuclear medicine imaging (NM).

Radiography is commonly the first modality employed and is of varying utility as the presence of osseous abnormalities depends on the duration of symptoms. More so, evaluating the involvement of the unossified epiphyses in younger children with radiography can be very difficult if not impossible, even with advanced disease [6]. Initially, only soft tissue swelling with loss of fat planes may be appreciated. After several days of symptoms, periosteal reaction may be evident. Lytic foci or a permeative appearance of the bone follows after 7–21 days (Fig. 2). In early CNO/CRMO, lytic metaphyseal foci that abut the growth plates of tubular bones can be seen (Fig. 3). These foci become sclerotic with time.

US is not typically employed to evaluate osseous structures. However, it may be useful for identifying superficial osseous findings including subperiosteal collections and periosteal reaction. It may also demonstrate adjacent soft tissue changes, such as sinus tracts and soft tissue abscess, as well as neighboring joint effusions that may indicate secondary septic arthritis [2, 6, 11]. The fibrous layer of the periosteum appears as a smooth, echogenic linear structure adjacent to the cortex. In the presence of a subperiosteal collection, fluid separates this structure from the underlying cortex (Fig. 4) [2].

MRI is the most useful modality for evaluating osteomyelitis, as it is quite sensitive for depicting marrow changes, even in early disease. The typical findings of osteomyelitis consist of diminished signal on T1-weighted sequences, markedly increased signal on fluid-sensitive sequences, and increased enhancement [6] (Fig. 5). CNO/CRMO foci in the axial skeleton, in contrast, tend to show milder marrow edema on MRI, without soft tissue involvement [2]. In addition to demonstrating primary bone findings, MRI beautifully depicts subperiosteal abscess, intraosseous abscess, associated soft tissue or intramuscular abscesses, and joint effusions

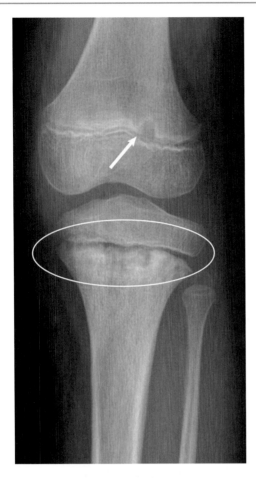

**Fig. 3** An 8-year-old girl with chronic nonbacterial osteomyelitis/ chronic recurrent multifocal osteomyelitis. Anteroposterior radiograph of the right knee demonstrates old, sclerotic disease foci within the proximal tibia metaphysis, along the growth plate (white oval). A focal lucency at the lateral aspect of the distal femoral metaphysis (white arrow), not appreciated on the prior radiographic examination (not shown), is consistent with new disease

(Figs. 6 and 7). Characteristic of subacute osteomyelitis is the "penumbra sign" which refers to the increased T1 signal of the granulation tissue which lines the intraosseous abscess cavity (Fig. 8) [12]. CNO/CRMO foci may also demonstrate small intraosseous fluid collections on MRI [10].

In the setting of marrow edema, primary bone tumors may be considered in the differential. There are important imaging characteristics that allow differentiation between osteomyelitis and the top two most common pediatric primary bone tumors, Ewing's sarcoma and osteosarcoma. Both entities are associated with a soft tissue mass (Fig. 9). Aggressive periosteal reaction, classically a "sunburst pattern" in osteosarcoma and "onion skin" pattern in Ewing's sarcoma, is best appreciated on CT or radiography (Fig. 10). Additionally, Ewing's sarcoma typically affects long bone diaphysis, in contrast to osteomyelitis which most commonly affects the metaphyses of long bones [13].

Most MRI findings of osteomyelitis are evident without intravenous contrast. However, intravenous contrast may be needed to diagnose isolated epiphyseal infection in young children, whose epiphyses are entirely or predominantly cartilaginous. In these children, who are typically less than 4 years old, fluid-sensitive sequences (such as T2 and short-tau inversion recovery (STIR) may have limited sensitivity, as normal epiphyseal cartilage appears hyperintense, partly masking edema that may result from infection (Fig. 11) [2].

CT has more utility in depicting osseous changes that occur in chronic osteomyelitis—not typically encountered in the emergency setting. These changes include heterogenous sclerosis and sequestra, regions of devitalized bone that are separated from the surrounding bone by granulation tissue (Fig. 12). Sequestra can be challenging to visualize on MRI, especially when small. Soft tissue involvement can be assessed with CT, particularly with the use of IV contrast, but MRI provides more optimal soft tissue evaluation [6, 11, 14, 15].

NM imaging is also an option. Bone scintigraphy, positron emission tomography-computed tomography (PET-CT), and tagged white blood cell scanning all demonstrate increased activity in the setting of acute osteomyelitis. However, these tests may not be as readily available. Additionally, bone scans and tagged white blood cell scans have limited anatomic detail. The strength of these modalities lies in determining the precise location when symptoms do not localize, as well as potential multifocality. NM imaging has largely been replaced with MRI, as the latter modality offers a detailed evaluation of the osseous structures and soft tissues in the acute setting without the use of ionizing radiation.

## Conclusion/Summary

Osteomyelitis is a disease process that can affect all pediatric patients. However, there is variation in causative pathogens and clinical presentation among younger and older children. Severe disease has become more common over the years due to the increased prevalence of infections with *MRSA*. Imaging is essential for making the diagnosis, determining disease extent, and revealing complications that would require surgical interventions.

### Key Points

1. *MRSA* osteomyelitis can result in severe multifocal disease with extensive soft tissue involvement and subperiosteal abscess.
2. Due to their developing immune systems, neonates are more at risk for osteomyelitis and often show mild clinical symptoms in the setting of an acute infection.

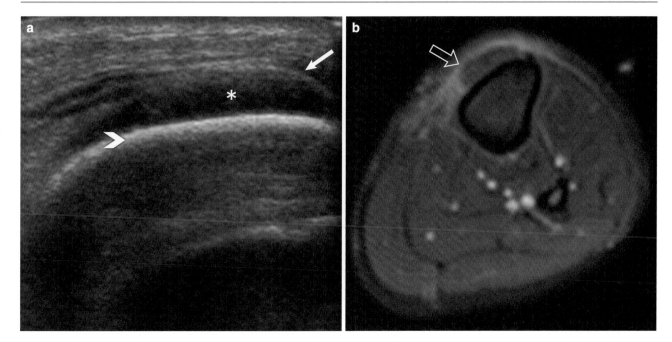

**Fig. 4** Subperiosteal abscess and osteomyelitis in a 16-year-old male. The left tibia was noted to be necrotic upon incision and drainage. (**a**) Transverse gray-scale US image of the anterior left tibia shows a complex subperiosteal fluid collection (asterisk) which is elevating the curvilinear, echogenic periosteum (arrow). The anterior tibia cortex is denoted by the arrowhead. (**b**) Axial post-contrast T1-weighted MR image with fat saturation demonstrates the peripherally enhancing subperiosteal abscess (open arrow)

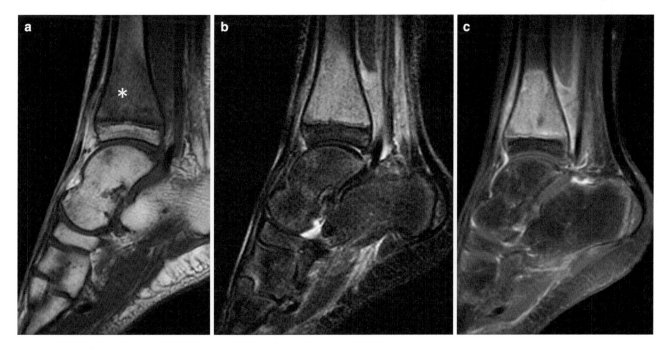

**Fig. 5** A 9-year-old boy with left tibial osteomyelitis. (**a**) Sagittal T1-weighted MR image of the left ankle shows diminished marrow signal at the tibial metaphysis (asterisk). (**b**) Sagittal STIR image of the left ankle shows increased signal at the tibial metaphysis corresponding to marrow edema. (**c**) Sagittal T1-weighted post-contrast MR image with fat saturation shows increased enhancement at the tibial metaphysis

3. CNO/CRMO demonstrates relatively little soft tissue abnormality and preferentially involves the periphyseal regions of tubular bones.

4. *K. kingae* is the most common pathogen involved in osteomyelitis and septic arthritis in young children.

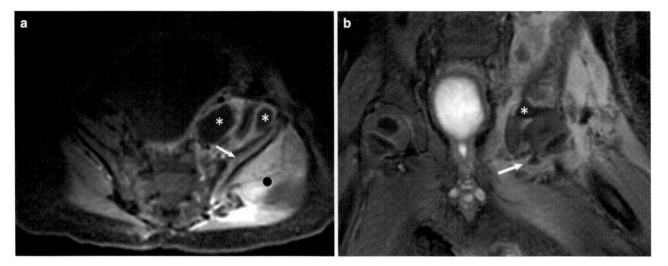

**Fig. 6** Septic arthritis complicated by osteomyelitis in an 11-month-old boy (same patient as shown in Fig. 2). (**a**) Axial T1-weighted post-contrast MR image with fat saturation shows extensively increased enhancement of the left iliac bone (arrow) and left gluteal muscles (black circle). Also noted are psoas and iliacus intramuscular abscesses (asterisks). (**b**) Coronal T1-weighted post-contrast MR image with fat saturation shows a left hip joint effusion with hyperenhancement of the synovium (arrow), as well as focally diminished enhancement of the left anterior acetabulum (asterisk), suggesting devitalized bone. The contra-lateral hip and surrounding muscles are unremarkable

**Fig.7** A 6-year-old boy with osteomyelitis. (**a**) Coronal T1-weighted post-contrast MR image with fat saturation shows a peripherally enhancing intraosseous abscess in the proximal tibial metaphysis (arrow). (**b**) Coronal T2-weighted, fat-saturated MR image shows hyperintense signal within the abscess cavity

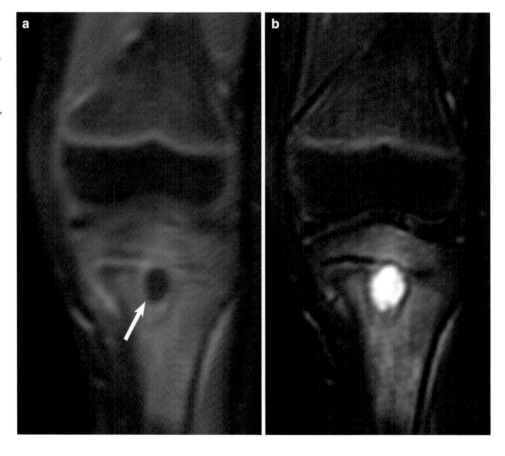

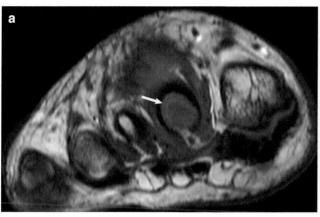
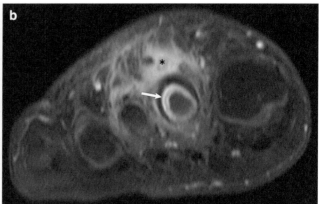

**Fig. 8** Intraosseous abscess and cellulitis in a 12-year-old girl with right foot pain. (**a**) Axial T1-weighted MR image demonstrates hyperintense signal of the intraosseous abscess wall (arrow), referred to as "penumbra sign." (**b**) Axial T1-weighted post-contrast MR image with fat saturation shows enhancement of the intraosseous abscess wall (arrow), as well as enhancement of the overlying dorsal soft tissues (asterisk)

**Fig. 9** A 6-year-old boy with Ewing's sarcoma. (**a**) Coronal T2-weighted fat-saturated MR image shows a predominantly hyperintense mass arising from the left mid tibial diaphysis (oval). (**b**) Coronal T1-weighted MR image demonstrates corresponding hypointense marrow signal. (**c**) Axial T1-weighted post-contrast MR image with fat saturation demonstrates an associated soft tissue mass (asterisk) extending beyond the cortex. Also noted is extensive cortical destruction (arrow)

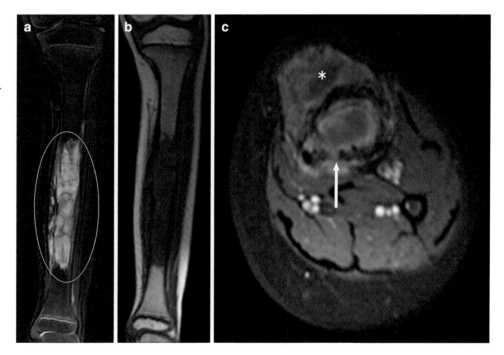

## Septic Arthritis

### Epidemiology

Septic arthritis, defined as an infection of the joint, has an annual incidence between 4 and 12 per 100,000 children. It is more common in younger children, peaking at age 3 years [1, 5]. It is considered a surgical emergency, as delays in diagnosis can lead to devastating joint destruction from proteolytic enzymes within the purulent joint fluid. Thus, the threshold for clinical suspicion of this entity should be low to trigger the cascade of appropriate diagnostic testing. As with osteomyelitis, hematogenous spread is the most common mechanism of infection, although the joint may also be seeded by direct spread from osteomyelitis or soft tissue infection, as well as direct intra-articular trauma. The most common causative pathogens are *S. aureus* and group A *Streptococcus* [8].

## Clinical Features

Septic arthritis and osteomyelitis may have similar clinical presentations and commonly coexist. Thus, it is important to

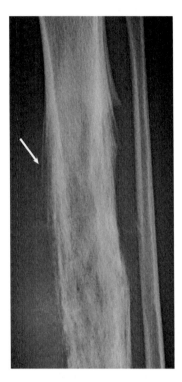

**Fig. 10** A 6-year-old boy with Ewing's sarcoma (same patient as Fig. 9). Anteroposterior radiograph of the left tibia shows layered periosteal reaction, which creates the "onion skin" pattern (arrow). Also demonstrated is a permeative appearance of the tibial diaphysis due to tumor infiltration

exclude concomitant osteomyelitis to avoid inadequate treatment. The following are associated with increased risk of concurrent osteomyelitis: infancy, adolescence, symptoms lasting more than 6 days, and infections with either methicillin-susceptible *Staphylococcus aureus* (*MSSA*) *or MRSA* [5]. The cartilaginous epiphyses and epiphyseal equivalents in neonates receive blood supply from metaphyseal vessels prior to the appearance of secondary ossification centers. Because of this, septic arthritis commonly follows osteomyelitis in this age group, especially in joints with an intracapsular metaphysis, such as the hip [1].

## Diagnostic Investigations

Radiography is typically the first modality employed to address musculoskeletal concerns, but this modality is of limited utility in the diagnosis of septic arthritis. The presence of a joint effusion is a sensitive though nonspecific indicator of joint infection. Elbow and knee effusions are readily diagnosed on radiographs, although very small effusions may be missed. However, radiographs are insensitive for the diagnosis of effusions elsewhere, especially at the hip—a relatively common location of septic arthritis.

US is, by contrast, a sensitive modality for the detection of joint effusions and is able to demonstrate small effusions in a variety of locations (Figs. 13 and 14). The presence of a joint effusion, however, does not automatically signify septic arthritis. Unfortunately, septic arthritis, transient synovitis, and other causes of effusion cannot be diagnosed simply by the presence of joint fluid. In the appropriate clinical setting, aspiration and fluid analysis are required to determine if an

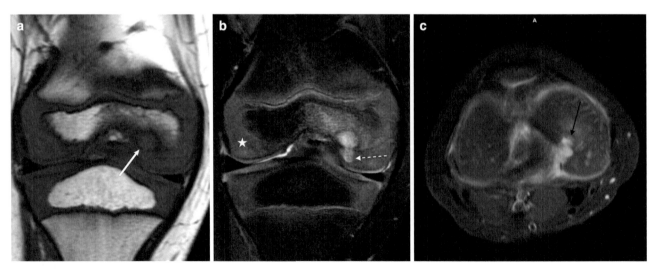

**Fig. 11** A 4-year-old boy with epiphyseal osteomyelitis. (**a**) Coronal T1-weighted MR image of the right knee demonstrates focally diminished signal within the ossification center. (**b**) Coronal T2-weighted MR image with fat-saturation demonstrates involvement of the epiphyseal cartilage (dashed arrow). Note the intrinsically high T2 signal of the uninvolved epiphyseal cartilage (asterisk). (**c**) Axial post-contrast T1-weighted MR image with fat saturation shows enhancement of the involved epiphyseal cartilage (black arrow). Courtesy of Herman J. Kan, MD, Texas Children's Hospital

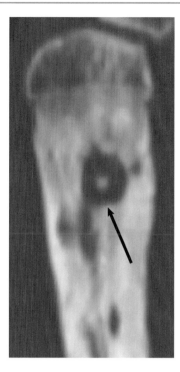

**Fig. 12** A 14-year-old male with chronic osteomyelitis. Coronal CT image of the right fibula demonstrates a sequestrum (arrow) and surrounding heterogenous sclerosis

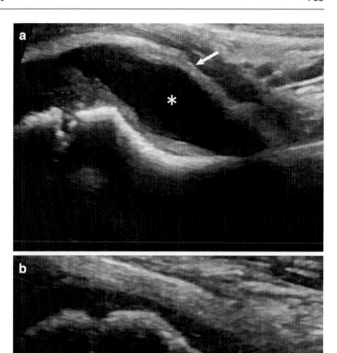

**Fig. 13** Septic arthritis in a 3-year-old girl with inability to bear weight. (**a**) Sagittal gray-scale US image of right the hip reveals a large joint effusion (asterisk) which causes bulging of the joint capsule (arrow). (**b**) Normal left hip for comparison

infection is present. Infected joint fluid is characterized as purulent or turbid with an increased white blood cell count above 200,000/mm3 or positive gram stain [16].

Like US, MRI is highly sensitive for the depiction of joint effusions. Synovial fluid demonstrates high STIR/T2 signal. In the setting of inflammation, the synovium will appear thickened and hyperenhancing on post-contrast images (Fig. 15). Marked synovial and surrounding soft tissue abnormalities are highly suggestive of septic arthritis. Additionally, signal alterations in the bone marrow, specifically ill-defined regions of low T1 signal and corresponding increased T2 signal on fat-suppressed images, as well as hyperenhancement, limited to the adjacent articular surfaces, make septic arthritis more likely than transient or noninfectious synovitis. Marrow edema extending beyond the adjacent articular surfaces is associated with coexistent osteomyelitis [16].

## Conclusion/Summary

Septic arthritis is a surgical emergency for which clinical suspicion is necessary in order not to delay diagnosis. Imaging, specifically US, while not diagnostic, can readily demonstrate joint effusions and then should trigger additional diagnostic testing required to confirm the diagnosis. Additionally, it is important to assess for concomitant osteomyelitis using MRI to avoid undertreatment.

## Key Points
1. Septic arthritis is a surgical emergency and can occur concomitantly with osteomyelitis.
2. Septic arthritis often follows osteomyelitis in neonates due to epiphyseal blood supply via metaphyseal vessels prior to the appearance of secondary ossification centers.
3. Septic arthritis is not an imaging diagnosis and must be confirmed with joint fluid analysis.

## Skin and Soft Tissue Infections

## Epidemiology

*S. aureus* is responsible for most skin and soft tissue infections in childhood, accounting for 70% of infections, predominantly folliculitis, cellulitis, impetigo, and surgical and traumatic soft tissue infections. Some *S. aureus* infections may be encountered in a polymicrobial setting. This is more likely with puncture wounds of the foot and decubitus ulcers, particularly in the perianal region [17]. As with osteomyelitis

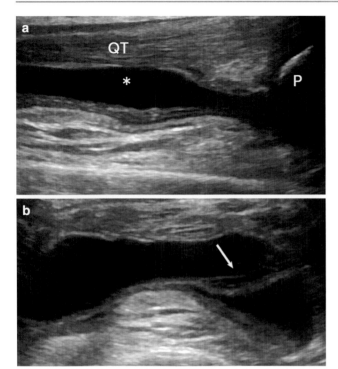

**Fig. 14** A 13-year-old female with septic arthritis. (**a**) Sagittal gray-scale US image of the right knee demonstrates a suprapatellar joint effusion (asterisk). The patella is denoted by "P." The quadriceps tendon is denoted by "QT." (**b**) Transverse view of the suprapatellar bursa shows septa (arrow) that raised concern for septic arthritis, which was later proven with joint aspiration

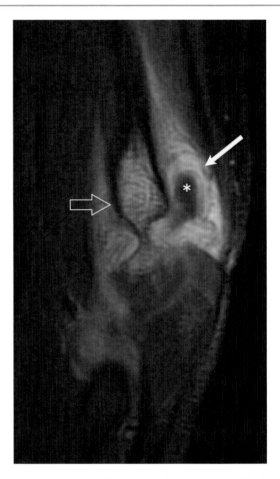

**Fig. 15** Osteomyelitis and septic arthritis in a 4-year-old girl with 3 days of fever and left elbow pain. Sagittal T1-weighted post-contrast MR image with fat saturation shows a large left elbow joint effusion (asterisk) and posterior bulging of the hyperenhancing joint capsule (arrow). Distal humeral marrow hyperenhancement (open arrow) indicates osteomyelitis

and septic arthritis, *MRSA* is increasingly prevalent with soft tissue infections, and the disease tends to be more severe and have a worse clinical outcome [18]. The specific disease entities that will be discussed in this section are cellulitis, soft tissue abscess, pyomyositis, and necrotizing fasciitis.

Cellulitis is a skin infection that involves the dermis and subcutaneous tissues. *S. aureus* and group A *Streptococcus* are the most common causative pathogens. *S. aureus* is a commensal bacterium that does not typically cause disease in healthy skin. However, infection in the skin with no obvious barrier disturbance can occur; this is referred to as a primary infection. Infections are more often secondary, occurring when the skin barrier is previously disturbed [17]. Less commonly, cellulitis may be secondary to hematogenous spread [19]. Causative pathogens vary somewhat by patient age and infection site. For example, *H. influenza* type B is a relatively common cause of facial infections in children under 3 years old, since children in this age group commonly carry the organism as a part of their normal pharyngeal flora [20].

Soft tissue abscesses are defined as organized fluid collections comprised of necrotic tissue. They often follow bacterial soft tissue infections and thus can be a result of preexisting cellulitis. The importance of diagnostic evaluation in cases of suspected cellulitis is identifying abscess formation. If present, an abscess would shift the course of treatment.

Pyomyositis is a skeletal muscle infection often accompanied by an abscess. Pyomyositis is common in tropical climates but encountered relatively infrequently in temperate regions. Hematogenous spread is the primary mechanism of infection. Bacteria usually seed previously traumatized muscle as healthy muscle usually resists infection. Systemic predisposing factors are typically present when pyomyositis develops in normal tissue. Underlying malnutrition and immunodeficiency are more commonly encountered in the pediatric population, whereas diabetes and intravenous drug usage predispose to pyomyositis in the adult population [11, 19, 21, 22].

Necrotizing fasciitis is a serious, rapidly progressive soft tissue infection involving the deep soft tissues. The mortality rate is high if not treated promptly and aggressively with extensive and early surgical debridement [23, 24]. This disease is rare in children, only reported in 0.08 per 100,000 per year [23]. Although highly uncommon in children, it is important to keep necrotizing fasciitis on the clinical radar, as the condition is often misdiagnosed in its early stages.

Overall, necrotizing fasciitis in children differs from that in adults. The disease usually occurs in previously healthy children, resulting from minor soft tissue trauma and/or minor skin abnormalities, whereas in adults the infection commonly occurs in immunosuppressed or diabetic individuals. Monomicrobial infections are typically responsible for necrotizing fasciitis in children, with *S. pyogenes* being the most commonly involved bacterium. Others include *S. aureus*, *E. coli*, and *Pseudomonas*. In contrast, with adults, necrotizing fasciitis is typically a polymicrobial infection [23, 25].

## Clinical Features

Skin and soft tissue infections in the pediatric population can present with nonspecific clinical findings, such as soft tissue induration and redness. Cellulitis is typically characterized by localized erythema, pain, and edema. It may be accompanied by systemic findings such as fever and malaise [19]. The legs and digits are frequently involved, but cellulitis can occur anywhere. Cellulitis and soft tissue abscess may have a similar presentation. If an abscess is developing, the clinical examination classically becomes notable for point tenderness and fluctuance [26]. However, it can sometimes be difficult to determine whether or not an abscess complicates soft tissue infection.

The nonspecific symptoms of pyomyositis, which include fever and localized swelling, may simulate other more common processes. For example, pyomyositis of the pelvic muscles surrounding the sciatic nerve may clinically simulate pelvic osteomyelitis or septic arthritis. Both entities are encountered much more often than pyomyositis [22].

Pyomyositis tends to be unifocal, although multifocality has been documented in up to 40% of cases. The quadriceps musculature is most commonly involved, followed by the gluteal muscles and iliopsoas [19]. There are three stages of pyomyositis. The first is the invasive stage, defined by muscle edema and pain. The suppurative stage follows, during which there is intramuscular abscess formation and fever. Most cases are diagnosed during the second stage. Finally, the late stage is characterized by multi-organ failure, septicemia, and a high mortality rate [11, 19].

Necrotizing fasciitis, like cellulitis, presents with induration, edema, and erythema in its early stages. More marked skin changes, including ecchymosis, crepitus, and vesiculation, are present with advanced disease. Characteristics that favor necrotizing fasciitis over a simple soft tissue infection are pain that is disproportionate to skin findings, rapid spread of skin involvement, and sepsis [23]. The trunk is most often affected in children, whereas the extremities are usually involved in adults [23, 24].

## Diagnostic Evaluation

The importance of imaging lies in determining the extent of soft tissue involvement and the presence or absence of an abscess to guide treatment decisions [8]. In the pediatric population, US is often employed due to its lack of ionizing radiation, potential for targeted evaluation, and most importantly ability to demonstrate fluid collections. US is also particularly useful for identifying foreign bodies that may serve as a nidus for infection. CT and MRI have specific advantages as well. Both provide a larger field of view, useful when assessing the extent and depth of an infection. MRI overall offers better soft tissue resolution than CT but is suboptimal for demonstrating soft tissue gas and foreign bodies. CT, in contrast, better depicts foreign bodies and soft tissue gas [19].

In cases of cellulitis, imaging can be utilized to exclude the presence of a superimposed abscess that might require aspiration or incision and drainage. US is often the initial imaging route for the evaluation of soft tissue infection. US shows increased echogenicity and thickening of the skin and subcutaneous tissues. Anechoic strands traverse echogenic fat lobules, creating a cobblestone appearance (Fig. 16) [11, 19].

On MRI, diffuse, ill-defined, or linear regions of subcutaneous thickening with diminished signal on T1 and increased signal on fluid-sensitive sequences are characteristic of cellulitis (Fig. 17) [19]. The affected regions also demonstrate enhancement on post-contrast imaging. CT shows indistinctness between soft tissue planes, soft tissue stranding, and thickening of the soft tissues. The muscles, deep fascial

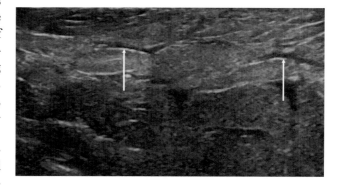

**Fig. 16** Cellulitis in a 17-year-old female with hyper Ig-E syndrome, presenting with localized left buttock tenderness and fever. Transverse gray-scale US image of the left buttock reveals increased echogenicity of the subcutaneous fat with interspersed curvilinear, hypoechoic foci (arrows)

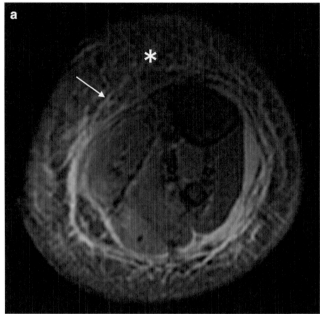

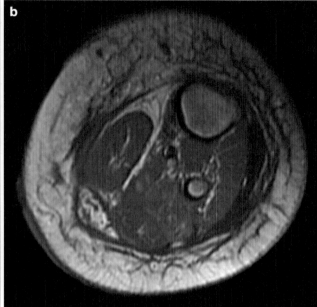

**Fig. 17** A 19-month-old boy with cellulitis of the left lower extremity. (**a**) Axial STIR image through the left tibia and fibula shows diffuse thickening throughout the subcutaneous fat (asterisk) and several linear and curvilinear hyperintense foci (arrow) consistent with edema. (**b**) Axial T1-weighted MR image shows corresponding hypointensity of the curvilinear foci

compartments, and bones appear normal on all imaging modalities, as the infection is by definition superficial [8].

In scenarios of suspected cellulitis where there is rapidly progressing disease and/or negligible response to antimicrobial therapy, imaging may be very useful [11, 19, 27]. A lower threshold for imaging utilization may be employed with immunocompromised patients who carry a greater risk of developing severe, deep, and rapidly progressing infections [28]. US is most often the initial modality used to evaluate for soft tissue abscess. An abscess appears as an anechoic or diffusely hypoechoic focal fluid collection (Fig. 18). Increased through transmission may also be appreciated. The abscess contents may on occasion appear hyperechoic or isoechoic compared to the surrounding tissues. Its liquefactive nature may be appreciated only with compression, which demonstrates the mobility of abscess contents. Color Doppler depicts the absence of blood flow centrally. Abscess margins may be well defined or poorly defined, blending with the surrounding soft tissues. Internal septa and echogenic foci, representing either debris or gas, may also be apparent [26].

The imaging appearance of pyomyositis corresponds with the previously discussed disease stages, specifically the first and second stages. On US, the invasive stage is characterized by a hypoechoic, ill-defined region within the involved muscle. An intramuscular fluid collection, compatible with an abscess, is found in the suppurative stage (Fig. 19) [11]. Similar correlates are seen on cross-sectional imaging. CT shows

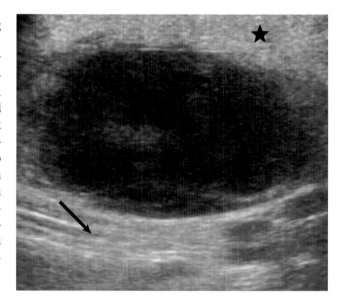

**Fig. 18** Soft tissue abscess in a 3-year-old boy. Sagittal gray-scale US image of the right thigh demonstrates an ovoid fluid collection within the subcutaneous fat. Markedly echogenic surrounding subcutaneous fat (star) indicates inflammatory change. Also noted is posterior acoustic enhancement deep to the fluid collection (arrow)

expansion of the muscle and hypoattenuation, corresponding with phlegmon and muscle edema during the first stage. Later in the infection, a well-defined, rim-enhancing fluid collection forms (Fig. 20). On MRI, muscle edema is characterized by increased T2 signal throughout the muscle. The abscess

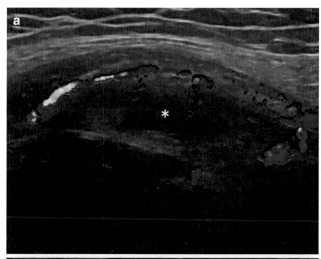

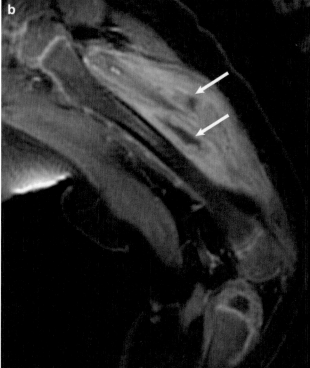

**Fig. 19** Pyomyositis in a 6-month-old boy with a left anterior thigh mass, fever, and leukocytosis. (**a**) Sagittal gray-scale US image with Doppler shows an intramuscular, hypoechoic fluid collection (asterisk) with peripheral vascularity. (**b**) Coronal post-contrast T1-weighted MR image with fat saturation shows diffuse hyperenhancement of the muscles of the anterior compartment of the left thigh, with focal, rim-enhancing fluid collections (arrows) which are highly consistent with intramuscular abscesses

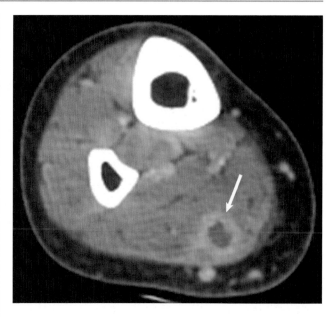

**Fig. 20** A 16-year-old male with pyomyositis. Axial CT image with IV contrast through the distal right lower extremity demonstrates an intramuscular, peripherally enhancing fluid collection representing an abscess (arrow)

that forms in the second stage demonstrates rim enhancement similar to CT, with the abscess contents usually displaying low to intermediate T1 signal and high T2 signal [19].

Given the high morbidity and mortality of necrotizing fasciitis, it is unfortunate that the diagnosis often cannot be made with certainty on cross-sectional imaging, since imaging findings are sensitive but not specific. One clue is the involvement of the deep and intramuscular fascia, which is strongly associated with the disease. In contrast, superficial involvement is typically seen with simple skin infections. T2-weighted MRI reveals hyperintense fluid signal in the affected fascia, associated fascial thickening measuring 3 mm or more, and involvement of three or more compartments (Fig. 21). Fluid signal may be evident within the musculature. Variable fascial enhancement patterns have been reported, ranging from increased to complete absence of enhancement. The latter pattern is more common and correlates with necrosis [19].

CT may show similar soft tissue changes, such as fatty infiltration, which appears as increased attenuation of the involved region, and fascial thickening. When compared to MRI, CT is more sensitive for the depiction of soft tissue gas, which presents clinically as crepitus. Unfortunately, this finding, while highly suggestive of necrotizing fasciitis, is rare and indicates advanced disease.

## Conclusion/Summary

Skin and soft tissue infections are relatively common within the pediatric population. The diagnosis of many of these entities is often made using clinical data. However, in confusing clinical scenarios and when dealing with high-risk groups, imaging can be of tremendous help in making the diagnosis, determining complications, and guiding treatment.

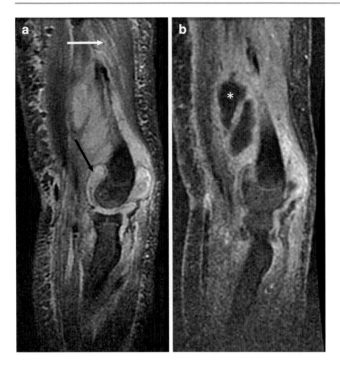

**Fig. 21** A 3 year-old boy with necrotizing fasciitis of the right upper extremity treated with multiple debridements. (**a**) Sagittal T2-weighted MR image with fat saturation and (**b**) sagittal T1-weighted post-contrast MR image with fat saturation. Extensive soft tissue inflammatory changes with increased T2 signal of the fascia (arrow) are noted. Also noted is an intramuscular abscess involving the brachialis muscle (asterisk) and a large elbow joint effusion (black arrow) due to septic arthritis. Courtesy of Elka Miller, MD, Children's Hospital of Eastern Ontario

### Key Points

1. *H. influenza* type B is a common cause of facial soft tissue infections in children under the age of 3.
2. In contrast to the polymicrobial infection commonly affecting the extremities in adults, necrotizing fasciitis is typically a monomicrobial infection that affects the trunk in children.
3. Muscle edema identified on imaging corresponds to the invasive stage of pyomyositis, while the presence of an intramuscular abscess corresponds to the suppurative stage of pyomyositis.

### References

1. Offiah AC. Acute osteomyelitis, septic arthritis and discitis: differences between neonates and older children. *Eur J Radiol.* 2006;60 (2):221–232. https://doi.org/10.1016/j.ejrad.2006.07.016
2. Jaramillo D, Dormans JP, Delgado J, Laor T, St Geme JW 3rd. Hematogenous Osteomyelitis in Infants and Children: Imaging of a Changing Disease. *Radiology.* 2017;283(3):629–643. https://doi.org/10.1148/radiol.2017151929
3. Burnett MW, Bass JW, Cook BA. Etiology of osteomyelitis complicating sickle cell disease. *Pediatrics.* 1998;101(2):296–297. https://doi.org/10.1542/peds.101.2.296
4. Fontalis A, Hughes K, Nguyen MP, et al. The challenge of differentiating vaso-occlusive crises from osteomyelitis in children with sickle cell disease and bone pain: A 15-year retrospective review. *J Child Orthop.* 2019;13(1):33–39. https://doi.org/10.1302/1863-2548.12.180094
5. Monsalve J, Kan JH, Schallert EK, Bisset GS, Zhang W, Rosenfeld SB. Septic arthritis in children: frequency of coexisting unsuspected osteomyelitis and implications on imaging work-up and management. *AJR Am J Roentgenol.* 2015;204(6):1289–1295. https://doi.org/10.2214/AJR.14.12891-1295; https://doi.org/10.2214/AJR.14.12891
6. van Schuppen J, van Doorn MM, van Rijn RR. Childhood osteomyelitis: imaging characteristics. *Insights Imaging.* 2012;3 (5):519–533. https://doi.org/10.1007/s13244-012-0186-8
7. Nixon GW. Hematogenous osteomyelitis of metaphyseal-equivalent locations. AJR *Am J Roentgenol.* 1978;130(1):123–129. https://doi.org/10.2214/ajr.130.1.123
8. Kothari NA, Pelchovitz DJ, Meyer JS. Imaging of musculoskeletal infections. *Radiol Clin North Am.* 2001;39(4):653–671. https://doi.org/10.1016/s0033-8389(05)70304-3
9. Peltola H, Pääkkönen M. Acute osteomyelitis in children. N Engl J Med. 2014;370(4):352–360. https://doi.org/10.1056/NEJMra1213956
10. Khanna G, Sato TS, Ferguson P. Imaging of chronic recurrent multifocal osteomyelitis. *Radiographics.* 2009;29(4):1159–1177. https://doi.org/10.1148/rg.294085244
11. Bureau NJ, Chhem RK, Cardinal E. Musculoskeletal infections: US manifestations. *Radiographics.* 1999;19(6):1585–1592. https://doi.org/10.1148/radiographics.19.6.g99no061585
12. Davies AM, Grimer R. The penumbra sign in subacute osteomyelitis. *Eur Radiol.* 2005;15(6):1268–1270. https://doi.org/10.1007/s00330-004-2435-9
13. Vartevan A, May C, Barnes CE. Pediatric Bone Imaging: Differentiating benign lesions from malignant. *Applied Radiology.* 2018. www.appliedradiology.com
14. Jennin F, Bousson V, Parlier C, Jomaah N, Khanine V, Laredo JD. Bony sequestrum: a radiologic review. *Skeletal Radiol.* 2011;40(8):963–975. https://doi.org/10.1007/s00256-010-0975-4
15. Desimpel J, Posadzy M, Vanhoenacker F. The Many Faces of Osteomyelitis: A Pictorial Review. *J Belg Soc Radiol.* 2017;101 (1):24. https://doi.org/10.5334/jbr-btr.1300
16. Lee SK, Suh KJ, Kim YW, et al. Septic arthritis versus transient synovitis at MR imaging: preliminary assessment with signal intensity alterations in bone marrow. *Radiology.* 1999;211 (2):459–465. https://doi.org/10.1148/radiology.211.2.r99ma47459
17. Ladhani S, Garbash M. Staphylococcal skin infections in children: rational drug therapy recommendations. *Paediatr Drugs.* 2005;7 (2):77–102. https://doi.org/10.2165/00148581-200507020-00002
18. Williams DJ, Cooper WO, Kaltenbach LA, et al. Comparative effectiveness of antibiotic treatment strategies for pediatric skin and soft-tissue infections. *Pediatrics.* 2011;128(3):e479–e487. https://doi.org/10.1542/peds.2010-3681
19. Hayeri MR, Ziai P, Shehata ML, Teytelboym OM, Huang BK. Soft-Tissue Infections and Their Imaging Mimics: From Cellulitis to Necrotizing Fasciitis. *Radiographics.* 2016;36 (6):1888–1910. https://doi.org/10.1148/rg.2016160068
20. Oumeish I, Oumeish OY, Bataineh O. Acute bacterial skin infections in children. *Clin Dermatol.* 2000;18(6):667–678. https://doi.org/10.1016/s0738-081x(00)00156-5
21. Gubbay AJ, Isaacs D. Pyomyositis in children. *Pediatr Infect Dis J.* 2000;19(10):1009–1013. https://doi.org/10.1097/00006454-200010000-00015
22. Hernandez RJ, Strouse PJ, Craig CL, Farley FA. Focal pyomyositis of the perisciatic muscles in children. *Am J Roentgenol.* 2002;179 (5):1267–71. https://doi.org/10.2214/ajr.179.5.1791267

23. Bingöl-Koloğlu M, Yildiz RV, Alper B, et al. Necrotizing fasciitis in children: diagnostic and therapeutic aspects. *J Pediatr Surg*. 2007;42 (11):1892–1897. https://doi.org/10.1016/j.jpedsurg.2007.07.018

24. Pfeifle VA, Gros SJ, Holland-Cunz S, Kämpfen A. Necrotizing fasciitis in children due to minor lesions. *J Pediatr Surg Case Rep*. 2017;25:52–5. https://doi.org/10.1016/j.epsc.2017.08.005

25. Fugitt JB, Puckett ML, Quigley MM, Kerr SM. Necrotizing Fasciitis. *Radiographics*. 2004;24(5):1472–1476. https://doi.org/10.1148/rg.245035169

26. Loyer EM, DuBrow RA, David CL, Coan JD, Eftekhari F. Imaging of superficial soft-tissue infections: sonographic findings in cases of cellulitis and abscess. *AJR Am J Roentgenol*. 1996;166 (1):149–152. https://doi.org/10.2214/ajr.166.1.8571865

27. Marin JR, Dean AJ, Bilker WB, Panebianco NL, Brown NJ, Alpern ER. Emergency ultrasound-assisted examination of skin and soft tissue infections in the pediatric emergency department. *Acad Emerg Med*. 2013;20(6):545–553. https://doi.org/10.1111/acem.12148

28. Ramakrishnan K, Salinas RC, Agudelo Higuita NI. Skin and Soft Tissue Infections. *Am Fam Physician*. 2015;92(6):474–483.

# Imaging of Pediatric Traumatic and Non-traumatic Chest Emergencies

Katya Rozovsky, Martin Bunge, Hayley Moffatt, Jens Wrogemann, and Martin H. Reed

## Contents

K. Rozovsky (✉) · M. Bunge · H. Moffatt · J. Wrogemann
Section of Pediatric Radiology, Children's Hospital, Department of
Radiology, University of Manitoba, Winnipeg, MB, Canada
e-mail: krozovsky2@hsc.mb.ca; mbunge@hsc.mb.ca;
hmoffatt@hsc.mb.ca; JWrogemann@hsc.mb.ca

M. H. Reed
Section of Pediatric Radiology, Children's Hospital, Departments of
Radiology and of Pediatrics and Child Health, University of Manitoba,
Winnipeg, MB, Canada
e-mail: MReed@hsc.mb.ca

© Springer Nature Switzerland AG 2022
M. N. Patlas et al. (eds.), *Atlas of Emergency Imaging from Head-to-Toe*,
https://doi.org/10.1007/978-3-030-92111-8_49

### Abstract

Chest emergencies are common in children, and early diagnosis and treatment are important to prevent potential complications. While imaging is essential in the diagnosis of most pediatric chest emergencies, the interpretation can be challenging as the same entities may vary in different pediatric age groups and are often different from adults. The choice of imaging techniques is an important part of management. Frontal and lateral plain radiographs remain the main initial imaging tool, while fluoroscopy and ultrasound can play a role in the workup of some chest emergencies and their complications. Computed tomography should be reserved for cases that require the highest imaging resolution. This chapter discusses the imaging features of most common pediatric chest emergencies, including infection, air leaks, foreign body aspiration, trauma, congenital abnormalities, and neoplasms. Familiarity with different thoracic emergencies in children of different ages and their radiological presentation will allow a prompt diagnosis.

### Keywords

Children · Emergencies · Chest · Imaging · Pneumothorax · Foreign body · Trauma · Infection · Thoracic

## Introduction

Thoracic and respiratory emergencies are common in the pediatric population and can be caused by infection, foreign body aspiration, air leaks, trauma, and congenital abnormalities, or in rare cases, neoplasms. Prompt and correct diagnosis is essential as young patients are especially prone to acute respiratory decompensation due to the specific features of developing lungs and airways.

In comparison to adults, children's airways have a smaller diameter, are more compliant, and produce more mucous which can lead to rapid development of airflow disturbance. The collateral pathways of lung ventilation are underdeveloped until the age of 7–8 years. Closer relationship of the organs in the thoracic cavity may lead to more complex injuries in cases of trauma.

In imaging of thoracic emergencies, frontal and lateral chest radiographs are the examination of choice and frequently are the only imaging modality required to establish a correct diagnosis. Computed tomography (CT) provides superior anatomic resolution and allows better evaluation of lung parenchyma, airways, and mediastinum. Contrast-enhanced CT (CECT) helps to differentiate vascular structures, lymph nodes, and mediastinal findings. CT carries a potential risk of added ionizing radiation and should be reserved for challenging cases such as complicated lung infection, thoracic trauma, and masses. Thoracic ultrasound is a radiation-free tool which is indicated for better characterization of pleural effusion and empyema, among other potential uses. The advantages of ultrasound have been described in the diagnosis of pneumothorax, lung infections, and neonatal lung pathologies. However, in the emergency setting, the routine use of ultrasound for these indications is somewhat limited. MRI of the thorax is used for the characterization of extrapulmonary soft tissues, such as mediastinal masses, and is rarely used in pediatric emergencies [1, 2].

In this chapter, we present examples of frequent and less frequent pediatric chest emergencies and provide the reader with key facts for the interpretation of thoracic imaging of pediatric emergencies. The most common pediatric chest emergences by age are presented in Table 1.

## Normal Chest

The normal radiological appearance of the pediatric chest varies widely depending on age, mainly because of the changing size and shape of the thymus. The thymus is a normal lymphatic organ in the anterior mediastinum that is fully developed at birth and may increase in size during infancy. It gradually involutes after the age of 2 but can be prominent in size during the first 4–5 years of life [3].

The normal thymus has a smooth, curvilinear border, is homogeneous and slightly lucent, and should not cause mass effect on surrounding structures. The anterior reflections of the ribs can produce a wavy contour ("wave sign") (Fig. 1). The normal thymus may have different shapes such as a bilobed with convex margins, or triangular ("sail sign") (Fig. 2). In older children, the margins become more concave.

**Table 1** Most common pediatric chest emergences in relation to age

| Pathology Age | Congenital | Air leaks | Infection | FB | Trauma | Neoplasms |
|---|---|---|---|---|---|---|
| **Neonate** (0–1 month) | Yes Cardiac, vascular, airways anomalies, CLO, CPAM, CDH | Yes | Yes Bacterial pneumonia (Group B Streptococcus and gram-negative enteric bacteria) | Infrequent | Yes Be aware of NAT | Infrequent |
| **Infant** (1–23 month) | Yes Cardiac, vascular, airways anomalies, CLO, CPAM, CDH | Yes | Yes Viral and bacterial | Yes From 6 months of age | Yes Be aware of NAT | Yes Neuroblastoma Germ cell tumors |
| **Preschool** (2–5 years) | Infrequent | Infrequent | Yes 95% viral (especially RSV) Bacterial | Yes Peak up to 3.5 years | Yes | Yes Leukemia Lymphoma Neuroblastoma |
| **School age child** (5–12 years) | Infrequent | Infrequent | Yes Viral Bacterial (Streptococcus) Mycoplasma | Infrequent | Yes | Yes Leukemia Lymphoma |
| **Adolescent** (13–18 years) | Infrequent | Yes | Yes Viral Bacterial (Streptococcus) Mycoplasma | Infrequent | Yes | Yes Leukemia Lymphoma Germ cell tumors |

*FB* Foreign bodies; *CLO* Congenital lobar overinflation; *CPAM* Congenital pulmonary airway malformation; *CDH* Congenital diaphragmatic hernia; *NAT* non-accidental trauma; *RSV* Respiratory syncytial virus

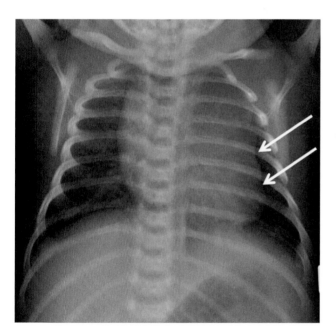

**Fig. 1** PA radiograph in a 2-week-old boy shows a normal thymus with a smooth undulating border – the "wave sign" (arrows). The normal thymus is homogeneous and slightly lucent. The thymus is located within the anterior mediastinum, which is best visualized on lateral view (not shown)

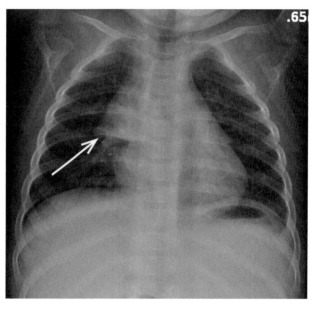

**Fig. 2** PA radiograph in a 10-month-old girl shows a normal thymus with a triangular shape – the "sail sign" (arrow). The normal thymus is lucent, and vessels can be seen through it

After 7–8 years, the thymus is difficult to visualize on radiographs but usually remains visible on CT and MRI [3–5].

The radiologists should routinely look for the presence of a thymic silhouette on each radiograph, especially in newborns and young children. Absence of the thymic silhouette on chest radiographs of a newborn or infant indicates thymic hypoplasia or aplasia, which may be seen in immunodeficiencies such as DiGeorge syndrome. The thymus can involute in response to stress, such as a severe disease or surgery.

After the resolution of stress, the thymus usually returns to normal size, a phenomenon known as thymic rebound.

Ectopic or accessory thymic tissue can be found in the neck and, in some cases, can be palpable. On ultrasound, the accessory or ectopic thymus is visualized as a homogeneous well-defined structure with multiple echogenic foci.

It is important to differentiate a normal thymus from upper mediastinal mass which can mimic thymus in young children. Unlike the normal thymus, a mediastinal mass usually produces mass effect displacing adjacent structures and may occupy different mediastinal compartments (Fig. 3) [3–5].

**Fig. 3** Nine-month-old boy admitted with increased work of breathing, cough, and desaturations. Neuroblastoma. PA (**a**) and lateral (**b**) radiographs demonstrate a space-occupying mass within the left posterior-upper mediastinum (asterisk), causing mass effect on the trachea with contralateral shift and narrowing (arrow)

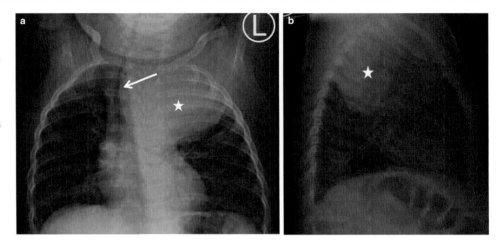

**Fig. 4** Seven-year-old boy choked on peanut. Cough. A left upper lobe bronchus foreign body (peanut) was retrieved on bronchoscopy. On the frontal inspiratory (**a**) view, the lung aeration is symmetric. The frontal expiratory view (**b**) reveals air trapping within the left hemithorax with increased lucency on the left, mediastinal shift to the right, and paradoxical movement of the ipsilateral hemidiaphragm during expiration (arrows)

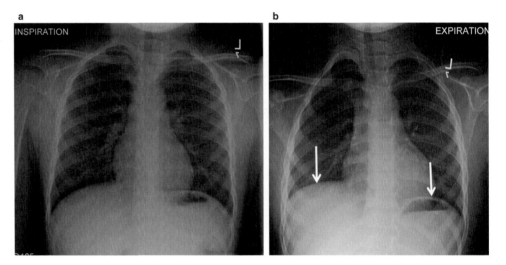

## Foreign Body Inhalation

### Epidemiology

Foreign body (FB) aspiration is a life-threatening emergency. The majority of cases occur between the ages of 1 and 3 years [6]. In many patients, the FB aspiration is unwitnessed. Most aspirated FBs are food particles. Nonorganic FBs are usually pins or small toy parts. The most common site of an inhaled FB is the thoracic inlet, followed by the carina and right bronchus [6, 7].

### Clinical Features

The classic clinical trial is a choking episode, followed by cough and wheezing. Other signs are dyspnea and asymmetrical air entry. An FB in the laryngeal inlet or trachea causes a barking cough and stridor [6, 8].

## Diagnostic Investigations

Frontal radiographs of the chest and neck should be used as the initial imaging approach and can help to identify radiopaque FBs, including their presence, their location, and their shape and density. However, up to 90% of inhaled FBs are not radiopaque, and initial radiographs are often normal [9].

The most common nondirect radiographic sign of an FB in the lower airways is unilateral lung hyperinflation caused by a "ball-valve" mechanism, which is best assessed on expiration views. With inspiration, the air bypasses the FB within the bronchus, and on expiration, the bronchus collapses against the FB, causing air trapping [7]. On expiration, the volume of the normal lung decreases, while the affected lung remains inflated and thus hyperlucent (Fig. 4) [10]. Fluoroscopy is an alternative dynamic approach to evaluate mediastinal shift and paradoxical movements of the ipsilateral hemidiaphragm during expiration [9]. Low-dose chest CT obtained during free-breathing without sedation and IV

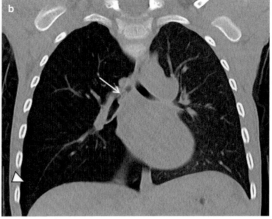

**Fig. 5** Twenty-month-old boy chocked on an orange peel. A foreign body was found within the right main bronchus: (**a**) The frontal chest radiograph showed an overinflated right lung. No radiopaque foreign body was identified. There is a small right pneumothorax (arrowhead). Coronal reconstruction of chest CT shows well-defined foreign body of soft tissue attenuation within the right main bronchus (arrow). The right lung is overinflated. There is a small right pneumothorax (arrowhead)

contrast is sensitive and specific for the diagnosis of FB aspiration, avoiding unnecessary bronchoscopy (Fig. 5). CT also helps to assess complications following removal of an FB: esophageal leak, mediastinitis/abscess, or injury of adjacent structures [11].

The management of children with suspected FB aspiration is determined by clinical symptoms and location of the FB. Unstable patients undergo emergency bronchoscopy.

## Summary

- Consider foreign body aspiration in a child with acute onset of cough, wheezing, and/or unilateral lung hyperinflation.
- Frontal neck and chest radiographs are the best initial examination.
- Expiratory view or fluoroscopy reveals the air trapping.
- Low-radiation dose chest CT can be used to assess foreign body location and to search for complications.

## Foreign Body Ingestion

### Epidemiology

The majority of ingested FBs are coins, crayons, small toys, pen caps, and batteries [9]. 80–90% FBs that reach the stomach can pass further through the digestive tract and do not require intervention. Esophageal impaction usually occurs at the upper esophageal sphincter, at the level of the distal aortic arch, or at the lower esophageal sphincter [9].

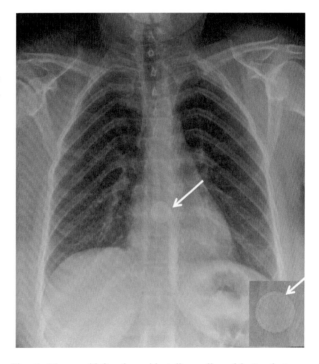

**Fig. 6** 14-year-old female accidentally swallowed button battery and presented with chest discomfort and drooling. Frontal chest radiograph demonstrates button battery within the distal esophagus. Notice the "double ring" which is characteristic for button batteries

### Clinical Features

Clinical presentation of an FB in the esophagus may include drooling, refusal to eat, choking, or gagging. Rarely the patients present with symptoms of airway obstruction because of compression of the trachea. Ingestion of batteries (Fig. 6) deserves particular attention because of the potential leakage of the toxic content that can rapidly lead to corrosive injury, mucosal burning, and perforation [7].

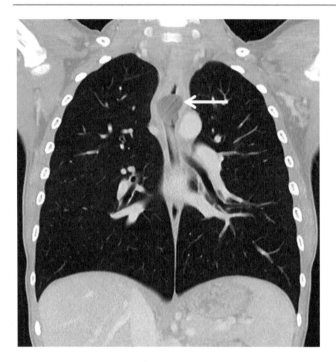

**Fig. 7** Five-year-old girl accidentally swallowed a heart-shaped wooden craft part. She presented with drooling, refusal to eat. The foreign body (FB) was not visualized on radiographs (not shown). The lung window coronal reconstructions from a subsequent chest CT demonstrate a heart-shaped foreign body of low density at the level of T4 (arrow)

## Diagnostic Investigations

The initial imaging includes frontal radiographs of the neck, chest, and abdomen. Fluoroscopy with water-soluble contrast or CT could be performed when the clinical history is clear and radiographs are negative (Fig. 7) [7, 9]. Important findings to report are the presence, number, and type of radiopaque FBs. Batteries, magnets, or sharp objects, and any signs of obstruction or perforation, require immediate attention. Contrast-enhanced CT(CECT) should be considered if there is a suspicion for complications (esophageal perforation, mediastinitis, or vascular injury). After endoscopic removal of the impacted battery, CECT or MRI of the mediastinum can be used to exclude aortic injury [12].

## Summary

- The initial imaging examination is frontal neck, chest, and abdomen radiographs.
- CT is helpful to assess for nonradiopaque FBs, and to search for complications.
- Batteries, magnets, or sharp objects should be immediately reported to the referring clinical team.

## Air-Leaks

### Pneumothorax

#### Epidemiology
The cause of pneumothorax can be often determined by clinical history, such as recent trauma, asthma exacerbation, or surgical intervention [13]. In the newborn period, prematurity, respiratory distress, and meconium aspiration are common reasons for a pneumothorax. It should be noted that in term infants about 25% of symptomatic pneumothorax occurs spontaneously [14]. Most cases of primary spontaneous pneumothorax occur in adolescents and often are caused by the rupture of an apical bleb [13, 15]. Children with connective tissue disorders such as Marfan, Ehlers-Danlos syndrome, or cystic fibrosis are at risk for pneumothorax [15, 16].

#### Clinical Features
Neonates and infants may present with sudden respiratory distress, unilaterally reduced breath sounds, and over-distention of the chest wall. Older children and teenagers present with chest pain and dyspnea. The severity of clinical presentation ranges from mild symptoms to severe respiratory failure. Tension pneumothorax is a respiratory emergency, presenting with tachycardia, hypotension, and cyanosis. It may cause rapid deterioration due to the compression of cardiovascular structures and should be immediately treated by needle thoracentesis [16].

#### Diagnostic Investigations
Chest radiography is the appropriate initial imaging modality. A PA upright radiograph shows the visceral pleural margin and absence of lung markings peripheral to it (Fig. 8). Neonates, infants, and critically ill patients are usually imaged in the supine position. Cross-table radiographs should be added to assess for an anteromedial air collection. Expiratory and decubitus views may aid in the diagnosis of equivocal cases [13, 14, 16, 17].

Signs of pneumothorax on a supine AP radiograph are the following:

- Radiolucency of the ipsilateral costophrenic angle – the "deep sulcus sign."
- Sharp ipsilateral border of the cardiothymic silhouette.
- Hyperlucency of the ipsilateral hemithorax.
- Sharply outlined medial superior pleural edge that may herniate across the midline and interface with the opposite lung.
- Collapsed ipsilateral lung.
- Downward shift of the ipsilateral hemidiaphragm [13, 17] (Fig. 9).

Tension pneumothorax is characterized by shift of the mediastinum toward the contralateral side with the deviation of the carina (Fig. 10). It is a life-threatening emergency and should be immediately communicated to the referring team [16]. Chest CT should be reserved for patients with chest trauma, or in complicated cases to exclude underlying pathology.

Bedside lung ultrasound has been described for diagnosis and follow-up of pneumothorax, especially in the setting of trauma or neonatal pneumothorax. The ultrasound diagnosis of pneumothorax is based on the following sonographic signs: the absence of lung sliding (rhythmic movement of parietal versus visceral pleura) and lung point (transition between normal lung sliding to no lung sliding) [2]. The routine use of lung ultrasound regarding pneumothorax remains controversial to our knowledge.

## Pneumomediastinum

### Epidemiology

Pneumomediastinum can be primary or secondary. Secondary causes include spontaneous (asthma, pneumonia, FB, vigorous cough, and croup), or traumatic/iatrogenic. In children <6 years, spontaneous pneumomediastinum often follows FB aspiration or asthma exacerbation [12, 13, 18].

### Clinical Features

Most patients present with retrosternal chest and neck pain, which increases with respirations, and dyspnea. Usually, pneumomediastinum is a self-limited condition. Traumatic pneumomediastinum and pneumomediastinum caused by an esophageal leak can become life-threatening.

### Diagnostic Investigations/Tips

The diagnosis is usually made on frontal and lateral radiographs of the chest by identifying lucent lines surrounding

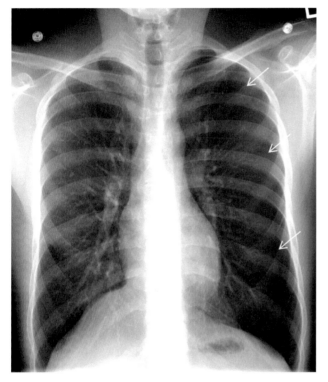

**Fig. 8** Fifteen-year-old boy with Marfan syndrome. Chest pain. Spontaneous left pneumothorax. PA upright chest radiograph demonstrates the visceral pleural edge as a thin white line within the left hemithorax (arrows), with the absence of lung markings peripheral to it

**Fig. 9** One-day-old term boy infant with respiratory distress. Bilateral pneumothorax: (**a**) Supine frontal view. There is a "deep sulcus sign" (arrows). There is a sharp border of the left cardiomediastinal silhouette (solid arrow). Note the visible pleural edge (arrowhead). (**b**) Cross-table lateral view. Retrosternal air (anterior pneumothorax) is present, displacing the anterior lung edge posteriorly (asterisk)

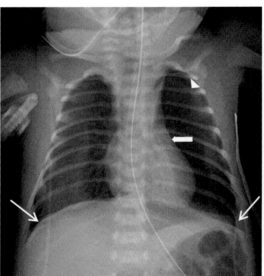
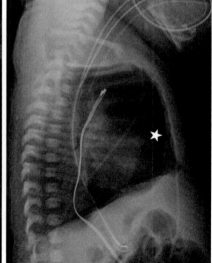

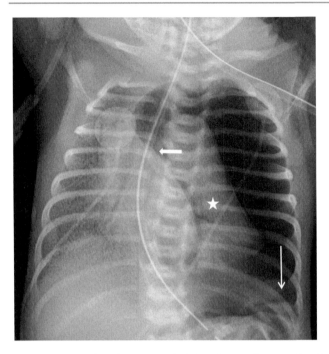

**Fig. 10** Term newborn boy presented with respiratory distress, reduced breath sounds on the left, and overdistention of the left chest wall. Tension pneumothorax. There is hyperlucency of the left hemithorax, with severe contralateral shift of the mediastinum (solid arrow), and downward shift of the left hemidiaphragm (arrow). The left lung is collapsed (asterisk)

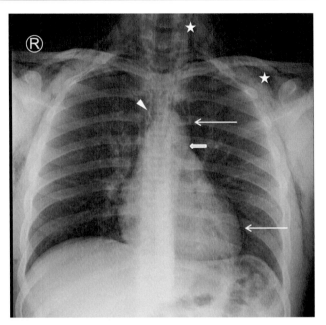

**Fig. 11** Eight-year-old girl presented with left neck and chest pain and cough. Spontaneous pneumomediastinum. Portable AP radiograph in a sitting position demonstrates areas of lucency within the soft tissues of the lower neck and chest wall (asterisks), streaky lucencies within the mediastinal fat (arrows), and a lucent line along the lateral aspect of the descending aorta (solid arrow), with air along the proximal airways – the "double-wall sign" (arrowhead)

the trachea, heart border, and aortic arch. Helpful radiographic signs include the following (Fig. 11):

- Streaks of air within the mediastinal fat.
- Air within the tissues of the lower neck.
- Linear band of air along the lateral aspect of the descending aorta.
- "Double-wall sign": air along the proximal airways
- "Continuous diaphragmatic sign": lucency that extends between the pericardium and diaphragm
- "Artery sign": air surrounding the pulmonary artery [19]
- "Thymic spinnaker sail sign" in neonates and infants: elevated medial and inferior surface of thymic lobes (Fig. 12) [13 19].

## Summary

- Cross-table or decubitus radiographs should be added routinely in neonates, infants, and critically ill children to assess for pneumothorax.
- Be aware that air leaks can occur at any age, including in newborns.
- Tension pneumothorax is a life-threatening emergency and should be immediately reported to the referring team.

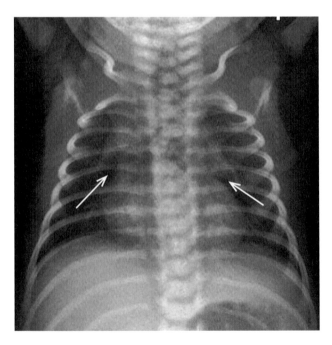

**Fig. 12** One-month-old boy with a history of prematurity. Respiratory distress. Pneumomediastinum in an infant. Portable AP supine chest radiograph demonstrates an elevated medial and inferior surface of thymic lobes – the "spinnaker sail sign" (arrows)

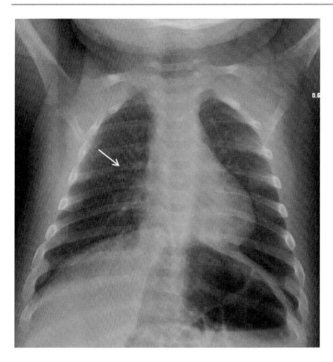

**Fig. 13** Three-month-old girl presented with fevers, cough, and wheezing. RSV bronchiolitis. PA radiograph demonstrates bilateral lung hyperinflation with flattening of the diaphragm. There is bilateral peribronchial thickening (arrow) within the perihilar areas

## Infection

Respiratory tract infections are a leading cause of illness in children [20, 21].

## Lower-Respiratory Tract Infection/Inflammation (LRTI)

LRTI usually has a viral etiology, frequently respiratory syncytial virus (RSV). Children present with fever, cough, and signs of respiratory distress such as wheezing. Routine imaging is not recommended. A radiograph is only indicated if the diagnosis is unclear. Radiographs may be normal or show hyperinflation, peribronchial thickening, and patchy atelectasis (Fig. 13) [22].

## Infections of Lung Parenchyma

### Pneumonia

#### Etiology
The causative agents vary by age (Table 1) [20, 23].

## Clinical Features

Typically, symptoms include fever and respiratory distress, such as increased work of breathing, cough, and tachypnea [24]. The presentation of a child with pneumonia is variable and sometimes nonspecific. For example, neonates may present with fussiness and difficulty in feeding, and older children may present with abdominal pain [20].

## Diagnostic Investigations

Frontal and lateral chest radiographs remain the first-line-imaging modality to confirm pneumonia when the clinical presentation is ambiguous, in cases of failure to respond to treatment, to help predict the infectious agent, and to assess for complications [20–24]. Radiographs are not usually indicated in the ambulatory settings as they cannot be used to distinguish between viral and bacterial infections, and have a limited role in the management of the disease [25, 26].

Pneumonia can be described by its radiographic pattern as lobar pneumonia or bronchopneumonia. Lobar pneumonia is a homogeneous air-space consolidation with air bronchograms predominantly involving one or multiple lobes. It is usually caused by a bacterial infection such as Group B Streptococcus, *Hemophilus influenza* type B, and *Klebsiella pneumoniae* [21, 25]. Imaging findings are similar to that of an adult, except for the radiologic entity known as round pneumonia. Round pneumonia occurs in children under the age of 8 years and is characterized by a well-defined, rounded opacity. It is attributed to poorly developed pores of Kohn (small passageways between adjacent alveoli) which result in a more compact area of consolidation (Fig. 14) [27]. Bronchopneumonia presents on radiographs as a diffuse peribronchial thickening and poorly defined air-space opacities or patchy areas of consolidation (Fig. 15). It is usually associated with gram-negative bacteria or *Staphylococcus aureus* [21, 25].

Chest CT is not warranted in the imaging of children with uncomplicated pneumonia and should be reserved to assess its complications. Lung ultrasound is an important tool to assess a pleural effusion but has limited value in the evaluation of lung parenchyma [24, 25].

## Complications of Pneumonia

**Empyema** is the presence of pus in the pleural space. Children with pneumonia may develop pleural effusions, but fewer than 5% of these effusions progress to empyema [24]. Ultrasound is effective in demonstrating septations, loculations, and debris within the effusion (Fig. 16).

**Necrotizing pneumonia** is an uncommon but serious acute complication of pneumonia, characterized by progressive pneumonic illness despite appropriate antibiotic therapy.

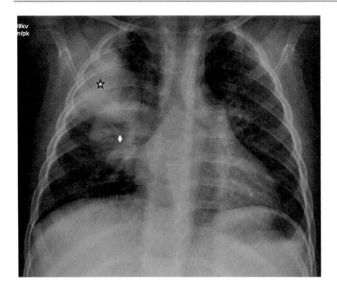

**Fig. 14** Sixteen-month-old girl presented with fevers, cough, and abnormal sounds on right lung auscultation. Round pneumonia. PA chest radiograph demonstrates two well-circumscribed rounded areas of opacification with air bronchograms, one located within the superior segment of the right lower lobe (diamond), and the second located within the posterior segment of the right upper lobe (asterisk). The opacifications completely resolved after 10 days of antibiotic treatment (not shown)

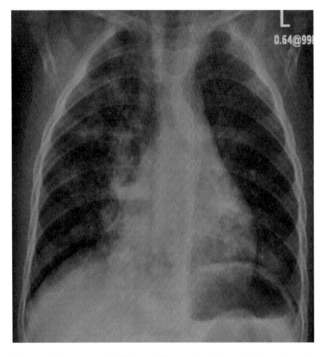

**Fig. 15** Eleven-month-old boy with cough and fever. Bilateral crepitation on auscultation. Bronchopneumonia. AP chest radiograph demonstrates bilateral patchy lung opacification and peribronchial thickening

CECT shows loss of normal pulmonary architecture, decreased parenchymal enhancement, and multiple thin-walled cavities [24].

**Lung abscess** – Destruction or necrosis of lung parenchyma that produces one or more large cavities (Fig. 17). CECT can be used to distinguish larger thick-walled cavities of the lung abscesses from smaller, multiple cavities of necrotizing pneumonia [23, 24].

**Pulmonary tuberculosis** rarely presents as an emergency. Primary tuberculosis in children most often presents with paratracheal and perihilar lymphadenopathy. In postprimary tuberculosis, which can occur in children as young as 8 years of age, consolidation can be typically seen in the apical and posterior segments [28].

**The coronavirus disease of 2019** (COVID-19) was declared a pandemic by the World Health Organization in March 2020. According to the recommendations of the American College of Radiology, in pediatric patients imaging is indicated if the child is not responding to outpatient treatment, requires hospitalization, or if hospital-acquired pneumonia is suspected. Chest radiograph is the first imaging choice. In children with mild respiratory symptoms, imaging findings could be absent, or may be present as patchy opacification with peripheral and lower lobe predominance (Fig. 18). CT should be considered in children with worsening clinical symptoms and/or lack of response to supportive therapy. On CT, the most common findings are bilateral peripheral ground-glass or confluent opacities with lower lobe predominance, as in affected adults. The radiological signs of COVID-19 are not pathognomonic [29, 30].

## Summary

- Chest radiographs are not indicated in ambulatory non-complicated cases.
- Imaging should be limited to ambiguous clinical presentation, failure to respond to treatment, and assessment of complications.
- IV contrast-enhanced chest CT should be reserved for complications of pneumonia.
- Chest ultrasound helps to characterize pleural effusion and to guide therapy.

## Pediatric Chest Trauma

### Epidemiology

Up to 8% of pediatric trauma cases involve injury to the chest [31]. Pulmonary contusions are the most common intrathoracic injuries. Rib fractures, pneumothorax, and hemothorax are less common than in adults, increasing in frequency with age. Injuries to the great vessels, heart, diaphragm, and central airway are uncommon in children [26–30].

**Fig. 16** One and a half-year-old girl with bacterial pneumonia, not improving with antibiotic treatment. Empyema: (**a**) PA chest radiograph demonstrates right upper and left lower lung consolidations (arrows). There is a large left pleural effusion, which appears loculated (asterisk). (**b**) Gray-scale ultrasound image of the left chest demonstrates large pockets of pleural fluid (asterisks) with echogenic debris, and thick septations (arrow)

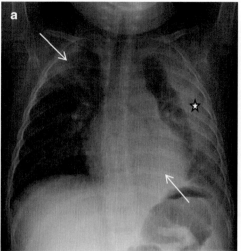
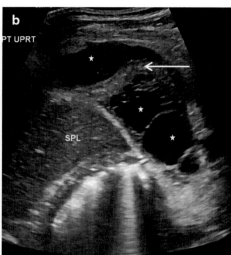

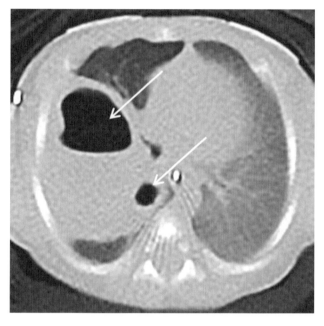

**Fig. 17** Three-month-old boy with a history of prematurity, recurrent aspirations, and previous right lung consolidation not responding to antibiotic treatment. Lung abscess. AP chest radiograph demonstrates large right lung opacification with well-defined central lucencies (not shown). Axial lung window chest CT image shows a large cavity with air-fluid level and a smaller cavity posterior to it (arrows)

## Clinical Features

The child with thoracic injury may present with chest pain, tachypnea, tachycardia, and hypotension. The plasticity of the rib cage and the smaller body mass of the child's chest wall results in the greater transmission of external forces to the lungs and mediastinum. Substantial injury to the lungs and mediastinum can occur with relatively minor damage to the chest wall [32]. Mediastinal structures in children are

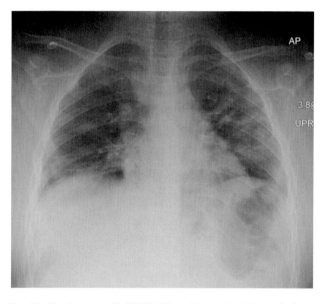

**Fig. 18** Twelve-year-old COVID-19-positive male with cough, fever, and shortness of breath. AP chest radiograph demonstrates bilateral patchy and confluent opacification with peripheral and lower lobe predominance

more mobile than in adults. Consequently, children are at greater risk for tension pneumothorax, airway compression, and caval compression and are at lower risk of mediastinal vascular injury [31–34].

All chest radiographs in children less than 3 years of age, whether or not there is a history of trauma, should be scrutinized for the presence of rib fractures [35]. Healing rib fractures, fractures at different stages of healing, and fractures inconsistent with the given mechanism of injury should prompt evaluation for nonaccidental injury. In contrast to high-energy chest trauma, where the increasing number of rib fractures is associated with increasing severity of the intrathoracic injury, rib fractures due to nonaccidental injury are often multiple, typically are the result of squeezing of the thorax, and are rarely associated with major intrathoracic injury (Fig. 19) [35, 36].

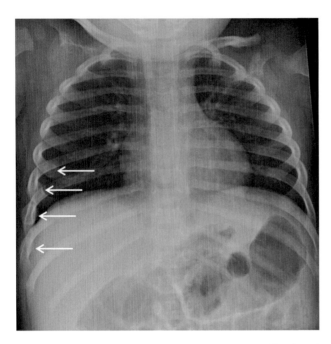

**Fig. 19** Twelve-month-old girl with irritability and suspicion for seizures. Healing rib fractures. Nonaccidental trauma (child abuse). AP supine chest radiograph demonstrates multiple healed fractures of the right sixth to ninth ribs (arrows)

## Diagnostic Investigations

Chest radiographs are the initial image modality, and the evaluation should include assessment of the following:

– Shape, width, and position of the mediastinum. The mediastinum will deviate toward atelectasis, and away from a large pneumothorax or hemothorax. The chest radiograph is abnormal in the majority of children with mediastinal great vessel injury (Fig. 20) [34, 36].
– Lungs for evidence of consolidation or atelectasis.
– Chest wall for fractures and deformities.
– The position of all internal catheters/support devices.

Chest CT should be used selectively in pediatric chest trauma to avoid unnecessary radiation [29]. CT is indicated for:

• Mediastinal widening on chest radiography
• High-energy trauma, including falls higher than 10 feet
• Penetrating trauma [31, 32]

CECT is necessary to assess potential injury to the great vessels. CT is more sensitive for rib fractures, pulmonary contusions, hemothorax, and pneumothorax than a chest radiograph, but when these injuries are not visible on a radiograph, they rarely require intervention [34].

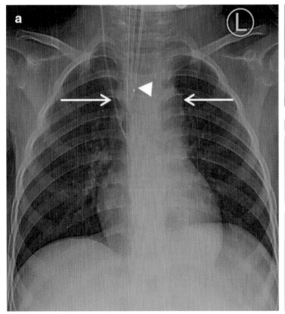
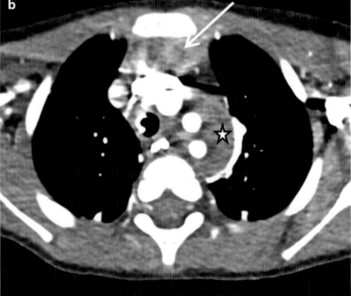

**Fig. 20** 3-year-old boy, penetrating injury to the left chest inlet. Mediastinal hematoma: (**a**) AP supine chest radiograph shows widening of the upper mediastinum (white arrows). The trachea and esophagus containing the endotracheal and nasogastric tubes are shifted to the right (arrowhead). (**b**) Axial CECT demonstrates left upper mediastinal hematoma (asterisk) surrounding the main blood vessels, and causing the rightward shift of the mediastinum. There is a normal thymic tissue within the anterior mediastinum (arrow)

Focused assessment with sonography for trauma (FAST) ultrasound is useful for the evaluation of pericardial and pleural fluid [36, 37].

## Summary

- The chest radiograph is the initial imaging modality in pediatric chest trauma.
- IV contrast-enhanced CT should be reserved for patients with substantial radiographic abnormalities, a high-energy mechanism of injury, or penetrating trauma.
- All chest radiographs in young children should be scrutinized for the presence of unexplained rib fractures, which may indicate a nonaccidental injury.

## Congenital Abnormalities

### Epidemiology

Congenital anomalies of lungs and airways are rare, and they do not always present with acute symptoms. In some cases, the diagnosis is known prenatally. In other cases, a young patient may present with acute respiratory distress of unknown etiology which requires prompt and accurate diagnosis. The most common congenital abnormalities include congenital diaphragmatic hernias, congenital lobar overinflation, and congenital pulmonary airway malformation (CPAM) or hybrid processes (CPAM and bronchopulmonary sequestration).

**Congenital diaphragmatic hernias** (CDH) are usually diagnosed prenatally (60–80%), but occasionally they present after birth, or later in childhood with respiratory distress.

### Diagnostic Investigations

Chest and abdominal radiographs are the initial images of choice. Chest findings will depend on the hernia contents. In the first radiographs after birth, herniated bowel may appear "solid," mimicking a mass until air enters the bowel. After the air enters the bowel, the hernia is easier to diagnose. Other radiographic findings are mediastinal shift away from the hernia, low lung volume due to lung hypoplasia, abnormal position of support devices, and paucity of intra-abdominal bowel gas (Fig. 21). Chest ultrasound is useful for the assessment of solid herniated structures and can help to identify the bowel loops within the thoracic cavity [38]. CT is not indicated routinely.

**Congenital lobar overinflation** (CLO) (congenital lobar emphysema or infantile lobar emphysema) is a rare abnormality caused by the weakening of the bronchial wall, resulting in bronchial collapse, or obstruction with unilateral air trapping and progressive overexpansion of a pulmonary lobe. CLO presents with respiratory distress, cyanosis, and progressive respiratory failure [39, 40].

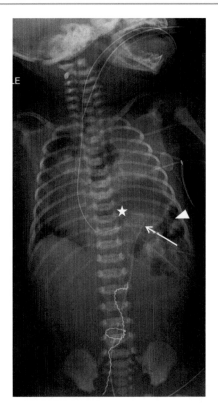

**Fig. 21** Newborn with severe respiratory distress, no prenatal assessment. Left diaphragmatic hernia. AP radiograph of the chest and abdomen demonstrates the right mediastinal shift. There is opacification of the left hemithorax, with lucent areas (arrowhead) representing bowel. There is a gasless abdomen. The stomach (indicated by the tip of the nasogastric tube) is projected over the left lower thorax (asterisk). Note the abnormal position of the umbilical venous central line (arrow)

### Diagnostic Investigations

On the first days of life, radiographs may show a nonspecific mass-like opacity due to the trapped fetal lung fluid. Progressively, the affected area becomes air-filled, and then hyperinflated and lucent, causing mass effect on normal lung and mediastinum (Fig. 22) [34]. The presence of vascular markings within the affected hemithorax helps to differentiate CLO from tension pneumothorax.

**Congenital pulmonary airway malformation** (CPAM) – A heterogeneous group of cystic and noncystic lung abnormalities resulting from airway maldevelopment [41].

### Diagnostic Investigations

A multicystic lung mass can contain variable large, small, or microcytic cavities. Microcystic type or fluid-filled larger cysts may mimic a solid mass on initial images (Fig. 23). Pneumothorax and mass effect may occur and cause acute respiratory symptoms. If the etiology remains uncertain, CECT should be obtained. In the case of a hybrid process, intravenous contrast will help to detect the systemic feeding vessel of the malformation [39, 42].

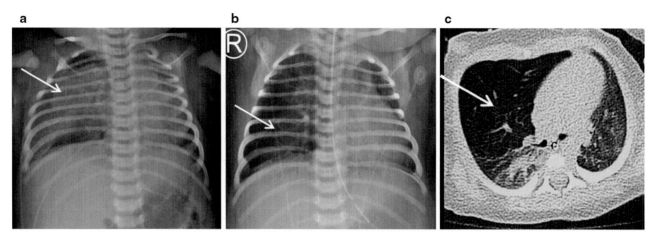

**Fig. 22** Newborn with respiratory distress. Congenital lobar over-inflation: (**a**) The first day of life. AP radiograph shows nonspecific opacification of the right upper and middle lung (arrow), and mild left shift of the mediastinum. (**b**) The third day of life. Overinflation of the right hemothorax (arrow) with the disappearance of the opacification. (**c**) Axial plane of chest CT confirms the overinflation of the right middle lobe (arrow) with small vascular markings

**Fig. 23** Newborn with antenatal diagnosis of CPAM. (**a**) AP radiograph obtained immediately after birth demonstrates opacification of the left lower lobe. (**b**) Axial plane of chest CT obtained at the age of 1 month shows multicystic lung mass contains small air-filled cavities. There is a mild rightward shift of the mediastinum

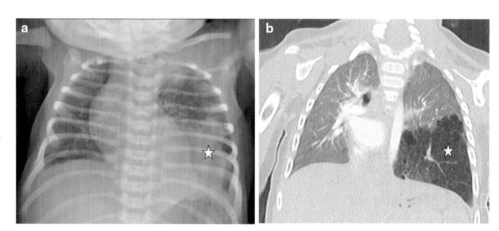

## Summary

- Congenital abnormalities should be considered in newborns and infants with respiratory distress and abnormal chest radiographs.
- On radiographs obtained shortly after birth, congenital diaphragmatic hernia, congenital lobar emphysema, and congenital pulmonary airway malformation may present as nonspecific lung opacification, which becomes lucent on follow-up radiographs.

## Thoracic Pediatric Neoplasms Presenting Emergently

### Mediastinal Masses

#### Epidemiology and Clinical Features

Mediastinal masses may present acutely with compression of the trachea or the superior vena cava. Most common mediastinal masses in children include the following:

**Lymphoma** (Hodgkin and non-Hodgkin) is the most common cause of an anterior mediastinal mass in children.

**Neurogenic tumors** cause 90% of posterior mediastinal masses.

**Germ cell tumors (GCT)** account for 6–18% of mediastinal masses. The age peaks for GCT are around 2 years and adolescents [43].

#### Diagnostic Investigations

On radiographs, most symptomatic mediastinal masses present with increased density and widening or distortion of the mediastinal silhouette. It is important to look for displacement or narrowing of the trachea. Lymphoma presents with infiltration of the thymus and mediastinal lymphadenopathy. There may be an associated pleural effusion. Neurogenic tumors such as neuroblastoma present as a paravertebral mass (Fig. 24). GCTs may contain calcifications and fat. CECT is indicated for better differentiation of the mass and assessment of airways, lung, and abdominal involvement. MRI of the spine should be obtained in neuroblastoma, to assess the intraspinal involvement [43, 44].

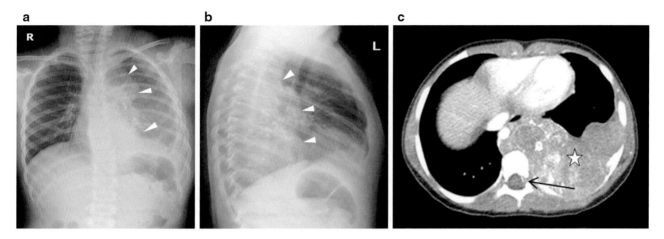

**Fig. 24** Mediastinal neuroblastoma. Three and a half-year old female presented with shortness of breath and thoracic scoliosis. PA (**a**) and lateral (**b**) chest radiographs demonstrate the widening of the left mediastinum, and opacification of the left posterior hemithorax, with lobulated borders (arrowheads). Axial plain of CECT (**c**) shows large partially enhancing and calcified well-defined mass (asterisk) within the left perivertebral area and posterior mediastinum, with mass effect on the thoracic aorta. The mass is extending into one of the left neurofiramen (arrow)

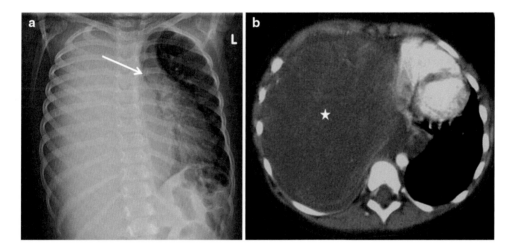

**Fig. 25** Pleuropulmonary blastoma. Five-year-old boy presented with shortness of breath, desaturations, and no fever: (**a**) PA chest radiograph shows dense opacification of the right hemithorax with mass effect on the mediastinum, leftward shift of the trachea (arrow), and opacification of the right diaphragm. (**b**) Axial plain of CECT confirmed the presence of large partially enhancing hypodense mass (asterisk) occupying the right hemithorax, with marked mass effect on the mediastinum

## Pulmonary Neoplasms

### Epidemiology

Pulmonary neoplasms are rare in children and rarely present as an emergency. The majority are metastatic, usually from Wilm's tumor or sarcoma. The most common primary malignancies in children are pleuropulmonaryblastoma and carcinoid tumor [45, 46].

### Clinical Features

Lung neoplasm usually presents with nonspecific symptoms such as cough, chest pain, shortness of breath, recurrent pneumonia, or wheezing.

**Pleuropulmonaryblastoma (PPB)** – rare malignant mesenchymal neoplasm of lung and pleura. There are three types:

Type 1 – cystic tumors, Type 2 – cystic and solid tumor, and Type 3 – solid tumors. The diagnosis of cystic PPB is challenging as it may mimic developmental lung processes.

### Diagnostic Investigations

PPB may present on plain radiographs as a solid mass, spontaneous pneumothorax (up to 30%), pleural effusion (up to 36%), or with air-filled lung cysts [47].

The Type 1 tumors are difficult to distinguish from CPAM. The Type 3 tumors may present as a large opacification of the hemithorax and often cause a mediastinal shift (Fig. 25). Chest ultrasound is recommended to differentiate the mass from a large region of consolidation or pleural effusion. CECT is required to better delineate and diagnose these tumors [46–48].

## Summary

- Pediatric chest masses are rare but should be considered in the differential diagnosis in cases of thoracic opacification, narrowing of airways, or mediastinal shift.
- Chest ultrasound helps to differentiate a chest mass from a large pleural effusion.
- IV contrast-enhanced CT should be obtained for better delineation of the mass extension and to assess for metastases.

## References

1. Hart A, Lee EY. Pediatric chest disorders: practical imaging approach to diagnosis. In: Hodler J, Kubik-Huch RA, von Schulthess GK, editors. Diseases of the chest, breast, heart and vessels 2019–2022: diagnostic and interventional imaging. Cham: Springer; 2019. p. 107–25.
2. Rea G, Sperandeo M, Di Serafino M, Vallone G, Tomà P. Neonatal and pediatric thoracic ultrasonography. J Ultrasound. 2019;22(2):121–30.
3. Menashe SJ, Iyer RS, Parisi MT, Otto RK, Stanescu AL. Pediatric chest radiographs: common and less common errors. AJR Am J Roentgenol. 2016;207(4):903–11.
4. Manchanda S, Bhalla AS, Jana M, Gupta AK. Imaging of the pediatric thymus: Clinicoradiologic approach. World J Clin Pediatr. 2017;6(1):10–23.
5. Winant AJ, Cho J, Alyafei TS, Lee EY. Pediatric thoracic anatomic variants: what radiologists need to know. Radiol Clin N Am. 2017;55(4):677–91.
6. Sahin A, Meteroglu F, Eren S, Celik Y. Inhalation of foreign bodies in children: experience of 22 years. J Trauma Acute Care Surg. 2013;74(2):658–63.
7. Pugmire BS, Lim R, Avery LL. Review of ingested and aspirated foreign bodies in children and their clinical significance for radiologists. Radiographics. 2015;35(5):1528–38.
8. Johnson K, Linnaus M, Notrica D. Airway foreign bodies in pediatric patients: anatomic location of foreign body affects complications and outcomes. Pediatr Surg Int. 2017;33(1):59–64.
9. Laya BF, Restrepo R, Lee EY. Practical imaging evaluation of foreign bodies in children: an update. Radiol Clin N Am. 2017;55(4):845–67.
10. Brown JC, Chapman T, Klein EJ, Chisholm SL, Phillips GS, Osincup D, Sakchalathorn P, Bittner R. The utility of adding expiratory or decubitus chest radiographs to the radiographic evaluation of suspected pediatric airway foreign bodies. Ann Emerg Med. 2013;61(1):19–26.
11. Ahmed OG, Guillerman RP, Giannoni CM. Protocol incorporating airway CT decreases negative bronchoscopy rates for suspected foreign bodies in pediatric patients. Int J Pediatr Otorhinolaryngol. 2018;109:133–7.
12. Kramer RE, Lerner DG, Lin T, et al. Management of ingested foreign bodies in children: a clinical report of the NASPGHAN endoscopy committee. J Pediatr Gastroenterol Nutr. 2015;60(4):562–74.
13. Johnson NN, Toledo A, Endom EE. Pneumothorax, pneumomediastinum, and pulmonary embolism. Pediatr Clin N Am. 2010;57(6):1357–83.
14. Duong HH, Mirea L, Shah PS, Yang J, Lee SK, Sankaran K. Pneumothorax in neonates: trends, predictors and outcomes. J Neonatal Perinatal Med. 2014;7(1):29–38.
15. Boone PM, Scott RM, Marciniak SJ, Henske EP, Raby BA. The genetics of pneumothorax. Am J Respir Crit Care Med. 2019;199(11):1344–57.
16. Robinson PD, Cooper P, Ranganathan SC. Evidence-based management of paediatric primary spontaneous pneumothorax. Paediatr Respir Rev. 2009;10(3):110–7.
17. Alford BA, McIlhenny J. An approach to the asymmetric neonatal chest radiograph. Radiol Clin N Am. 1999;37(6):1079–92.
18. Wong KS, Wu HM, Lai SH, Chiu CY. Spontaneous pneumomediastinum: analysis of 87 pediatric patients. Pediatr Emerg Care. 2013;29(9):988–91.
19. Zylak CM, Standen JR, Barnes GR, Zylak CJ. Pneumomediastinum revisited [published correction appears in Radiographics 2001;21(6):1616]. Radiographics. 2000;20(4):1043–57.
20. Donnelly LF. Fundamentals of pediatric radiology. Philadelphia: Saunders; 2001. p. 5–54.
21. World Health Organization. Pneumonia. [homepage on the internet]. 2019. Available from: https://www.who.int/news-room/fact-sheets/detail/pneumonia
22. Subcommittee on Diagnosis and Management of Bronchiolitis. Diagnosis and management of bronchiolitis. Pediatrics. 2006;118(4):1774–93.
23. Ostapchuk M, Roberts DM. Haddy r. community-acquired pneumonia in infants and children. Am Fam Phys. 2004;70(5):899–908. Available from https://www.aafp.org/afp/2004/0901/p899.html
24. Choy G, Yager PH, Noviski N, Westra SJ. Imaging of chest infections in children. In: Medina LS, Applegate KE, Blackmore CC, editors. Evidence-based imaging in pediatrics. New York: Springer Science + Business Meida; 2010. p. 401–17.
25. O'Grady KF, Torzillo PJ, Fawley K, Chang AB. The radiological diagnosis of pneumonia in children. Pneumonia. 2014;5:38–51.
26. Swingler GH. Radiologic differentiation between bacterial and viral lower respiratory infection in children: a systematic literature review. Clin Pediatr (Phila). 2000;39(11):627–33.
27. Kim YW, Donnelly LF. Round pneumonia: imaging findings in a large series of children. Pediatr Radiol. 2007;37:1235–40.
28. Concepcion NDP, Laya BF, Andronikou S, Daltro PAN, Sanchez MO, Uy JAU, et al. Standardized radiographic interpretation of thoracic tuberculosis in children. Pediatr Radiol. 2017;47:1237–48.
29. Foust AM, Phillips GS, Chu WC, Daltro P, Das KM, Garcia-Peña P, Kilborn T, Winant AJ, Lee EY. International expert consensus statement on chest imaging in pediatric COVID-19 patient management: imaging findings, imaging study reporting and imaging study recommendations. Radiol Cardiothorac Imaging. 2020;2(2):e200214. https://doi.org/10.1148/ryct.2020200214. PMCID: PMC7233446.
30. Shelmerdine SC, Lovrenski J, Caro-Domínguez P, Toso S, Collaborators of the European Society of Paediatric Radiology Cardiothoracic Imaging Taskforce. Coronavirus disease 2019 (COVID-19) in children: a systematic review of imaging findings [published online ahead of print, 2020 Jun 18]. Pediatr Radiol. 2020;50(9):1217–1230.
31. Herrera P, Langer JC. Thoracic trauma in children. In: Mikrogianakis A, Valani R, Cheng A, editors. The Hospital for sick children manual of pediatric trauma. Lippincott, Williams and Wilkins; 2008. Accessed 22 May 2020.
32. Pediatric trauma. In: ATLS advanced trauma life support student course manual, 10th edn. The Committee on Trauma, American College of Surgeons, Chicago; 2018. Accessed 7 May 2020.
33. Piccolo CL, Ianniello S, Trinci M, et al. Diagnostic imaging in pediatric thoracic trauma. Radiol Med. 2017;122:850–65.
34. Holscher CM, Faulk LW, Moore EE, et al. Chest computed tomography imaging for blunt pediatric trauma: not worth the radiation risk. J Surg Res. 2013;184:352–7.
35. Weirich Paine C, Fakeye O, Christian CW, Wood JN. Prevalence of abuse among young children with rib fractures. Pediatr Emerg Care. 2019;35(2):96–103.

36. Pearson EG, Fitzgerald CA, Santore MT. Pediatric thoracic trauma: current trends. Semin Pediatr Surg. 2017;26:36–42.

37. Moore MA, Wallace C, Westra SJ. The imaging of paediatric thoracic trauma. Pedatr Radiol. 2009;39:485–96.

38. Taylor GA, Atalabi OM, Estroff JA. Imaging of congenital diaphragmatic hernias. Pediatr Radiol. 2009;39(1):1–16.

39. Demir OF, Hangul M, Kose M. Congenital lobar emphysema: diagnosis and treatment options. Int J Chron Obstruct Pulmon Dis. 2019;14:921–8.

40. Cataneo DC, Rodrigues OR, Hasimoto EN, Schmidt AF Jr, Cataneo AJ. Congenital lobar emphysema: 30-year case series in two university hospitals. J Bras Pneumol. 2013;39(4):418–26.

41. Dillman JR, Sanchez R, Ladino-Torres MF, Yarram SG, Strouse PJ, Lucaya J. Expanding upon the unilateral hyperlucent hemithorax in children. Radiographics. 2011;31(3):723–41.

42. Sood S, Rissmiller J, Hryhorczuk A. Pediatric chest: a review of the must-know diagnoses. Appl Radiol. 2018. www.appliedradiology.com

43. Jaggers J, Balsara K. Mediastinal masses in children. Semin Thorac Cardiovasc Surg. 2004;16(3):201–8.

44. McCarville MB. Malignant pulmonary and mediastinal tumors in children: differential diagnoses. Cancer Imaging. 2010;10 Spec no A (1A):S35–41.

45. Cohen MC, Kaschula RO. Primary pulmonary tumors in childhood: a review of 31 years' experience and the literature. Pediatr Pulmonol. 1992;14:222–32.

46. Dishop MK, Kuruvilla S. Primary and metastatic lung tumors in the pediatric population: a review and 25-year experience at a large children's hospital. Arch Pathol Lab Med. 2008;132(7):1079–103.

47. Messinger YH, Stewart DR, Priest JR, et al. Pleuropulmonaryblastoma: a report on 350 central pathology-confirmed pleuropulmonaryblastoma cases by the International Pleuropulmonary Blastoma registry. Cancer. 2015;121(2):276–85.

48. Lichtenberger JP 3rd, Biko DM, Carter BW, Pavio MA, Huppmann AR, Chung EM. Primary lung tumors in children: radiologic-pathologic correlation from the radiologic pathology archives. Radiographics. 2018;38(7):2151–72.

# Imaging of Pediatric Traumatic and Nontraumatic Abdominal and Pelvic Emergencies

**50**

Margherita Trinci, Marco Di Maurizio, Enrica Rossi, Ginevra Danti, and Vittorio Miele

## Contents

### Abstract

Abdominal pain is one of the most frequent causes of emergency department (ED) visits in pediatric patients. The role of diagnostic imaging is to help the pediatric emergency physician and pediatric surgeon to clarify the cause of pain and whether it needs medical or surgical treatment. The differential diagnosis includes many entities, with often overlapping presentations. Therefore, it is essential to know the diagnostic findings which can be obtained with current techniques. Ultrasound (US) is presently the modality of choice for the initial evaluation of acute abdominal pain due to its diagnostic value and lack of ionizing radiation exposure. In nontraumatic abdominal and pelvic acute pain, computed tomography (CT) must be reserved for special cases only and magnetic resonance imaging (MRI) is a possible alternative to CT. However, the cost and availability of MRI limit its utilization. Abdominal trauma is an additional common cause for ED imaging in children. CT is the reference standard method for victims of high-energy trauma. In minor trauma, mainly indirect low-energy trauma, ultrasound is also used. It is currently possible to improve the diagnostic accuracy of ultrasound with the use of IV contrast-enhanced ultrasound (CEUS). MRI is a method for patients who have had high-energy trauma in some

M. Trinci
Department of Emergency Radiology, Azienda Ospedaliera S. Camillo-Forlanini, Rome, Italy

M. Di Maurizio · E. Rossi
Department of Radiology, Azienda Ospedaliero Universitaria Meyer, Florence, Italy
e-mail: marco.dimaurizio@meyer.it

G. Danti · V. Miele (✉)
Department of Radiology, Azienda Ospedaliero Universitaria Careggi, Florence, Italy
e-mail: vmiele@sirm.org

© Springer Nature Switzerland AG 2022
M. N. Patlas et al. (eds.), *Atlas of Emergency Imaging from Head-to-Toe*,
https://doi.org/10.1007/978-3-030-92111-8_50

selected, specific conditions such as pancreatic trauma and the follow-up of traumatic injuries.

**Keywords**

Emergency radiology · Pediatric acute abdomen · Pediatric trauma · Computed tomography · Ultrasound · Contrast-enhanced ultrasound · Magnetic resonance imaging

## Introduction

Since infants cannot localize pain and preschool children are often imprecise in their responses, accurate clinical information and physical examination of children is often a challenge for the pediatrician and pediatric surgeon. In children, especially under 3 years of age, periumbilical pain is the most common presentation regardless of the underlying etiology, and it does not contribute to a specific diagnosis. When children refer to pain in the abdominal or pelvic quadrants, a working diagnosis can be related to one or more pathologies (Drawing 1). Pediatric abdominal pain manifests differently in the various age groups and, therefore, three groups of patients are classically distinguished. The first group is newborns. Neonatal acute abdominal entities will not be covered in this chapter. The second group includes 2- to 6-year-old children. The third group is children 6 year old and older. It is estimated that within the first 15 years of life, approximately 15% of children are referred to the pediatrician for abdominal/pelvic pain. In this population, only about one-third will need hospital treatment: The cause of the pain is often benign, and frequently is gaseous colic at all ages. The role of imaging is to help distinguish the causes of medical and surgical pain by triaging patients toward conservative or nonconservative treatment. Ultrasound (US) is undoubtedly now the initial imaging test for evaluating nontraumatic abdominal and pelvic pain in the pediatric patient.

In this chapter, we will discuss the most frequent medical and surgical causes of abdominal and pelvic pain in children and adolescents, and their differential diagnoses and complications. The topics covered will include intussusception, Henoch-Schonlein purpura, appendicitis, and its main differential diagnoses including terminal ileitis and Meckel's diverticulum, ovarian torsion, hematocolpos/hematometra, pyelonephritis, and renal abscess. Finally, the chapter will conclude with a discussion on pediatric trauma.

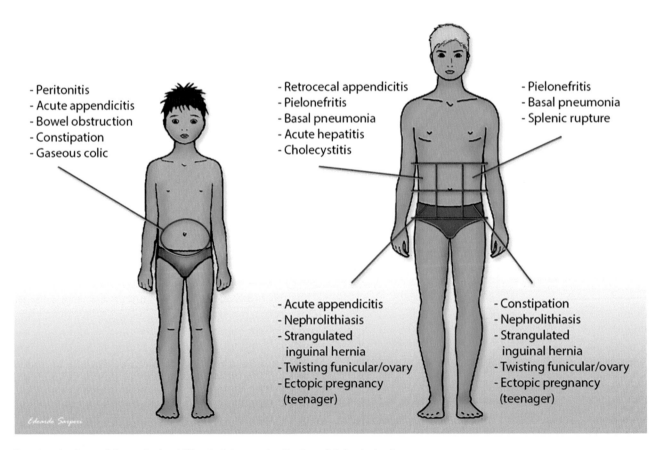

- Peritonitis
- Acute appendicitis
- Bowel obstruction
- Constipation
- Gaseous colic

- Retrocecal appendicitis
- Pielonefritis
- Basal pneumonia
- Acute hepatitis
- Cholecystitis

- Pielonefritis
- Basal pneumonia
- Splenic rupture

- Acute appendicitis
- Nephrolithiasis
- Strangulated inguinal hernia
- Twisting funicular/ovary
- Ectopic pregnancy (teenager)

- Constipation
- Nephrolithiasis
- Strangulated inguinal hernia
- Twisting funicular/ovary
- Ectopic pregnancy (teenager)

**Drawing 1.** Acute abdomen in the child and adolescent: localization of abdominal pain

## Acute Nontraumatic Abdominal Emergencies

In children between 2 and 6 years old, the main surgical causes of abdominal pain include intussusception, acute appendicitis, and frequently intestinal volvulus, while less common is Henoch-Schonlein purpura [1].

## Intussusception

Intussusception is one of the main causes of the acute abdomen after the first 3 months of life up to 3 years, with a seasonal incidence (winter and spring) related to the main viral infections [2]. Intussusception is an intestinal hernia caused by the penetration of a proximal portion of the intestine into an adjacent distal segment (colic, ileal, or both), with an antegrade telescopic mechanism. The most common location is ileocecal, where the starting point of the invaginated segment is represented by the ileocecal valve, and it is often related to mesenteric lymphoid hyperplasia due to an infection. The forms most frequently associated with an acute abdomen are the ileo-colic and ileo-ileocolic ones, which appear as a rounded mass in the right abdomen, crossing the midline in the epigastrium or behind the umbilicus. The ileoileal form is less common in children (1.7–17% of all types), but given its limited clinical relevance and frequent spontaneous resolution, it is often misdiagnosed or mistaken for gastroenteritis. Colocolic intussusceptions are rare in the pediatric population, often associated with a preexisting colonic pathologic process which acts as a leading point [3, 4]. In children older than three years, it is often possible to identify a leading point, which can be appendicitis, Meckel's diverticulum, polyp, hemangioma, or conditions which cause hypertrophy of the Peyer patches

(including Henoch-Schönlein purpura, lymphoma, and rotavirus infection) [4, 5].

Ultrasound is considered the technique of choice for diagnosis, due to its high sensitivity (97.9%) and specificity (97.8%). Imaging findings on US include the *target sign*, a single hypoechoic ring with a hyperechoic center, and the *pseudokidney* sign which is the superimposition of hypo- and hyperechoic areas representing the edematous walls of the intussusceptum and layers of compressed mucosa (Fig. 1) [6, 7]. The role of ultrasound does not end in the diagnostic phase, but remains central also in the therapeutic one. There are different techniques to reduce the invagination with compressed air technique under fluoroscopic guidance most commonly, or under ultrasound guidance (following the retrograde progression of the air or water introduced by the rectal catheter, until the resolution of the ileocolic obstruction) [8, 9]. With color Doppler, diminished or absent vascularity increases the probability of intestinal necrosis and the failure rate of reduction.

Both the ileoileal and ileocolic intussusception are complications associated with Henoch-Schonlein purpura (HPS), a systemic small-vessel vasculitis in childhood (Fig. 2) [10]. Gastrointestinal sequelae can include bowel infarction, perforation, obstruction, and intussusception (uncommon in adults and children under the age of 3 years). The sites of intussusception with HSP are most frequently ileoileal (51%), followed by ileocolic (39%), and rarely jejunojejuneal and colocolic. [11, 12].

## Malrotation and Volvulus

Intestinal malrotation occurs because of failure of the normal rotation and fixation of the bowel, determining the etiopathogenetic substrate for an acute intestinal obstruction,

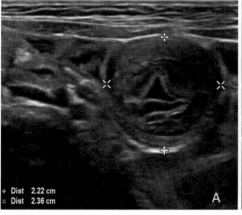
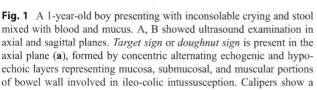
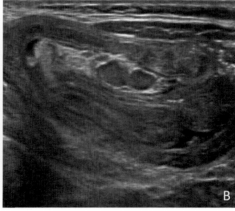

**Fig. 1** A 1-year-old boy presenting with inconsolable crying and stool mixed with blood and mucus. A, B showed ultrasound examination in axial and sagittal planes. *Target sign* or *doughnut sign* is present in the axial plane (**a**), formed by concentric alternating echogenic and hypoechoic layers representing mucosa, submucosal, and muscular portions of bowel wall involved in ileo-colic intussusception. Calipers show a

large diameter of the intussusception mass (2.3 cm) and the fat core–to-wall index >1 (this is calculated as the ratio of the fat core diameter to the wall thickness of involved bowel). B. *Pseudokidney sign* is present in the sagittal plane (**b**), results from the entrance of the intussuscepted bowel loop, fat, and several lymph nodes into the intussuscipiens

**Fig. 2** A 9-year-old boy with melena and severe abdominal pain, associated with bilateral knee pain and reddish splotches on his buttocks. Ultrasound (US) demonstrates bowel abnormalities caused by Henoch-Schonlein purpura. There is concentric bowel wall thickening with ill-defined layers (**a**, axial plane) of echogenic mucosa, hypoechoic submucosa, and an echogenic muscular layer (**b**, sagittal plane). Color Doppler US (**c, d**, axial, and sagittal plane) shows diffuse peripheral hyperemia and typical mesenteric vascular engorgement related to the underlying inflammatory process. In HSP, these signs can be seen as multifocal findings with skip areas, in contrast to other types of vasculitis. No US signs of HSP complications, such as intussusception or ascites, were seen in this patient

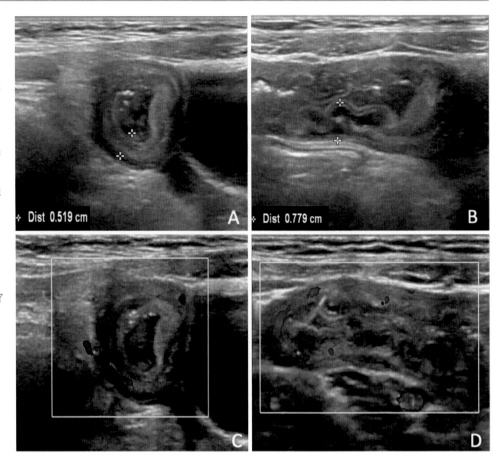

particularly related to Ladd's band and volvulus. Symptomatic malrotation is a diagnosis usually made in the newborn and young infant, and up to 90% of cases occur within the first year of life. Small bowel volvulus can lead to ischemia of the midgut from superior mesenteric artery (SMA) occlusion and irreversible intestinal necrosis. Midgut volvulus is the most marked potential result of intestinal malrotation, which is potentially life threatening, and any duodenal obstruction presenting at birth must be considered as a midgut volvulus until proved otherwise. In an infant with bilious vomiting, a fluoroscopic examination with contrast is the image of choice to assess the position of the ligament of Treitz. Contrast examination can be performed with air or diluted water-soluble nonionic contrast agent, in particular when there is the risk of potential perforation. In more recent years, US has been used for the assessment of the anatomic position reversed between the superior mesenteric vein (SMV) and the superior mesenteric artery (SMA), as a probable sign of malrotation, and the presence of a *whirlpool sign* (WS) (wrapping of the SMV and the mesentery around the SMA), as a sign of midgut volvulus [13, 14].

Colonic volvulus and in particular sigmoid volvulus is very uncommon in children, and is usually associated with a long-standing history of constipation or pseudo-obstruction [14–15] (Fig. 3) .

## Acute Appendicitis

Acute appendicitis is the most common abdominal surgical emergency in children, with an incidence that reaches a peak during adolescence (29.2/10,000 to 19.3/10,000 in children aged 10–14 years). It is less frequent in preschool children (2–9%), and it is rare in infants [16]. Despite its high incidence, the diagnosis of acute appendicitis often presents a challenge, especially in children under 5 years old in whom the symptoms are often atypical, with consequent delay in diagnosis and increase in complications.

Ultrasound (US) is currently the first-line modality in the diagnosis of acute appendicitis in children of all ages, with sensitivity and specificity values respectively between 78–99 and 83–99%, and a diagnostic accuracy of 70–99% [17–19]. Ultrasound signs of acute appendicitis include a tubular structure with no compressibility, lack of peristalsis, transverse diameter equal to or greater than 6 mm, wall thickness greater than 2 mm, loss of wall layering with a widely hypoechoic appearance, inflammatory changes in the surrounding mesenteric fat, and distension of the appendicular lumen (fluid with or without an appendicolith(s)) (Fig. 4) [20, 21].

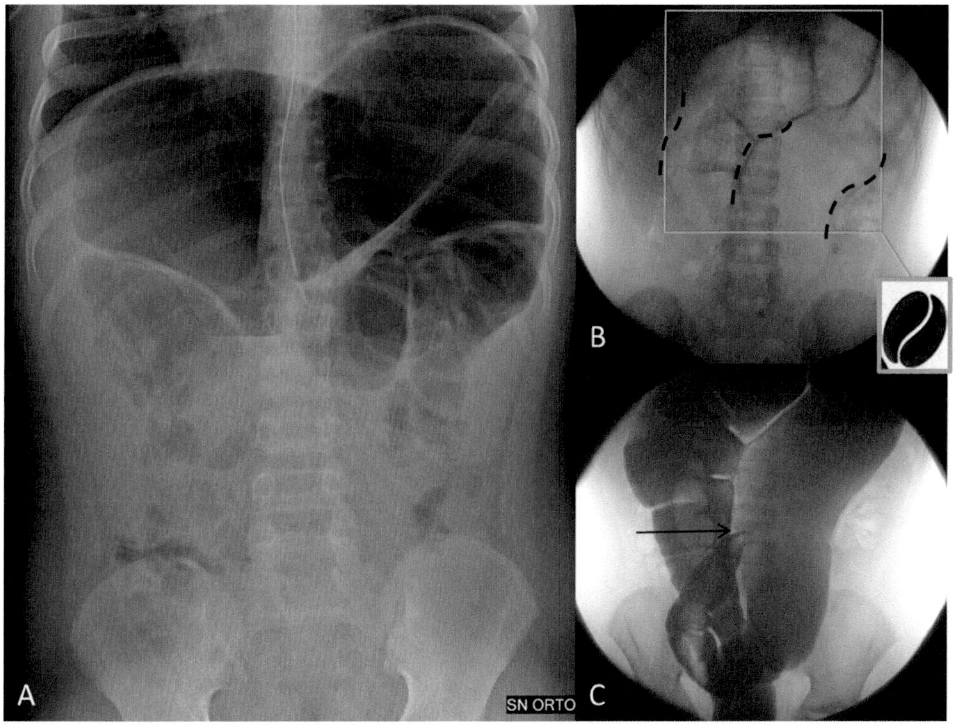

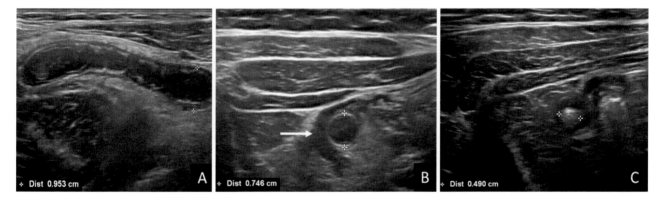

**Fig. 3** A 11-year-old boy with recurrent constipation, vomiting, and diarrhea. Abdominal radiograph shows findings of bowel obstruction, with marked distension of a loop of a large bowel in the upper abdomen (**a**). The radiographic features of a sigmoid volvulus are the left position of the dilated loop, the presence of a few air-fluid levels, and the loss of the normal *colonic haustral pattern* (**a**). Other specific signs of sigmoid volvulus are *the coffee bean sign* (**b**) and the *Frimann-Dahl sign* representing the sigmoid wall (three dense lines converging to the site of obstruction, usually in the pelvis; three dashed lines in **b**). **c**, Fluoroscopy shows another typical sign described as the *coffee bean sign* associated with a *beak sign* (black arrow), representing the point of the closed-loop obstruction

**Fig. 4** A 9-year-old boy, with abdominal pain, vomiting, and fever. Ultrasound shows the spectrum of findings in pediatric acute appendicitis. (**a**), (sagittal plane) an a-peristaltic, enlarged (9.5 mm), and noncompressible appendix, with preserved layers of the wall at an early *stage*; (**b**), on axial section, calipers define a target fluid-filled structure, with an ill-defined appearance of the appendiceal wall (*phlegmonous stage*), associated with a small peri-appendicular fluid collection (white arrow). (**c**), (axial plane) hyperechoic appendicolith at the appendix's apex

The natural evolution of appendicular inflammation can lead to perforation with progressive phlegmonous appearance and development of a peri-appendicular abscess, defined by an organized fluid collection with mass effect. In perforated appendicitis (gangrenous stage), there is a decrease in the rate of detection of the appendix, which is usually decompressed. Ultrasound remains the modality of choice to evaluate associated findings of perforated appendicitis, which can include dilated or thick-wall bowel loops, extraluminal fluid (simple or complex), and the presence of phlegmons or collections [22]. The development of complications, both as an evolution of appendicitis and postsurgical, should be evaluated with cross-sectional imaging [23]. Computed tomography of the abdomen/pelvis is often considered. However, the use of ionizing radiation must impose judicious management according to the ALARA principle, and therefore in many centers fast-sequence MR has been adopted for evaluation of equivocal findings in ultrasound and for the assessment of children with known or suspected complications of appendicitis.

## Meckel's Diverticulitis

Meckel's diverticulum is the most common congenital anomaly of the gastrointestinal tract, caused by the failure of the regression of the omphalomesenteric duct that normally occurs from the fifth to the eighth week of gestation [24]. Most Meckel's diverticula are located within 40–100 cm of the ileocecal valve, and originate from the anti-mesenteric side of the distal small intestine, affecting about 2% of the population [25]. The inflamed diverticulum can present with bleeding, inflammation, intussusception, bowel obstruction, or perforation, or a combination of these, and can mimic appendicitis (Fig. 5). In terms of incidence, however, the main complication is acute or chronic intestinal bleeding, representing the primary cause of anemia in children due to occult bleeding, followed by intestinal obstruction from secondary invagination.

## Inflammatory Bowel Disease

Among the intestinal pathologies in the differential diagnosis of appendicular inflammation, one of the main differential consideration is an acute flare-up of inflammatory bowel disease, in particular Crohn disease, which has a typical location in the terminal ileum. The "target sign" is the classic US finding in Crohn disease, and consists of a hypoechoic border, concentric thickening of the distal small intestinal wall, and central echogenic intestinal content within the narrowed lumen; another common sign of the acute phase is a prominence of vessels adjacent to the involved intestinal wall (comb sing) (Fig. 6). The affected intestinal segment is relatively noncompressible, with reduced or absent peristalsis in the small bowel [26, 27]. Although these ultrasound signs are typical for Crohn's disease, many other conditions, including infectious, ischemic, neoplastic, and radiation induced, can show completely overlapping sonographic findings in the distal small bowel. Transmural inflammation can lead to perivisceral edema and fibrosis, involving the adjacent mesentery, creating mass effect and associated inhomogeneous hyperechogenicity of the adjacent fat (the so-called "creeping" fat). Fibro-fatty proliferation is predictive of active inflammation, whereas mesenteric and locoregional lymphadenopathy is discovered in both the acute and chronic phases [28].

## Ovarian Pathology

In female patients, the main differential diagnosis of appendicitis is ovarian torsion, representing approximately up to 2–3% of all visits for abdominal pain in emergency departments. It can occur at any age, but it is more frequent between 9 and 14 years, with an average age of 12 years [29]. Ovarian torsion is caused by twisting of the vascular pedicle of the ovary, fallopian tube, or both, with venous obstruction, edema, arterial impairment, and ischemia. If untreated, infarction occurs. Developmental anomalies of the fallopian tubes or mesosalpinx (excessive length or absence), as well as the presence of intrinsic ovarian or tubal pathology (tumors, cysts, trauma, or recent surgery), are the main predisposing factors [29, 30].

Ultrasound findings which are highly concerning for ovarian/adnexal torsion include an enlarged, edematous, and

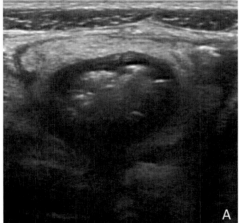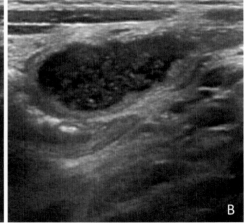

**Fig. 5** A 5-year-old girl with abdominal pain and dysuria. Sonographic findings (**a, b**, axial, and sagittal planes) of an inflamed Meckel's diverticulum show a tubular structure with a thickened wall. The structure is filled with fluid and debris

**Fig. 6** An 11-year-old boy with right lower quadrant pain. MR enterography shows focal concentric wall thickening of the distal-most portion of the terminal ileum (**a**, white arrow), with wall hyperenhancement after IV gadolinium injection (**b**), and restricted water diffusion on the ADC map (**c**, dashed arrow)

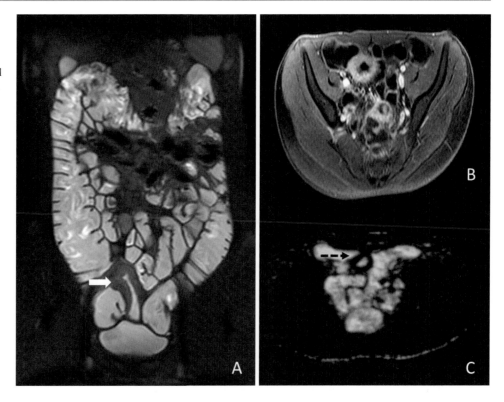

abnormally positioned ovary, with prominent follicles which are peripherally located. Although the presence of arterial and venous flow does not exclude the possibility of torsion, the identification of a twisted vascular pedicle (33%) is highly specific, but there are variable flow patterns (from normal to completely absent, or with asymmetry in the flow between the two ovaries) (Fig. 7). There is conflicting data, to our knowledge, about the diagnostic value of color Doppler in the diagnosis of ovarian torsion. In general, the predictive values, positive and negative (with the transabdominal approach), are relatively low [31]. The presence of a mass or cyst can create a diagnostic dilemma. In patients where a mass is present on ultrasound, MR can be helpful for further delineation of the findings [32].

Apart from ovarian torsion, the differential diagnosis of acute right lower quadrant abdominal pain in girls includes not only appendicitis, but also other adnexal masses, in particular after menarche hemorrhagic ovarian cysts, and less frequent pelvic inflammatory disease and ectopic pregnancy.

Hematometrocolpos refers to a blood-filled distended uterus and vagina, usually due to an anatomical mechanical obstruction stopping the evacuation of the menstrual blood. This condition encompasses different pathologies including imperforated hymen, Mullerian duct anomaly (unicornuate, bicornuate, and didelphys uterus), cloacal malformation, and cervical/vaginal stenosis. Girls, usually between 9 and 13 years, will most frequently present with primary

amenorrhea, cyclical pelvic pain, and pressure and low back pain. Ultrasound is usually the first imaging modality utilized, and will demonstrate a distended uterine/vaginal cavity with heterogeneous avascular material. Computed tomography is not usually utilized in these patients, however, sometimes contrast-enhanced CT is useful to establish correct diagnosis in patients with equivocal sonographic findings. MRI is helpful to confirm blood products, the absence of a solid mass, and to clarify the anatomy [33].

## The Distal Urinary Tract Infections (UTI)

The distal UTI mainly involves the distal tract, but frequently the same pathogens can lead to the involvement of the upper tract with possible long-term consequences [34]. Urinary flow obstruction is one of the main predisposing conditions in both infants and older children, in particular, if caused by urethral stricture or posterior urethral valves. Although with some limitations in revealing noncomplicated distal UTI, US is the method of choice to identify patients predisposed to renal obstruction and to initially diagnose pyelitis, pyelonephritis, and renal abscesses. Ultrasound also guides other diagnostic investigations (cystourethrography and radionuclide cystography) in those at risk of kidney scarring, recurrence, or chronicity. In particular, imaging plays a role to help identify patients with high risk of pyelonephritis recurrence (with anatomic or functional genitourinary tract

**Fig. 7** Ovarian torsion in a 14-year-old girl is shown. Ultrasound examination (axial planes). There is edema and enlargement of the right ovary (maximal diameter > 4 cm; right ovarian volume is 26 ml in comparison to 3.8 ml of the left one), with peripheral displaced follicles (in the upper half of the Figure **a**). By Color Doppler, there is a lack of vascularization in the right ovary compared with the left, where it is normal (in the lower half of the Figure **b**)

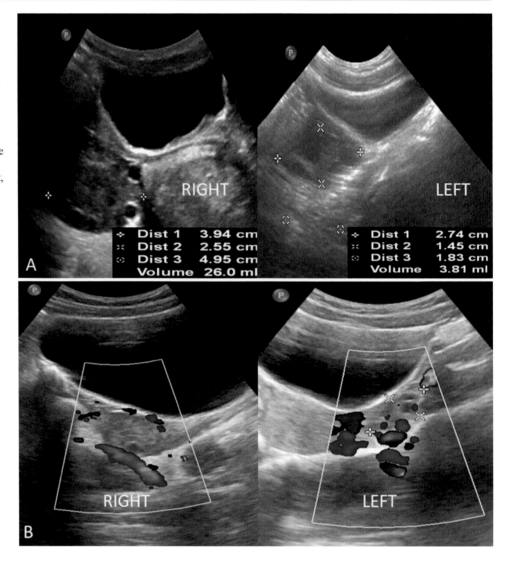

## Traumatic Abdominal Emergencies

Traumatic nonintentional or intentional injuries are the main causes of death in children and teenagers aged 1–18 [36]. Blunt abdominal injuries account for approximately 90% of all pediatric trauma. Although most traumatic events are mild or moderate in severity, children can also experience multiorgan trauma, even from low-energy traumatic mechanisms. In fact, unlike what happens in the adult, in the child the proximity of the abdominal organs to each other and the reduced quantity of connective and adipose tissue cause more frequently substantive injuries to a variety of internal organs [37]. Management of the injured child needs special

abnormalities) and in patients at risk for renal scar development and consequently permanent renal damage with possibly chronic hypertension and renal failure [35] (Fig 8).

considerations such as reducing diagnostic radiation exposure, family presence during the examinations, dedicated equipment, and specific pain management, as well as an understanding of the anatomy, physiology, and psychology of children [36–38].

Diagnostic imaging plays a key role in the management of trauma patients, allowing the demonstration of organ injury, and the need for interventional radiology treatment. As in adults, we distinguish two different kinds of trauma, which are managed differently. They are high-energy or major trauma, and low-energy or minor trauma. In any trauma case, the hemodynamic stability and cardiorespiratory conditions are the main parameters in the management of trauma patients. In the case of major trauma and hemodynamic instability, an extended-to-thorax focused assessment with sonography for trauma (E-FAST) must be performed in the emergency room during the resuscitation/stabilization maneuvers. The examination of the thorax with the technique

**Fig. 8** Axial (**a**) and sagittal (**b**) US images in a 4-year-old boy with known vesicoureteral reflux determining a condition of pyonephrosis. He had fever and a positive urinary culture. The US shows renal collecting system and calyceal dilatation by complex fluid, with debris associated with thickening of the renal pelvis and ureteral wall

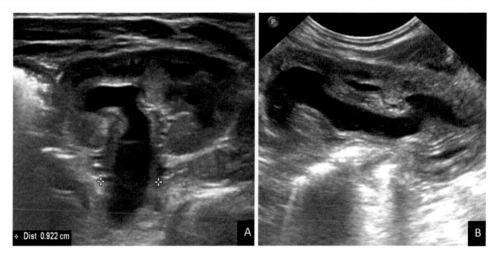

E-FAST depicts the presence of hemothorax and pneumothorax, including the presence of hemopericardium whose evaluation is already performed with FAST scan, through the execution of some rapid standard scanning with a convex and linear probe. Thoracic ultrasound (E-FAST) is a rapid and accurate first-line, bedside diagnostic modality for the diagnosis of pneumothorax in unstable patients with major chest trauma during the primary survey in the emergency room. The ultrasound signs of pneumothorax are loss of lung "sliding," absence of B lines, presence of "lung point" (this is the junction between sliding lung and absent sliding and gives an indication of pneumothorax size by its location), and absence of "lung pulse" (this is the movement of the pleura determined by cardiac activity). This assessment has a sensitivity of 90.9% and a specificity of 98.2% in the detection of pneumothorax, compared to a sensitivity and specificity of conventional radiography, respectively, of 50.2% and 99.0% [39].

The examination does not interrupt the primary survey, and allows the resuscitator to continue to stabilize the patient (Drawing 2) [40–42].

Similar to adult trauma patients, hemodynamically stable pediatric patients with major trauma total-body IV contrast-enhanced CT (CECT) is usually performed. CECT is the current reference standard in the evaluation of trauma patients, allowing in a very short time frame an overall assessment of solid and hollow organs, vascular structures, and bones, and to highlight any findings that will potentially change patient's management from conservative to operative [43].

In cases of minor trauma, there is no consensus on the management of the pediatric patient, to our knowledge. The use of CT as a first-choice examination does not seem justified in children, because it leads to overexposure to radiation.

In low-energy trauma and isolated trauma, the first diagnostic approach in the child can be performed by radiography, and, if necessary, by abdominal sonography.

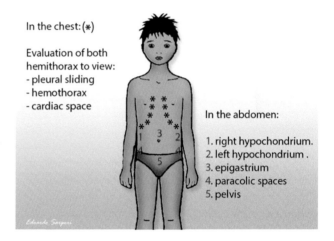

In the chest: (∗)

Evaluation of both hemithorax to view:
- pleural sliding
- hemothorax
- cardiac space

In the abdomen:

1. right hypochondrium.
2. left hypochondrium .
3. epigastrium
4. paracolic spaces
5. pelvis

**Drawing 2.** E-FAST: the ultrasound exploration sites

However, while US has a high sensitivity for the evaluation of the presence of abdominal fluid, reported from 63 to 99%, [44–46], its ability to reveal any organ injury, and particularly to the bowel/retroperitoneum, is limited to < 50% due to patient constitution, operator dependence, and patient condition/inability to cooperate with the examination.

In the abdomen, parenchymal organs are most frequently affected in traumatic injuries. The liver and spleen are the most affected organs, due to their relatively larger size, proximity to the rib arches, and the reduced protection offered by the muscles of the abdominal wall, which are less developed in children than in adults. However, in the child, the retroperitoneal organs can also be easily traumatized. Both the kidneys and the pancreas have poor protection due to the reduced amount of retroperitoneal fat tissue, and the pancreas can be compressed against the bony structure of the spine. The CT findings of traumatic injuries to the abdominal and pelvic organs in children are quite similar to those of adult patients [47] (Fig.9).

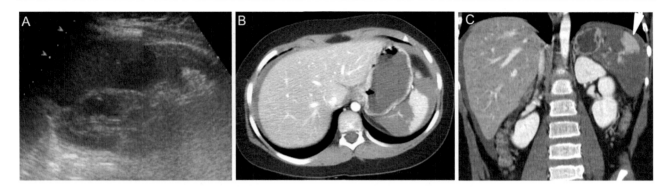

**Fig. 9** A 9-year-old boy with high-energy trauma, caused by a crash between a car and a motorbike. Splenic injury. (**a**), US shows extended disruption of the spleen. Healthy splenic parenchyma is not recognizable. (**b**), IV axial contrast-enhanced CT image and (**c**), coronal IV contrast-enhanced CT reconstruction demonstrate the extended disruption of the spleen. A minimal amount of normal parenchyma is noted (arrowhead)

On baseline US, the finding of a nonhomogeneous parenchymal abnormality with poorly defined margins and a hyperechoic appearance in comparison to the surrounding parenchyma strongly suggests acute injury. Such a finding, however, is not always easily detectable. This occurs both in traumatic injuries to the liver and kidneys, while in the spleen more often a recent injury can have the same echogenicity as the normal splenic parenchyma, and, therefore, can be easily missed. Moreover, approximately 30% of injuries to solid organs do not reach the organ capsule and do not cause hemoperitoneum and/or hemo-retroperitoneum, and this increases the risk of nonrecognition of injuries [48].

These limitations can be overcome by completing the baseline US examination with IV contrast-enhanced ultrasound (CEUS). With exclusive use in low-energy or isolated trauma, this technique has increased the detection of abdominal injuries compared with basic ultrasound, reaching sensitivity and specificity values similar to those of a CECT, which is the reference standard [49–52].

In case of free fluid in the abdomen at baseline ultrasound, or in case of evidence of parenchymal heterogeneity, the CEUS will allow detection of otherwise unrecognized or questionable injuries. The goal of CEUS examination is to discharge the healthy patient without further investigations or unnecessary hospitalization, and to carry out all the necessary investigations only in the injured patient. The CEUS imaging features are comparable to that of CECT: A laceration is represented as a linear area without IV contrast enhancement. The margins of laceration and its relationship with the organ capsule can be detected using CEUS (Fig.10). The presence of parenchymal foci of contrast medium in the laceration or leakage of extracapsular contrast indicates intraparenchymal or intraperitoneal active bleeding. A pseudoaneurysm is represented by pooling of contrast medium that does not change its shape over time [53].

Before performing CEUS informed consent from the patient's parents/guardians must be obtained; this is generally possible since the use of CEUS is performed only on low-energy or isolated trauma. The main potential advantages of CEUS are several, including its rapid performance, which can be done at the patient's bedside, and the possibility of avoiding unnecessary CECT examinations, reducing ionizing radiation exposure [54].

In order to avoid unnecessary radiation exposure of the patient, in the context of low-energy trauma both CEUS and MRI are valid tools in the follow-up of abdominal and pelvic injuries [55].

The limitations of the CEUS are same as with basic US, but has other specific limits, in particular: difficulties in depicting intestinal and mesenteric traumatic injuries; it is not possible to evaluate the presence of injury to renal excretory system because ultrasound contrast media has only a vascular phase and no renal excretion; and there are limitations in assessing for active bleeding, since it has lower sensibility than CECT [53–55].

## Conclusions

Diseases of the abdominal organs are among the most frequent causes of visits to the emergency department in children. In the case of nontraumatic emergencies, the greatest difficulty is that of narrowing down the diagnosis between conditions which often have a very similar clinical presentation and which can be differentiated only with careful knowledge of pathology and the possible findings of diagnostic imaging. All cross-sectional imaging modalities have their diagnostic utility, and must be adequately used to support the diagnostic process.

In patients with abdominal trauma, the diagnostic algorithms are different in the case of high and low kinetic energy trauma. In patients with high-energy trauma, the use of CT, preceded by E-FAST in the emergency department, is mandatory for the correct and complete triage of patients. In the

**Fig. 10** A 9-year-old girl with isolated trauma, fell beating the left flank. Renal injury. (**a**), Color Doppler US image demonstrates extensive injury to the middle third of the kidney (white arrow). At the upper and lower poles, there is an intraparenchymal flow signal on Doppler interrogation. (**b**), CEUS depicts the full-thickness injury of the kidney (white arrow) and an extensive perirenal collection (asterisk). (**c**) and (**d**), axial IV contrast-enhanced CT scan and 3D MIP reconstruction show the perirenal fluid collection (asterisk in **c**) and the urine leakage (arrowheads in **c**, **d**)

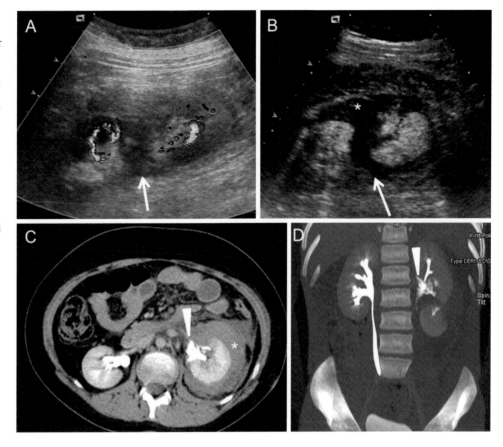

case of direct trauma, with low kinetic energy, the use of ultrasound is more applicable, possibly with the addition of CEUS. In any case, the correct use of diagnostic imaging must be aimed not only at identifying the causative process, but also at helping to choose the most appropriate therapeutic strategy.

# References

1. Naffaa L, Barakat A, Baassiri A, et al. Imaging acute non-traumatic abdominal pathologies in pediatric patients: a pictorial review. J Radiol Case Rep. 2019;13:29–43.
2. Rogers TN, Robb A. Intussusception in infants and young children. Surgery. 2010;28:402–5.
3. LeeHS CJY, Koo JW, et al. Clinical characteristics of intussusception in children: comparison between small bowel and large bowel type. Korean J Gastroenterol. 2006;47:37–43.
4. Siaplaouras J, Moritz JD, Gortner L, et al. Small bowel intussusception in childhood. Klin Padiatr. 2003;215:53–6.
5. Bartocci M, Fabrizi G, Valente I, et al. Intussusception in childhood, role of sonography on diagnosis and treatment. J Ultrasound. 2014;18:205–11.
6. Wong CW, Chan IH, Chung PH, et al. Childhood intussusception: 17-year experience at a tertiary referral centre in Hong Kong. Hong Kong Med J. 2015;22(1):15.
7. Cogley JR, O'Connor SC, Houshyar R, et al. Emergent pediatric US: what every radiologist should know. RadioGraphics. 2012;32: 651–65.
8. Kim YG, Choi BI, Yeon KM, et al. Diagnosis and treatment of childhood intussus ception using real time ultrasonography and saline enema: preliminary report. J Korean Soc Med Ultrasound. 1982;1:66–70.
9. Sadigh G, Zou KH, Razavi SA, et al. Meta-analysis of air versus liquid enema for intussusception reduction in children. AJR Am J Roentgenol. 2015;205:W542–9.
10. Lioubashevsky N, Hiller N, Rozovsky K, et al. Ileocolic versus small-bowel intussusception in children: can US enable reliable differentiation. Radiology. 2013;269:266–71.
11. Chang WL, Yang YH, Lin YT, et al. Gastrointestinal manifestations in Henoch-Schönlein purpura: a review of 261 patients. Acta Paediatr. 2004;93:1427–31.
12. Chen SY, Kong MS. Gastrointestinal manifestations and complications of Henoch-Schönlein purpura. Chang Gung Med J. 2004;27:175–81.
13. Berrocal T, Lamas M, Gutieerrez J, et al. Congenital anomalies of the small intestine, colon, and rectum. Radiographics. 1999;19: 1219–36.
14. Torres AM, Ziegler MM. Malrotation of the intestine. World J Surg. 1993;17:326–31.
15. Bhandari TR, Shahi S. Volvulus of sigmoid colon in a challenged adolescent: an unusual case report. Ann Med Surg (Lond). 2019;44: 26–8.
16. Almaramhy HH. Acute appendicitis in young children less than 5 years: review article. Ital J Pediatr. 2017;43:15.
17. Chan I, Bicknell SG, Graham M. Utility and diagnostic accuracy of sonography in detecting appendicitis in a community hospital. AJR Am J Roentgenol. 2005;184:1809–12.
18. Lee JH, Jeong YK, Park KB, et al. Operator-dependent techniques for graded compression sonography to detect the appendix and diagnose acute appendicitis. AJR Am J Roentgenol. 2005;184:91–7.

19. Kessler N, Cyteval C, Gallix B, et al. Appendicitis: evaluation of sensitivity, specificity, and predictive values of US, Doppler US, and laboratory findings. Radiology. 2004;230:472–8.

20. Jeffrey RB Jr, Jain KA, Nghiem HV. Sonographic diagnosis of acute appendicitis: interpretive pitfalls. AJR Am J Roentgenol. 1994;162: 55–9.

21. Di Giacomo V, Trinci M, Van der Byl G, et al. Ultrasound in newborns and children suffering from nontraumatic acute abdominal pain: imaging with clinical and surgical correlation. J Ultrasound. 2015;18:385–93.

22. Mittal MK, Dayan PS, Macias CG, et al. Performance of ultrasound in the diagnosis of appendicitis in children in a multicenter cohort. Acad Emerg Med. 2013;20:697–702.

23. Tseng P, Berdahl C, Kearl YL, et al. Does right lower quadrant abdominal ultrasound accurately identify perforation in pediatric acute appendicitis? J Emerg Med. 2016;50:638–42.

24. Gezer HÖ, Temiz A, Ince E, et al. Meckel diverticulum in children: evaluation of macroscopic appearance for guidance in subsequent surgery. J Pediatr Surg. 2015;51:1177–80.

25. Sanchez TR, Corwin MT, Davoodian A, et al. Sonography of abdominal pain in children: appendicitis and its common mimics. J Ultrasound Med. 2016;35:627–35.

26. Dong J, Wang H, Zhao J, et al. Ultrasound as a diagnostic tool in detecting active Crohn's disease: a meta-analysis of prospective studies. Eur Radiol. 2014;24:26–33.

27. Fraquelli M, Colli A, Casazza G, et al. Role of US in detection of Crohn disease: meta-analysis. Radiology. 2005;236(1):95–101.

28. Maconi G. Crohn's disease. In: Maconi G, Porro GB, editors. Ultrasound of the gastrointestinal tract. German: Springer-Verlag, Berlin; 2014. p. 95–108.

29. Schmitt ER, Ngai SS, Gausche-Hill M, et al. Twist and shout! Pediatric ovarian torsion clinical update and case discussion. Pediatr Emerg Care. 2013;29:518–23.

30. Rey-Bellet Gasser C, Gehri M, Joseph GM, et al. Is it ovarian torsion? a systematic literature review and evaluation of prediction signs. Pediatr Emerg Care. 2016;32:256–61.

31. Naiditch JA, Barsness KA. The positive and negative predictive value of transabdominal color Doppler ultrasound for diagnosing ovarian torsion in pediatric patients. J Pediatr Surg. 2013;48: 1283–7.

32. Rougier E, Mar W, Della Valle V, et al. Added value of MRI for the diagnosis of adnexal torsion in children and adolescents after inconclusive ultrasound examination. Diagn Interv Imaging. 2020;101(11):747–56.

33. Maneschi F. Le malformazioni uterine. Roma: CIC Edizioni Internazionali; 1994.

34. Okarska-Napierała M, Wasilewska A, Kuchar E. Urinary tract infection in children: diagnosis, treatment, imaging – comparison of current guidelines. J Pediatr Urol. 2017;13:567–73.

35. Bocquet N, Biebuyck N, Lortat Jacob S, et al. Imaging strategy for children after a first episode of pyelonephritis. Arch Pediatr. 2015;22(5):547–53.

36. Committee on pediatric emergency medicine, council on injury; violence, and poison prevention, section on critical care, section on orthopaedics, section on surgery, section on transport medicine, pediatric trauma society, and society of trauma nurses pediatric committee. Management of pediatric trauma. Pediatrics. 2016;138(2):e20161569.

37. Lee LK, Fleisher GR Trauma management: approach to the unstable child. 2020

38. Miele V, Di Giampietro I, Ianniello S, et al. Diagnostic imaging in pediatric polytrauma management. Radiol Med. 2015;120:33–49.

39. Alrajhi K, Woo MY, Vaillancourt C. Test characteristics of ultrasonography for the detection of pneumothorax: a systematic review and meta-analysis. Chest. 2012 Mar;141(3):703–8.

40. Montoya J, Stawicki SP, Evans DC, et al. From FAST to E-FAST: an overview of the evolution of ultrasound-based traumatic injury assessment. Eur J Trauma Emerg Surg. 2016;42(2):119–26.

41. Manka M Jr, Moscati M, Raghavendran K, et al. Sonographic scoring for operating room. West J Emerg Med. 2010;11:138–43.

42. Piccolo CL, Trinci M, Pinto A, et al. Role of contrast-enhanced ultrasound (CEUS) in the diagnosis and management of traumatic splenic injuries. J Ultrasound. 2018;21:315–27.

43. Miele V, Piccolo CL, Trinci M, et al. Diagnostic imaging of blunt abdominal trauma in pediatric patients. Radiol Med. 2016;121:409–30.

44. Brown MA, Sirlin CB, Hoyt DB, et al. Screening ultrasound in blunt abdominal trauma. J Intensive Care Med. 2003;18:253–60.

45. Branney SW, Wolfe RE, Moore EE, et al. Quantitative sensitivity of ultrasound in detecting free intraperitoneal fluid. J Trauma. 1995;39: 375–80.

46. Latteri S, Malaguarnera G, Mannino M, et al. Ultrasound as point of care in management of polytrauma and its complication. J Ultrasound. 2017;20:171–7.

47. Lynch T, Kilgar J, Al Shibli A. Pediatric abdominal trauma. Curr Pediatr Rev. 2018;14(1):59–63.

48. Chiu WC, Cushing BM, Rodriguez A, et al. Abdominal injuries without hemoperitoneum: a potential limitation focused abdominal sonography trauma (FAST). J Trauma. 1997;42:617–23.

49. Miele V, Piccolo CL, Galluzzo M, et al. Contrast-enhanced ultrasound (CEUS) in blunt abdominal trauma. Br J Radiol. 2016;89: 20150823.

50. Pinto F, Miele V, Scaglione M, et al. The use of contrast-enhanced ultrasound in blunt abdominal trauma: advantages and limitations. Acta Radiol. 2014;55:776–84.

51. Menichini G, Sessa B, Trinci M, et al. Accuracy of Contrast-Enhanced Ultrasound (CEUS) in the identification and characterization of traumatic solid organ lesions in children: a retrospective comparison with baseline-US and CE-MDCT. Radiol Med. 2015;120:989–1001.

52. Sidhu PS, Cantisani V, Deganello A, et al. Role of Contrast-enhanced Ultrasound (CEUS) in paediatric practice: an EFSUMB Position statement. Ultraschall Med. 2017;38:33–43.

53. Sessa B, Trinci M, Ianniello S, et al. Blunt abdominal trauma: role of Contrast-Enhanced Ultrasound in the detection and staging of abdominal traumatic lesions compared with US and CE-MDCT. Radiol Med. 2015;120:180–9.

54. Yusuf GT, Sellars ME, Deganello A, et al. Analysis of the safety and cost implications of pediatric contrast-enhanced ultrasound at a single center. AJR Am J Roentgenol. 2017;208:446–52.

55. Miele V, Piccolo CL, Sessa B, et al. Comparison between MRI and CEUS in the follow-up of patients with blunt abdominal trauma managed conservatively. Radiol Med. 2016;121:27–37.

# Pediatric Emergencies: Role of the Interventional Radiologist

# 51

Gali Shapira-Zaltsberg, Michael Temple, and Joao Amaral

## Contents

**Abstract**

Emergency image-guided interventions in pediatric patients frequently require different interventional skills and techniques to accommodate the patient's size and a spectrum of anatomical and developmental variants. In this chapter, we describe pediatric interventions which are commonly performed emergently, divided into anatomical areas. The procedures in the chest include aspiration or drainage of pleural effusion, pneumothorax, and lung abscess, catheter-directed thrombolysis (CDT) of massive or sub-massive pulmonary embolism (PE), and bronchial artery embolization (BAE) for the treatment of massive hemoptysis. Abdominal procedures described include abscess drainage; management of gastrostomy tubes, gastrojejunostomy tubes, and cecostomy tubes; embolization for the management of massive gastrointestinal (GI) bleeding; and embolization for splenic or hepatic trauma. The renal procedures include nephrostomy tube placement and embolization for renal trauma. Musculoskeletal procedures, including arthrocentesis for suspected septic joint and bone biopsy for osteomyelitis, will also be reviewed. We also describe issues related to emergent vascular access in children.

G. Shapira-Zaltsberg (✉)
Department of Medical Imaging, CHEO, Ottawa, University of Toronto, Toronto, ON, Canada
e-mail: GShapira@cheo.on.ca

M. Temple · J. Amaral
Division of Image-Guided Therapy (IGT), Department of Diagnostic Imaging, The Hospital for Sick Children, Medical Imaging department, University of Toronto, Toronto, ON, Canada
e-mail: michael.temple@sickkids.ca; joao.amaral@sickkids.ca

© Springer Nature Switzerland AG 2022
M. N. Patlas et al. (eds.), *Atlas of Emergency Imaging from Head-to-Toe*,
https://doi.org/10.1007/978-3-030-92111-8_51

**Keywords**

Interventional pediatric radiology · Chest tubes · Catheter-directed thrombolysis · Abscess drainage · Embolization · Nephrostomy tube · G tubes · Vascular access · PICC · CVL

## Introduction

Compared to adults, emergency image-guided interventions in pediatric patients frequently require different interventional skills and techniques to accommodate for patient size and a potential spectrum of anatomical and developmental variants while minimizing ionizing radiation according to the ALARA ("as low as reasonably achievable") principle. Weighing the risk versus benefit of a proposed procedure must include considerations such as the need for general anesthesia or sedation due to the lack of compliance in many pediatric patients. In addition, children can decompensate quickly; hence, emergent interventions may be undertaken in patients who are relatively clinically well.

In this chapter, we describe the pediatric interventions which are most commonly performed emergently, divided into anatomical areas, and subdivided into vascular and nonvascular procedures.

## Chest

The indications for emergency thoracic interventions in the pediatric population, similar to the adult counterpart, include nonvascular procedures, such as pneumothorax drainage and pleural effusion/empyema drainage and abscess drainage, and vascular interventions such as catheter-directed thrombolysis (CDT) of massive or sub-massive PE and bronchial artery embolization (BAE).

## Nonvascular Thoracic Interventions

### Pleural Effusion and Empyema

Parapneumonic effusions are common in pediatric bacterial pneumonia, with a frequency of 21–91%, evolving into empyema in a range of 28–53% of cases [1]. The need for drainage is dictated by the severity of respiratory distress and the effusion size. Effusion size is classified similar to that in adults (i.e., small effusion, <10mm or opacifies <25% of the hemithorax; moderate effusion, >10mm rim of fluid but opacifies <50% of the hemithorax; and large effusion, opacifies >50% of the hemithorax). Small effusions often respond to antibiotic therapy without the need for intervention. Moderate to large effusions more likely cause respiratory compromise, do not resolve quickly, and benefit from drainage [2]. Prior to drainage, an ultrasound (US) should be done to confirm the presence of an effusion, assess its nature (e.g., septations, debris), and identify an optimal site for tube placement [2]. Typically, the effusion is accessed under US guidance with an IV cannula/needle that will allow insertion of a 0.018- or a 0.035-inch guidewire. The tract is then dilated under fluoroscopy or US guidance to avoid kinking of the wire, followed by placement of a pigtail-type draining catheter, ranging in size from 6 to 14 French, depending on the size of the child and the viscosity of the fluid (Fig. 1). Alternatively, large effusions may be accessed using a trocar technique (see description in Sect. 2.1.3). The drain is then

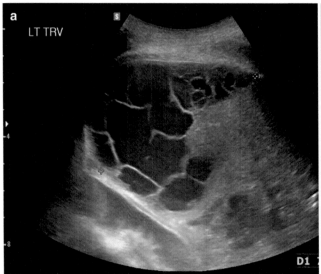
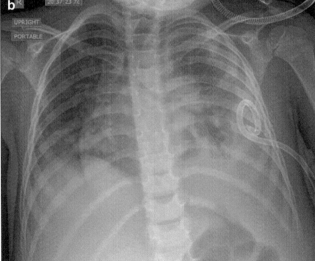

**Fig. 1** A 5-year-old-girl with complicated pneumonia. Frontal AP chest radiograph showed nearly complete opacification of the left hemithorax with mediastinal shift to the right. The presence of a complex effusion was confirmed on chest US (**a**), subsequently drained under US guidance. Follow-up chest radiograph (**b**) and chest US (not shown) shows residual complex effusion, treated with tPA

attached to a dry suction water seal draining system under gravity or with low-pressure suction ($-10$ to $-40$ cm $H_2O$) [3]. Tissue Plasminogen Activator (tPA) can be administered if there is poor drainage with evidence of significant residual effusion/empyema, likely with internal septations and debris, on repeat US.

## Pneumothorax

The therapeutic approach to pneumothorax primarily depends on its size and clinical presentation. Small pneumothoraces do not usually require intervention, whereas large pneumothoraces require hospitalization and often necessitate placement of small-bore catheters [4]. In adults, the presence of a visible rim of $>2$ cm between the lung margin and the chest wall on a chest radiograph is considered a "large" pneumothorax [5]. However, there is no consensus, to our knowledge, regarding the classification of pneumothoraces in the pediatric age range [6], and the size is often assessed subjectively. If the placement of a chest tube is warranted, access to the pleural cavity is typically obtained under fluoroscopy guidance, and a chest tube is then placed similarly to that described above for pleural effusion drainage. A pneumothorax drainage with immediate lung re-expansion is depicted in Fig. 2.

## Lung Abscess Drainage

Pulmonary abscesses and infected congenital pulmonary airway malformations (CPAM) can be drained via percutaneous catheters. As the tube passes through the pleural space into lung parenchyma, associated bronchopleural fistula formation can result in the need for prolonged drainage. As such, careful communication regarding the necessity of lung drainage needs to be undertaken with the referring service. Likewise, discussion with the anesthesiologist before draining intraparenchymal lung abscesses is very important due to the risk of dissemination of the abscess contents into the ipsilateral or contralateral lung, potentially resulting in significant morbidity and even mortality. Small collections may be aspirated, whereas larger abscesses will usually require indwelling drain placement. Catheter insertion can be performed using a trocar or Seldinger technique. In the trocar technique, the catheter is loaded onto a sharp introducer, and under imaging guidance, it is used to puncture the abscess cavity. The catheter is then advanced over the introducer into the cavity. The primary advantage of the trocar technique is that it is quick and avoids multiple wire and catheter manipulations. The main disadvantage is that the trocar technique can result in a less-than-optimal catheter position and increased complication risk of bleeding and tissue damage with the larger introducer/catheter, if the correct trajectory is not chosen. In the Seldinger technique, the abscess cavity is punctured under image guidance with a needle which allows for the passage of a guidewire into the fluid collection. After serial dilatation of the tract, the catheter is placed over the wire and formed within the collection using US or fluoroscopic guidance. The Seldinger technique is more controlled and can result in less risk to nearby structures; however, it is lengthier, and it can also result in more leakage of body fluids around the indwelling wire. A lung abscess with normal lung surrounding it usually cannot be readily visualized under US and may require CT guidance for drainage [7].

## Vascular Thoracic Interventions

## Massive and Sub-massive Pulmonary Embolism (PE): CDT

PE in the pediatric population is relatively rare when compared to adults; however, the incidence is increasing, and timely diagnosis and treatment are critical [8]. Given the lack of specificity of non-imaging diagnostic tests (e.g., D-dimer) and the vague clinical presentation, imaging serves a primary role in the evaluation of pediatric PE [9]. Pulmonary artery CDT has long been considered as a first-line treatment option for adult patients with acute massive PE [10] when emergent surgical intervention is not necessary or possible. However, pharmacological and/or mechanical CDT has only recently emerged as a safe, alternative treatment in the setting of sub-massive and massive PE in pediatric and adolescent patients [11, 12]. Dosing for pediatric thrombolysis has not been scientifically determined, to our knowledge. Dabin et al. suggest a dose of tPA delivered through the infusion catheters into the pulmonary arteries (PA) of $0.03–0.06$ mg/kg/hr, with a maximum dose of 1 mg/hr based on published recommendations [13, 14]. If infusion catheters are placed in both pulmonary arteries, then the dose is to be split between the two catheters [11]. Figure 3 shows a case of a pharmacological and mechanical CDT in a 16-year-old patient.

## Massive Hemoptysis: BAE

Hemoptysis is an unusual condition in children, with tuberculosis, fungal infections, and bronchiectasis, mainly due to cystic fibrosis (CF), being the most common causes. Most cases of hemoptysis in children are mild and self-limiting. Hemoptysis in a child of a volume of $>8$ ml/kg in 24 hours is considered life-threatening [15]. BAE has become an established procedure in the management of massive and recurrent hemoptysis, in both adult and pediatric patients [15, 16]. Embolization is successful in controlling hemoptysis in over 90% of the cases but with recurrence rates as high as 60% in CF [3]. Before BAE, an attempt is made to localize the site of hemorrhage, using CTA and/or bronchoscopy. CTA is also valuable in demonstrating the appearance of the bronchial arteries prior to intervention (Fig. 4a). In children, BAE is typically performed under general anesthesia. Femoral access is gained under US guidance, and a 4 or 5 French sheath is placed. Selective bronchial artery

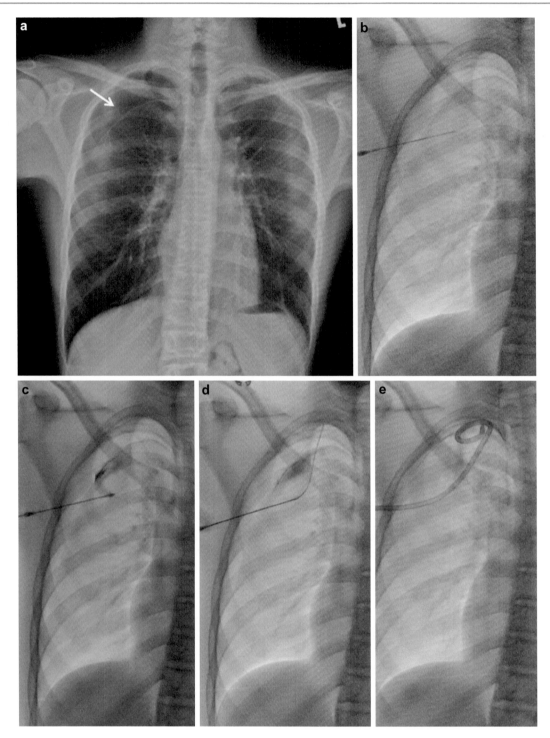

**Fig. 2** Chest radiograph (**a**) of a 15-year-old male with history of two previous spontaneous pneumothoraces, presenting with a 2-day history of shortness of breath, shows a right pneumothorax (arrow) with mild mediastinal shift. The pneumothorax was accessed under fluoroscopy guidance with a 16G needle (**b**), and an appropriate position in the pleural space was confirmed with contrast injection (**c**). A 0.035-inch guidewire was passed through the needle (**d**), and subsequently a 12 French drainage catheter was inserted over the wire into the pleural space. Air was evacuated from the chest and the lung re-expanded (**e**)

angiography can be the initial step; however, some authors advocate initially targeting the subclavian artery and its branches and occluding any collaterals that may be revealed

[15], thus reducing the risk of inadvertent embolization of the vertebral arteries. The abnormal appearing bronchial arteries are subsequently selected and embolized, preferably using

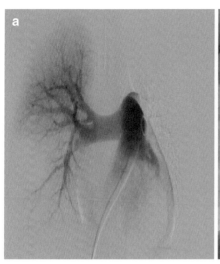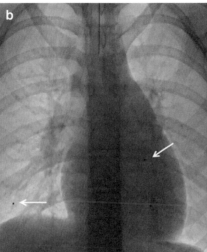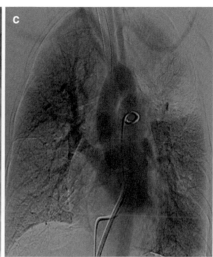

**Fig. 3** CTA of a 16-year-old female on oral contraceptives showed bilateral massive PE (not shown). A subsequent conventional pulmonary angiogram demonstrated no flow to the left lung and the lower lobe of the right lung (**a**). A 4 French multi-sidehole infusion catheters (arrows) were placed for tPA infusion (**b**). The following day, a conventional pulmonary angiogram obtained at the level of the pulmonary trunk demonstrated interval improvement in the perfusion of the left lung, although still markedly hypoperfused, with no definite improvement in perfusion of the right lung (not shown). Mechanical thrombolysis was then done. An aspiration catheter was advanced to multiple sites in the pulmonary vessels bilaterally, and the clot was aspirated (not shown). Repeat angiograms showed marked interval improvement in the perfusion to the left lung and right lower lobe (**c**). A repeat CTA 2 days after the mechanical CDT showed substantial interval improvement in the clot load and right-heart strain (not shown)

polyvinyl alcohol (PVA) particles, typically 300–500 microns in size, to reduce the passage of embolic agent through bronchopulmonary shunts and to avoid distal embolization of normal bronchial branches which may lead to bronchial wall, esophageal wall, or aortic wall necrosis (Fig. 4) [3, 15, 16].

## Abdomen/Pelvis

### Nonvascular Abdominal/Pelvic Interventions

#### Abscess Drainage

In children, the most common cause of intra-abdominal abscesses is perforated appendicitis. Primary drainage of one or more collections is frequently performed and is preferred as an alternative to surgery, which allows the patient to recover from their acute infection [17, 18]. Interventions are primarily performed using real-time US for needle guidance and fluoroscopy to monitor wire manipulation and optimize drain placement [18] (Fig. 5). Seldinger or trocar techniques are used for introducing a catheter into an abscess [7].

Drainage of deep pelvic collections is performed via a transrectal or transgluteal approach. The transrectal approach, with the patient in a left lateral decubitus position, is preferred. Using a Seldinger technique, an 18-G needle is advanced through an US guide into the abscess (Fig. 6). Then a 0.035-inch guidewire is advanced through the needle into the abscess, the needle and the transrectal probe are removed, and, subsequently, a multipurpose drainage catheter (8–12 Fr) is advanced over the guidewire into the abscess. Fluoroscopy is used to ensure a straight course of the guidewire, avoiding kinking or buckling [19]. The collection is drained, and, in some cases, saline lavage is performed.

Similar to complex pleural effusions, if drainage of the abscess ceases but a residual complex collection is identified on imaging, intracavitary tPA can be administered to liquefy the abscess contents and promote drainage [17].

### Gastrotomy and Gastrojejunostomy Tubes

Gastrostomy tubes (G tubes) and gastrojejunostomy tubes (GJ tubes) are commonly placed in children who require long-term nutritional support. High rates of emergency department (ED) visits and hospital readmissions after G/GJ tube placement have been reported (approximately 8% of patients visit the ED within 90 days post G/GJ tube placement) [20]. The most common complications presenting in the ED are tube dislodgement, tube malposition, and/or tube obstruction.

Dislodged Tubes: All patients and/or their caregivers should receive education regarding urgently replacing completely dislodged tubes with a temporary tube (e.g., Foley catheter) to maintain and protect the stoma tract. If efforts to place a temporary tube fail, patients should present to the ED for assistance. If the ED physician or other clinician initially evaluating the patient is not able to reestablish access to the stoma, the interventional radiology team should be contacted to attempt to salvage the gastrointestinal (GI) access. If it is a GJ tube that is dislodged, feeds should

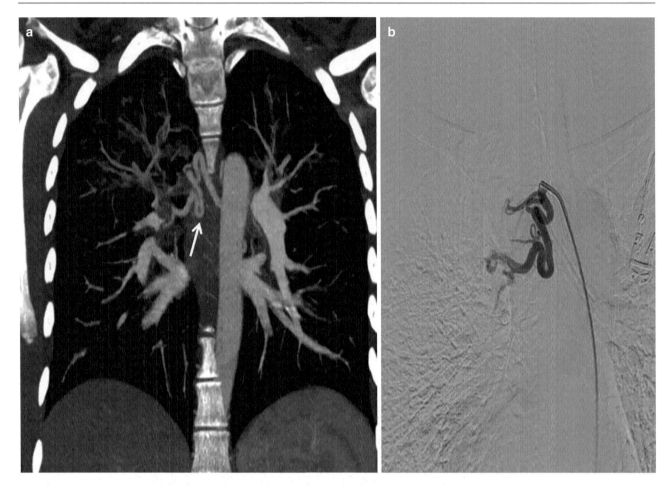

**Fig. 4** Coronal (**a**) CTA image of a 16-year-old female with a history of CF and massive hemoptysis shows a markedly dilated and tortuous right-sided bronchial artery (arrow). Bronchiectasis, predominantly in the right upper lobe, and focal consolidation, in the right middle lobe (not shown), were also seen. The patient was referred for embolization. Access was gained into the right common femoral artery. A 5 French catheter was advanced into the enlarged right bronchial artery. Angiograms demonstrated large tortuous bronchial arteries. The anterior spinal artery was not opacified (**b**). A bronchial branch into the right lower lobe was cannulated and angiogram performed showing some tortuosity (not shown). No abnormal shunts or connections were identified. This branch was embolized with 1 ml of particles 355–500 microns (diluted with 10 ml of contrast and 10 ml of saline) (not shown). A right upper lobe bronchial branch angiogram demonstrated potential communication with a subclavian vessel (not shown). Given the controlled symptoms, no embolization was performed on this branch

be held until the GJ tube is replaced. In these cases, the patient may need to be admitted for temporary IV hydration or IV medication, depending on the patient's clinical status and the availability of the interventional radiology team.

Malpositioned GJ Tubes: Patients with GJ tubes which are malpositioned (Fig. 7) often present with vomiting of feeds, feeding intolerance, or feeds injected through the jejunostomy port coming out through the stoma or the gastrostomy port [21]. As for completely dislodged GJ tubes, feeds should be held until the GJ tube is reinserted and adequately positioned.

Tube Obstruction: G tubes and GJ tubes can become clogged with repeated usage or with instillation of material incompatible with the catheter [21]. This will present with resistance to injection of fluids, feeds, or medications. Methods of chemical (i.e., enzymes) unclogging should be implemented, and if the obstruction persists, mechanical unclogging with a wire and/or tube exchange is warranted.

Intussusception (Fig. 8) can occur in patients with GJ tubes, typically presenting with bilious vomiting, abdominal distension, and pain during feeds. The diagnosis is made with US. In case of a persistent intussusception, the tube should be retracted so the tip is proximal to the region of intussusception. Sometimes temporary bowel rest is necessary, requiring GJ tube removal and insertion of a temporary G tube that should not be used for feeding. The GJ tube is readvanced/replaced after 24 to 48 hours of bowel rest [3]. In distinction to ileocolic intussusception, bowel hypoperfusion and perforation is uncommon with GJ-associated intussusception.

## Cecostomy Tubes

A percutaneous cecostomy tube (C tube) is a safe and effective method to provide access for antegrade enemas that help children become "socially continent" [22, 23]. Similar to G/GJ tubes, the C tube may dislodge, break, or block. The caregiver

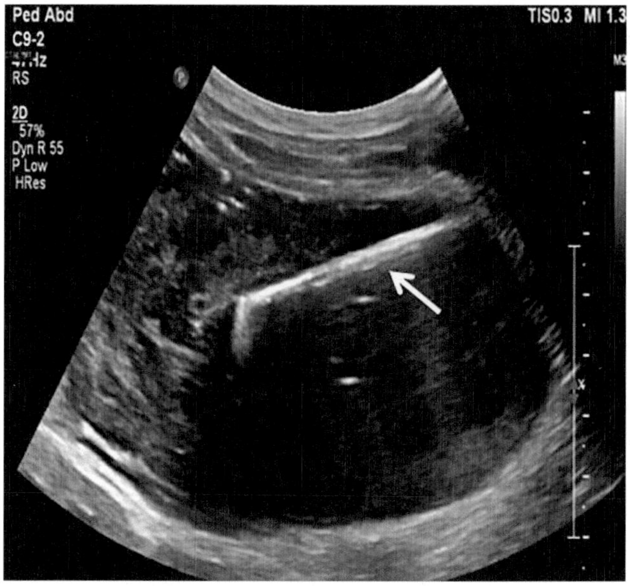

**Fig. 5** A 9-year-old girl with perforated appendicitis. Under US guidance, a large right lower quadrant collection was accessed with a 12 French drain using a trocar technique (arrow). A 450 ml of pus was drained

is instructed to irrigate with warm water in case of blockage and to place a temporary tube (e.g., Foley catheter) to protect the stoma tract in case of dislodgement. If unsuccessful, the interventional radiology team should be contacted.

## Vascular Abdominal/Pelvic Interventions

### Massive GI Bleeding

Emergent angiographic intervention for GI bleeding is generally reserved for unstable patients with massive bleeding. Stable patients will benefit more from abdominal CT angiography and/or Tc-99m RBC scintigraphy, providing a higher detection rate in localizing the source of bleeding [24] and allowing for a more targeted angiographic intervention. Although selective catheter angiography can be used to detect GI bleeding rates as low as 0.5 mL/min, the intermittent nature of bleeding in some patients may result in false-negative examinations [24]. Before the procedure, coagulation factors and the hemoglobin level should be optimized as much as possible, and blood products need to be

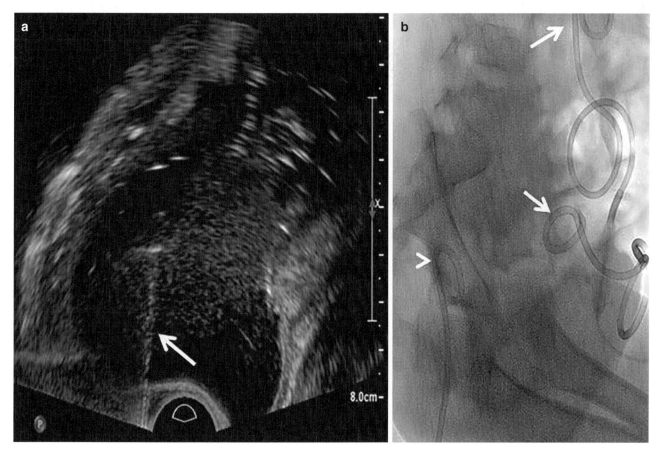

**Fig. 6** A 9-year-old girl with perforated appendicitis. Under transrectal US guidance, a large collection in the retro-vesical area was accessed with an 18-gauge needle (arrow) (**a**). A 0.035-inch guidewire was passed through the needle, and the tract was dilated under fluoroscopy.

A 12 French drainage catheter was inserted over the guidewire into the collection (arrowhead) (**b**). 250 ml of pus was drained. Note the two previously placed percutaneous drains (arrows) (**b**)

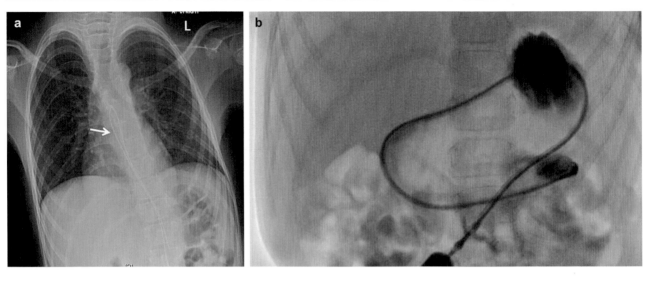

**Fig. 7** Chest radiograph of a 9-year-old boy showing a GJ tube projecting over the esophagus (arrow) in a child presenting with feeding intolerance (**a**). The GJ tube was repositioned using fluoroscopy (**b**)

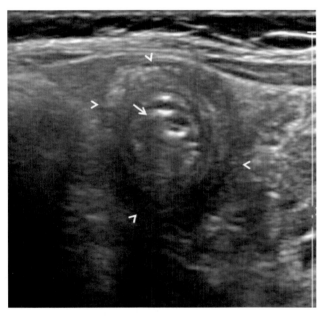

**Fig. 8** A 5-year-old girl with GJ tube presented with abdominal pain. Intussusception (arrowheads) around the tube (arrow) noted on US. The GJ tube was removed, and a temporary G tube was placed. Intragastric position was confirmed with contrast injection (not shown)

## Splenic Trauma

The spleen is the most common solid organ injured in pediatric blunt abdominal trauma. In children, initial nonoperative management is the current standard of care. Even though angioembolization appears to be a safe intervention, the vast majority of retrospective observational data show that very few pediatric patients with contrast extravasation may benefit from embolization. Therefore, proximal splenic artery embolization is typically reserved for patients with high-grade injuries, transient response to resuscitation, and/or persistent blood requirements [25]. It decreases the arterial flow to the spleen, thereby lowering the pressure within the splenic capsule, allowing healing without infarction, and preserving the splenic parenchyma [26].

## Hepatic Artery Embolization

In adults with blunt hepatic trauma, the use of hepatic angioembolization is recommended when there is ongoing bleeding demonstrated by the presence of an arterial blush on CT [27]. The rationale for this is that emergency laparotomy and perihepatic packing often stops hepatic venous bleeding, but mechanical pressure may not be adequate to stop intraparenchymal arterial bleeding. Although only a few cases of pediatric hepatic angioembolization have been described in the literature for treatment of active arterial bleeding, as in adults, it appears to be a safe alternative to open laparotomy to arrest hepatic hemorrhage in children [28] (Fig. 10). The portal blood supply to the liver protects the parenchyma from ischemia if hepatic arterial embolization is needed. Embolization is usually done with Gelfoam, PVA particles, coils, or glue, reducing perfusion pressure to stop the hemorrhage.

available in the room. A 4 or 5 French arterial sheath is placed in the common femoral artery. Selective catheterization of the celiac artery, superior mesenteric artery (SMA), and inferior mesenteric artery (IMA) should be done regardless of upper versus lower GI bleeding, to account for the rich collateral supply of the GI tract. If contrast extravasation is identified, embolization with temporary (Gelfoam) or more permanent agents (PVA particles, coils, or glue) is currently the preferred method for decreasing perfusion pressure to stop the hemorrhage [24] (Fig. 9).

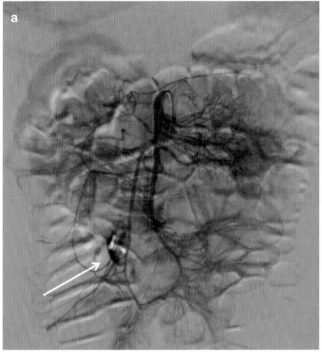
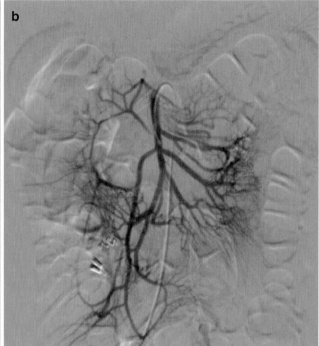

**Fig. 9** A 16-year-old male with Peutz-Jeghers syndrome who presented with GI hemorrhage following polypectomy. SMA angiography demonstrated contrast extravasation at the site of arterial hemorrhage adjacent to the endoscopic clips (arrow) (**a**). A microcatheter system was used to obtain access selectively to the branches supplying the area of active hemorrhage, coils were deployed, and repeat SMA angiography demonstrated no further active bleeding (**b**).

## Renal

### Nonvascular Genitourinary Interventions

#### Renal Obstruction: Nephrostomy

The clinical indications for percutaneous nephrostomy (PCN) in children include urinary obstruction (e.g., UPJ, UVJ, or PUV calculi), especially when complicated by infection or sepsis, and temporary urinary diversion in patients with obstructive uropathies, urinary fistulas, leaks, or hemorrhagic cystitis. PCN has been shown to have a high technical success rate (99%) in children when performed by dedicated pediatric interventional radiologists [29]. Seldinger or trocar technique can be used for PCN. If the patient presents with signs of infection, contrast should be used only to confirm catheter position due to the risk of reflux of infected urine/contrast into the renal parenchyma and the development of overwhelming sepsis. PCN placement in neonates and young infants is particularly challenging due to the small renal size and lack of support of the thin renal parenchyma and adjacent tissues. The collecting system can rapidly decompress during the procedure. In these cases, it is suggested to avoid serial dilatations [3] (Fig. 11).

## Vascular Genitourinary Interventions

### Renal Hemorrhage: Renal Artery Embolization

The kidney is the most common organ affected by blunt abdominal trauma in children [30]. It can also sustain iatrogenic damage from renal biopsies. Similar to pediatric splenic and hepatic trauma, the majority of cases of renal parenchyma trauma are effectively treated by conservative treatment. When indicated, renovascular interventions in genitourinary trauma include embolization for hemorrhage or reestablishment of flow with angioplasty and stenting [26] (Fig. 12).

## Musculoskeletal

### Septic Joint

The presence of joint effusion and clinically suspected septic arthritis is an interventional/surgical emergency. The most involved joint in the pediatric population is the hip, with transient synovitis as the main differential diagnosis. US is used to assess for the presence of effusion and to guide arthrocentesis if needed [31] (Fig. 13).

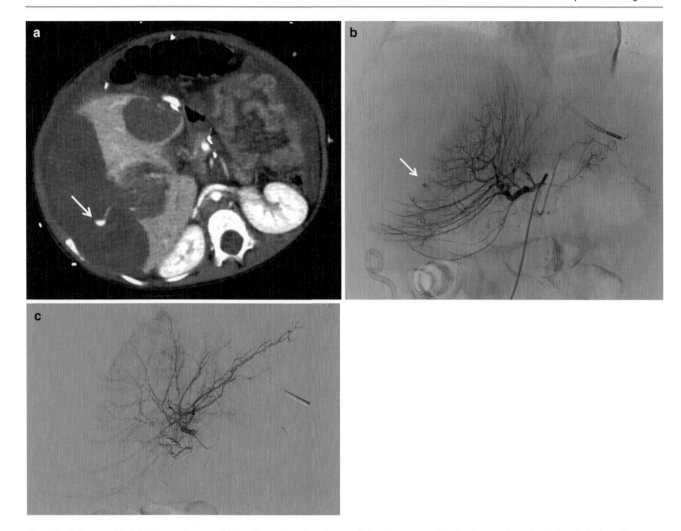

**Fig. 10** A 2-year-old girl with an obstructed Meso-Rex shunt (autologous graft extending from the superior mesenteric vein into the Rex recess of the left portal vein) following extrahepatic portal venous obstruction secondary to umbilical venous line, 1 week following transhepatic intervention for multiple portal vein dilatations and thrombolysis with tPA, presented with hemoperitoneum on US and hemorrhagic shock. CTA in the arterial phase (**a**) shows a focus of active contrast extravasation (arrow) within a large hematoma occupying the right lobe of the liver, most likely from a branch of the right hepatic artery. Common hepatic artery DSA was then performed emergently, demonstrating peripheral focal contrast extravasation in the right lobe of the liver (arrow) (**b**). The right hepatic artery and its branches were embolized utilizing multiple coils. Repeat DSA performed immediately after the embolization demonstrated no residual contrast extravasation to suggest active bleeding (**c**).

## Osteomyelitis

The bacteriology of pediatric osteomyelitis has changed due to increased virulence of *Staphylococcus aureus*, primarily of the methicillin-resistant strains [32]. Early cultures from the site of infection in acute hematogenous osteomyelitis (AHO) can help target therapy and decrease complications [32]. US-guided aspiration of joint, periosteal, or soft tissue fluid can help establish an organism. Image-guided percutaneous bone biopsy has been shown to be safe and effective in obtaining bone for cultures in children with AHO not requiring open surgical drainage [33] (Fig. 14).

## Vascular Access

In many pediatric centers, interventional radiologists provide US-guided venous access, placing a variety of devices including port-a-catheters (port), tunnelled and non-tunnelled central venous lines (CVLs), and peripherally inserted central catheters (PICCs). Establishing venous access in infants and children is often technically challenging and requires patience, practice, and experience. As such, the interventional radiology service is often the final resource for peripheral IV access [34]. US-guided venous access is typically

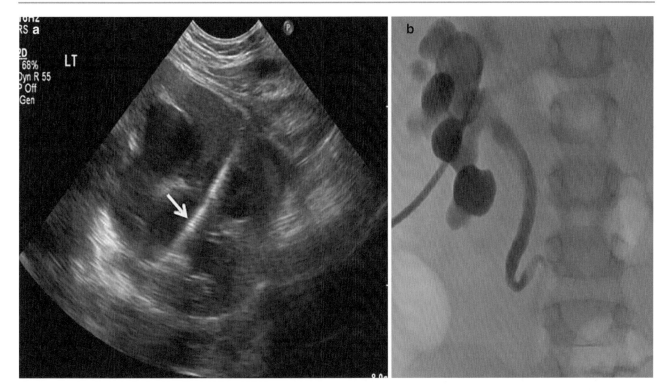

**Fig. 11** PCN in a 7-year-old boy with left-sided pyelonephritis and a complex urology history including bladder exstrophy repair with bilateral ureterosigmoidostomy. The lower calix was accessed with a 19-gauge needle under US guidance, and a 0.035" guidewire was passed through the needle (arrow) (**a**). Under fluoroscopy (prone position), the tract was dilated, a 10 French drainage catheter was inserted, and adequate position in the renal pelvis was confirmed with contrast injection (**b**)

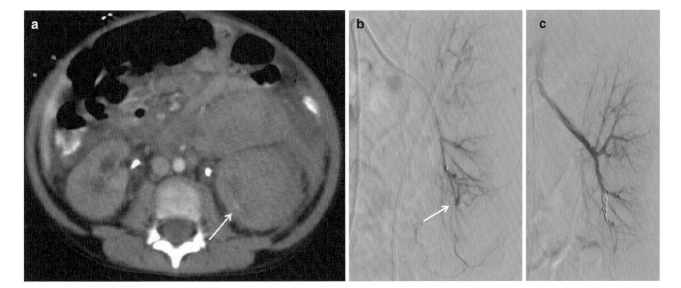

**Fig. 12** A 5-year-old girl with substantial hemorrhage following renal biopsy. CTA shows an arterial blush (arrow) in the lower pole of the left kidney (**a**) with associated perirenal hematoma. A selective left renal angiogram showed an area of contrast extravasation in the left kidney (arrow) (**b**), which was embolized using coils (**c**)

obtained using a high-frequency linear array transducer ("hockey stick"-type transducer) in a transverse orientation. A single-wall puncture is generally preferable; however, it is not always feasible, especially in very small veins. In those circumstances, a two-walled puncture, in which the needle transfixes the vessel and then it is slowly withdrawn until a flashback of blood is seen, is necessary. The puncture is often performed with a micropuncture needle or a sheathed needle which allows placement of a guidewire (e.g., 22- or 24-gauge angiocatheter and a 0.018- or 0.014-inch wire, respectively), over which a longer and larger cannula can be placed [35].

The urgent need for CVL placement from the ED is relatively uncommon, with possible indications including lack of success in obtaining peripheral access, in which case a temporary, non-tunneled femoral or jugular CVL can be placed. Another indication for urgent central venous access is the need for hemodialysis (HD). HD catheters have two lumens and must provide high flow rates for their intended use of circulating venous blood. Therefore, large catheters must be inserted. Larger catheters mean increased difficulty of catheter insertion and increased rate of complications [36]. Both tunneled and non-tunneled CVL insertions are performed in a strictly sterile manner [37]. Ideally, access is gained to the right jugular vein under US guidance, and a guidewire is manipulated to the IVC. In more urgent situations, femoral HD catheters are placed. For tunneled CVLs, a small incision is made at the anterior chest wall, and the catheter is tunneled through the subcutaneous tissues to the venotomy site. A peel-away sheath introducer is subsequently inserted over the guidewire to allow for the insertion of the CVL into the venous system.

Patients with port-a-catheters (ports), PICCs, and CVLs may present to the ED with a variety of issues, with central line-associated bloodstream infection (CLABSI) being the most common serious complication. The typical presentation of fever and chills immediately after accessing a catheter that has been locked for some time is not always present, and most episodes are not associated with any visible abnormality at the site of the catheter. As such, the catheter may not always be immediately considered as the source of fever, and unless an alternative source is identified, all bloodstream infections in patients with a port, CVL, or PICC are classified as CLABSI [37]. Timely removal of the catheter is indicated if (1) the line is no longer needed; (2) infection is complicated by sepsis, tunnel, or port-a-catheter pocket infection or by endocarditis or suppurative thrombophlebitis; (3) there is relapse of CLABSI with an identical organism; or (4) there is infection with *Staphylococcus aureus*, mycobacteria, fungi such as *Candida, Bacillus cereus,* and some multiresistant bacteria. After removal of an infected catheter, reinsertion of a new long-term CVL should ideally be delayed until blood cultures (collected after removal) are negative to prevent immediate contamination of the new device [39].

Patients may also present to the ED due to mechanical line dysfunction of the port, CVL, or PICC. If a catheter is blocked, a thrombus/clot is likely. If it can be flushed but will not aspirate, malposition of the tip or, more commonly, a fibrin sheath enveloping the intravascular portion of the catheter should be suspected. If the problem is not resolved with the infusion of tPA, the interventional radiology team should

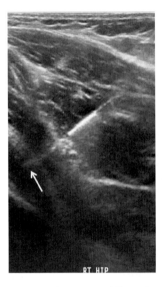

**Fig. 13** US of the right hip of a 10-year-old boy who presented with hip pain and fever showed joint effusion with internal debris. Under US guidance, a 20-gauge needle (arrow) was advanced into the right hip capsule, and thick straw-colored fluid was aspirated and sent to the laboratory for analysis.

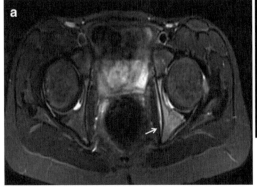
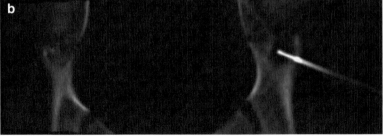

**Fig. 14** Axial STIR MR image of the pelvis of an 11-year-old girl with a 3-week history of persistent left hip pain, fevers, and weight loss, showing increased signal intensity involving the left acetabulum (arrow), with mild adjacent soft tissue edema (**a**). A bone biopsy was requested to confirm the diagnosis and guide therapy. The patient was positioned on the lateral decubitus position with the left hip up. A bone biopsy was obtained under cone-beam CT guidance, using a 15-gauge biopsy needle via a 14-gauge coaxial needle (**b**)

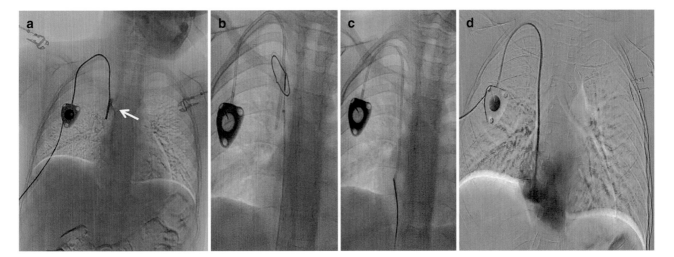

**Fig. 15** A 4-year-old girl with a right chest wall port malfunction. A linogram was obtained, showing contrast around the tube with retrograde flow, indicating a fibrin sheath (arrow, **a**). Access was obtained to the right femoral vein and via a 6 French vascular sheath (not shown), a snare wire was advanced around the catheter, and the line was stripped several times (**b-c**). Post-stripping linogram was done showing a straight jet of contrast, with no evidence of reflux of contrast around the tube to suggest a residual fibrin sheath (**d**).

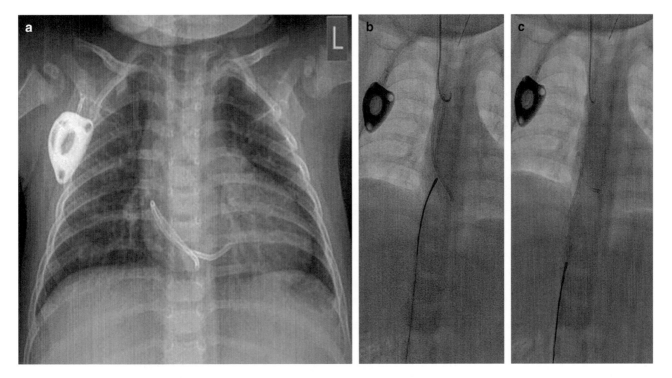

**Fig. 16** Chest radiograph of a 1-year-old boy shows a broken port-a-catheter, with the displaced catheter looping in the right atrium and extending into the right ventricle (**a**). Access was obtained to the right jugular vein and the right common femoral vein. A 4 French pigtail catheter was inserted using the jugular approach and was used to pull the catheter into the right atrium (**b**). A 2.5-cm snare wire was inserted into the femoral sheath and was manipulated into the right atrium. The free catheter fragment was engaged and secured with the snare, and it was entirely removed through the right femoral sheath (**b-c**). The port chamber was then removed, with no residual fragment seen at the end of the procedure (not shown).

be contacted to attempt catheter rewiring, fibrin stripping (Fig. 15), or line exchange/replacement if needed [39].

A line can also be fully or partially pulled out. In these cases, the catheter is ideally exchanged over a wire. If not feasible and the access site cannot be salvaged, de novo placement of a line is warranted.

Local swelling, pain, and skin site leakage on injection are symptoms suggestive of line breakage. Other signs are resistance to injection, inability to withdraw blood, cough, and chest pain. In these cases, a chest radiograph should be done to identify any migrated broken fragment. Fractured PICC and CVL fragments are retrieved from the heart and pulmonary arteries by using a snare to entrap the fragment (Fig. 16), via a femoral, brachial, basilic, cephalic, or jugular approach. A vascular sheath is used to prevent tearing of the vein during the final removal of the fragment. The fragment should be removed sooner than later, due to the increased risk of cardiac arrhythmia, thrombus formation, and incorporation into the vessel wall [36].

## Take-Home Points:

- Emergency image-guided interventions in pediatric patients frequently require different interventional skills and techniques than in the adult population, including the need for general anesthesia or sedation in most patients.
- The use of multiple imaging modalities, primarily US and fluoroscopy, is key in many pediatric interventional procedures including drainage of pleural effusion, pneumothorax, lung abscess, abdominal/pelvic fluid collections, and nephrostomy tube placement.
- Complications related to radiologically placed gastrotomy tubes, gastrojejunostomy tubes, and cecostomy tubes in children are common. While some issues can be handled in the ED, tube replacement by interventional radiology may be required in other cases.
- Interventional radiology plays a critical role in the treatment of acute pediatric trauma or hemorrhage, often mitigating the need for surgical intervention.
- Obtaining pediatric venous access (including peripheral IVs, PICCs, Ports, and CVLs) and managing venous access-related complications (e.g., stripping of a fibrin sheath, fragmented catheters) are often challenges met with image-guided techniques by interventional radiologists.

## References

1. Islam S, Calkins CM, Goldin AB, et al. APSA outcomes and clinical trials committee, 2011–2012. The diagnosis and management of empyema in children: a comprehensive review from the APSA outcomes and clinical trials committee. J Pediatr Surg. 2012;47:2101–10.
2. Feola GP, Hogan MJ, Baskin KM, et al. Quality improvement standards for the treatment of pediatric empyema. JVIR. 2018;29 (10):1415–22.
3. Temple M, Marshalleck FE. Pediatric interventional radiology: handbook of vascular and non-vascular interventions. New York, NY: Springer; 2014. p. 307.
4. Posner K, Needleman JP. Pneumothorax. Pediatr Rev. 2008;29(2): 69–70.
5. MacDuff A, Arnold A, Harvey J. On behalf of the BTS Pleural Disease Guideline Group. Management of spontaneous pneumothorax: British Thoracic Society pleural disease guideline 2010. Thorax. 2010;65(Suppl 2):ii18eii31. https://doi.org/10.1136/thx.2010. 136986.
6. Robinson PD, Cooper P, Ranganathan SC. Evidence-based management of paediatric primary spontaneous pneumothorax. Paediatr Respir Rev. 2009;10:110–7.
7. Hogan MJ, Marshalleck FE, Sidhu MK, et al. Quality improvement guidelines for pediatric abscess and fluid drainage. JVIR. 2012;23: 1397–402.
8. Zaidi AU, Hutchins KK, Rajpurkar M. Pulmonary embolism in children. Front Pediatr. 2017;5:170.
9. Thacker PG, Lee EY. Pulmonay embolism in children. AJR. 2015;204:1278–88.
10. Kuo WT, Gould MK, Louie JD, Rosenberg JK, Sze DY, Hofmann LV. Catheter-directed therapy for the treatment of massive pulmonary embolism: Systematic review and meta-analysis of modern techniques. J Vasc Interv Radiol. 2009;20:1431–40.
11. Dabin J, Gill AE, Durrence WW, et al. Catheter-directed pharmacologic thrombolysis for acute submassive and massive pulmonary emboli in children and adolescents—an exploratory report. Pediatr Crit Care Med. 2020;21(1):e15–22. https://doi.org/10.1097/PCC. 0000000000002172.
12. Bavare AC, Naik SX, Lin PH, et al. Catheter-directed thrombolysis for severe pulmonary embolism in pediatric patients. Ann Vasc Surg. 2014;28(7):1794.
13. Tarango C, Manco-Johnson MJ. Pediatric thrombolysis: a practical approach. Front Pediatr. 2017;5:260. https://doi.org/10.3389/fped. 2017.00260.
14. Wang M, Hays T, Balasa V, et al. Low-dose tissue plasminogen activator thrombolysis in children. J Pediatr Hematol Oncol. 2003;25(5):379–86.
15. Roebuck DJ, Barnacle AM. Haemoptysis and bronchial artery embolization in children. Paediatr Respir Rev. 2008;9:95–104.
16. Yoon W, Kim JK, Kim YH, Chung TW, Kang HK. Bronchial and nonbronchial systemic artery embolization for life-threatening hemoptysis: a comprehensive review. Radiographics. 2002;22(6): 1395–409.
17. McCann JW, Maroo S, Wales P, et al. Image-guided drainage of multiple intraabdominal abscesses in children with perforated appendicitis: an alternative to laparotomy. Pediatr Radiol. 2008;38: 661–8.
18. Gervais DA, Brown SD, Connolly SA, Brec SL, Harisinghani MG, Mueller PR. Percutaneous imaging-guided abdominal and pelvic abscess drainage in children. Radiographics. 2004;24(3):737–54.
19. Mubarak WM, Sheikh N, John P, Temple MJ, Amaral JG, Connolly BL. Use of the transrectal ultrasound probe in aspiration and drainage in pediatric patients: a retrospective observational study. JVIR. 2019;30:908–14.
20. Berman L, Hronek C, Raval MV, et al. Pediatric gastrostomy tube placement: lessons learned from high-performing institutions through structured interviews. Pediatr Qual Saf. 2017;2:e016.
21. Kumbhar SS, Plunk MR, Nikam R, Boyd KP, Thakrar PD. Complications of percutaneous gastrostomy and gastrojejunostomy tubes in children. Pediatr Radiol. 2020;50:404–14.
22. Chait PG, Shlomovitz E, Connolly BL, Temple MJ, Restrepo R, Amaral JG, Muraca S, Richards HF, Ein SH. Percutaneous cecostomy: updates in technique and patient care. Radiology. 2003;227(1)
23. Donkol RH, Al-Nammi A. Percutaneous cecostomy in the management of organic fecal incontinence in children. World J Radiol. 2010;2(12):463–7.
24. Wells ML, Hansel SL, Bruining DH, Fletcher JG, Froemming AT, Barlow JM, Fidler JL. CT for evaluation of acute gastrointestinal bleeding. Radiographics. 2018;38(4):1089–107.
25. Coccolini F, Monotori G, Catena F, et al. Splenic trauma: WSES classification and guidelines for adult and pediatric patients. World J Emerg Radiol. 2017;12(40). https://doi.org/10.1186/s13017-017-0151-4.
26. Sidhu MK, Hogan MJ, Shaw DW, Burdick T. Interventional radiology for paediatric trauma. Pediatr Radiol. 2009;39:506–15.
27. Kozar RA, McNutt MK. Management of adult blunt hepatic trauma. Curr Opin Crit Care. 2010. https://doi.org/10.1097/MCC. 0b013e32833f5cd5.

28. Ong CP, Toh L, Lo RHG, Yapa T, Narasimhan K. Primary hepatic artery embolization in pediatric blunt hepatic trauma. J Pediatr Surg. 2012;47:2316–20.
29. Shellikeri S, Daulton R, Sertic M, Connolly B, Hogan M, Marshalleck F, Cahill AM. Pediatric percutaneous nephrostomy: a multicenter experience. JVIR. 2018;29:328–34.
30. Lin W-C, Lin C-H. The role of interventional radiology for pediatric blunt renal trauma. Ital J Pediatr. 2015;41:76.
31. Tsung JW, Blaivas M. Emergency department diagnosis of pediatric hip effusion and guided arthrocentesis using point-of-care ultrasound. J Emerg Med. 2009;35(4):393–9.
32. Jaramillo D, Dormans JP, Delgado J, Laor T, St. Geme JW. Hematogenous osteomyelitis in infants and children: imaging of a changing disease. Radiology. 2017;283(3):629–43.
33. McNeil JC, Forbes AR, Vallejo JG, Flores AR, Hultén KG, Mason EO, Kaplan SL. Role of operative or interventional radiology-guided cultures for osteomyelitis. Pediatrics. 2016;137(5). https://doi.org/10.1542/peds.2015-4616.
34. Krishnamurthy G, Keller MS. Vascular access in children. Cardiovasc Intervent Radiol. 2011;34:14–24.
35. Donaldson JS. Pediatric vascular access. Pediatr Radiol. 2006;36:386–97.
36. Chait PG, Temple M, Connolly B, John P, Restrepo R, Amaral JG. Pediatric interventional venous access. Tech Vasc Interv Radiol. 2002;5(2):95–102.
37. Connolly B. Pediatric hemodialysis interventions. In: Rajan DK, editor. Essential of percutaneous dialysis interventions. New York: Springer; 2011. p. 398–412.
38. Wolf J, Curtis N, Worth LJ, Flynn P. Central line–associated bloodstream infection in children: an update on treatment. Pediatr Infect Dis J. 2013;32(8):905–10.
39. Nayeemuddin M, Pherwani AD, Asquith JR. Imaging and management of complications of central venous catheters. Clin Radiol. 2013;68(5):529–44.

# Index

Printed by Printforce, the Netherlands